MAGILL'S
MEDICAL GUIDE

MAGILL'S
MEDICAL GUIDE

Fourth Revised Edition

Volume III
Heimlich maneuver — Nervous system

Medical Consultants

Anne Lynn S. Chang, M.D.
Stanford University

Laurence M. Katz, M.D.
University of North Carolina, Chapel Hill

H. Bradford Hawley, M.D.
Wright State University

Nancy A. Piotrowski, Ph.D.
University of California, Berkeley

Connie Rizzo, M.D., Ph.D.
Columbia University

Project Editor
Tracy Irons-Georges

SALEM PRESS, INC.
Pasadena, California   Hackensack, New Jersey

Editor in Chief: Dawn P. Dawson

Editorial Director: Christina J. Moose *Production Editor:* Joyce I. Buchea
Project Editor: Tracy Irons-Georges *Acquisitions Editor:* Mark Rehn
Editorial Assistant: Dana Garey *Page Design:* James Hutson
Photo Editor: Cynthia Breslin Beres *Layout:* William Zimmerman

Cover Design: Moritz Design
Illustrations: Hans & Cassady, Inc., Westerville, Ohio

Magill's Medical Guide: Health and Illness, 1995
Supplement, 1996
Magill's Medical Guide, revised edition, 1998
Second revised edition, 2002
Third revised edition, 2005
Fourth revised edition, 2008

∞ The paper used in these volumes conforms to the American National Standard for Permanence of Paper for Printed Library Materials, Z39.48-1992 (R1997).

Note to Readers

The material presented in *Magill's Medical Guide* is intended for broad informational and educational purposes. Readers who suspect that they suffer from any of the physical or psychological disorders, diseases, or conditions described in this set should contact a physician without delay; this work should not be used as a substitute for professional medical diagnosis or treatment. This set is not to be considered definitive on the covered topics, and readers should remember that the field of health care is characterized by a diversity of medical opinions and constant expansion in knowledge and understanding.

Library of Congress Cataloging-in-Publication Data

Magill's medical guide. — 4th rev. ed. / medical consultants, Anne Lynn S. Chang . . . [et al.] ; project editor, Tracy Irons-Georges.
    p.   ;   cm.
   Includes bibliographical references and index.
   ISBN 978-1-58765-384-1 (set : alk. paper)
   ISBN 978-1-58765-385-8 (vol. 1 : alk. paper)
   ISBN 978-1-58765-386-5 (vol. 2 : alk. paper)
   ISBN 978-1-58765-387-2 (vol. 3 : alk. paper)
   ISBN 978-1-58765-388-9 (vol. 4 : alk. paper)
   ISBN 978-1-58765-407-7 (vol. 5 : alk. paper)
  1. Medicine—Encyclopedias. I. Chang, Anne. II. Title: Medical guide.
  [DNLM: 1. Medicine — Encyclopedias — English. W 13 M194 2008]
RC41.M34   2008
610.3—dc22
                                                          2007033818

First Printing

PRINTED IN THE UNITED STATES OF AMERICA

CONTENTS

COMPLETE LIST OF CONTENTS

VOLUME 1

VOLUME 2

VOLUME 3

VOLUME 4

Volume 5

MAGILL'S
MEDICAL GUIDE

HEIMLICH MANEUVER

PROCEDURE

ANATOMY OR SYSTEM AFFECTED: Chest, lungs, mouth, neck, respiratory system, throat

SPECIALTIES AND RELATED FIELDS: Emergency medicine

DEFINITION: An emergency technique used to prevent suffocation when the airway becomes blocked.

INDICATIONS AND PROCEDURES

The Heimlich maneuver is an emergency technique, introduced in 1974 by Dr. Henry J. Heimlich, that guides a rescuer through a set of manipulative procedures to prevent suffocation when a victim's airway (windpipe) becomes blocked by food, water, or other foreign material. The maneuver lifts the diaphragm and forces enough air from the lungs to create an artificial cough. This cough intends to move the obstructive foreign body from the windpipe in order to resume normal and functional breathing (ventilation).

The Heimlich maneuver should be performed only if a choking victim cannot speak, cough, or breathe. Several indications may signal such a situation: frantic gestures to the throat, a face that turns blue in color because of lack of oxygen, and the production of loud noises in an attempt to take in breaths of air.

Before attempting the Heimlich maneuver, permission in the form of an affirmative nod or gesture should be given by a conscious victim to the intended administrator of the maneuver. When performing the technique, the rescuer is usually positioned behind the sitting or standing victim, with his or her arms around the victim's waist. The rescuer makes a fist with one hand and places that hand, with the thumb toward the victim, just above the victim's navel or below the rib cage and above the waist. The free hand should clasp the fisted hand tightly. Then, in a series of sharp thrusts upward and inward, the rescuer attempts to develop enough air pressure in the airway to force the lodged foreign object back up the trachea. The procedure may

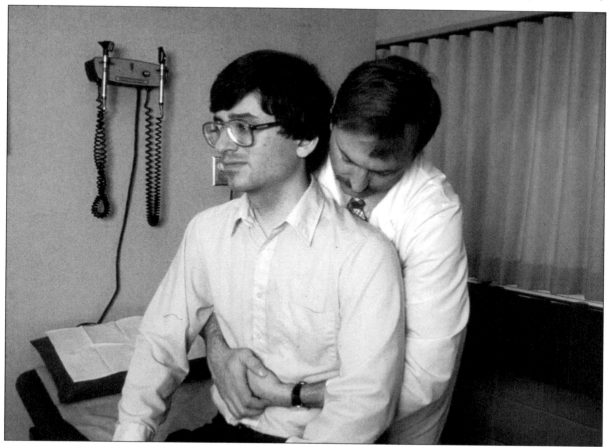

A doctor demonstrates the Heimlich maneuver. (Custom Medical Stock Photo)

have to be repeated several times before the foreign object is expelled. Once the airway is cleared, the victim should start coughing and/or regain normal breathing. In cases when breathing is not resumed, then cardiopulmonary resuscitation (CPR) may have to be administered. In more serious choking cases in which the airway is not cleared of the obstruction, a small incision to the windpipe called a tracheostomy may have to be completed.

USES AND COMPLICATIONS

In addition to choking victims, the Heimlich maneuver may be administered to asthmatics and drowning victims. While it can be performed on all people, modifications should be adapted when executed upon infants (it is not recommended for infants less than one year old), children, and very obese, pregnant, or unconscious adults. The Heimlich maneuver may also be self-administered.

The Heimlich maneuver is one of the best courses to follow for the prevention of asphyxiation during a choking episode, but it does come with several precautions. In addition to modifications depending on the age and situation of the victim, incorrect administration of the Heimlich maneuver by incorporating techniques such as chest thrusts, back slaps, and abdominal thrusts can cause bruised ribs, broken bones, damage to internal organs, and even death. If all the guidelines are effectively followed by the administrator, however, then the victim should feel little or no bodily discomfort and should recover quickly.

—*Nicholas Lanzieri*

See also Asphyxiation; Asthma; Cardiopulmonary resuscitation (CPR); Choking; Drowning; Emergency medicine; Emergency medicine, pediatric; Lungs; Pulmonary medicine; Pulmonary medicine, pediatric; Respiration; Resuscitation.

FOR FURTHER INFORMATION:

American Medical Association. *Handbook of First Aid and Emergency Care.* Rev. ed. New York: Random House, 2000.

"Heimlich Maneuver." In *Everything You Need to Know About Medical Treatments.* Springhouse, Pa.: Springhouse, 1996.

Icon Health. *Heimlich Maneuver: A Medical Dictionary, Bibliography, and Annotated Research Guide to Internet References.* San Diego, Calif.: Author, 2004.

Tintinalli, Judith E., ed. *Emergency Medicine: A Comprehensive Study Guide.* 6th ed. New York: McGraw-Hill, 2004.

White, R. D. "Foreign Body Airway Obstruction: Considerations in 1985." *Circulation* 74, no. 6, pt. 2 (1986): IV60-62.

HEMATOLOGY

SPECIALTY

ANATOMY OR SYSTEM AFFECTED: Blood, circulatory system, immune system, liver, musculoskeletal system, spleen

SPECIALTIES AND RELATED FIELDS: Cardiology, cytology, forensic medicine, genetics, immunology, oncology, pathology, serology, vascular medicine

DEFINITION: The study of the blood, including its normal constituents, and such blood disorders as anemia, leukemia, and hemophilia.

KEY TERMS:

anemia: a condition characterized by a deficiency of red blood cells or hemoglobin

bone marrow: the soft substance that fills the cavities within bones and that is the site of blood cell production

clotting factors: chemicals circulating in the blood which are necessary for the process of blood clotting

hematologist: one who specializes in the study of blood, its components and disorders

hemoglobin: the iron-containing molecule within red blood cells responsible for oxygen and carbon dioxide transport

leukemia: a condition characterized by the presence of numerous immature white blood cells in the circulating blood

plasma: the fluid portion of blood, containing water, proteins, minerals, nutrients, hormones, and wastes

platelets: specialized cell fragments that initiate blood clotting

red blood cell: a flexible, biconcave blood cell that contains hemoglobin

white blood cell: one of several types of colorless, large blood cells that work together to combat infections

SCIENCE AND PROFESSION

Most branches of medical science study a particular organ that is made of specific tissues and is located in a definite part of the body. Hematology is unique because its subject, the blood, is a liquid tissue constantly in motion and therefore in constant contact with every other tissue and organ of the body.

It has been estimated that blood travels about 16 kilometers (10 miles) an hour. It takes six seconds for blood to travel from the heart to the lungs, about eight seconds from the heart to the brain, and only fourteen seconds from the heart all the way to the toes. Hematologists studying these shifting currents of the blood are able to detect patterns that allow the early discovery of many disorders of the blood itself and of the organs that it supplies.

Blood is a complex material composed of approximately 55 percent plasma and 45 percent cells, which are also called formed elements. The plasma, or liquid portion of the blood, is about 90 percent water and 10 percent substances dissolved or suspended in that water. Part of that 10 percent consists of a remarkable array of substances, including nutrients, gases, salts, wastes, and hormones being transported around the body. The other, larger part of the 10 percent is another remarkable array—plasma proteins such as fibrinogen, albumin, and globulins with a great diversity of functions to accomplish. The modern hematologist's ability to measure and monitor all these plasma components precisely has greatly aided physicians in the treatment of innumerable diseases.

Beyond an analysis of the ingredients of the plasma, hematologists focus on the normal and abnormal conditions of the blood's cells. An individual has 25 trillion red blood cells; 10 million of these cells die or are destroyed each second, and 200 billion new ones need to be made each day. Hematologists discovered that these tiny, biconcave discs packed with hemoglobin transport the vast majority of the oxygen needed constantly by every cell of every organ for energy production.

Before each red blood cell is released from the bone marrow where it is produced, the bulk of its living nucleus is expelled. A small amount of nuclear material remains, as a fine network, in these young cells called reticulocytes. The number of reticulocytes released into the blood is an indication of the activity of the bone marrow. Hematologists use this number in both the diagnosis and the assessment of the response to treatment, in conditions such as the various forms of anemia.

Not only the total number and maturity but also the shape, diameter, and flexibility of red blood cells can give the hematologist important information. For years, such information was gathered by laborious manual methods. Electronic counters can now obtain this information with great speed and even greater accuracy.

Hematologists can also gauge the effectiveness of red blood cells by seeing how much hemoglobin they contain. The amount of this red pigment present—and therefore functioning—was once estimated by being matched against progressively darker-colored glass "standards." Now this figure too is accurately perceived using a precise, photoelectric technique.

Another useful test is called the packed cell volume (PCV) test. It not only reveals the proportion of the red blood cells to the plasma but also allows the calculation of their average size and their hemoglobin content.

An equally common blood investigation is the erythrocyte sedimentation rate (ESR). The erythrocytes, the term that hematologists use to describe red blood cells, normally fall slowly down through the plasma in a standard tube. A very rapid sedimentation rate demonstrates a disturbance in the plasma proteins that may be very dangerous. Usually, the faster they settle out, the sicker the patient, with a wide variety of inflammations as possible causes.

Beginning in the middle of the twentieth century, an increasing number of radioactive tests were developed by which hematologists can assess more accurately total blood volume and the survival time of red blood cells or platelets in circulation. Assessing total volume is important. A loss of more than 1 liter (2 pints) is quite dangerous because it can cause a total collapse of the blood vessels.

This reaction gives a clue about the importance of a second kind of blood cell, the platelet, and its work in stopping bleeding. When a blood vessel is first cut, platelets (or thrombocytes) rush to the site. They swell into irregular shapes, become sticky, clog the cut, and create a plug. The smallest blood vessels rupture hundreds of times a day, and platelets alone are able to make the necessary repairs. If the cut is too large, platelets—which are like sponges filled with diverse and biologically active compounds—disintegrate. Their ingredients react with numerous clotting factors in the plasma to initiate clot formation.

Hematologists check blood samples carefully to ascertain whether their patients possess the normal number of platelets—more than a trillion for the average adult. Since platelets live only about ten days, it is necessary to monitor those patients who exhibit significantly low amounts of these cells. If their bone marrow is not constantly replacing these platelets, these patients might bleed to death from a small cut. On the other hand, doctors must monitor any tendency toward the formation of too many platelets because of the danger of thrombophlebitis, the blockage of a vein by a blood clot.

As with red blood cells, the widespread use of electronic counters has made the measurement of the numbers of platelets and of white blood cells (the third type of blood cell) rapid, efficient, and extremely accurate.

White blood cells are hardest to count because they are the least numerous, making up only 0.1 percent of the total blood. Their number also varies dramatically from 4,000 to 11,000 per cubic centimeter of blood, according to the individual, the time of day, the outside temperature, and many other ordinary factors.

Hematologists can deduce the degree of maturity of circulating white blood cells from the appearance of their nuclei. There are five kinds of white blood cells (or leukocytes), whose normal proportions in the blood are quite specific and change drastically if an infection is present. The number of monocytes, for example, is normally 5 percent. If typhus, tuberculosis, or Rocky Mountain spotted fever organisms are present, the number will rise to 20 or 30 percent. The normal 60 percentage of neutrophils will increase to 75 percent or more in the presence of pneumonia or appendicitis.

DIAGNOSTIC AND TREATMENT TECHNIQUES

Blood to be tested by a hematologist is withdrawn from a vein. A thin smear or film of the blood is placed on a glass slide and stained to bring out identifying features more prominently. The microscope then reveals the proportion of different cell types and any variation from the normally expected amount. This examination alone may give an immediate diagnosis of a particular blood disorder. For example, a red blood cell count that is less than 4 million or more than 6 million per cubic centimeter of blood is considered unusual and is probably an indication of disease.

It often becomes necessary to study not only the circulating blood cells but also the original cells within the bone marrow which produce the erythrocytes, thrombocytes, and leukocytes. The hematologist must then use a long, thin needle to remove a sample of the marrow from within the tibia (shinbone) of a child or the pelvis (hipbone) or sternum (breastbone) of an adult. This test can provide a reliable diagnosis of a specific blood disorder.

The blood disorders that hematologists are routinely called on to diagnose and treat include diseases of the red blood cells, white blood cells, platelets, and clotting factors and failures of correct blood formation.

The disorders involving a deficiency of red blood

cells or their hemoglobin are called anemias. There are many types of anemia, which are named, distinguished, and treated according to their causes. Some anemias exist because of a lack of the materials needed to build red blood cells: iron, vitamin B_{12}, and folic acid. Other anemias are caused by a shortening of the life span of red blood cells or by inherited abnormalities in hemoglobin. Still others are attributable to chronic infections or cancer.

Iron-deficiency anemia is by far the most common; it is particularly prevalent in women of childbearing age and in children. In young children who are growing rapidly, constant increase in muscle mass and blood volume will cause anemia unless a high enough level of iron is present in the diet. All women between puberty and the menopause lose iron with the menstrual flow of blood and, therefore, are always prone to iron-deficiency anemia. A pregnant woman is even more likely to develop this condition; iron is literally removed from her body and transferred through the placenta to the developing fetus.

The symptoms of iron-deficiency anemia may include a reduced capacity for physical work, paleness, breathlessness, increased pulse and, possibly, a sore tongue. The hematologist witnessing small, misshapen red blood cells deficient in hemoglobin will recommend an increase in iron in the diet. The hematologist will also send this patient for various gastrointestinal tests because of the possibility of internal bleeding or failure of the intestine to absorb iron properly.

Another class of anemias involves a lack of vitamin B_{12} or of folic acid. Without the help of these two substances, the bone marrow cannot build red blood cells correctly. These anemias are diagnosed when the hematologist finds bizarre cells called megaloblasts in the patient's bone marrow. Both vitamin B_{12} and folic acid can be added to the diet or given by injection. The problem may stem, however, not from an insufficient amount of vitamin B_{12} in the diet but from the inability of the stomach lining to produce a substance called intrinsic factor. In this case, the patient will never be able to absorb this vitamin properly and is said to suffer from pernicious anemia.

Those anemias characterized by the early and too frequent destruction of red blood cells are grouped together as hemolytic anemias. Some of these disorders are acquired, while others are inherited. In both types, hemoglobin from the destroyed red blood cells can be detected by the hematologist in the plasma, the urine, or the skin, where it causes the yellowing called jaundice.

Because the many types of anemia are so common, hematologists find that the diagnosis and treatment of these diseases form a large part of their everyday practice. All types of leukemia, on the other hand, are quite rare. They are caused by a change in one kind of primitive blood cell in the bone marrow. The result is uncontrolled growth of these cells, which do not mature but which invade the blood as badly functioning cells. Leukemia is often thought of as cancer of the blood.

Although it is not known what causes leukemia in a particular person, the disease seems to be associated with certain factors, including injury by chemicals or radiation, viruses, and genetic predisposition. Many cases of acute leukemia occur either in children who are under fourteen or in adults who are between fifty-five and seventy-five years of age. In children, it is almost always a disorder in the bone marrow cells that produce the white blood cells, called lymphocytes. This disorder is called acute lymphoblastic leukemia, or ALL. Adult leukemia usually occurs in the bone marrow that forms some other type of white blood cell and is called acute nonlymphoblastic leukemia, or ANLL.

Hematologists diagnose both conditions by their shared symptoms: abnormal bone marrow tissue and a lack of normal white blood cells and platelets in the circulating blood. The patient will often have been referred to the hematologist because of an uncontrollable infection (from a lack of normal white blood cells) or uncontrollable bleeding (from a lack of normal platelets). In both children and adults, anemia usually accompanies acute leukemia because defective bone marrow is not able to produce red blood cells properly either.

Less rare than acute leukemia are the various chronic types. One type called chronic granulocytic leukemia (CGL) occurs most often after the age of fifty. Unfortunately, its early symptoms are few and vague, so that the disease may have progressed greatly before its presence would even be suspected. By such time, an enormous enlargement of the spleen, along with elevations in both white blood cell and platelet counts, can be noted.

Two stages are usually seen in chronic granulocytic leukemia. Early treatment can relieve all symptoms, shrink the spleen, and return all blood cells to normal values. Eventually, however, the leukemic condition recurs, and the patient usually lives an average of only three years. Bone marrow transplantation from a suitable donor or a more recent process by which one's own marrow is removed, irradiated, and returned to the bones have become the increasingly common recommendations of the hematologist confronted with this condition.

A second type of chronic leukemia is known as chronic lymphatic leukemia (CLL). Unlike most of the other leukemias, CLL has no known cause, but it is most often found in male patients over the age of forty. Often quite symptomless, it is only discovered by chance. The hematologist is able to diagnose CLL by an increased proportion of abnormal white blood cells present in the blood. Surprisingly, this form of leukemia can vary from a case that remains symptomless, with the patient surviving twenty years or more, to a rapidly progressing case with increasing anemia and constant infections.

The third major class of disorders diagnosed and treated by hematologists consists of those involving abnormal bleeding. The diagnosis is quite simple. The hematologist notes whether bleeding from a tiny puncture in the ear lobe stops within three minutes, as it should. If the bleeding does not stop, the determination of the cause may be difficult: It may involve too few platelets or abnormal or missing clotting factors.

Very precise tests of an increasingly sophisticated nature are now used by hematologists to determine whether a bleeding disorder is attributable to inheritance (as with hemophilia), a vitamin K deficiency, or a side effect of medication or is secondary to a type of leukemia.

PERSPECTIVE AND PROSPECTS

That blood and the vessels that carry it are important to life and health was evident even to ancient peoples. Around 500 B.C.E., Alcmaeon, a Greek, was the first to discover that arteries and veins are different types of vessels. A century later, Hippocrates observed that blood, left to stand, settles into three distinct layers. The top or largest layer is a clear, straw-colored liquid that is now called plasma. The middle layer is a narrow white band that is now known to contain white blood cells. The bottom, quite large layer, he observed to be red; it contains the cells that are now called red blood cells.

Very little else of value seems to have been learned about the blood until the seventeenth century, which witnessed many discoveries in medical science. In 1628, William Harvey, an English doctor, demonstrated scientific evidence of circulation. He found proof of a circular route and of the purpose of circulation. By 1661, the Italian scientist Marcello Malpighi reported seeing the tiny vessels called capillaries in the lungs of the frog.

Another giant step toward modern hematology occurred in the 1660's because of the efforts of Richard Lower of England and Jean-Baptiste Denis of France. Almost simultaneously, they accomplished blood transfusions from dog to dog and, soon after, from animal to human. Some transfusions were very successful; others were fatal to the patient. Almost 250 years would pass before the reason for success or failure would be learned.

In 1688, the Dutch scientist Antoni van Leeuwenhoek was able to describe and measure red blood cells accurately. He also observed that they changed shape to squeeze through tiny blood vessels. It was almost a hundred years later, in the 1770's, that Joseph Priestley, in England, found that the oxygen in the air changed dark blood from the veins into a bright red color. Only in the 1850's did the German researcher Otto Funke find within those red blood cells the compound hemoglobin, which is affected by the presence or absence of oxygen.

Although the first research on blood clotting, by William Hewson, occurred in 1768, the disease called hemophilia, or the failure of the blood to clot, was not described until 1803, by John Otto.

In the United States in the early 1900's, Karl Landsteiner discovered why certain blood can be safely transfused: the existence of the ABO blood types. This renowned hematologist was still advancing his science forty years later when he discovered the Rh system of blood types.

Another renowned hematologist, Max Perutz, worked steadily from 1939 to 1978 to understand fully the structure and function of the hemoglobin molecule. The 1940's had seen another breakthrough when Edwin Cohn, another American, discovered how to separate and purify the various plasma proteins. His work gave fellow hematologists the tools to study individual plasma components in order to learn the exact role of each in the blood. Since that time, scores of hematologists have so advanced this medical science that blood seems to have yielded most of its secrets. The ability of hematologists to treat so many types of anemia, leukemia, and other blood disorders successfully is the fruit of their tireless work.

—Grace D. Matzen

See also Acquired immunodeficiency syndrome (AIDS); Anemia; Bleeding; Blood and blood disorders; Blood testing; Bone marrow transplantation; Cholesterol; Circulation; Cytology; Cytopathology; Dialysis; Disseminated intravascular coagulation (DIC); Ergogenic aids; Fluids and electrolytes; Forensic pathology; Hematology, pediatric; Hemolytic disease of the newborn; Hemophilia; Histiocytosis; Histology; Hodgkin's disease; Host-defense mechanisms; Hypercholesterolemia; Hyperlipidemia; Immune system; Immunology; Infection; Ischemia; Jaundice; Kidney disorders; Kidneys; Laboratory tests; Leukemia; Liver; Lymphadenopathy and lymphoma; Lymphatic system; Nephrology; Nephrology, pediatric; Phlebotomy; Rh factor; Septicemia; Serology; Sickle cell disease; Thalassemia; Thrombocytopenia; Thrombolytic therapy and TPA; Thrombosis and thrombus; Transfusion; Vascular medicine; Vascular system; Von Willebrand's disease; Wiskott-Aldrich syndrome.

FOR FURTHER INFORMATION:

Avraham, Regina. *The Circulatory System.* Philadelphia: Chelsea House, 2000. Contains a brief but excellent description of the blood: its many components and their diverse functions. Includes a useful glossary and a lengthy appendix listing other sources of information about blood and circulatory disorders.

Bick, Roger L. *Disorders of Thrombosis and Hemostasis: Clinical and Laboratory Practice.* 3d ed. Philadelphia: Lippincott Williams & Wilkins, 2002. An excellent introduction to the diagnosis and management of clotting and bleeding disorders.

Lichtman, Marshall A., et al., eds. *Williams Hematology.* 7th ed. New York: McGraw-Hill, 2006. An accessible handbook that covers the pathogenetic, diagnostic, and therapeutic essentials of blood cell and coagulation protein disorders.

Rodak, Bernadette, ed. *Hematology: Clinical Principles and Applications.* 2d ed. Philadelphia: W. B. Saunders, 2002. A comprehensive textbook covering all aspects of hematology and hemostasis.

Tortora, Gerard J., and Sandra Reynolds Grabowski. *Introduction to the Human Body: The Essentials of Anatomy and Physiology.* 6th ed. Hoboken, N.J.: John Wiley & Sons, 2004. A general textbook of anatomy and physiology. Contains comprehensive information about the blood, the vessels in which it travels, the heart that pumps it, and the relationship of blood to immunity.

HEMATOLOGY, PEDIATRIC
SPECIALTY

ANATOMY OR SYSTEM AFFECTED: Blood, bones, circulatory system, immune system, liver, musculoskeletal system, spleen

SPECIALTIES AND RELATED FIELDS: Cytology, genetics, immunology, neonatology, pathology, pediatrics, perinatology, serology, vascular medicine

DEFINITION: The diagnosis and treatment of blood disorders in infants and children.

KEY TERMS:

anemia: a red blood cell deficiency caused by a decrease in hemoglobin or red cell production, an increase in cell destruction, or blood loss

erythrocytes: red blood cells

hematology: the scientific, medical study of blood and blood-forming tissues

hematopoiesis: the production of red and white cells and platelets, which occurs mainly in bone marrow

hemorrhage: the loss of a large amount of blood in a short period of time

leukemia: the presence of an increased number of leukocytes in the blood, with the specific disorder classified according to the predominant proliferating cells, the clinical course, and the duration of the disease

leukocytes: white blood cells

leukopenia: an abnormal decrease in white blood cells

neonate: a newborn infant

pediatric: pertaining to neonates, infants, and children up to the age of twelve

polycythemia: an abnormal increase in red blood cells

thrombocytes: platelets

venipuncture: a method of obtaining blood from a vein using a tourniquet, needle, and syringe

SCIENCE AND PROFESSION

Blood, the body's life-sustaining fluid, is composed of red and white cells and platelets floating in plasma. Blood transports oxygen from the lungs to the tissues; removes waste products such as carbon dioxide, urea, and lactic acid; transports hormones and nutrients; removes body heat from central to peripheral parts of the body; clots in order to seal hemorrhages; transports leukocytes and antibodies to fight injury and infection; and stores and circulates elements such as calcium and iron. The diagnosis of hematologic disorders requires the comparison of blood and bone marrow values to established reference ranges. These ranges can vary considerably during a child's growing years, with such im-

portant changes as polycythemia in the neonatal period followed by physiologic anemia of infancy, which is maximal at two and a half to three months.

Pediatric hematology involves the ongoing assessment of an infant's or child's blood and bone marrow. This specialty requires such skills as the identification of problems, the setting of goals, the use of appropriate interventions (including diet, teaching, and medication), and an evaluation of the outcome of this care. Routine blood screening involves the removal of blood by a medical laboratory phlebotomist using venipuncture in children and heel or finger stick in infants to assess the following: a complete coronary risk profile with lipid fractionation, a complete blood count (CBC), a chemistry 27 profile, an iron-deficiency profile, and diabetes mellitus screening.

A complete coronary risk profile with lipid fractionation is an assessment of total serum cholesterol, high-density lipoprotein cholesterol, low-density lipoprotein cholesterol, very-low-density lipoprotein cholesterol, total cholesterol/high-density lipoprotein cholesterol ratio, triglycerides, chylomicrons, and possibly apolipoproteins. A CBC involves an analysis of hemoglobin, hematocrit, and red and white blood cell counts with white blood cell differential, including granulocytes (neutrophils, eosinophils, and basophils) and agranulocytes (lymphocytes and monocytes). A chemistry 27 profile assesses important blood constituents such as iron and protein storage, uric acid, several electrolytes, and enzymes. An iron-deficiency profile includes measurements of total iron-binding capacity, percentage of transferrin saturation, and serum ferritin. Diabetes mellitus screening, an assessment of glucose and protein-bound glucose (indicative of the previous seven to fifteen days), is important because only an estimated one-half of all diabetics are diagnosed.

Some of the major manifestations of hematologic disease in infants and children are disorders in the function of red blood cells, white blood cells, or hemostasis. Red blood cell disorders include anemia caused by the inadequate production of erythrocytes and/or hemoglobin as a result of genetic disease or iron deficiency, anemia caused by excessive loss of erythrocytes as a result of hemorrhage or hemolytic problems, polycythemia, erythrocytosis, erythremia, and blood transfusion. Disorders of white blood cells include leukopenia, agranulocytosis, periodic neutropenia, Chediak-Higashi syndrome, and leukemias. Blood diseases associated with defects in hemostasis include disturbances in the mechanism for clotting, such as hemophilia, Von Willebrand's syndrome, deficiencies in factor II (prothrombin), factor XII deficiency, and disorders involving fibrinogen and fibrin; and defects in hemostasis in small vessels, such as thrombocytopenia, Aldrich's syndrome, and thrombopoietin deficiency.

DIAGNOSTIC AND TREATMENT TECHNIQUES

The diagnosis of pediatric hematological disorders begins with a routine blood chemistry analysis, leading to more specific tests and a medical history of the infant or child and family members to determine if the problem is congenital or acquired, chronic or episodic, and static or progressive. Iron deficiency (also called anemia) is probably the most common nutritional problem in the world today. Anemia decreases work capacity by restricting oxygen and carbon dioxide transport and reducing aerobic energy production via the inhibition of iron-dependent muscle enzymes. Therapy for anemia generally involves diet manipulation and medication but is highly variable and depends on the specific causative factors. Since the prevalence of anemia correlates strongly with socioeconomic status, screening intervals and therapy must be planned individually for each child. Up to 20 percent of children from poor homes may be anemic at one year of age, while only 4 percent of children from higher-income homes will be anemic. Anemia becomes less common between three and five years of age, thus diminishing the need for regular screening.

PERSPECTIVE AND PROSPECTS

Future research in pediatric hematology will probably include further investigation of reticulocytes, immature red blood cells that are larger than mature erythrocytes yet nonnucleated, that circulate in the blood for one to two days while maturing. Research into the causes of and prevention techniques for the development of anemia will continue to be a major focus.

Public health authorities have recommended routine screening of the entire newborn population for a variety of hereditary diseases, including acquired immunodeficiency syndrome (AIDS). This recommendation is likely to generate considerable controversy. Many states have recently required screening for phenylketonuria (PKU), a condition which can be toxic to brain tissue, even though it occurs in fewer than 1 in 16,000 neonates.

—Daniel G. Graetzer, Ph.D.

See also Acquired immunodeficiency syndrome (AIDS); Anemia; Bleeding; Blood and blood disorders; Blood testing; Bone marrow transplantation; Circulation; Cytology; Cytopathology; Dialysis; Disseminated intravascular coagulation (DIC); Fluids and electrolytes; Hematology; Hemolytic disease of the newborn; Hemophilia; Histiocytosis; Histology; Host-defense mechanisms; Immune system; Immunology; Infection; Ischemia; Jaundice; Kidney disorders; Kidneys; Laboratory tests; Leukemia; Liver; Lymphadenopathy and lymphoma; Lymphatic system; Nephrology, pediatric; Pediatrics; Phlebotomy; Rh factor; Septicemia; Serology; Sickle cell disease; Thalassemia; Thrombocytopenia; Transfusion; Vascular medicine; Vascular system; Von Willebrand's disease; Wiskott-Aldrich syndrome.

FOR FURTHER INFORMATION:

Greer, John, et al., eds. *Wintrobe's Clinical Hematology.* 11th ed. Philadelphia: Lippincott Williams & Wilkins, 2004. Includes good information on laboratory hematology, with emphasis on interpretation, immunodiagnosis, flow cytometry, clusters of differentiation, cytogenetics, and molecular genetics.

Keene, Nancy. *Childhood Leukemia: A Guide for Families, Friends and Caregivers.* 3d ed. Cambridge, Mass.: O'Reilly and Associates, 2002. Keene uses the story of her daughter's battle with leukemia as a vehicle to explore the physical and emotional impacts of the disease. Offers guidance on coping with procedures, hospitalizations, school, and associated social, emotional, and financial problems.

Kimball, Chad T. *Childhood Diseases and Disorders Sourcebook: Basic Consumer Health Information About Medical Problems Often Encountered in Preadolescent Children.* Detroit: Omnigraphics, 2003. Offers basic facts about cancer, sickle cell disease, diabetes, and other chronic conditions in children and discusses frequently used diagnostic tests, surgeries, and medications. Long-term care for seriously ill children is also presented.

Miller, Denis R., et al., eds. *Blood Diseases of Infancy and Childhood: In the Tradition of C. H. Smith.* 7th ed. St. Louis: Mosby-Year Book, 1995. A thorough text on all aspects of pediatric hematology. Includes bibliographical references and an index.

Nathan, David G., and Stuart H. Orkin, eds. *Nathan and Oski's Hematology of Infancy and Childhood.* 6th ed. Philadelphia: W. B. Saunders, 2003. This textbook will undoubtedly be useful to many readers not directly involved in clinical or research pediatric hematology. First, it provides basic scientists with a clinical perspective. Second, pediatric and adult subspecialists will occasionally need it to read about rare conditions, and it should be included in the reference collection of every library on adult hematology or general pediatrics.

HEMIPLEGIA
DISEASE/DISORDER

ANATOMY OR SYSTEM AFFECTED: Arms, brain, head, joints, legs, muscles, musculoskeletal system, nervous system, tendons

SPECIALTIES AND RELATED FIELDS: Exercise physiology, family medicine, neurology, orthopedics, physical therapy

DEFINITION: Paralysis of one side of the body, usually caused by brain damage.

CAUSES AND SYMPTOMS

Hemiplegia is paralysis or partial paralysis of one side of the body, typically involving the leg, arm, and trunk. It is caused by damage or disease of the part of the brain that controls the motor nervous system. The damage may occur prior to birth, during birth, or after birth as a result of an accident, illness, or stroke. The most common cause is a cerebrovascular disease that leads to clotting of the cerebral arteries or bleeding from the diseased arterial wall, eventually producing a stroke. The site most often affected is the internal capsule, where packed nerve fibers descend from the cortex of the brain into the spinal cord.

INFORMATION ON HEMIPLEGIA

CAUSES: Brain damage or disease as a result of accident, illness, or stroke

SYMPTOMS: Paralysis on one side of body, muscle weakness and spasticity, poor balance, speech difficulties, epileptic seizures, visual field defects, emotional and behavioral problems, gait problems

DURATION: Long-term

TREATMENTS: Depends on severity; may include physical therapy, speech therapy, occupational therapy, braces or orthotics, electrical stimulation, drugs, Botox injections, surgery, acupuncture

---

Immediately after a stroke, the affected body parts are initially limp. In a few days or weeks, the limbs become stiff and spastic. Symptoms of hemiplegia can include paralysis on one side of the body, muscle weakness and spasticity, poor balance, speech difficulties, epileptic seizures, visual field defects, emotional and behavioral problems, and gait problems, including limping and toe drop. Increased energy expenditure results from compensatory adjustments during walking that produce abnormal movements of the body's center of gravity.

TREATMENT AND THERAPY

Treatments for hemiplegia are designed to improve strength and range of motion, increase bodily functions, and reduce or prevent spasticity. Long-term care is very important. Depending on the severity of the disorder, physical therapy, speech therapy, occupational therapy, braces or orthotics, electrical stimulation, drugs, Botox injections, and surgery may be used as corrective procedures. Acupuncture and electroacupuncture procedures may be promising treatments for hemiplegia. Children who suffer from hemiplegia may also receive special educational services to help improve specific learning difficulties caused by the disorder. Affected children should involve the weaker side of the body in everyday activities so that they become as two-sided as possible.

PERSPECTIVE AND PROSPECTS

The side of the body affected by hemiplegia depends on which side of the brain has been damaged. The left side of the brain controls the right side of the body, while the right side controls the left side of the body. Depending on which side of the body is affected, the disease is often referred to as right hemiplegia or left hemiplegia.

Childhood hemiplegia affects up to one child per one thousand. An associated rare neurological disorder, alternating hemiplegia of childhood (AHC), produces periodic transient attacks of hemiplegia that affect one side of the body or the other. An attack of AHC may last from a few minutes up to days. The attacks may alternate from one side of the body to the other. The symptoms are usually relieved with bed rest and proper sleep.

—*Alvin K. Benson, Ph.D.*

See also Brain; Brain damage; Brain disorders; Nervous system; Neuroimaging; Neurology; Neurology, pediatric; Paralysis; Paraplegia; Physical rehabilitation; Quadriplegia; Strokes.

FOR FURTHER INFORMATION:

Bobath, Berta. *Adult Hemiplegia: Evaluation and Treatment*. 3d ed. London: Heinemann Medical Books, 1990.

Davies, Patricia M. *Steps to Follow: The Comprehensive Treatment of Patients with Hemiplegia*. 2d ed. New York: Springer, 2004.

Neville, Brian, and Robert Goodman, eds. *Congenital Hemiplegia*. London: MacKeith, 2001.

Spivack, Barney S., ed. *Evaluation and Management of Gait Disorders*. New York: Marcel Dekker, 1995.

HEMOCHROMATOSIS

DISEASE/DISORDER

ALSO KNOWN AS: Bronze diabetes

ANATOMY OR SYSTEM AFFECTED: Genitals, heart, liver, pancreas

SPECIALTIES AND RELATED FIELDS: Cardiology, endocrinology, gastroenterology, internal medicine

DEFINITION: A multisystem disease characterized by increased iron absorption and storage.

INFORMATION ON HEMOCHROMATOSIS
CAUSES: Genetic defect in iron production
SYMPTOMS: Damage to pancreas, skin, testes, and heart, causing diabetes mellitus, bronze-like skin pigmentation, loss of libido and erectile dysfunction, and abnormal heart rhythms or heart failure
DURATION: Chronic
TREATMENTS: Phlebotomy (blood removal) to create mild anemia

CAUSES AND SYMPTOMS

Iron is used by the body for various processes, such as making hemoglobin, the oxygen-carrying molecule in blood. Hemochromatosis is an inherited disorder characterized by the excessive absorption and accumulation of iron from the diet. This excess iron is deposited in various organs. Damage to these organs from years of iron accumulation results in the symptoms of hemochromatosis. The most commonly affected organs are the pancreas (causing diabetes), the skin (causing bronzelike skin pigmentation), the testes (causing loss of libido and erectile dysfunction), and the heart (causing abnormal heart rhythms or heart failure). The pituitary gland, which regulates sex hormones and metabolism, can also be affected. Although the liver is commonly involved as well, this usually results in mild abnormalities in blood tests of liver enzymes rather than liver failure. However, cirrhosis of the liver can occur, and these patients are at risk for developing liver cancer. Unfortunately, most of the above warning symptoms occur late in the disease, after decades of iron accumulation and organ damage have already taken place.

TREATMENT AND THERAPY

Ideally, hemochromatosis should be detected and treated before the onset of symptoms. Screening for patients with a family history of this disease can be performed via blood tests, such as the iron saturation index. More recently, a genetic test for a common mutation that causes hemochromatosis has been developed. Liver biopsy is sometimes needed to confirm the diagnosis. Treatment consists of repeated phlebotomy, or the removal of blood. Typically one unit of blood is removed per week until the patient becomes mildly anemic. Hemochromatosis may require the removal of up to 150 units of blood over several years. Subsequently, phlebotomy is repeated every three to four months, and the patient's iron stores (ferritin) are monitored. If phlebotomy is started before liver cirrhosis develops, then many complications can be avoided.

PERSPECTIVE AND PROSPECTS

Hemochromatosis was initially described in 1865 as a triad of glucose in the urine, dark pigmentation of the skin, and liver cirrhosis. Research into the disease has resulted in tremendous advances in the understanding of iron metabolism. The gene responsible for hemochromatosis has been mapped to chromosome 6. Although the genetic defect is present in both men and women, men develop the disease much more often, since menstruation removes excess iron in women. A test to screen for one common mutation in this gene is available, but its usefulness is limited since several other mutations may cause the disease, especially in non-Caucasian ethnic groups.

—*Ahmad Kamal, M.D.*

See also Hematology; Hematology, pediatric; Liver disorders; Metabolic disorders; Metabolism; Nephrology; Nephrology, pediatric.

FOR FURTHER INFORMATION:

Barton, James C., and Corwin Q. Edwards, eds. *Hemochromatosis: Genetics, Pathophysiology, Di-*

agnosis, and Treatment. New York: Cambridge University Press, 2000.

Burke, Wylie, P. D. Phatak, and E. D. Weinberg, eds. *Iron Disorders Institute Guide to Hemochromatosis.* Nashville: Cumberland House, 2001.

Everson, Gregory T., and Marilyn Olsen. *Living with Hemochromatosis.* New York: Hatherleigh Press, 2003.

Parker, James N., and Philip M. Parker, eds. *The Official Patient's Sourcebook on Hemochromatosis.* San Diego, Calif.: Icon Health, 2002.

Weinberg, E. D., and Cheryl D. Garrison. *Exposing the Hidden Dangers of Iron: What Every Medical Professional Should Know About the Impact of Iron on the Disease Process.* Nashville: Cumberland House, 2004.

HEMOLYTIC DISEASE OF THE NEWBORN
DISEASE/DISORDER

ALSO KNOWN AS: Erythroblastosis fetalis, Rh incompatibility, ABO incompatibility

ANATOMY OR SYSTEM AFFECTED: Blood, brain, liver, skin

SPECIALTIES AND RELATED FIELDS: Hematology, neonatology, neurology

DEFINITION: The destruction of red blood cells in a fetus by antibodies transferred from the mother.

KEY TERMS:

antibodies: proteins produced by the immune system to destroy invading organisms or those perceived as foreign to the body

bilirubin: a pigment derived from the breakdown of red blood cells

Coombs' test: a test used to determine whether sensitization has occurred

---

INFORMATION ON HEMOLYTIC DISEASE OF THE NEWBORN

CAUSES: Blood incompatibilities between mother and fetus

SYMPTOMS: Pale skin, enlarged liver and spleen, progressive jaundice and anemia within twenty-four hours of birth, deafness

DURATION: Varies

TREATMENTS: Light therapy, drug therapy, blood transfusions, iron and folic acid supplementation

---

exchange transfusion: the exchange of all or most of a patient's blood for donor blood; in a baby with hemolytic disease, usually performed through the umbilical vein

hemolysis: the rapid destruction of red blood cells

jaundice: yellow pigmentation resulting from the deposition of bilirubin in the skin

kernicterus: brain damage produced by the deposition of bilirubin in the brain

Rhogam: a protein that destroys Rh-positive cells

sensitization: the development of antibodies to a substance

CAUSES AND SYMPTOMS

Hemolytic disease of the newborn is a disorder in which maternal antibodies induce hemolysis of the red blood cells of the fetus or newborn, producing jaundice. The most common causes are ABO or Rh incompatibilities. ABO incompatibility occurs when the mother's blood is type O and the baby's blood is either type A or type B. The newborn develops jaundice within the first forty-eight hours of birth as a result of increasing bilirubin levels in the blood. Rh incompatibility can arise when an Rh-negative woman is carrying a second Rh-positive fetus. During the delivery of the first Rh-positive baby, blood from the newborn may pass into the mother's circulation. If no treatment is given, the woman may develop anti-Rh antibodies, which will remain in her circulation. If the fetus in her next pregnancy is also Rh-positive, the anti-Rh antibodies will cross over into the baby's blood, causing hemolysis of the red blood cells. In severe cases, the hemolysis starts in utero and the fetus will develop anemia, progressing to generalized edema with heart failure (hydrops fetalis) and death if the anemia is not corrected.

During the pregnancy, a positive Coombs' test indicates that the woman has been exposed and thus sensitized to Rh factor. A woman who is Rh-negative can become sensitized in three ways: by having delivered an Rh-positive baby following a previous pregnancy and not having received the protein Rhogam; by receiving an erroneous infusion of Rh-positive blood; and by having a spontaneous or induced abortion of an Rh-positive embryo or fetus. A rising concentration of antibodies during the course of the pregnancy indicates that hemolysis is occurring in the fetus. A small amount of amniotic fluid is obtained through a needle inserted through the mother's abdomen to determine the severity of the disease in the fetus. At birth, the baby may have pale skin and an enlarged liver and spleen. Progressive jaundice and anemia develop within the first twenty-four hours. High levels may cause the bilirubin to enter the brain and produce kernicterus. The baby with kernicterus shows little activity (hypoactivity), refuses to suck milk, and experiences seizures that can progress to permanent neurologic damage or to coma and death. Deafness may be a consequence of high bilirubin levels during the newborn period.

TREATMENT AND THERAPY

There is no preventive treatment for ABO incompatibility. Phototherapy, or light therapy, is used to decrease the level of bilirubin. Phototherapy acts on the bilirubin deposited in the skin and makes it water soluble, so that the pigment can be excreted through the gastrointestinal tract. An exchange transfusion may be required to decrease the concentration of bilirubin if it rises to dangerous levels. These levels will depend on the baby's maturation and clinical condition.

Preventive treatment for Rh incompatibility consists of giving Rhogam to all Rh-negative pregnant women at twenty-eight weeks of gestation and within the first seventy-two hours after the delivery of an Rh-positive baby. All Rh-negative women who have experienced an abortion or who have erroneously received a transfusion of Rh-positive blood should also receive Rhogam.

An Rh-negative pregnant woman with a positive Coombs' test needs to have periodic Coombs titers, or antibody concentration measurements, to determine what type of intervention, if any, is required. This test should first be done between sixteen and eighteen weeks of gestation. Rising Coombs titers indicate that hemolysis is occurring in the fetus. Prenatal interventions may include correcting fetal anemia by giving red blood cells directly to the fetus, either into the abdomen or into the umbilical vein. The fetus must be observed with sonography for the development of fetal edema, an ominous sign. At birth, the baby may have severe anemia requiring immediate correction. Phototherapy and an exchange transfusion may be needed if bilirubin rises above acceptable levels. Other modes of therapy, such as phenobarbital, agar gel, and rectal suppositories, are of limited value in reducing bilirubin in infants with hemolytic disease.

Before discharge from the hospital nursery, a hearing test must be done for all infants who have had jaundice during the neonatal period. Anemia may develop during the first six weeks of life as a result of the persistence of antibodies in the baby's blood. Close follow-up of hemoglobin levels must be done after discharge from the hospital. Blood transfusions may be indicated, as well as iron and folic acid supplementation.

PERSPECTIVE AND PROSPECTS

The incidence of Rh incompatibility has decreased remarkably since the advent of Rhogam. Nevertheless, it still occurs, particularly when unidentified miscarriages have occurred. Rh-negative fetuses can be identified early using special techniques available only in large medical centers. Therapy for hydrops fetalis has improved with the use of cordocentesis. This therapy, which consists of obtaining and transfusing blood directly into the umbilical cord while the fetus is in utero, is available in specialized medical centers and has helped many sensitized babies to survive. Immunoglobulin has been used to block hemolysis, but it cannot be used for treatment. Agents that can metabolize bilirubin are currently under investigation.

—*Gloria Reyes Báez, M.D.*

See also Anemia; Blood and blood disorders; Critical care, pediatric; Emergency medicine, pediatric; Hearing loss; Immune system; Jaundice; Neonatology; Rh factor; Umbilical cord.

FOR FURTHER INFORMATION:

Behrman, Richard E., Robert M. Kliegman, and Hal B. Jenson, eds. *Nelson Textbook of Pediatrics.* 17th ed. Philadelphia: Saunders, 2004. Text covering all medical and surgical disorders in children with authoritative information on genetics, endocrinology, etiology, epidemiology, pathology, pathophysiology, clinical manifestations, diagnosis, prevention, treatment, and prognosis.

Kemper, Kathi J. *The Holistic Pediatrician: A Pediatrician's Comprehensive Guide to Safe and Effective Therapies for the Twenty-five Most Common Ailments of Infants, Children, and Adolescents.* New York: HarperCollins, 2002. Integrates mainstream and alternative medicine to aid parents in dealing with the most common childhood health problems such as fever, diaper rash, ear infections, and allergies.

Levy, Joseph. "Newborn Jaundice." *Parents Magazine* 69, no. 7 (July, 1994): 59-60. Jaundice is a fairly common condition in newborns because many do not have mature enough livers to process and excrete bilirubin, which causes the yellow color of jaundiced babies. The different types of jaundice, symptoms, and treatments for the disease are discussed.

Martin, Richard J., Avroy A. Fanaroff, and Michele C. Walsh, eds. *Fanaroff and Martin's Neonatal-Perinatal Medicine: Diseases of the Fetus and Infant.* 2 vols. 8th ed. Philadelphia: Mosby Elsevier, 2006. Contains a chapter called "Erythroblastosis Fetalis." An exhaustive resource covering all the major diseases of the infant and fetus. Includes bibliographical references and an index.

Nathanson, Laura Walther. *The Portable Pediatrician: A Practicing Pediatrician's Guide to Your Child's Growth, Development, Health, and Behavior from Birth to Age Five.* 2d ed. New York: HarperCollins, 2002. An engaging, easy-to-read guide for parents to assess their child's development, medical symptoms, and behavioral problems.

HEMOLYTIC UREMIC SYNDROME
DISEASE/DISORDER
ALSO KNOWN AS: Gasser syndrome

ANATOMY OR SYSTEM AFFECTED: Blood, circulatory system, gastrointestinal system, kidneys, nervous system, urinary system

SPECIALTIES AND RELATED FIELDS: Family medicine, gastroenterology, hematology, nephrology, nutrition, pediatrics, urology

DEFINITION: A predominantly childhood disorder produced primarily by a strain of *Escherichia coli* bacteria and characterized by acute kidney failure, hemolytic anemia, and a low platelet count.

CAUSES AND SYMPTOMS
In the majority of cases, hemolytic uremic syndrome develops after the digestive system has been infected by the O157:H7 strain of *Escherichia coli* (*E. coli*). Undercooked meats, contaminated fresh vegetables and fruits, unpasteurized dairy products and juices, and contaminated water are the primary sources of this bacterium. Hemolytic uremic syndrome can be passed from person to person. Less common sources include *Shigella*, *Salmonella*, *Yersinia*, and *Campylobacter* bacteria.

Following a siege of gastroenteritis that typically lasts for three to ten days and usually includes vomiting, fever, cramping, and diarrhea, hemolytic uremic syndrome develops when the *E. coli* produce toxins that enter the bloodstream and begin destroying red blood cells and platelets. The damaged red blood cells block tiny blood vessels in the kidneys, making it more and more difficult for the kidneys to function. Resulting symptoms can include reduced urine output,

---

INFORMATION ON HEMOLYTIC UREMIC SYNDROME

CAUSES: Infection with *E. coli* or other bacteria that produce toxins which enter the bloodstream

SYMPTOMS: Initially, vomiting, fever, cramping, and diarrhea; progressing to red blood cell destruction, poor kidney function, reduced urine output, paleness, bruises, blood in urine and feces, extreme fatigue, irritability, seizures, increased blood pressure, swollen limbs

DURATION: Acute

TREATMENTS: Supportive measures; in severe cases, dialysis or kidney transplantation

---

paleness, small body bruises, blood in the urine and stool, extreme fatigue, irritability, seizures, increased blood pressure, and swollen limbs.

TREATMENT AND THERAPY
Once an individual is diagnosed with hemolytic uremic syndrome, the typical treatment is mostly supportive. Maintaining normal electrolyte and water levels in the body eases the immediate symptoms and helps prevent further complications. Vital signs are monitored frequently, as is the weight of the patient. Blood transfusions are necessary only when there is severe anemia.

Depending on urine output and electrolyte abnormalities, dialysis may be used. On rare occasions, the victim may require a kidney transplant. Administration of antimotility agents, antibiotics, or platelet transfusions seems to worsen the outcome. Approximately 85 percent of children with hemolytic uremic syndrome recover fully without further complications.

PERSPECTIVE AND PROSPECTS
Hemolytic uremic syndrome was first described by Swiss hematologist Conrad von Gasser in 1955. Although it is an uncommon illness, striking examples exist in which many individuals have been infected during a particular time frame. In 2000, more than two thousand people developed hemolytic uremic syndrome symptoms after drinking contaminated water in Walkerton, Ontario, Canada; seven died. Three months later, forty individuals experienced hemolytic uremic syndrome symptoms after eating at a Sizzler restaurant in Milwaukee, Wisconsin; one died. In 2006, more than 180 individuals were identified with hemo-

lytic uremic syndrome symptoms in the United States as a result of contaminated spinach grown in California; three died.

Research into treating hemolytic uremic syndrome has focused on preventing its onset by using chemical agents that bind the toxins produced by *E. coli* O157:H7 within the intestines. Strategies involving immunization are also being developed.

—*Alvin K. Benson, Ph.D.*

See also Bacterial infections; Bacteriology; Blood and blood disorders; Childhood infectious diseases; Dialysis; *E. coli* infection; Food poisoning; Hematology; Hematology, pediatric; Kidney disorders; Kidney transplantation; Kidneys; Nephrology; Nephrology, pediatric.

FOR FURTHER INFORMATION:

Hoffman, Ronald, et al., eds. *Hematology: Basic Principles and Practice*, 4th ed. Philadelphia: Churchill Livingstone, 2005.

Kaper, James B., and Alison D. O'Brien, eds. *Escherichia coli O157:H7 and Other Shiga Toxin-Producing E. coli Strains*. Washington D.C.: ASM Press, 1998.

Parker, James N., and Philip M. Parker, eds. *The Official Patient's Sourcebook on Hemolytic Uremic Syndrome: A Revised and Updated Directory for the Internet Age*. San Diego, Calif.: Icon Health, 2002.

HEMOPHILIA

DISEASE/DISORDER

ANATOMY OR SYSTEM AFFECTED: Blood

SPECIALTIES AND RELATED FIELDS: Genetics, hematology, serology

DEFINITION: A genetic disorder characterized by the blood's inability to form clots as a result of the lack or alteration of certain trace plasma proteins.

KEY TERMS:

clotting factors: substances present in plasma that are needed for the coagulation of blood

hemophilia A: a genetic blood disease characterized by a deficiency of clotting factor VIII

hemophilia B: a genetic blood disease characterized by a deficiency of clotting factor IX

hemostasis: the process of stopping the flow of blood at an injury site

von Willebrand's disease: a genetic blood disease characterized by a deficiency of the von Willebrand clotting factor

CAUSES AND SYMPTOMS

The circulatory system must be self-healing; otherwise, continued blood loss from even the smallest injury would be life-threatening. Normally, all except the most catastrophic bleeding is rapidly stopped in a process known as hemostasis. Hemostasis takes place through several sequential steps or processes. First, an injury stimulates platelets (unpigmented blood cells) to adhere to the damaged blood vessels and then to one another, forming a plug that can stop minor bleeding. This association is mediated by what is called the von Willebrand factor, a protein that binds to the platelets. As the platelets aggregate, they release several substances that stimulate vasoconstriction, or a reduction in size of the blood vessels. This reduces the blood flow at the injury site. Finally, the aggregating platelets and damaged tissue initiate blood clotting, or coagulation. Once bleeding has stopped, the firmly adhering clot slowly contracts, drawing the edge of the wounds together so that tough scar tissue can form a permanent repair on the site.

Formation of a blood clot involves the participation of nearly twenty different substances, most of which are proteins synthesized by plasma. All but two of these substances, or factors, are designated by a roman numeral and a common name. A blood clot will be defective if one of the clotting factors is absent or deficient in the blood, and clotting time will be longer. The clotting factors, with some of their alternative names, are factor I (fibrinogen), factor II (prothrombin), factor III (tissue factor or thromboplastin), factor IV (calcium), factor V (proaccelerin), factor VII (proconvertin), factor VIII (antihemophilic factor), factor IX (Christmas factor), factor X (Stuart factor), factor XI (plasma thromboplastin antecedent), factor XII (Hageman factor), and factor XIII (fibrin stabilizing factor).

Several of the clotting factors have been discovered by the diagnosis of their deficiencies in various clotting disorders. The inherited coagulation disorders are uncommon conditions with an overall incidence of probably no more than 10 to 20 per 100,000 of the population. Hemophilia A, the most common or classic type of coagulation disorder, is caused by factor VIII deficiency. Hemophilia B (or Christmas disease) is the result of factor IX deficiency. It is quite common for severe hemophilia to manifest itself during the first year of life. Hazardous bleeding occurs in areas such as the central nervous system, the retropharyngeal area, and the retroperitoneal area. Bleeding in these areas requires admission to the hospital for observation and

INFORMATION ON HEMOPHILIA

CAUSES: Genetic blood defect
SYMPTOMS: Loss of large amounts of blood from even small injuries, hemorrhaging without apparent cause, bruising, pain, swelling, joint lesions, urinary bleeding, pseudotumors
DURATION: Chronic
TREATMENTS: Fresh frozen plasma, clotting factor concentrates, drug therapy

therapy. Joint lesions are very common in hemophilia because of acute spontaneous hemorrhage in the area, specially in weight-bearing joints such as ankles and knees. Urinary bleeding is often present at some time. The appearance of pseudotumors, caused by swelling involving muscle and bone produced by recurrent bleeding, is also common.

Hemophilia is transmitted entirely by unaffected females (carriers) to their sons in a sex-linked inheritance deficiency. Congenital deficiencies of the other coagulation factors are well recognized, even though bleeding episodes in these cases are uncommon. Deficiency of more than one factor is also possible, although documentation of such cases is very rare, perhaps because only patients with milder variations of the disease survive.

Von Willebrand's disease, unlike the hemophilias that mainly involve bleeding in joints and muscles, involves mainly bleeding of mucocutaneous tissues or skin. It affects both men and women. This disease shares clinical characteristics with hemophilia A, or classic hemophilia, including decreased levels of clotting factor VIII. This similarity made the differentiation between the two diseases very difficult for a long time. It has now been established that there are two different factors involved in von Willebrand's disease, each with a different function. The von Willebrand factor is involved in the adhesion of platelets to the injured blood vessel wall and to one another and, together with factor VIII, circulates in plasma as a complex held by electrostatic and hydrophobic forces. The von Willebrand factor is a very large molecule, consisting of a series of possible multimeric structures. The bigger and heavier the multimer, the better it works against bleeding. Von Willebrand's disease is one of the least understood clotting disorders. Three types have been identified, with at least twenty-seven variations. With type I, all the multimers needed for successful clotting are present in the blood, but in lesser amounts than in healthy individuals. In type II, the larger multimers, which are more active in hemostasis, are lacking, and type III patients exhibit a severe lack of all multimers.

TREATMENT AND THERAPY

The normal body is continually producing clotting factors in order to keep up with natural loss. Sometimes the production is stepped up to cover a real or anticipated increase in the need for these factors, such as in childbirth. Hemophiliacs, lacking some of these clotting factors, may lose large amounts of blood from even the smallest injury and sometimes hemorrhage without any apparent cause. The symptoms of their diseases may be alleviated by the intravenous administration of the deficient clotting factor. How this is done depends on the specific factor deficiency and the magnitude of the bleeding episode, the age and size of the patient, convenience, acceptability, cost of product, and method and place of delivery of care.

There are many sources for clotting factors. Fresh frozen plasma contains all the clotting factors, but since the concentration of the factors in plasma is relatively low, a large volume is required for treatment. Therefore, it can be used only when small amounts of clotting factor must be delivered. Its use is the only therapy for deficiencies of factors V, XI, and XII. Plasma is commonly harvested from single donor units to minimize the risk of infection by the hepatitis virus or human immunodeficiency virus (HIV), thus eliminating the risk involved in using pooled concentrates from many donors. Cryoprecipitates are the proteins that precipitate in fresh frozen plasma thawed at 4 degrees Celsius. The precipitate is rich in factors VIII and XIII and in fibrinogen, and carries less chance of infection with hepatitis. Its standardization is difficult, however, and is not required by the Food and Drug Administration. As a result, dosage calculation can be a problem. In addition, there is no method for the control of viral contamination. Therefore, cryoprecipitates are not commonly used unless harvested from a special known and tested donor pool. Clotting factor concentrates present many advantages. They are made from pooled plasma obtained from plasmapheresis or a program of total donor unit fractionation and are widely available. Factors VIII and IX can also be produced from plasma using monoclonal methods. Porcine factor VIII presents an alternative to patients with a naturally occurring antibody to human factor VIII.

Other substances can replace missing clotting factors as well. The synthetic hormone desmopressin acetate (also known by the letters DDAVP) has been used to stimulate the release of factor VIII and von Willebrand factor from the endothelial cells lining blood vessels. It is commonly used for patients with mild hemophilia and von Willebrand's disease. DDAVP has no effect on the concentration of the other factors, and aside from the common side effect of water retention, it is a safe drug. Antifibrinolytic drugs prevent the natural breakdown of blood clots that have already been formed. Although such drugs are not useful for the primary care of hemophiliacs, they are useful for use after dental extractions and in the treatment of other open wounds, after a clot has formed.

Between 10 and 15 percent of the patients affected with severe hemophilia develop factor VIII inhibitors (antibodies), which prevents their treatment with the usual methods. Newer therapeutic approaches have provided additional options for the management and control of bleeding episodes. The use of prothrombin complex concentrates or porcine factor VIII concentrates is indicated for low responders (those with a low amount of antibodies present in their system). An option for high responders is to try to eradicate the inhibitor present in their systems. One way to do this is with a regimen of immunosuppressive drugs. These are very limited in value, however, and cannot be used with HIV-positive hemophiliacs. The drugs used in this approach include substances such as cyclophosphamide, vincristine, azathioprine, and corticosteroids. Another approach utilizes intravenous doses of gamma globulin to suppress, but not eradicate, the inhibitors. Yet another strategy is an immune tolerance regimen, in which factor VIII is administered daily in small amounts. This method causes the inhibitors to decrease and, in some cases, disappear. The regimen can also involve the prophylactic use of factor VIII (or factor VIII in combination with immunosuppressive drugs).

The introduction of plasma clotting factor concentrates has changed the treatment of patients with clotting factor deficiencies. It has brought about a remarkable change in the longevity of these patients and their quality of life. The availability of cryoprecipitates and concentrates of factors II, VII, VIII, IX, X, and XIII has made outpatient treatment for bleeding episodes routine and home infusion or self-infusion a possibility for many patients. Hospitalization for inpatient treatment is rare, and early outpatient therapy of bleeding episodes has decreased the severity of joint deformities.

Nevertheless, other problems are apparent in hemophiliac patients. Viral contamination of the factor concentrates has allowed the development of chronic illnesses, infection with HIV, immunologic diseases, liver and renal diseases, joint disorders, and cardiovascular diseases. While the use of heat for virus inactivation, beginning in 1983, resulted in a reduction in HIV infections, the majority of patients exposed to the virus had already been infected. The strategies to prevent contraction of hepatitis from these concentrates include vaccination against the contaminating viruses and the elimination of viruses from the factor replacement product. The non-A, non-B hepatitis virus is very difficult to remove, however, and the use of monoclonal factors seems to be the only solution to this problem. In general, difficulties associated with treatment have been largely eliminated through the production of the required clotting factors using recombinant DNA techniques, a process performed independent of human blood.

Treatment of von Willebrand's disease also includes pressure dressing, suturing, and oral contraceptives. A pasteurized antihemophiliac concentrate that contains substantial amounts of von Willebrand factor is used in severe cases.

Hematomas, or hemorrhages under the skin and within muscles, can frequently be controlled by application of elastic bandage pressure and ice. The ones that cannot be controlled easily within a few hours may cause muscle contraction and require factor replacement therapy. Exercise is recommended for joints after bleeding, as it helps protect joints by increasing muscle bulk and power and can also help relieve stress. Devices to protect joints, such as elastic bandages and splints, are commonly used. In extreme cases, orthopedic surgical procedures are readily available.

Analgesics, or painkillers, play an important part in the alleviation of chronic pain. Because patients cannot use products with aspirin and/or antihistamines, which inhibit platelet aggregation and prolong bleeding time, substances such as acetaminophen, codeine, and morphine are used. Chronic joint inflammation is reduced by the use of anti-inflammatory agents such as ibuprofen and of drugs used in rheumatoid arthritis patients.

The need for so many specialties and disciplines in the management of hemophilia has led to the development of multidisciplinary hemophilia centers. Genetic education (information on how the disease is transmitted), genetic counseling (the discussion of an individual's genetic risks and reproductive options), and genetic testing have provided great help to patients and affected families. Early and prenatal diagnosis and carrier detection have provided options for family planning.

PERSPECTIVE AND PROSPECTS

Descriptions of hemophilia are among the oldest known accounts of genetic disease. References to a bleeding condition highly suggestive of hemophilia go back to the fifth century, in the Babylonian Talmud. The first significant report in medical literature appeared in 1803 when John C. Otto, a Philadelphia physician, described several bleeder families with only males affected and with transmission through the mothers. The literature of the nineteenth century contains many descriptions of the disease, particularly the clinical characteristics of the hemorrhages and family histories. The disease was originally called haemorrhaphilia, or "tendency toward hemorrhages," but the name was later contracted through usage to hemophilia ("tendency toward blood"), the accepted name since around 1828.

Transfusion therapy was proposed as early as 1832, and the first successful transfusion for the treatment of a hemophiliac patient was reported in 1840 by Samuel Armstrong Lane. The use of blood from cows and pigs in the transfusions was explored but abandoned because of the numerous side effects. It was not until the beginning of the twentieth century that serious studies on clotting in hemophilia were started. Attention was directed to the use of normal human serum for treatment of bleeding episodes. Some of the patients responded well, while others did not. This result is probably attributable to the fact that some had hemophilia A—these patients did not respond because factor VIII, in which they are deficient, is not present in serum— while some others had hemophilia B, for which the therapy worked. In 1923, harvested blood plasma was used in transfusion, and it was shown to work as well as whole blood. With blood banking becoming a reality in the 1930's, transfusions were performed more frequently as a treatment for hemophilia.

The history of the fractionation of plasma began around 1911 with Dr. Addis, who prepared a very crude fraction by acidification of plasma. In 1937, Drs. Patek and Taylor produced a crude fraction which, on injection, lowered the blood-clotting time in hemophiliacs. In the period from 1945 to 1960, a number of plasma fractions with antihemophiliac activity were developed. The use of fresh frozen plasma increased as a result of advances in the purification of the fractions. Some milestones can be identified in the production of the plasma fractions: the development of quantitative assays for antihemophiliac factors, the discovery of cryoprecipitation, and the development of glycine and polyethylene precipitation.

In 1952, four significant and independent publications indicated that there is a plasma-clotting activity separate from that concerned with classic hemophilia—in other words, that there are two types of hemophilia. One (hemophilia A) is characterized by a deficiency in factor VIII, while the other (hemophilia B) is characterized by deficiency in factor IX. Carriers of hemophilia A can have a mean factor VIII level that is 50 percent lower than that of normal females, while carriers of hemophilia B show levels of factor IX that are 60 percent below normal. The two diseases have the same pattern of inheritance, are similar in clinical appearance, and can be distinguished only by laboratory tests.

Hemophilias are caused by a disordered and complex biological mechanism that continues to be explored. Recombinant DNA techniques have now revealed the molecular defect in factor VIII or factor IX deficiencies in some families, demonstrating that a variety of gene defects can produce the classic phenotype of hemophilia. These techniques have also provided new tools for carrier detection and prenatal diagnosis.

Current treatment of hemophilia has converted the hemophiliac from an in-hospital patient to an individual with more independent status. Crucial in this development has been the creation of comprehensive care centers and of the National Hemophilia Foundation, which provide comprehensive treatment for the hemophilia patient. With the advancement of recombinant DNA technology, the future looks brighter for the sufferers of this disease.

—*Maria Pacheco, Ph.D.*

See also Acquired immunodeficiency syndrome (AIDS); Bleeding; Blood and blood disorders; Genetic diseases; Genetics and inheritance; Transfusion; Von Willebrand's disease.

FOR FURTHER INFORMATION:

Bellenir, Karen, ed. *Genetic Disorders Sourcebook: Basic Consumer Information About Hereditary Diseases and Disorders.* 3d ed. Detroit: Omnigraphics, 2004. This nontechnical sourcebook offers basic information about lifestyle expectations, disease management techniques, and current research initiatives for the most common types of genetic disorders, including a resource list of three hundred genetic disorders and related topics.

Bloom, Arthur L., ed. *The Hemophilias*. New York: Churchill Livingstone, 1982. The series presents accounts of methods for the study of blood and its disorders. This book concentrates on hemophilia, presenting a description of available assay methods, purification methods, and prenatal diagnosis.

Hilgartner, Margaret W., and Carl Pochedly, eds. *Hemophilia in the Child and Adult*. 3d ed. New York: Raven Press, 1989. A compilation of the thoughts and experiences of clinicians who deal with hemophilia, as well as some practical approaches to patient care. A well-organized and informative book.

Jones, Peter. *Living with Haemophilia*. 5th ed. New York: Oxford University Press, 2002. An excellent book for the layperson, it was written specifically for patients and their families. In an easy-to-read, understandable format, explains the transmission of bleeding disorders through families, their manifestations, and their management.

King, Richard A., Jerome I. Rotter, and Arno G. Motulsky, eds. *Genetic Basis of Common Diseases*. 2d ed. New York: Oxford University Press, 2002. Covers advances in the understanding of molecular processes involved in genetic susceptibility and disease mechanisms. Examines a range of diseases in detail and includes a chapter on genetic counseling.

National Hemophilia Foundation. http://www.hemophilia.org/. A Web site that promotes education, research and advocacy on behalf of people with bleeding disorders.

Parker, James N., and Philip M. Parker, eds. *The 2002 Official Patient's Sourcebook on Hemophilia*. San Diego, Calif.: Icon Health, 2002. Draws from public, academic, government, and peer-reviewed research to provide a wide-ranging handbook for patients with hemophilia.

Rodak, Bernadette, ed. *Hematology: Clinical Principles and Applications*. 2d ed. Philadelphia: W. B. Saunders, 2002. A comprehensive textbook covering all aspects of hematology and hemostasis.

Voet, Donald, and Judith G. Voet. *Biochemistry*. 3d ed. Hoboken, N.J.: John Wiley & Sons, 2004. A comprehensive biochemistry textbook with an excellent section on blood and blood-clotting mechanisms.

HEMORRHOID BANDING AND REMOVAL

PROCEDURE

ANATOMY OR SYSTEM AFFECTED: Anus, blood vessels, circulatory system, gastrointestinal system, intestines

SPECIALTIES AND RELATED FIELDS: Family medicine, gastroenterology, general surgery, proctology

DEFINITION: The surgical ligation and removal of protruding veins from the lower rectum.

INDICATIONS AND PROCEDURES

Hemorrhoids, or piles, result from the protrusion or varicosity of veins found within the mucous membranes of the rectum. Hemorrhoids may develop either inside or outside the rectum, and they are among the more common of human afflictions.

Hemorrhoids generally develop as a result of increased pressure placed on veins within the rectum. The pressure may be attributable to straining as a result

The Removal of Hemorrhoids

A proctoscope applying a band to a hemorrhoid

A hemorrhoid being withdrawn by a clamp and cut off with a scalpel

Severe and distended hemorrhoids may be removed in one of two ways: through the placement of a rubber band around the base of the hemorrhoid, which constricts its blood supply and causes it to wither and drop off; or through surgical excision.

of constipation or to prolonged sitting. In women, they often develop during pregnancy and following childbirth. Treatment depends on the severity of discomfort and location of the hemorrhoid.

External hemorrhoids are often not painful, and they may respond to the application of cool compresses or over-the-counter astringent creams. Creams and suppositories containing steroids may be prescribed by a physician. Internal hemorrhoids may not be noticeable unless a vein ruptures, causing some bleeding, pain, and itching. Since bacteria regularly pass through the rectal area, infection may increase the itching and pain, eventually requiring treatment. If discomfort continues and is not relieved through simple medication, the hemorrhoids may require surgical removal. Several methods exist for removal. Often, the vein is stretched and cut off at its base. Local anesthetics may be necessary, and there may be bleeding and discomfort. Internal hemorrhoids may also be eliminated through cryosurgery, the application of subfreezing temperatures to eliminate tissue. The complete surgical removal of the hemorrhoid, hemorrhoidectomy, may be warranted under certain circumstances.

Hemorrhoid banding, also referred to as rubber band ligation and Barron ligation, involves the placement of a tight rubber band at the base of the hemorrhoid. Over the next few days, the vein will degenerate and slough off. The procedure is relatively simple and can be performed on an outpatient basis. Aside from some discomfort for several days, there are few side effects associated with the banding procedure. Warm sitz baths and local astringents may be helpful in reducing any swelling or pain, and the patient should eat a diet conducive to a soft stool.

—*Richard Adler, Ph.D.*

See also Colon and rectal surgery; Colonoscopy and sigmoidoscopy; Constipation; Cryosurgery; Hemorrhoids; Pregnancy and gestation; Proctology; Varicose veins; Vascular medicine; Vascular system.

For Further Information:

Becker, Barbara. *Relief from Chronic Hemorrhoids.* New York: Dell, 1992.

The Hemorrhoid Book: A Look at Hemorrhoids—How They're Treated and How You Can Prevent Them from Coming Back. San Bruno, Calif.: Krames Communications, 1991.

Parker, James N., and Philip M. Parker, eds. *The Official Patient's Sourcebook on Hemorrhoids.* San Diego, Calif.: Icon Health, 2002.

Peikin, Steven R. *Gastrointestinal Health.* Rev. ed. New York: HarperCollins, 1999.

Sachar, David B., Jerome D. Waye, and Blair S. Lewis, eds. *Pocket Guide to Gastroenterology.* Rev. ed. Baltimore: Williams & Wilkins, 1991.

Wanderman, Sidney E., with Betty Rothbart. *Hemorrhoids.* Yonkers, N.Y.: Consumer Reports Books, 1991.

HEMORRHOIDS
DISEASE/DISORDER

ANATOMY OR SYSTEM AFFECTED: Anus, blood vessels, circulatory system, gastrointestinal system, intestines

SPECIALTIES AND RELATED FIELDS: Family medicine, gastroenterology, proctology

DEFINITION: Blood-swollen enlargements of specialized tissues that help close the anus, as a result of intravenous pressure in the hemorrhoidal plexus; sometimes called piles.

KEY TERMS:

anus: the valve at the end of the rectum that prevents waste matter from leaking out until a person is ready to defecate

cauterize: to sear tissue with heat or a corrosive substance

dentate line: the junction in the anus where the external skin meets the internal mucosa

gastroenterologist: a physician who specializes in the gastrointestinal tract and related organs

mucosa: the mucus-secreting membrane that lines the surface of internal organs directly exposed to elements from outside the body, such as the lungs and intestines

proctologist: a physician who specializes in diseases of the rectum

rectum: the storage compartment at the end of the colon where wastes collect before defecation

stool: the excreted waste products of digestion

thrombosis: the condition of having a clot in a blood vessel

CAUSES AND SYMPTOMS

Hemorrhoids, some physiologists suggest, are one of the prices that humans pay for walking upright. The vascular system—the veins and arteries that circulate blood—evolved in an animal that walked on all fours. Now that humans spend most of their time standing, gravity puts awkward pressure on the system, and at the bottom of major parts of the system, as in the tissue

---

INFORMATION ON HEMORRHOIDS

CAUSES: Increased pressure in lower abdomen resulting from constipation, diarrhea, long periods of sitting, pregnancy and childbirth

SYMPTOMS: Burning, itching, bleeding around anus

DURATION: Often short-term but can be chronic

TREATMENTS: Change in dietary and/or lifestyle habits; use of ointments, creams, medicated pads, and suppositories; surgery if needed

---

around the anus, the column of blood above weighs heavily on the network of small blood vessels there. It does not take much additional pressure to cause a vessel's wall to balloon out. When it does, the result is a hemorrhoid, a little pouch protruding on the surface of the anus, similar to a hernia or varicose vein. Most people have hemorrhoids, even if they do not realize it, and the major symptoms are rarely dangerous, although they can be extremely annoying. Sometimes, however, hemorrhoids develop into or mask life-threatening diseases.

The term "hemorrhoid" derives from Greek words meaning "blood flowing," an apt description of the circulatory activity in the anal walls and an inadvertently apt warning of what most alarms people—hemorrhoids occasionally bleed. (The alternative, and now obsolescent, term "piles" comes from Latin *pila*, a ball, apparently a metaphor for the appearance of hemorrhoids.) Specifically, the "blood flowing" refers to the supple blood vessels of the internal rectal plexus, a series of pouches that act as cushions to help seal the anus shut. When these pouches become enlarged, they turn into hemorrhoids, which jut from the anus wall and swell up to 3 centimeters in length.

Because of the sphincter that controls defecation, not all hemorrhoids are visible without the aid of special instruments. The anus, an oval opening about 3 centimeters in front of the spine, is the valve ending the digestive tract. Like the mouth's lips, which begin the tract, the anus can purse shut, a state made possible by two concentric, circular sphincter muscles which act like drawstrings on a cloth bag. When sensors in the rectum signal the time to defecate, these muscles relax to pass stool and then immediately contract to close the anus again. As in the mouth, external skin meets the internal mucosal membrane in the anus; the meeting place is a

corrugated joint called the dentate line (or, alternatively, the anorectal juncture or pectinase line). It is in this area—between the skin covering the external (or lower) sphincter and the mucosa over the internal (or upper) sphincter—that hemorrhoids form. Those that bulge out from the dentate line or above are hidden from sight by the closed anus and are called internal hemorrhoids; those that protrude below the closed anus, and so can be seen or felt, are called external hemorrhoids.

External hemorrhoids are the ones famed for vexing people. When the skin is stretched over swelled hemorrhoids, its sense receptors are activated, making the hemorrhoids burn and itch, sometimes so intolerably that the urge to scratch them is uncontrollable. Scratching, especially with abrasive materials such as toilet paper, often scrapes and tears the tissue. The bright red blood from these lesions is easily noticeable on the toilet paper and may even drip into the toilet bowl or onto underclothes. Likewise, the passage of a hard, dry stool often abrades hemorrhoids to the point of bleeding.

Internal hemorrhoids do not itch or burn and rarely cause pain because the mucosal tissue over them has no nerve endings, but they can also bleed when a passing stool damages them. (Pain may be "referred," however, from a damaged internal hemorrhoid to the sciatic nerve, bladder, lower back, or genitals; that is, a person feels little or no pain in the anorectal area, but suddenly pain flares in one of these other areas.) An especially elongated internal hemorrhoid at times can protrude through the anus, a condition called prolapse. Usually, it spontaneously recedes or can be pushed back inside with a finger, but upon rare occasion a group of internal hemorrhoids prolapse, swelling and sending the internal sphincter into painful spasms. A doctor's help may then be required to reduce the pain and fit the hemorrhoids inside.

The blood vessels in the internal rectal plexus swell so easily because they lack valves. Without valves to regulate the local flow of blood, the walls are vulnerable to any sudden increase in pressure. Even a small, transient increase above the normal pressure of blood circulation can cause the vessels to bulge. Often, these bulges disappear when the excess pressure disappears or remain swollen only briefly afterward. If the increased pressure is high enough, however, a permanent protrusion results, drooping from the anal wall like lumps of melted wax on a candle. Even then, if the hemorrhoid is internal, the patient may feel no discomfort and may not realize that a hemorrhoid has formed.

Some people are more susceptible to chronic hemorrhoids than others because of a hereditary lack of elasticity in the blood vessels. In such people, standing for long periods of time can add enough pressure to make hemorrhoids swell. Nevertheless, anyone can get hemorrhoids; all that is needed is enough pressure in the lower abdomen. Straining on the toilet to pass stool is the most common cause. People strain when they are constipated or have diarrhea, and since a poor diet can lead to these conditions, hemorrhoids can be a secondary effect of poor eating habits. Those who like to sit on the toilet a long time, reading or watching television while waiting for a bowel movement, also increase pressure on the anus because of the posture and the compressing effect of the toilet ring; they are likely to develop hemorrhoids. People who regularly lift heavy weights as part of their jobs or for recreation are especially susceptible if they hold their breath while lifting: This action pushes the diaphragm downward on organs below it, including the anus, putting pressure on them. Similarly, during pregnancy women can develop hemorrhoids as the expanding womb crowds and increases pressure on nearby organs; these hemorrhoids are exacerbated by delivery, but they usually go away afterward. Psychologists add to these causes the guilt that some people feel about eating and excreting, guilt spawned by overindulgence in food or bad toilet training; they bear down on their bowels to defecate as quickly as possible and by doing so stress the hemorrhoidal vessels. Finally, hemorrhoids occasionally develop because of some serious diseases, such as heart failure and cirrhosis of the liver, which elevate pressure in the veins, and rectal cancer, which can create a false sense of fullness so that the person strains to pass a stool that is not really there.

Although they seldom do more than itch, external hemorrhoids can thrombose—develop clots of coagulated blood from a burst or swollen vessel under the skin—and grow as large as a grape. A doctor can relieve the pain by slicing open the hemorrhoid and squeezing out the clot. Left alone, a thrombosed hemorrhoid may rupture, causing a painful and bloody mess that is ripe for infection. Yet the greatest threat of hemorrhoids lies not in the symptoms themselves but in how they might be confused with those of other, deadly diseases. Colorectal cancer, inflammatory bowel disease, and sexually transmitted diseases such as syphilis, gonorrhea, and herpes can lead to discharges of blood, as can anal fissures (cracks in the anal canal), fistulas (tunnel-like passages between an infected gland and mucosa or

skin), and abscesses (pus-filled sacs under the mucosa). A person who dismisses the bloody discharge as simply a flare-up of hemorrhoids may be delaying treatment for the real cause. In the case of colorectal cancer, one of the most common cancers in the United States, such a delay can be fatal. Only a doctor has the tools and vantage point to distinguish between the relatively benign hemorrhoids and a dangerous disorder.

TREATMENT AND THERAPY

Since hemorrhoid-like symptoms can be produced by deadly diseases, a thorough checkup at the doctor's office includes an examination of the anus and rectum, especially if the patient has noticed bleeding. In addition to the visual inspection and "digital" examination, during which the doctor inserts a finger and feels around for enlarged hemorrhoids or other masses, patients provide clues by describing the color, amount, and time of bleeding. If the blood is bright red and occurs in small quantities during or just after defecation, hemorrhoids are most likely to blame. If dark red blood or clots appear in the stool or seep out randomly, however, the doctor will look for other causes, inspecting the anus, rectum, and colon with various types of endoscopes, fiber-optic-filled flexible tubes that can also collect tissue samples. Once the doctor rules out other diseases, the patient has three basic choices: change

Hemorrhoids

Internal hemorrhoid

Rectum

External hemorrhoids

Anus

habits, rely on therapy, or have the hemorrhoids removed.

If a person's hemorrhoids do not cause severe discomfort, the doctor will likely recommend a diet with high fiber and water intake. Fiber and water together make stools bulky and soft. They pass more easily during defecation than small, hard, dry stools. The patient does not have to strain, and so no further pressure is put on existing hemorrhoids. Furthermore, soft stools do not scrape hemorrhoids and cause them to bleed. The doctor will also suggest regular exercise, since this helps the bowels work more efficiently and reduces the chance of constipation. Finally, the patient may receive instructions on the proper way to breathe during heavy exertion so as to lessen the stress on the hemorrhoids. With a better diet, more exercise, and less physical straining, patients may find that hemorrhoids have disappeared completely.

Until hemorrhoids shrink, they plague the patient, and to reduce the itching and burning a number of therapies prove effective, if only temporarily. An ice compress eases the discomfort, as does a sitz bath (sitting for at least fifteen minutes in shallow warm water), which also cleanses the site of potentially infecting wastes and promotes healing in damaged tissue. Should these relatively simple and cheap measures be impracticable, a variety of ointments, creams, medicated pads, and suppositories, either prescription or nonprescription, may provide relief. Some are inert, such as petroleum jelly, and coat and lubricate the hemorrhoids, protecting them from irritation. Some have an astringent effect, tightening and sealing tissue and thereby protecting it. Others have anesthetic ingredients, numbing the tissue, or anti-inflammatory effects, decreasing swelling. None of these medications has a proven capacity to make swelling go away entirely, and those with active ingredients may cause an allergic response. For patients with constipation, doctors may prescribe stool softeners to eliminate straining during defecation. Laxatives are usually to be avoided because the chemicals in them irritate hemorrhoids, and the resulting diarrhea often causes urgency and pressure in the rectal area.

When hemorrhoids become chronically and unusually swollen or the patient can no longer endure the discomfort, removing them is the last resort. This cure is certain, although not necessarily permanent, but it has its cost in pain and recovery time. There are seven basic methods, six that cause the target hemorrhoid to shrivel, to drop off on its own, or both, and one, surgery, that removes it directly.

The surgical removal of hemorrhoids, called hemorrhoidectomy, is a relatively simple operation; nevertheless, it is usually reserved for those patients who for one reason or another cannot undergo one of the other methods. The patient is given a local anesthetic to deaden the tissue in the anus, although some patients are rendered unconscious with a general anesthetic; the surgeon cuts off the hemorrhoid at its base and then sews the wound closed with absorbable sutures. The recovery period may require hospitalization for up to a week, during which pain medication, stool softeners, and anal pads are necessary until the tissues heal. Bed rest after hospitalization and sitz baths may also be necessary. Because of this recovery time—as much as a month all together—hemorrhoidectomies are not widely popular among patients or physicians. Moreover, urine retention, infection, and hemorrhaging after the operation are possible complications.

The remaining methods avoid the trauma of cutting, and the first of them, ligation, is the oldest of all the methods, referred to in the writings of Hippocrates (c. 460-c. 370 B.C.E.). Ancient Greek physicians tied a thread around a hemorrhoid to strangle its blood supply; modern gastroenterologists or proctologists use special rubber bands. The effect is the same: The hemorrhoid dries up, shrivels, and falls off. Little pain accompanies the procedure, which is done in the doctor's office. Ligation, however, can only be used for internal hemorrhoids.

Likewise, sclerotherapy, cryosurgery, and infrared coagulation are only for internal hemorrhoids because the pain would be too intense on external hemorrhoids. In sclerotherapy, the doctor injects a liquid—usually phenol in oil or quinine in urea—that seals closed the blood vessels at the base of the hemorrhoid. With no blood in them, the vessels eventually shrink to normal dimensions and, if stressing pressure on them is not resumed, the hemorrhoid disappears. In cryosurgery, super cold liquid nitrogen or nitrous oxide is applied to the hemorrhoid, freezing it and killing the tissue. The hemorrhoid slowly melts and, as it does, shrinks and finally sloughs off. Popular in the 1970's and early 1980's, cryosurgery lost favor because of the messy and extended recovery time. Useful for mild, small hemorrhoids, infrared coagulation involves a beam of infrared light that, aimed at the hemorrhoid, shrinks it by cauterizing the tissue. The heat of the beam can cause pain in other parts of the anus during the procedure.

The remaining methods, laser surgery and electric

current coagulation, can be used on external hemorrhoids. Like infrared coagulation, laser surgery trains a beam of light—in this case intense visible light—that burns and shrinks the hemorrhoid to a stub. Since the laser cauterizes as it destroys tissue and therefore seals off blood vessels, its main advantage over regular surgery lies in reduced bleeding. Recovery time is shorter, about a week, and hospitalization is usually not necessary. This procedure is much more expensive than a hemorrhoidectomy or ligation, however, because of the cost of laser technology. In electric current coagulation, electrodes pass either direct or alternating current through the hemorrhoids. Because tissue is a poor conductor, the resistance to the current creates heat, which cooks the hemorrhoid, coagulating and shrinking it.

Which method the surgeon, gastroenterologist, or proctologist uses depends partly upon the physician's and patient's preferences and partly upon the size and location of the hemorrhoid. Ligation remains the most frequently used method because it is relatively cheap and fast.

PERSPECTIVE AND PROSPECTS

According to Napoleon's personal physician, piles cost the emperor the Battle of Waterloo, which ended his reign. His hemorrhoids were so inflamed and painful on the morning of the battle that he could not get out of bed, much less sit on his horse. Without his personal direction, the French lost. Popular writers often cite this dramatic example, sometimes with humorous overtones, to demonstrate how seriously hemorrhoids can interfere with the lives of even the great.

Certainly, hemorrhoids are no laughing matter. Yet the long-standing taboo in the United States about excretion and the anus has prompted many Americans either to laugh nervously about their hemorrhoids or to keep silent, preferring to suffer stoically rather than to risk becoming the target of jokes. For this reason, it is nearly impossible to say how many sufferers there are in the United States. Estimates vary from several million people to the entire population over the age of thirty.

Whatever the exact statistic, clearly many people share a problem that embarrasses them too much to discuss openly or that they believe is too trivial for medical attention. If they need relief from the itching and pain, they treat themselves. A large industry in home remedies and over-the-counter medications serves them: Rectal medications alone earned drug companies $178 million in 1999, according to the Consumer

Healthcare Products Association. The benefits of such medications are difficult to assess, and some authorities claim that petroleum jelly eases the itching and burning as much as any preparation specifically intended for hemorrhoids. Folk remedies, such as suppositories made of tobacco or compresses soaked in papaya juice, can damage tissue outright, making the problem worse. Moreover, throughout the United States specialized clinics offer surgical cures for hemorrhoids, promising patients quick relief on an outpatient basis and using expensive methods, particularly laser surgery.

Therefore, many people spend considerable money and time, often wasting both, to tend a chronic discomfort that can as readily be prevented or palliated by a change in habits, doctors claim. Like colon cancer and many other intestinal ailments, hemorrhoids are most common in populations whose diet includes a high number of processed foods, which are low in fiber. While fiber is no panacea, people in cultures whose diet contains significant fiber have larger stools and fewer intestinal complaints in general.

Because hemorrhoids are in most cases preventable or controllable without treatment, they have been cited, along with deadly maladies such as colon cancer and inflammatory bowel disease, in criticisms of both the American diet and Americans' eagerness to rely on medical intervention to save them from their own unhealthy habits. In the case of hemorrhoids—while they are not exclusively a malady of Western civilization—the fast pace and pressures of life, the attitudes about defecation, and the eating habits of industrial cultures help give them a distracting prominence.

—Roger Smith, Ph.D.

See also Colon and rectal polyp removal; Colon and rectal surgery; Colon cancer; Colon therapy; Colonoscopy and sigmoidoscopy; Cryosurgery; Endoscopy; Hemorrhoid banding and removal; Intestinal disorders; Intestines; Pregnancy and gestation; Thrombosis and thrombus.

FOR FURTHER INFORMATION:

Becker, Barbara. *Relief from Chronic Hemorrhoids.* New York: Dell, 1992. An excellent book for general readers, it gives advice on every aspect of diagnosis, treatment, removal procedures, and alternative therapies. Special attention is given to improving the patient's diet, and extensive, very specific tables on proper foods accompany the argument for this self-help approach.

"Help for Hemorrhoids Includes Fiber, Fluids, and Fitness." *Environmental Nutrition* 23, no. 4 (April, 2000): 7. Hemorrhoids are a common medical problem, especially for people over age fifty. The best way to prevent hemorrhoids is to avoid constipation by combining a high-fiber diet with plenty of fluids and regular physical activity.

Litin, Scott C., ed. *Mayo Clinic Family Health Book*. 3d ed. New York: HarperResource, 2003. Perhaps the best general medical text for the layperson, this book covers the entire medical field. While the information is derived from a wide variety of highly technical sources, the articles are written to be easily understood by a general audience.

Minkin, Mary Jane. "Prevent Hemorrhoids." *Prevention* 50, no. 6 (June, 1998): 76. Pushing or straining too hard due to constipation is a major reason hemorrhoids develop. Tips on how to prevent constipation are offered.

Okie, Susan. "Colon Susceptible to Other Woes Besides Cancer: The Basics on Everything from Crohn's Disease to Hemorrhoids." *The Washington Post*, February 10, 1998, p. Z19. Between 10 and 20 percent of American adults suffer from irritable bowel syndrome, a set of symptoms that can be painful, inconvenient, and at times disabling.

Peikin, Steven. *Gastrointestinal Health*. Rev. ed. New York: HarperCollins, 1999. Concerned almost wholly with the effect of nutrition on GI maladies, the author offers a self-help guide for the afflicted. After explaining the GI tract's workings and describing common symptoms, Peikin specifies diets that he argues will relieve symptoms.

Sachar, David B., Jerome D. Waye, and Blair S. Lewis, eds. *Pocket Guide to Gastroenterology*. Rev. ed. Baltimore: Williams & Wilkins, 1991. This diagnosis-oriented handbook gives information on all gastroenterological ailments in outline form, making it valuable for quick studies on major problems. The section on hemorrhoids, though superficial, lays out the basic symptoms and treatments.

Wanderman, Sidney E., with Betty Rothbart. *Hemorrhoids*. Yonkers, N.Y.: Consumer Reports Books, 1991. Providing a simple but thorough overview of anatomical problems, causes, medications, therapies, and removal methods, this short book also discusses related complaints, such as fissures and fistulas, and dangerous diseases whose symptoms can be mistaken for those of hemorrhoids.

HEPATITIS

DISEASE/DISORDER

ANATOMY OR SYSTEM AFFECTED: Liver

SPECIALTIES AND RELATED FIELDS: Epidemiology, internal medicine, toxicology, virology

DEFINITION: An inflammatory condition of the liver, characterized by discomfort, jaundice, and enlargement of the organ and bacterial, viral, or immunological in origin; may also result from use of alcohol and other toxic drugs.

KEY TERMS:

alanine aminotransferase: a liver enzyme associated with the metabolism of the amino acid alanine; elevated levels are an indication of liver damage

aspartate aminotransferase: a liver enzyme associated with metabolism of the amino acid aspartate; elevated levels are an indication of liver damage

cirrhosis: chronic degeneration of the liver, in which normal tissue is replaced with fibroid tissue and fat; commonly associated with alcohol abuse but can also result from hepatitis

hepatitis A virus: the virus associated with certain forms of hepatitis; generally contracted through fecal contamination of food and water

hepatitis B virus: the agent associated with severe forms of viral hepatitis; contracted through contaminated blood or hypodermic needles or through contaminated body fluids, and sometimes found in association with hepatitis D virus

hepatitis C virus: formerly referred to as the etiological agent for non-A, non-B viral hepatitis; most often passed in contaminated blood

hepato: a prefix denoting anything associated with the liver—for example, a hepatocyte is a liver cell

jaundice: a symptom of a variety of liver disorders which manifests as yellowish discoloration of the skin, the whites of the eyes, and other tissues; hepatocellular jaundice results from hepatitis

CAUSES AND SYMPTOMS

Hepatitis, a pathology referring to inflammation of the liver, may result from any of a variety of causes but commonly follows bacterial or viral infection. Hepatitis may be associated with an autoimmune phenomenon in which the body produces antibodies against liver tissue. Liver inflammation may also be an aftereffect of the use of alcohol or various hepatotoxic chemicals, either through the taking of illegal drugs or as a side effect of the legal use of pharmacological agents. Among the pharmaceuticals that can cause liver damage are antibiotics such as isoniazid and rifampin and the pain-killer acetaminophen.

Symptoms associated with hepatitis are a reflection of the function of the liver. The liver is arguably the most complex organ in the body. More than five hundred different functions have been associated with the organ, including the production of bile for emulsification of fats and the secretion of glucose, proteins, or vitamins for use elsewhere in the body. The liver plays a major role in the detoxification of the blood, removing alcohol, nicotine, and other potentially poisonous substances. The Kupffer cells in the liver function in the removal of infectious agents or foreign material from the blood. More than 10 percent of the blood supply in the body is found within the liver at any time.

Among the functions of the liver is the removal of hemoglobin in the blood, released as a result of the lysis (disintegration) of red blood cells. A breakdown product of hemoglobin is the yellowish compound bilirubin. It is the buildup of bilirubin in blood that results in the appearance of jaundice in cases of inadequate liver function, such as during hepatitis.

Although hepatitis may develop from a variety of causes, it most commonly results from infection of the liver. Nearly any infectious agent may potentially damage the liver, but generally these involve one of several types of viruses, bacteria, fungi, or amoebas. Liver disease may also be significantly exacerbated by alcohol abuse, as is seen in patients with cirrhosis. Regardless of the specific cause, symptoms of liver disease remain similar in most cases. The liver is often enlarged and tender to physical examination. The person may feel tired and run a low-grade fever. It is not unusual for the person to feel nauseous and lose weight. Jaundice is common in most patients; the concentrations of the enzymes alanine aminotransferase (ALT) and aspartate aminotransferase (AST) may rise. Levels of these enzymes, however, are not necessarily indications of the severity of liver disease; in any event, their levels often fall over the course of the disease.

Three particular viruses have been associated with most forms of viral hepatitis (types A, B, and C), while a fourth (type D) appears as a passenger during some cases of hepatitis B. Several additional viruses, designated hepatitis E (HEV) through hepatitis G (HGV), have also been linked to forms of the disease. Hepatitis A results from infection with hepatitis A virus (HAV), a virus classified in the same group as the poliovirus and rhinoviruses (cold viruses). The disease is transmitted through a fecal-to-oral method and is self-limited (running a definite and limited course). Often the disease is subclinical (undetectable), particularly as seen in children. Replication of the virus occurs in hepatocytes (liver cells); the virus then passes into the intestine and is eliminated with the feces. A long incubation period following ingestion may occur, sometimes as long as a month, and during much of this period the person is capable of transmitting the disease. In otherwise healthy individuals, recovery is complete and occurs over several weeks. Anti-HAV antibodies are present in the blood of about 30 to 40 percent of the general population, reflecting the widespread nature of the disease.

Hepatitis B (HBV), formerly called serum hepatitis, is a potentially much more severe form of the disease. The disease in young children is frequently asymptomatic, with appearance of symptoms in older individuals being more common. In general, however, the most frequent result of primary infection with HBV is a mild or subclinical course of infection. The disease is most commonly seen in the fifteen-to-thirty-five age group, in part reflecting its method of transmission (through blood or body fluids).

Persistent infection with HBV, occurring in approximately 1 to 3 percent of patients, can be associated with either an asymptomatic carrier state or chronic hepatitis. The chronic state may be severe, with progression to cirrhosis and cellular degeneration or inflammation. In fact, it is the immune response to the presence of HBV that may contribute to liver degeneration. HBV infection results in the expression of viral antigens, which stimulate an immune response, on the surface of liver cells. Among the inflammatory cells present at the sites of infection are a large proportion of lymphocytes. These include cytotoxic T cells, lymphocytes associated with the killing of virally infected cells. Because immunologically impaired individuals infected with HBV often suffer a mild form of the disease, the possi-

---

INFORMATION ON HEPATITIS

CAUSES: Bacterial or viral infection, immunological disorder, abuse of alcohol and other toxic drugs
SYMPTOMS: Jaundice, liver enlargement, discomfort, fatigue, low-grade fever, nausea, weight loss
DURATION: Ranges from short-term to chronic
TREATMENTS: Antibiotics, hospitalization

bility exists that it is the immune response itself that contributes to the ensuing liver damage.

Hepatitis B transmission occurs through blood or bodily fluids, including semen and vaginal secretions. Because HBV is also found in saliva, the disease may be transmitted among family members through non-sexual contact. Maternal-neonatal transmission may occur, occasionally while the fetus is in the uterus but more likely during the labor or birth process. There is, however, no evidence for transmission through food or water or by an airborne means.

Clinical features of HBV infections are similar to those associated with other forms of hepatitis. In the asymptomatic form of type B disease, AST or ALT levels may be elevated, but jaundice is absent. Adults with symptomatic hepatitis B may suffer jaundice (icteric hepatitis), or they may not (nonicteric hepatitis). There is generally a mild fever, fatigue, and weakness.

Accompanying an indeterminant number of HBV infections is a second virus, designated the hepatitis D virus (HDV). HDV is a defective virus, capable of replication only in the presence of HBV. Not surprisingly, its geographic distribution and mode of transmission are similar to those of HBV. The prevalence of HDV has been found to be as high as 70 percent in some outbreaks of HBV and nonexistent in others. In most cases, HDV infection results in subclinical or mild hepatitis. In about 15 percent of cases, the disease may progress to a more severe form. HDV may itself be cytopathic (causing pathological changes) for hepatocytes, but this remains to be established firmly.

Based on the exclusion of other types of etiologic agents, including HAV, HBV, Epstein-Barr virus, and cytomegalovirus, non-A, non-B (NANB) hepatitis was considered a clinical entity. During the late 1980's, NANB hepatitis was determined to be caused by a newly isolated infectious agent, designated hepatitis C virus (HCV). The study of HCV was hampered by the inability to grow the virus in cell culture. Ironically, the virus was cloned and characterized before it was even physically observed, allowing for the development of a screening assay used for the detection of contaminated serum. In the United States, approximately 25 percent of hepatitis is associated with HCV. Before screening procedures were put into place in 1992, HCV infection was the major complication of blood transfusions or transfusions of blood products. Infection now occurs through sexual intercourse, the sharing of intravenous needles, and accidental needle punctures among health care workers. HCV has been increasingly recognized as a major health threat. It creates serious liver damage and is the leading cause of liver transplants. It is all the more dangerous because patients are often asymptomatic and learn of the infection when the blood is screened for other reasons. As a result, many people are unknowing carriers of the virus.

Outbreaks of an enterically transmitted NANB hepatitis (NANB hepatitis transmitted through the intestines), designated hepatitis E, have also been found in some parts of the world. Though hepatitis E has been around at least since 1955 (and no doubt earlier, but undocumented), it was only in the late 1980's that it was determined to be a unique form of the disease. Transmission occurs through eating or drinking contaminated food or water, though there is evidence that household contact with infected persons may also transmit the disease. Hepatitis E is most common in the poor countries of Asia, with sporadic outbreaks elsewhere. The few cases found in the United States have involved travelers to these areas.

Acute hepatitis is less commonly associated with infection by other viruses. These include the herpes family of viruses, such as herpes simplex, cytomegalovirus, and Epstein-Barr virus. Because the prevalence of these viruses is quite high, immunosuppressed or immunodeficient patients may be at particular risk.

Certain forms of hepatitis are associated with an autoimmune response. In these cases, the cause is not an infectious agent but rather a form of rejection by the body of its own liver tissue. Autoimmune hepatitis is suspected in individuals in which the disease persists for at least six months with no evidence of exposure to an infectious agent or hepatotoxin. In nearly one-third of these individuals, other immunological diseases such as lupus or arthritis may be present. The clinical manifestations of autoimmune hepatitis are similar to those of other forms of the disease. Most patients exhibit jaundice, a mild fever, weakness, and weight loss. The liver is often enlarged and tender. Unlike other forms of hepatitis, found equally in men and women, autoimmune hepatitis is most commonly found in women. Prognosis of the disease is unclear, as an unknown percentage of cases are subclinical. Severe forms have a high fatality rate.

TREATMENT AND THERAPY

Treatment for the various forms of viral hepatitis is, for the most part, symptomatic and supportive. Hospitalization may be required in severe cases, but, in general, any restriction of activity is left up to the patient. This is particularly convenient, since recovery often involves a long convalescence. As long as a healthy diet is maintained, no special dietary requirements exist, but a high-calorie diet is often preferable. Drugs or chemicals that are potentially damaging to the liver, including alcohol and certain antibiotics or painkillers, should be avoided.

Hepatitis induced by other forms of infectious agents such as bacteria or fungi may be treated using an appropriate course of antibiotic therapy. In cases of drug-induced disease, avoidance of the chemical is a key to recovery. Bacterial infections of the liver are often associated with patients who are malnourished, such as the elderly or alcoholics, or who may be immunosuppressed. These problems must also be addressed during the course of treatment.

Prevention of the disease is preferable, however, and because the means of viral spread has been well established in most cases, appropriate measures can often be taken. For the most part, the viruses associated with hepatitis have little in common with one another aside from their predilection for hepatocytes. Thus, preventing their spread involves different strategies.

HAV is almost always spread through a fecal-oral means of transmission. Often the source is an infected person involved in the preparation of uncooked foods. Common sense dictates that the person should wash after every use of a toilet, but this is often not the case. Not surprisingly, children attending day care centers frequently become infected. Contaminated groundwater is also a potential source of outbreaks in areas in which proper sewage treatment does not take place. Less commonly, HAV is spread directly from person to person through sexual contact. A method called immunoprophylaxis can prevent the development of symptoms in individuals exposed to hepatitis A by utilizing a form of passive immunity. Developed during World War II, the procedure involves the pooling of serum from immune individuals. Inoculation of the serum into exposed persons is effective in prevention of the disease in most cases.

In 1994, SmithKline Beecham Pharmaceuticals developed and received Food and Drug Administration (FDA) approval for the first vaccine shown to be safe and effective in preventing HAV infection. Manufactured under the trade name Havrix, the vaccine consists of a formalin-inactivated strain of HAV, to be administered in three doses to children. In 1996, a similar vaccine was developed by Merck and Co., to be sold under the trade name Vagta.

The transmission of HBV generally involves passage via contaminated blood or body secretions. In the period prior to the screening of blood, transfusions were the most common means of spreading the disease—hence the designation "serum hepatitis." Since the 1980's, the most common means of documented spread has been through either sexual contact or the sharing of contaminated hypodermic needles. Semen, vaginal secretions, and saliva from infected individuals all contain the active virus, and limiting exchange of these fluids is key to prevention of transmission. Even so, the means of infection in nearly one-third of symptomatic cases remains unknown.

An effective vaccine for prevention of HBV infection was first developed during the 1970's and early 1980's. The vaccination procedure was later modified to create an effective combined active-passive vaccine. Passive immunization utilizes antibodies purified from the blood of donors who have recovered from HBV infection. This hepatitis B immune globulin (HBIG) is combined with a recombinant yeast vaccine that contains hepatitis virus proteins but lacks the genetic material necessary for the virus to replicate. Because HBIG already contains a high level of anti-HBV antibody, it is effective as a postexposure preventive for an individual who has come in contact with the disease. For example, a person exposed to the virus through an accidental needle stick, such as an unimmunized health care worker, may not have time to proceed through the regimen of treatment. The use of HBIG provides a short-term means of protection. The combined vaccine is used as a method of pre-exposure immunization. In the early 1990's, vaccination was recommended to only those persons at high risk for exposure to HBV. This group is composed of homosexual or bisexual men, health care workers (including physicians and dentists), and persons dealing with individuals in whom the disease is commonly found.

Because hepatitis D virus is defective in replication, requiring the presence of HBV, no specific measures of prevention are necessary. Immunization against HBV is sufficient to prevent the spread of HDV.

The deadly HCV is treated with antiviral agents, such as ribavirin and shots of interferon. A longer-acting form called pegylated interferon (Pegasys) is still in the experimental stage but is showing some promise against this liver-destroying infection.

The transmission of the hepatitis E virus is also through a fecal-oral route. The drinking of water contaminated by sewage has been the most common source of transmission. Because no active means of prevention has been developed, prevention of exposure requires that the individual avoid any food or water potentially contaminated with sewage. This is particularly true in areas of the world in which hepatitis E is found. Though the precaution may seem obvious, the safety of the water, as well as any object washed in the water, is not always readily apparent.

Autoimmune hepatitis results from an aberrant immune system rather than from an infectious agent. Treatment generally involves the use of immunosuppressive drugs to limit the immune response. Corticosteroids such as prednisone, sometimes in combination with azathioprine, have proven effective in the therapy of many patients. Still, in some cases the disease progresses to cirrhosis and results in death. Treatment generally is carried out over a long period of time, at least a year, and relapses are common. Often, the patient requires lifetime therapy. The immunosuppressive activity of the therapy may also leave the patient more susceptible to infection. In some cases, liver transplantation has proven effective, at least in the short term. Because the liver rejection was caused by an autoimmune response in the first place, the transplant may also be subject to the same phenomenon.

PERSPECTIVE AND PROSPECTS

Inflammation of the liver resulting in hepatitis can develop from a variety of mechanisms. Most often, these mechanisms are associated with either a chemical injury or infection by a microbiological agent.

Infections of the liver generally involve one of several viral agents. The association of liver disease, or at least jaundice, with an infectious agent was suspected as early as the time of Hippocrates (the fifth century B.C.E.). Hippocrates described a syndrome which was undoubtedly viral hepatitis. The disease was also described in the Babylonian Talmud about eight hundred years later. Epidemics of the disease have been reported since the Middle Ages; these most likely involved outbreaks of hepatitis A. The spread of this disease through personal contact was confirmed in the 1930's.

Type B, or serum hepatitis, was described as a clinical entity by A. Lurman in 1855. Lurman observed that 15 percent of shipyard workers in Bremen, Germany, who received a smallpox vaccine containing human lymph developed jaundice within the following six months. In the early years of the twentieth century, jaundice frequently developed among patients who received vaccines prepared from convalescent serums or who underwent procedures such as venipuncture using instruments which had not been properly sterilized. By 1926, the blood-borne nature of the disease had been confirmed. In 1942, more than twenty-eight thousand American soldiers developed jaundice after vaccination with a yellow fever vaccine prepared from pooled human serums. By then it had become obvious that at least two forms of infectious agents were associated with viral hepatitis.

The isolation of HBV occurred as a result of studies initiated by Baruch Blumberg in 1963. Blumberg was actually attempting to correlate the development of diseases such as cancer with particular patterns of proteins found in the serum of individuals. His approach was to collect blood from persons in various parts of the world and then analyze their serum proteins. Blumberg found an antigen, a protein, in the blood of Australian aborigines which reacted with antibodies in the blood of an American hemophiliac. Blumberg called the protein the Australia (Au) antigen. It later became apparent that the Au antigen could be isolated from the blood of patients with serum hepatitis. By 1970, it was established that what Blumberg had referred to as the Au antigen was in fact the HBV particle.

HBV is associated with more than simply viral hepatitis. Chronic hepatitis associated with HBV can often develop into hepatocellular carcinoma, or cancer of the liver. The precise reason is unclear; the cancer may result from the chronic damage to liver tissue associated with long-term infection by HBV.

An effective vaccine for the prevention of HBV infection was licensed in 1982. By the late 1990's, the effectiveness of a worldwide vaccination program, under the auspices of the World Health Organization, had led to the possibility that hepatitis resulting from HBV infection, as well as hepatocellular carcinoma, could be controlled within another decade.

Cases of HCV continue to climb because of the high numbers of asymptomatic carriers. In 2003, it was estimated that four million Americans were infected with HCV and that approximately ten thousand would die from it each year, with that number expected to triple by 2010. About 170 million people were infected worldwide. As a result, HCV may prove to be one of the next important threats to global health.

—Richard Adler, Ph.D.;
updated by Tracy Irons-Georges

See also Addiction; Alcoholism; Autoimmune disorders; Cirrhosis; Immunization and vaccination; Jaundice; Liver; Liver cancer; Liver disorders; Liver transplantation; Nonalcoholic steatohepatitis (NASH); Viral infections.

FOR FURTHER INFORMATION:

Boyer, Thomas D., Teresa L. Wright, and Michael P. Manns, eds. *Zakim and Boyer's Hepatology: A Textbook of Liver Disease*. 5th ed. Philadelphia: Saunders Elsevier, 2006. A thorough compendium on most aspects of liver disease. The section on hepatitis contains a complete clinical description of the disease and of the biology of the hepatitis viruses.

Everson, Gregory T., and Hedy Weinberg. *Living with Hepatitis C: A Survivor's Guide*. 3d ed. New York: Hatherleigh Press, 2002. An invaluable resource that reviews the latest clinical trials; updates all of the organizations, resources, and information that has changed since the last edition; and offers chapters on research trends, liver transplants, children, coinfection with HIV/AIDS or hepatitis B, and the nutritional, emotional, and financial challenges that accompany infection with hepatitis C.

Frank, Steven A. *Immunology and Evolution of Infectious Disease*. Princeton, N.J.: Princeton University Press, 2002. Blends research from molecular biology, immunology, pathogen biology, and population dynamics to discuss how and why parasites vary to escape recognition by the immune system, vaccine design, and the control of epidemics.

Gorbach, Sherwood L., John G. Bartlett, and Neil R. Blacklow, eds. *Infectious Diseases*. 3d ed. Philadelphia: W. B. Saunders, 2004. A thorough discussion of infectious diseases. Included is a brief history, an account of the mechanisms of disease and immunity, and a concise discussion of a broad range of infectious agents. The section on hepatitis viruses is well written and not particularly detailed.

Hepatitis Foundation International. http://www.hepfi.org/. A foundation that teaches the public and hepatitis patients how to prevent, diagnose, and treat viral hepatitis and supports research into prevention, treatment, and cures for the disease.

Humes, H. David, et al., eds. *Kelley's Textbook of Internal Medicine*. 4th ed. Philadelphia: Lippincott Williams & Wilkins, 2000. A medical textbook on the subject. The book contains an extensive section on liver diseases, including a concise description of viral hepatitis. The discussion of hepatitis viruses is thorough, clear, but not overly detailed.

Levine, Arnold. *Viruses*. New York: W. H. Freeman, 1992. A well-written outline of viruses and their his-tory. Some basic knowledge of biology is helpful in certain areas of the book, but overall the format and style should reach nearly all general readers. The book is profusely and colorfully illustrated. Several sections deal specifically with viral hepatitis.

Palmer, Melissa. *Dr. Melissa Palmer's Guide to Hepatitis and Liver Disease*. Rev. ed. Garden City Park, N.Y.: Avery, 2004. Palmer, a nationally recognized hepatologist, provides plainly written medical information explaining how the liver is integral to every aspect of daily functioning and well-being. Includes "The Basics," "Understanding and Treating Viral Hepatitis," "Understanding and Treating Other Liver Diseases," and "Treatment Options and Lifestyle Changes."

Shaw, Michael, ed. *Everything You Need to Know About Diseases*. Springhouse, Pa.: Springhouse Press, 1996. This well-illustrated consumer reference, compiled by more than one hundred doctors and medical experts, describes five hundred illnesses and conditions, their causes, symptoms, diagnosis, treatment, and prevention. Of particular interest is chapter 6, "Liver and Gallbladder."

Spector, Steven. *Viral Hepatitis: Diagnosis, Therapy, and Prevention*. Totowa, N.J.: Humana Press, 1999. This clearly written and readable review of viral hepatitis provides useful information for family physicians interested in this protean disorder. Each chapter is divided into sections, allowing the reader to quickly access desired information.

HERBAL MEDICINE
TREATMENT
ALSO KNOWN AS: Plant medicine
ANATOMY OR SYSTEM AFFECTED: All
SPECIALTIES AND RELATED FIELDS: All
DEFINITION: The traditional and scientific application of chemicals directly derived from any part of plants for medicinal purposes. The medicinal uses of plants are for both preventive and curative purposes.

KEY TERMS:

alkaloid: a large group of compounds that contain nitrogen and usually have a basic reaction (for example, cocaine, caffeine, nicotine, quinine, and morphine)

antiseptic: a chemical substance that inhibits the growth of bacteria

glycoside: a compound containing a carbohydrate molecule (sugar) that yields glucose on hydrolysis and a nonsugar component called aglycone *hormone:* chemical messengers produced by the tissues of an organism to act as signaling compounds for the regulation of functions

hypertension: persistent high blood pressure

hypotension: low blood pressure

leukemia: a cancer of the blood-forming organs, marked by the abnormal multiplication and development of leukocytes

pathogen: any agent or microorganism capable of producing disease

pharmaceutical: a medicinal drug

purgative: referring to substances that promote the rapid elimination of material from the digestive tract

THE CHEMICALS OF PLANT-DERIVED MEDICINES

Plants synthesize a wide array of secondary compounds that play a role in the physiology of plants but do not usually constitute an important part of the basic metabolism of plants. Secondary compounds enable plants to attract animals and also help plants to avoid or overcome their natural enemies of infection, parasitism, and predation. These secondary compounds are the main chemicals in plants that humans use as medicinal herbs. Fatty acids, essential oils, gums, resins, alkaloids, and steroids are the most common secondary compounds in plants.

Humans use oils and gums as purgatives and as carriers or emulsifiers in many drug preparations. Volatile oils and resins are often used to help processes that seek to penetrate tissues of the body and are also used as antiseptics. Alkaloids and steroids are the two major classes of plant-derived compounds used in human medicine today. These chemical compounds can occur in different forms that have one or more sugar molecules attached. Such forms, called glycosides, are often the medicinally active form of a compound.

All forms of steroids are complex chemical compounds that have the same fundamental structure of four carbon rings, called the backbone. When different chemical groups are added at different places on the backbone, a variety of steroidal compounds are produced as a result. For example, when sugar molecules are added to the carbon rings, steroidal glycosides are produced. Various cardiac glycosides and steroid hormones are produced by the addition of specific side chains or extra rings to the steroid backbone.

The second major group of medicinally important chemicals synthesized in plants is the alkaloids. They contain nitrogen and usually exhibit an alkaline reaction. Alkaloids were formerly considered secondary products, but unlike steroids, they have recently been shown occasionally to enter into the primary metabolism of plants. Many alkaloids are extremely poisonous to humans, and many have been used as poisons in many cultures around the world. Several of these plant chemicals possess antimicrobial properties and are used to kill harmful microorganisms that are pathogenic. A number of them are used as dietary supplements for balanced human nutrition and good health.

MEDICINAL PLANTS OF IMPORTANCE

In the past, some natural chemicals and oils were of tremendous medicinal use in treating diseases. Quinine was used for the treatment of malaria, cocaine was used as a calming agent and a local anesthetic, and chaulmoogra oil was employed for the treatment of leprosy. Although these herbal medicines are rarely used today, many plants are still of great importance as sources of medicinal compounds. Both steroids and glycosides occur in many angiosperms.

To cite a few examples, certain members of the yam genus *Dioscorea* contain particular kinds of steroids in their tubers called saponins that are similar to human sex hormones. The chemical diosgenin can be extracted from the tubers, which is a good starting point for the chemical synthesis of saponins. The majority of the hormones synthesized from diosgenin are used in birth control pills, for the production of hormones that regulate the menstrual cycle, or as a component of fertility drugs. Cortisone and hydrocortisone are two other important hormones that are synthesized from diosgenin. They are used for the treatment of severe allergic reactions, arthritis, and Addison's disease, which is caused by malfunctioning of the adrenal glands.

Opium poppy, *Papaver somniferum*, is one of the oldest and still predominant sources of analgesics, which relieve pain. More than twenty-six different alkaloids have been isolated from opium, but only three of them—morphine, codeine, and papaverine—are used extensively. Morphine and codeine are used as painkillers, and papaverine is used primarily in drugs for the treatment of internal spasms, particularly those of the intestinal tract.

Another group of alkaloids is obtained from members of the potato family. They are considered analgesics and are used for controlling a variety of muscle spasms and in psychiatry. Alkaloids from *Atropa belladonna* are prescribed for stomach and bladder cramps and to prevent nausea and vomiting caused by motion sickness. They are prescribed for victims of Parkinson's disease to decrease stiffness and tremors and are often given to patients before surgery as a relaxant and to reduce salivation. These alkaloids, especially atropine, are helpful in cases of nerve gas (organophosphate insecticides) or mushroom poisoning. Alkaloids of the North American lily such as American false hellebore, *Veratrum viride*, have hypotensive properties and are used to treat high blood pressure.

Cinchona, the genus known primarily as a source of quinine, produces about thirty other alkaloids, including the compound quinidine, which is useful in treating heart disease. Quinidine inhibits abnormal rapid contractions of the upper right chamber of the heart and corrects improper heart rhythms.

Rauwolfia serpentina was used in the past for treating snakebites. It was later found to be useful in the treatment of hypertension by relaxing the heart muscle and thus lowering blood pressure, but it produced the side effects of depression and tremors, and its use was therefore discontinued. In 1952, the important alkaloid reserpine was isolated in Switzerland from the root where it is concentrated, although it occurs everywhere in the plant. The dramatic effects of reserpine completely altered practices in mental institutions because of its pronounced calming effect on schizophrenics without producing undesirable side effects. A relatively New World species, *R. tetraphylla*, is also a source of the alkaloid.

The few known substances that are able to arrest cancer cells are plant alkaloids. The common periwinkle, *Catharanthus reseus*, has been used in its native range in Europe for hundreds of years as a folk treatment for diabetes. It is now used effectively to treat some leukemias, especially those that commonly afflict children. The two active alkaloids are vinblastine and vincristine. Mayapple, *Podophylum peltatum*, contains antitumor alkaloids. Today mayapple alkaloids are used as the basis of VM-26 (teniposide), a drug used to treat testicular tumors and, with other agents, breast and lung cancer. The alkaloid colchicine is extracted from the corms of the autumn crocus, *Colchicum autumnale*. Colchicine is primarily used for the reduction of inflammation and pain caused by gout

but is also used in the treatment of cancer. Taxol, a compound most abundant in the bark of the Pacific yew, *Taxus brevifolia*, has been a major success in the treatment of breast and uterine cancer.

Several mucilaginous compounds of plant origin are used in soothing ointments and as carriers for other medicines. Species of *Aloe*, primarily *A. barbadensis*, have been used for their soothing gels. Chymopapain, an enzyme that exhibits specificity in its dissolution of proteins, is obtained from papaya, *Carica papaya*. It is injected by doctors into the soft central area of a deformed disk in humans to dissolve a large part of it and relieve the pressure on adjacent nerves.

PERSPECTIVE AND PROSPECTS

The medicinal uses of plants by humans have been known since ancient times and can be said to predate written history. Every culture on earth has used plants to cure disease, ease pain, and heal the ills and discomforts of the human body. People first started to keep records of herbal medicine about five thousand to seven thousand years ago in China and Mesopotamia. Sumerian drawings of opium poppy capsules from 2500 B.C.E. suggest that considerable knowledge of medicinal plants was in place. A substantial record of the use of herbs in medicine comes from the Code of Hammurabi, a series of tablets carved under the direction of the king of Babylon in about 1770 B.C.E. These tablets mention plants, such as henbane, licorice, and mint, that are still used in medicines at the present time. The Egyptians later recorded their knowledge of illnesses and cures on temple walls and in the Ebers papy-

A variety of herbs can be used to prevent and treat illnesses. (PhotoDisc)

rus (1550 B.C.E.), which contains more than seven hundred medicinal formulas.

In Greece, Hippocrates (c. 460-c. 370 B.C.E.) prescribed sound nutrition, purgatives, and botanical drugs for humans. He consequently earned the reputation as the father of medicine by being the first person to document illnesses and their treatment in a rational and orderly fashion. The most significant contribution made by Greeks toward the documentation of plants with healing properties was made by Dioscorides in his five-volume work entitled *De Materia Medica*. His encyclopedia described the preparation of about one thousand simple drugs. For several centuries afterward, it was the foundation text for practitioners of herbal medicine throughout Europe.

A stronger link was established between the studies of botany and medicine during the Middle Ages, and printed herbals became more available with the invention of the printing press in 1439. More herbs were added to the list from the New World when Europeans arrived in North America and learned Native American herbal uses. In the fourteenth century, the Renaissance led Europe into the determination of the medicinal uses of plants.

In the seventeenth and eighteenth centuries, science and philosophy advanced to the stage of experiments and hypothesis testing. It was not until the early 1800's, however, that scientists first began to isolate and extract healing compounds from plants. This experimental approach to medicine led to an improved understanding of physiology and provided a framework for the careful testing of medical treatments, including medicinal herbs.

The first half of the twentieth century saw tremendous advancements in medicine as more causes of diseases were discovered and new effective drugs were produced. Several modern medicines were produced as isolated and purified products of traditional plant-derived extracts, including morphine, quinine, and ephedrine. Medical chemists then began to determine the structures of these compounds and the possibility of their synthesis. In addition, they explored the chances of using the knowledge of the active ingredients of a natural healing herb to synthesize chemically related compounds that were potentially better medicines than the original one.

In the latter part of the twentieth century and the beginning of the twenty-first century, the prevalence of some diseases in some parts of the world and the emergence of diseases such as acquired immunodeficiency syndrome (AIDS) and severe acute respiratory syndrome (SARS) have challenged scientists, botanists, and doctors to explore plant sources for drugs that will offer possible or better cures.

Medicinal herbs are central to alternative therapies, which are gaining popularity in the twenty-first century. This trend is partly attributable to modern research into plant medicine and the remarkable healing results of herbal application to some diseases. For example, years of studies have shown that garlic can help control blood pressure and cholesterol. Yet few mainstream doctors recommend it, even though garlic is cheaper than pharmaceuticals and causes fewer side effects. This situation is beginning to change, however, because of a growing interest in natural sources of medicine. An estimated 80 percent of the world's population still rely on herbs for treating and preventing disease. In the United States, an estimated 25 percent of pharmaceuticals are still derived from plant sources. Native American herbs are still used by North American doctors in the twenty-first century. Many people do not realize that medical herbs are a key link between alternative therapies and mainstream medicine. Scientists around the world depend on herbs to develop new, more potent medications, and the search continues for plants with healing properties.

In 2004, researchers found that 20 percent of Aruvyedic supplements contained heavy metals, such as arsenic, lead, and mercury, exceeding safe levels as determined by the Environmental Protection Agency (EPA). Herbal remedies do not require testing before use by the public, and the Dietary Supplement Health and Education Act (DSHEA) does not require proof of safety or efficacy.

—Samuel V. A. Kisseadoo, Ph.D.;
updated by LeAnna DeAngelo, Ph.D.

See also Alternative medicine; Antioxidants; Food biochemistry; Homeopathy; Marijuana; Nutrition; Over-the-counter medications; Pharmacology; Pharmacy; Self-medication; Supplements; Toxicology.

FOR FURTHER INFORMATION:

Castleman, Michael. *Blended Medicine: How to Integrate the Best Mainstream and Alternative Remedies for Maximum Health and Healing.* Emmaus, Pa.: Rodale Press, 2002. Provides comprehensive knowledge on the use of medicinal plants as the center of alternative medicine. Discusses how different forms of treatment can be "blended" for different diseases.

Maleskey, Gale, and the editors of Prevention Health

Books. *Nature's Medicines: From Asthma to Weight Gain, from Colds to High Cholesterol—The Most Powerful All-Natural Cures.* Emmaus, Pa.: Rodale Press, 1999. Contains a detailed account of health supplements and the use of natural herbs to prevent and cure several common ailments. Includes an index, charts, and elaborate information on the names of many plants and natural supplements, plus steps that one can follow in order to use them effectively.

Simpson, Beryl Brintnall, and Molly Conner Ogorzaly. *Economic Botany: Plants in Our World.* 3d ed. Boston: McGraw-Hill, 2001. Gives an excellent account of the history and use of medicinal plants in different cultures over the centuries. Highlights modern utility and research into herbal medicine. Contains good illustrations, photographs, references, the scientific and common names of plants, a glossary, and an index.

White, B. Linda, and Steven Foster. *The Herbal Drugstore.* Emmaus, Pa.: Rodale Press, 2003. Provides one of the best natural alternatives to over-the-counter and prescription medicines. Contains charts, illustrations, scientific names, and an index.

Yeager, Selene. *The Doctor's Book of Food Remedies.* Emmaus, Pa.: Rodale Press, 2000. Gives a very detailed account of the healing properties of most common food items and herbs. Contains outlines of various preparations, charts, illustrations, and an index.

HERMAPHRODITISM AND PSEUDOHERMAPHRODITISM
DISEASE/DISORDER

ANATOMY OR SYSTEM AFFECTED: Genitals, reproductive system, urinary system

SPECIALTIES AND RELATED FIELDS: Embryology, endocrinology, genetics, gynecology, urology

DEFINITION: Abnormal primary sexual characteristics caused by developmental defects.

CAUSES AND SYMPTOMS

Hermaphroditism is a condition in which testicular and ovarian tissues are found in the same person and their urogenital development is ambiguous. A baby with an enlarged clitoris resembling a penis and fused labial-scrotal folds is often designated a male, whereas a baby with a normal clitoris and open labial folds might be considered a female. Generally, inappropriate levels of male and female hormones during fetal development are responsible for ambiguous genitals at birth.

Pseudohermaphroditism is a condition in which ei-

> ## INFORMATION ON HERMAPHRODITISM AND PSEUDOHERMAPHRODITISM
>
> **CAUSES:** Genetic defect of sex organs
> **SYMPTOMS:** Abnormal appearance of primary sexual characteristics
> **DURATION:** Chronic unless corrected
> **TREATMENTS:** Hormonal therapy, surgery

ther testicular tissues or ovarian tissues, but not both, are found in an individual with ambiguous urogenital development. XY pseudohermaphrodites develop internal testes, but their external genitals and appearance at birth are female. They lack ovaries, Fallopian tubes, and a uterus, but they have a blind (dead-end) vagina. There are two types of XY pseudohermaphrodites, those with testicular feminization syndrome (TFS) and those with *huevodoce* (or *guevedoces*) syndrome (HDS).

As individuals with TFS enter puberty, they begin to grow genital hair and breasts and have the appearance of normal females because they are unable to respond to any form of testosterone. When individuals with HDS begin puberty, the clitoris enlarges into a penis-like structure without a urethra. The urethral opening is at the base of the enlarged clitoris. One or both of the internal testes descend into scrotal sacs, and the teenager begins to develop masculine body and facial hair, but there is no breast development. In some cases, the voice deepens, and muscle mass and body shape become more masculine. Individuals with *huevodoce* syndrome develop as they do because they are unable to convert testosterone to 5-alpha-dihydrotestosterone (DHT), the inducer necessary for the early development of male tissues. At puberty, the testes produce very large amounts of testosterone, which is able to make up for the lack of DHT and to stimulate some tissues to develop further.

TREATMENT AND THERAPY

Hormone therapy or even operations to remove vestigial testes at birth might be of value in promoting the development of normal external genitals in hermaphroditic babies. In children with HDS, hormone therapy helps to resolve the ambiguous development of external genitalia at puberty. There are no treatments or therapies for individuals with TFS because these individuals are not responsive to testosterone.

PERSPECTIVE AND PROSPECTS

In general, persons with TFS think of themselves as females. They are sexually attracted to men and usually marry. No treatment should be considered for these individuals. Many individuals with HDS remain in a female role, but some take on the male role as they change at puberty. Hormone therapy might be of value in helping to establish the roles they desire in their culture.

—Jaime S. Colomé, Ph.D.

See also Genetic diseases; Genetics and inheritance; Puberty and adolescence; Reproductive system; Sexual differentiation.

FOR FURTHER INFORMATION:

Dreger, Alice Domurat. *Hermaphrodites and the Medical Invention of Sex.* Cambridge, Mass.: Harvard University Press, 2000.

Fausto-Sterling, Anne. *Sexing the Body: Gender Politics and the Construction of Sexuality.* New York: Basic Books, 2000.

Hellinga, Gerhardus. *Clinical Andrology: A Systematic Approach, with a Chapter on Intersexuality.* London: Heinemann, 1976.

Hunter, R. H. F. *Sex Determination, Differentiation, and Intersexuality in Placental Mammals.* New York: Cambridge University Press, 1995.

Kessler, Suzanne. *Lessons from the Intersexed.* New Brunswick, N.J.: Rutgers University Press, 1998.

Moore, Keith L., and T. V. N. Persaud. *The Developing Human.* 7th ed. Philadelphia: W. B. Saunders, 2003.

HERNIA

DISEASE/DISORDER

ANATOMY OR SYSTEM AFFECTED: Abdomen, gastrointestinal system, intestines, reproductive system, stomach

SPECIALTIES AND RELATED FIELDS: Gastroenterology, internal medicine

DEFINITION: A pouchlike mass consisting of visceral material encased in properitoneal tissue (the hernial sac) protruding through an aperture in the abdomen—a result of a weakening in the abdominal wall.

KEY TERMS:

Bassini technique: the most widely accepted surgical method for treating hernias; named after the Italian surgeon Edoardo Bassini

hernioplasty: the surgery performed to treat hernia patients

incarceration: an advanced and dangerous hernial stage which occurs when the hernial sac protrudes

---

INFORMATION ON HERNIA

CAUSES: Presence of scar tissue, heavy physical exertion in work or athletics, obesity, aging, congenital abnormality

SYMPTOMS: Heartburn, swallowing difficulty, chest pain, belching

DURATION: Acute or chronic

TREATMENTS: Surgery

---

well beyond the abdominal aperture and is constricted at the neck

inguinal hernia: the most common form of hernia, in which the hernial sac protrudes into the lower groin area

reducible hernia: a hernia that has not advanced significantly beyond the weakened aperture in the abdomen; such hernias were formerly treated by means of the externally applied pressure of a truss

CAUSES AND SYMPTOMS

A hernia condition exists when either tissues from, or actual portions of, vital internal organs protrude beyond the enclosure of the abdomen as a result of an abnormal opening in several possible areas of the abdominal wall. In most hernias, the protruding material remains encased in the tissue of the peritoneum. This saclike extension forces itself into whatever space can be ceded by neighboring tissues outside the abdomen. Because of the swelling effect produced, the hernia is usually visible as a lump on the surface of the body. As there are several types of hernias that may occur in different areas of the abdomen, the place of noticeable swelling and the internal organs affected may vary. With the single exception of the pancreas, hernia cases have been recorded involving all other organs contained in the abdomen. The most common hernial protrusions, however, involve the small intestine and/or the omenta, folds of the peritoneum. Another category of hernia, referred to as hernia adipose, consists of a protrusion of peritoneal fat beyond the abdominal wall.

Generally speaking, the cause of hernial conditions involves not only an internal pressure pushing portions of the viscera against the abdominal wall (hence the danger of bringing on a hernia through heavy physical exertion in work or athletics) but also a point of weakness in the abdominal wall itself. Two such points of potential weakness exist in all normal, healthy individuals: the original umbilical ring, which should normally "heal" over after the umbilical cord is severed; and the groin tissues in the lower portion of the abdomen—the region where the most common hernia, the inguinal hernia, occurs. Another possible source of vulnerability to hernia protrusions is connected to the individual's prior surgical history: Scar tissue may prove to be the weakest point of resistance to pressures originating anywhere in the abdominal region.

It should be noted that, because the abdominal tissues of infants and young children are particularly delicate, there is a proportionately higher occurrence of hernial conditions among babies and toddlers. If the hernia is diagnosed and treated early enough, complete healing is almost certain in such cases, most of which do not develop beyond the preliminary, or reducible, stage.

The several stages, or degrees, of hernial development usually begin with what doctors call a reducible hernia condition. At this stage, a patient suffering from hernia, sensing the onset of the disorder, may be able to obtain temporary relief from a developing protrusion by changing posture angle when upright or by lying down. Until the late twentieth century, some physicians preferred to treat reducible hernias by means of an externally attached pressure device, or truss, rather than resorting to surgical intervention. This form of treatment was gradually dropped in favor of increasingly effective hernioplasty operations.

When a hernial condition enters what is called the stage of incarceration, the advanced protrusion of the sac containing portions of viscera through the opening, or ring, in the abdominal wall can cause very severe complications. If, as is frequently the case, the protruding hernia sac passes through the ring as a fingerlike tube and then assumes a globular form outside the abdominal wall, a state of incarceration exists. As this state advances, the patient runs the risk of hernial strangulation. The constricting pressure of the ring's edges on the hernial sac interferes with circulatory functions in the herniated organ, causing destruction of tissues and, unless surgical intervention occurs, rapid spread of gangrene throughout the affected organ. It was the sixteenth century French surgeon Pierre Franco who carried out the first operation to release a strangulated hernia by inserting a thin instrument between the incarcerated bowel and the herniated sac, then incising the latter without touching the extruded vital organ.

A surprisingly wide range of hernial conditions have been noted and studied. These include hernias in the umbilical, epigastric (upper abdominal), spigelian (transversus abdominal muscle), interparietal, and groin regions. Hernias in the groin can be either femoral or inguinal. Inguinal hernias affecting the groin area have always been by far the most common, accounting for more than three-quarters of hernial cases, particularly among males.

Inguinal hernias share a number of common characteristics with one another and with the other closely associated form of groin hernia, the femoral hernia. Inguinal hernias are all caused by the abnormal introduction of a hernial sac into one of the four-centimeter-long inguinal canals located on the sides of the abdomen. These canals originate in the lower portion of the abdomen at an aperture called the inguinal ring. They have an external exit point in the rectus abdominal tissue. Located inside each inguinal canal are the ilioinguinal nerve, the genital branch of the genitofemoral nerve, and the spermatic cord. A comparable passageway from the abdomen into the groin area is found at the femoral ring, through which both the femoral artery and the femoral vein pass.

It may take a long period, sometimes years, for the sac to engage itself fully in the inguinal or femoral ring. Once the ring is passed, however, pressures from inside the abdomen help it descend through the canal rather quickly. If the external inguinal ring is firm in structure, and particularly if the narrow passageway is largely

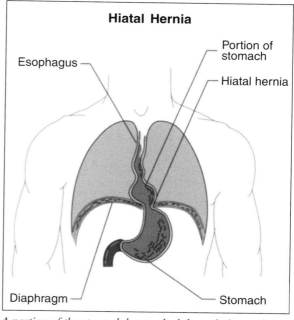

A portion of the stomach has pushed through the weakened abdominal wall.

filled with the thickness of the spermatic cord, the inguinal hernia may be partially arrested at this point. In men, once it passes beyond the external inguinal ring, however, it quickly descends into the scrotum. In women, the inguinal canal contains the round ligament, which may also temporarily impede the further descent of the hernial sac beyond the external inguinal opening.

Treatment and Therapy

Given the widespread occurrence of hernia conditions at all age levels in most societies, physicians receive extensive training in the diagnosis and, among those with surgical training, the treatment of hernia patients. Near-total consensus among doctors now demands surgery (external trusses having been largely abandoned), but different schools support different surgical methods. With the exception of operations involving the insertion of prosthetic devices to block the extension of hernia damage, most recent inguinal hernioplasty methods derive from the model finalized by the Italian Edoardo Bassini in the late nineteenth century.

Bassini believed that the surgical methods of his time fell short of the goal of complete hernial repair, since most postoperational patients were required to wear a truss to guard against recurring problems. In the simplest of surgical terms, his solution involved the physiological reconstruction of the inguinal canal. The operation provided for a new internal passageway to an external opening, as well as strengthened anterior and posterior inguinal walls. After initial incisions and ligation of the hernial sac, Bassini's method involved a separation of tissues between the internal inguinal ring and the pubis. A tissue section referred to as the "triple layer" (containing the internal oblique, the transversus abdominal, and the transversalis fascia tissue layers) was then attached by a line of sutures to the Poupart ligament, with a lowermost suture at the edge of the rectus abdominal muscle. Such local reconstruction of the inguinal canal proved to strengthen the entire zone against the recurrence of ruptures.

Physicians operating on indirect, as opposed to direct, inguinal hernias confront a relatively uncomplicated set of procedures. In the former case, a high ligation of the peritoneal sac (a circular incision of the peritoneum at a point well inside the abdominal inguinal ring) usually makes it possible to remove the sac entirely. Complications can occur if the patient is obese, since a large mass of peritoneal fatty material may be joined to the sac, obstructing access to the inguinal ring. For normal indirect inguinal hernias, the next ba-

sic step, after ensuring that no damage has occurred to the viscera either during formation of the hernia or in the process of relocating the contents of the hernial sac inside the abdomen, is to use one of several surgical methods to reduce the opening of the inguinal ring to its normal size. The physician must also ensure that no damage to the posterior inguinal wall has occurred and that its essential attachment to Cooper's ligament does not require additional surgical attention.

One must contrast the relative simplicity of indirect inguinal hernia surgery to treatment of direct inguinal hernias. In these cases, the hernia does not protrude through the existing inguinal aperture, but, as a result of a weakening of local tissues, passes directly through the posterior inguinal wall. The direct inguinal hernia is usually characterized by a broad base at the point of protrusion and a relatively short hernial sac. When a physician recommends surgical treatment of such hernias, the surgeon must be prepared for the extensive task of surgical reconstruction of the posterior inguinal wall as part of the operation.

Two additional reasons tend to discourage an immediate decision to operate on direct inguinal hernias. First, this form of hernia rarely strangulates the affected viscera, since the aperture stretches to allow protrusion of the hernial sac. Second, once physicians find obvious symptoms of a direct inguinal hernia (a ceding of the weakened posterior inguinal wall to pressures originating in the abdomen), they may decide to examine the patient more thoroughly to determine whether the cause behind the symptoms demands an entirely different prognosis. Such causes of abdominal pressures may range from the effects of a chronic cough to much more serious problems, including inflammation of the prostate gland or other forms of obstruction in the colon itself.

Perspective and Prospects

Because the phenomenon of hernias has been the subject of scientific observation since the onset of formal medical writing itself, a stage-by-stage development of prognoses has been associated with this condition. A main dividing line appears between the mid-eighteenth and mid-nineteenth centuries, however, between the extremely rudimentary surgical treatments of the late Middle Ages and Renaissance and what can be called modern prognoses.

Without doubt the surgical contribution of the sixteenth century Frenchman Pierre Franco, who performed the first operation to release an incarcerated hernia, must be considered a landmark. The major general cause for advancement in knowledge of hernias, however, is tied to the birth of a new era in medical science, characterized by the use, from about 1750 onward, of anatomical dissection to investigate the essential characteristics of a number of common diseases.

Before the relatively long line of contributions that led to general adoption of the Bassini technique of operating on hernias, surgeons tended to follow the so-called Langenbeck method, named after the German physician who pioneered modern hernioplasty. This method held that simple removal of a hernial sac at the point of its protrusion from the abdomen and closing the external aperture would lead to a closing of the sac by "adhesive inflammation." Such spontaneous closing occurs when a severed artery "recedes" to the first branching-off point.

It took contributions by at least two lesser-known late nineteenth century forerunners to Edoardo Bassini to convince the surgical world that hernia operations must involve a high incision of the hernial sac. Both the American H. O. Marcy (1837-1924) and the Frenchman Just Marie Marcellin Lucas-Championnière (1843-1913) have been recognized for their insistence on the necessity of high-incision operations. Their hernia operations, by incising the external oblique fascia, were the first to penetrate well beyond the external ring to expose the entire hernial sac. Following removal of the sac, it was then possible for surgeons to close the transversalis fascia and to repair the higher interior tissues that might have been damaged by the swollen hernia.

Following initial acceptance of the technique of high-incision hernial operations, a number of physicians recommended a variety of methods that might be used to repair internal tissue damage. These methods ranged from simple ligation of the sac at the internal ring, without more extensive surgery involving either the abdominal wall or the spermatic cord, to the much more extensive method practiced by Bassini. Even after the Bassini method succeeded in gaining almost universal recognition, other adaptations (but nothing that represented a full innovation) would be added during the middle decades of the twentieth century. One such method, which borrowed from the German physician Georg Lotheissen's use of Cooper's ligament to serve as a foundation for suturing damaged layers of lower abdominal tissues, earned its proponent, the American Chester McVay, the honor of having the operation named after him.

Finally, one should note that, although few significant changes have occurred in most doctors' view of what must be done surgically to treat hernia patients, surgical use of laser beams in the 1990's began to affect the techniques of hernioplasty, particularly in terms of recovery time.

—*Byron D. Cannon, Ph.D.*

See also Abdomen; Abdominal disorders; Gastroenterology; Gastroenterology, pediatric; Gastrointestinal disorders; Gastrointestinal system; Hemorrhoids; Hernia repair; Intestinal disorders; Intestines.

FOR FURTHER INFORMATION:

Bendavid, Robert, et al., eds. *Abdominal Wall Hernias: Principles and Management.* New York: Springer, 2000. A comprehensive examination of advances in hernia repair surgery.

Fitzgibbons, Robert J., Jr., and A. Gerson Greenburg, eds. *Nyhus and Condon's Hernia.* 5th ed. Philadelphia: Lippincott Williams & Wilkins, 2002. Widely recognized and updated joint contribution by a large number of specialized physicians. Examines such topics as the etiology, history, and anatomy of hernias; conventional, laparoscopic, and endoscopic groin hernia repairs; complications of groin hernia; and pediatric hernias.

Hernia Resource Center. http://www.herniainfo.com/. Provides FAQs about hernias, latest medical news and research, information on surgical treatment options, and tools to help find a doctor specializing in hernias.

Kurzer, Martin, Allan E. Kark, and George W. Wantz, eds. *Surgical Management of Abdominal Wall Hernias.* Malden, Mass.: Blackwell Science, 1999. Although surgeons generally agree that hernias should be treated surgically, which surgical approach is the most appropriate for hernia repair is a much-debated issue. This book examines the various approaches.

Ponka, Joseph L. *Hernias of the Abdominal Wall.* Philadelphia: W. B. Saunders, 1980. A general medical textbook containing excellent illustrative plates.

HERNIA REPAIR
PROCEDURE

ANATOMY OR SYSTEM AFFECTED: Abdomen, gastrointestinal system, intestines, stomach

SPECIALTIES AND RELATED FIELDS: Gastroenterology, general surgery

DEFINITION: Surgery to correct organ or tissue protrusions.

INDICATIONS AND PROCEDURES

A hernia is an abnormal protrusion of an organ or organ part from its normal body cavity, most often tissue protruding through the abdominal wall. Abdominal hernias may occur in the groin (inguinal hernia), upper thigh (femoral hernia), navel (umbilical hernia), and diaphragm (hiatal hernia). They may be congenital or acquired in later life. Herniated tissue is most often part of the small or large intestine. It can also be part of the bladder or the stomach in femoral and hiatal hernias, respectively. Most hernias occur as a result of strain to the abdominal wall or its injury. For example, they are often caused by athletic overexertion or hard labor. Consequently, men are more subject to acquired hernias than women.

Congenital inguinal hernias in male infants can occur when the testicles of a developing fetus work their way down the inguinal canal to the scrotum. If the tissue sac accompanying them does not close off correctly, congenital hernia occurs. In men, acquired inguinal hernias occur when excess abdominal strain ruptures the intestinal wall and releases a loop of intestine. Inguinal hernias are less common in women and are associated with the canal that holds the round ligament of the uterus. Femoral hernias in both sexes lie on the inner sides of the blood vessels of the thighs and are always acquired, often by overexertion. Umbilical hernias, which may be congenital or acquired, protrude from the navel.

Incisional hernia is caused by the incomplete healing of surgical wounds of the abdomen. A fifth hernia type is hiatal hernia, which occurs at the opening where the esophagus passes through the diaphragm (the hiatus). Such hernias, in which part or all of the stomach passes through the diaphragm, may cause no external symptoms and be diagnosed only when chest X rays are taken for other reasons. If symptoms do occur, they usually include heartburn and chest pain.

Hernias are classified according to severity. Reducible hernias are those which can be resolved by pushing herniated tissue back into its proper position. Irreducible hernias are more serious. They cannot be pushed back manually because of their position, or because of the presence of adhesions that bind them in place. Such

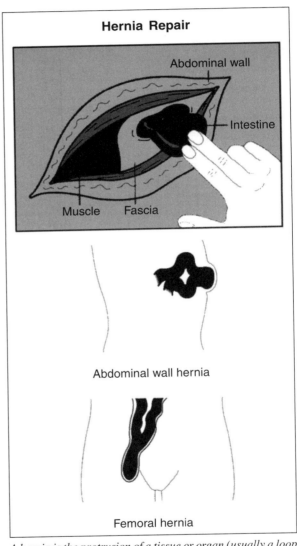

Hernia Repair

Abdominal wall

Intestine

Muscle   Fascia

Abdominal wall hernia

Femoral hernia

A hernia is the protrusion of a tissue or organ (usually a loop of intestine) into another area of the body. With abdominal wall hernias, which include inguinal and umbilical hernias, the intestine protrudes through a weakness in the abdomen; with femoral hernias, the intestine passes down the canal containing the major blood vessels to the thigh and appears as a bulge in the groin area. When a hernia presents a danger to the patient, the intestine must be surgically returned to its proper position.

hernias can only be corrected with surgery. Strangulated hernias are those whose size and location pinch herniated tissue, cutting off blood flow. They require immediate surgical treatment to prevent the development of gangrene or peritonitis, both of which can be fatal.

Surgical repair is the suggested treatment for most hernias. If the patient is temporarily too ill for surgery, a truss may be used to diminish pain and swelling for inguinal, femoral, umbilical, and incisional hernias. Trusses, however, provide only temporary, symptomatic relief, except perhaps in umbilical hernias of very young children. Extreme caution is necessary: Reducible hernias treated with trusses can become irreducible or strangulated.

Standard hernia surgery can be accomplished in several ways. For the correction of inguinal or umbilical hernias, first the muscle wall is opened. Then, after the herniated loop is moved into an appropriate position, the muscle wall is closed as normally as possible. In more severe types of hernia repair involving visible protrusions, the abdominal wall is opened, adhesions are cut away, and the tissue is returned to a normal position. Then, the muscle wall is closed to restore normal muscle layers. When strangulation occurs, damaged tissue is cut away, normal sections are joined together, and viable tissue is returned to the abdomen, followed by abdominal closure. Incisional hernias are treated similarly, in a fashion dependent on the extent of the external damage and the degree of herniation.

Hiatal hernias are treated medically, whenever possible, because they tend to recur after surgery. Medical treatment includes restriction of activity, weight loss, and diet modification. Surgery is carried out when these efforts fail or if severe adhesions and/or strangulation occurs. The goal of this surgery is to strengthen the closure at the junction between the diaphragm and the esophagus.

USES AND COMPLICATIONS

The surgeries to correct inguinal, femoral, umbilical, and incisional hernias are straightforward. In all cases, but especially in strangulation, patients are checked before release to ensure that normal bowel movement occurs, that incisions have not become infected, and that fever has not developed. At this time, patients are also shown how to protect their incisions before coughing, are advised to maintain a high fluid intake to engender normal bowel function, are warned against overex-

ertion, and are made aware of signs of incision infection. Furthermore, they are advised to resume work or physical activity only after consulting the physician involved.

Patients who have undergone surgery to correct a hiatal hernia are given much the same advice. Their surgery, however, is more extensive and prone to more complications. Therefore, they are provided with recommendations concerning which foods and activities to avoid. Furthermore, they are advised of the extended time period required before they can return to normal function and are told that without careful compliance, the problem will recur.

PERSPECTIVE AND PROSPECTS

Major advances in the treatment of hernias have included better diagnosis of their extent and the necessary means of their correction. Computed tomography (CT) scanning and other imaging techniques can make possible very accurate diagnoses. Progress in the surgical techniques used in hernia repair includes laparoscopy, in which a fiber-optic tube is used to visualize the chest cavity and thus to minimize incision size in the correction of hiatal hernias. All these methodologies are expected to improve in the future.

—*Sanford S. Singer, Ph.D.*

See also Abdomen; Abdominal disorders; Gangrene; Gastroenterology; Gastroenterology, pediatric; Gastrointestinal disorders; Gastrointestinal system; Hernia; Internal medicine; Intestinal disorders; Intestines; Pediatrics; Peritonitis.

FOR FURTHER INFORMATION:

Beers, Mark H., et al. *The Merck Manual of Diagnosis and Therapy.* 18th ed. Whitehouse Station, N.J.: Merck Research Laboratories, 2006. Contains a useful exposition of the characteristics, etiology, diagnosis, and treatment of hernia. Designed for physicians, the material is also useful for less specialized readers. Information on related topics is also included.

Fitzgibbons, Robert J., Jr., and A. Gerson Greenburg, eds. *Nyhus and Condon's Hernia.* 5th ed. Philadelphia: Lippincott Williams & Wilkins, 2002. Widely recognized and updated joint contribution by a large number of specialized physicians. Examines such topics as the etiology, history, and anatomy of hernias; conventional, laparoscopic, and endoscopic groin hernia repairs; complications of groin hernia; and pediatric hernias.

Mulholland, Michael W., et al., eds. *Greenfield's Surgery: Scientific Principles and Practice.* 4th ed. Philadelphia: Lippincott Williams & Wilkins, 2006. Covers the scope and practice of surgery and includes reviews of wound biology, immunology, the management of trauma and transplantation, surgical practice according to anatomic region and specialty, and musculoskeletal, neurologic, genitourinary, and reconstructive surgery.

Tierney, Lawrence M., Stephen J. McPhee, and Maxine A. Papadakis, eds. *Current Medical Diagnosis and Treatment 2007.* New York: McGraw-Hill Medical, 2006. This text, updated yearly, is the point of reference for physicians and other health care practitioners. It incorporates each year's biomedical research discoveries that have immediate, relevant, and applicable use for the patient.

Zinner, Michael J., et al., eds. *Maingot's Abdominal Operations.* 10th ed. Stamford, Conn.: Appleton & Lange, 1997. This textbook has long been considered the classic work on all surgical disciplines.

HERNIATED DISK. *See* SLIPPED DISK.

HERPES

DISEASE/DISORDER

ANATOMY OR SYSTEM AFFECTED: Genitals, mouth, nerves, reproductive system, skin

SPECIALTIES AND RELATED FIELDS: Dermatology, family medicine, gynecology, urology, virology

DEFINITION: A family of viruses that cause such diseases as cold sores, genital herpes, chickenpox, shingles, and mononucleosis. The term "herpes" is also used to refer to an infection with herpes simplex, either type 1 or type 2.

KEY TERMS:

antiviral agent: a drug that acts against a virus, usually by preventing it from reproducing itself; may be used at the first evidence of symptoms to reduce the severity and length of an episode or continually to prevent episodes from occurring

cold sore: also known as a fever blister; a sore, frequently on the lips but sometimes on the chin, cheeks, nostrils, and occasionally the gums or palate, that causes itching, burning, or tenderness, followed by crusting over

ganglia: clusters of nerves

genitalia: the internal and external reproductive organs

gingivostomatitis: inflammation of the gums and mouth

Kaposi's sarcoma: a rare cancer of connective tissue, found primarily in persons with acquired immunodeficiency syndrome (AIDS)

latent: inactive

lymphoma: one of a number of cancers of the lymphatic system

recurrent: repeated

vesicle: also called a blister; a collection of fluid under the epidermis, or topmost layer of the skin

virus: a tiny disease-causing organism that invades living cells and uses their processes in order to reproduce itself

whitlow: a herpes infection on the finger; it is found commonly in health care workers who must put their fingers into others' mouths and can occur even with the use of protective gloves

CAUSES AND SYMPTOMS

Eight different herpesviruses cause infection in humans. Herpes simplex types 1 and 2 (HHV1 and HHV2) cause cold sores and genital herpes, while herpes zoster or varicella-zoster virus (HHV3) causes chickenpox (varicella) and shingles. HHV4, also known as Epstein-Barr virus, causes infectious mononucleosis. A variant of this virus has also been implicated in a rare type of lymphoma. Cytomegalovirus (HHV5) causes a wide variety of health problems, including serious illness in newborn babies, an illness that strongly resembles infectious mononucleosis, and, in persons with AIDS and other immune deficiencies, disease of the retina, stomach, bowels, liver, lungs, and nervous system. Roseola, one of the many rash-and-fever diseases of childhood, is caused by HHV6. HHV7 is associated with seizures and encephalitis, while HHV8 is associated with Kaposi's sarcoma and some lymphomas.

Most commonly, however, the term "herpes" refers to infection with HHV1 and HHV2. A characteristic of both HHV1 and HHV2 infection is blisters clustered on reddened skin or mucous membranes. These blisters then either dry up or break, forming a shallow ulcer, and then crust over and gradually resolve. Another important characteristic is the tendency of infections to recur. This happens because the virus never truly goes away. Rather, it settles in ganglia under the skin and remains latent until some trigger causes it to become active again, resulting in a less severe outbreak at the same site of the body as the primary (first) infection. The trigger may be something physical such as sunburn or a fever, a change in the immune system as with ag-

INFORMATION ON HERPES

CAUSES: Viral infection
SYMPTOMS: Painful or itchy blisterlike lesions, fever, headache, tiredness, nerve pain, sore throat, swollen lymph nodes, sometimes enlarged liver and spleen
DURATION: Varies from short-term to recurrent
TREATMENTS: Antiviral drugs, supportive care

ing, or psychological stress. Recurrences tend to be heralded by itching, tingling, or burning at the site of the original outbreak for hours or days before the blisters occur. Recurrences may be rare or frequent.

Some people are infected with the virus but never have any symptoms. On the other hand, the first infection may cause a person to become very ill. The oral form, called herpetic gingivostomatitis, usually occurs in childhood. Symptoms include painful sores in the mouth, swollen and bleeding gums, swollen glands, and fever. The sores in the mouth may be so severe that it is difficult to eat or drink, and dehydration may become a problem. The genital form of herpes causes painful blisters in the genital area, swollen glands in the groin, fever, and other flulike symptoms. The blisters may make urination extremely painful. Regardless of the site, the first infection usually lasts about two weeks. The blisters themselves may last longer, but they typically scab over without leaving a scar.

Recurrent infections tend to be milder, with a single or small cluster of blisters erupting very close to the original site of infection. Recurrences typically last a shorter time than did the primary infection.

The diagnosis of herpes infection is usually made by observing the characteristic rash. During the first three days of an outbreak, it is possible to culture the virus from the base of one of the ulcers. Blood tests in a person with no current symptoms are not helpful because they do not distinguish between recent infection and one that occurred years before.

TREATMENT AND THERAPY

The best treatment for herpes infections is prevention. HHV1 is spread in air droplets, so covering coughs and sneezes is essential. Direct contact with the fluid from the blisters or ulcers can also pass HHV1 or HHV2 from one person to another. Once the blisters have

dried up or crusted over, they are much less contagious. Some people with herpes shed low levels of the virus even when they have no blisters. They may not even know they have the infection.

No treatment eliminates the virus from the body, but antiviral drugs will help shorten the length and severity of an outbreak. Continuous antiviral treatment will suppress the virus and prevent recurrences in most cases. Effective antiviral medications are available by prescription. Of these, oral medications are generally more effective than ointments applied directly to the blister. The common antiviral drugs include acyclovir, famciclovir, valaciclovir, and penciclovir. Over-the-counter lysine supplements seem to be helpful for some people, although scientific studies have not proven their effectiveness.

PERSPECTIVE AND PROSPECTS

A wide variety of vaccines, antibodies, and drugs that stimulate the immune system have been tested in the treatment of herpes, but they have either been ineffective or have caused unacceptable side effects. Researchers in the early twenty-first century, however, have found a new type of drug that works to suppress enzymes produced by the virus that seems to be effective in animal models.

—*Rebecca Lovell Scott, Ph.D., PA-C*

See also Canker sores; Cervical, ovarian, and uterine cancers; Chickenpox; Chronic fatigue syndrome; Cold sores; Epstein-Barr virus; Genital disorders, female; Genital disorders, male; Gynecology; Mononucleosis; Reye's syndrome; Sexually transmitted diseases (STDs); Shingles; Skin disorders; Viral infections; Warts.

FOR FURTHER INFORMATION:

American Medical Association. *American Medical Association Family Medical Guide*. 4th rev. ed. Hoboken, N.J.: John Wiley & Sons, 2004.

Herpes Resource Center. http://www.herpesresource center.com/.

Komaroff, Anthony, ed. *Harvard Medical School Family Health Guide*. New York: Free Press, 2005.

Parker, James N., and Philip M. Parker, eds. *The Official Patient's Sourcebook on Genital Herpes*. San Diego, Calif.: Icon Health, 2002.

Stoppard, Miriam. *Family Health Guide*. New York: DK, 2004.

HICCUPS

DISEASE/DISORDER

ALSO KNOWN AS: Hiccoughs

ANATOMY OR SYSTEM AFFECTED: Chest, lungs, muscles, respiratory system, throat

SPECIALTIES AND RELATED FIELDS: Family medicine, gastroenterology, neurology

DEFINITION: Involuntary, spasmodic contractions of the diaphragm and the simultaneous closure of the glottis.

CAUSES AND SYMPTOMS

A hiccup is caused by an involuntary, spasmodic contraction of the diaphragm, the large partition of muscles and tendons that separates the chest from the abdomen. The diaphragm draws air into the lungs through rhythmic contractions. When it contracts suddenly, an opening located toward the top of the trachea (windpipe) between the vocal cords in the larynx (voice box) called the glottis snaps shut abruptly. The combination of air being forced through the vocal cords in the larynx and the abrupt closure of the glottis causes the sound associated with hiccups.

There are a number of causes of hiccups, the most common being overdistension of the stomach. Other causes include gastric irritation from spicy or rich foods and nerve spasms. There is some indication that hiccups are controlled by the central nervous system.

Hiccups generally last for a very short time, usually stopping within minutes. People who suffer from hiccups for more than twenty-four hours or who have repetitive attacks are said to suffer from chronic hiccups. This condition is very rare.

People of all ages can suffer from hiccups. Pregnant women report that fetuses sometimes have hiccups in the womb.

INFORMATION ON HICCUPS

CAUSES: Overdistension of stomach, gastric irritation from spicy or rich foods, nerve spasms

SYMPTOMS: Involuntary, spasmodic contractions of diaphragm and simultaneous closure of glottis; stomach upset

DURATION: Ranges from short-term to chronic

TREATMENTS: Varies; can include holding one's breath, drinking a glass of water, breathing deeply or into a paper bag

---

TREATMENT AND THERAPY

An attack of hiccups is not serious and is generally self-limiting. A number of techniques to stop are practiced, including holding one's breath, drinking a glass of water, breathing deeply, or breathing into a paper bag.

Babies often suffer from hiccups, particularly during nursing. Some mothers report that feeding the baby a quarter of a teaspoon of sugar mixed in 4 ounces of water calms the hiccups. Doctors suggest that hiccup-prone babies be fed before they are overly hungry and when they are calm.

—*Diane Andrews Henningfeld, Ph.D.*

See also Abdomen; Breast-feeding; Coughing; Respiration.

FOR FURTHER INFORMATION:

Gluck, Michael, and Charles E. Pope II. "Hiccups and Gastrointestinal Reflux Disease: The Acid Perfusion Test as a Provocative Maneuver." *Annals of Internal Medicine* 105 (1996): 219-220.

Heuman, Douglas M., A. Scott Mills, and Hunter H. McGuire, Jr. *Gastroenterology.* Philadelphia: W. B. Saunders, 1997.

Launois, J. L., W. A. Bizec, J. C. Whitelaw et al. "Hiccup in Adults: An Overview." *European Respiratory Journal* 6 (1993): 563-575.

Shay, Steven D. S., Robert L. Myers, and Lawrence F. Johnson. "Hiccups Associated with Reflux Esophagitis." *Gastroenterology* 87 (1984): 204-207.

HIP FRACTURE REPAIR

PROCEDURE

ANATOMY OR SYSTEM AFFECTED: Bones, hips, joints, legs, musculoskeletal system

SPECIALTIES AND RELATED FIELDS: Geriatrics and gerontology, orthopedics

DEFINITION: The repair or replacement of a broken hip joint.

KEY TERMS:

arthroplasty: joint replacement

osteoporosis: a loss of bone mass accompanied by increasing fragility and brittleness

INDICATIONS AND PROCEDURES

Hip fracture repair constitutes one of the most common procedures performed by orthopedic surgeons. The human hip consists of two bones, the hipbone and the thighbone (femur), and their point of intersection, a cup-shaped cavity called the acetabulum. This hip joint forms a ball-and-socket mechanism that allows the leg to move in different directions. As a major weight-bearing joint, the hip is vulnerable both to sudden trauma, such as sports injuries, and to degenerative disorders of aging, such as osteoporosis. If the loss of bone mass associated with osteoporosis is sufficiently advanced, a simple fall from a standing position can shatter the hip joint. The most common fracture involves the femur snapping or cracking just below the rounded end that fits into the acetabulum.

PERSPECTIVE AND PROSPECTS

The repair of hip fractures involves the realignment of the bone fragments and the insertion of a long nail into the bone to hold them together. A plate is attached to the nail and to the healthy bone surrounding the fracture in order to give support.

Because broken bones heal slowly in the elderly, in the past a broken hip almost inevitably resulted in these patients becoming permanent invalids restricted to wheelchairs or, at best, forced to rely on walkers and enjoying only limited mobility. This bleak prognosis changed in the 1960's when orthopedic specialists working with biomedical engineers developed artificial hip joints. The combination of prosthetic devices and surgical techniques known as total hip arthroplasty (THA) allows physicians to return patients to active, independent lives. In THA, the weakened end of the femur is removed and an artificial replacement installed. The replacement can consist of any of a variety of materials, but typically it is constructed of a chromium steel alloy coated with a ceramic polymer that helps resist corrosion as well as providing a surface with which the patient's bone can bond. The end of the prothesis and the surface of the acetabulum are coated with plastic polymers to reduce friction. Research indicates that artificial hip joints last fifteen years or longer before wear and tear on the lining of the ball-and-socket joint creates problems.

—*Nancy Farm Mannikko, Ph.D.*

See also Aging: Extended care; Arthroplasty; Arthroscopy; Bone disorders; Bone grafting; Bones and the skeleton; Emergency medicine; Fracture and dislocation; Fracture repair; Geriatrics and gerontology; Hip replacement; Orthopedic surgery; Orthopedics; Osteoporosis; Physical rehabilitation.

FOR FURTHER INFORMATION:

Brunicardi, F. Charles, et al., eds. *Schwartz's Principles of Surgery*. 8th ed. New York: McGraw-Hill, 2005.
Currey, John D. *Bones: Structures and Mechanics*. Princeton, N.J.: Princeton University Press, 2002.
Doherty, Gerard M., and Lawrence W. Way, eds. *Current Surgical Diagnosis and Treatment*. 12th ed. New York: Lange Medical Books/McGraw-Hill, 2006.
Morrey, Bernard, ed. *Joint Replacement Arthroplasty*. 3d ed. Philadelphia: Churchill Livingstone, 2003.
Nelson, Miriam, and Sarah Wernick. *Strong Women, Strong Bones: Everything You Need to Know to Prevent, Treat and Beat Osteoporosis*. New York: Berkley, 2001.
Townsend, Courtney M., Jr., et al., eds. *Sabiston Textbook of Surgery*. 17th ed. Philadelphia: Elsevier Saunders, 2005.
Wilmore, Douglas W., et al., eds. *Scientific American Surgery 2006*. New York: Scientific American, 2007.

HIP REPLACEMENT
PROCEDURE

ANATOMY OR SYSTEM AFFECTED: Bones, hips
SPECIALTIES AND RELATED FIELDS: Orthopedics, rheumatology
DEFINITION: The removal of diseased bone tissue in the hip and its replacement with an artificial device.

INDICATIONS AND PROCEDURES

The most common reason for hip replacement surgery is the decline in efficiency of the hip joint that often results from osteoarthritis. Osteoarthritis is a common form of arthritis that causes joint and bone deterioration, which may lead to the wearing down of cartilage and cause the underlying bones to rub against each other. This may result in severe pain and stiffness in the affected areas. Other conditions that may lead to the need for hip replacement include rheumatoid arthritis (a chronic inflammation of the joints), avascular necrosis (loss of bone caused by insufficient blood supply), and injury.

Generally, physicians may be more inclined to choose less invasive techniques such as physical therapy, medication, or walking aids before resorting to surgery. In some cases, exercise programs may help reduce hip pain. In addition, if preliminary treatment does not improve the patient's condition, doctors may use corrective surgery that is not as invasive as hip replacement. However, when these efforts do not reduce pain or increase mobility, hip replacement may be the best option. In addition, the age of the patient may be an important factor in the decision to replace the hip. The majority of hip replacements are performed on individuals over the age of sixty-five. One of the reasons for this is that the activity level of older adults is lower than that of younger adults, therefore reducing the concern that the new hip will wear out or fail. However, technological advances have improved the quality of the artificial hip, making hip replacement surgery a more likely intervention for younger adults as well.

Generally, a candidate for total hip replacement surgery (THR) possesses a hip that has worn out from arthritis, falls, or other conditions. The hip consists of a ball-and-socket joint where the head of the femur (thigh bone) fits into the hip socket, or acetabulum. In a normal hip, this arrangement provides for a relatively wide range of motion. For some older adults, however, deterioration caused by arthritis and other conditions reduces the effectiveness of this arrangement, compromising the integrity of the hip socket or the femoral head. This state can lead to extreme discomfort.

Total hip replacement may provide the best long-term relief for these symptoms. Total hip replacement involves the removal of diseased bone tissue and the replacement of that tissue with prostheses (artificial devices used to replace missing body parts). Usually, both the femoral head and hip socket are replaced. The femoral head is replaced with a metal ball that is attached to a metal stem and placed into the hollow marrow space of the femur. The hip socket is lined with a plastic socket. Other materials have been used effectively as hip replacements.

In some cases, the surgeon will use cement to bond the artificial parts of the new hip to the bone tissue. This approach has been the traditional method of ensuring that the artificial parts hold. One problem with this method is that over time, cemented hip replacements may lose their bond with the bone tissue. This may result in the need for an additional surgery. However, a cementless hip replacement has been developed. This approach includes a prosthesis that is porous so that bone tissue may grow into the metal pores and keep the prosthesis in place.

Both procedures have strengths and weaknesses. In general, recovery time may be shorter with cemented prostheses since one does not have to wait for bone growth to attach to the artificial prostheses. However, the potential for long-term deterioration of the replaced hip must be considered. A cemented hip generally lasts about fifteen years. With this in mind, physicians may be more likely to use a cemented prosthesis for patients over the age of seventy. Cementless hip replacement may be more advisable for younger and more active patients. Some physicians have used a combination of approaches, known as a "hybrid" or "mixed" hip. This combination relies on an uncemented socket and a cemented femoral head.

USES AND COMPLICATIONS

Total hip replacements are generally quite successful, with about 96 percent of surgeries proceeding without complications. In rare instances, however, complications occur, including blood clots and infections during surgery, and hip dislocation or bone fracture after surgery. In addition, in some cases, bone grafts may be used to assist in the restoration of bone defects. In these instances, bone may be obtained from the pelvis or the discarded head of the femur. Other postoperative complications may include some pain and stiffness.

Patients recovering from total hip replacement usually remain in the hospital up to ten days if there are no complications. However, physical therapists may initiate therapy as soon as the day after surgery. Physical therapy involves the use of exercises that will improve recovery. Many patients are able to sit on the edge of their bed, stand, and even walk with assistance as early as two days after surgery. Patients must remember that their artificial hip may not provide the same full range of motion as an undiseased hip. Physical therapists teach patients how to perform daily activities without placing an undue burden on their new hips. This may require learning a new method of sitting, standing, and performing other activities.

While many factors may affect recovery time, full recovery from surgery may take up to six months. At that point, many patients enjoy such activities as walking and swimming. Doctors and physical therapists may discourage patients from participating in such high-impact activities as jogging or playing tennis, which may burden the new hip. Despite these restrictions, many patients are able to perform normal activities without pain and discomfort. Nonetheless, people who have undergone hip replacement surgery are advised to consult with their doctor about proper exercise and activity levels.

PERSPECTIVE AND PROSPECTS

Total hip replacement is one of the most common surgical interventions that older adults face. The American Academy of Orthopedic Surgeons estimates that more than 120,000 hip replacement surgeries are performed in the United States each year. The average age of the patient who undergoes hip replacement surgery is sixty-seven years, while 67 percent of total hip replacements are performed on individuals age sixty-five or older. Approximately 60 percent of hip replacement surgeries are performed on women.

—*H. David Smith, Ph.D.*

See also Arthritis; Bone disorders; Bones and the skeleton; Hip fracture repair; Orthopedics; Osteonecrosis.

FOR FURTHER INFORMATION:

Bucholz, Robert, and Joseph A. Buckwalter. "Orthopedic Surgery." *Journal of the American Medical Association* 275, no. 23 (June 19, 1996). The research focus of orthopedic surgery is discussed, including research on the use of recombinant growth factors to induce bone repair and the regeneration of cartilaginous surfaces.

Duffey, Timothy P., Elliott Hershman, Richard A. Sanders, and Lori D. Talarico. "Investigating the Subtle and Obvious Causes of Hip Pain." *Patient Care* 31, no. 18 (November 15, 1997). A delay in diagnosing the cause of a patient's acute hip pain could lead to significant impairment of the hip. Talarico explains how to maximize one's investigative effort and make the most of treatment.

Dunkin, Mary Anne. "Hip Replacement Surgery." *Arthritis Today* 12, no. 2 (March/April, 1998). Two types of joint prostheses are discussed. Illustrations by Kevin A. Somerville show the difference between a healthy hip joint and cartilage that is damaged.

Finerman, Gerald A. M., et al., eds. *Total Hip Arthroplasty Outcomes.* New York: Churchill Livingstone, 1998. Discusses topics such as the anatomic medullary looking prosthesis, the porous-coated anatomic prosthesis, the anatomic porous replacement system, long-term results of hybrid prostheses, and the hybrid total hip replacement.

Lane, Nancy E., and Daniel J. Wallace. *All About Osteoarthritis: The Definitive Resource for Arthritis Patients and Their Families.* New York: Oxford University Press, 2002. A comprehensive look at the degeneration of bones and joints accompanied by detailed illustrations of key joints—knees, hips, fingers, backs, hands, and necks. Covers the steps of diagnosis, how the body is affected, and ways to manage the disease, including new medications and surgical options.

MacWilliam, Cynthia H., Marianne U. Yood, James J. Verner, Bruce D. McCarthy, and Richard E. Ward.

"Patient-Related Risk Factors That Predict Poor Outcome After Total Hip Replacement." *Health Services Research* 31, no. 5 (December, 1996). A study identifies factors associated with poor outcome after total hip replacement (THR) surgery. It is the first to present results from the American Medical Group Association (AMGA) THR consortium.

Morrey, Bernard, ed. *Joint Replacement Arthroplasty.* 3d ed. Philadelphia: Churchill Livingstone, 2003. Reviews arthroplasty of all joints. Each section concludes with chapters on alternatives and future directions of research and practice.

Silber, Irwin. *Patient's Guide to Knee and Hip Replacement: Everything You Need to Know.* New York: Simon & Schuster, 1999. Written by a hip-replacement patient, guides readers through the complete joint-replacement process, from the initial diagnosis and the decision whether to have surgery, the hospital stay, and the full recovery period.

Trahair, Richard C. S. *All About Hip Replacement: A Patient's Guide.* Oxford, England: Oxford University Press, 1999. Includes bibliographical references and an index.

Van De Graaff, Kent M., and Stuart Ira Fox. *Concepts of Human Anatomy and Physiology.* 5th ed. Dubuque: Iowa: Wm. C. Brown, 2000. Chapters 8 through 11 present a first-rate introduction to bones, the skeleton, and joints. The many clear illustrations, photographs, clinical commentaries, and X rays, as well as a pronunciation guide, a complete index, and a glossary, make this a very accessible book for the nonspecialist reader.

HIPPOCRATIC OATH

ETHICS

DEFINITION: A document, written in the fifth century B.C.E., to offer guidelines for the emerging medical profession, which continues to be the subject of debate in modern practice because of the ethical issues that it addresses.

KEY TERMS:

euthanasia: the practice (particularly in cases involving patients of advanced age) of withholding medical treatments that might sustain life that would otherwise expire "naturally"; in a more controversial form, it is associated with the administration of drugs by physicians in order to avert prolonged suffering

living will: a legally binding document instructing a physician not to prolong life by externally administered life support systems if the patient is unable to express his or her decision concerning forms of medical treatment recommended by a physician

malpractice insurance: insurance policies held by physicians in order to protect them financially in the event of a patient-initiated lawsuit alleging incidents of improper medical decisions or incompetence

MEDICAL CODES OF ETHICS

Western civilization has long held the writings of the fifth century B.C.E. Greek physician Hippocrates, and in particular the Hippocratic oath, as a model of ethical values to be followed in the medical profession. As the nature of Western civilization itself has changed over the centuries, interpretations of the ethical values behind the Hippocratic oath have also changed. The circumstances of modern medical practice and ethical values, however, have ironically made certain elements of the classical Hippocratic tradition even more relevant than they may have appeared in previous eras.

In fact, the Hippocratic oath is only the introductory section of the *Corpus Hippocraticum* (Hippocratic Collection) traditionally attributed to Hippocrates. (There is debate about whether he is the author of all the books or only some.) The actual medical observations of Hippocrates were studied and applied for many centuries, until scientific research rendered many of them recognizably obsolete. A number of sections of the corpus, however, reflect the Greek physician's recurring concern for rules to guide the medical profession. Hippocrates' chapters on "The Art," "Decorum," and "The Law" complement the more famous ethical precepts contained in the oath.

The first part of the oath itself covers the physician's lifelong commitment to his or her teachers. This commitment extends not only to the symbolic bonds of respect but also to obligation to share one's medical practice and even to provide financial assistance to one's teachers, if requested. Additionally, the physician is committed to train, free of charge, the families of his or her teachers in the art of medicine.

The second part of the Hippocratic oath contains the more general pledges that would contribute to its value as an ethical guide for the medical profession. The physician is bound, in a very general way, to help the sick according to his or her ability and judgment in a manner that can never be interpreted as involving injury or wrongdoing. The physician is bound both to confidentiality concerning direct experiences in the patient-doctor relationship and to extreme discretion to avoid

the circulation of professional knowledge that is not appropriate for publication abroad.

In addition to these general precepts, all of which have an ethical timelessness that would survive the centuries, there were two points in the oath that refer to specific issues that cannot be separated from the modern debate over medical ethics. Addressing the questions of euthanasia ("mercy killing") and abortion, Hippocrates stated: "I will give no deadly drug to any, though it be asked of me, nor will I counsel such, and especially I will not aid a woman to procure abortion."

Anyone searching for wider guidelines can glean many items of timeless wisdom from other sections of Hippocrates' writings. In the pieces titled "The Physician" and "Decorum," for example, the personal behavior of doctors is discussed. In all cases, Hippocrates exhorted physicians to maintain even levels of dignity and patience, to practice exemplary personal hygiene, and to avoid excesses in living habits that could introduce an element of distance between themselves and the patients who depend on them. Many centuries later, as in the eighteenth century English essay by Samuel Bard titled "A Discourse upon the Duties of a Physician," one can see similar concerns for behavioral propriety toward the defenseless: for example, "Never affect to despise a man for the want of a regular education, and treat even harmless ignorance with delicacy and compassion" and protect against the effects of "foolhardiness and presumption." These admonitions are indicative of the defining boundaries of the views of Hippocrates and those of the later, Christian era on the practice of medicine. The main attention of commentators on the Hippocratic corpus in recent generations has been directed to two broad divisions in the main ethical issues that he formulated: the physician's role in abortion and in the decision to end life by either withholding or administering certain treatments. It took many centuries, however, for degrees of emphasis in analyzing the Hippocratic oath to take form. In the interim, and after a delay that separated the classical world from the late medieval world, different interpretations of the Hippocratic oath would appear, each reflecting the cultural environment to which it was meant to apply.

Several factors may explain why centuries passed before systematic attention was given to the rules of medicine first broached in the classical Greek and Roman worlds. The first of these was the general decline of political and economic conditions after the fall of Rome (fifth century C.E.), which had repercussions in a variety of cultural areas. Medical practices tended to revert to quite crude levels until the rediscovery of early medical texts, including those of Hippocrates, sparked interest in improving conditions of medical treatment in the late Middle Ages.

One can say that, in addition to editing elements of Hippocratic teachings to Christianize the pagan references that they contained, a second important redirection occurred in setting down medieval rules for the practice of medicine. It was Holy Roman Emperor Frederick II, around 1241, who specified for the first time that the higher authority of the state alone should define institutional procedures for certifying physicians. This was to be done through formal training and examinations in the universities of Naples or Salerno, and later in universities throughout the Western world.

In addition to rules leading to physicians' certification, Frederick II stipulated that doctors must take an oath binding them to obligations that, in comparison to the Hippocratic oath or modern codes of medical ethics, covered very specific issues. One of these was an obligation to report any irregularities in an apothecary's preparation of drugs that were to be dispensed to patients. Another enjoined doctors to provide free medical services to the poor.

If one looks at more modern standards for the regulation of relations between physician and patient, it is possible to suggest that—until some very major changes took place in society's views on delicate questions previously reserved for ecclesiastical law—similar operatives continued to govern the guidelines for medical ethics. In the "Code of Medical Ethics" (1846-1847) by the American Medical Association (AMA), for example, primary focus is still visibly on the physician's obligation to place the patient's interest before his or her own, particularly in terms of prospects for material or other forms of personal gain. Defense of the public's interest against quackery or the distribution of drugs that are either dangerous or illegally prepared follows, as well as avoidance of "crude hypotheses" or "magnification of the importance of services" sought, merely for the purpose of "temporary effect and popularity." Although there are enormous time spans between the classical Hippocratic model, the medieval variant offered by Frederick II, and the mid-nineteenth century AMA code, all are comparable in their focus on what, in the terminology of the 1847 code, would be called "Duties for Support of Professional Character" (part 1, article 1) or "Duties of the Profession to the Public" (part 2, article 1).

One hundred years later, however, different societal attitudes toward medical ethics would establish themselves in most Western nations, including the United States. Generally stated, the basic changes reflected in ethical debates emphasized (or questioned the rising emphasis on) the protection of individual rights and privacy in matters relating to human life and the intervention of physicians. On one hand, changing directions in the expression of ethical orientations stemmed from advances made in key areas of medical science in the twentieth century, such as technologies for combating terminal disease, saving the lives of severely preterm infants, and prolonging life in old age. On the other hand, and in an even broader context, extraordinary scientific discoveries concerning the genetic keys behind life itself introduced an entirely different dimension to medical ethics, that of responsibility for monitoring or "engineering" life that has not yet been conceived.

MODERN APPLICATIONS

Although neither the original nor edited versions of the Hippocratic oath are applied today as a condition for becoming a doctor, the medical profession in the United States has definitely formalized publication of what it considers to be a necessary code of medical ethics. Evolving versions of this "Code of Medical Ethics" date from the original (1847) text of the AMA as revised by specific decisions in 1903, 1912, and 1947.

When the AMA adopted a statement under the title "Guide to Responsible Professional Behavior" in 1980, it assigned to a formal body within its organization, the Council on Ethical and Judicial Affairs, the task of publishing, on a yearly basis, updated paragraphs that reflect ethical guidelines for the profession as a whole. These evolving guidelines are organized under such subheadings as "Social Policy Issues," "Interprofessional Relations," "Hospital Relations," "Confidentiality," and "Fees and Charges."

At the turn of the twenty-first century, the public's growing uncertainty about a doctor's role in a market-oriented health care delivery system and increasing mistrust in the face of malpractice suits prompted physicians to question their professional responsibilities and roles within modern medicine. In 2002, a joint effort between the American Board of Internal Medicine (ABIM), the American College of Physicians-American Society of Internal Medicine (ACP-ASIM), and the European Federation of Internal Medicine (EFIM) introduced a new professional code of conduct designed to address these issues and help physicians meet the needs of patients in the twenty-first century. The charter incorporated traditional understanding of professional norms into the unique circumstances of modern medicine by addressing issues such as patient autonomy and choice, working in physician teams and respecting other professionals, managing conflicts of interest, social justice and equality in health care access, and market forces—issues not relevant during the time of Hippocrates. The American-British team noted that they hoped their efforts reaffirmed to a wary public the profession's commitment to putting the needs of the patient first and offered guidelines to physicians for coping with the ethical problems in the modern world.

Along with such modern-day charters, physicians are bound to respect the ethical guidelines provided to them by their professional association. Failure to respect these guidelines is tantamount to breaking one's binding ethical obligations and can lead to expulsion from the medical profession.

Several major changes, both in levels of medical technology and in social attitudes toward issues relating to medical practice, have played key roles in several spheres of an ongoing debate concerning medical ethics. In two cases, those of abortion and euthanasia, debate has focused on the ethics of deciding to end life; in the third, referred to generally as genetic engineering, the central question involves both the living and those yet to be born. In all these spheres, the legal and ethical debates have revolved around potential conflicts between physicians and patients but also in the context of wider social values.

Movement from the historical domain of idealized codes or oaths to the more practical and contemporary realm of changing societal reactions to what constitutes injury or breach of professional ethics in several areas of modern medicine is facilitated by reference to landmark legal decisions that have given a modern and quite different meaning to Hippocratic concepts.

Probably the most widely recognized issue reflecting such ethical conflicts, and one that received specific attention in the Hippocratic oath itself, involves abortion. In the United States, the climate of public opinion toward doctor-assisted pregnancy terminations was altered considerably by the landmark 1973 Supreme Court decision *Roe v. Wade*. In this decision, the Court judged that state laws defining abortion as a criminal offense were unconstitutional. The main thrust of the argument in *Roe v. Wade* was that, although the Constitution does not provide a specific guarantee of a civil right of privacy that could be applied to questions of life and death in medical care, parallels exist in Supreme Court decisions on other matters of individual rights with respect to procreation. These rights tend to fall under the Fourteenth Amendment's concept of personal liberty and restrictions on state action. These rights, in the Court's words, are "broad enough to encompass a woman's decision whether or not to terminate her pregnancy."

Reference to the fundamental right of "personal privacy" in *Roe v. Wade* granted individual women and their physicians recourse against specific state laws criminalizing abortion. It did not, however, consider the right to have an abortion to be unqualified. Nor did it extend beyond the domain of pregnancy termination to cover a general assumption that constitutional protection of the right of privacy included the individual's right to "do with one's body as one pleases." In fact, there was an explicit suggestion that the legal definition of protection of an individual's right to privacy where critical medical decisions affecting vital life processes are concerned is "not unqualified and must be considered against important state interests in regulation."

As time passed in the evolving debate over abortion, definitions of what this could mean became colored by the inevitable introduction of religious conceptions of defense of the unborn individual—the fetus—as a possessor of life separate from that of the pregnant woman. This was a precursor to the "right to life" versus "right to choice" debate that would place physicians between two poles of opinion as to where their final obligations should lie.

What seemed most important in the beginnings of the abortion debate (and then, a few years later, the euthanasia debate) was the Supreme Court's inclusion of commentary on Hippocratic ethical precepts as part of its argument justifying recognition of individual rights to final responsibility for the disposition of someone else's "future" life or the disposition of one's own life. The *Roe v. Wade* brief actually argued that the strict Hippocratic injunction against abortion must be recognized as a reflection of only one segment of opinion and values (specifically Pythagorean) at a particular time in history. By underlining the fact that other views and practices were known to be current throughout antiquity, and that later Christian ethics chose to ignore diversity of interpretations of medical ethics in such matters, *Roe v. Wade* implied that diversity of ethical opinion within a social environment must be recognized in order to avoid too narrow a definition of what standards should be followed by physicians in dealing with their patients.

The implications of these two directions in interpreting the ethical bonds between patient and physician—the right to privacy in reaching individual decisions and recognition of a degree of social relativity in defining guidelines for medical ethics—are equally visible in the debate concerning the ultimate source of authority for deciding when to terminate life and the presumed authority of the Hippocratic oath in this process.

Two issues, one involving the ethics of sustaining life by means of advanced medical technology and the other involving the "engineering" of lives according to genetic predictions, fall under the provisions of the Hippocratic oath. As one approaches more contemporary statements of professional obligations of medical doctors, such as the "Principles of Medical Ethics" (1957) of the American Medical Association, one finds that, as certain areas of specificity in classical Hippocratic or Christian medical ethics (the illegality of abortions or the administration of deadly potions) tend to decline in visibility, another area begins to come to the forefront—namely, striving continually to improve medical knowledge and skills to be made available to patients and colleagues.

This more modern concern for the application of advancements in medical knowledge, especially in the technology of medical lifesaving therapy, has introduced a new focus for ethical debate: not "lifesaving" but "life-sustaining" techniques, particularly in cases judged to be otherwise terminal or hopeless. As with the issue of abortion, the question of a doctor's responsibility to use every means within his or her reach to sustain life, even when there is no hope of a meaningful future for the patient, reflects a dilemma regarding Hippocratic injunctions. This debate is more important now than in any earlier era because advanced medical technology has made it possible either to extend the lives of aged patients who would die without life-sustaining machines or—in the case of younger persons afflicted by brain damage, for example—to sustain life although the patient remains in a comatose state.

A prototype in the latter case was a 1976 Supreme Court decision that allowed the parents of New Jersey car accident victim Karen Quinlan to instruct her physician to remove life support systems so that their comatose daughter would die. At issue in this complicated case, which also rested on legal discussions of the con-

stitutional right of privacy, was the question of who should decide that inevitable natural death is preferable to prolongation of life by externally administered means. When the Court took this decision away from an appointed court guardian and gave it to those closest to the patient, the question became whose privacy was being protected. This dilemma is not unlike that inherent in the abortion debate, where the privacy of the pregnant woman is weighed against that of the as-yet-unconscious, unborn child. To whom does the physician's oath to avoid doing injury actually apply?

Legal solutions to subareas of the euthanasia debate were attained in stages, especially in cases of the very aged or patients afflicted with known terminal diseases. A living will, for example, allows individuals to instruct their physicians not to sustain their lives by artificial means if, beyond a certain point, they are unable to express their own will to die. In some cases, this discretion is assigned to the next of kin. In both cases, the objective is to remove ultimate responsibility for inevitable natural death from the physician's shoulders and to place it as closely as possible to within the private sphere of the patient.

A final area of contemporary debate over medical ethics illustrates how far conceptions of ultimate responsibility for the protection of life have gone beyond frames of reference that might have been familiar not only in Hippocrates' time but also as recently as the generation of doctors trained before the 1980's. Impressive advances in the research field of human genetics by the mid-1980's began to make it possible to predict, through analysis of deoxyribonucleic acid (DNA) structures, the likelihood that certain genetic traits (specifically debilitating chronic diseases) might be transmitted to the offspring of couples under study. Inherent in the rising debate over the ethics of such studies, which range from the prediction of reproductive combinations (genetic counseling) through actual attempts to detach and splice DNA chains (genetic engineering), was the delicate question of who, if anyone, should hold the responsibility of determining if individuals have ultimate control over their genes. In the most extreme hypothetical argument, a notion of scientific exclusion of certain gene combinations, or planning of desirable gene pools in future generations, began to appear in the 1980's and 1990's. These notions represent potential problems for medical ethics that, because of exponential changes in technological possibilities, surpass the entire realm of Hippocratic principles.

PERSPECTIVE AND PROSPECTS

Despite the introduction of certain legal precedents that tried to protect both physicians and their patients against dilemmas stemming from the assumed immutable ethical principles of the Hippocratic oath, society continues to witness practical shortcomings in modern understanding of who needs to be protected and how such protection should be institutionalized.

Malpractice insurance offers legal protection to physicians against personal damage claims levied by aggrieved patients or those surviving deceased patients; by the late twentieth century in the United States, these rates had soared. The larger debate regarding whether what physicians have done in individual cases was right or wrong rests on the assumption that his or her judgment can be put to the test by private parties defending their rights against professional incompetence. Therefore, the issue, as well as the institutional and/or legal devices pursued to resolve it, lies beyond the strict realm of a patient's privacy vis-à-vis a physician's responsibilities.

More characteristic examples of the contemporary social-ethical dilemma of whether doctors are fulfilling their appropriate professional responsibilities in recognizing patients' rights to certain types of treatment continue to fall into legally unresolved categories. The most obvious appears to be the ongoing debate concerning the legality of physician-assisted abortions. The considerations that have been introduced clearly go beyond the black-or-white principles that simple comparison with the content of the Hippocratic oath might involve. Courts and legislators involved in the ethics of abortion have had to devote extensive attention to the considerations of how pregnancies were induced (with attention to the anomalies of incest or rape, for example) or to questions of whether tax-appropriated funds gathered from an ethically divided public body can be dispensed to pay for medically approved abortions.

Still other dimensions of contemporary physician-patient relationships reveal that new forms of legislation will be needed before debates over the applicability of Hippocratic principles to modern society will recede from front-page prominence. With living wills having more or less resolved the question of individuals' right to instruct physicians or families to make decisions for them when personal capacities decline to incoherence, signs of new legal dilemmas began to emerge in the 1990's concerning fully coherent, terminally ill patients. Despairing of future suffering that can come well before any question of life support devices arises, some patients contracted their physicians— initially one physician in particular, Jack Kevorkian of Detroit, Michigan—to perform "mercy killing" by the administration of lethal poisons. Thus, one of the specific negative injunctions of the original Hippocratic oath returned the question of individual physicians' ethical and legal obligations to the forefront of public attention and court proceedings more than two millennia after its initial statement.

—*Byron D. Cannon, Ph.D.*

See also Abortion; American Medical Association (AMA); Cloning; Education, medical; Ethics; Euthanasia; Genetic engineering; Law and medicine; Malpractice.

FOR FURTHER INFORMATION:

Campbell, Alistair V., Grant Gillett, and Gareth Jones. *Medical Ethics.* 4th ed. New York: Oxford University Press, 2005. A text that takes an interdisciplinary approach in examining major ethical questions in medical practice, including issues in genetics, prenatal and neonatal care, AIDS, mental health, geriatrics, and end-of-life care.

Casarett, David J., Frona Daskal, and John Lantos. "Experts in Ethics? The Authority of the Clinical Ethicist." *The Hastings Center Report* 28, no. 6 (November/December, 1998): 6-11. This article examines the work of Jurgen Habermas, which provides a basis for a model of clinical ethics consultation in which consensus, grounded in moral theory, assumes a central theoretical role.

Devine, Richard J. *Good Care, Painful Choices: Medical Ethics of Ordinary People.* 2d ed. New York: Paulist Press, 2000. An accessible survey of medical ethics for the layperson. Covers moral concepts such as personhood and conscience, abortion, genetics, organ transplants, end-of-life issues, and social health issues, including informed consent and health care access and reform.

Fletcher, John C., et al., eds. *Introduction to Clinical Ethics.* 2d ed. Frederick, Md.: University Publishing Group, 1997. This group of essays by contributing authors addresses the topic of ethics in contemporary medicine. Includes a bibliography.

Harron, Frank. *Biomedical-Ethical Issues: A Digest of Law and Policy Development.* Binghamton, N.Y.: Vail-Ballou Press, 1983. New Haven, Conn.: Yale University Press, 1983. A collection of key contemporary documents, including court decisions, state and federal laws, and policy statements by a number of professional associations regarding the most-debated ethical issues in medicine.

Jonsen, Albert R., Mark Siegler, and William J. Winslade. *Clinical Ethics: A Practical Approach to Ethical Decisions in Clinical Medicine.* 6th ed. New York: McGraw-Hill, 2006. Discusses the whole range of medical ethics, including legal issues, confidentiality, care of the dying patient, and euthanasia and assisted suicide.

Munson, Ronald, comp. *Intervention and Reflection: Basic Issues in Medical Ethics.* 7th ed. Belmont, Calif.: Thomson/Wadsworth, 2004. An undergraduate text that combines social context, case studies, readings, and decision scenarios for topics that include abortion, advances in gene therapy, genetic discrimination, and health care rights.

Pence, Gregory. *Classic Cases in Medical Ethics: Accounts of Cases That Have Shaped Medical Ethics, with Philosophical, Legal, and Historical Backgrounds.* 4th ed. Boston: McGraw-Hill, 2004. Surveys important cases that have defined and shaped the field of medical ethics. Each case is accompanied by careful discussion of pertinent philosophical theories and legal and ethical issues.

HIRSCHSPRUNG'S DISEASE

DISEASE/DISORDER

ALSO KNOWN AS: Congenital megacolon

ANATOMY OR SYSTEM AFFECTED: Anus, intestines, nerves

SPECIALTIES AND RELATED FIELDS: Cytology, family medicine, obstetrics, pediatrics, proctology

DEFINITION: A disease of the large intestine that makes bowel movements difficult or impossible.

CAUSES AND SYMPTOMS

Hirschsprung's disease is caused when the lower part of the large intestine (colon), including the rectum, does not have the ganglion nerve cells to control the muscles that produce the contractions necessary for a bowel movement. Occasionally, the whole large intestine and even portions of the small intestine may be missing these nerve cells. The disease develops prior to birth. In the normal development of a fetus, the ganglion nerve cells grow from the top of the intestine down to the anus. For some unknown reason, the nerve cells stop growing at some distance down the intestine in children who experience Hirschsprung's disease.

> **INFORMATION ON HIRSCHSPRUNG'S DISEASE**
>
> **CAUSES:** Lack of ganglion nerve cells for muscle control in lower colon
> **SYMPTOMS:** Severe constipation, vomiting of bile, swollen abdomen, enterocolitis
> **DURATION:** Acute
> **TREATMENTS:** Surgery to remove affected area of colon

The disease manifests itself most often in young children, although it can appear when an individual is a teenager or an adult. In an individual with Hirschsprung's disease, the healthy upper portion of the colon pushes stool down until it reaches the affected part. The stool then stops. New stool backs up behind it. Severe constipation results. In some cases, the victim may not be able to have any bowel movements at all. Babies with Hirschsprung's disease often vomit up bile and experience swollen abdomens after eating. Infections, particularly enterocolitis, may develop in the intestines, which could even burst the colon.

TREATMENT AND THERAPY

Diagnosis of the disorder is confirmed by a barium enema X ray and a biopsy of the rectum. Barium makes the intestine show up better on an X ray. Manometry is also often used by the doctor to diagnose the disease. In this procedure, a small balloon is inflated inside of the rectum. If the anal muscle does not relax, the patient may have Hirschsprung's disease.

A pull-through operation removes the affected area of the intestine. The remaining ends are joined together. After this surgery, 85 to 90 percent of the patients pass feces normally, although some may experience diarrhea or constipation for a period of time. Eating high-fiber foods can help reduce diarrhea and constipation. Since the intestine is shortened by the surgery, not as much fluid is absorbed by the body. Consequently, the patient will need to drink plenty of fluids.

PERSPECTIVE AND PROSPECTS

Hirschsprung's disease occurs in approximately 1 out of every 5,000 births. About 80 percent of patients are boys. Children with Down syndrome are at a high risk for developing the disorder.

Hirschsprung's disease has been found to be hereditary, with the risk greater if the mother has the condition. Even if the parents have not had the disorder develop in their own lives, they may pass it on to their children. If one child in a family has the disease, other children are at greater risk to be born with it.

—*Alvin K. Benson, Ph.D.*

See also Constipation; Enterocolitis; Gastroenterology; Gastroenterology, pediatric; Gastrointestinal system; Genetic diseases; Intestinal disorders; Intestines; Neonatology; Peristalsis; Surgery, pediatric.

For Further Information:

Eichenwald, Heinz F., Josef Ströder, and Charles M. Ginsburg, eds. *Pediatric Therapy*. 3d ed. St. Louis: Mosby Year Book, 1993.

Holschneider, Alexander M., and Prem Puri, eds. *Hirschsprung's Disease and Allied Disorders*. 3d ed. New York: Springer, 2007.

Icon Health. *Hirschsprung's Disease: A Medical Dictionary, Bibliography, and Annotated Research Guide to Internet References*. San Diego, Calif.: Author, 2004.

Histiocytosis
Disease/disorder

Also known as: Langerhans cell histiocytosis (LCH), histiocytosis X, eosinophilic granuloma, Hand-Schüller-Christian disease, Letterer-Siwe disease

Anatomy or system affected: Blood, bones, ears, gastrointestinal system, immune system, liver, lungs, nervous system, skin, throat

Specialties and related fields: Hematology, immunology

Definition: A group of relatively rare blood disorders characterized by the abnormal accumulation of white blood cells called histiocytes, leading to a wide range of adverse bodily responses.

Causes and Symptoms

There is no clear understanding of the exact etiology of histiocytoses, blood disorders characterized by an accumulation of white blood cells called histiocytes, including monocytes and macrophages. Langerhans cell histiocytosis (LCH) is the most common type. At least four or five people per million are affected, with more males affected than females. The disorder affects both children and adults.

LCH may develop in response to underlying immunodeficiency or as a secondary effect from a viral infection. Symptoms vary based on the severity of the dis-

---

> ### Information on Histiocytosis
>
> **Causes:** Response to underlying immunodeficiency or secondary effect from viral infection
>
> **Symptoms:** Depends on severity; may include bone lesions (especially skull), rashes, respiratory problems (cough, shortness of breath), gastrointestinal problems (bleeding, elevated liver enzymes)
>
> **Duration:** Short-term or long-term
>
> **Treatments:** Depends on the severity; may include chemotherapy

---

ease, and patients may be relatively symptom-free. LCH may be localized to one area or organ, or it may be more diffuse, involving multiple organs. It can cause lesions on bone, especially skull bones, or it may manifest itself as a skin rash. Respiratory symptoms such as cough or shortness of breath may signify that LCH has affected the lungs. Gastrointestinal manifestations of the disease include bleeding within the gastrointestinal tract or elevated liver enzymes. LCH can also affect the lymph nodes or the central nervous system and may contribute to the development of diabetes insipidus, growth hormone deficiency, and hypopituitarism (underactive pituitary gland).

Definitive diagnosis requires a biopsy, and the differential diagnosis (other diseases similar to it) is broad. Making the diagnosis requires a high index of suspicion because it is rare and easily missed. Helpful radiologic tests might include a chest X ray or a skeletal survey.

Treatment and Therapy

Treatment options vary widely based on the severity of the disease. On one hand, minimal treatment may be needed for symptom-free, single-system involvement, especially as LCH affecting only one system often remits completely. On the other hand, more severe disease affecting many systems may warrant chemotherapy, with characteristic remissions and relapses.

Perspective and Prospects

The histiocytoses are classified into three types: LCH, hemophagocytic lymphohistiocytosis (HLH), and malignant histiocytosis. The impacts of LCH can be many, some with short-term and others with long-term consequences: stunted growth, dental problems, hearing loss, and hepatic fibrosis, to name a few. Though caregivers from a variety of medical specialties are often involved in caring for LCH patients and tremendous strides in diagnosis and treatment have been made, many patients still suffer from problematic, recurrent disease.

—*Leonard Berkowitz, D.O.,*
and Paul Moglia, Ph.D.

See also Blood and blood disorders; Hematology; Hematology, pediatric; Immune system; Immunology; Immunopathology.

For Further Information:

Arceci, Robert J., B. Jack Longley, and Peter D. Emanuel. "Atypical Cellular Disorders." *Hematology*, 2002, 297-314.

Egeler, R. Maarten, and Giulio J. D'Angio, eds. *Langerhans Cell Histiocytosis*. Philadelphia: W. B. Saunders, 1998.

Histiocytosis Association of America. http://www .histio.org/.

Osband, Micheal E., and Carl Pochedly, eds. *Histiocytosis-X*. Philadelphia: Saunders, 1987.

HISTOLOGY

Specialty

Anatomy or system affected: All

Specialties and related fields: Biochemistry, cytology, dermatology, hematology, internal medicine, oncology, pathology, vascular medicine

Definition: The study of the body's tissues—epithelial, connective, muscle, and nerve tissues—to find the changes in structure that can be induced by disease.

Key terms:

collagen: a fibrous protein occurring in many types of connective tissue

connective tissues: tissues containing large amounts of matrix outside the cells

epithelia: tissues that originate in broad, flat surfaces

matrix: organic or inorganic material occurring in connective tissues but located outside the cells

muscle tissues: tissues specialized in such a manner that they respond to stimulation by contracting along their long axes

nerve tissues: tissues specialized in such a manner that they respond to stimulation by conducting nerve impulses along their surfaces

tissues: groups of similar cells that are closely interrelated in function and organized together spatially

Types of Tissues

Histology is the study of tissues, which are groups of similar cells that are closely interrelated in their function and are organized together by location and structure. The four major types of tissues are epithelial tissue, connective tissue, muscle tissue, and nervous tissue.

Epithelial tissue (or epithelia) includes those tissues that originate in broad, flat surfaces. Their functions include protection, absorption, and secretion. Epithelia can be one-layered (simple) or multilayered (stratified). Their cells can be flat (squamous), tall and thin (columnar), or equal in height and width (cuboidal). Some simple epithelia have nuclei at two different levels, giving the false appearance of different layers; these tissues are called pseudostratified. Some simple squamous epithelia have special names: The inner lining of most blood vessels is called an endothelium, while the lining of a body cavity is called a mesothelium. Kidney tubules and most small ducts are also lined with simple squamous epithelia. The pigmented layer of the retina and the front surface of the lens of the eye are examples of simple cuboidal epithelia. Simple columnar epithelia form the inner lining of most digestive organs and the linings of the small bronchi and gallbladder. The epithelia lining the Fallopian tube, nasal cavity, and bronchi are ciliated, meaning that the cells have small hairlike extensions called cilia.

The outer layer of skin is a stratified squamous epithelium; other stratified squamous epithelia line the inside of the mouth, esophagus, and vagina. Sweat glands and other glands in the skin are lined with stratified cuboidal epithelia. Most of the urinary tract is lined with a special kind of stratified cuboidal epithelium called a transitional epithelium, which allows a large amount of stretching. Parts of the pharynx, larynx, urethra, and the ducts of the mammary glands are lined with stratified columnar epithelia.

Glands are composed of epithelial tissues that are highly modified for secretion. They may be either exocrine glands (in which the secretions exit by ducts that lead to targets nearby) or endocrine glands (in which the secretions are carried by the bloodstream to targets some distance away). The salivary glands in the mouth, the glandular lining of the stomach, and the sebaceous glands of the skin are exocrine glands. The thyroid gland, the adrenal gland, and the pituitary gland are endocrine glands. The pancreas has both exocrine and endocrine portions; the exocrine parts secrete digestive enzymes, while the endocrine parts, called the islets of Langerhans, secrete the hormones insulin and glucagon.

Connective tissues are tissues containing large amounts of a material called extracellular matrix, located outside the cells. The matrix may be a liquid (such as blood plasma), a solid containing fibers of collagen and related proteins, or an inorganic solid containing calcium salts (as in bone).

Blood and lymph are connective tissues with a liquid matrix (plasma) that can solidify when the blood clots. In addition to plasma, blood contains red cells (erythrocytes), white cells (leukocytes), and the tiny platelets that help to form clots. The many kinds of leukocytes include the so-called granular types (basophils, neutrophils, and eosinophils, all named according to the staining properties of their granules), the monocytes, and the several types of lymphocytes. Lymph contains lymphocytes and plasma only.

Most connective tissues have a solid matrix that includes fibrous proteins such as collagen and also elastic fibers, in some cases. If all the fibers are arranged in the same direction, as in ligaments and tendons, the tissue is called regular connective tissue. The dermis of the skin, however, is an example of an irregular connective tissue in which the fibers are arranged in all directions. Loose connective tissue and adipose (fat) tissue both have very few fibers. The simplest type of loose connective tissue, with the fewest fibers, is sometimes called areolar connective tissue. Adipose tissue is a connective tissue in which the cells are filled with fat deposits. Hemopoietic (blood-forming) tissue, which occurs in the bone marrow and the thymus, contains the immature cell types that develop into most connective tissue cells, including blood cells. Cartilage tissue matrix contains a shock-resistant complex of protein and sugarlike (polysaccharide) molecules. Cartilage cells usually become trapped in this matrix and eventually die, except for those closest to the surface. Bone tissue gains its supporting ability and strength from a matrix containing calcium salts. Its typical cells, called osteocytes, contain many long strands by means of which they exchange nutrients and waste products with other osteocytes, and ultimately with the bloodstream. Bone also contains osteoclasts, large cells responsible for bone resorption and the release of calcium into the bloodstream.

Mesenchyme is an embryonic connective tissue made of wandering amoebalike cells. During embryological development, the mesenchyme cells develop into many different cell types, including hemocyto-blasts, which give rise to most blood cells, and fibroblasts, which secrete protein fibers and then usually differentiate into other cell types.

Muscle tissues are tissues that are specially modified for contraction. When a nerve impulse is received, the overlapping fibers of the proteins actin and myosin slide against one another to produce the contraction. The three types of muscle tissue are smooth muscle, cardiac muscle, and skeletal muscle.

Smooth muscle contains cells that have tapering ends and centrally located nuclei. Muscular contractions are smooth, rhythmic, and involuntary, and they are usually not subject to fatigue. The cells are not cross-banded. Smooth muscle occurs in many digestive organs, reproductive organs, skin, and many other organs.

The term "striated muscle" is sometimes used to refer to cardiac and skeletal muscle, both of which have cylindrical fibers marked by cross-bands, which are also called cross-striations. The striations are caused by the lining up of the contractile proteins actin and myosin.

Cardiac muscle occurs only in the heart. Its cross-striated fibers branch and come together repeatedly. Contractions of these fibers are involuntary and rhythmic, and they occur without fatigue. Nuclei are located in the center of each cell; the cell boundaries are marked by dark-staining structures called intercalated disks.

Skeletal muscle occurs in the voluntary muscles of the body. Its cylindrical, cross-striated fibers contain many nuclei but no internal cell boundaries; a multinucleated fiber of this type is called a syncytium. Skeletal muscle is capable of producing rapid, forceful contractions, but it fatigues easily. Skeletal muscle tissue always attaches to connective tissue structures.

Nervous tissues contain specialized nerve cells (neurons) that respond rapidly to stimulation by conducting nerve impulses. All neurons contain RNA-rich granules, called Nissl granules, in the cytoplasm. Neurons with a single long extension of the cell body are called unipolar, those with two long extensions are called bipolar, and those with more than two long extensions are called multipolar. There are two types of extensions: Dendrites conduct impulses toward the cell body, while axons generally conduct impulses away from the cell body. Many axons are surrounded by a multilayered fatty substance called the myelin sheath, which is actually made of many layers of cell membrane wrapped around the axon.

Nervous tissues also contain several types of neuroglia, which are cells that hold nervous tissue together. Many neuroglia have processes (projections) that wrap around the neurons and help nourish them. Among the many types of neuroglia are the tiny microglia and the larger protoplasmic astrocytes, fibrous astrocytes, and oligodendroglia.

Two major tissue types make up most of the brain and spinal cord, or central nervous system. The first type, gray matter, contains the cell bodies of many neurons, along with smaller amounts of axons, dendrites, and neuroglia cells. The second type, white matter, contains mostly the axons, and sometimes also the dendrites, of neurons whose cell bodies lie elsewhere, along with the myelin sheaths that surround many of the axons. Clumps of cell bodies are called nuclei within the brain and ganglia elsewhere. Bundles of axons are called tracts within the central nervous system and nerves in the peripheral nervous system.

HISTOLOGY AS A DIAGNOSTIC TOOL

Many diseases produce changes in one or more body tissues; these changes are so characteristic that the diagnosis of a disease often depends on the microscopic observation of changes in tissues. In order for such a diagnosis to be made, the tissue must be sliced very thin on a machine called a microtome. Some tissues are sliced while frozen; others must be hardened (or "fixed") in chemical solutions. After being sliced, the tissue is usually stained with chemical dyes that make viewing easier. Some tissues are viewed under the light microscope; others are sliced even thinner for viewing by electron microscopy.

Most hospitals have a pathology department that is responsible for these operations. After the tissues are sliced and examined, the pathologist makes a report that usually includes a diagnosis of the disease shown by the tissue samples.

Many diseases result in marked changes in the tissue at the microscopic level. Adaptively altered changes, which are usually reversible, include an increase in cell size (hypertrophy), increase in cell numbers (hyperplasia), a change from one cell or tissue type to another (metaplasia), and a decrease in size by withering (atrophy). Prolonged or repeated insults to the tissue may result in altered or atypical growth patterns (dysplasia). Overwhelming or sustained injury results in irreversible changes such as tissue degeneration or death. Tissue degeneration often includes the accumulation of abnormal amounts of fatty, fibrous, or pigmented tissue. Tissue death in a body that goes on living is called necrosis, and it may be of several types. If tissue death exceeds a certain limit, then the death of the organism results. Once this occurs, the tissues usually release protein-digesting enzymes that digest their own cell contents, a process known as autolysis.

Changes to cellular organelles can often be seen with an electron microscope before they become apparent at the light microscope level. Disturbances of the cell membrane may alter the flow of fluids (especially water) and cause changes to occur in the fluid composition of the cytoplasm. Too much fluid may result in swelling and eventually in bursting of the cells; too little fluid results either in shrinkage or in the coagulation of proteins. Swelling may also be induced by the lack of oxygen flow to the mitochondria, which can also result in the deposition of fats or calcium. The increase in the water content of the cells can also cause swelling in the endoplasmic reticulum and the detachment of ribosomes from the surfaces of the rough endoplasmic reticulum. Most damaging of all are the disturbances of the lysosomes, which can release their protein-digesting enzymes and cause autolysis.

At the light microscope level, other changes that may result from disease processes include the coalescence of numerous dropletlike vacuoles into a single, large, fluid-filled space. Other changes that may indicate disease are abnormal cell shapes, changes in the proportion of blood cells, and the rupture of cell membranes or other structures. Substances that may accumulate in diseased cells include glycogen (a sugar storage product), fibrous deposits of collagen and other proteins, and mineral deposits such as calcium salts. Abnormalities of the nucleus may include nuclear fragmentation, loss of the staining properties of the nucleus, or pyknosis, a shrinkage of the nucleus that also includes the clumping of its chromosomal material.

Edema, or tissue swelling, is a condition that can easily be confirmed by microscopic examination of histological sections. The swelling is marked by an increase in the amount of extracellular fluid. In the case of pulmonary edema, the fluid stains pink and fills the usually empty lung spaces (alveoli).

A different type of change is seen in Barrett's esophagus, a condition caused by the repeated backflow (or reflux) of gastric fluids into the esophagus. The inner lining of the esophagus is usually a stratified squamous epithelium, but in Barrett's esophagus the surface cells become taller, and the lining is changed into a columnar epithelium resembling that of the stomach.

Most cancers are recognized by abnormalities of the affected tissues, usually including more cells in the process of cell division (mitosis). The most dangerous cancers are marked by large tumors with ill-defined, irregular margins. If the cancer tumor is well-defined, small, and has a smooth, circular margin, the cancer is much less of a threat.

In juvenile diabetes, histological examination of the pancreas reveals a greatly reduced number of pancreatic islets, and those that remain are smaller and more fibrous. Herpes simplex infection causes the epidermal cells of the skin to undergo a buildup of fluid and a consequent balloonlike swelling. Warts of the skin are marked by a thickening of the outermost layer (stratum corneum) of the epidermis. Pernicious anemia, or vitamin B_{12} deficiency, results in a deterioration of the glands in the stomach lining. Crohn's disease produces swelling of the affected parts of the intestine, deposition of fat and lymphoid tissue, and ultimately tissue loss and deposition of fibrous scar tissue; the affected parts typically alternate with healthy regions. Cirrhosis of the liver, which is most commonly the result of chronic alcohol abuse, proceeds through a fatty stage (marked by deposition of fatty tissue), a fibrotic stage (marked by small nodules and scars), and an end stage marked by abnormal shrinkage (atrophy) of liver tissue, scars, and larger nodules up to 1 centimeter in diameter. Emphysema, a lung disease found in many smokers, is recognizable histologically by an enlargement of the air spaces and by the presence of black, tarlike deposits within the lung tissue. Fibrocystic changes of the breast may be marked by the deposition of fibrous tissue, by increasing cell numbers, and by the enlargement of the glandular ducts.

Systemic lupus erythematosus (SLE), a connective tissue disease, often produces red skin lesions marked by degeneration and flattening of the lower layers of the epidermis, drying and flaking of the outermost layer, dilation of the blood vessels under the skin, and the leakage of red blood cells out of these vessels, adding to the red color. (The word "erythematosus" means "red.")

Muscular dystrophy has several forms; the most common form is marked in its advanced stages by enlarged muscles in which the muscle tissue is replaced by a fatty substance. Another muscular disease, myasthenia gravis, is often marked by overall enlargement of the thymus and an increase in the number of thymus cells. Myocardial infarction (heart attack), a form of heart disease marked by damage to the heart muscle, is indicated in histological section by dead, fibrous scar tissue replacing the muscle tissue in the heart wall. In patients with arteriosclerosis, the usually elastic walls of the arteries become thicker and more fibrous and rigid. Many of the same patients also suffer from atherosclerosis, a buildup of deposits on the inside of the blood vessels that partially or completely blocks the flow of blood.

In nervous tissue, damage to peripheral nerves often results in a process called chromatolysis in the cell bodies of the neurons from which these axons arise. The nuclei of these cells enlarge and are displaced to one side, while the Nissl granules disperse and the cell body as a whole undergoes swelling. Increased deposits of fibrous tissue characterize multiple sclerosis and certain other disorders of the nervous system. Some of these diseases are also marked by a degeneration of the myelin sheath around nerve fibers. In the case of a cerebrovascular stroke, impaired blood supply to the brain causes degeneration of the neuroglia, followed by general tissue death and the replacement of the neuroglia by fibrous tissue. Cranial hematoma (abnormal bleeding in any of several possible locations) results in the presence of blood clots (complete with blood cells and connective tissue fibers) in abnormal locations. Alzheimer's disease is marked by granules of a proteinlike substance called amyloid, often containing aluminum, surrounded by additional concentric layers of similar composition. Advanced stages of alcoholism are marked in brain tissue by the destruction of certain neurons and neuroglia. Poliomyelitis, or polio, is marked by the destruction of nervous tissue in the anterior horn of the spinal cord.

PERSPECTIVE AND PROSPECTS

The microscopic study of tissues began historically with Robert Hooke's *Micrographia* (1665) and the studies of Marcello Malpighi (1628-1694), but early microscopes were low in quality by today's standards. As microscopes improved, so did their use in studying tissues. During the 1830's, the Scottish botanist Robert Brown (1773-1858) discovered the cell nucleus. Soon, German biologists Matthias Jakob Schleiden (1804-1881) and Theodor Schwann (1810-1882) developed the so-called cell theory, a theory which proclaimed that all living things are constructed of cells and that all biological processes are rooted in processes occurring at the level of cells and tissues. The greatest advances in microscopic optics were made between 1870 and 1900, mostly in Germany, and the study of histology benefited greatly.

The great pathologist Rudolph Virchow (1821-1902) was the first to emphasize the structural changes in cells caused by the disease process; he showed that many diseases could be detected at the cellular level under the microscope. This claim, coupled with the enthusiasm for the cell theory, aroused great interest in the study of cells throughout Europe and later in America. Advances in tissue-staining techniques in microanatomy were made in various countries over a long period; the Czech histologist and physiologist Jan Evangelista Purkinje (1787-1869) was one of the leaders of this early period. Early in the twentieth century, histologists Santiago Ramón y Cajal (1852-1934) of Spain and Camillo Golgi (1844-1926) of Italy shared the 1906 Nobel Prize in Physiology or Medicine for their detailed work on the tissue structure of the nervous system. In the decades after World War II, the electron microscope became a standard instrument for the ultrafine study of tissue details at and even below the cellular level. Today, pathology laboratories routinely use the microscopic examination of tissues as an important tool in diagnosis.

—*Eli C. Minkoff, Ph.D.*

See also Alzheimer's disease; Arteriosclerosis; Biopsy; Bleeding; Blood and blood disorders; Bones and the skeleton; Cells; Cirrhosis; Crohn's disease; Cytology; Dermatology; Emphysema; Glands; Herpes; Lymphatic system; Multiple sclerosis; Muscles; Muscular dystrophy; Nervous system; Neurology; Orthopedics; Pathology; Poliomyelitis; Skin; Strokes; Systemic lupus erythematosus (SLE).

FOR FURTHER INFORMATION:

Fawcett, D. W. *A Textbook of Histology*. 12th ed. New York: Chapman & Hall, 1994. A classic standard, well illustrated with a variety of light micrographs (often in color) and electron micrographs. Most thorough in its descriptions of physiological functions.

Junqueira, Luiz Carlos, and José Carneiro. *Basic Histology: Text and Atlas*. 11th ed. New York: McGraw-Hill, 2005. A leading text that describes the structure and function of cells and the function and specialization of the four tissue groups: epithelial, connective, adipose, and nerve. Also includes chapters on the cytoplasm and cell nucleus that review recent discoveries in cell biology.

Kerr, Jeffrey B. *Atlas of Functional Histology*. St. Louis: Mosby, 1999. This volume includes discussion of histology as it applies to the major biological systems, such as the endocrine, respiratory, reproductive, gastrointestinal, nervous, and circulatory systems.

Kessel, Richard G. *Basic Medical Histology: The Biology of Cells, Tissues, and Organs*. New York: Oxford University Press, 1998. This textbook is derived from Kessel's notes, figures, and references accumulated over thirty-five years of teaching histology at the University of Iowa. Suitable for advanced undergraduate students in biology or possibly first-year medical students.

Lewin, Benjamin. *Genes IX*. 9th rev. ed. Sudbury, Mass.: Jones & Bartlett, 2007. A college textbook that discusses the entire field of molecular biology and genetics, with many references to the structure and activity of the cell nucleus. Although written at the college level, it is readable and accessible to a general audience. Many highly informative illustrations and diagrams are included.

Ross, Michael H., and Wojciech Pawlina. *Histology: A Text and Atlas*. 5th ed. Baltimore: Lippincott Williams & Wilkins, 2006. Introductory text on histology that covers vast array of topics, including methods, the cell, the classification of tissues, epithelial tissue, connective tissue, cartilage, bone, blood, muscle, nerves, cardiovascular tissue, lymphatic tissue, and the esophagus and gastrointestinal tract.

HIV. *See* HUMAN IMMUNODEFICIENCY VIRUS (HIV).

HIVES

DISEASE/DISORDER

ALSO KNOWN AS: Urticaria

ANATOMY OR SYSTEM AFFECTED: Immune system, skin

SPECIALTIES AND RELATED FIELDS: Dermatology, family medicine, immunology, internal medicine, pediatrics

DEFINITION: Pink swellings called wheals that may occur in groups on any part of the skin.

CAUSES AND SYMPTOMS

Hives are produced by blood plasma leaking through tiny gaps between the cells lining small vessels in the skin. A natural chemical called histamine is released from mast cells, which lie along the blood vessels in the skin. Allergic reactions, foods, drugs, or other chemicals can cause histamine release.

INFORMATION ON HIVES

CAUSES: Allergic reactions, foods, drugs, environmental toxins, infections, insect bites, internal diseases, physical stimuli (*e.g.*, heat, cold)
SYMPTOMS: Inflammation, itchiness
DURATION: Acute or chronic
TREATMENTS: Antihistamines

Hives can vary in size from as small as a pencil eraser to as large as a dinner plate, and they may join together to form larger swellings. When hives are forming, they are usually very itchy; they may also burn or sting. Nearly 20 percent of the general population will have at least one episode of hives in their lifetime. Acute hives may last for a few days to weeks. If they last for more than six weeks, they are called chronic hives.

The most common causes of acute hives are foods, drugs, infections, insect bites, and internal diseases. Other causes are physical stimuli, including pressure, cold, and sunlight.

TREATMENT AND THERAPY

The best treatment for hives is to find the cause and then eliminate it. Unfortunately, this is not always an easy task. Even if a cause cannot be found, antihistamines are usually prescribed to provide some relief. Antihistamines work best if taken on a regular schedule. It may be necessary to try more than one or use different combinations of antihistamines to find out what works best. In severe cases of hives, an injection of epinephrine (adrenalin) or a cortisone preparation can bring dramatic relief.

PERSPECTIVE AND PROSPECTS

In 1927, Sir Thomas Lewis reported the association between wheals and small blood vessel dilation, which later confirmed the importance of histamine as a cause of hives. Years of research showed that apart from allergy, nonimmunological stimuli can cause hives as well. A recent report that some patients with chronic hives may have formed antibodies against the immunoglobulin IgE receptor suggests that the cause of hives could be multifactorial.

—*Shih-Wen Huang, M.D.*
See also Allergies; Antihistamines; Bites and stings; Dermatology, pediatric; Immune system; Itching; Over-the-counter medications; Rashes; Skin; Skin disorders.

FOR FURTHER INFORMATION:

Adelman, Daniel C., et al., eds. *Manual of Allergy and Immunology.* 4th ed. Philadelphia: Lippincott Williams & Wilkins, 2002.

Delves, Peter J., et al. *Roitt's Essential Immunology.* 11th ed. Malden, Mass.: Blackwell, 2006.

Joneja, Janice M. V., and Leonard Bielory. *Understanding Allergy, Sensitivity, and Immunity.* New Brunswick, N.J.: Rutgers University Press, 1990.

Kindt, Thomas J., Richard A. Goldsby, and Barbara A. Osborne. *Kuby Immunology.* 6th ed. New York: W. H. Freeman, 2007.

Middlemiss, Prisca. *What's That Rash? How to Identify and Treat Childhood Rashes.* London: Hamlyn, 2002.

Young, Stuart, Bruce Dobozin, and Margaret Miner. *Allergies.* Rev. ed. New York: Plume, 1999.

HODGKIN'S DISEASE
DISEASE/DISORDER

ANATOMY OR SYSTEM AFFECTED: Lymphatic system
SPECIALTIES AND RELATED FIELDS: Hematology, internal medicine, oncology, serology
DEFINITION: A neoplastic disorder originating in the tissues of the lymphatic system, recognized by distinctive histologic changes and defined by the presence of Reed-Sternberg cells.

KEY TERMS:

chemotherapy: a modality of cancer treatment consisting of the administration of cytotoxic drugs

combination chemotherapy: the use of multiple chemical agents in the treatment of cancer, each in a lower dosage so that the overall toxicity, but not the effectiveness, is reduced

neoplastic: pertaining to cancerous growths

prognosis: a prediction of the outcome of treatment for a disease on the basis of clinical and pathologic parameters, such as pathology, clinical stage, and presence or absence of symptoms such as fever, night sweats, and unexplained weight loss

radiotherapy: the use of radiation to kill cancer cells or shrink cancerous growth; when high and full doses of radiation (measured in units called rads) are used, the patient is said to be given a "megavoltage"

CAUSES AND SYMPTOMS

Malignant lymphomas are neoplasms of lymphoid tissues and are of two general categories: those related to Hodgkin's disease and others that are collectively called non-Hodgkin's lymphomas. The lymphoid tissues represent the structural expressions of the immune system, which defends the body against microbes. This system is widely spread throughout the body, is highly complex, and interacts closely with other physiologic systems of the body—especially the mucosa that lines the airways and digestive tract, where there is direct exposure to environmental microbes and other foreign substances. The components of this system are aggregations of lymphocytes in the mucosal linings (such as tonsils and adenoids), lymph nodes, and the spleen. The components of the lymphatic system connect with one another via small lymphatic vessels. The lymph nodes, which are situated in anatomical regions all over the body, interconnect and drain centrally toward the great veins of the body. The cellular components of the immune system are the lymphocytes, also called immunocytes. These account for about 20 percent of blood cells; lymphocytes make up the bulk of the lymphoid tissue that makes up the lymphatic system. The blood cells have a finite life and are disposed of in the spleen, which is the largest lymphoid organ in the body.

There are two major functional immunologic classes of lymphocytes and several other subclasses. Nevertheless, all share similar morphologic appearance, being small round cells almost completely occupied by a round nucleus. The B lymphocyte (the B refers to its bone marrow derivation) can, under proper antigenic stimulation, transform and mature into a plasma cell, which is the cell in charge of producing antibodies. Antibodies are the protein products of the immune system that act by capturing and removing foreign substances, called antigens. The other major class of lymphocytes is the T lymphocyte (the T refers to its thymus derivation). T lymphocytes are of at least two major functional subclasses, which either help or suppress the B lymphocytes in their transformation into plasma cells; thus they are termed helper and suppressor T

cells, respectively. Other cellular components of the immune system, cellular monocytes and macrophages, play an important role in carrying and transferring specific immunologic information between the various cellular components of the immune-lymphatic system. This, then, is a highly organized and complex system, with positive and negative biofeedback that maintains optimal, balanced proportions of all the cellular components that make up the system.

Hodgkin's disease is a neoplasm of the lymphoid tissues that usually arises in lymph nodes, often in the neck, and has a varied histologic appearance characterized by the presence of Reed-Sternberg cells. The Reed-Sternberg cell is a giant cell having two nuclei that are situated in a mirror-image fashion. Treatment and prognosis in Hodgkin's disease are determined by two parameters: the histopathologic classification, whereby the morphologic appearance is evaluated by the pathologist, and the clinical staging classification, whereby the extent of spread of the disease and its localization are determined by clinical studies. The pathology is studied by reviewing thinly cut sections of diseased lymph nodes removed from the patient. This study is most important for establishing a diagnosis of Hodgkin's disease and ruling out other conditions that may closely simulate its clinical and/or pathologic features. At times, peer consultations are used to confirm the diagnosis.

Reed-Sternberg cells have a characteristic appearance and must be identified to make a diagnosis of Hodgkin's disease. The pathologic classification of this disease, based on microscopic study, recognizes four different types, each with its own clinical implications regarding survival and prognosis. The classification is based on the relative dominance of lymphocytes when compared to the number of the neoplastic Reed-Sternberg cells. In the most favorable type, the lymphocytes predominate and Reed-Sternberg cells are sparse; this type is called lymphocyte predominance. In the worst type, the lymphocytes are very sparse and there are many more Reed-Sternberg cells and their variants; this type is called lymphocyte depletion. In between these two extremes are the mixed-cellularity type, in which there is an even mixture of lymphocytes and Reed-Sternberg cells, and nodular sclerosis, which forms nodules of fibrous scar tissue that surround the mixture of lymphocytes and Reed-Sternberg cells.

This classification has important prognostic implications. It correctly presumes that the neoplastic cells are the Reed-Sternberg cells and their variants, and that the lymphocytes are induced by the immune system to multiply and to fight the spread of the neoplastic cells. It follows that the more the process is successful, the better is the prognosis. Hence lymphocyte predominance carries a more favorable outlook than lymphocyte depletion, with mixed-cellularity types somewhere in between. Nodular sclerosis also carries a good prognosis. Other inflammatory cells are invariably mixed with the lymphocytes and Reed-Sternberg cells; these cells are also part of the body's immune response against cancer cells.

The clinical staging classification of Hodgkin's disease was formulated by a group of experts who met at a workshop in Ann Arbor, Michigan, in 1971. It is based on the proposition that the disease begins in a single group of lymph nodes (usually in the neck) and then spreads to the next adjacent group of lymph nodes, on the same side, before it crosses over to the other side of the body. The disease then advances farther across the diaphragm muscle, which separates the thorax from the abdominal cavity, and finally disseminates into the blood to involve the bone marrow and other distant sites. In this schema, stage I represents early stage, with involvement of only a single lymph node region, and stage II is the condition in which two or more such regions are involved on the same side of the diaphragm (that is, either above or below the diaphragm).

In the United States, Hodgkin's disease is an uncommon neoplasm accounting for an estimated 7,600 cases, or fewer than 1 percent of all new cases of cancer, a year. In 2002, the disease resulted in approximately 1,300 deaths according to American Cancer Society statistics. The incidence in the United States is slightly higher in males than females, and in whites than blacks. Incidence trends show a mild rise for the nodular sclerosis type in young adults and a mild decrease of Hodgkin's disease over the age of forty.

Hodgkin's disease can occur at any age, although the highest peak incidence occurs in adolescents and young adults, and smaller peaks occur in the fifth and sixth decades of life. Most patients come to clinical attention because of painless, nontender, enlarged lymph nodes in the neck or armpits (above the diaphragm) or, less commonly, in the groin. In the young adult or adolescent, a mass in the chest may press against the airways to produce a dry, hacking cough and shortness of breath, which may be the patient's first symptoms. Some patients may have anemia or severe itching. At times, especially when the disease is aggressive and extensive, the patient may have a fever, which may run

for a few days and then disappear, only to recur after a week or two; there can also be night sweats and weight loss. These symptoms—fever, night sweats, and weight loss—indicate a less favorable prognosis. Younger patients and those with lymphocyte predominance and nodular sclerosis histologic types (favorable histologic types) tend to have limited disease—that is, stages I and II—found primarily above the diaphragm. Older patients and those with mixed-cellularity or lymphocyte depletion types are more likely to have extensive disease involving lymph nodes on both sides of the diaphragm (stage III) or even involving the liver, spleen, and bone marrow (stage IV).

When a patient with persistent lymph node enlargement seeks medical attention, a lymph node biopsy is usually made to make sure of the diagnosis. Other cancers that may simulate Hodgkin's disease must be excluded, as well as a long list of benign conditions such as infectious mononucleosis and tuberculosis. A series of blood tests, X-ray and other imaging studies, and a bone marrow biopsy are done in order to evaluate the spread of disease and to assign the proper clinical stage. At times, even surgical exploration of the abdomen, with biopsies of abdominal lymph nodes, the liver, and the spleen, is done to assign an accurate stage of Hodgkin's disease; this procedure is called staging laparotomy.

TREATMENT AND THERAPY

Modern cancer therapy has achieved its greatest triumph in the treatment of Hodgkin's disease. The advent of a generally acceptable histopathologic classification, accurate staging, improved radiotherapy, effective chemotherapy, and supportive care, such as antibiotics and the transfusion of platelets, have contributed to the impressive 80 percent overall cure rate. The therapy is enhanced by an effective teamwork of medical experts in oncology, radiation therapy, surgery, pathology, and diagnostic radiology.

Because Hodgkin's disease spreads in an orderly fashion through adjacent lymph node groups, effective high-dose radiation can be directed at affected lymph nodes and at their neighboring, uninvolved nodes. Irradiation, with a full dose of 3,500 to 4,000 rads in three to four weeks, can eradicate Hodgkin's disease in involved nodes within the treatment field more than 95 percent of the time. In addition, extended-field irradiation of the adjacent uninvolved nodes is a standard practice used to eradicate minimal or early disease in these lymph nodes.

Stages I and II can be treated with radiotherapy alone by an extended field to include all areas above the diaphragm bearing lymph nodes (the axilla, neck, and chest), and in most cases the lymph nodes in the abdomen. Such treatment cures about 90 percent of patients. For patients in which the disease is found extensively in the chest, chemotherapy is added to the radiotherapy and results in prolonged, relapse-free survival in 85 percent of patients.

A variety of cytotoxic drugs (those that kill cells) are available to treat Hodgkin's disease. Such drugs are similar to nitrogen mustard (which was once used in war) and are toxic to the body. It has been found that when more than one drug is used, each in a smaller dose, the toxicity can be reduced without diminishing effectiveness. Thus combination chemotherapy has evolved. There are many effective regimens of combination chemotherapy that are called by the initials of the individual components; the most widely used is MOPP (mechlorethamine, Oncovin, procarbazine, and prednisone). In stage III, chemotherapy with or without radiotherapy is used, depending upon specific variations within the stage, with cure rates achieved in 75 to 80 percent of patients. Even in stage IV disease, combination chemotherapy (particularly with MOPP) has produced a complete remission in about 75 percent of patients, with a cure rate of more than 50 percent.

Bone marrow transplantation, which is the intravenous infusion of normal marrow cells into the patient shortly after treatment in order to protect the patient from toxicity, has permitted the use of much higher doses of certain drugs. It allows the therapist to irradiate all the patient's bone marrow, eradicating both "good" and "bad" cells, with the hope that the normal marrow cells that are infused will populate the bone marrow and grow there. Bone marrow transplantation has been successfully used mainly in young patients who were resistent to conventional chemotherapy.

PERSPECTIVE AND PROSPECTS

Thomas Hodgkin of Guy's Hospital in London was the first to recognize the disease that would bear his name. In 1832, he described the gross autopsy findings and clinical features of seven patients who had simultaneous enlargement of grossly diseased lymph nodes and spleens, and he considered the condition to be a primary affliction of these organs. This condition, he himself records, was vaguely outlined by Marcello Malpighi in 1665. Four years earlier than Hodgkin, David Craige had described the autopsy findings of a simi-

lar case. Subsequent histologic examination of tissues from Hodgkin's original cases confirmed the disease in three of them. In 1865, Sir Samuel Wilks elaborated on the autopsy studies of similar cases and published the findings on fifteen patients, calling the condition Hodgkin's disease.

Important histopathologic observations were contributed by William Greenfield in 1878 and E. Goldman in 1892. George Sternberg described the giant cells but believed the condition to be a peculiar form of tuberculosis. The recognition that these cells were an integral part of the disease awaited the careful pathologic observation of Dorothy Reed of The Johns Hopkins Hospital in Baltimore. These cells, appropriately named Reed-Sternberg cells, are the hallmark of Hodgkin's disease.

Controversy as to the nature of this disease led early investigators to study infectious agents as possible etiologic causes, especially the tuberculosis bacillus, but to no avail. More recent studies have examined the roles of other viral infectious agents, especially the agent of infectious mononucleosis, but with no consistent results. At present, the condition is accepted as neoplastic, probably triggered by some unknown environmental agent or agents.

Between 1930 and 1950, major advances included the recognition of meaningful histologic subtypes of Hodgkin's disease correlating with prognosis, and the development by Vera Peters of a clinical staging system. Impressive responses to X-ray therapy were reported at the beginning of the twentieth century, and treatment with megavoltage therapy was further developed. By World War II, it became realistic to speak of curing some patients with early Hodgkin's disease. The potential for a cure meant that accurate histologic diagnosis and estimation of the extent and localization of disease were imperative in planning treatment; a multidisciplinary approach to diagnosis and treatment was developed. Modern concepts of histologic classification became codified at a conference held in Rye, New York, in 1965, and the clinical staging system was refined into its present form at a workshop held at Ann Arbor, Michigan, in 1971.

Modern effective chemotherapy was developed concurrently with these advances in classification, staging, and radiotherapy. The alkylating agents, created as an outgrowth of studies on nitrogen mustard gas during World War II, provided the first drugs to produce impressive shrinkage of the tumor and significant palliation of the disease. The subsequent developments in modern pharmacology and therapeutics enabled Vince DeVita and his coworkers, in 1970, to design the first effective combination chemotherapy regimen, MOPP.

Today, many more such regimens are being tested; the possibility for cure has become a realistic hope for every patient with Hodgkin's disease. This is the case because of the refinement of ancillary therapies with antibiotics (for infections that may occur during the necessary phases of suppression of the immune system by these powerful toxic drugs) and platelet transfusion technology. Bone marrow transplantation technology also offers strong hope of curing patients with advanced cases who are resistant. The bone marrow is harvested and then reintroduced into a patient whose marrow has been effectively disabled. Immunotherapy is also being investigated. It can boost the patient's ability to combat disease by modulating the body's responses. The drawback to aggressive combinations of chemotherapy and radiotherapy, however, is the emergence of therapy-related leukemia and leukemia-like malignancies several years after the completion of successful therapy for Hodgkin's disease.

—*Victor H. Nassar, M.D.*

See also Bone marrow transplantation; Cancer; Chemotherapy; Lymphadenopathy and lymphoma; Lymphatic system; Malignancy and metastasis; Oncology; Radiation therapy.

FOR FURTHER INFORMATION:

CA: A Cancer Journal for Clinicians 43, no. 1. January/February, 1993. A journal published by the American Cancer Society. This special issue is devoted to a discussion of cancer statistics, including those regarding Hodgkin's disease.

Dollinger, Malin, et al. *Everyone's Guide to Cancer Therapy.* 4th ed. Kansas City, Mo.: Andrews McMeel, 2002. An excellent source of medical information about cancer, written for the general public. A helpful glossary of medical terminology is provided.

Eyre, Harmon J., Dianne Partie Lange, and Lois B. Morris. *Informed Decisions: The Complete Book of Cancer Diagnosis, Treatment, and Recovery.* 2d ed. Atlanta: American Cancer Society, 2002. This text from the American Cancer Society is intended for the layperson. It is exemplary in its discussion of cancer.

Greer, John, et al., eds. *Wintrobe's Clinical Hematology.* 11th ed. Philadelphia: Lippincott Williams & Wilkins, 2004. A textbook of hematologic disorders,

with an excellent review of Hodgkin's disease. Written for clinicians and students of medicine.

Lichtman, Marshall A., et al., eds. *Williams Hematology.* 7th ed. New York: McGraw-Hill, 2006. An up-to-date textbook that offers an authoritative review of all aspects of Hodgkin's disease.

Lymphoma Information Network. http://www.lymphomainfo.net/hodgkins/. Offers information on the diagnosis and treatment options for adult and childhood Hodgkin's disease and resources for further research.

Parker, James N., and Philip M. Parker, eds. *The Official Parent's Sourcebook on Childhood Hodgkin's Disease.* San Diego, Calif.: Icon Health, 2002. Draws from public, academic, government, and peer-reviewed research to provide a wide-ranging handbook for families of children with Hodgkin's disease.

_____. *Official Patient's Sourcebook on Adult Hodgkin's Disease.* San Diego, Calif.: Icon Health, 2002. Draws from public, academic, government, and peer-reviewed research to provide a wide-ranging handbook for adult patients with Hodgkin's disease.

Williams, Stephanie F., Ramez Farah, and Harvey M. Golomb, eds. *Hodgkin's Disease.* Philadelphia: W. B. Saunders, 1989. A volume in the series Hematology/Oncology Clinics of North America. A thorough review of this disease—its diagnosis, pathology, and treatment. Includes bibliographical references and an index.

HOLISTIC MEDICINE

SPECIALTY

ANATOMY OR SYSTEM AFFECTED: All

SPECIALTIES AND RELATED FIELDS: Alternative medicine, environmental health, nursing, osteopathic medicine, preventive medicine, psychology

DEFINITION: The practice of medicine to maintain both physical and psychological health as a natural deterrent to disease and as a way of realizing one's highest potential.

KEY TERMS:

hospice care: an alternative to hospitalization for the terminally ill or aged that allows for the dignified acceptance of impending death

stress management: the alleviation of stress, a form of preventive medicine borrowed from holistic approaches to common emotional disorders

SCIENCE AND PROFESSION

Although the phenomenon of holistic medicine gained increased attention in the latter half of the twentieth century, most of the principles associated with it have appeared in various forms and in various cultures over the centuries. Ironically, it may have been the progress of medical science generally and the widespread use by doctors of new drugs to treat disease that sparked what some would call holistic medicine's call for a return to basics. For example, some proponents of holism oppose automatic reliance on surgical methods of treating some ailments for not recognizing either their causes or more beneficial modes of treatment. In addition, holists oppose a reliance on drugs not only because they hold certain maladies to be curable (or indeed totally avoidable) without them but also because of possible negative side effects.

A number of quite sophisticated principles could fall under the presumed "basics" of the holistic approach to health. Primary among these is a conviction that—short of obvious conditions involving attacks by virus, bacteria, or chronic debilitation of certain organs of the body, including the nervous system—increased awareness of the nature of bodily functions can help maintain a healthy level of balance within the total organism. Essential to the principle of balance is recognition of the importance of the mind in influencing one's reactions, both psychological and physical, to circumstances in the surrounding environment. Some holists adhere to the Abraham Maslow school of psychology, which places strong emphasis on questions of drive toward "need fulfillment" in both the physical and psychological domains. Certain bodily states can easily be linked to biologically stimulated drives, including hunger and sexuality. Less apparent psychological drives, however, may also trigger physical reactions. Imbalances in fulfilling the natural drives for love or success are held responsible for many forms of physical disorder that could be averted, such as anorexia nervosa, ulcers, and stress.

Several approaches to holistic medicine consider the end goal of good physical health to be not only the avoidance of disease but also the realization of a positive, life-enhancing experience. In some cases, the inspiration for such theories comes from long traditions in Asian philosophies and religions that assume close links between the psychic and the physical realms of life. An assumption that may or may not be shared between such philosophies and holists is that a "true" state of health leads to superior levels of awareness in both spheres.

Physicians interested in holistic medicine need not, however, be tied solely to disease-specific or "consciousness-heightening" aspects of what can be a very general field. Some specialists in geriatrics, for example, adopt holistic approaches to counseling the elderly about natural stages of aging, preparing them to accept, with a minimum of anxiety, the gradual decline that accompanies the end of life. Growing emphasis on hospice care for the terminally ill or aged, as opposed to hospitalization, is connected with this aspect of holistic medicine.

DIAGNOSTIC AND TREATMENT TECHNIQUES

Although individual physicians may espouse holistic approaches, many persons without formal medical training choose to practice it themselves to maintain their bodies and minds in the healthiest state possible. Such practices may be individual and personal, ranging from exercise and dietary habits to meditation. They may also involve group associations supported by the participation of trained physicians or laypersons. It has become possible to find method-specific holistic centers specializing in a range of techniques. These range from, for example, very general holistic health and nutrition institutes to highly specialized centers that strive to treat those suffering from chronic pain through localized electrical nerve stimulation.

Essential to almost all holistic approaches to treatment is an emphasis on the physician's role as a facilitator—someone who is able to help the patient recognize what he or she should do to adopt various attitudes and actions that can alleviate all or part of the observed disorder. In this connection, a number of general practitioners maintain auxiliary personnel to provide various therapies (massages, controlled breathing, and so on) to supplement, or sometimes to replace, such standard treatments as drug prescriptions or minor surgery.

PERSPECTIVE AND PROSPECTS

It was the South African political figure Jan Smuts who, in 1926, first used the specific word "holism" to describe, not holistic medicine per se, but the philosophical principle which holds that whole systems (and therefore whole organisms) involve entities that are greater than, and different from, the sum of their component parts. In medicine, the idea that external factors intervene to affect the way that an organism functions is almost as old as medicine itself. Hippocrates, for example, is known to have been concerned about environmental causes for certain disorders and to have included emotional and nutritional considerations in diagnosing patients.

Two aspects of holistic approaches to health and daily life in the postindustrial world are likely to increase in importance in coming generations: concern over improving dietary habits and exercise patterns. The discovery of the possible long-term harm that can come from poorly balanced diets (particularly those with a high fat content or excessive chemical additives) has made such specialized practices of holists as vegetarianism and fasting more familiar and at least partly attractive to the wider public. Likewise, the holistic emphasis on regular physical exercise for people of all ages has increasingly become part of many general practitioners' standard advice to their patients.

—*Byron D. Cannon, Ph.D.*

See also Aging; Aging: Extended care; Alternative medicine; Death and dying; Environmental diseases; Environmental health; Exercise physiology; Family medicine; Meditation; Nutrition; Osteopathic medicine; Preventive medicine; Psychiatry; Psychiatry, child and adolescent; Psychiatry, geriatric; Telemedicine; Terminally ill: Extended care.

FOR FURTHER INFORMATION:

American Holistic Health Association. http://www .ahha.org/. A Web site dedicated to honoring the whole person and encouraging people to actively participate in their own health and health care.

Kemper, Kathi J. *The Holistic Pediatrician: A Pediatrician's Comprehensive Guide to Safe and Effective Therapies for the Twenty-five Most Common Ailments of Infants, Children, and Adolescents.* New York: HarperCollins, 2002. Integrates mainstream and alternative medicine to aid parents in dealing with the most common childhood health problems such as fever, diaper rash, ear infections, and allergies.

Nordenfelt, Lennart. *On the Nature of Health.* Rev. 2d ed. Boston: Kluwer, 1995. Deals with the relationship between good health and the welfare of individuals and society as they interact.

Pelletier, Kenneth R. *The Best Alternative Medicine.* New York: Fireside, 2002. Surveys alternative therapies such as homeopathy, Western herbal medicine, traditional Chinese medicine, acupuncture, and naturopathy and provides definitions, background, and examples of specific treatments.

_____. *Holistic Medicine: From Stress to Optimum Health.* New York: Delacorte Press, 1979. A general text that seeks to strengthen the public image of holistic medicine, both for the prevention and for the treatment of disease, while discounting some popular myths.

Salmon, J. Warren, ed. *Alternative Medicines: Popular and Policy Perspectives.* New York: Tavistock, 1984. Offers comparative views of Western and Chinese approaches to holistic medicine but also includes other, less widely recognized alternatives, ranging from chiropractic to psychic healing.

Trivieri, Larry, Jr., and John W. Anderson, eds. *Alternative Medicine: The Definitive Guide.* 2d ed. Berkeley, Calif.: Ten Speed Press, 2002. An encyclopedic volume with contributions from four hundred alternative physicians who review safe, affordable, and effective remedies for more than two hundred medical conditions.

Woodham, Anne, and David Peters. *The Encyclopedia of Healing Therapies.* New York: DK, 1997. This book explains holistic and complementary medicine and offers a guide to well-being. Also contains information on finding practitioners, a directory of associations, a glossary, and a bibliography.

HOMEOPATHY

SPECIALTY

ANATOMY OR SYSTEM AFFECTED: All

SPECIALTIES AND RELATED FIELDS: Immunology, pathology, pharmacology

DEFINITION: A system of medicine based on the principle that an ill patient can be provided effective and nontoxic treatment through the use of weak or very small doses of a substance that would cause similar symptoms in a healthy individual.

KEY TERMS:

antidote: anything that counteracts the effect of a substance, such as a homeopathic remedy

Materia Medica: the homeopathic pharmacopoeia, a list of remedies with their associated symptoms and uses

potency: the strength of a homeopathic remedy, according to the number of times it has been diluted and succussed

proving: the testing of a substance or remedy on healthy volunteers (provers), who take repeated doses and record in detail any symptoms produced by it

Repertory: an index of symptoms, each heading listing the drugs known to cause the symptom *succussion:* violent shaking at each stage of dilution in the preparation of a remedy

tincture: a remedy in liquid form, normally with alcohol and water as a solvent; the most concentrated form is called the mother tincture, from which all dilutions are made

SCIENCE AND PROFESSION

In conventional medicine, diseases, or changes from the normal physiological state, are diagnosed on the basis of symptoms and physical signs. This enables the physician to find a cause for which there is a specific treatment, or to treat the patient's symptoms. There are few treatments, however, that cure the patient as a whole. Sometimes, symptoms are assumed to be the disease, and the method of action is to try to fix the symptoms and not the disease. Suppressing or removing symptoms does not necessarily constitute a cure. Curing patients means restoring them to a sense of well-being that is physical, emotional, and mental. Homeopathic medicine is a form of treatment that studies the person as a whole, with particular interest in the patient as an individual. Homeopathy is a therapeutic method that consists of prescribing for a patient weak or infinitestimal doses of a substance which, when administered to a healthy person, causes symptoms similar to those exhibited by the ill patient. Homeopathic remedies stimulate the defense mechanisms of the body, causing them to work more effectively and making them capable of curing the individual. While controversial and not accepted by most physicians, homeopathy is not intended to substitute for conventional medicine. Rather, it is a system of therapeutics which is meant to enlarge and broaden the physician's outlook, and in some cases, it might bring about a cure not possible with the usual drugs.

The word "homeopathy" is derived from the Greek words *homoios,* meaning "like" or "similar," and *pathos,* meaning "suffering." A symptom is defined as the changes felt by the patient or observed by another individual that may be associated with a particular disease. When a homeopathic drug or remedy is administered in repeated doses to a group of healthy persons, certain symptoms and signs of toxicity are produced. These symptoms are carefully annotated in what is called the proving of a remedy. In some cases, there are accidental provings—cases in which the symptoms produced by a drug in a healthy person are observed because of an accident, such as being bitten by a snake. Other sources for the proving of a remedy are the cases in which, after

Homeopathy

The principle underlying homeopathy is that taking small amounts of a substance that normally produces a certain symptom will stimulate the immune system to counteract that very symptom. For example, a patient suffering from diarrhea may be given an infinitesimally small dose of a laxative which has been ground into a fine powder with a mortar and pestle.

a remedy has been successfully prescribed, symptoms cured by it that were not present in the provings are noted. Some of these symptoms are common to many drugs, and a few are characteristic of particular ones. It is then possible to build a symptom-complex picture which is unique to each drug or remedy. In many cases, when the symptom-complex presented by the patient is compared to the symptom-complex produced by a certain remedy, there will be a resemblance—often a close one—between the patient's symptom picture and the effects of a given drug on healthy persons.

The first and fundamental principle of homeopathy is the selection and use of the similar remedy, based on the patient's symptoms and characteristics and the drug's toxicology and provings. A second principle is the use of remedies in extremely small quantities. The most successful remedy for any given occasion will be the one whose symptomatology presents the clearest and closest resemblance to the symptom-complex of the sick person in question. This concept is formally presented as the Law of Similars, which expresses the similarity between the toxicological action of a substance and its therapeutic action; in other words, the same things that cause the disease can cure it. For example, the effects of peeling an onion are very similar to the symptoms of acute coryza (the common cold). The remedy prepared from *Allium cepa* (red onion) is used to treat the type of cold in which the symptoms resemble those caused by peeling onions. In the same way, the herb white hellebore, which toxicologically produces cholera-like diarrhea, is used to treat cholera.

The homeopathic principle is being applied whenever a sick person is treated using a method or drug that can cause similar symptoms in healthy persons. For example, conventional medicine uses radiation therapy, which causes cancer, to treat this disease. Orthodox medicine, however, does not follow other fundamental principles of homeopathy, such as the use of infinitesimal doses.

Homeopathy stimulates the defense mechanism to make it work more effectively and works on the concept of healing instead of simply treating a disease, combating illness, or suppressing symptoms. Individualization plays a crucial role in homeopathic treatment. Even when two individuals have the same ailment, their symptoms can be different. Remedies are therefore selected on an individual basis, depending on the specific, complete symptom picture of the individual. Homeopathic physicians must develop a different approach to their patients, which involves a diagnosis as well as a study of the whole individual. The way in which some homeopathic remedies work is still unknown, but the persistence of homeopathy since the mid-nineteenth century would seem to suggest its effectiveness in helping sick people.

Some conditions do not respond well to homeopathy, such as those requiring surgery, immediately life-threatening situations such as severe asthma attacks, or situations for which an improvement requires a change in diet (such as iron deficiency) or reduced exposure to environmental stress (a change in lifestyle). Nevertheless, homeopathy appears to help in these cases. For example, it can be useful for faster, complete healing after surgery or after the necessary change in lifestyle has been made. In the United States, both the Food and Drug Administration (FDA) and traditional homeopaths have been concerned about the use of homeopathic remedies to treat serious problems, such as cancer, and their use by unlicensed practitioners. In some cases, the ability to prescribe homeopathic remedies has been restricted to osteopaths, naturopaths, and medical doctors. In some cases, homeopathy does not work; the reason is unknown.

Individuals who have benefited from these remedies may not care whether homeopathy can be scientifically explained or whether research has proven its effectiveness. Nevertheless, some facts suggest that homeopathic medicines are not placebos and that the infinitesimal doses produce true biological action. For example, homeopathic medicines work on animals and are also commonly and successfully used on infants; it is doubtful that psychological suggestion can explain their success in these cases. Moreover, homeopathic microdoses have the capacity to cause symptoms in healthy individuals, and the experience of what is called a healing crisis—temporary exacerbation of symptoms that is sometimes observed during the healing process—cannot be produced by placebos or psychological suggestion. The major drawback to most homeopathic research, however, is that it is rarely published in respected scientific journals, and whatever little has been published has been received with much skepticism from the medical community.

The action of homeopathic medicines supports the theory that each organism expresses symptoms in an effort to heal itself. This homeopathic action can augment, complement, and sometimes replace present medical technologies. For example, abuse of strong medications can lead to resistance to the drugs themselves, allergies, and other unpleasant side effects. In homeopathy, small drug doses have been shown to be more effective than larger ones, which in itself can reduce the undesired side effects associated with the use of common medications.

DIAGNOSTIC AND TREATMENT TECHNIQUES

The first step in treating an illness using homeopathy is taking the case history or symptom picture (the detailed account of what is wrong with the patient as a whole). This is carried out in a similar way by classical doctors and homeopathic practitioners, since most homeopaths are doctors or have some conventional medical training. The symptoms are divided into three categories: general, mental/emotional, and physical.

The homeopath then consults the *Materia Medica* (the encyclopedia of drug effects) and/or the *Repertory* (an index of symptoms from the *Materia Medica* listed in alphabetical order, used as a cross-reference between symptoms and remedies) to decide on the remedy to be used. The professional homeopath works with a number of *Materia Medica* texts compiled by different homeopaths.

The classical homeopath will give only one remedy at a time in order to gauge its effect more efficiently. The best-known unconventional usage of homeopathic medicines is of combination medicines or complexes, normally a mixture of between three and eight low-potency remedies. This approach is useful when the correct remedy is not available or when the practitioner is unsure as to which one to use. These mixtures are commonly sold in health food stores and are named for the disease or symptom that they are supposed to cure. Another unconventional use is what is called pluralism, which is the application of two or more medicines at a time, each of which is taken at a different time of day. This approach is most commonly used in Europe.

Homeopathy is a natural pharmaceutical system that utilizes microdoses of substances to arouse a healing response by stimulating the patient's immune system. Homeopathic remedies are always nontoxic because of the small concentrations used. They do not act chemically but rather according to a particular physical state linked to the way in which they are prepared. They have the capacity of making the ill subject react to his or her disease, and in this way they are considered specific stimulants.

Homeopathic remedies come from the plant, mineral, and animal kingdoms. Plants are the source of more than half of the remedies. They are harvested in their natural state according to strict norms by qualified specialists and are used fresh after thorough botanical inspection. Mineral remedies include natural salts and metals, always in their purest state. Animal remedies may contain venoms, poisonous insects, hormones, or physiological secretions such as musk or squid ink.

In all cases, the starting remedy is made from a mixture of the substance itself, which has been steeped in alcohol for a period of time and then strained. This starting liquid is called a tincture or mother tincture. In the decimal scale, a mixture of one-tenth tincture and nine-tenths alcohol is shaken vigorously, a process known as succession; this first dilution is called a 1X. (The number in the remedy reveals the number of times that it has been diluted and succussed; thus, 6X means diluted and succussed six times.) In the centesimal scale, the remedy is diluted using one part tincture in a

hundred, and the letter *C* is used after the number. The number indicates the degree of the dilution, while the letter indicates the technique of preparation (decimal or centesimal). Insoluble substances are diluted by grinding them in a mortar with lactose to the desired dilution. The greater the dilution of a remedy, the greater its potency, the longer it acts, the deeper it heals, and the fewer doses are needed.

A medicine is chosen for its similarity to the person's symptoms, so that the person's bioenergetic processes are hypersensitive to the substance. One theory used to explain the success of homeopathic remedies, even when they are used in such small concentrations, is that they work through some kind of resonance within the individual's system. There are other examples of high sensitivity to small amounts of substances in the animal kingdom, such as in the case of pheromones, sex attractants that affect only animals of the same species in very small amounts and at a very long distance.

Constantine Hering (1800-1880), the founder of American homeopathy, was the first to make note of the specific features of the healing process to create a

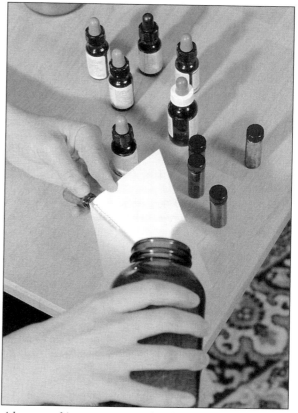

A homeopathist prepares remedies for a patient. (PhotoDisc)

holistic assessment tool that can be used to evaluate a patient's progress. His observations are summarized in Hering's Law of Cure: First, the human body seeks to externalize disease, to dislodge it from more serious, internal levels to more superficial ones; for example, in the healing of asthma the patient may exhibit an external skin rash before complete cure is achieved. Second, the healing progresses from the top of the body to the bottom; someone with arthritis will feel better in the upper part of the body earlier than in the lower part. Third, the healing proceeds in the reverse order of the appearance of the symptoms; that is, the more recent symptoms will heal first, and old symptoms may reappear before complete healing.

Homeopathic remedies are most commonly available in tablet form, combined with sugar from cow's milk. The tablets can be soft (so that they dissolve easily under the tongue and are easy to crush) or hard (so that they must be chewed and held in the mouth for a few seconds before being swallowed), or they can be prepared as globules (tiny round pills). The liquid remedies are dissolved in alcohol. Also available are powders that are wrapped individually in small squares of paper (convenient if the remedy is needed for only a few doses or is to be sent by mail), wafers, suppositories, and liniments. Homeopathic tablets will keep their strength for years without deteriorating, but they must be stored in a cool, dark, and dry place with their bottle tops screwed on tightly, away from strong-smelling substances.

The prescribed quantities are the same for babies, children, adults, and older people. The size of a dose is immaterial; it is how often it is taken that counts. The strength (potency) that is needed changes with the circumstances. The greater the similarity between the symptoms and the remedy, the greater the potency to be used (that is, the more dilute the remedy).

The following substances all counteract the effects of a homeopathic remedy to some extent (and as such are considered antidotes): camphor, coffee, menthol/eucalyptus, peppermint, recreational drugs, and any strong-smelling or strong-acting substance.

As with all treatments, there are some dangers associated with homeopathic cures, such as unintentional provings. These take place when, after an initial improvement, the symptoms characteristic of the remedy appear, creating a worse situation for the patient. Sometimes, this reaction takes place because the individual has been taking the remedy for too long, and it can be stopped by discontinuing the remedy or by using

an antidote. In other cases, there is a confused symptom picture, the effect being that the remedy is working in a limited way or curing a restricted number of symptoms.

Homeopathy is important in the treatment of bacterial infections (where resistance to antibiotics can develop) and viral conditions. Homeopathic remedies stimulate the person's resistance to infection without the side effects of antibiotics, and they help the body without suppressing the organism's self-protective responses. The remedies used are safer than regular medicines because they exhibit minimal side effects, and counterreactions between medicines can be prevented.

Homeopathic remedies are exempt from federal review in the United States. In 1938, any drug listed in the *Homeopathic Pharmacopoeia of the United States* was accepted by the FDA. Consequently, prescribed homeopathics do not have to undergo the rigorous safety and effectiveness testing the regulating agency requires of drugs used in orthodox medicine. Nonprescription homeopathics are also exempt and can be purchased in pharmacies, greengroceries, and health food stores throughout the country. The FDA requires that, as with any over-the-counter drug, a remedy be sold only for a self-limiting condition (such as headaches, menstrual cramps, or insomnia) and that the indications be printed on the label. The ingredients and their dilution must also be listed. Nonhomeopathic active ingredients cannot be included in the preparation.

PERSPECTIVE AND PROSPECTS

The Law of Similars was observed twenty-five centuries ago by Hippocrates and was utilized by people of many cultures, including the Mayans, Chinese, Greeks, and American Indians. In the following centuries, other doctors made similar observations, but they did not come to any practical conclusions. It was not until the end of the eighteenth century that a German physician, Christian Friedrich Samuel Hahnemann, studied the matter further, developed it, and gave it a scientific basis.

Hahnemann recruited a group of healthy subjects to take the remedies and report in a diary the symptoms that they caused, a process called proving the substance. He and his subjects proved more than a hundred remedies and produced a very accurate collection for use by other homeopathy practitioners. He also found that the remedies worked better in very small doses. Homeopathy was initially rejected by the medical profession, but its methods became more accepted when Hahnemann obtained astonishing results with his patients. In 1810, he published a book called *Organon der rationellen Heilkunde* (*The Organon of Homœopathic Medicine*, 1836), in which he presented the philosophy of homeopathy. He also published *Materia Medica pura* in six volumes between 1811 and 1821. These volumes contain the compilations of his provings. As new remedies are discovered, they are added to the compilation. By the time of Hahnemann's death in 1843, homeopathy was established around the world.

In the 1820's, homeopathy arrived in the United States at a time when the state of orthodox medicine was worse than in Europe. Many ordinary people consulted herbalists and bonesetters, so homeopathy was easily accepted and soon flourished. In 1844, the American Institute of Homeopathy was founded. In 1846, however, the American Medical Association (AMA) was founded, and it adopted a code of ethics which forbade its members to consult homeopaths. Nevertheless, public demand continued. The 1860's through the 1880's saw the heyday of homeopathy in the United States, with the institution of training programs, hospitals, and asylums and the training of thousands of homeopaths in the country.

Developments in orthodox medicine around the end of the nineteenth century strengthened this camp, however, while the homeopathic establishment was weakened by internal division. In 1911, the AMA moved to close many homeopathic teaching institutions because they were considered to provide a poor standard of education. By 1950, all the homeopathic colleges in the United States were either closed or no longer teaching homeopathy. By the 1990's, it was roughly estimated that only five hundred to one thousand medical doctors used homeopathics in their practices, though the number of homeopaths and osteopaths prescribing them had probably increased. Although the AMA has no official statement on homeopathy, it is no longer part of the medical school curriculum.

Homeopathy has exhibited a renaissance, and it is popular throughout the world, especially in France. Perhaps the reasons for this revived popularity include both skepticism surrounding conventional medicine and a need for alternatives in the face of challenging health problems: Homeopathy offers a safe alternative as it seeks to improve the general level of health of the whole person, emotionally as well as physically. It must not be forgotten, however, that this brand of medicine has a long way to go before its curative powers are proven.

—*Maria Pacheco, Ph.D.*

See also Alternative medicine; Disease; Herbal medicine; Immune system; Immunology; Pathology; Pharmacology; Toxicology.

FOR FURTHER INFORMATION:

Aubin, Michel, and Philippe Picard. *Homeopathy: A Different Way of Treating Common Ailments*. Translated by Pat Campbell and Robin Campbell. Bath, Avon, England: Ashgrove Press, 1989. An easy-to-read book which includes a critical analysis of orthodox medicine from the perspective of an orthodox doctor turned homeopath, a description of homeopathy, and a section on self-treatment with homeopathy.

Castro, Miranda. *The Complete Homeopathy Handbook: A Guide to Everyday Health Care*. Rev. ed. New York: Pan Press, 1996. Examines the principles underlying the theory of homeopathy, as well as how to prescribe and learn the best use of homeopathic medicines that are available over the counter.

Josephson, Laura. *Homeopathic Handbook of Natural Remedies: Safe and Effective Treatment of Common Ailments and Injuries*. New York: Random House, 2002. Gives an overview of the healing principles and history of homeopathy, guidelines for identifying and treating symptoms, and instructions for preparing and stocking your home kit. Includes an entire section on childhood conditions, an extensive directory of homeopathic pharmacies, and a list of articles and other publications that provide further information.

McCabe, Vinton. *Practical Homeopathy: A Comprehensive Guide to Homeopathic Remedies and Their Acute Uses*. New York: St. Martin's Press, 2000. McCabe, president of the Connecticut Homeopathic Association and a member of the faculty and board of the Hudson Valley School of Classical Homeopathy, joins philosophy and pharmacy in a practical way in this resource. Includes homeopathic remedies.

National Center for Homeopathy. http://www.homeopathic.org/. Offers resources on research, training, and how to find a homeopath.

Ullman, Dana. *Discovering Homeopathy: Medicine for the Twenty-first Century*. 2d rev. ed. Berkeley, Calif.: North Atlantic Books, 1991. Includes sections on the history and research methods of homeopathy and an excellent section on sources (books, computer programs, tapes) and general information on homeopathy. Lists pharmacies, organizations, schools, and training programs in the United States.

_____. *Essential Homeopathy: What It Is and What It Can Do for You.* Novato, Calif.: New World Library, 2002. Provides answers to frequently asked questions, introduces readers to the practice, and explains which conditions respond best to homeopathic treatment. Surveys treatments for common ailments including digestive troubles, colds, flus, allergies, and headaches.

Hormone replacement therapy (HRT)

Treatment

Anatomy or system affected: Blood vessels, bones, brain, breasts, circulatory system, genitals, heart, psychic-emotional system, reproductive system, skin, urinary system, uterus

Specialties and related fields: Cardiology, endocrinology, family medicine, geriatrics and gerontology, gynecology, hematology, internal medicine, oncology, orthopedics, preventive medicine, vascular medicine

Definition: Estrogens, with or without progestogens, given to women in the perimenopause to treat or prevent a variety of conditions.

Key terms:

hypothalamus: a part of the brain that controls many body functions; its releasing hormones stimulate the pituitary to secrete hormones of its own

incontinence: inability to control the bladder or bowel

menopause: the last menstrual period that a woman experiences

osteoporosis: thinning of the bones, which occurs in all people as they age

perimenopause: a period of years around the menopause, during which changes occur in the balance among the reproductive hormones, leading to the cessation of menses and the end of fertility; this time of transition from reproductive to postreproductive life is also known as the climacteric

pituitary gland: the body's master gland that produces various hormones which in turn stimulate other glands in the body to produce their own hormones; in women, the pituitary produces follicle-stimulating hormone and luteinizing hormone, which stimulate the ovary to produce estrogens and progesterone

progestogen: any of a number of substances (natural or synthetic) that have a progesterone-like effect

prolapse: the slipping out of place of an internal organ, such as the uterus

transdermal: through the skin; transdermal medications are those which are applied as creams, gels, or patches and are then absorbed through the skin

Indications and Procedures

During a woman's reproductive years, a complex feedback loop among the hypothalamus, pituitary gland, and ovaries causes the ovaries to produce various sex hormones, the major ones being estrogens and progesterone. These hormones are responsible for developing the secondary sexual characteristics such as breasts and pubic hair, for governing the menstrual cycle, and for maintaining a pregnancy should one occur. They also have profound effects on a woman's skin, heart, blood vessels, lipids (blood fats, such as cholesterol), bones, blood, and other systems.

As women approach the menopause, changes begin to occur in the hormone feedback loop. The menstrual cycle typically becomes shorter and more irregular, and then menses cease altogether. As hormone levels decline and the ratio between the estrogens and progesterone changes, the woman's body undergoes other changes such as thinning of the mucous membranes in the reproductive and urinary tract, drying of the skin, thinning of the bones, and alterations in cholesterol levels. Perimenopausal women may also experience hot flashes, night sweats, insomnia, mood swings, and other uncomfortable symptoms. Postmenopausal women do continue to produce sex hormones, although in smaller amounts. The adrenal glands are responsible for much of the postmenopausal hormone production, and some production occurs by conversion of other hormones in the body tissues.

The menopause normally occurs between the ages of forty-five and fifty-five. If a woman undergoes the menopause before age forty, it is called premature menopause. A woman who stops menstruating because of a total hysterectomy, in which not only the uterus but also the Fallopian tubes and ovaries are removed, undergoes what is called a surgical menopause. Women who undergo radiation of the ovaries will also experience an artificial menopause. The discomforts associated with the menopause may be exaggerated in these women.

Health care providers have used hormone replacement therapy (HRT) to treat uncomfortable perimenopausal symptoms and to prevent or treat a number of conditions associated with the postmenopausal state. HRT may include estrogen alone or a combination of estrogen and progesterone. At times, other hormones such as testosterone may be used to treat symptoms, but it is the estrogen-progesterone combination that comprises what is commonly thought of as HRT. Estrogen replacement therapy by itself is known as ERT.

USES AND COMPLICATIONS

A variety of estrogens and progestogens are available for the treatment of menopausal symptoms and for the prevention of health problems that accelerate after the menopause. They include oral estrogens and progestins, transdermal estrogens, injectable estrogens and progestins, and topical estrogens. Available oral estrogens for HRT include conjugated estrogens, micronized estradiol, piperazine estrone, ethinyl estradiol, quinestrol, and chlorotrianisene. Of these, the conjugated equine estrogens have been most extensively studied over a long period of time. They are usually well tolerated by patients. Various estrogens are also available as transdermal patches or vaginal creams. The oral progestogens used for HRT include medroxyprogesterone acetate and micronized progesterone.

At various periods throughout the twentieth century, health care providers and researchers have recommended that all women in the perimenopause begin hormone replacement. However, important questions about the safety and effectiveness of HRT have subsequently limited its use. In the first decade of the twenty-first century, recommendations from major medical organizations were generally that the decision whether to use HRT and for how long should be individualized. It should be used only to provide relief for severe symptoms and to prevent or treat specific conditions in women at high risk for problems.

Serious potential side effects and contraindications must be considered before making the decision to begin HRT. First, women who take estrogen supplementation without a progestogen are at increased risk for developing excessive thickening of the lining of the uterus. This situation can ultimately result in carcinoma (cancer) of the uterus. For this reason, women who have not had a hysterectomy are advised to take combination estrogen-progestogen HRT. If the combination is given on a cyclical basis, however, the woman will most likely experience monthly withdrawal bleeding. This is not always acceptable to postmenopausal women. About 90 percent of women who take a continuous dose of a lower-dose progestogen will not bleed at all after a year of its continuous use; the remainder will bleed occasionally.

Another risk to be considered is the possible development of breast cancer. Scientific studies have produced conflicting results about this risk. Some studies have shown a small increased risk of breast cancer with postmenopausal estrogen replacement used for extended periods of time. Adding a progestogen does not appear to change this risk.

Women who take oral estrogen supplements have an increased tendency to develop blood clots. This is not the case, however, for women who used transdermal formulations. Estrogen replacement therapy is also associated with an increased risk of gallbladder disease.

Women who should not take estrogen-containing hormone replacement at all include those with unexplained vaginal bleeding, a history of uterine or breast cancer, liver disease, or a history of blood clots in the veins. HRT should be used with caution in women with seizure disorders, high blood pressure, diabetes mellitus, migraines, gallbladder disease, and certain other conditions.

Minor adverse effects of hormone treatment include swelling, breast tenderness, bloating, headaches, and increased cervical mucus.

Some specific changes associated with the menopausal state that may be altered or prevented through the use of HRT are reproductive tract changes, urinary tract changes, vasomotor instability, osteoporosis, cardiovascular changes, skin and hair changes, and psychological changes, including dementia.

As the supply of estrogen decreases, women experience thinning and drying of the vaginal tissues. The cervix, uterus, and ovaries become smaller in size, and the cervix stops producing mucus. In addition, the ligaments that support the reproductive organs become more relaxed. These changes may lead to painful sexual intercourse, bleeding with minor trauma, itching, vaginal discharge, and prolapse of the uterus. The Food and Drug Administration (FDA) recommends vaginal cream formulations if vaginal thinning and dryness are the woman's only problem, rather than oral medications which affect the entire body.

The tissues of the bladder and urethra also become thinner, which may lead to urinary urgency, painful urination, or increased frequency. Some women even become incontinent. The evidence is not entirely clear about the usefulness of estrogen replacement therapy in this setting.

Vasomotor instability refers to the changes that lead to hot flashes and increased sweating. These flushes may be accompanied by heart palpitations, weakness, fatigue, dizziness, or lightheadedness. The episodes may cause nighttime awakening or insomnia, which in turn may lead to memory problems or irritability. The major treatment for vasomotor instability is the administration of estrogen, although progestogens have been used in women who cannot take estrogen. Some women find relief from a different type of drug called clonidine. Other treatments, which have not been studied as thoroughly as estrogen and progesterone, include various vitamin and mineral supplements, tranquilizers, and antidepressants.

All people gradually lose bone mass as they age, but in the years following the menopause this process accelerates in women, particularly in the type of bone known as trabecular bone. Postmenopausal women's risk for hip fracture becomes two to three times that of men. For this reason, estrogen has been recommended for prevention of osteoporosis, particularly in women who are thin, smoke cigarettes, have a strong family history of osteoporosis, drink large amounts of alcohol, or have some other risk factor. Studies have shown that women who take postmenopausal estrogen decrease their risk of hip fracture by up to 50 percent. The risk for fracture of the vertebrae in the spine decreases by about half as well.

With concerns about the safety of estrogens, however, other drugs are increasingly used to prevent or treat osteoporosis, including drugs from the classes known as bisphosphonates and selective estrogen receptor modulators (SERMs). Calcitonin and progestogens may also be used but do not seem to be as effective as the estrogens, bisphosphonates, or SERMs. All menopausal women should probably take supplemental calcium and vitamin D, exercise regularly, stop smoking if needed, and limit alcohol, caffeine, salt, and animal proteins in order to minimize their risk of developing osteoporosis.

Before the menopause, very few women have heart attacks. This state changes rapidly after the menopause, and by age seventy women have the same risk of heart attack as men. The conclusion has been that the higher levels of estrogen in premenopausal women must have a beneficial effect on the heart. Medical studies, however, have provided contradictory evidence about the effect of postmenopausal HRT on cardiovascular disease, with some studies indicating that HRT protects women and others indicating no effect or even an increased risk for heart disease with HRT.

From a theoretical standpoint, postmenopausal estrogen could affect cardiovascular health in two ways. First, estrogen supplementation increases the type of cholesterol that protects the heart (high-density lipoprotein, or HDL) and decreases the amount of harmful cholesterol (low-density lipoprotein, or LDL). Second, estrogen seems to have a direct effect on the blood vessels, helping to prevent atherosclerotic plaques from building up and narrowing the arteries.

In actual practice, however, no studies have clearly shown a benefit in terms of reduced heart attack or cardiac death rates in women who take HRT. One section of a long-term study funded by the National Institutes of Health (NIH), called the Women's Health Initiative, compared thousands of women who took combination HRT to women who received a placebo (sugar pill). Those on the combination treatment had an increased risk for heart disease, stroke, and blood clots in the lung. Major medical organizations, including the American Heart Association (AHA), the American College of Obstetricians and Gynecologists (ACOG), and the North American Menopause Society (NAMS), have recommended that combination therapy not be used for the prevention of cardiac disease.

As people age, they experience changes in the skin and hair. The skin becomes thinner and less elastic, particularly in sun-exposed areas. There is some loss of pubic hair and hair in the armpits. Some women experience balding, and some develop coarse facial hair. Body hair may either increase or decrease. The skin has estrogen receptors, so those changes are thought to be caused by decreased estrogen. Hair changes are more likely to result from a change in the ratio of estrogen to testosterone in the body after the menopause. Testosterone levels remain nearly the same before and after the menopause, while estrogen levels drop drastically. HRT does seem to improve or prevent skin changes.

Some studies have found that women in the early menopause experience more irritability, depression, and feelings of anxiety. It is not clear if these changes are attributable to some change in brain chemistry as a result of decreased estrogen, societal expectations about aging, or some other factor. Some researchers have suggested that the lack of sleep caused by hot flashes and night sweats is the source of mood changes, rather than being a function of the menopause itself. Furthermore, many perimenopausal women have multiple stressors, such as caring for aging parents, that may contribute to depression and anxiety. On the other hand, some researchers found that women who did not have hot flashes but did experience depression improved with the administration of estrogen. Some evidence exists that the areas of the brain responsible for memory are affected by estrogen, leading to the suggestion that Alzheimer's disease and other dementias may be prevented or treated by HRT.

In summary, the clearest indications for HRT are severe menopausal symptoms and the prevention of osteoporosis in women at high risk. For women with severe vasomotor symptoms, a fairly high dose of estrogen is probably indicated at first but this amount should be reduced as soon and as rapidly as possible. If the primary problem is vaginal dryness or discomfort, then estrogen cream may be helpful and have fewer side effects than oral estrogen. Other treatment modalities may limit further the use of estrogen in the prevention of osteoporosis.

PERSPECTIVE AND PROSPECTS

Feminist thinkers and researchers have periodically raised important questions about the use of sex hormones in women. They point out that many of the conditions that are treated with hormones are a part of women's normal life experience. By declaring such events as pregnancy and the menopause as "problems" and treating them with hormones, normal life events become "medicalized"—a condition to be treated at great expense and some risk to health and well-being. A second important issue raised by feminists is that hormones have been administered to women for various conditions without adequate testing and with serious consequences. For example, in the mid-twentieth century, physicians encouraged perimenopausal women to take estrogen to remain "forever young." Because these women were given estrogen without the progesterone needed to protect against the development of uterine cancer, cancer rates rose dramatically and estrogen alone was withdrawn as a treatment for the menopause.

—*Rebecca Lovell Scott, Ph.D., PA-C*

See also Aging; Arteriosclerosis; Breast cancer; Cervical, ovarian, and uterine cancers; Endocrinology; Endometrial cancer; Gynecology; Heart disease; Herbal medicine; Hormones; Hot flashes; Hysterectomy; Infertility, female; Menopause; Menstruation; Midlife crisis; Osteoporosis; Sweating; Women's health.

FOR FURTHER INFORMATION:

Love, Susan, and Karen Lindsey. *Dr. Susan Love's Menopause and Hormone Book: Making Informed Choices.* Rev. ed. New York: Random House, 2003. An excellent overview of the menopause and the pros and cons of hormone replacement therapy with alternative treatments.

National Women's Health Network. *The Truth About Hormone Replacement Therapy: How to Break Free from the Medical Myths of Menopause.* Roseville, Calif.: Prima, 2002. A feminist, strongly anti-HRT argument.

Seaman, Barbara. *The Greatest Experiment Ever Performed on Women: Exploding the Estrogen Myth.* New York: Hyperion, 2003. A history of the medicalization of the menopause and other normal stages of a woman's life and the use of estrogen. Offers a strong critique and details about the dangers of estrogen.

HORMONES
BIOLOGY

ANATOMY OR SYSTEM AFFECTED: Circulatory system, endocrine system, glands, psychic-emotional system

SPECIALTIES AND RELATED FIELDS: Biochemistry, endocrinology, pharmacology

DEFINITION: Chemical substances that are secreted by endocrine glands or specialized secretory cells into the blood or nearby tissues to act on those tissues and affect its function.

KEY TERMS:

adrenal glands: endocrine organs located on top of the kidneys; their function is to produce steroid hormones such as cortisol and sex hormones

deoxyribonucleic acid (DNA): the basic building block of life, which bears encoded genetic information; it is found mainly in chromosomes and can reproduce

messenger ribonucleic acid (mRNA): a single-stranded RNA that arises from and is complementary to double-stranded DNA; it passes from the nucleus to the cytoplasm, where its information is translated into proteins

prohormone: a hormone that must be cut or modified in a specific way in order to achieve full activity

receptor: a molecular structure at the cell surface or inside the cell that is capable of combining with hormones and causing a change in cell metabolism or function

STRUCTURE AND FUNCTIONS

The definition of the term "hormone" has continued to change over the years. The classic definition is that of an endocrine hormone—that is, one secreted by ductless glands directly into the blood and acting at a distant site. The definition can be expanded to include any chemical substance secreted by any cell of the body that has a specific effect on another cell. A hormone can affect a nearby cell (paracrine action) or the cell that secretes it (autocrine action). Certain hormones are produced by the brain and kidneys, which are not thought of as classic endocrine glands. In fact, the largest producer of hormones is the gastrointestinal tract, which is not usually thought of as an endocrine gland.

Hormones fall into two major categories: peptide hormones, which are derived from amino acids, and steroid hormones, which are derived from cholesterol. The different classes of hormones have different mechanisms of action. Peptide hormones work by interacting with a specific receptor located in the plasma membrane of the target cell. Receptors have different regions, or domains, that perform specialized functions. One part of the receptor has a specific three-dimensional structure similar to a keyhole into which a certain hormone can fit. This design allows a specific action of a hormone despite the fact that the hormone is often circulating in minute quantities in the bloodstream along with myriad other hormones.

There are different classes of plasma membrane receptors. One class is that of the receptor kinases. The insulin receptor is an example. In this case, the part of the receptor molecule that faces the cytoplasm, or inside of the cell, is able to perform a specific function. When insulin interacts with its receptor, a chemical change occurs on the receptor that allows it to activate proteins within the cell. Many hormones use a similar cascade of chemical reactions to control and amplify signals from outside the cell and effect change within the cell itself.

Another class of membrane receptors includes the G-protein coupled receptor. An example is the beta-2 adrenergic receptor. Epinephrine interacts with this receptor, causing the activation of a signal transducer or G protein. This activated G protein then leads to the modification of a specific protein, which leads to a cascade of biochemical events within the cell. This is another example of an amplification mechanism.

Steroid hormones exert their effects by means of a different mechanism. For example, glucocorticoids exert their effects by entering the cell and binding to specific glucocorticoid receptors in the cell nucleus. The glucocorticoid-receptor complex is able to bind specific regulatory DNA sequences, called glucocorticoid response elements. This binding is able to activate gene transcription, which causes an increase in mRNA and, ultimately, the translation of the mRNA to deliver a newly secreted protein. The protein can then act to change the cell's metabolism in some way. Cortisol, a type of glucocorticoid, is produced by the adrenal glands when a person is under stress. It can lead to changes in blood sugar levels, affect immune system function, and, at high levels, increase fat deposition in characteristic areas of the body.

Most hormones that circulate in the blood are attached to binding proteins. The general binding proteins in the body are albumin and transthyreitin. These two proteins bind many different hormones. There are also specific binding proteins, such as thyroid-binding globulin, which binds thyroid hormone, and insulin-like growth factor-binding proteins, which bind to the family of insulin-like growth factors. The bound hormone is considered the inactive hormone, and the free hormone is the active hormone. Therefore, binding proteins make it possible to control an active hormone precisely, without having to synthesize a new hormone.

Hormones can be secreted in a variety of time frames. Some hormones, such as testosterone, are secreted in a pulsatile fashion that changes over minutes or hours. Other hormones, such as cortisol, are secreted in a diurnal pattern, with levels varying depending on the time of day. Cortisol levels are highest at about 8 A.M. and fall throughout the day, with the lowest levels occurring between midnight and 2 A.M. The menstrual cycle is an example of the weekly to monthly variation of hormone production. For instance, progesterone (a steroid hormone) levels rise throughout the menstrual cycle and fall prior to the onset of menses. The exact control mechanisms that determine the rhythmicity of hormone production are unknown.

The ability to study and utilize hormones in treating human disease has been revolutionized by molecular biology. The first hormone to be synthesized for clinical use was insulin. The need for a secure and steady supply of insulin prompted scientists to look for alternative sources of this hormone in the 1970's. At that time, insulin was isolated and purified from animal pancreas glands, mostly those of cows and pigs. It was suspected, however, that insulin could be made in the laboratory via genetic engineering. Native insulin is produced from a prohormone, proinsulin. Recombinant DNA human insulin is currently made by encoding for the proinsulin molecule and then using enzymes to cut the molecule in the proper places, yielding insulin and a piece of protein called C peptide. This process, which is very similar to the process that the body uses to create insulin, produces high yields of active hormone.

Modern molecular biology techniques were used to identify a hormone and receptor involved in weight regulation. Originally discovered in mice, a gene called *ob* was identified in human beings which produced a hormone called leptin. Leptin and its receptor are believed to play a role in signaling satiety to the brain. If the leptin signal does not reach the brain as the result of a faulty receptor, the brain will not produce the satiety signal. Appetite will remain high. Thus, a defective leptin system may contribute to obesity in human beings. The functioning of leptin may also be responsible for cycles of weight loss and gain in dieters. As obese individuals lose adipose tissue, less leptin is synthesized and the brain may not send out sufficient signals to indicate satiety, thus increasing appetite and food consumption. The leptin-obesity connection is under intensive study.

THE MEDICAL USE OF HORMONES

The biological roles of hormones are numerous and critical to the normal function of important organ systems in human beings, and there are many examples of medical uses for hormones. In general, any derangements in the amount of hormones made, or in the timing of their production, can result in significant human disease or discomfort. For example, in women who reach the menopause, declining levels of estrogen and progesterone from the ovaries can lead to undesirable consequences such as hot flushes, vaginal dryness, and bone mineral density loss. Taking exogenous estrogen and progesterone, in the form of hormone replacement therapy, can reduce or stop these consequences. Another example of exogenous hormone use in human disease is thyroid hormone. People with thyroid disease, such as Hashimoto's thyroiditis, do not produce adequate levels of thyroid hormone. This condition can lead to intense fatigue and weight gain. These symptoms may be relieved by taking a synthetic thyroid hormone called levothyroxine.

Another example of the medical use of hormones is the role of synthetic erythropoietin in treating and preventing anemia. Normally, erythropoietin is made by the kidneys. It is essential for the differentiation and development of stem cells from the bone marrow into red blood cells. Most patients who develop kidney failure also suffer from severe anemia because the ability to synthesize erythropoietin is lost as the kidneys are de-stroyed by disease. Giving this hormone to a patient with kidney disease can lead to the restoration of that patient's red blood cell mass. Correcting the anemia that accompanies chronic renal disease can improve the exercise tolerance and overall quality of life of kidney disease patients. The hormone must be given by injection several times per week. It has been made available to the almost 50,000 Americans with chronic renal failure who require dialysis. Erythropoietin can also be given to renal failure patients who do not yet require dialysis but who do have anemia.

Another example of a hormone that has been synthesized for treatment of human disease is calcitonin. Calcitonin is a polypeptide hormone secreted by specialized C cells of the thyroid gland (also called parafollicular cells). The parafollicular cells make up about 0.1 percent of the total mass of the thyroid gland, and the cells are dispersed within the thyroid follicles. Calcitonin has been isolated from several different animal species, including the salmon, eel, rat, pig, sheep, and chicken. The main physiologic function of the hormone is to lower the serum calcium level. It does this by inhibiting calcium resorption from bone. Calcitonin has been used to treat patients with Paget's disease, a disorder of abnormal bone remodeling that can lead to deformities, bone pain, fractures, and neurological problems. Calcitonin has also been used in the past to treat patients with osteoporosis, a condition of bone density depletion associated with aging which can lead to bone fractures.

The first and most commonly used form of the hormone in the United States is salmon calcitonin. This form is a more potent inhibitor of bone resorption than the human form. A small number of patients given the drug will develop a resistance to it. The etiology of this resistance may be the development of antibodies to the salmon calcitonin. Subsequently, calcitonin was synthesized via recombinant DNA technology. Although the human form is somewhat less potent, the fact that its amino acid structure is identical to that of the native hormone makes it much less immunogenic than salmon calcitonin, and theoretically less likely to produce resistance. In fact, patients who were resistant to salmon calcitonin may be switched to human calcitonin and achieve a therapeutic effect.

An example of a hormone with multiple medical uses is vasopressin, also known as antidiuretic hormone. Normally, vasopressin is produced in the posterior pituitary gland (located in the brain); it is responsible for water conservation. An increase in plasma osmolality or a decrease in circulating blood volume will normally cause its release. Central diabetes insipidus, a disorder involving an absence or abnormal decrease of vasopressin, is characterized by an inappropriately dilute urine. Central diabetes insipidus can be caused by a variety of factors, including trauma, neurosurgery, brain tumors, brain infections, and autoimmune disorder. The clinical symptoms of the disease are polyuria and polydipsia. The patient may put out up to 18 liters of urine per day. If such large volume deficits are not remedied, more serious symptoms will ensue, including dangerously low blood pressure and coma. The acute treatment of any patient with central diabetes insipidus involves the replacement of body water with intravenous fluids. The chronic therapy involves replacement of the hormone vasopressin.

Several different forms of the hormone may be used, depending on the clinical situation. Aqueous vasopressin is useful for diagnostic testing and for acute management following trauma or neurosurgery. For diagnostic testing, it is often given subcutaneously at the end of the water deprivation test to determine whether the patient will respond to the hormone with a decrease in urine output and an increase in urine osmolality greater than 50 percent. After surgery, vasopressin can be given either intramuscularly, with a duration of action of about four to six hours, or by continuous intravenous infusion to ensure a steady level of the hormone.

In obstetrics, vasopressin is also known as pitocin, a hormone that can cause powerful uterine contractions. It is commonly used to augment labor, as when the mother's own uterine contractions are not adequate to expel the baby. It is given intravenously and titrated up until regular contractions of the uterus occur. Another use of vasopressin is in the acute setting of advanced cardiac life support, also known as a code situation. A patient noted to have a cardiac arrhythmia such as ventricular fibrillation may receive vasopressin as well as shocks from a defibrillator in an attempt to restore a perfusing cardiac rhythm.

One of the most important uses of hormones in medicine is for contraception, specifically in the form of birth control pills. In the early 1900's, the observation was made that mice that were fed extracts from ovaries could be rendered infertile. In the 1920's, the critical substance responsible for this infertility was discovered to be sex steroid hormones. The production of birth control pills dates back to the 1920's and 1930's, when steroid hormones such as progesterone were isolated from animal sources, such as pigs. By the 1940's,

progesterone could be isolated in large quantities from Mexican yams, which caused the prices for progesterone to fall dramatically. With the fall in prices, the idea that progesterone could be sold in the mass market as a birth control pill became more feasible. The first clinical trial of the birth control pill in human beings occurred in 1956. Since then, several generations of progesterones have been mass produced for the purposes of birth control. Each successive generation of progesterone has caused fewer undesirable side effects, and the dosage necessary to achieve a contraceptive effect has been found to be much lower than those found in the original birth control pills.

Birth control pills and the progesterone contained within them have other medical uses besides contraception. Birth control pills can be used to regulate menstrual cycles in women who suffer from irregular menstrual cycles or abnormal vaginal bleeding. They can be used to decrease heavy menstrual periods. They can even be useful in decreasing acne, which can lead to permanent scarring when it is severe.

PERSPECTIVE AND PROSPECTS

The study of hormones has been instrumental in understanding how human beings adapt to and live in their environment. Hormones are involved in the regulation of body homeostasis and all critical aspects of the life cycle. The study of hormones has expanded as scientists have produced large amounts of synthetic hormones in the laboratory for use in research.

The history of insulin discovery and production is an example of the rapid scientific progress made in the field of hormone research. In 1889, Joseph von Mering and Oskar Minkowski demonstrated that dogs whose pancreases had been removed exhibited abnormalities in glucose metabolism that were similar to those seen in human diabetes mellitus patients. This fact suggested that some factor made by the pancreas lowered the blood glucose. The search for this factor led to the discovery of insulin in 1921 by Frederick C. Banting and Charles H. Best. They were able to extract the active substance from the pancreas and to demonstrate its therapeutic effects in dogs and humans. The chemistry of insulin progressed with the establishment of the amino acid sequence and three-dimensional structure in the 1960's. In 1960, insulin became the first hormone to be measured by radioimmunoassay. With advances in laboratory techniques in the 1970's, it became the first hormone to be commercially available via recombinant DNA technology, thus ensuring the availability of pure hormone without the need for animal sources.

The ability to synthesize hormones and their receptors has increased greatly. In fact, scientists can clone genes, or parts of genes, and synthesize the associated protein in order to make hormones that are encoded by the body. This method involves amplifying small amounts of DNA isolated from the cell using the technique of polymerase chain reaction (PCR). This allows large amounts of the same piece of DNA to be made in a matter of hours, which can then be transcribed into RNA and translated to yield the hormone. These powerful techniques, developed in the research laboratory, have been applied on a commercial basis and have provided enormous benefits to people. One such example is the production of growth hormone.

—*RoseMarie Pasmantier, M.D.;*
Karen E. Kalumuck, Ph.D.;
updated by Anne Lynn S. Chang, M.D.

See also Addison's disease; Corticosteroids; Cushing's syndrome; Diabetes mellitus; Dwarfism; Endocrine disorders; Endocrinology; Endocrinology, pediatric; Genetic engineering; Gigantism; Glands; Goiter; Growth; Hormone replacement therapy (HRT); Hyperhidrosis; Hyperparathyroidism and hypoparathyroidism; Hypoglycemia; Insulin resistance syndrome; Leptin; Melatonin; Menopause; Metabolism; Obesity; Paget's disease; Pancreas; Pancreatitis; Pregnancy and gestation; Puberty and adolescence; Steroid abuse; Steroids; Sweating; Thyroid disorders; Weight loss and gain.

FOR FURTHER INFORMATION:
Barinaga, Marcia. "Obesity: Leptin Receptor Weighs In." *Science* 271 (January 5, 1996): 29. This article presents a summary of leptin receptor research accessible to the nonspecialist, as well as a discussion of the prospects for obesity drug research.
Bliss, Michael. *The Discovery of Insulin*. 3d ed. Toronto: University of Toronto Press, 2000. Very stimulating reading that re-creates the excitement surrounding the discovery of insulin. This novel gives the reader a feeling for the circumstances leading up to that momentous event.
Griffin, James E., and Sergio R. Ojeda, eds. *Textbook of Endocrine Physiology*. 5th ed. New York: Oxford University Press, 2004. A well-written book that presents an excellent summary of how hormones work and affect the body.
Larsen, P. Reed, et al., eds. *Williams Textbook of Endo-*

crinology. 10th ed. Philadelphia: W. B. Saunders, 2003. This extensive book on endocrinology covers all different aspects of the field. It is written by recognized experts in endocrinology in a very readable style.
Marieb, Elaine N. *Essentials of Human Anatomy and Physiology*. 8th ed. San Francisco: Pearson/Benjamin Cummings, 2006. This introductory anatomy and physiology textbook, easily accessible to those with little science background, is richly illustrated with diagrams and photographs that help to illuminate body systems and processes.
Tierney, Lawrence M., Stephen J. McPhee, and Maxine A. Papadakis, eds. *Current Medical Diagnosis and Treatment 2007*. New York: McGraw-Hill Medical, 2006. Contains a good chapter on endocrinology that describes common diseases which are a result of hormone abnormalities. Concisely and clearly written, with a medical focus.

HOSPICE
HEALTH CARE SYSTEM
DEFINITION: Hospice care is a holistic approach to caring for the dying and their families by addressing their physical, emotional, and spiritual needs.

Hospice is a philosophy of care directed toward persons who are dying. Hospice care uses a family-oriented holistic approach to assist these individuals in making the transition from life to death in a manner that preserves their dignity and comfort. This approach, as Elisabeth Kübler-Ross would say, allows dying patients "to live until they die." Hospice care encourages patients to participate fully in determining the type of care that is most appropriate for their comfort. By creating a secure and caring community sensitive to the needs of the dying and their families and by providing palliative care that relieves patients of the distressing symptoms of their disease, hospice care can aid the dying in preparing mentally as well as spiritually for their impending death.

Unlike traditional health care, where the patient is viewed as the client, hospice care, with its holistic emphasis, treats the family unit as the client. There are usually specific areas of stress for the families of the dying. In addition to the stress of caring for the physical needs of the dying, family members often feel tremendous pressure maintaining their own roles and responsibilities within the family itself. The conflict of caring for their own nuclear families while caring for dying relatives places a huge strain on everyone involved and can be a source of anxiety and guilt for the patient as well. Another area of stress experienced by family members involves concern for themselves, that is, having to put their own lives on hold, keeping from getting physically run down, dealing with their newly acquired time constraints, and viewing themselves as isolated from friends and family. Compounding this is the guilt that many caregivers feel over not caring for the dying relative as well or as patiently as they might, or secretly wishing for the caregiving experience to reach an end.

Due to the holistic nature of the care provided, the hospice team is actually an interdisciplinary team composed of physicians, nurses, psychological and social workers, pastoral counselors, and trained volunteers. This medically supervised team meets weekly to decide on how best to provide physical, emotional, and spiritual support for dying patients and to assist the surviving family members in the subsequent grieving process.

This type of care can be administered in three different ways. It can be home-health-agency based, delivered in the patient's own home. It can be dispensed in an institution devoted solely to hospice care. It can even be administered in traditional medical facilities (such as hospitals) that allot a certain amount of space (perhaps a wing or floor, or even a certain number of beds) to this type of care. Fewer than 20 percent of hospices are totally independent and unaffiliated with any hospitals.

PRINCIPLES

Hospice care attempts to enhance the quality of dying patients' final days by providing them with as much comfort as possible. It is predicated on the belief that death is a natural process with which humans should not interfere. The principles of hospice care, therefore, revolve around alleviating the anxieties and physical suffering that can be associated with the dying process, and not prolonging the dying process by using invasive medical techniques. Hospice care is also based on the assertion that dying patients have certain rights that must be respected. These rights include a right to absent themselves from social responsibilities and commitments, a right to be cared for, and the right to continued respect and status. The following seven principles are basic components of hospice care.

The first principle is highly personalized and holistic care of the dying, which includes treating dying patients emotionally and spiritually as well as physically.

This interpersonal support, known as bonding, helps patients in their final days to live as fully and as comfortably as possible, while retaining their dignity, autonomy, and individual self-worth in a safe and secure environment. This one-on-one attention involves what can be called therapeutic communication. Knowing that someone has heard, that someone understands and is concerned, can be profoundly healing.

Another principle is treating pain aggressively. To this end, hospice care advocates the use of narcotics at dosages that will alleviate suffering while, at the same time, enabling patients to maintain a desired level of alertness. Efforts are made to employ the least invasive routes to administer these drugs (usually orally, if possible). In addition, pain medication is administered before the pain begins, thus alleviating the anxiety of patients waiting for pain to return. Since it has been shown that fear of pain often increases the pain itself, this type of aggressive pain management gives dying patients more time and energy to respond to family members and friends and to work through the emotional and spiritual stages of dying. This dispensation of pain medication before the pain actually occurs, however, has proven to be perhaps the most controversial element in hospice care, with some critics charging that the dying are being turned into drug addicts.

A third principle is the participation of families in caring for the dying. Family members are trained by hospice nurses to care for the dying patients and even to dispense pain medication. The aim is to prevent the patients from suffering isolation or feeling as if they are surrounded by strangers. Participation in care also helps to sustain the patients' and the families' sense of autonomy.

The fourth principle is familiarity of surroundings. Whenever possible, it is the goal of hospice care to keep dying patients at home. This eliminates the necessity of the dying to spend their final days in an institutionalized setting, isolated from family and friends when they need them the most. It is estimated that close to 90 percent of all hospice care days are spent in patients' own homes. When this is not possible and patients must enter institutional settings, rules are relaxed so that their rooms can be decorated or arranged in such a way as to replicate the patients' home surroundings. Visiting rules are suspended when possible, and visits by family members, children, and sometimes even pets are encouraged.

The fifth principle is emotional and spiritual support for the family caregivers. Hospice volunteers are specially trained to use listening and communicative techniques with family members and to provide them with emotional support both during and after the patient's death. In addition, because the care is holistic, the caregivers' physical needs are attended to (for example, respite is provided for exhausted caregivers), as are their emotional and spiritual needs. This spiritual support applies to people of all faith backgrounds, as impending death tends to put faith into a perspective where particular creeds and denominational structures assume less significance. In attending to this spiritual dimension, the hospice team is respectful of all religious traditions while realizing that death and bereavement have the ability to both strengthen and weaken faith.

The sixth principle is having hospice services available twenty-four hours a day, seven days a week. Because of its reliance on the assistance of trained volunteers, round-the-clock support is available to patients and their families.

The seventh principle is bereavement counseling for the survivors. At the time of death, the hospice team is available to help families take care of tasks such as planning the funeral and probating the will. In the weeks after the death, hospice volunteers offer their support to surviving family members in dealing with their loss and grief and the various phases of the bereavement process, always aware of the fact that not all bereaved need or want formal interventions.

History

The term "hospice" comes from the Latin *hospitia*, meaning "places of welcome." The earliest documented example of hospice care dates to the fourth century, when a Roman woman named Fabiola apparently used her own wealth to care for the sick and dying. In medieval times, the Catholic Church established inns for poor wayfarers and pilgrims traveling to religious shrines in search of miraculous cures for their illnesses. Such "rest homes," usually run by religious orders, provided both lodging and nursing care, since the medieval view was that the sick, dying, and needy were all travelers on a journey. This attitude also reflects the medieval notion that true hospitality included care of the mind and spirit as well as of the body. During the Protestant Reformation, when monasteries were forcibly closed, the concepts of hospice and hospital became distinct. Care of the sick and dying was now considered a public duty rather than a religious or private one, and many former hospices were turned into state-run hospitals.

The first in-patient hospice establishment of modern times (specifically called "hospice") was founded by Mary Aitkenhead and the Irish Sisters of Charity under her leadership in the 1870's in Dublin, Ireland. Cicely Saunders, a physician at St. Joseph's Hospice in London, which was founded by the English Sisters of Charity in 1908, began to adapt the ancient concept of hospice to modern palliative techniques. While there, Saunders became extremely close to a Holocaust survivor who was dying of cancer. She found that she shared his dream of establishing a place that would meet the needs of the dying. Using the money he bequeathed her at his death as a starting point, Saunders raised additional funds and opened St. Christopher's Hospice in Sydenham, outside London, in 1967. Originally it housed only cancer patients, but with the financial support of contracts with the National Health Service in England and private donations, it later expanded to meet the needs of all the dying. In fact, no patient has ever been refused because of inability to pay. St. Christopher's has served as a model for the hospices to be built later in other parts of the world.

Even though hospice care did not originate with Cicely Saunders, she is usually credited with founding the first modern hospice, since she introduced the concept of dispensing narcotics at regular intervals in order to preempt the pain of the dying. She was also the first to identify the need to address other, nonphysical sources of pain for dying patients.

Two years after St. Christopher's Hospice was opened, Kübler-Ross wrote *On Death and Dying*, which validated the hospice movement by relating stories of the dying and their wishes as to how they would be treated. In 1974, the United States opened its first hospice, Hospice, Inc. (later called the Connecticut Hospice), in New Haven, Connecticut. Within the next twenty-five years, over three thousand hospice programs would be implemented in the United States. In Canada, the first "palliative care" unit (as hospices are referred to in Canada) was opened in 1975 by Dr. Balfour M. Mount at the Royal Victoria Hospital in Montreal. This is considered to be the first hospital-based hospice in North America.

Cost

Because of hospice care's reliance on heavily trained volunteers and contributions, and because death is seen as a natural process that should not be prolonged by invasive and expensive medical techniques, hospice care is much less costly than traditional acute care facilities.

Because hospice care is a philosophy of care rather than a specific facility, though, legislation to provide monetary support for hospice patients took a great deal of time to be approved. In 1982, the U.S. Congress finally added hospice care as a Medicare benefit. In 1986, it was made a permanent benefit. Medicare requires, however, that there be a prognosis of six months or less for the patient to live. Hospice care is also reimbursable by many private insurance companies.

The National Hospice Organization (NHO) originated in 1977 in the United States as a resource for the many groups across the country who needed assistance in establishing hospice programs in their own communities. The purpose of this organization is to provide information about hospice care to the public, to establish conduits so that information may be exchanged between hospice groups, and to maintain agreed-upon standards for developing hospices around the country. The NHO publishes *Guide to the Nation's Hospices* on an annual basis.

—Mara Kelly-Zukowski, Ph.D.

See also Death and dying; Euthanasia; Grief and guilt; Hospitals; Medicare; Terminally ill: Extended care.

FOR FURTHER INFORMATION:

Buckingham, Robert W. *The Handbook of Hospice Care*. New York: Prometheus Books, 1996. Covers the history and philosophy of hospice care while providing practical information as to its cost, how to find hospice programs in your own community, and how to manage grief. Focuses on two target populations for hospice care: children and AIDS victims.

Byock, Ira, ed. *Dying Well: Peace and Possibilities at the End of Life*. New York: Riverhead Books, 1998. President of the American Academy of Hospice and Palliative Medicine at the time he wrote this book, Dr. Byock uses the personal stories of his patients to show the best ways to die. Provides information for the families of the dying who wish to make their loved ones' final days as comfortable and meaningful as possible.

Connor, Stephen R. *Hospice: Practice, Pitfalls, and Promise*. Washington, D.C.: Taylor & Francis, 1998. This book provides a useful outline of the history, structure, and function of hospice programs in the United States, with understandably less emphasis on medical issues. There is clear evidence of wide experience and consideration of the real world of hospice care, not second-hand distillation from the literature.

Corr, Charles A., Clyde M. Nabe, and Donna M. Corr. *Death and Dying, Life and Living*. 5th ed. Belmont, Calif.: Wadsworth, 2005. This book provides perspective on common issues associated with death and dying for family members and others affected by life-threatening circumstances.

Forman, Walter B., et al., eds. *Hospice and Palliative Care: Concepts and Practice*. 2d ed. Sudbury, Mass.: Jones and Bartlett, 2002. A text that examines the theoretical perspectives and practical information about hospice care. Other topics include community medical care, geriatric care, nursing care, pain management, research, counseling, and hospice management.

Lattanzi-Licht, Marcia, John J. Mahoney, and Galen W. Miller. *The Hospice Choice: In Pursuit of a Peaceful Death*. New York: Simon & Schuster, 1998. Definitive resource from the National Hospice Organization. Provides practical information such as range of hospice services, methods of payment, and so on. Intersperses stories of families who have received hospice care with a thorough explanation of its history, principles, and benefits.

Meyer, Maria M., and Paula Derr. *The Comfort of Home: A Complete Guide for Caregivers*. 3d ed. Portland, Oreg.: CareTrust, 2007. A very useful guide to caregiving in the home. Provides a chronological structure to define preparation for caregiving and the day-to-day expectations, and gives a listing of numerous research resources.

National Hospice and Palliative Care Organization. http://www.nhpco.org/. A group that advocates for the terminally ill and their families, develops public and professional educational programs and materials to enhance understanding and availability of hospice and palliative care, and conducts research, among other activities.

Sendor, Virginia F., and Patrice M. O'Connor. *Hospice and Palliative Care: Questions and Answers*. Lanham, Md.: Scarecrow, 1997. The user-friendly question-and-answer style of this volume allows for use as a quick reference. The purpose is to address the questions often asked by individuals faced with a terminal illness and those involved in the care of the terminally ill.

HOSPITALS

HEALTH CARE SYSTEM

DEFINITION: Institutions focused on the management, prevention, and treatment of illness; utilizing a staff of medical and allied health professionals, hospitals provide medical, surgical, and psychiatric treatment along with emergency care and evaluation.

KEY TERMS:

emergency room: a place where rapid evaluation and treatment of sudden illnesses, accidents, and traumas occur

intensive care: continuous medical treatment involving vigilant monitoring of the vital signs of patients with grave physical conditions

outpatient care: evaluation and treatment services not requiring an overnight stay

triage: a process in which patient needs are evaluated by a health care team and preliminary treatment plans are made

ORGANIZATION AND FUNCTIONS

Hospitals are run both privately and under public auspices, such as a local, state, or federal government. In general, they can be classified in three ways: nonprofit versus for-profit, general versus specialty, and short-term versus long-term care. Typically, they are organized in a hierarchical fashion: A governing body, such as a board of directors and its committees, oversees an administrator who, in turn, oversees a variety of departmental managers. While the governing body is responsible for defining and fostering the hospital's mission, the administrator guides the implementation of the mission, and the managers enact it. As such, hospitals have feedback mechanisms from the departments and chief administrator back to the board to ensure quality and progress.

STAFF AND SERVICES

Most hospitals have five primary departments for service management: financial, support, nursing, medical, and ancillary. The first two, financial and support, provide nonmedical services, while the remainder provide direct and indirect medical services. The financial department relies on office personnel and manages business functions, such as admissions, data management, accounting, and collections. In contrast, the support department manages administrative functions (such as volunteer services, medical records, purchasing, personnel), environmental concerns (such as maintenance and housekeeping), and nonmedical patient services

(such as dietary needs and social services). This department hosts a diverse service staff, ranging from janitors to dietitians to social workers.

As patients, individuals typically enter hospitals through admissions, the emergency room, or a hospital clinic, or via referral from a private doctor. Thus, depending on a patient's route of admission, his or her interaction with different departmental service staff may vary considerably. In any hospital, however, the nursing service has perhaps the greatest visibility, as it fulfills functions in the emergency and operating rooms, outpatient clinics, and inpatient units. In fact, nurses may perform any of the following duties, depending on their level of training and where they work within a hospital: triage, charting, medical room preparation, medication administration, vital signs monitoring, assistance of patients with meals and hygiene, and staff training. In addition, the nursing service typically dominates short-term special care units, such as intensive care and the emergency room, and nonacute care units, such as renal dialysis centers, psychiatric and substance abuse units, and long-term care centers for chronic illnesses.

Equally well known is the medical service, consisting of physicians, osteopathic physicians, podiatrists, dentists, and psychologists. Typically, this service manages the delivery of care for general medicine, surgery, obstetrics and gynecology, pediatrics, and psychiatry. While the nursing service historically has dominated the emergency room, more recently medical staff are leading in this service area. Many different classes of emergency rooms exist, however, ranging from highly staffed by physicians and specialists (twenty-four-hours on site) to minimally staffed (an on-call emergency nurse or technician who transfers patients to hospitals with life support equipment). Consequently, this balance between nursing and medical services may vary considerably among hospital emergency rooms.

Finally, ancillary service professionals assist the medical service staff in rendering diagnoses and treating patients. These staff members are highly trained and commonly use sophisticated equipment and methods. Subdepartments composing this service include the laboratory, pharmacy, anesthesiology, physical therapy, electrocardiography (ECG or EKG), electroencephalography (EEG), magnetic resonance imaging (MRI), and inhalation therapy departments. Radiology is also included and has three divisions: diagnostic radiology, therapeutic radiology, and nuclear medicine.

PERSPECTIVE AND PROSPECTS

The word "hospital" was derived from the Greek word *hospitum*, meaning a place for the reception of pilgrims, and the Latin word *hospes*, meaning "guest" or "host." Originally, hospitals existed as temples or churches in ancient Greece and Rome, where priest-physicians performed healing miracles on the mind, body, and spirit. Later, hospitals were run by Christians and church bishops in Europe and served primarily as places of refuge and service for travelers. It was not until 600 C.E. that European hospitals specifically began caring for the sick. Similarly, in America, hospitals were not established until the eighteenth century—and then, only in larger cities. At that time, they primarily functioned as places where the urban poor could receive care and where individuals with contagious diseases could be confined during epidemics. With the advent of modern medicine and developments such as anesthesia and antibiotic drugs, hospitals were seen less as places to be sick and more as places to get well. As a result, they began to take in patients from all sectors of society and with a broader diversity of medical needs.

Today, hospitals are large, financially driven institutions that focus not only on the provision of emergency medical services and healing the very sick but also on the prevention of illness. Increasingly, specialty hospitals are addressing specific groups of patients, such as children, women, elders, and individuals with particular illnesses, such as cancer. In addition, specialty hospitals are taking on identities as centers for research and teaching as they improve treatment methods and strategies. With improved drug therapies and medical procedures, there is also a trend in general hospitals toward outpatient and day care for chronic illnesses replacing a long history of inpatient services. In the future, these trends toward service specialization and outpatient service are expected to continue, with hospitals increasing their use of illness prevention strategies, as well as continuing to improve their delivery of critical care and emergency services for diverse groups of patients.

—Nancy A. Piotrowski, Ph.D.

See also Anesthesiology; Critical care; Critical care, pediatric; Emergency care; Geriatrics and gerontology; Malpractice; Nursing; Obstetrics; Oncology; Para-

Older adults may find themselves hospitalized for acute illnesses, chronic illnesses, or injuries—all of which present higher risks for the elderly than for younger adults. (Digital Stock)

medics; Pediatrics; Physician assistants; Psychiatry; Psychiatry, child and adolescent; Psychiatry, geriatric; Surgery, general; Surgery, pediatric; Terminally ill: Extended care.

FOR FURTHER INFORMATION:

Birenbaum, Aaron. *Wounded Profession: American Medicine Enters the Age of Managed Care.* Westport, Conn.: Greenwood Press, 2002. Traces the evolution of health care in the United States during the 1990's and examines the rising costs, consumer backlash, and new legislation.

Christman, Luther, and Michael A. Counte. *Hospital Organization and Health Care Delivery.* Boulder, Colo.: Westview Press, 1981. Details guidelines and rationale for health care risk management, looking beyond conventional hospital-based, clinical initiatives to encompass a variety of health care settings.

Clifford, Joyce C. *Restructuring: The Impact of Hospital Organization on Nursing Leadership.* Chicago: AHA Press, 1998. An examination of the evolution of the role of the chief nursing officer in hospitals responding to a dramatically changing health care environment. Clifford examines the impact of change on the management and administration of clinical nursing services and considers the opportunities and ramifications of how present actions can affect the future of nursing.

Dranove, David. *The Economic Evolution of American Health Care: From Marcus Welby to Managed Care.* Princeton, N.J.: Princeton University Press, 2002. Traces the economic, technological, and historical forces that have transformed the health care field.

Melnick, Glenn, Emmett Keeler, and Jack Zwanziger. "Market Power and Hospital Pricing: Are Nonprofits Different?" *Health Affairs* 18, no. 3 (June, 1999): 167-173. This study shows that nonprofit and government hospitals have steadily become more willing to raise prices to exploit market power and discusses the implications for antitrust regulators and agencies that must approve nonprofit conversions.

Sloane, Robert M., and Beverly LeBov Sloane. *A Guide to Health Facilities: Personnel and Management.* 3d ed. Ann Arbor, Mich.: Health Administration Press, 1992. Offers an overview of health facilities, with a look at hospital administration. Includes bibliographical references and an index.

HOST-DEFENSE MECHANISMS

BIOLOGY

ANATOMY OR SYSTEM AFFECTED: Blood, cells, gastrointestinal system, immune system, skin, urinary system

SPECIALTIES AND RELATED FIELDS: Hematology, immunology, preventive medicine, serology

DEFINITION: Immunological methods that the body uses to protect against external infectious agents and to maintain internal homeostasis, such as those rooted in the skin, sweat, urine, tears, phagocytes, and "helpful" bacteria.

KEY TERMS:

antibodies: proteins produced by immune cells called lymphocytes; antibodies bind to targets called antigens in a highly specific manner

antigen: any substance that causes the formation of a specific antibody; generally a protein

complement: a series of serum proteins that, when activated, carry out a variety of immune functions; the most notable complement function is the lysis of a target

granulocyte: a white blood cell characterized by large numbers of cytoplasmic granules, including neutrophils, eosinophils, and basophils

innate immunity: nonspecific immunity in the sense that prior contact with an infectious agent is not required for proper innate immune response

interferons: a family of proteins; some of these proteins induce an antiviral state within a cell, while others serve to regulate aspects of the immune response

lymphocyte: either of two kinds of small white blood cells; B lymphocytes function to secrete antibodies, while T lymphocytes function to destroy virus-infected cells

macrophage: any of several forms of either circulating or fixed phagocytic cells of the immune system

neutrophil: a circulating white blood cell that serves as one of the principal phagocytes for the immune system

phagocyte: any cell capable of surrounding, ingesting, and digesting microbes or cell debris; in a certain sense, phagocytes function as scavengers

STRUCTURE AND FUNCTIONS

Humans exist in an environment that contains a wide variety of potentially infectious agents. These agents range in size from microscopic viruses—such as rhinoviruses, which cause the common cold—to a wide variety of bacteria and even macroscopic agents such as parasitic worms. In the absence of a functioning immune system, as is observed in persons with acquired immunodeficiency syndrome (AIDS) or congenital immune deficiencies, a person will eventually succumb to overwhelming infections.

Host-defense mechanisms consist of two major components: an innate system that is not dependent on prior exposure to an infectious agent and an acquired immunity that is stimulated by exposure to an agent. In general, the innate system functions in a nonspecific manner, while the acquired immune responses are highly specific.

The first major lines of host defense are the physical barriers to infection. These include the intact skin and the mechanical or physical barriers that serve to protect body openings. Few infectious agents are capable of penetrating intact skin. Numerous sweat glands and follicles are also associated with skin, and their secretion of fatty acids or lactic acid serves to produce an acid environment that inhibits the growth of bacteria. In addition, the high salt content found on the surface of the body also serves to inhibit growth. Bacteria that can resist the high levels of salt and acid, such as *Staphylococcus* or *Streptococcus*, tend to cause skin-related problems such as acne or boils.

Openings of the body, such as the mouth, anus, and vagina, exhibit both the physical barrier of skin and a variety of other defense strategies. Secreted mucus serves to trap foreign particles, which can then be expelled, depending on the tissue, by the ciliary action of the cells, coughing or sneezing, or the washing action of saliva, urine, or tears. Many of these secretions also contain antibacterial or antiviral agents. Gastric juices contain hydrochloric acid, while the enzyme lysozyme, found in tears and saliva, serves to cause the breakdown of certain bacteria.

The normal flora of organisms found within the body also plays an important role in defense. Bacteria in the mouth and gut serve to suppress any external agents that may find their way to those regions. Removal of the innate flora with antibiotics may result in yeast infections of the mouth or vaginal tract, or ulceration by "opportunistic" organisms of the gut.

Penetration of the host by infectious agents initially brings into action other aspects of the innate immune system. This can take the form of a series of "professional" phagocytes, cells that literally eat foreign particles such as bacteria; also included are chemical agents found in tissue and blood.

Two major forms of phagocytes are found in blood and tissues: neutrophils and monocytes/macrophages. Neutrophils represent the most numerous white cells in blood, approximately 60 to 70 percent of the total. They can be recognized by their multilobed nuclei, which confer the ability to pass between the endothelial cells of capillaries into sites of tissue infections. When neutrophils locate a target, such as an infectious agent or a dead cell, they surround that target with membranous arms called pseudopods and ingest it. Once the particle

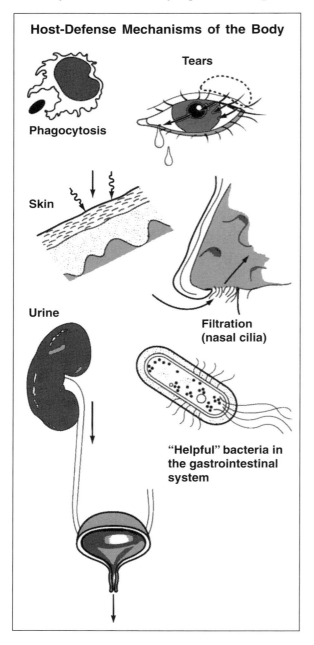

Host-Defense Mechanisms of the Body

Phagocytosis

Tears

Skin

Urine

Filtration
(nasal cilia)

"Helpful" bacteria in
the gastrointestinal
system

is incorporated within this "phagosome," it is ready for killing and digestion.

The killing of ingested organisms such as bacteria involves a series of complicated reactions, the major products of which are highly reactive oxidizing agents such as peroxides or metabolic by-products such as acid. At the same time, digestive organelles within the phagocyte, called lysosomes, fuse with the phagosome. Lysosomes contain numerous digestive enzymes, and these function to digest the engulfed particle. In effect, the particle now ceases to exist.

Monocytes, which are most often observed in their differentiated macrophage stage, function in a similar manner. Unlike circulating cells such as neutrophils, however, macrophages constitute the mononuclear phagocytic system that is associated with many tissues in the body. Examples of tissue-associated macrophages are the Kupffer cells of the liver, the microglia of the brain, and certain alveolar cells of the lungs. In addition to serving a nonspecific phagocytic function, macrophages serve as antigen-presenting cells (APCs) for specific immune responses.

A variety of blood chemicals also can be associated with innate immunity. Complement represents a series of some twenty blood proteins, activated in a cascade fashion, which exhibit a variety of pharmacologic activities. The complement pathway can be initiated upon exposure to certain bacteria. Components of the pathway can serve as chemoattractants for neutrophils. They can increase the efficiency of phagocytosis (opsonization), and they can form a membrane attack complex on the surface of a target, resulting in lysis.

Another type of blood cell may play a role in certain types of parasitic infections: the eosinophil. Granulocytes like the neutrophils, eosinophils contain within their granules digestive enzymes capable of being released against targets such as parasitic worms. The binding of these enzymes on the surface of a target damages the parasite's membrane, resulting ultimately in death of the parasite.

Acquired host defenses, while involving mechanisms similar to those of the innate systems, differ in one important way: They require prior exposure to the antigen. Acquired immunity consists of two major arms: humoral immunity, which represents substances soluble in the blood; and cellular immunity, which utilizes cells targeted against agents in a specific manner.

Humoral immunity centers primarily on proteins called antibodies. Exposure to foreign antigens triggers a series of reactions among three separate types of blood cells: antigen-presenting cells, T lymphocytes, and B lymphocytes. It is the B cell that actually secretes the antibodies.

The process starts when an APC encounters and phagocytizes an antigen. The antigen is digested, and pieces, or determinants, of the antigen are expressed on the surface of the cell. The most common APC is the macrophage, but antigen presentation can also be carried out by dendritic cells found in the dermis of the skin. This portion of the process is analogous to the series of events associated with innate immunity. At this point, however, the determinant is "presented" to appropriate T and B lymphocytes. Only those lymphocytes that possess specific receptors for that antigenic determinant can interact with the APC; it is this aspect that represents the specificity of the reaction. In association with a subclass of T lymphocytes called T helper cells (also known as CD4+ cells), the B cell is stimulated to begin the secretion of large quantities of antibodies. The antibodies recognize and bind only those antigens against which they were produced.

The formation of antigen-antibody complexes is the key to the humoral response. The result of the reaction depends upon the form taken by the antigen. The binding of antibodies to a bacterium or virus results in opsonization, a significantly enhanced ability of phagocytes to engulf the target. Antibody binding to a virus may also inhibit the agent's binding to a target cell, rendering the virus inactive. If the antigen is a toxin, antibody binding will neutralize the molecule.

The other arm of acquired immunity directly utilizes cellular defenses. The key cell here is the T lymphocyte. T lymphocytes mature in an organ called the thymus, which is located in humans near the thyroid in the neck and which provides the basis for the cells' name. T cells are often referred to as "killer cells" (or CD8+ cells) because of their function. They possess receptors on their surfaces that bind to specific target cells, which are generally cells infected with viruses, though T cells are also associated with rejection of foreign grafts. Once the T cell binds to the target, pharmacologically active granules are released that bind to and disrupt the membrane of the target. Thus, the humoral response is directed primarily against extracellular agents such as bacteria, while the cellular response is directed primarily against internal parasites.

DISORDERS AND DISEASES

In their most obvious form, the mechanisms of host defense protect against disease. Humans exist in an environment that is a sea of microorganisms. Most infections, while often uncomfortable, are not life-threatening. It is only when the immune system fails to function properly or is overwhelmed that illness results in the death of the individual. Ironically, the study of these circumstances has provided much knowledge of the functioning of the immune system.

Throughout history, diseases have periodically plagued humanity. Epidemics of viral diseases such as polio and bacterial infections such as bubonic plague or cholera have killed untold millions of persons. Among the most important advances in medicine since the eighteenth century has been the development of vaccination as a means of preventing disease. In the case of passive immunity, host defenses are temporarily augmented, while active immunity, mimicking an actual infection, often provides lifelong protection.

Passive immunity involves the acquisition of preformed antibodies by an individual. Since colostrum, or milk from a nursing mother, contains a form of antibody, this is the most common form of passive immunization. Preformed antibodies may also be given to a person exposed to potentially lethal toxins under circumstances in which there may be insufficient time for a proper immune response. These can include persons exposed to snake venom or tetanus toxin. While temporarily providing protection, passively acquired antibodies survive in the individual only for a short period.

More commonly, vaccines are utilized to provide active immunization by stimulating the acquired host defenses. These vaccines generally utilize inactivated or attenuated parasites that stimulate specific cellular or humoral responses. The prototypes of active immunization are the polio vaccines developed by Jonas Salk and Albert Sabin in the 1950's. Salk's vaccine utilizes a formalin-inactivated poliovirus, while Sabin's consists of attenuated virus. While controversy exists regarding which is superior, both vaccines act in basically the same manner. Exposure to either vaccine results in the production of protective antibodies in the circulation of the individual. In the event of actual infection by poliovirus, the agent would be neutralized before it could reach its target in the central nervous system. Analogous vaccines have been developed against previously common viral diseases such as smallpox, measles, and mumps, and against bacterial diseases such as pertussis (whooping cough) and diphtheria.

The process by which the acquired immune process functions is in part defined by the nature of the antigen. It is also important to remember that the humoral and cellular defense systems are not self-exclusive; each functions in conjunction with the other. If the antigen in question is a bacterium, it is primarily the role of the humoral system to deal with the infection. This can take several forms. The antibody may bind to the surface of the cell, inactivating the cell wall or membrane enzymes, resulting in the death of the cell. The antibody-antigen (bacterium) complex may also activate the complement pathway, resulting in either opsonization or the formation of a membrane attack complex by complement components. Indeed, antibody binding by itself may result in opsonization.

If the antigen is a virus-infected cell, the cellular portion of the response comes into play. Cytotoxic T cells can bind to the target through specific receptors, causing the death of the virus-infected cell. If an antibody binds to viral receptors on the infected cell, cytotoxic cells with receptors for the antibody may show increased affinity for the target in a process called antibody-dependent cell-mediated cytotoxicity (ADCC). The result is the death of the target. The antibody may also serve to neutralize a cell-free virus before the particle can even infect the target cell. Certain bacteria, however, such as the mycobacteria associated with tuberculosis and leprosy, are actually found as intracellular parasites. In such cases, it is the cellular immune system that plays a major role in defense. In this manner, the humoral and cellular defense mechanisms complement each other.

Failure of the immune system to function is clearly illustrated in persons infected with the human immunodeficiency virus (HIV), the virus that causes AIDS. HIV infects the subclass of T lymphocytes called T helper cells. The eventual result is the death and depletion of this subclass of cells. As briefly described earlier, T helper cells are central to the function of both the humoral and the cellular arms of acquired immunity. The interaction of these cells with B lymphocytes is necessary for both antibody production by these cells and their proliferation. The T helper cell is also required for activation and proliferation of the CD8+ cytotoxic T cells.

As AIDS progresses in the individual, the T-helper subclass becomes increasingly depleted. As a result, both the cellular and humoral immune systems become progressively less functional. The person becomes more susceptible to opportunistic organisms in the environment and eventually succumbs to any of a wide variety of diseases.

In rare congenital cases, only certain aspects of the

immune system are nonfunctional. These often tragic examples serve to illustrate the role of various cells within the host defense. For example, children with B-cell deficiencies suffer from repeated bacterial infections, while yeast and viral infections rarely result in problems. Children in whom the thymus fails to develop (DiGeorge or Nezelof syndromes), however, suffer from repeated viral infections but rarely from bacterial infections.

Severe combined immunodeficiency syndrome (SCID) affects approximately one of every 150,000 live births. This genetic disorder is the result of a lack of the enzyme adenosine deaminase (ADA), which ultimately causes a lack of functioning T cells. For years, patients with this disorder had been doomed to living in sterile bubble environments and would die at a young age because of their inability to fight even the mildest infection. Bone marrow transplants for patients with compatible donors can sometimes strengthen the immune system; however, this option is not available for everyone.

In 1990, two unrelated girls with SCID, four and nine years old, were the subject of the first clinical trial of gene therapy. T cells in their blood were isolated and cultured, and normal copies of the ADA gene were introduced into the cells. The genetically engineered T cells were then infused back into the patients over a period of approximately two years. Both girls showed remarkable improvement, with near normal levels of ADA and functioning immune systems, and were thereafter able to lead normal lives. These positive results remained several years after cessation of the actual gene therapy, indicating that this first clinical trial of gene therapy was a success. The door is now open for using gene therapy on other disorders, including those of the immune system.

Host defenses are also utilized within the homeostatic process, which can be defined as maintaining the status quo. An example of such a process is the role of the immune system in protecting humans against various forms of cancer. Although immunosuppressed individuals appear to be at no greater risk for most cancers than normal persons, certain types of skin cancers, as well as certain types of B-cell lymphomas, arise more frequently in these persons. Thus, it is likely that the immune system plays at least some role in protecting the individual from certain forms of cancer. Artificial stimulation of the immune system has, however, been utilized in an attempt to treat sundry forms of advanced cancers. The process involves the removal of immune cells from the patient and the incubation of those cells with a form of interferon generally secreted by T helper cells during their regulation of the immune response. The cells are then returned to the patient. The theory is that, by nonspecifically stimulating cytotoxic cells, some of those cells may serve to destroy the cancer. In some instances, patients have shown improvement.

Clearly, the immune system functions by means of a complex process of cellular interactions. The initial encounter with a foreign infectious agent utilizes an innate system that serves as a first line of defense. Then, through a type of learning process, a specific immune response is generated that provides a more rapid, more efficient means of generating protection.

PERSPECTIVE AND PROSPECTS

Manipulating the host's immune system in order to protect against disease dates back more than a thousand years. In order to protect themselves against smallpox, the Chinese carried out a practice called variolation, in which dried crusts obtained from the pocks of mild cases were inhaled. The practice was copied by early Arabic physicians and eventually made its way to eighteenth century Europe. In the late eighteenth century, an English country physician, Edward Jenner, observed that dairy maids who had recovered from a mild disease called cowpox rarely exhibited the scars associated with smallpox. Jenner reasoned that a person who had been exposed to the cowpox agent would be protected against smallpox. Jenner tested his theory and was proved correct. Smallpox became the first disease that could be prevented by vaccination.

Competition between French and German scientists during the late nineteenth century resulted in much of the existing basic knowledge of host defenses. A Russian, Élie Metchnikoff, working with Louis Pasteur in Paris during the 1880's, developed the views of cellular immunity that are still current. In that same period, the work of Emil von Behring and Paul Ehrlich in Berlin established the role of humoral immunity in protecting against disease.

Active immunization remains the primary method by which an individual may be protected from disease, but the process lends itself to a variety of problems. Not all antigenic determinants of the bacterium or parasite in question are equally important. A response to some antigens may actually hinder the immune response to more important determinants. Furthermore, some individuals react inappropriately to some vaccines, resulting in severe allergic reactions.

For these reasons, much research involves the attempt to isolate only the desired antigen for the vaccine. This has taken several approaches. Purified components, rather than the entire organism, have been used in some vaccines. In some cases, the gene that encodes the desired antigen has been isolated and spliced into the genetic material of a harmless organism. Such an approach has been used to produce a modified hepatitis B vaccine. The gene encoding the surface antigen of the virus has been spliced into the genome of vaccinia, long used for vaccination against smallpox. When the individual is vaccinated, the hepatitis gene is expressed (though no virus can be made), and the person becomes immune to the disease. In theory, whole cocktails of vaccines can be prepared in a similar manner.

New illnesses and other environmental hazards that affect host defenses continue to arise. AIDS may be unusually lethal, but as a previously unknown disease, it is by no means unique. Nevertheless, the ability of the host immune system to respond to new infectious agents remains a bulwark for maintaining the health of an individual.

—Richard Adler, Ph.D.;
updated by Karen E. Kalumuck, Ph.D.

See also Bacterial infections; Bacteriology; Blood and blood disorders; Cells; Glands; Immune system; Immunization and vaccination; Immunology; Immunopathology; Infection; Skin; Sweating; Urinary system; Viral infections.

FOR FURTHER INFORMATION:

Adelman, Daniel C., et al., eds. *Manual of Allergy and Immunology.* 4th ed. Philadelphia: Lippincott Williams & Wilkins, 2002. Examines research developments and the clinical diagnosis and treatment of allergies and immune disorders. Topics include asthma, disorders of the eye, diseases of the lung, anaphylaxism, insect allergies, drug allergies, rheumatic diseases, transplantation immunology, and immunization.

Bibel, Debra Jan, ed. *Milestones in Immunology.* New York: Springer-Verlag, 1988. A compendium of historic articles related to the development of immunology. In association with each original article is an outline explaining the significance of the material. The book presents the evolution of thought in the field in a clear manner, illustrating how knowledge builds upon previous information.

Delves, Peter J., et al. *Roitt's Essential Immunology.* 11th ed. Malden, Mass.: Blackwell, 2006. Though the chapters explaining the technical aspects of the subject become quite detailed, the introductory material dealing with basic host defense is clear and concise. Numerous photographs are included.

Frank, Steven A. *Immunology and Evolution of Infectious Disease.* Princeton, N.J.: Princeton University Press, 2002. Blends research from molecular biology, immunology, pathogen biology, and population dynamics to discuss how and why parasites vary to escape recognition by the immune system, vaccine design, and the control of epidemics.

Hall, Stephen S. *A Commotion in the Blood: Life, Death, and the Immune System.* New York: Henry Holt, 1997. Discusses the revolution in immunotherapy, traces the story of how doctors have learned to use the immune system to develop a wide array of cutting-edge therapies, details the politics of discovery, and explains the complexities of human blood.

Murray, Patrick R., Ken S. Rosenthal, and Michael A. Pfaller. *Medical Microbiology.* 5th ed. Philadelphia: Elsevier/Mosby, 2005. Focuses on microbes that cause disease in humans. Each chapter consistently presents the etiology, epidemiology, host defenses, identification, diagnosis, prevention, and control of each disease.

Paul, William E., ed. *Immunology: Recognition and Response.* New York: W. H. Freeman, 1991. Paul has assembled a collection of readings from *Scientific American* that deal with the indicated subject. Most of the articles are written at a level that can be understood by persons with a background in basic science.

Playfair, J. H. L., and B. M. Chain. *Immunology at a Glance.* 8th ed. Malden, Mass.: Blackwell, 2005. A collection of short chapters dealing with various aspects of host defense. The material, which is abbreviated, clearly defines the described subjects. The book is written in an introductory manner, though its coverage is extensive.

HOT FLASHES

DISEASE/DISORDER

ALSO KNOWN AS: Hot flushes

ANATOMY OR SYSTEM AFFECTED: Endocrine system, reproductive system

SPECIALTIES AND RELATED FIELDS: Endocrinology, gynecology

DEFINITION: Temporary sensations of warmth experienced by perimenopausal and postmenopausal women in which the upper body feels hot, the skin turns red, and sweating occurs.

KEY TERMS:

complete hysterectomy: surgical removal of the uterus and ovaries

hormone replacement therapy (HRT): estrogen/progesterone given to postmenopausal women to alleviate symptoms associated with the menopause

natural menopause: the point at which a woman has not had her menstrual cycle for twelve consecutive months

night sweats: hot flashes that occur at night, typically during sleep

vasomotor symptoms: symptoms relating to nerves and muscles that cause blood vessels to constrict or dilate

CAUSES AND SYMPTOMS

Hot flashes are the most common complaint of perimenopausal and postmenopausal women, whether the menopause occurs naturally as a function of age or is artificially induced, either surgically (by complete hysterectomy) or chemically (using chemotherapy or medication that interferes with ovarian function). Hot flashes are a vasomotor response to decreased levels of estrogen circulating in the bloodstream. When hot flashes occur, skin temperature rises, causing the face and upper body (or in some cases the entire body) to become hot, red, and sweaty. Flushing may also be accompanied by feelings of palpitations, anxiety, and irritability.

While the underlying physiology of hot flashes is not fully understood, it is believed to involve a disturbance in thermoregulation. Normally, the thermoregulatory mechanism in the brain, called the hypothalamus, responds to any increase in body temperature above approximately 100 degrees by sweating in order to cool off. Postmenopausal women instead sweat in response to any rise in temperature, even if it is from 96 to 97 degrees while sleeping. It appears that with declining circulating estrogen levels, norepinephrine levels rise in the brain, resulting in a downward resetting of the normal thermoregulatory set point, falsely causing women to believe that they are overheating. In response, blood vessels dilate, producing the vasomotor symptoms experienced as hot flashes.

TREATMENT AND THERAPY

Women suffering from hot flashes should wear cool clothing; keep room temperatures cool; sleep with light blankets; drink cold beverages; limit intake of caffeine, alcohol, and spicy foods; avoid smoking; use relaxation techniques; and get regular exercise.

INFORMATION ON HOT FLASHES

CAUSES: Vasomotor response to decreased levels of estrogen with menopause

SYMPTOMS: Elevated temperature in face and upper body, red skin, sweating, palpitations, anxiety, irritability

DURATION: Temporary

TREATMENTS: Lifestyle factors (cool room temperatures, light blankets at night, cool clothing, relaxation techniques, regular exercise, avoidance of smoking, cold beverages, limited intake of caffeine, alcohol, or spicy foods; hormone replacement therapy; alternative medicine (soy, phytoestrogens)

If these measures do not alleviate hot flashes, then medical treatment is available. The most effective treatment involves estrogen (or estrogen/progesterone) replacement, which serves to reset the thermoregulatory mechanism to a higher (normal) level, so that hot flashes no longer occur. While hormone replacement therapy (HRT) is effective in alleviating hot flashes, recent research has shown that it may have undesirable long-term effects relating to cancer, heart disease, and cognitive function. Alternative treatments, including the use of soy and phytoestrogens, are becoming increasingly popular. Current research indicates that paroxetine, a selective serotonin reuptake inhibitor (SSRI), appears to be effective in alleviating hot flashes.

PERSPECTIVE AND PROSPECTS

Approximately 80 percent of women experience hot flashes during the menopause. Symptoms are most frequent and intense for the first two to four years following the cessation of menstruation. Ongoing research is attempting to identify effective treatment modalities that do not lead to long-term adverse effects.

—*Robin Kamienny Montvilo, R.N., Ph.D.*

See also Aging; Endocrinology; Gynecology; Hormone replacement therapy (HRT); Hormones; Hyperhidrosis; Menopause; Menstruation; Sweating; Women's health.

FOR FURTHER INFORMATION:

Budoff, Penny. *No More Hot Flashes—and Even More Good News.* New York: Warner Books, 1999.

Northrup, Christiane. *The Wisdom of Menopause: Cre-

ating Physical and Emotional Health and Healing During the Change. New York: Bantam, 2006.

Stenchever, Morton A., et al. *Comprehensive Gynecology.* 4th ed. St. Louis: Mosby, 2006.

HUMAN GENOME PROJECT. *See* GENOMICS.

HUMAN IMMUNODEFICIENCY VIRUS (HIV)

DISEASE/DISORDER

ANATOMY OR SYSTEM AFFECTED: Immune system

SPECIALTIES AND RELATED FIELDS: Immunology, microbiology, virology

DEFINITION: A retrovirus that attacks cells of the immune system, leading to a loss of immune function and the development of acquired immunodeficiency syndrome (AIDS).

Human immunodeficiency virus (HIV), the pathogen that causes AIDS. (PhotoDisc)

CAUSES AND SYMPTOMS

HIV is a human retrovirus containing two copies of a 9,749-base ribonucleic acid (RNA) molecule as its genetic material. Among the proteins carried by retrovirus particles is an enzyme called reverse transcriptase, which upon infection of the cell transcribes the RNA genome into a DNA copy. The DNA copy then integrates into a human chromosome and is maintained in a form called a provirus. The provirus acts as a template to produce copies of the HIV RNA genome. Once the provirus has integrated, infection is irreversible.

> ### INFORMATION ON HUMAN IMMUNODEFICIENCY VIRUS (HIV)
>
> **CAUSES:** Transmission through exchange of body fluids (semen, vaginal fluid, blood, human milk)
>
> **SYMPTOMS:** Flulike or mononucleosis-like symptoms upon initial transmission; later, various opportunistic infections
>
> **DURATION:** Chronic, eventually fatal
>
> **TREATMENTS:** Highly active antiretroviral therapy (HAART) with nucleoside or nucleotide analogues, reverse transcriptase inhibitors, protease inhibitors, inhibitors of cellular entry

HIV falls into the subgroup of retroviruses called lentiviruses, "slow viruses" that do not cause a disease state until many years after infection. For example, the period of time between HIV infection and development of disease averages between five and ten years in untreated persons. Despite the absence of symptoms, the person may be infectious during this period.

There are two forms of HIV. HIV-1, which arose in Central Africa, is the predominant form throughout most of the world, including the United States. HIV-2, a less common form found in western Africa, is less harmful and reproduces more slowly. These viruses evolved from related agents called simian immunodeficiency viruses (SIV) in apes and monkeys. HIV-1 is believed to have arisen from SIV found in chimpanzees in either the Republic of Congo or Cameroon, while HIV-2 is believed to have arisen from SIV of the Sootey Mangabey monkey of western Africa.

HIV is transmitted only through the exchange of body fluids, including semen, vaginal fluid, blood, and human milk. Therefore, the primary routes are sexual transmission, the use of dirty needles by intravenous drug users, and HIV-positive mother-to-child transmission during childbirth or from HIV-contaminated breast milk. Transmission through dirty needles used in body piercing or tattooing may occur. Early in the AIDS epidemic, infection was also acquired through the transfusion of contaminated blood or blood products, leading to a very high rate of transmission to hemophiliacs. Today, such transmission is extremely rare, as the blood supply is routinely tested for HIV.

TREATMENT AND THERAPY

The lack of fidelity associated with replication of HIV results in a high number of mutations, making it difficult for the immune system of the infected host to respond as it would to infections by other viruses. Consequently, no effective vaccine to prevent infection with HIV has been developed. The Food and Drug Administration (FDA) has approved some two dozen drugs to treat HIV infection; more are in clinical trials. These drugs fall into four categories: nucleoside or nucleotide analogues, which act as direct inhibitors of reverse transcriptase; inhibitors that indirectly inhibit reverse transcriptase by binding to the enzyme; protease inhibitors that interfere with the processing of HIV proteins and assembly of progeny viruses; and inhibitors of entry of HIV into the cell. Because the virus has a very high rate of mutation, resistance to individual anti-HIV drugs may appear quickly. Present therapy, called highly active antiretroviral therapy (HAART), involves the use of three or four anti-HIV drugs simultaneously. HAART therapy, also termed "cocktail therapy," increases efficacy and reduces the probability of developing simultaneous resistance of HIV to all three or four drugs being used.

—*Ralph R. Meyer, Ph.D.;*
updated by Richard Adler, Ph.D.

See also Acquired immunodeficiency syndrome (AIDS); Autoimmune disorders; Immune system; Immunodeficiency disorders; Immunology; Immunopathology; Sexually transmitted diseases (STDs); Viral infections.

FOR FURTHER INFORMATION:

Fan, Hung, Ross F. Conner, and Luis P. Villarreal. *The Biology of AIDS.* 4th ed. Sudbury, Mass.: Jones & Bartlett, 2000.

Matthews, Dawn D., ed. *AIDS Sourcebook.* 3d ed. Detroit: Omnigraphics, 2003.

Stine, Gerald J. *AIDS Update 2007.* Upper Saddle River, N.J.: Prentice Hall, 2007.

Strauss, James, and Ellen Strauss. *Viruses and Human Disease.* San Diego, Calif.: Academic Press, 2002.

HUMAN PAPILLOMAVIRUS (HPV)
DISEASE/DISORDER

ALSO KNOWN AS: Papovaviruses

ANATOMY OR SYSTEM AFFECTED: Anus, genitals, reproductive system, skin

SPECIALTIES AND RELATED FIELDS: Epidemiology, gynecology, oncology, public health, virology

DEFINITION: A group of viruses, some of which are sexually transmitted and associated with genital warts and genital cancer.

KEY TERMS:

cervical cancer: cancer of the cervix that is associated with human papillomavirus

Gardasil: a vaccine against the common forms of human papillomavirus that cause cervical cancer

genital warts: warts occurring in the genital and anal areas and often associated with cancer of the reproductive tract

Pap smear: a screening test to detect precancerous and cancerous cells of the cervix

CAUSES AND SYMPTOMS

Papillomaviruses are deoxyribonucleic acid (DNA) viruses than infect the skin and mucous membranes. Human papillomaviruses belong to a group of papillomaviruses that consists of nearly 120 strains. Most strains are virtually harmless, causing nothing more than benign skin warts (papillomas), while others cause genital warts (condyloma acuminate) and may cause cancer.

Sexual contact is the primary mechanism by which the virus is acquired. About thirty HPV strains are sexually transmitted and can infect the external genitalia, urethra, anus, rectum, and sometimes the mouth and throat. Some low-risk strains cause genital warts, while the ten more virulent, high-risk strains cause abnormal

---

INFORMATION ON HUMAN PAPILLOMAVIRUS (HPV)

CAUSES: Viral infection spread through skin (usually sexual) contact

SYMPTOMS: Warts or cancer in genital and anal areas

DURATION: Acute in initial infection, then chronic and often recurrent

TREATMENTS: For warts, topical ointments, creams, resins, or gels and electrocautery, cryosurgery, or laser surgery; for cancer, chemotherapy, radiation, surgery; prevention possible with vaccine

Papanicolaou (Pap) smears and can in some instances cause cancer of the cervix, vagina, vulva, penis, scrotum, anus, and/or the mouth and pharynx. Almost all cases of cervical cancer are the result of persistent HPV infection.

HPV is one of the most common sexually transmitted diseases (STDs). It has been estimated that more than 50 percent of sexually active people and up to 75 percent of sexually active women will develop an HPV infection during their lifetimes. Although the active viral infection is usually cleared by the immune system within a few months, it often remains dormant and can later cause a reinfection. Babies of infected women may contract potentially life-threatening HPV infections during delivery.

Women are more susceptible to developing genital warts. Many infected people, however, do not have genital warts. Infected women who are asymptomatic are often diagnosed by an abnormal Pap smear. In 2003, the Food and Drug Administration (FDA) approved the use of testing for high-risk HPV DNA as a routine screening procedure. DNA testing is also used as a confirmatory test for HPV after an abnormal Pap test.

Frequent Pap tests are the best way to diagnose HPV infections in asymptomatic women. About 10 percent of HPV-infected women will develop precancerous changes in their cervix, and about 8 percent of these women will develop the early stages of cervical cancer. Since persistent HPV infection is a hallmark of developing cervical cancer and since the cancer usually develops slowly over five to ten years, early diagnosis and treatment can be effective in preventing cervical cancer.

Genital warts are highly contagious and are transmitted through skin-to-skin contact from sexual activity. Risk reduction for HPV infection can be achieved by reducing the frequency of sexual contact. Condom use may partially reduce the risk of HPV infection in women. Since condoms do not cover all infected areas, however, their use does not eliminate the risk of infection. Research has suggested that microbicides may prevent infection if they are applied before sexual activity.

TREATMENT AND THERAPY

Since there is no cure for an HPV infection, the primary treatments are for warts. Some treatments involve the use of topical ointments, creams, resins, and gels such as imiquimod (Aldara), podophyllin and podofilox (Condylox), and 5-fluorouracil, as well as trichloroacetic acid. Alternatively, warts may be removed by electrocautery, cryosurgery, laser, or conventional surgery.

In 2006, the FDA approved Gardasil, developed by Merck, for use as a preventive vaccine for the most prevalent HPV strains that cause cervical cancer and genital warts. Gardasil is active against two low-risk HPV strains that are the leading cause of genital warts and two high-risk strains that cause up to 70 percent of cervical cancers in the United States. Gardasil is recommended for females between the ages of nine and twenty-six. Routine Pap testing is still recommended, since Gardasil does not protect against all strains of HPV. GlaxoSmith Kline is also developing an HPV vaccine known as Cervarix.

PERSPECTIVE AND PROSPECTS

HPV was first described as a cause of skin warts in 1907. The relationship between sexual activity and cervical cancer was noted when it was discovered that women who have or who have had multiple sexual partners have a greater risk of developing cervical cancer than do women who have had few or no sexual partners. It was not until the 1980's that HPV was linked to cervical cancer.

The mechanism by which HPV causes cancer has recently been determined. Two proteins encoded by HPV DNA attach to and inactivate cellular proteins that control cell division. With these cellular proteins inactivated, the cell multiplies uncontrollably. Current research is directed toward the development of a vaccine that would inactivate the viral proteins that bind to and inhibit the proteins controlling cell division.

Since sisters of women with cervical cancer have a higher risk of developing cervical cancer, it is thought that genetics may be involved in the progression of the disease.

—*Charles L. Vigue, Ph.D.*

See also Cancer; Carcinogens; Cervical, ovarian, and uterine cancers; Genital disorders, female; Genital disorders, male; Gynecology; Immunization and vaccination; Pap smears; Reproductive system; Screening; Sexually transmitted diseases (STDs); Skin; Skin cancer; Skin disorders; Viral infections; Warts; Women's health.

FOR FURTHER INFORMATION:

Crum, Christopher P., and Gerard J. Nuovo. *Genital Papillomaviruses and Related Neoplasms.* New

York: Raven Press, 1991. An overview of HPV and its role in disease.

Eifel, Patricia J., and Charles Levenback, eds. *Cancer of the Female Lower Genital Tract.* Hamilton, Ont.: B. C. Becker, 2001. Several chapters are dedicated to cervical cancer. Well illustrated with numerous color photographs.

Gross, Gerd, and Geo von Krogh, eds. *Human Papillomavirus Infections in Dermatovenereology.* Boca Raton, Fla.: CRC Press, 1997. An overview of skin diseases caused by HPV. Each chapter is by a different expert. Illustrated with black-and-white photographs.

McCance, Dennis J., ed. *Human Papilloma Viruses.* New York: Elsevier Science, 2002. An overview of HPV including its role in causing disease. Each chapter was written by an expert in the field.

Mindel, Adrian, ed. *Genital Warts: Human Papillomavirus Infection.* Boston: Arnold, 1995. Each chapter is by a different expert. Several chapters are devoted to HPVs association with cancer. Illustrated with several black-and-white photographs.

Sterling, Jane C., and Stephen K. Tyring, eds. *Human Papillomaviruses: Clinical and Scientific Advances.* New York: Arnold, 2001. An excellent book illustrated with numerous colored photographs. Each chapter is by a different investigator in the field.

HUNTINGTON'S DISEASE
DISEASE/DISORDER

ALSO KNOWN AS: Huntington's chorea

ANATOMY OR SYSTEM AFFECTED: Brain, nerves, nervous system

SPECIALTIES AND RELATED FIELDS: Biotechnology, genetics, neurology, psychiatry, psychology

DEFINITION: In this autosomal dominant genetic neurodegenerative disease, patients have uncoordinated movements as a result of neuron degeneration.

CAUSES AND SYMPTOMS

The mutated gene responsible for Huntington's disease is located on one arm of chromosome 4 and produces the protein huntingtin. The gene contains repeats of the triplet nucleotide sequence CAG. Normal individuals have between nine and thirty-five (on average eighteen or nineteen) CAG repeats in their genes; affected individuals have forty or more repeats, with an average of forty-six repeats. Individuals with between thirty-six and thirty-nine repeats may or may not develop Hun-

> ### INFORMATION ON HUNTINGTON'S DISEASE
> **CAUSES:** Genetic protein defect
> **SYMPTOMS:** Uncoordinated movements (chorea), loss of muscle control (dystonias), personality changes, gradual loss of cognition, death
> **DURATION:** Progressive, eventually fatal
> **TREATMENTS:** Tricyclic antidepressants for psychological problems and neuroleptics for chorea

tington's disease. The disease always occurs if the expansion is forty or more repeats. The larger the number of repeats above forty, the earlier the onset of the disease. The disease-causing gene is dominant, so those who inherit the mutated gene develop the disease and have a 50 percent chance of passing the defective gene on to their children.

The triplet CAG codes for the amino acid glutamine. Mutant forms of the huntingtin proteins have forty or more glutamines in the protein. Huntington's disease appears to be caused by a mutation involving a gain of function, in which the expanded polyglutamine region makes the mutant huntingtin protein toxic. Aggregates of mutant huntingtin are observed in the neurons of those who died from Huntington's disease. Normal huntingtin appears to keep neurons alive by stopping programmed cell death.

The neuropathology of Huntington's disease is primarily the degeneration of neurons of the striatum (part of the basal ganglia) and the motor cortex. Clinical manifestations of Huntington's disease typically begin in midlife (thirties and forties), with characteristic motor abnormalities such as uncoordinated movements (chorea) and loss of muscle control (dystonias), personality changes, a gradual loss of cognition, and eventually, death. Huntington's disease primarily affects the central nervous system, but most patients actually die of heart or respiratory complications from long confinement to bed or from head injuries caused by frequent falls.

TREATMENT AND THERAPY

The present treatment for Huntington's disease is the use of drugs such as tricyclic antidepressants to control psychological problems and neuroleptics to treat the associated chorea. In 2003, clinical trials were examining the effects of implanting fetal neurons into the brains of Huntington's disease patients.

PERSPECTIVE AND PROSPECTS

In 1872, George Huntington first reported this hereditary disease that he observed in a Long Island, New York, family. Because of the uncoordinated movements of patients, he termed the condition "chorea," from the Greek word for "dance." In 1981, Nancy Wexler began to study a large extended family with Huntington's disease in an isolated village on Lake Maracaibo, Venezuela. Studies of this family aided the work of localizing the gene responsible for this disease. In 1993, that gene was identified by the collaborative work of fifty-eight scientists, led by James R. Gusella and Francis S. Collins.

—Susan J. Karcher, Ph.D.

See also Brain; Brain disorders; Genetic diseases; Motor neuron diseases; Nervous system; Neuralgia, neuritis, and neuropathy; Neurology; Neurology, pediatric; Tics.

FOR FURTHER INFORMATION:

Baréma, Jean. *The Test: Living in the Shadow of Huntington's Disease.* New York: Franklin Square Press, 2005.

Bates, Gillian, Peter S. Harper, and Lesley Jones, eds. *Huntington's Disease.* 3d ed. New York: Oxford University Press, 2002.

Cattaneo, Elena, Dorotea Rigamonti, and Chaiara Zuccato. "The Enigma of Huntington's Disease." *Scientific American* 287 (December, 2002): 92-97.

Lewis, Ricki. *Human Genetics: Concepts and Applications.* 7th ed. New York: McGraw-Hill, 2007.

Nussbaum, Robert L., Roderick R. McInnes, and Willard F. Huntington. *Thompson and Thompson Genetics in Medicine.* Rev. 6th ed. Philadelphia: W. B. Saunders, 2004.

Rubinsztein, David C. "Lessons from Animal Models of Huntington's Disease." *Trends in Genetics* 18 (April 4, 2002): 202-209.

HYDROCELECTOMY

PROCEDURE

ANATOMY OR SYSTEM AFFECTED: Genitals, reproductive system

SPECIALTIES AND RELATED FIELDS: General surgery, urology

DEFINITION: The removal of a hydrocele, a collection of fluid between the lining membranes protecting the testicle in the scrotum.

INDICATIONS AND PROCEDURES

Hydrocelectomy is primarily indicated for hydroceles in adults which produce discomfort, objectionable scrotal enlargement, or an uncertainty regarding underlying testicular abnormalities upon scrotal ultrasound or physical examination. The presence of a hydrocele does not necessarily require surgical intervention, drainage, or other intervention; it must be accompanied by some significant abnormality to require surgery.

Hydroceles occur in 1 percent of adult males. In patients between the ages of eighteen and thirty-five, the presence of an underlying testicular tumor must be ruled out. Accurate diagnosis can be carried out through physical examination. A hydrocele is a smooth, cystlike mass completely surrounding the testicle such that only the mass can be palpated; the testis, inside, cannot be felt. Hydroceles do not involve the spermatic cord. When a light is shined through the cyst, the light is readily transmitted. If the hydrocele is large or tense and the testis cannot be examined, ultrasound examination can eliminate the diagnosis of a testicular abnormality.

Surgical excision is the most effective method for treatment and can be done on an outpatient basis. A 5.0- to 7.6-centimeter (2.0- to 3.0-inch) incision is made in the scrotum, and the wall of the hydrocele is identified and dissected free. The hydrocele sac is removed and its edges sewn or cauterized to eliminate bleeding. The testis is then returned to the scrotum, and the incision is closed. For large hydroceles, a small drainage tube is introduced into the scrotum to limit swelling.

USES AND COMPLICATIONS

The most frequent complication of hydrocele surgery is scrotal swelling, which may continue for eight weeks. Most patients return to full activity within seven to ten days of surgery, however, and recurrences are rare.

In addition to surgical removal, other treatment options include needle aspiration and aspiration with the injection of sclerosing agents. Needle aspiration is rarely effective and increases infection risk. Fluid usually reaccumulates within three months of aspiration. Aspiration with the injection of sclerosing agents such as tetracycline is successful in fewer than 50 percent of patients and usually requires multiple treatments.

—Culley C. Carson III, M.D.

See also Abscess drainage; Cyst removal; Men's health; Reproductive system; Testicular surgery.

FOR FURTHER INFORMATION:

Graham, Sam D., Jr. et al., eds. *Glenn's Urologic Surgery*. 6th ed. Philadelphia: Lippincott Williams & Wilkins, 2004.

Kay, K. W., R. V. Clayman, and P. H. Lange. "Outpatient Hydrocele and Spermatocele Repair Under Local Anesthesia." *Journal of Urology* 130, no. 2 (August, 1983): 269-271.

Sherwood, Lauralee. *Human Physiology: From Cells to Systems*. 6th ed. Belmont, Calif.: Thomson/Brooks/Cole, 2007.

HYDROCEPHALUS
DISEASE/DISORDER

ALSO KNOWN AS: "Water on the brain"

ANATOMY OR SYSTEM AFFECTED: Brain, head, nervous system, psychic-emotional system

SPECIALTIES AND RELATED FIELDS: Critical care, general surgery, neonatology, neurology, perinatology

DEFINITION: A collection of excessive amounts of cerebrospinal fluid (CSF) within the cranial cavity, which can cause increased pressure within the brain and skull, leading to brain tissue damage and, in infants, enlargement of the skull.

KEY TERMS:

cerebrospinal fluid (CSF): the fluid that bathes and nourishes the inner and outer surfaces of the brain and spinal cord

shunt: a tube that is surgically inserted to drain excess fluid away from an area such as the brain

"water on the brain": a common term for hydrocephalus

CAUSES AND SYMPTOMS

Frequently referred to as "water on the brain," hydrocephalus is a disorder most commonly seen in newborns and infants but sometimes occurring in older children and adults. The water is actually a relatively small amount (about 10 cubic centimeters for every kilogram of body weight) of cerebrospinal fluid (CSF), which surrounds and cushions the brain and spinal cord on both the inside and the outside. Within the brain are four CSF-filled spaces called ventricles. The CSF is continuously formed here and then moves down through the central canal, a tube that runs the length of the spinal cord. From the base of the spine, the fluid moves upward on the outside of the spinal cord, returning to the skull, where it covers the outer surfaces of the

INFORMATION ON HYDROCEPHALUS

CAUSES: Congenital defect, head injury, infection, brain hemorrhage, tumor
SYMPTOMS: Enlarged head, lethargy, vomiting, irritability, epilepsy, rigidity of legs, loss of normal reflexes
DURATION: Typically chronic
TREATMENTS: Surgery

brain. Here it is absorbed by the brain's outer lining. If interference occurs in any part of this process, CSF continues to accumulate in the brain. This usually causes increased pressure to develop within the skull. Abnormally high pressure can lead to permanent brain damage and even death. In the infant, this accumulation also causes the skull to enlarge, since the growth regions of the skull have not yet become firm.

Excessive CSF may develop due to overproduction of fluid in the brain, a blockage of the fluid's circulation, or a blockage of fluid reabsorption on the brain's surface. Hydrocephalus can be congenital or may develop as a result of a head injury, infection, brain hemorrhage, or tumor. Congenital hydrocephalus and most hydrocephalus that begins in infancy are characterized by an enlarged head, which continues to grow at an abnormally rapid pace.

Symptoms and signs that accompany congenital hydrocephalus include lethargy, vomiting, irritability, epilepsy, rigidity of the legs, and the loss of normal reflexes. If left untreated, the condition causes drowsiness, seizures, and severe brain damage, leading to death possibly within days or weeks. Hydrocephalus is also often associated with other anomalies of the brain and nervous system, such as spina bifida.

When hydrocephalus develops in older children and adults, the head size will not increase since the growth lines in the bones of the skull have hardened. If the CSF pressure increases, resulting symptoms include headaches, vomiting, vision problems, problems with muscle coordination, and a progressive decrease in mental activity.

TREATMENT AND THERAPY

Diagnosis of hydrocephalus and related nervous system defects sometimes can be made before birth, either by fetal ultrasound or by testing for the presence of an abnormal amount of a brain-associated protein, alpha-fetoprotein, in the pregnant woman's blood. However,

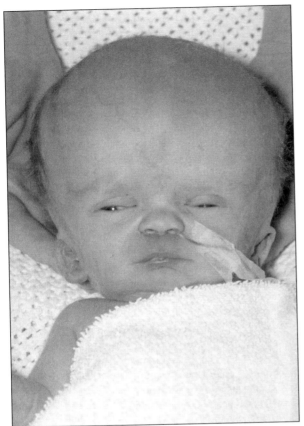

A baby with hydrocephalus. (Custom Medical Stock Photo)

even with early diagnosis and surgical intervention promptly after birth, the prognosis is guarded.

Older children and adults suspected of having hydrocephalus should be examined by a neurologist. A computed tomography (CT) scan or magnetic resonance imaging (MRI) of the brain can visualize the structure of the brain and the extent of the hydrocephalus.

Surgical correction is the primary treatment for hydrocephalus. The excess pressure must be drained from within the brain, or a balance between the production and elimination of CSF must be established. In some cases, a combination of surgery and medication is successful. For example, the drugs furosemide (Lasix) and acetazolamide (Diamox), when used for increased CSF pressure from brain hemorrhage, may reduce the amount of CSF fluid produced and thereby decrease the amount of swelling.

Relieving the CSF pressure within the brain is generally achieved by the surgical insertion of a tube, called a shunt, through brain tissue into one of the cerebral ven-tricles. A one-way valve is attached to the tube; this allows CSF to escape from the skull cavity when the pressure exceeds a certain level. The tubing is then passed beneath the skin into either the right side of the heart or the abdominal cavity, where the excessive CSF can be absorbed safely. Complications of this procedure are fairly common and include repeated infections, septicemia, peritonitis, or meningitis.

PERSPECTIVE AND PROSPECTS

The outcome of treated patients with hydrocephalus has improved over the years, but the condition is still associated with long-term problems. A modest percentage of newborns with congenital hydrocephalus will survive and achieve normal intelligence.

—*Cynthia Breslin Beres*

See also Birth defects; Brain; Brain damage; Brain disorders; Childbirth complications; Critical care, pediatric; Fetal surgery; Meningitis; Mental retardation; Neonatology; Nervous system; Neuroimaging; Neurology, pediatric; Pediatrics; Shunts; Spina bifida; Spinal cord disorders; Surgery, pediatric.

FOR FURTHER INFORMATION:

Behrman, Richard E., Robert M. Kliegman, and Hal B. Jenson, eds. *Nelson Textbook of Pediatrics.* 17th ed. Philadelphia: Saunders, 2004. Text covering all medical and surgical disorders in children, with authoritative information on genetics, endocrinology, etiology, epidemiology, pathology, pathophysiology, clinical manifestations, diagnosis, prevention, treatment, and prognosis.

Cinalli, G., W. J. Maixner, and C. Sainte-Rose, eds. *Pediatric Hydrocephalus.* New York: Springer, 2004. Discusses how genetic research, the use of MRI, neuroendoscopic surgery, and other therapies have had an impact on the diagnosis and treatment of hydrocephalus.

Hydrocephalus Association. http://www.hydroassoc .org/. A Web site that provides information and resources, support, and educational help for patients with hydrocephalus.

Leikin, Jerrold B., and Martin S. Lipsky, eds. *American Medical Association Complete Medical Encyclopedia.* New York: Random House Reference, 2003. A concise presentation of numerous medical illnesses. A good general reference.

Merenstein, Gerald B., and Sandra L. Gardner, eds. *Handbook of Neonatal Intensive Care.* 6th ed. St. Louis: Mosby Elsevier, 2006. A text covering clinical issues such as nutritional and metabolic support and diseases of the neonate.

Parker, James N., and Philip M. Parker, eds. *The Official Parent's Sourcebook on Hydrocephalus.* Rev. ed. San Diego, Calif.: Icon Health, 2002. Draws from public, academic, government, and peer-reviewed research to provide a wide-ranging handbook for families of children with hydrocephalus.

Toporek, Chuck, and Kellie Robinson. *Hydrocephalus: A Guide for Patients, Families, and Friends.* Sebastopol, Calif.: O'Reilly & Associates, 1999. Provides clear advice on living with hydrocephalus.

HYDROTHERAPY

TREATMENT

ANATOMY OR SYSTEM AFFECTED: All

SPECIALTIES AND RELATED FIELDS: Alternative medicine, physical therapy, rheumatology, sports medicine

DEFINITION: Exercise in warm water, which can aid in the treatments of several disorders.

INDICATIONS AND PROCEDURES

Hydrotherapy is one of the oldest therapies still in use. A procedure with origins in ancient Greece has today found a place in alternative medicine. In many hospitals across the United States, physicians advocate hydrotherapy, or water treatment.

One use of hydrotherapy is as an alternative method of exercising for patients with chronic heart failure, since the buoyancy effect reduces loading. Exercises to improve mobility, strength, and cardiovascular fitness can be provided easily in water. Immersion in warm water has been used in bathing resorts in Europe since the beginning of the twentieth century to reduce heart failure symptoms as well as to enhance heart function.

Systemic diseases such as diabetes mellitus, peripheral heart disease, neuropathy, steroid dependence, and venous stasis are major contributing factors to forming chronic wounds. The consequence is a nonhealing wound with hypoxia, infection, edema, and metabolic abnormalities. Patients with such wounds, in need of extensive debridement, are usually advised to be immersed in a full-body whirlpool. The reason behind whirlpool therapy is that whirling and agitation of the water, with injected air, removes contaminants and toxic debris and dilutes bacterial contents. The common therapeutic protocol is a twenty- to thirty-minute session, three to four times per week. Typically, this regimen is continued for a brief period.

Physical therapists have always recommended hydrotherapy to relieve extreme pain. Therefore it is not surprising that it has found a place in providing relief for patients with fibromyalgia.

Another area where hydrotherapy has found popularity is in labor and childbirth. Studies indicate using hydrotherapy for relief of rapid pain and anxiety in labor. Subjective maternal responses to bathing in labor have been favorable. No maternal or infant infections have been attributed to bathing with intact or ruptured membranes. Maternal bathing in labor does not appear to affect Apgar scores or stress hormones at birth.

A recent study indicates that hydrotherapy has proven to be beneficial in treating Rett's syndrome. An

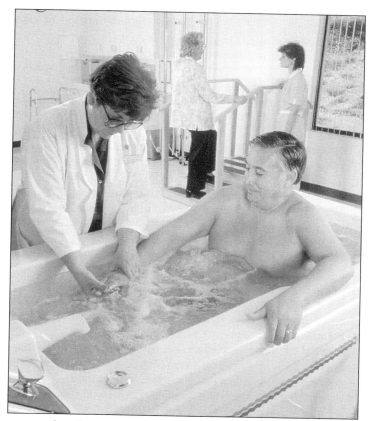

A patient receives a therapeutic bath. (Digital Stock)

eleven-year-old girl with stage III Rett's syndrome was treated with hydrotherapy in a swimming pool twice a week for eight weeks. In conclusion, after the application of hydrotherapy, stereotypical hand movements had decreased and purposeful hand functions and feeding skills had increased.

PERSPECTIVE AND PROSPECTS

Ancient Greek literature contains a considerably large volume of published articles concerning different types of baths and hydrotherapy. These topics were addressed for preventive, hygienic, or therapeutic purposes. These Greek baths were classified in two categories: cold water baths and hot water baths. Cold water baths were said to slow down blood circulation; decrease the amount of sweat; increase muscular strength, the ability to work, and a sense of well-being; and improve physical, mental, and moral balance. The hot water baths were reported to be relaxing, antispasmodic, and beneficial for treating nervous disturbances.

—*Giri Sulur, Ph.D.*

See also Alternative medicine; Cardiac rehabilitation; Childbirth; Colon therapy; Exercise physiology; Fibromyalgia; Healing; Heart failure; Pain management; Physical rehabilitation; Sports medicine.

FOR FURTHER INFORMATION:

Buchman, Dian Dincin. *The Complete Book of Water Healing*. 2d ed. New York: McGraw-Hill/Contemporary Books, 2001.

Cole, Andrew J., and Bruce E. Becker, eds. *Comprehensive Aquatic Therapy*. 2d ed. Philadelphia: Butterworth Heinemann, 2004.

Ruoti, Richard G., David M. Morris, and Andrew J. Cole, eds. *Aquatic Rehabilitation*. Philadelphia: Lippincott, 1997.

Ryrie, Charlie. *The Healing Energies of Water*. North Clarendon, Vt.: Charles Tuttle, 1999.

HYPERADIPOSIS

DISEASE/DISORDER

ALSO KNOWN AS: Severe obesity, extreme obesity
ANATOMY OR SYSTEM AFFECTED: All
SPECIALTIES AND RELATED FIELDS: Biochemistry, endocrinology, family medicine, genetics, nutrition
DEFINITION: Having excess body fat; exceeding 200 percent of standard body weight as defined on a height-weight table.

INFORMATION ON HYPERADIPOSIS

CAUSES: Sedentary lifestyle, genetic predisposition, diet, emotional disorders
SYMPTOMS: Shortness of breath, difficulty breathing, sleep disruption, low back pain, osteoarthritis, skin disorders, excessive sweating, fluid accumulation in the ankles and feet
DURATION: Often chronic
TREATMENTS: Clinical programs combining supervised weight loss, behavior modification, and exercise; surgery if needed

---

CAUSES AND SYMPTOMS

Obesity results from consuming more calories than the body uses. Severe obesity accounts for less than 1 percent of all obesity in the United States but is linked to a large number of deaths each year, many of them due to heart disease or diabetes. Genetics, socioeconomic status, and emotional disturbances may all contribute to severe obesity.

One leading theory proposes that body weight is regulated by a set point in the hypothalamus (a section of the brain), similar to a thermostat setting. A higher-than-normal set point would explain why some people are obese and why losing weight and maintaining weight loss are difficult for them. It is also well established that an increase in the size and/or number of fat cells adds to the amount of fat stored by the body. Those who become obese during early childhood may have up to five times as many fat cells as people of normal weight. Because the number of cells cannot be reduced, weight loss can come about only by decreasing the amount of fat stored in each cell.

Accumulation of excess fat below the diaphragm and in the chest wall places pressure on the lungs, leading to shortness of breath and difficulty in breathing, even with minimal exertion. This may also seriously interfere with sleep. Low back pain and osteoarthritis, especially in the hips, knees, and ankles, may be seen, and skin disorders are common, owing to moisture retention in the folds of the fatty skin. Because of a low ratio of surface area to body weight in severe obesity, the body has a hard time getting rid of excess body heat, leading to excessive sweating and fluid accumulation in the ankles and feet.

Fat tends to accumulate in the abdomen in males, and in the thighs and buttocks in females. Abdominal obesity in particular is linked with a high incidence of coronary artery disease, high blood pressure, adult onset diabetes, hyperlipidemia, and gallbladder disease. In addition, an increase in menstrual disorders and in breast, uterine, and ovarian cancer is seen in women. Men have higher rates of colorectal and prostate cancer.

TREATMENT AND THERAPY

Self-help and nonclinical weight loss programs rarely work in individuals with severe obesity. Clinical programs that combine supervised weight loss, behavior modification, and exercise have shown good results. Drugs such as amphetamines (ephedrine) have questionable value in cases of severe obesity. Total fasting produces a risk of ketonemia and electrolyte imbalances, leading to cardiac arrhythmias.

Surgery has become an increasingly popular form of treatment. Vertical banded gastroplasty (stomach stapling) and gastric bypass are the most common procedures. Both produce satiety with small food intake and, if coupled with exercise, can result in weight losses approximating one-half of the excess weight (80 to 160 pounds). Jejunoileal bypass is also effective but produces a permanent malabsorption syndrome that may lead to other metabolic problems. Liposuction, where a small incision is made and fatty deposits are suctioned out, produces only moderate results in the severely obese. Because of potential risks to blood vessels and nerves, only a small amount of fat can be removed from each location.

Leptin, the protein hormone product of the ob gene, has been suggested as a useful new treatment for severe obesity. However, only about 5 percent of obese individuals fail to produce leptin on their own, and in those individuals either daily injections of leptin or gene therapy to correct the chromosomal defect would be required. Neither is currently considered a practical solution.

PERSPECTIVE AND PROSPECTS

Since 1900, the incidence of severe obesity in the United States has more than doubled, despite the fact that the average number of calories consumed per day has decreased by 10 percent. The most likely explanation is a decrease in physical activity among the population at large. While everyone needs to be conscious of dietary intake and exercise needs, parents of young children in particular need to be careful not to use food as either reward or punishment, as the early years of development appear to be most crucial in setting the stage for later obesity.

—*Kerry L. Cheesman, Ph.D.*

See also Bariatric surgery; Eating disorders; Glands; Leptin; Malnutrition; Nutrition; Obesity; Obesity, childhood; Weight loss and gain; Weight loss medications.

FOR FURTHER INFORMATION:

American Obesity Association. http://www.obesity .org/. A comprehensive Web site with information on the disease, research resources, advocacy, disability issues, community action, and personal stories, among many other topics.

Bjorntorp, Per, ed. *International Textbook of Obesity*. New York: Wiley, 2001. Text that examines the epidemiology, causes, and current research and management.

Brownell, Kelly D., and Katherine Battle Horgen. *Food Fight: The Inside Story of America's Obesity Crisis, and What We Can Do About It*. Chicago: Contemporary Books, 2004. A critical examination of the United States' "toxic environment" of obesity. Explores the roots of the obesity epidemic and its impact on the country's health and productivity.

Goldman, Lee, and Dennis Ausiello, eds. *Cecil Textbook of Medicine*. 22d ed. Philadelphia: W. B. Saunders, 2004. This textbook offers a brief review of all aspects of the problem of obesity by a recognized authority in the field.

Smith, J. Clinton. *Understanding Childhood Obesity*. Tuscaloosa: University of Mississippi Press, 1999. A handbook explaining the basic body processes and the research under way to combat childhood obesity.

Waddon, Thomas A., and Albert J. Stunkard. *Handbook of Obesity Treatment*. Rev. ed. New York: Guilford Press, 2004. A comprehensive text that examines the epidemiology, prevalence, and health consequences of obesity. Topics include binge-eating disorder and night-eating syndrome, energy metabolism, genetics, exercise, behavioral weight control, drug and surgical treatment, and treatment in minorities and children.

HYPERBARIC OXYGEN THERAPY
TREATMENT

ANATOMY OR SYSTEM AFFECTED: Blood, circulatory system, lungs, respiratory system

SPECIALTIES AND RELATED FIELDS: Anesthesiology, biotechnology, critical care, emergency medicine, pulmonary medicine, serology

DEFINITION: In hyperbaric oxygen therapy, patients are placed in a chamber where pure oxygen is circulated in an environment whose air pressure is two or three times higher than that at sea level.

KEY TERMS:

decompression sickness: also called the bends; a condition in which bubbles of nitrogen are introduced into the bloodstream

hypoxia: low oxygen in the tissues

ischemia: loss of blood flow

osteomyelitis: bone infection

INDICATIONS AND PROCEDURES

Hyperbaric oxygen therapy is used in cases that compromise the ability of a person's red blood cells to distribute oxygen throughout the body. This situation usually results in hypoxia, a condition in which the tissues are starved of the life-giving oxygen that they require.

Adult humans consume about three pounds of food and three pounds of water every day. Through respiration, however, they routinely consume twice that amount of oxygen daily. At least one-third of this oxygen enters the bloodstream for distribution to tissues. If these tissues are deprived of oxygen, a condition called ischemia, then they may be destroyed, making people with lowered oxygen levels vulnerable to diseases and infections.

When the oxygen content of the tissues becomes dangerously low, as in cases of hypoxia, immediate treatment is essential. If such treatment is not given, then the results can be fatal. The most effective treatment, often provided in emergency situations, is to place the patient in a hyperbaric chamber, a sealed container in which the atmosphere is gradually increased to a level two or three times greater than that at sea level. Pure (100 percent) oxygen is pumped into the chamber. Patients are confined to such chambers from one hour to an hour and a half.

The air that humans usually breathe contains about 21 percent oxygen and 78 percent nitrogen. The air pressure within the hyperbaric chamber can increase the number of oxygen molecules in the bloodstream by up to 2,000 percent. With this dramatic increase, oxygen begins to enter oxygen-starved tissue and bone cells.

The hyperbaric chamber was initially used to save the lives of deep-sea and scuba divers who ascended too fast from the ocean's depths, causing them to suffer

A patient prepares to enter a hyperbaric oxygen chamber. (Custom Medical Stock Photo)

from decompression sickness (the bends), a potentially fatal condition caused by the formation of nitrogen gas bubbles in the bloodstream. Those suffering from the bends are deprived of the life-sustaining oxygen that the body requires to function effectively. It was found that immersing sufferers in a pressurized environment enabled their red blood cells to absorb sufficient oxygen to nourish their tissues and bones.

Most hospitals set aside rooms into which pure (100 percent) oxygen is piped. Patients in need of hyperbaric oxygen therapy are placed in such rooms and may, through tubes in their noses, be fed the oxygen that they need directly. Such treatment is intermediate. When it proves insufficient, placing patients in pressurized atmospheres for specific lengths of time can result in dramatic increases in the amount of oxygen that they can absorb and in subsequent improvement in their conditions.

USES AND COMPLICATIONS

Besides its use in treating people suffering from the bends, the hyperbaric chamber is employed to treat several other life-threatening conditions. Such therapy is routinely used to treat injuries incurred in automobile or motorcycle accidents in which parts of the body are crushed. Treatment in a hyperbaric chamber heightens the delivery of oxygen to damaged tissues and bones. It can control swelling and limit infection.

Some people have wounds that refuse to heal, such as foot ulcers in diabetic patients whose circulatory systems are compromised, resulting in low oxygen levels. Hyperbaric treatment can increase the amount of oxygen in their bloodstreams and promote healing.

Similarly, such bone infections as osteomyelitis that do not respond to conventional treatment are sometimes controlled by hyperbaric oxygen therapy. The oxygen that such treatment delivers to the bloodstream can control bacterial infections and increase the effectiveness of the body's defensive white blood cells.

Cancer patients undergoing radiation may suffer from scarring and compression of important blood vessels, thereby inhibiting the circulation of oxygen throughout the body. Hyperbaric oxygen therapy aids in increasing such circulation, permitting oxygen to reach damaged cells and keep them from dying. This treatment is often used in treating patients with head and neck cancers.

Carbon monoxide poisoning is a pernicious and potentially fatal form of poisoning. Because carbon monoxide is colorless and odorless, it can affect whole fam-

ilies confined in closed houses with defective heating systems. When victims of such poisoning are rescued, immediate hyperbaric oxygen treatment is essential. Such treatment pumps essential oxygen into the bloodstream and aids the body in expelling carbon monoxide. If treatment is given without delay, then damage to the central nervous system and red blood vessels can be circumvented.

This therapy is being used increasingly in the treatment of burn victims, in whom it may reduce swelling, limit infection, and decrease the effects of lung damage resulting from inhaling smoke and overheated air. Because hyperbaric oxygen therapy is often a choice of last resort for people who are dangerously ill, the risks are high and the rate of fatalities is considerable.

PERSPECTIVE AND PROSPECTS

With the remarkable growth of new procedures in medicine, the outlook for hyperbaric oxygen therapy is bright. Once used almost exclusively to treat the bends, such therapy currently is being found effective in dealing with any health problem in which the circulation of oxygen throughout the body is compromised.

—*R. Baird Shuman, Ph.D.*

See also Altitude sickness; Burns and scalds; Cancer; Circulation; Embolism; Healing; Lungs; Osteomyelitis; Oxygen therapy; Poisoning; Pulmonary medicine; Radiation therapy; Respiration; Ulcers; Vascular medicine; Vascular system; Wounds.

FOR FURTHER INFORMATION:

Jain, K. K. *Textbook of Hyperbaric Medicine.* 4th ed. Cambridge, Mass.: Hogrefe & Huber, 2004.

Oregon Health and Science University Evidence-Based Practice Center. *Hyperbaric Oxygen Therapy for Brain Injury, Cerebral Palsy, and Stroke.* Rockville, Md.: U.S. Dept. of Health and Human Services, Public Health Service, Agency for Healthcare Research and Quality, 2003.

Sheldon, Lisa Kennedy. *Oxygenation.* Thorofare, N.J.: Slack, 2001.

HYPERCHOLESTEROLEMIA
DISEASE/DISORDER

ANATOMY OR SYSTEM AFFECTED: Blood, blood vessels, circulatory system, heart, liver

SPECIALTIES AND RELATED FIELDS: Cardiology, hematology, nutrition, pharmacology, vascular medicine

DEFINITION: A high level of cholesterol in the bloodstream, which is considered a major risk factor for heart attack or stroke.

CAUSES AND SYMPTOMS

It has been difficult for the medical profession to establish a clear, causal connection between high cholesterol in the blood and heart disease. Only by studying a large number of patients over an extended time, as was done at Framingham, Massachusetts, was it possible to establish a now widely accepted statistical correlation between high cholesterol and cardiovascular problems. Cholesterol is a fatty material similar to animal fats, which are called lipids. In the bloodstream, cholesterol lipids combine with proteins to form either a low-density lipoprotein (LDL) or high-density lipoprotein (HDL). LDL transports cholesterol from the liver and intestines to other parts of the body where it is needed. HDL transports excess cholesterol back to the liver, where it is metabolized and excreted. HDL prevents excess fat from being deposited on the walls of arteries and therefore is commonly called the "good" cholesterol. Research has established that LDL in blood should be less than 200 milligrams per deciliter, whereas HDL should be greater than 50 milligrams per deciliter, with a ratio of LDL to HDL of preferably four or less. A person is not aware of having high cholesterol. If the condition is not treated, however, then the likelihood of plaque buildup on artery walls and a possible blockage, causing a stroke or heart attack, is increased.

TREATMENT AND THERAPY

The first step to reduce excess cholesterol in the bloodstream is a change in diet. As a general guideline, the consumption of vegetables, fruits, and grains should be increased, while red meat, egg yolks, and high-fat dairy products should be decreased. Vegetable oils made from corn, olives, or soybeans, which are low in saturated fats, are preferable to butter and animal fats. The next step is to increase physical exercise, which generally raises HDL, the good cholesterol. Several prescription medications, such as Zocor or Lipitor, have been shown to be effective in lowering LDL. A physician needs to monitor a patient's liver function to verify that no harmful side effects are occurring.

PERSPECTIVE AND PROSPECTS

The 1985 Nobel Prize in Medicine was awarded to Drs. Michael Brown and Joseph Goldstein for their study of cell-surface receptors that control the entry of LDL into

> ### INFORMATION ON HYPERCHOLESTEROLEMIA
>
> **CAUSES:** Diet, high levels of low-density lipoproteins (LDLs) and low levels of high-density lipoproteins (HDLs)
> **SYMPTOMS:** Plaque buildup on artery walls and possible blockage, causing stroke or heart attack
> **DURATION:** Chronic
> **TREATMENTS:** Dietary changes (increase in vegetables, fruits, and grains and decrease in red meat, egg yolks, and high-fat dairy products); increased physical exercise; medications (Zocor, Lipitor)

cells. They showed that some people have a deficiency of these receptors. As a result, LDL does not enter cells at the normal rate but continues to circulate in the bloodstream, where it then can adhere to artery walls. In the future, it may be possible to produce drugs that stimulate the body to make more LDL receptors, which would remove excess LDL from the bloodstream.

—*Hans G. Graetzer, Ph.D.*

See also Arteriosclerosis; Blood and blood disorders; Cholesterol; Heart disease; Hyperlipidemia; Lipids; Steroids.

FOR FURTHER INFORMATION:

American Medical Association. *American Medical Association Family Medical Guide*. 4th rev. ed. Hoboken, N.J.: John Wiley & Sons, 2004.
Cooper, Kenneth H. *Controlling Cholesterol the Natural Way*. New York: Bantam Books, 1999.
Kowalski, Robert E. *The New Eight-Week Cholesterol Cure*. New York: Harper & Row, 2006.

HYPERHIDROSIS
DISEASE/DISORDER

ALSO KNOWN AS: Excessive sweating, excessive perspiration
ANATOMY OR SYSTEM AFFECTED: Glands, skin
SPECIALTIES AND RELATED FIELDS: Dermatology, internal medicine, neurology
DEFINITION: Excessive sweating, which may be generalized or limited to certain areas of the body, particularly the hands and feet. The paroxysmal form of this disorder affects approximately 1 percent of the population of the United States.

CAUSES AND SYMPTOMS

The purpose of perspiration is to keep the body at an ideal temperature. The sweat glands are affected by the sympathetic branch of the autonomic nervous system. Two types of sympathetic nerve fibers affect sweat glands: the noradrenergic, which respond to emotional stimuli, and the cholinergic, which respond to temperature. Hyperhidrosis refers to sweating that is greater than is needed to keep the body at a normal temperature.

Hyperhidrosis may be due to a secondary cause, such as hyperthyroidism, hormonal treatments, obesity, the menopause, or severe psychiatric disorders. The immediate cause of primary hyperhidrosis (not attributable to another disorder or condition) is dysfunction of the sympathetic branch of the autonomic nervous system; however, the underlying cause of the dysfunction is not clear.

Hyperhidrosis may affect the entire body (general), or it may affect only specific areas, such as the armpits (axillary), palms of the hands (palmar), soles of the feet (plantar), or face (facial). General hyperhidrosis may be a variation on normal sweating. Paroxysmal localized hyperhidrosis, periodic excessive perspiration in a particular area of the body, may also occur. A genetic predisposition may be present. Persons who are obese are more likely to be affected, as are people with certain forms of eczema. Hyperhidrosis can also occur following frostbite.

Hyperhidrosis can vary in severity from being merely embarrassing to quite disabling. It tends to begin in adolescence and gradually improve with age.

TREATMENT AND THERAPY

Topical antiperspirants applied to the affected areas may control the symptoms. Drugs that block the sympathetic portion of the autonomic nervous system may also be used. Some people with localized sweating respond to iontophoresis, a technique in which the affected area is placed in an electrolyte solution and stimulated with low-level electrical current. Some success has been shown with injections of botulinum toxin (Botox) into the affected areas. This technique has considerable disadvantages, however. Repeated injections are needed, and they are both painful and costly. Furthermore, the injections may cause temporary weakness of the hand muscles. Surgery to the affected areas of the nervous system has a 90 percent success rate for excessive sweating of the palms but is accompanied by numerous complications, including wound infection,

---

INFORMATION ON HYPERHIDROSIS

CAUSES: Hyperthyroidism, hormonal treatments, obesity, menopause, severe psychiatric disorders
SYMPTOMS: Excessive sweating of the armpits, palms, soles, face, or entire body
DURATION: Acute episodes
TREATMENTS: Topical antiperspirants, iontophoresis, Botox injections

---

sweating with eating (gustatory sweating), and recurrent hyperhidrosis. Little evidence exists for the effectiveness of psychotherapy, hypnosis, acupuncture, and herbal or homeopathic remedies.

—*Rebecca Lovell Scott, Ph.D., PA-C*
See also Botox; Dermatology; Glands; Hormones; Host-defense mechanisms; Nervous system; Neurology; Obesity; Skin; Sweating; Thyroid disorders.

FOR FURTHER INFORMATION:

American Medical Association. *American Medical Association Family Medical Guide*. 4th rev. ed. Hoboken, N.J.: John Wiley & Sons, 2004.

Haider, Aamir. "Hyperhidrosis: An Approach to Diagnosis and Management." *Dermatology Nursing* 16, no. 6 (December 1, 2004): 515-518.

Komaroff, Anthony, ed. *Harvard Medical School Family Health Guide*. New York: Free Press, 2005.

Kreyden, O. P., R. Böni, and G. Burg, eds. *Hyperhidrosis and Botulinum Toxin in Dermatology*. New York: S. Karger, 2002.

Stoppard, Miriam. *Family Health Guide*. New York: DK, 2004.

HYPERLIPIDEMIA
DISEASE/DISORDER

ANATOMY OR SYSTEM AFFECTED: Blood
SPECIALTIES AND RELATED FIELDS: Family medicine, hematology, internal medicine, serology, vascular medicine
DEFINITION: The presence of abnormally large quantities of lipids (fats) in the blood.

CAUSES AND SYMPTOMS

Although elevated triglyceride levels have been implicated in clinical ischemic diseases, most investigators believe that cholesterol-rich lipids are a more significant risk factor. Although measurements of both cholesterol and triglyceride levels have been used to predict coronary disease, studies suggest that the determination of the alpha-lipoprotein/beta-lipoprotein ratio is a more reliable predictor. Because the alpha-lipoprotein has a higher density than the beta-lipoprotein, they are more often designated as high-density lipoprotein (HDL) and low-density lipoprotein (LDL), respectively. HDL is often referred to as "good cholesterol," and LDL is referred to as "bad cholesterol." The latter is implicated in the development of atherosclerosis.

Atherosclerosis is a disease that begins in the innermost lining of the arterial wall. Its lesions occur predominantly at arterial forks and branch openings, but they can also occur at sites where there is injury to the arterial lining. The initial lesion usually appears as fatty streaks or spots, which have been detected even at birth. With passing years, more of these lesions appear, and they may develop into elevated plaques that obstruct the flow of blood in the artery. The lesions are rich in cholesterol derived from beta-lipoproteins in the plasma. In addition to elevated blood lipids, other risk factors associated with atherosclerosis include hypertension, faulty arterial structure, obesity, smoking, and stress.

TREATMENT AND THERAPY

The treatment of hyperlipidemia involves both dietary and drug therapies. Although studies in nonhuman primates indicate that the reduction of hyperlipidemia results in decreased morbidity and mortality rates from arterial vascular disease, studies in humans are less conclusive. Initial treatment involves restricting the dietary intake of cholesterol and saturated fat. Drug therapy is instituted when further lowering of the serum lipids is desired. Among the drugs that have been used as antihyperlipidemic agents are lovastatin and its analogues, clofibrate and its analogues (particularly gemfibrozil), nicotinic acid, D-thyroxine, cholestyramine, probucol, and heparin. A simplified diagram of the endogenous biosynthesis and biotransformation of cholesterol is given below.

acetate → C acetyl SCoA → HMGCoA → MVA → squalene → desmosterol → cholesterol → bile acids

Lovastatin blocks the synthesis of cholesterol by inhibiting the enzyme (HMGCoA reductase) that catalyzes the conversion of beta-hydroxy-beta-methyl glutaryl coenzyme A (HMGCoA) to mevalonic acid (MVA), the regulatory step in the biosynthesis of cho-

---

INFORMATION ON HYPERLIPIDEMIA

CAUSES: Hypertension, faulty arterial structure, obesity, smoking, stress
SYMPTOMS: Development of atherosclerosis
DURATION: Varies; often chronic
TREATMENTS: Dietary changes, drug therapy

---

lesterol. Both lovastatin and MVA are beta, delta-dihydroxy acids, but lovastatin has a much more lipophilic (fat-soluble) group attached to it. Clofibrate and gemfibrozil block the synthesis of cholesterol prior to the HMGCoA stage. For this reason, they are likely to inhibit triglyceride formation as well. Nicotinic acid inhibits the synthesis of acetyl coenzyme A (acetyl SCoA) and thus would be expected to block the synthesis of both cholesterol and the triglycerides. To be effective in lowering the serum level of lipids, nicotinic acid must be taken in large amounts, which often produces an unpleasant flushing sensation in the patient. A way to inhibit the synthesis of cholesterol at the post-MVA stages has also been sought. Agents such as triparanol, which inhibit biosynthesis near the end of the synthetic sequence, have been developed. Although they are effective in lowering serum cholesterol, they had to be withdrawn from clinical use because of their adverse side effects on the muscles and eyes. Moreover, the penultimate product in the biosynthesis of cholesterol proved to be atherogenic. Investigations are being conducted on the inhibition of cholesterol synthesis at both the immediate presqualene and immediate postsqualene stages. The effects of such inhibitors on the production of steroid hormones and ubiquinones, as well as on cholesterol and triglycerides, are expected to be of considerable interest.

D-thyroxine promotes the metabolism of cholesterol in the liver, transforming it into the more hydrophilic (water-soluble) bile acids, thereby facilitating its elimination from the body. An approach to reducing the serum level of cholesterol by a process involving the sequestering of the bile acids utilizes the resin cholestyramine as the sequestrant. The sequestered bile acids cannot be reabsorbed into the enterohepatic system and are eliminated in the feces. Consequently, more cholesterol is oxidized to the bile acids, resulting in the reduction of the serum level of cholesterol. Unfortunately, a large quantity of cholestyramine is required. Sequestration of cholesterol with beta-sitosterol prevents both the absorption of dietary cholesterol and the reabsorption of endogenous cholesterol in the intestines. Here, too, a large quantity of the sequestrant needs to be administered.

Probucol is an antioxidant. Because, structurally, it is a sulfur analogue of a hindered hydroquinone, it acts as a free radical scavenger. Evidence suggests that the antihyperlipidemic effect of probucol is attributable to its ability to inhibit the oxygenation of LDL. The oxygenated LDL is believed to be the atherogenic form of LDL. Heparin promotes the hydrolysis of triglycerides as it activates lipoprotein lipase, thereby reducing lipidemia. Because of its potent anticoagulant properties, however, its use in therapy must be closely monitored. Cholesterol that is present in atherosclerotic plaques is acylated, generally by the more saturated fatty acids. The enzyme catalyzing the acylation process is acyl-CoA cholesterol acyl transferase (ACAT). The development of regulators of ACAT and the desirability of reducing the dietary intake of saturated fatty acids are based on this rationale.

Cholesterol within the cell is able to inhibit further synthesis of cholesterol by a feedback mechanism. Cholesterol that is associated with LDL is transported into the hepatic cell by means of the LDL receptor on the surface of the cell. In individuals who are afflicted with familial hypercholesterolemia, an inherited disorder that causes death at an early age, the gene that is responsible for the production of the LDL receptor is either absent or defective. Studies in gene therapy have shown that transplant of the normal LDL receptor gene to such an individual results in a dramatic decrease in the level of the "bad cholesterol" in the serum. Cholesterol derivatives that are oxygenated at various positions have also been found to regulate the serum level of cholesterol by either inhibiting its synthesis or promoting its catabolism. More studies need to be done, however, in order to demonstrate their effectiveness in humans and to establish that they themselves do not induce atherosclerosis.

—*Leland J. Chinn, Ph.D.*

See also Arteriosclerosis; Blood and blood disorders; Cholesterol; Heart disease; Hypercholesterolemia; Hypertension; Insulin resistance syndrome; Lipids; Metabolic syndrome; Metabolism; Obesity.

FOR FURTHER INFORMATION:

Anderson, J. W. "Diet First, Then Medication for Hypercholesterolemia." *JAMA: The Journal of the American Medical Association* 290, no. 4 (July 23, 2003): 531-533. Examines the therapeutic use of anticholesteremic agents and diet therapy as treatment for hyperlipidemia.

Ball, Madeleine, and Jim Mann. *Lipids and Heart Disease: A Guide for the Primary Care Team.* 2d ed. New York: Oxford University Press, 1994. Topics include the function of lipids, plasma lipids and coronary heart disease, atherosclerosis, and hyperlipidemia.

Farnier, Michel, and Jean Davignon. "Current and Future Treatment of Hyperlipidemia: The Role of Statins." *The American Journal of Cardiology* 82, no. 4B (August 27, 1998): 3J-10J. Hyperlipidemia is recognized as one of the major risk factors for the development of coronary artery disease and progression of the atherosclerotic lesions. Dietary therapy together with hypolipidemic drugs is central to the management of hyperlipidemia.

Haffner, Steven M. "Diabetes, Hyperlipidemia, and Coronary Artery Disease." *The American Journal of Cardiology* 83, no. 9B (May 13, 1999): 17F-21F. Type II diabetes is associated with a marked increase in the risk of coronary artery disease. Dyslipidemia is believed to be a major source of this increased risk.

Hirsch, Anita. *Good Cholesterol, Bad Cholesterol: An Indispensable Guide to the Facts About Cholesterol.* New York: Avalon, 2002. Examines the facts on all the varieties of cholesterol, including HDL, LDL, and VDL. Also discusses how to determine what your blood cholesterol test results mean and how to manage cholesterol levels through diet, exercise, and stress management.

McGowan, Mary P., and Jo McGowan Chopra. *Fifty Ways to Lower Cholesterol.* New York: McGraw-Hill, 2002. Provides explanations of both "good" and "bad" cholesterol and the latest information on key treatments, medication, and lifestyle issues.

Rifkind, Basil M., ed. *Drug Treatment of Hyperlipidemia.* New York: Marcel Dekker, 1991. Discusses such topics as hyperlipoproteinemia and antilipemic agents. Includes bibliographical references and an index.

Safeer, Richard S., and Cynthia L. Lacivita. "Choosing Drug Therapy for Patients with Hyperlipidemia." *American Family Physician* 61, no. 11 (June 1, 2000): 3371-3382. Almost thirteen million American adults require drug therapy to meet the low-density lipoprotein goals set by the National Cholesterol Education Program.

Witiak, D. T., H. A. I. Newman, and D. R. Feller, eds. *Antilipidemic Drugs: Medicinal, Chemical, and*

Biochemical Aspects. New York: Elsevier, 1991. Discusses such topics as antilipemic agents, lipids, and lipoproteins. Includes bibliographical references.

HYPERPARATHYROIDISM AND HYPOPARATHYROIDISM
DISEASE/DISORDER

ANATOMY OR SYSTEM AFFECTED: Endocrine system, glands, musculoskeletal system, neck

SPECIALTIES AND RELATED FIELDS: Endocrinology

DEFINITION: Excessive, uncontrolled secretion (hyperparathyroidism) or reduced secretion (hypoparathyroidism) of parathyroid hormone.

CAUSES AND SYMPTOMS

The precise regulation of calcium is vital to the survival and well-being of all animals. Approximately 99 percent of the calcium in the body is found in bones and teeth. Of the remaining 1 percent, about 0.9 percent is packaged within specialized organelles inside the cell. This leaves only 0.1 percent of the total body calcium in blood. Approximately half of this calcium is either bound to proteins or complexed with phosphate. The other half of blood calcium is free to be utilized by cells. For this reason, it is critical that calcium inside the cell be rigorously maintained at extremely low concentrations. Even a slight change in calcium outside the cell can have dramatic consequences.

The function and regulation of calcium. Calcium plays a vital role in many different areas of the body. For example, the entry of calcium into secretory cells, such as nerve cells, triggers the release of neurotransmitters into the synapse. A fall in blood calcium results in the overexcitability of nerves, which can be felt as a tingling sensation and numbness in the extremities. Similarly, calcium entry into cells is essential for muscle contraction in both heart and skeletal muscle.

Free calcium is thus one of the most tightly regulated substances in the body. The key player in the moment-to-moment regulation of calcium is parathyroid hormone (PTH). PTH is synthesized in the parathyroid glands, a paired gland located in the neck, and released in response to a fall in blood calcium. PTH serves several functions: to increase blood calcium, to decrease blood phosphate, and to stimulate the conversion of vitamin D into its active form, which can then stimulate the uptake of calcium across the digestive tract. Together these actions result in an increase in free calcium, which returns calcium concentrations in the blood to normal.

PTH binds to specific receptors located primarily in bone and kidney tissue. Since most calcium is stored in bone, it serves as a bank for withdrawal of calcium in times of need. Activation of a PTH receptor on osteoclasts, or bone-cutting cells, results in the production of concentrated acids that dissolve calcium from bone, thereby making more free calcium available to the blood supply. PTH also acts on the kidney, where it stimulates calcium uptake from the urine while promoting phosphate elimination. As a result, more calcium is made available to the blood and less phosphate is available to form complexes with the free calcium.

By exerting these effects on its target organs, PTH can restore low calcium concentrations in the blood to normal. Once calcium has returned to a particular set point, PTH secretion is slowed dramatically. If PTH release is not controlled, however, the imbalance in calcium can lead to life-threatening situations. These conditions are termed hyperparathyroidism and hypoparathyroidism.

Hyperparathyroidism. This disorder is defined as the excessive and uncontrolled secretion of PTH. The release of a closely related substance, PTH-related protein, from cancer cells can also cause this condition. Hyperparathyroidism is found in 0.1 percent of the population and is more common in the elderly, who have an incidence rate of approximately 2 percent.

There are two types of hyperparathyroidism, primary and secondary. Primary hyperparathyroidism is caused by disease or damage to the parathyroid glands. For example, cancer of the parathyroid gland can result in the uncontrolled release of PTH and is charac-

---

INFORMATION ON HYPERPARATHYROIDISM AND HYPOPARATHYROIDISM

CAUSES: Endocrine disorder, aging, disease, accidental removal of parathyroid gland or damage to its blood supply

SYMPTOMS: Osteoporosis, muscle weakness, nausea, kidney stones, peptic ulcers, muscle cramps, seizures, paranoia, depression

DURATION: Often chronic

TREATMENTS: Drug therapy, hormonal therapy (*e.g.*, estrogen), surgery, vitamin D supplements, calcium restriction or supplements

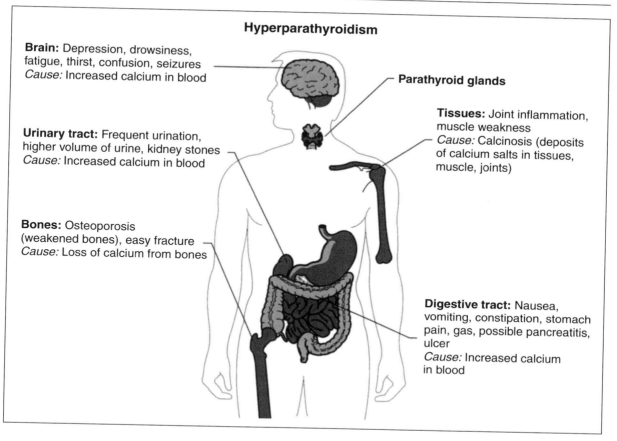

Hyperparathyroidism

Brain: Depression, drowsiness, fatigue, thirst, confusion, seizures
Cause: Increased calcium in blood

Parathyroid glands

Tissues: Joint inflammation, muscle weakness
Cause: Calcinosis (deposits of calcium salts in tissues, muscle, joints)

Urinary tract: Frequent urination, higher volume of urine, kidney stones
Cause: Increased calcium in blood

Bones: Osteoporosis (weakened bones), easy fracture
Cause: Loss of calcium from bones

Digestive tract: Nausea, vomiting, constipation, stomach pain, gas, possible pancreatitis, ulcer
Cause: Increased calcium in blood

terized by an increase in blood calcium. The symptoms associated with primary hyperparathyroidism include osteoporosis, muscle weakness, nausea, and increased incidence of kidney stones and peptic ulcers. These symptoms can all be linked to the presence of excess calcium, which is a result of the oversecretion of PTH.

Secondary hyperparathyroidism often results when PTH cannot function normally, such as in kidney failure or insensitivity of target tissues to PTH. Secondary hyperparathyroidism is usually characterized by an overall decrease in blood calcium levels, even though there is a marked increase in the amount of PTH being released. Its symptoms may include muscle cramps, seizures, paranoia, depression, and, in severe cases, tetany (the tonic spasm of muscles). These symptoms are a direct result of the decline in available calcium.

Hypoparathyroidism. Less common than hyperparathyroidism, hypoparathyroidism is defined by a reduction in the secretion of PTH. This condition is normally characterized by low calcium levels and elevated phosphate levels in response to the lack of PTH. Not only are calcium levels unusually low, but phosphate

levels are unusually high as well, which complicates this condition because phosphate ties up some of the free calcium.

Hypoparathyroidism can also have primary and secondary causes. Primary hypoparathyroidism is known to have two separate origins. The most common is a decrease in PTH release caused by accidental removal of the parathyroid gland. The other is damage of the blood supply around the parathyroid glands. Both occur after there has been some type of surgery or other medical procedure in the neck area. Consequently, the decline in PTH results in low calcium and elevated phosphate concentrations.

Secondary hypoparathyroidism is a frequent complication of cirrhosis and is characterized by a decrease in both calcium and magnesium concentration. Because magnesium is essential for the release of PTH, this condition can be corrected with magnesium replacement.

Complications associated with all types of hypoparathyroidism include hyperventilation, convulsions, and in some cases tetany of the muscle cells.

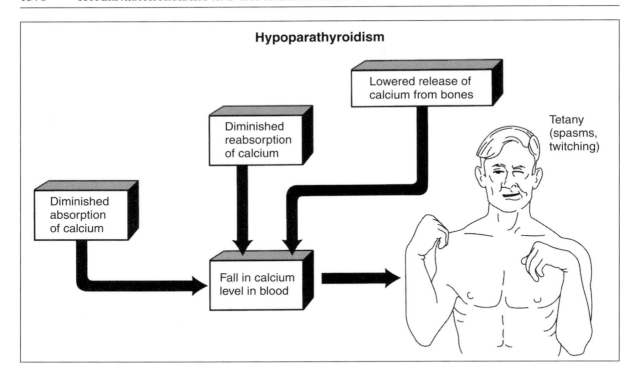

Hypoparathyroidism

Lowered release of calcium from bones

Diminished reabsorption of calcium

Diminished absorption of calcium

Fall in calcium level in blood

Tetany (spasms, twitching)

TREATMENT AND THERAPY

The treatments for primary hyperparathyroidism vary and are dependent on the severity of the condition. Specific drugs can be prescribed that lower elevated blood calcium. Hormone therapy, which includes the administration of estrogen, also acts to restore calcium to normal. Other treatments include dietary calcium restriction and/or surgery to remove the abnormal parathyroid tissue.

Treatment of secondary hyperparathyroidism often involves correcting the problems associated with kidney failure. This can be done by administration of a dietary calcium supplement to restore plasma calcium levels or, in more severe cases, by kidney transplantation. Vitamin D therapy has also been attempted for those patients diagnosed in the early stages of renal failure.

Hypoparathyroidism is usually treated with dietary calcium and vitamin D supplementation. Both of these treatments promote calcium absorption and decrease calcium loss. The duration of the treatment depends on the severity of the condition and may last a lifetime.

—Jeffrey A. McGowan and Hillar Klandorf, Ph.D.

See also Endocrine disorders; Endocrinology; Endocrinology, pediatric; Glands; Hashimoto's thyroiditis; Hormones; Osteoporosis; Stones; Vitamins and minerals.

FOR FURTHER INFORMATION:

Al Zarani, Ali, and Michael A. Levine. "Primary Hyperparathyroidism." *The Lancet* 349, no. 9060 (April 26, 1997): 1233-1238. The authors discuss primary hyperparathyroidism (PHP), a common endocrine disorder characterized by excessive secretion of parathyroid hormone and consequent hypercalcemia.

Bar, Robert S., ed. *Early Diagnosis and Treatment of Endocrine Disorders.* Totowa, N.J.: Humana Press, 2003. Reviews the early signs and symptoms of common endocrine diseases, surveys the clinical testing needed for a diagnosis, and presents recommendations for therapy.

Burch, Warner M. *Endocrinology.* 3d ed. Baltimore: Williams & Wilkins, 1994. A handbook of endocrine diseases designed for the house officer. Includes bibliographical references and an index.

Gardner, David G., and Dolores Shoback, eds. *Greenspan's Basic and Clinical Endocrinology.* 8th ed. New York: McGraw-Hill, 2007. This resource superbly reviews contributions of molecular biology to endocrinology and the practical implications of these advances. Each chapter includes advances in molecular biology and the diagnosis and management of the various syndromes.

Larsen, P. Reed, et al., eds. *Williams Textbook of Endocrinology.* 10th ed. Philadelphia: W. B. Saunders,

2003. Text that covers the spectrum of information related to the endocrine system, including thyroid disorders, diabetes, endocrinology and aging, female reproduction and fertility control, sexual function and dysfunction, kidney stones, and endocrine hypertension.

Neal, J. Matthew. *Basic Endocrinology: An Interactive Approach.* Malden, Mass.: Blackwell Science, 2000. Meant to supplement existing textbooks, this guide to the basic clinical principles and physiology of clinical endocrinology is for medical students, residents, and others needing a review of clinical endocrinology.

Ruggieri, Paul, and Scott Isaacs. *A Simple Guide to Thyroid Disorders: From Diagnosis to Treatment.* Omaha, Nebr.: Addicus Books, 2003. A user-friendly guide that covers how the thyroid gland works and explains common disorders. Special attention is given to how thyroid diseases affect specific populations such as women, children, and the elderly.

HYPERTENSION
DISEASE/DISORDER

ANATOMY OR SYSTEM AFFECTED: Blood vessels, brain, circulatory system, heart, kidneys, urinary system

SPECIALTIES AND RELATED FIELDS: Cardiology, family medicine, internal medicine

DEFINITION: An abnormally high blood pressure, an often silent cardiovascular condition that may lead to heart attack, stroke, and major organ failures.

KEY TERMS:

cardiovascular: of, relating to, or involving the heart and blood vessels

cerebrovascular: of, or involving, the brain and the blood vessels supplying it

diastolic blood pressure: the pressure of the blood within the artery while the heart is at rest

hypertension: abnormally high blood pressure, especially high arterial blood pressure; also the systemic condition accompanying high blood pressure

peripheral vascular: of, relating to, involving, or forming the vasculature in the periphery (the external boundary or surface of a body); usually referring to circulation not involving cardiovascular, cerebrovascular, or major organ systems

side effect: a secondary and usually adverse effect (as of a drug); also known as an adverse effect or reaction

---

INFORMATION ON HYPERTENSION

CAUSES: Stress, genetic factors, obesity, diabetes mellitus, physiological factors
SYMPTOMS: Often asymptomatic
DURATION: Often long-term
TREATMENTS: Drug therapy (diuretics, beta-blockers, calcium-channel blockers, ACE inhibitors); lifestyle changes (weight reduction, alcohol restriction, regular exercise)

---

sphygmomanometer: a device that uses a column of mercury to measure blood pressure force; pressure is measured in millimeters of mercury

systolic blood pressure: the pressure of the blood within the artery while the heart is contracting

CAUSES AND SYMPTOMS

Hypertension is a higher-than-normal blood pressure (either systolic or diastolic). Blood pressure is usually measured using a sphygmomanometer and a stethoscope. The stethoscope is used to hear when the air pressure within the cuff of the sphygmomanometer is equal to that in the artery. When taking a blood pressure, the cuff is pumped to inflate an air bladder secured around the arm; the pressure produced will collapse the blood vessels within. As cuff pressure decreases, a slight thump is heard as the artery snaps open to allow blood to flow. At this point, the cuff pressure equals the systolic blood pressure. As the cuff pressure continues to fall, the sound of blood being pumped will continue but become progressively softer. At the point where the last sound is heard, the cuff pressure equals the diastolic blood pressure.

In hypertension, both systolic and diastolic blood pressures are usually elevated. Blood pressures are reported as the systolic pressure over the diastolic pressure, such as 130/80 millimeters of mercury. It is important to recognize there are degrees of seriousness for hypertension. The higher the blood pressure, the more rigorous the treatment may be. When systolic pressures are in the high normal range, the individual should be closely monitored with annual blood pressure checks. Persistently high blood pressures (greater than 140-159/90-99 millimeters of mercury) require closer monitoring and may result in a decision to treat the condition with medication or other types of intervention.

The blood pressure in an artery is determined by the relationship among three important controlling factors:

Blood Pressure

Systolic   Diastolic

Blood pressure is measured in two numbers: systolic pressure (the pressure of the blood as it flows out when the heart contracts) over diastolic pressure (the pressure of the blood within the artery as it flows in when the heart is at rest). Readings greater than 140 systolic over 90 diastolic indicate the presence of hypertension.

the blood volume, the amount of blood pumped by the heart (cardiac output), and the contraction of smooth muscle within blood vessels (arterial tone). To illustrate the first point, if blood volume decreases, the result will be a fall in blood pressure. Conversely, the body cannot itself increase blood pressure by rapidly adding blood volume; fluid must be injected into the circulation to do so.

A second controlling factor of blood pressure is cardiac output (the volume of blood pumped by the heart in a given unit of time, usually reported as liters per minute). This output is determined by two factors: stroke volume (the volume of blood pumped with each heartbeat) and the heart rate (beats per minute). As heart rate increases, output generally increases and blood pressure may rise as well. If blood volume is low, such as with excessive bleeding, the blood returning to the heart per beat is lower and could lead to decreased output. To compensate, the heart rate increases to prevent a drop in blood pressure. Therefore, as cardiac output changes, blood pressure does not necessarily change.

Last, a major controlling factor of blood pressure is arterial tone. Arteries are largely tubular, smooth muscles that can change their diameter based on the extent of contraction (tone). This contraction is largely under the control of a specialized branch of the nervous system called the sympathetic nervous system. An artery with high arterial tone (contracted) will squeeze the

blood within and increase the pressure inside. There is also a relaxation phase that will allow expansion and a decrease in blood pressure. Along with relaxation, arteries are elastic to allow some stretching, which may further help reduce pressure or, more important, help prevent blood pressure from rising.

There are two general types of hypertension: essential and secondary. Secondary hypertension is attributable to some underlying identifiable cause, such as a tumor or kidney disease, while essential hypertension has no identifiable cause. Therefore, essential hypertension is a defect that results in excessive arterial pressure secondary to poor regulation by any one of the three controlling factors discussed above. Each factor can serve as a focal point for treatment with medications.

The negative consequences of hypertension are mainly manifested in the deteriorating effect that this condition has on coronary heart disease (CHD). Cardiovascular risk factors for CHD are described as two types, unmodifiable and modifiable. Unmodifiable risk factors cannot be changed. This group includes gender, race, advanced age, and a family history of heart disease (hypertensive traits can be inherited). The modifiable risk factors are cigarette smoking (or other forms of tobacco abuse), high blood cholesterol levels, control over diabetes, and perhaps other factors not yet discovered. For example, additional factors are now recognized for their adverse effects on hypertension, including obesity, a lack of physical activity, and psychological factors.

There is no definitive blood pressure level at which a person is no longer at risk for CHD. While any elevation above the normal range places the person at increased risk for CHD, what are considered high normal blood pressures were previously defined as normal. (Looking back at older data, researchers noted that persons able to maintain pressures at or below 139/89 millimeters of mercury had less severe CHD.) The defini-

BLOOD PRESSURE AND HYPERTENSION	
Status	*Systolic/Diastolic*
Normal	>120/>80
Prehypertension	120-139/80-89
Stage I hypertension	140-159/90-99
Stage II hypertension	<160/100

tion of "normal" blood pressure may change again in the future as new information is discovered. There is a practical limit as to how low pressure can be while maintaining day-to-day function.

In coronary heart disease, the blood supply to the heart is reduced and the heart cannot function well. The common term for arteriosclerosis, "hardening of the arteries," indicates the symptom of reduced blood flow, which is a major component of CHD. When the heart cannot supply itself with the necessary amount of blood (a condition known as ischemia), a characteristic chest pain called angina may be produced. The hardening aspect of this disease is the result of cholesterol deposits in the vessel, which decrease elasticity and make the vessel wall stiff. This stiffness will force pressures in the vessel to increase if cardiac output rises. As pressures advance, the vessel may develop weak spots. These areas may rupture or lead to the development of small blood clots that may clog the vessel; either problem will disrupt blood flow, making the underlying CHD worse. Eventually, if the blood supply is significantly reduced, a myocardial infarction (heart attack) may occur. Where the blood supply to the heart muscle itself is functionally blocked, that part of the heart will die.

Besides contributing to an increased risk of heart attack and coronary heart disease, hypertension is a major risk for other vascular problems, such as stroke, kidney failure, heart failure, and visual disturbances secondary to the effects on the blood vessels within the eye. Hypertension is a major source of premature death in the United States and by all estimates affects more than sixty million Americans. Forty percent of all African Americans and more than half of those over the age of sixty are affected. Public awareness of hypertension is increasing, yet less than half of all patients diagnosed are treated. More important, only one in five identified hypertensives have the condition under control. This lack of control is particularly important when one considers the organs influenced by hypertension, most notably the brain, eyes, kidneys, and heart.

Although causative factors of hypertension cannot be identified, many physiological factors contribute to hypertension. They include increased sympathetic nervous activity (part of the autonomic nervous system), which promotes arterial contraction; overproduction of an unidentified sodium-retaining hormone or chronic high sodium intake; inadequate dietary intake of potassium or calcium; an increased or inappropriate secretion of renin, a chemical made by the kidney; defi-

ciencies of arterial dilators, such as prostaglandins; congenital abnormalities (birth defects) of resistance vessels; diabetes mellitus or resistance to the effects of insulin; obesity; increased activity of vascular growth factors; and altered cellular ion transport of electrolytes, such as potassium, sodium, chloride, and bicarbonate.

The kidneys are greatly responsible for blood pressure control. They have a key role in maintaining both blood volume and blood pressure. When kidney function declines, secondary to problems such as a decrease in renal blood flow, the kidney will release renin. High renin levels result in activation of the renin-angiotensin-aldosterone system. The resulting chemical cascade produces angiotensin II, a potent arterial constrictor. Another chemical released is aldosterone, an adrenal hormone which causes the kidney to retain water and sodium. These two actions add to blood volume and increase arterial tone, resulting in higher blood pressure. Normally, the renin-angiotensin-aldosterone system protects kidney function by raising blood pressure when it is low. In hypertensives, the controlling forces seem to be out of balance, so that the system does not respond appropriately. The renin-angiotensin-aldosterone system has a negative effect on bradykinin, a chemical which protects renal function by producing vasodilating prostaglandins that help maintain adequate renal blood flow. This protection is especially important in elderly individuals, who may depend on this system to maintain renal function. The system can be inhibited by medications such as aspirin or ibuprofen, resulting in a recurrence of hypertension or less control over the existing disease.

Arteries are largely smooth muscles under the control of the autonomic nervous system, which is responsible for organ function. Yet there is often no conscious control of organs; for example, one can "tell" the lungs to take a breath, but one cannot "tell" the heart to beat. The autonomic nervous system has two branches, sympathetic and parasympathetic, that essentially work against each other. The sympathetic system exerts much control over blood pressure. Many chemicals and medicines, such as caffeine, decongestants, and amphetamines, affect blood pressure by mimicking the effects of increased sympathetic stimulation of arteries.

Numerous factors associated with blood pressure elevations will affect one or more of the key determinants of blood pressure; they affect one another as well. An example will show the extent of their relationship. Sodium and water retention will increase blood volume returning to the heart. As this return increases, the heart will increase output (to a point) to prevent heart failure. This higher cardiac output may also raise blood pressure. If arterial vessels are constricted, pressures may be even higher. This elevated pressure (resistance) will force the heart to try to increase output to maintain blood flow to vital organs. Thus, a vicious cycle is started; hypertension can be perceived as a merry-go-round ride with no exit.

Treatment and Therapy

Blood pressure reduction has a protective effect against cardiovascular disease. Generally, as blood pressure decreases, arteries are less contracted and are able to deliver more blood to the tissues, maintaining their function. Further, this decreased blood pressure will help reduce the risk of heart attack in the patient with heart disease. With lower pressures, the heart does not need to work as hard supplying blood to itself or the rest of the body. Therefore, the demand for cardiac output to supply blood flow is less. This reduced workload lowers the incidence of angina.

Treatment of hypertensive patients may involve using one to four different medications to achieve the goal of blood pressure reduction. There are many types of medications from which to choose: diuretics, sympatholytic agents (also known as antiadrenergic drugs), beta-blockers (along with one combined-action alpha-beta blocker), calcium-channel blockers, peripheral vasodilators, angiotensin-converting enzyme inhibitors, and the newest class, angiotension receptor inhibitors. The list of available drugs is extensive; for example, there are fourteen different thiazide-type diuretics and another six diuretics with different mechanisms of action. So many choices may present the physician with a confusing set of alternatives.

Patients prone to sodium and water retention are treated with diuretics, agents that prevent the kidney from reabsorbing sodium and water from the urine. Diuretics are usually added to other medications to enhance those medications' activity. Research into thiazide-type diuretics has shown that these agents possess mild calcium-channel blocking activity, aiding their ability to reduce hypertension.

Beta-blocking agents are used less often than when they were first developed. They work by decreasing cardiac output through reducing the heart rate. Although they are highly effective, the heart rate reduction tends to produce side effects. Most commonly, patients complain of fatigue, sleepiness, and reduced exercise tolerance (the heart rate cannot increase to adapt to the increasing demand for blood in tissues and the heart itself). These agents are still a good choice for hypertensive patients who have suffered a heart attack. Their benefit is that they reduce the risk of a second heart attack by preventing the heart from overworking.

Calcium-channel blockers were originally intended to treat angina. These agents act primarily by decreasing arterial smooth muscle contraction. Relaxed coronary blood vessels can carry more blood, helping prevent the pain of angina. When calcium ions enter the smooth muscle, a more sustained contraction is produced; therefore, blocking this effect will produce relaxation. Physicians noted that this relaxation also produced lower blood pressures. The distinct advantage to these agents is that they are well tolerated; however, some patients may require increasing their fiber intake to prevent some constipating effects.

Peripheral vasodilators have been a disappointment. Theoretically, they should be ideal since they work directly to cause arterial dilation. Unfortunately, blood pressure has many determinants and patients seem to become "immune" to direct vasodilator effects. Peripheral vasodilators are useful, however, when added to other treatments such as beta-blockers or sympatholytic medications.

The sympatholytic agents are divided into two broad categories. The first group works within the brain to decrease the effects of nerves that would send signals to blood vessels to constrict (so-called constrict messages). They do this by increasing the relax signals coming out of the brain to offset the constrict messages. The net effect is that blood vessels dilate, reducing blood pressure. Many of these agents have fallen into disfavor because of adverse effects similar to those of beta-blockers. The second group of sympatholytics works directly at the nerve-muscle connection. These agents block the constrict messages of the nerve that would increase arterial smooth muscle tone. Overall, these agents are well tolerated. Some patients, especially the elderly, may be very susceptible to their effect and have problems with low blood pressure; this issue usually resolves itself shortly after the first dose.

The renin-angiotensin-aldosterone system is a key determinant of blood pressure. Angiotensin-converting enzyme inhibitors (ACE inhibitors) work by blocking angiotensin II and aldosterone and by preserving bradykinin. They have been found quite effective for reducing blood pressure and are usually well tolerated. Some patients will experience a first-dose effect, while others may develop a dry cough that can be corrected by dose reductions or discontinuation of the medication. The angiotension receptor inhibitors work, instead, by blocking the effects of this substance on the target cells of the arteries themselves. They are proving to be excellent substitutes for people who cannot tolerate the related class of ACE inhibitors.

Unfortunately, and contrary to popular belief, no one can reliably tell when his or her own blood pressure is elevated. Consequently, hypertension is called a "silent killer." It is extremely important to have regular blood pressure evaluations and, if diagnosed with hypertension, to receive treatment.

From 1950 through 1987, as advances in understanding and treating hypertension were made, the United States population enjoyed a 40 percent reduction in coronary heart disease and a more than 65 percent reduction in stroke deaths. (By comparison, noncardiovascular deaths during the same period were reduced little more than 20 percent.)

It is evident that blood pressure can be reduced without medications. Research in the 1980's led to a nonpharmacologic approach in the initial management of hypertension. This strategy includes weight reduction, alcohol restriction, regular exercise, dietary sodium restriction, dietary potassium and calcium supplementation, stopping of tobacco use (in any form), and caffeine restriction. Often, these methods can produce benefits without medication being prescribed. Using this approach, medication is added to the therapy if blood pressure remains elevated despite good efforts at nonpharmacologic control.

Other aspects of hypertension and hypertensive patients have been identified to help guide the clinician to the proper choice of medication. With this approach, the clinician can focus therapy at the most likely cause of the hypertension: sodium and water retention, high cardiac output, or high vascular resistance. This pathophysiological approach led to the abandonment of the rigid step-care approach described in many texts covering hypertension. The pathophysiological approach to hypertension management is based on a series of steps that are taken if inadequate responses are seen (see figure).

By far, the best strategy for controlling hypertension is to be informed. Each person needs to be aware of his or her personal risk for developing hypertension. One should have regular blood pressure evaluations, avoid eating excessive salt and sodium, increase exercise, and reduce fats in the diet. Maintaining ideal body

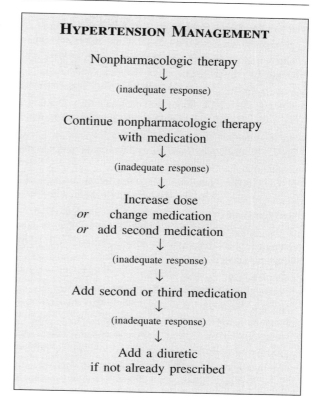

HYPERTENSION MANAGEMENT

Nonpharmacologic therapy
↓
(inadequate response)
↓
Continue nonpharmacologic therapy with medication
↓
(inadequate response)
↓
Increase dose
or change medication
or add second medication
↓
(inadequate response)
↓
Add second or third medication
↓
(inadequate response)
↓
Add a diuretic
if not already prescribed

weight may be a key control factor. Studies have shown that patients who have been successful at losing weight will require less stringent treatment. The benefits could be a need for fewer medications, reduced doses of medications, or both.

—*Charles C. Marsh, Pharm.D.;*
updated by Connie Rizzo, M.D., Ph.D.

See also Angina; Arteriosclerosis; Cardiology; Cholesterol; Circulation; Claudication; Embolism; Heart; Heart attack; Heart disease; Hyperadiposis; Hypercholesterolemia; Hyperlipidemia; Hypotension; Insulin resistance syndrome; Kidney disorders; Kidneys; Metabolic syndrome; Phlebitis; Physical examination; Preeclampsia and eclampsia; Pulmonary hypertension; Strokes; Thrombolytic therapy and TPA; Thrombosis and thrombus; Vascular medicine; Vascular system.

FOR FURTHER INFORMATION:

American Society of Hypertension. http://www.ash-us.org/. A group dedicated to promoting and encouraging the development, advancement, and exchange of scientific information in all aspects of research, diagnosis, and treatment of hypertension and related cardiovascular diseases.

McGowan, Mary P., and Jo McGowan-Chopra. *The Hypertension Sourcebook*. Chicago: Contemporary Books, 2001. An excellent guide to living with and managing hypertension.

Messerli, Franz H., ed. *Cardiovascular Disease in the Elderly*. 3d ed. Boston: Kluwer Academic, 1993. An excellent book for detailed discussions regarding cardiovascular disease in older persons. Issues such as aging, multiple illnesses, and the social challenges seen in the elderly are discussed.

_____. *The Heart and Hypertension*. New York: Yorke Medical Books, 1987. An excellent reference work edited by one of the most distinguished clinicians and researchers in hypertension. This text's strength is its discussion of the pathophysiology of hypertension.

Piscatella, Joseph, and Barry Franklin. *Take a Load Off Your Heart: 109 Things You Can Do to Prevent or Reverse Heart Disease*. New York: Workman, 2002. Easy-to-follow guide that details such preventive measures as managing stress, improving diet, and exercising and offers more than one hundred practical tips for preventing, stabilizing, and reversing heart disease.

Rowan, Robert L. *Control High Blood Pressure Without Drugs: A Complete Hypertension Handbook*. Rev. ed. New York: Simon & Schuster, 2001. A revised edition of a well-known book that details advances in medical research, guidelines for coping with hypertension if it occurs, and ways to lower your blood pressure through inexpensive natural means. Includes a list of Web sites and a fully updated bibliography.

Seeley, Rod R., Trent D. Stephens, and Philip Tate. *Anatomy and Physiology*. 7th ed. New York: McGraw-Hill, 2006. A well-illustrated, easy-to-read basic reference text for the general reader. The text's obvious strengths are its discussions of the heart, arteries, and veins and their roles in cardiovascular function.

Tierney, Lawrence M., Stephen J. McPhee, and Maxine A. Papadakis, eds. *Current Medical Diagnosis and Treatment 2007*. New York: McGraw-Hill Medical, 2006. This text, updated yearly, is the point of reference for physicians and other health care practitioners. It incorporates each year's biomedical research discoveries that have immediate, relevant, and applicable use for the patient.

Hyperthermia and hypothermia

DISEASE/DISORDER

ANATOMY OR SYSTEM AFFECTED: All

SPECIALTIES AND RELATED FIELDS: Anesthesiology, critical care, emergency medicine, environmental health, internal medicine

DEFINITION: Hyperthermia is the elevation of the body core temperature of an organism, while hypothermia is a decrease in that temperature; an extreme in either condition is a medical emergency. They both can be induced therapeutically in certain medical and surgical conditions.

KEY TERMS:

ambient temperature: the temperature of the surrounding environment

body temperature: the temperature that reflects the level of heat energy in an animal's body; a consequence of the balance between the heat produced by metabolism and the body's exchange of heat with the surrounding environment

frostbite: injury that results from exposure of skin to extreme cold, most commonly affecting the ears, nose, hands, and feet

hibernation: a condition of dormancy and torpor that occurs in poikilotherm vertebrates and invertebrates; as the environmental temperatures drop, the inner core temperature of such animals also drops to decrease the metabolic rate and physiological functions

homeotherms: animals, such as birds and mammals, that have the ability to maintain a high body core temperature despite large variations in environmental temperatures

---

INFORMATION ON HYPERTHERMIA AND HYPOTHERMIA

CAUSES: Extended exposure to heat or cold

SYMPTOMS: For hyperthermia, headache, nausea, dizziness, heat exhaustion or stroke, cessation of perspiration, hot and dry skin, rapid pulse, quick and shallow breathing; for hypothermia, tingling, pain, numbness, sometimes frostbite on nose, ears, hands, and feet

DURATION: Acute

TREATMENTS: For hyperthermia, cooling of body, replacement of body fluids, treatment of shock, emergency resuscitation; for hypothermia, warm water on affected body part, hospitalization in intensive care unit

CAUSES AND SYMPTOMS

Body temperature reflects the level of heat energy in the body of an animal or human being. It is the consequence of the balance between the heat generated by metabolism and the body's heat exchange with the surrounding environment (ambient temperature). Generally, animal life can be sustained in the temperature range of 0 degrees Celsius (32 degrees Fahrenheit) to 45 degrees Celsius (113 degrees Fahrenheit), but appropriate processes can store animal tissues at much lower temperature. Homeotherms, such as birds and most mammals, have the ability to maintain their high body core temperature despite large variations in environmental temperatures. Poikilotherms have slow metabolic rates at rest and, as a result, difficulty in maintaining their inner core temperatures. Such a form of thermal regulation is called ectothermic ("outer heated") and is directly affected by the uptake of heat from the environment; such organisms are often termed cold-blooded. On the other hand, homeotherms are endothermic ("inner heated") and depend largely on their fast and controlled rates of heat production; such organisms are termed warm-blooded. Thus, the lizard, an example of an ectotherm, maintains its body temperature by staying in or out of shade and by assuming a posture toward the sun that would maximize the adjustment for its body heat. At night, the lizard burrows, but its body temperature still drops considerably until the next morning, when it increases with the rising sun.

Body core temperatures vary considerably among mammals and birds. For example, the sparrow's inner core temperature is about 43.5 degrees Celsius (110.3 degrees Fahrenheit), the turkey's 41.2 degrees Celsius (106.2 degrees Fahrenheit), the cat's 36.4 degrees Celsius (97.5 degrees Fahrenheit), and the opossum's 34.7 degrees Celsius (94.5 degrees Fahrenheit). In humans, although the temperature of the inner organs varies by only 1 to 2 degrees Celsius (1.8 to 3.6 degrees Fahrenheit), the skin temperature may vary 10 to 20 degrees Celsius (18 to 36 degrees Fahrenheit) below the core temperature of 37 degrees Celsius (98.6 degrees Fahrenheit), depending on the ambient temperature. This is possible because the cells of the skin, muscles, and blood vessels are not as sensitive as are those of the vital organs.

An elevation in core temperature of homeotherms above the normal range is called hyperthermia, while a corresponding decrease is called hypothermia. Both can be brought about by extremes in the environment. Although the human body can withstand a lack of food for a number of weeks and that of water for several days, it cannot survive a lack of thermoregulation, which is the maintaining of the inner core temperature. The core temperature has to be kept within strict limits; otherwise, the brain and heart will be compromised and death will result. Clinically, the body's core temperature can be monitored by recording the temperature of the rectum, the eardrum, the mouth, the temporal artery, and the esophagus. In elderly people, the body's ability to cope with extreme temperatures may be impaired. Exposure to even mildly cold temperatures may lead to accidental hypothermia that can be fatal if not detected and treated properly.

All animals produce heat by oxidation of substrates to carbon dioxide. On the average, about 75 percent of food energy is converted to heat during adenosine triphosphate (ATP) formation and its transfer to the functional systems of the cells. In defense against heat, sweating is the primary physiological mechanism in mammals. Dogs, cats, and other furred carnivores increase evaporative heat loss by panting, while small rodents spread saliva. Human beings have two to three million glands that can produce up to 23 liters of sweat per hour for a short period of time.

Fever may occur for at least four main reasons. Infection by microorganisms is the most familiar because of its large variety of causes. An infection may be bacterial (as with septicemia and abscesses), viral (in measles, mumps, and influenza), protozoal (in malaria), or spirochaetel (in syphilis). Fever can also occur because of immunological conditions, such as a response to drug allergies or a blood transfusion reaction. Other causes are malignancy, such as Hodgkin's disease and leukemia, and noninfectious inflammation, as seen in gout or thrombophlebitis.

Antipyretics are medicines whose consumption results in the lowering of fever. Aspirin, acetaminophen, and ibuprofen are common, over-the-counter fever-reducing medications. The mechanism of action of the nonnarcotic antipyretics remains a subject of research. Two hypotheses are considered to justify the suppression of fever. One hypothesis suggests the drugs reset the temperature in the hypothalamus of the brain by potentially blocking certain brain chemical activity. The other postulates that a modification of the physiological membrane properties takes place, with subsequent incorporation of drug molecules into the tertiary structure of proteins.

Temperature regulation involves the hypothalamus of the brain and the spinal cord, which monitor the difference between the internal and peripheral (core and skin) temperature, with physiological and psychological adjustments to maintain a constant internal temperature. The brain records the various body temperatures via specialized nerve endings called thermoreceptors. Heat transfer occurs between the skin surface and the environment via radiation (which takes place when environmental temperature is lower than body temperature; 60 to 70 percent of body heat is lost through this method), conduction (which takes place by means of physical contact), convection (which occurs through the movement of air), or evaporation (perspiration or sweating).

During cold weather, hikers and climbers are particularly at risk for hypothermia; in extreme cases, body functions are depressed to the extent that victims may be mistaken for dead. Injuries that result from skin exposure to extreme cold are described as frostbite. Frostbite most commonly affects peripheral tissue such as the nose, ears, hands (especially the fingertips), and feet, which first turn unusually red and then unnaturally white. Early symptoms include feelings of coldness, tingling, pain, and numbness. Frostbite takes place when ice crystals form in the skin and (in the most serious cases) in the tissue beneath the skin. If not treated, frostbite may lead to gangrene, the medical term for tissue death. The freezing-thawing process causes mechanical disruption (from ice), intracellular and extracellular biochemical changes, and the disruption of the blood corpuscles. Frostbite treatment involves the removal of wet and restrictive clothing or jewelry. Warm water can be used on the involved body part to restore blood circulation, which will to be painful for the victim. Extreme care should be taken when moving the body part with frostbite. Massage of the area should never be done, as the skin and tissues are very fragile and may be further damaged.

There are several types of hypothermia. Immersion hypothermia occurs when a person falls into cold water. Any movement of the body leads to loss of heat, and the drastic temperature change may trigger a heart attack. Divers are equipped with wet suits to minimize heat loss, but they cool themselves rapidly when they move in cold water and, at the same time, breathe dry air mixtures. Submersion hypothermia is actual drowning in cold water. Often during drowning, the person experiences a spasm of the larynx or is able to hold his or her breath. However, the lack of oxygen forces the relaxation of these responses, and water is swallowed. The majority of this water goes into the stomach, but it only takes a very small amount of water in the lungs to cause enough oxygen deprivation to slow or even stop the heart. In cold water, the human body responds by lowering its metabolism, which will allow the individual (especially a child) to survive for a prolonged period without adequate oxygen before death occurs. The exact amount of time that a person can survive in cold water conditions is unknown. Reports have demonstrated survival in cases of submersion for more than an

First Aid for Hypothermia

Position patient on two blankets with arms raised.

Wrap lower blanket around patient's body.

Lower patient's arms and prepare upper blanket as shown.

Very Important: The patient's face should be left exposed, and blankets should be loose enough that the patient can move.

hour. Unless the person shows evidence of decay, attempts should be made to rescue the individual and involve emergency medical personnel. When removing a victim from the water, care should be taken to remove the individual in a prone (face down) position to avoid circulatory collapse from the sudden decrease in water pressure. This is a common cause of sudden death for a conscious individual who is rescued from the water.

Clinical reports also indicate hypothermia in alcohol-intoxicated individuals. Shivering is the brain's hypothalamic response to hypothermia. The hypothalamus stimulates reflexes in the spinal cord that trigger a sequence of skeletal muscle contractions which lead to an increase in body temperature. Other conditions that promote heat loss in the already hypothermic person include tight and wet clothing, injury causing hemorrhage, fatigue, and even psychosis.

Treatment and Therapy

Nature protects poikilotherm vertebrates and invertebrates in winter by means of hibernation. Hibernation, which is a condition of dormancy and torpor, occurs when the body temperatures of such animals drop in response to a decrease in environmental temperatures. Animals such as bears, raccoons, badgers, and some birds become drowsy in winter because ambient temperature drops of a few degrees considerably decrease their metabolic rates and physiological functions. For example, the body temperature of a bear is 35.5 degrees Celsius (95.9 degrees Fahrenheit) at an air temperature of 4.4 degrees Celsius (39.9 degrees Fahrenheit) and only 31.2 degrees Celsius (88.1 degrees Fahrenheit) at an air temperature of −4 degrees Celsius (24.8 degrees Fahrenheit).

In humans, however, a significant decrease in body temperature is always a medical emergency requiring immediate attention. The treatment for mild cases of hypothermia may consist only of removing wet clothing before providing additional clothing or blankets. Movement of the victim must be minimized to avoid causing abnormal heart rhythms. Providing warm fluids and attempts at rewarming beyond those mentioned are not recommended for laypersons. Severe hypothermia requires hospitalization in an intensive care unit (ICU), where the body temperature is returned to normal by placing the patient under special heat-reflecting blankets; by infusing warm intravenous (IV) fluids; by irrigating the stomach, abdominal cavity, and bladder with warm fluids; or by circulating the victim's blood through a machine to warm it.

Hyperthermia (an elevated core body temperature) can be in response to illness (fever) or environmental conditions (heat exhaustion or heat stroke). Heat stroke, defined as a core temperature above 40 degrees Celsius (104 degrees Fahrenheit), is a medical emergency that occurs when the thermoregulatory system fails. The victim is unable to cool the body's elevated temperature through normal mechanisms of sweating. A sustained elevated temperature can cause seizures in young children and infants. Adults, especially the elderly, are prone to experience confusion. Treatment while waiting for the arrival of emergency medical services includes placing the victim in a cool environment, removing the victim's clothing, and placing ice packs to the groin, neck, and underarm regions. Shivering should be avoided. Salt tablets or solutions should not be given by laypersons because of the risk of elevated sodium levels and the possibility of stomach upset.

Both hyperthermia and hypothermia have been used in medical treatments. Cancer treatment has consisted primarily of radiation therapy, surgery, and chemotherapy. More recent experimental approaches for cancer treatment include immunotherapy and hyperthermia. Hyperthermia has been used with chemotherapy or radiation therapy to improve blood flow to the targeted cancer cells, to increase the drug concentration inside the cancer cells, and to kill cancer cells. Hyperthermia has been used to damage and kill cancer cells while preserving the healthy nearby cells. This preservation is attributed to the differences in the structure of cancer cells, which are effectively damaged by heat. Further studies are needed to determine the temperature that is needed to damage or kill the cancer cells without harming other cells. Most body tissues can withstand temperature up to 44 degrees Celsius for up to one hour, with the exception of the brain, spinal cord, and nerves. These structures have been found to have irreversible damage at lower temperatures and shorter exposure time than other tissues.

Ultrasonic irradiation, which uses a thin, stainless steel tube to induce hyperthermia, is believed to be the promising technique of the future. The heat generated by the energy produced improves the local blood supply by dilating the blood vessels. This dilation, together with an acceleration of enzyme activity, helps cells to obtain fresh nutrients and, at the same time, rid themselves of waste products. The other advantage of ultrasonic irradiation is the vibrations that it creates. In a hardened and calcified brain tumor, for example, these

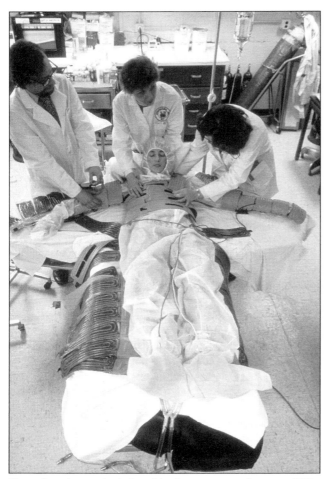

Hyperthermia may be induced in the treatment of cancer. (Mike Mitchell/National Cancer Institute)

vibrations can crush the tumor, which can then be removed via vacuum.

Induced hypothermia is selectively used in various heart and brain surgeries. The patient's body temperature is lowered by the use of cooling blankets and other devices. The core temperature is monitored by bladder and rectal electronic devices. The hypothermia is considered neuro-protective. It is uncertain if the brain protection is from lowered oxygen metabolism or prevention of harmful chemical reactions. The goal of the majority of surgical procedures is to keep the patient's temperature within the normal range. Hypothermia has been associated with increased blood loss, higher infection rates, and other poor outcomes in many surgical situations. Therapeutic hypothermia has also been used after cardiac arrest to preserve heart tissue by decreasing its oxygen demand.

PERSPECTIVE AND PROSPECTS

Both hypothermia and hyperthermia have had a commanding role in medicine. An Egyptian papyrus roll which can be dated back to 3000 B.C.E. describes the treatment of a breast tumor with hyperthermia. Heat has been used as a therapeutic agent since the days of Hippocrates (c. 460-c. 370 B.C.E.), who stated that a patient who could not be cured by heat was actually incurable. In the seventeenth century, the Japanese performed hyperthermia to treat syphilis, arthritis, and gout, using hot water to increase the body temperature to about 39 degrees Celsius.

The medical use of hyperthermia owes much of its modern-era development to Georges Lakhovsky (1880-1942), a Russian Jew who had a brilliant physics background and did most of his work in Paris, France. Although he is not generally given the credit for it, he was the first person to design and build a "short wave diathermy" machine, which created artificial fever for the first time in 1923. His work was done primarily on patients with malignant tumors at the Hospital de la Salpetriere and the Hospital Saint-Louis. The first machine that he developed used frequencies from 0.75 megahertz to 3,000 megahertz, a range very much in use in today's clinical hyperthermia. In 1931, he started using a new machine that emitted radio waves of multiple wavelengths. He had partial success with his treatment, as reported to the Pasteur Institute and the French Academy of Sciences. Other scientists in this field include the German physicians W. Busch and P. Bruns, who applied it to erysipelas infection in 1886, and the Swedish gynecologist N. Westermark, who applied it with partial success to nonoperable carcinomas of the cervix uteri in 1898. The combination of hyperthermia and immunotherapy was applied by William B. Coley, a New York surgeon who managed to cause complete regression of malignant melanoma in patients by inducing artificial fever created by inoculation of infected erysipelas cells.

The practice of hyperthermia in conjunction with chemotherapy, radiation, and surgery for the treatment of cancers is still in its infancy. Research has had mixed results in its outcomes. Studies have shown that heat is able to kill cancer cells left behind following surgery, and it can kill those cells that tend to be radiation resistant. Unlike radiation, hyperthermia has no known cumulative toxicity. The challenge is to determine the effectiveness of hyperthermia alone and with other treatments, the amount of heat needed to kill cancer cells and preserve normal cells, and the proper hyperthermia techniques, such as ultrasound-induced hyperthermia.

The application of hyperthermia in cases of acquired immunodeficiency syndrome (AIDS) has not yet provided decisively positive results. The process has involved circulating the patient's blood through a chamber heated to approximately 10 degrees Fahrenheit higher than the body temperature. Although the AIDS virus is killed, many of the patients' other enzymes are found to lose their activity. Consequently, United States health officials have opposed and criticized blood-heating therapy for this disease until more convincing results are produced.

The role of hyperthermia in treating metastatic cancer, in combination with radiation and drugs that are heat and radiation cell sensitizers, is increasing. This technique has been made feasible by the technological advancements in deep-heating machines, such as the Magnetrode and the BSO annular array, which allow the sequential regional hyperthermia of large body regions such as the thorax and the abdomen. The challenge becomes to prevent heat stroke during the procedure.

Hypothermia-induced brain surgery protects brain tissue. In stroke patients, a temperature elevation of 1 degree Celsius (1.8 degrees Fahrenheit) can increase the size of the damaged tissue by as much as 50 percent.

—*Soraya Ghayourmanesh, Ph.D.;*
updated by Amy Webb Bull, D.S.N., A.P.N.

See also Anesthesia; Anesthesiology; Critical care; Critical care, pediatric; Emergency medicine; Fever; Frostbite; Gangrene; Heat exhaustion and heat stroke; Hyperhidrosis; Surgery, general; Sweating.

FOR FURTHER INFORMATION:

Bloomfield, Molly M., and Lawrence J. Stephens. *Chemistry and the Living Organism.* 6th ed. New York: John Wiley & Sons, 1996.

Bucher, Linda. "Emergency Care Situations." In *Medical-Surgical Nursing*, edited by Sharon Lewis, Margaret Heitkemper, and Shannon Dirksen. 6th ed. St. Louis: Mosby, 2004.

Foltz, Patricia, Cheryl Wavrin, and Robert Sticca. "Heated Intraoperative Intraperitoneal Chemotherapy: The Challenges of Bringing Chemotherapy into Surgery." *Association of Operating Room Nurses Journal* 80, no. 6 (December, 2004): 1055-1063.

Futterman, Laurie G., and Louis Lemberg. "The Significance of Hypothermia in Preserving Ischemic Myocardium." *American Journal of Critical Care* 13, no. 1 (January, 2004): 79-84.

Harries, Mark. "Near Drowning: ABC of Resuscitation." *British Medical Journal* 327 (December 6, 2003): 1336-1338.

Morcom, Fiona. "Chill Out: Therapeutic Hypothermia Improves Survival." *Emergency Nurse* 11, no. 4 (August, 2003): 24-28.

Olson, DaiWai, and Carmelo Graffagnino. "Extremes of Hot or Cold Can Lead to Secondary Injuries." *Nursing* 35, no. 7 (July, 2005): 32cc1-32cc2.

Ross, Jennifer Lea. "Near Drowning: Swimming and Other Water Activities Are a Big Part of Summertime Fun, but They're Not Without Risk." *RN* 68, no. 7 (July, 2005): 36-41.

Sommer, Cynthia V., and Carol M. Porth. "Inflammation, Tissue Repair, and Fever." In *Essentials in Pathophysiology*, edited by Porth. 2d ed. Philadelphia: Lippincott Williams & Wilkins, 2007.

Van der Zee, J. "Heating the Patient: A Promising Approach?" *Annals of Oncology* 13, no. 8 (August, 2002): 1173-1184.

HYPERTROPHY

BIOLOGY

ANATOMY OR SYSTEM AFFECTED: All

SPECIALTIES AND RELATED FIELDS: Endocrinology, family medicine, internal medicine

DEFINITION: The growth of a tissue or organ as the result of an increase in the size of the existing cells within that tissue or organ; this process is responsible for the growth of the body as well as for increases in organ size caused by increased workloads on particular organs.

KEY TERMS:

atrophy: the wasting of tissue, an organ, or an entire body as the result of a decrease in the size and/or number of the cells within that tissue, organ, or body

compensatory hypertrophy: an increase in the size of a tissue or an organ in response to an increased workload placed upon it

growth: the increase in size of an organism or any of its parts during the developmental process; caused by increases in both cell numbers and cell size

hyperplasia: the increase in size or growth of a tissue or an organ as a result of an increase in cell numbers, with the size of the cells remaining constant

PROCESS AND EFFECTS

The growth and development of the human body and all its parts requires not only an increase in the number of body cells as the body grows, a process known as hyperplasia, but also an increase in the size of the existing cells, a process known as hypertrophy. It is true that as humans grow, they increase the number of cells in their bodies, resulting in an increase in the size of tissues, organs, systems, and the body. For some tissues, organs, and systems, however, the number of cells is genetically set; therefore, the number of cells will increase minimally if at all after birth. Thus, if growth is to occur in those tissues, organs, and systems, it must take place by means of an increase in the size of the existing cells.

The process of hypertrophy occurs in nearly all tissues in the body but is most common in those tissues in which the number of cells is set at the time of birth. Among such tissues are adipose tissue, which is composed of fat cells, and nervous tissue, which is found in the brain, in the spinal cord, and in skeletal muscle tissue. Other tissues, such as cardiac tissue and smooth muscle tissue, also show the ability to undergo hypertrophy.

It is generally true that the number of fat cells within the human body is set at birth. Therefore, an increase in body fat is thought to result primarily from an increase in the amount of fat stored within the fat cells. An increase in the amount of fat consumed in the diet increases the amount of fat that is placed inside a fat cell, resulting in an increase in the fat cell's size.

The number of nerve cells within the brain and spinal cord also is set at birth. The cerebellum of the human brain, however, increases in size about twentyfold from birth to adulthood. This increase is brought about by an increase in the size of the existing nerve cells, and particularly by an increase in the number of extensions protruding from each nerve cell and the length to which the extensions grow. Furthermore, there is an increase in the number of the components within the cell. Specifically, there is an increase in the number of mitochondria within the cell, which provide a usable form of energy so that the cell can grow.

The number of skeletal muscle cells is also, in general, preset at the time of birth. The skeletal muscle mass of the human body increases dramatically from birth to adulthood. This increase is accomplished primarily by means of individual skeletal muscle cell hypertrophy. This increase in the diameter of the individual muscle cells is brought about by increases in the amounts of the contractile proteins, myosin and actin,

as well as increases in the amount of glycogen and the number of mitochondria within individual cells. As each muscle cell increases in size, it causes an increase in the size of the entire muscle of which it is a part.

Each of the above-mentioned examples occurs naturally as part of the growth process of the human body. Some tissues, however, are capable of increasing in size as the result of an increased load or demand being placed upon them. This increased load or demand is usually brought about by an increased use of the muscle. This increase in the size of cells in response to an increased demand or use is called compensatory hypertrophy. The most common tissues that show the phenomenon of compensatory hypertrophy are the skeletal, cardiac, and smooth muscles.

Skeletal muscle is particularly responsive to being utilized. This response, however, is dependent upon the way in which the skeletal muscle is used. It is well known that an increase in the size of skeletal muscle can be brought about by such exercises as weight lifting. Lifting heavy weights or objects requires strong contractions of the skeletal muscle that is doing the lifting. If this lifting continues over a long period of time, it eventually results in an increase in the size of the existing muscle fibers, leading to an increase in the size of the exercised muscle. Because the strength of a muscle is dependent upon its size, the increase in the muscle's size results in an increase in its strength. The extent to which the size of the muscle increases is dependent upon the amount of time spent lifting the objects and the weight of the objects. The size that a muscle can reach is, however, limited.

Unlike exercises such as weight lifting, endurance types of exercise, such as walking, jogging, and aerobics, do not result in larger skeletal muscles. These types of exercise do not force the skeletal muscles to contract forcibly enough to produce muscle hypertrophy.

In the same way that an increased load or use will cause compensatory hypertrophy in skeletal muscle, a decreased use of skeletal muscle will result in its shrinking or wasting away. This process is referred to as muscle atrophy. This type of atrophy commonly occurs when limbs are broken or injured and must be immobilized. After six weeks of the limb being immobilized, there is a marked decrease in muscle size. A similar type of atrophy occurs in the limb muscles of astronauts, since there is no gravity present in space to provide resistance against which the muscles must work. If the muscles remain unused for more than a few months, there can be a loss of about one-half of the muscle mass of the unused muscle.

Cardiac muscle, like skeletal muscle, can also be caused to hypertrophy by increasing the resistance against which it works. Although endurance exercise does not cause hypertrophy in skeletal muscle, it does result in an increased size of the heart because of the hypertrophy of the existing cardiac muscle cells in this organ. In fact, the heart mass of marathon runners enlarges by about 40 percent as a result of the increase in endurance training. This increase occurs because the heart must work harder to pump more blood to the rest of the body when the body is endurance exercising. Only endurance forms of exercise result in the hypertrophy of the cardiac muscle. Weight lifting, which causes hypertrophy of skeletal muscle, has no effect on the cardiac muscle.

Smooth muscle also is capable of compensatory hypertrophy. Increased pressure or loads on the smooth muscle within arteries can result in the hypertrophy of the muscle cells. This in turn causes a thickening of the arterial wall. Smooth muscle, however, unlike skeletal and cardiac muscle, is capable of hyperplasia as well as hypertrophy.

COMPLICATIONS AND DISORDERS

Hypertrophy also occurs as a result of some pathological and abnormal conditions. The most common pathological hypertrophy is enlargement of the heart as a result of cardiovascular disease. Most cardiovascular diseases put an increased workload on the heart, making it work harder to pump the blood throughout the body. In response to the increased workload, the heart increases its size, a form of compensatory hypertrophy.

The left ventricle of the heart is capable of hypertrophying to such an extent that its muscle mass may increase four- or fivefold. This increase is the result of improper functioning of the valves of the left heart. The valves of the heart work to prevent the backflow of blood from one chamber to another or from the arteries back to the heart. If the valves in the left heart are not working properly, the left ventricle contracts and blood that should leave the ventricle to go out to the body instead returns to the left ventricle. The enlargement of the left ventricle increases the force with which it can pump the blood out to the body, thus reducing the amount of blood that comes back to the left ventricle despite the damaged heart valves. There is, however, a point at which the enlargement of the left ventricle can no longer help in keeping the needed amount of blood

flowing through the body. At that point, the left ventricle finally tires out and left heart failure occurs.

The same type of hypertrophy can and does occur in the right side of the heart as well. Again, this is the result of damaged valves that are supposed to prevent the backflow of blood into the heart. Should the valves of both sides of the heart be damaged, hypertrophy can occur on both sides of the heart.

High blood pressure, also known as hypertension, may also lead to hypertrophy of the ventricles of the heart. With high blood pressure, the heart must work harder to deliver blood throughout the body because it must pump blood against an increased pressure. As a result of the increased demand upon the heart, the heart muscle hypertrophies in order to pump more blood.

The hypertrophy of the heart muscle is beneficial in the pumping of blood to the body in individuals who have valvular disease and hypertension; however, an extreme hypertrophy sometimes leads to heart failure. One of the reasons this may occur is the inability of the blood supply of the heart to keep up with the growth of the cardiac muscle. As a result, the cardiac cells outgrow their blood supply, resulting in the loss of blood and thus a loss of oxygen and nutrients needed for the cardiac cells to survive.

Smooth muscle, like cardiac muscle, may also hypertrophy under the condition of high blood pressure. Smooth muscle makes up the bulk of many of the arteries and smaller arterioles found in the body. The increased pressure on the arterial walls as a result of high blood pressure may cause the hypertrophy of the smooth muscles within the walls of the arteries and arterioles. This increases the thickness of the walls of the arteries and arterioles but also decreases the size of the hollow spaces within those vessels, which are known as the lumina. In the kidneys, the narrowing of the lumina of the arterioles may result in a decreased blood supply to these organs. The reduced blood flow to the kidneys may eventually cause the kidneys to shut down, leading to renal failure.

Smooth muscle may also hypertrophy under some unique conditions. During pregnancy, the uterus will undergo a dramatic hypertrophy. The uterus is a smooth muscle organ that is involved in the housing and nurturing of the developing fetus during pregnancy. Immediately prior to the birth of the fetus, there is marked hypertrophy of the smooth muscle within this organ. This increase in the size of the uterus is beneficial in providing the strong contractions of this organ that are needed for childbirth.

Skeletal muscle also may be caused to hypertrophy in some diseases in which there is an increase in the secretion of male sex hormones, particularly testosterone. Men's higher levels of testosterone, a potent stimulator of muscle growth, are responsible for the fact that males have a larger muscle mass than do females. Furthermore, synthetic testosterone-like hormones have been used by some athletes to increase muscle size. These synthetic hormones are called anabolic steroids. The use of these steroids does result in the hypertrophy of skeletal muscle, but these steroids have been shown to have harmful side effects.

Obesity is another condition that results largely from the hypertrophy of existing fat cells. In children, however, obesity is thought to result not only from an increase in the size of fat cells but also from an increase in their number. In adults, when weight is lost, it is the result of a decrease in the size of the existing fat cells; the number of fat cells remains constant. Thus, it is important to prevent further weight increases in overweight children to prevent the creation of fat cells that will never be lost.

In the onset of diseases that result in muscle degeneration, such as muscular dystrophy, there is a hypertrophy of the affected muscles. This hypertrophy differs from other forms of muscle hypertrophy in that the muscle cells do not increase in size because of an increase in the contractile protein, mitochondria, or glycogen, but because the muscle cells are being filled with fat. As a result of the contractile protein being replaced with fat, the affected muscles are no longer useful.

PERSPECTIVE AND PROSPECTS

The exact mechanisms that bring about and control the hypertrophy of cells and tissues are not well understood. During the growth and developmental periods, however, the hypertrophy of many tissues is thought to be under the control of blood-borne chemicals known as hormones. Among these hormones is one that promotes growth and is thus called growth hormone. Growth hormone brings about an increase in the number and size of cells. Growth hormone causes the hypertrophy of existing cells by increasing the protein-making capability of these cells. Thus, there is an increase in the number of organelles, such as mitochondria, within the cell, which leads to an increase in cell size.

Growth hormone also causes the release of chemicals known as growth factors. There are several differ-

ent growth factors, but one of particular importance is nerve growth factor. Nerve growth factor is involved with the increase in number of cell processes of single nerve cells. Such chemicals have been shown to enhance the growth of damaged nerve cells in the brains of animals. As a result, it is possible that nerve growth factor could be used in the treatment of nerve damage in humans by causing the nerves to grow new cell processes and form new connections to replace those that were damaged. This may be of great importance for the treatment of those suffering from brain or spinal cord damage.

Other hormones may have similar effects on tissues other than nervous tissue. For example, the hypertrophy of the smooth muscle in the uterus is thought to be brought about hormonally. Immediately prior to birth, when the hypertrophy of the uterus is occurring, there is an increased amount of estrogen, the primary female hormone, in the blood. It is this increase in estrogen that is thought to lead to the great enlargement of the uterus during this time. Some hormones have the effect of preventing or inhibiting the hypertrophy of body tissues. The enlargement of the uterus prior to birth is brought about not only by an increase in estrogen but also as a result of a decrease in another hormone known as progesterone. Progesterone levels are high in the blood throughout pregnancy. Immediately prior to birth, however, there is a dramatic decrease in the level of progesterone in the blood. Thus, it is believed that the high level of progesterone prevents or inhibits the hypertrophy of the smooth muscle cells in the uterus, since the hypertrophy of this organ will not occur until estrogen levels are high and progesterone levels are low.

It has been suggested that compensatory hypertrophy, such as that which occurs in skeletal, smooth, and cardiac muscle, occurs as a result of the stretching of muscle. Some studies have shown that the stretching of skeletal, cardiac, and smooth muscle does lead to hypertrophy. American astronauts and Russian cosmonauts, however, showed a loss in muscle mass even though they exercised and stretched their muscles as much as three hours per day, seven days per week. This suggests that mechanisms other than the stretching of muscles may be involved in compensatory muscle hypertrophy.

Through an understanding of the mechanisms involved in muscle hypertrophy, it may one day be possible to prevent the atrophy that occurs during space flights, prolonged bed rest, and immobilization necessitated by the injury of limbs. Furthermore, the understanding of the mechanisms that control hypertrophy may help to alleviate the effects of disabling diseases such as muscular dystrophy by reversing the effects of muscle atrophy.

—David K. Saunders, Ph.D.

See also Endocrinology; Endocrinology, pediatric; Ergogenic aids; Exercise physiology; Growth; Hormones; Muscles; Muscular dystrophy; Obesity; Obesity, childhood; Pregnancy and gestation; Steroid abuse; Steroids.

FOR FURTHER INFORMATION:

Guyton, Arthur C., and John E. Hall. *Textbook of Medical Physiology.* 11th ed. Philadelphia: Elsevier Saunders, 2006. An easily read textbook that provides much information on compensatory hypertrophy and other forms of hypertrophy. Provides an in-depth look at hypertrophy and the mechanisms that bring it about, particularly the effects of exercise on the hypertrophy of skeletal and cardiac muscle.

Larsen, P. Reed, et al., eds. *Williams Textbook of Endocrinology.* 10th ed. Philadelphia: W. B. Saunders, 2003. Text that covers the spectrum of information related to the endocrine system, including thyroid disorders, human growth, diabetes, endocrinology and aging, female reproduction and fertility control, sexual function and dysfunction, kidney stones, and endocrine hypertension.

Marieb, Elaine N., and Katja Hoehn. *Human Anatomy and Physiology.* 7th ed. San Francisco: Pearson Benjamin Cummings, 2007. Provides an in-depth look at how obesity occurs as a result of both hypertrophy and hyperplasia. Also provides an overview of the hormones that can cause hypertrophy and the mechanisms by which they bring about changes in size.

Shier, David N., Jackie L. Butler, and Ricki Lewis. *Hole's Essentials of Human Anatomy and Physiology.* 9th ed. New York: McGraw-Hill, 2004. An introductory college anatomy and physiology text that is easily read and understood. Provides a good general overview of the processes of hypertrophy and atrophy.

Shostak, Stanley. *Embryology: An Introduction to Developmental Biology.* New York: HarperCollins, 1991. Provides an introduction to the growth and development of the human body. It provides a good discussion of the role that hypertrophy plays in the development of the human body. It also points out those tissues that grow primarily by hypertrophy rather than by hyperplasia.

Tortora, Gerard J., and Bryan Derrickson. *Principles of Anatomy and Physiology.* 11th ed. Hoboken, N.J.: John Wiley & Sons, 2006. This textbook does a good job of explaining hypertrophy in skeletal, cardiac, and smooth muscle. It provides several examples of pathological conditions in which hypertrophy occurs and may be harmful.

HYPERVENTILATION

DISEASE/DISORDER

ANATOMY OR SYSTEM AFFECTED: Lungs, respiratory system

SPECIALTIES AND RELATED FIELDS: Emergency medicine, pulmonary medicine

DEFINITION: Breathing at a faster rate than what is needed for metabolism, resulting in the exhalation of carbon dioxide faster than it is produced.

CAUSES AND SYMPTOMS

Hyperventilation is rapid deep or quick shallow breathing, both of which can result in a dramatic decrease in carbon dioxide levels and an increase in the pH of the blood. While its purpose is an attempt to get more oxygen, hyperventilation can actually result in feeling breathless or dizzy and, in extreme cases, fainting.

There are several possible causes or reasons for hyperventilation, including anxiety, panic attacks, agoraphobia (fear of open spaces), depression, anger, and overconsumption of caffeine. Hyperventilation can also be a symptom of an underlying disease process such as an infection, bleeding, or heart and lung disor-

---

INFORMATION ON HYPERVENTILATION

CAUSES: Anxiety, panic attacks, fear, depression, anger, caffeine overconsumption

SYMPTOMS: Rapid deep or quick shallow breathing causing shortness of breath, fast pulse, chest pain or tightening, dry mouth, numbness around lips and hands, blurred vision, seizures, loss of consciousness

DURATION: Acute or chronic

TREATMENTS: Reassurance, removal of cause of anxiety; for severe, recurrent cases, antidepressants, beta-blockers, stress management classes, breathing retraining der, as well as a response to altitude exposure. Hyperventilation syndrome (HVS) can be manifested either acutely or chronically.

Chronic HVS can cause a variety of physical problems involving respiratory, cardiac, neurologic, or gastrointestinal (GI) systems. Aerophobia, a fear of fresh air, brings on the GI problems such as flatulence, bloating, and belching. Besides rapid breathing, hyperventilation can cause a fast pulse, shortness of breath, chest pain or tightening, dry mouth (from mouth breathing), numbness around the lips and hands, and, in more severe cases, blurred vision, seizures, and loss of consciousness. The chest pain resembles typical angina but does not usually respond to nitroglycerine. Changes in the patient's electrocardiogram (ECG) are common, including ST segment elevation or depression, T-wave inversion, or a prolonged QT interval. Patients with mitral valve prolapse are particularly susceptible to HVS. On occasion, hyperventilation can also be manifested with extreme agitation, tingling in the extremities, or painful hand and finger spasms. The chief characteristic of chronic HVS is multiple complaints without supporting physical evidence. Hence, classic hyperventilation is not readily apparent, but frequent sighing may be evidenced, along with chest wall tenderness, numbness, and tingling sensations. To rule out more serious conditions, arterial blood gases, toxicology screens, and chest X rays are suggested.

Hyperventilation is a technique purposefully used by swimmers and deep-sea divers to enable prolonged breath-holding. Many drownings have been related to this practice, however, because it can cause delayed unconsciousness underwater and subsequent death.

TREATMENT AND THERAPY

Contrary to popular belief, breathing into a paper bag to slow down respiration and retain carbon dioxide is not recommended as a treatment for hyperventilation because of the potential life-threatening aggravation of a more serious medical problem such as hypoxia, a myocardial infarction (heart attack), pneumothorax, or pulmonary embolism.

After life-threatening causes of hyperventilation are eliminated, the most successful treatment for hyperventilation is reassurance, discussion of how hyperventilation is causing the patient's symptoms, and removal of the cause of the anxiety, if possible. Instructions from a respiratory therapist on proper abdominal diaphragmatic breathing are also helpful. A patient who faints should be placed flat on the floor with legs ele-

vated. For more severe recurrent cases, antidepressants, beta-blockers, stress management classes, or breathing retraining have all been proven effective in reducing hyperventilation episodes.

—*Bonita L. Marks, Ph.D.*

See also Altitude sickness; Anxiety; Asphyxiation; Caffeine; Choking; Dizziness and fainting; Lungs; Numbness and tingling; Panic attacks; Pulmonary medicine; Pulmonary medicine, pediatric; Respiration; Resuscitation; Unconsciousness; Wheezing.

FOR FURTHER INFORMATION:

Callaham, M. "Hypoxic Hazards of Traditional Paper Bag Rebreathing in Hyperventilating Patients." *Annals of Emergency Medicine* 18, no. 6 (1989): 622-628.

Cowley, D. S., and P. P. Roy-Byrne. "Hyperventilation and Panic Disorder." *American Journal of Medicine* 83, no. 5 (1987): 929-937.

Gardner, W. N. "The Pathophysiology of Hyperventilation Disorders." *Chest* 109, no. 2 (1996): 516-534.

McArdle, William, Frank I. Katch, and Victor L. Katch. *Exercise Physiology: Energy, Nutrition, and Human Performance.* 6th ed. Philadelphia: Lippincott Williams & Wilkins, 2007.

HYPNOSIS
PROCEDURE

ANATOMY OR SYSTEM AFFECTED: Brain, nervous system, psychic-emotional system

SPECIALTIES AND RELATED FIELDS: Alternative medicine, anesthesiology, immunology, psychiatry, psychology

DEFINITION: The induction of an altered state of consciousness.

KEY TERMS:

hypnotherapy: a therapeutic method in which hypnosis works in conjunction with the psychotherapeutic process

hypnotic depth: a state frequently measured by the degree of suggestibility possessed by a presumably hypnotized individual

hypnotic induction: the production of hypnosis by means of precise rules and patterns (formal) or rules and patterns that permit limited flexibility (informal)

operator: the person who induces a hypnotic state; synonymous with "hypnotist" and "suggestor"

suggestion: a communication that evokes a nonvoluntary response reflecting the ideational content of the communication

INDICATIONS AND PROCEDURES

The term "hypnosis" comes from the Greek word *hypnos*, meaning sleep. While scientists and researchers do not understand the exact nature of hypnosis, theorists agree that it is an altered state of consciousness occurring on a continuum of awareness. Hypnosis may occur naturally and spontaneously, as in the case of a daydream. The daydreamer is alert and awake but focuses attention inward rather than outward.

The trance state, often synonymous with the hypnotic state, is characterized by an altered psychological state and minimal motor functioning. A trance can be recognized by the individual's glassy-eyed stare, lack of mobility, and unresponsiveness to external stimuli. A person in a trance state has a heightened receptivity to suggestion. Hypnosis, then, is a natural state that can be induced by another or by oneself (self-hypnosis) for a specific purpose. As a method of treatment, hypnosis, which is often used in conjunction with other approaches to alter psychophysiological states, promotes an understanding that allows for creative problem solving.

In the hypnotic state, the subject is not necessarily docile or submissive and may, because of unconscious processes, reject a suggestion given by even the most expert hypnotist. Four basic types of suggestion have been described: verbal, which includes words and any kind of sound; nonverbal, which applies to body language and gestures; intraverbal, which relates to the intonation of words; and extraverbal, which utilizes the implications of words and gestures that facilitate the acceptance of ideas. Suggestions are also described as being direct or indirect. Suggestibility is a behavior that is not hindered by the individual's logical processes but is enhanced by the subject's motivation, expectation, and trust in the operator as well as by the frequency and manner in which a suggestion is given.

Typically, prior to hypnosis, a subject is seated comfortably opposite or alongside the operator. The operator and subject generally have already discussed what will occur during the hypnotic process. The subject is encouraged to talk about his or her attitudes regarding hypnosis and the operator, as well as any previous experience with hypnosis. If the situation is a clinical one, a full psychiatric history and evaluation will already have been completed. For a positive hypnotic experience to emerge, a comfortable and trusting relationship between subject and operator must exist. There must be a willingness to undergo the experience on the part of the subject and a sensitive, observant, and supportive attitude on the part of the operator. Not all subjects are hypnotizable, but it is believed that most individuals, under appropriate circumstances, can respond to simple suggestions.

The induction process can be one of many types, ranging from directing the subject to close his or her eyes and think of a peaceful scene to having the subject gaze at a particular spot, shiny object, or swinging pendulum until the subject's eyes become heavy and close. Focusing on an object or scene leads the subject to redistribute his or her attention so as to withdraw it from the general surroundings and focus it on a circumscribed area. In the meantime, the subject is encouraged to relax and to allow events to unfold naturally. This induction procedure is sometimes followed, or even replaced, by what are described as deepening techniques. The direction is given to imagine gradually descending a staircase or elevator, or drifting on a boat past a slowly disappearing landscape. Counting forward or backward is another deepening or induction technique. Throughout this procedure, the operator offers comments or suggestions in a slow, repetitive, monotonous voice, exhorting the subject to feel relaxed and calm or to float and drift.

After a period generally lasting from one to several minutes, the operator gives the subject motor and sensory suggestions. For example, the operator may ask the subject to concentrate on the feelings in his or her fingers and hand, to feel the small muscles in the fingers begin to twitch and the arm and forearm begin to feel light. The operator states that these muscles will eventually feel so light that they will lift up off the armrest of the chair and, continually floating upward, ultimately reach the side of the subject's face. The operator might add that the higher the hand floats, the deeper the hypnosis will become, and the deeper the hypnosis becomes, the higher the hand will float. The operator then adds that when the hand reaches the side of the face, the subject will be deeply hypnotized.

When this point is reached, and the hand and arm have "levitated," the operator assumes that the subject is well hypnotized and then adds suggestions that are appropriate to the situation. Not all subjects, however, respond to hypnosis to the same extent or at the same rate.

There is no evidence to support the view that the operator in hypnosis is able to control the experience and behavior of the subject against the latter's wishes. It is the subject's motivation to behave in accordance with the wishes and directions of the operator that creates that erroneous impression. Moreover, there is no evidence to support the idea that a hypnotized subject can transcend his or her normal volitional capacity because of the hypnosis; despite persuasive clinical reports of altered somatic structures in hypnosis, no physiological changes uniquely associated with hypnosis have been demonstrated. Hypnosis is not so much a way of manipulating behavior as of creating increased perception and memory.

USES AND COMPLICATIONS

Because the mind, body, and emotions are interdependent, factors that influence one influence the others as well. The roles of the mind and emotions in functional or psychophysiological (psychosomatic) illness are widely recognized, but in cases of organic illness, their importance is often underestimated.

Regardless of etiology (causes), there are physical and psychological components to all illness. Emotional states that continue over extended periods can produce physiological changes. The fear, resentment, or depression that often accompanies illness may prolong or exacerbate it and interfere with a patient's willingness or ability to participate in treatment. Addressing such issues through hypnosis can greatly improve the overall medical management of a patient, from the initial diagnosis through all forms of treatment, including the treatment of unconscious and critically ill patients.

One advantage of modern clinical hypnosis is that it requires the practitioner to approach the patient as a whole person rather than as a collection of parts, one or more of which may be diseased. For the physician using hypnosis, a medical history goes beyond a list of past illnesses, allergies, and hospitalizations. A more comprehensive picture is developed that includes an understanding of a patient's personality, present state of mind, and life history and the positive aspects as well as the stresses and strains of the patient's present environment.

The use of hypnosis in most, if not all, medical specialties has been well documented. Hypnosis can be used alone or in combination with other approaches to overcome a variety of habit disorders. While some problems, such as thumb-sucking, can be resolved relatively quickly, others, such as overeating, sometimes require extended treatment or a multidimensional approach. Smoking and bed-wetting are examples of habit disorders that can be managed through hypnosis.

There is much evidence that children as a group are more responsive to hypnosis than adults, and that in-

fants and young children frequently experience hypnosis as a natural part of their lives. Children can often be helped in a remarkably short period of time. Hypnosis has been used with children in the treatment of such diverse ailments as bed-wetting, soiling, asthma, epilepsy, learning difficulties, some behavioral and delinquency problems, stuttering, and nailbiting.

Hypnosis has been used effectively as an adjunct to the treatment of numerous problems with autonomic (internal) nervous system components. For example, there have been many controlled studies and successful case reports on the use of hypnosis in the treatment of asthma, which is the most common of the psychophysiological respiratory disorders. Through hypnosis, a patient can be helped to break the vicious cycle in which anxiety and emotional upsets can trigger an acute asthma attack, which in turn can produce anxiety and fear of other attacks.

Hypnosis has also been used effectively in the control and relief of pain. Because pain is experienced psychologically as well as physiologically, hypnosis can help people alter the perception of pain. A patient can learn to block pain to specific areas of the body, lessen the sensation of pain, or move pain from one area of the body to another. This ability is useful in the management of many types of pain, including chronic back pain, postoperative pain, and the pain associated with illness, migraine headache, burns, childbirth, and medical procedures.

In addition to being used to treat chronic conditions such as hypertension, hypnosis has been used to provide symptomatic relief of other chronic conditions, such as musculoskeletal disorders (for example, rheumatoid arthritis, osteoarthritis, fractures, and bursitis) and hemophilia.

Hypnosis has been used in dentistry for the relief of anxiety as well as pain and has been found to be helpful in teeth grinding (bruxism) and gagging. Modern hypnodontics is not primarily concerned with producing a surgical hypoanalgesia except in rare instances in which chemical anesthesia cannot be tolerated. The dentist is concerned with making visits to his or her office more tolerable and less threatening.

In obstetrics and surgery, hypnosis has been used to induce relaxation and relieve anxiety and to reduce the amount of anesthetic necessary. Occasionally, no anesthetic is required. This is sometimes desirable in childbirth, when the mother prefers to be aware of the birth process, or in other surgical procedures in which a minimum of anesthetic is desirable.

Hypnosis has also been utilized by the police in what has been termed "investigative hypnosis." Witnesses to crimes are interrogated in an effort to improve their memory retrieval.

Hypnosis has also been helpful in increasing athletic effectiveness. It has been utilized by both team and individual athletes to increase self-confidence and other factors such as self-image and the ability to assess the competition. Hypnosis thus applied to maximize performance in sports has been very effective, but the principles involved are essentially no different from those applied to other areas of living, such as increasing the efficiency of performance in the home, school, or workplace.

Since the mid-1970's, there has been much research into immune system functioning. Studies of the effects of stress on immune system functioning are lending scientific support to anecdotal reports that indicate that hypnosis may be effective in altering the disease process in cancer and AIDS patients. Researchers have found that unless treatments for these illnesses are based on the premise that the mind, body, and emotions are all striving to achieve health, physical intervention alone (radiation or chemotherapy, for example) will not be effective.

PERSPECTIVE AND PROSPECTS

Although medical hypnosis is considered to have had its beginnings with the Viennese physician Franz Anton Mesmer (1733-1815) in the latter half of the eighteenth century, hypnosis, or something very similar to it, has been practiced by religious and other healers in various ways for centuries in most cultures. The earliest evidence of its existence was found among shamans, who were also referred to as "witch doctors," "medicine men," or "healers."

In preparation for healing, a shaman adhered to certain practices that allowed his or her powers of concentration to be heightened. Placing himself or herself in isolation, the shaman began a descent into the "lower world." This often meant visualizing an opening in the earth and a journey downward into that opening. The journey was frequently accompanied by rhythmic drumming, chanting, singing, or dancing. The monotonous rhythm and constancy allowed the shaman's subconscious mind to become strongly focused, seek out the sick spirit of the patient, make it whole, and bring it back to the patient. The shaman actually engaged in a powerful process of visualization and suggestion during which the shaman willed the sick person to be healed.

In the eighteenth century, Mesmer recognized this ancient healing phenomenon and incorporated it into a theory of animal magnetism. Mesmer believed that a "cosmic fluid" could be stored in inanimate objects, such as magnets, and transferred to patients to cure them of illness.

Mesmer dressed flamboyantly. His consulting rooms were dimly lit and hung with mirrors, and he kept soft music playing in the background. The doctor's patients sat in a circle around a vat that contained such elements as powdered glass or iron filings. Then the patients grasped iron rods that were immersed in the vat and were believed to transmit a curing force.

Mesmer's first success was with a twenty-nine-year-old woman who suffered from a convulsive malady, a condition commonly called a "nervous disorder." Her symptoms consisted of blood rushing to her head and a tremendous pain in her ears and head. This state was followed by delirium, rage, vomiting, and fainting. During one of the woman's attacks, Mesmer applied three magnets to the patient's stomach and legs while she concentrated on the positive effects of the "cosmic fluid." In a short time, her symptoms subsided. When her symptoms resurfaced the next day, Mesmer gave her another treatment and achieved similar results. Mesmer believed that the "cosmic fluid," stimulated by the magnets, was directed through his patient's body. Her energy flow was restored, and as a result she regained her health.

Eventually Mesmer discarded the magnets. He began to regard himself as a magnet through which a fluid life force could be conducted and then transmitted to others as a healing force. This is what Mesmer described as "animal magnetism."

Despite the fact that no scientific evidence supported the existence of Mesmer's "cosmic fluids" or the concept of "animal magnetism," he had a tremendous rate of success. Thousands flocked to him for treatment. The only explanation for his success is that his patients were literally "mesmerized" into the belief and expectation that they would be cured. "Mesmerism" was a forerunner of the concept of hypnotic suggestion.

During this same period, a new slant on Mesmer's theories was introduced by one of his disciples, the Marquis de Puységur. He believed that the "cosmic fluid" was not magnetic but electric. This electric fluid was generated in all living things—in plants as well as animals. Puységur used the natural environment to fill his patients with the healing electric fluid that was expected to end their suffering. His clinic was held outdoors, where the sick were received under an elm tree in the center of the village green. Puységur believed that the tree had an innate healing power and that the force would travel through the trunk and branches to cords that he hung from the tree. At the foot of the tree, patients sat in a circle on stone benches with the cords wrapped around the diseased parts of their bodies. They were "connected" to one another when they touched their thumbs together, which made it possible for the "fluid" to circulate from person to person and to heal.

During this activity, Puységur noticed a strange phenomenon. Some of the patients entered a state of deep sleep as a result of being mesmerized. In this state, the patient could still communicate and be lucid and responsive to the suggestions of the mesmerist. The marquis had discovered the hypnotic trance but had not identified it as such.

In the mid-1800's, the hypnotic trance was used to relieve pain. An eminent London physician, John Elliotson (1791-1868), reported 1,834 surgical operations performed painlessly. In India, a Scottish surgeon named James Esdaile (1808-1859) performed many major operations, such as amputation of limbs, using mesmerism (or, as he called it, "magnetic sleep") as the sole anesthetic. One procedure involved conditioning the patient weeks prior to surgery. This was accomplished by inducing a trance state in the patient and offering posthypnotic suggestions to numb the part of the body on which the surgery was to be performed. In a second method, the hypnotist attended to the patient in the operating room, inducing a trance state and suggesting disassociation from any pain. It was possible for the patient to be completely lucid during this state and also to be oblivious to pain, as though completely anesthetized.

Mesmerism continued to provoke new theories and uses. During the late nineteenth century, an English physician, James Braid (1795-1860), gave mesmerism a scientific explanation. He believed mesmerism to be a "nervous sleep" and coined the word "hypnosis," which was derived from the Greek word *hypnos*, meaning sleep. Braid showed that hypnotized subjects are often abnormally susceptible to impressions on the senses and that much of the subjects' behavior was caused by suggestions made verbally.

Soon, other theories began to emerge. Jean Martin Charcot (1825-1893), a neurologist who taught in Paris, explained hypnosis as a state of hysteria and categorized it as an abnormal neurological activity.

In France, Auguste Ambroise Leibeault (1823-1904) and Hippolyte Bernheim (1837-1919) were the first to regard hypnosis as a normal phenomenon. They asserted that expectation is the most important factor in the induction of hypnosis, that increased suggestibility is its essential symptom, and that the hypnotist works on the patient by means of mental influences.

As hypnosis began to receive serious study and could be explained rationally, it began to gain acceptance in the scientific community. It was no longer relegated to the realm of the bizarre.

Sigmund Freud became interested in hypnosis at this same time and visited Leibeault and Bernheim's clinic to learn their induction techniques. As Freud observed patients enter a hypnotic state, he began to recognize the existence of the unconscious. Although he was not the first to make this observation, he was the first to recognize the unconscious as a major source of psychopathology. Early in his research, however, Freud rejected hypnosis as the tool to unlock repressed memories, favoring instead his technique of free association and dream interpretation. With the rise of psychoanalysis in the first half of the twentieth century, hypnosis declined in popularity.

Then, however, a reversal occurred. During World War II, interest in hypnosis was regenerated by the need for short-term therapy (it was often applied in cases of "battle fatigue") and by the combination of hypnosis and more traditional analytic approaches. Mind control and "brainwashing" techniques that surfaced during the Korean War again sparked interest in the power of suggestion, especially when the subject was under duress. In the late 1960's and early 1970's, with the rise of public interest in alternative forms of mental health (Transcendental Meditation, biofeedback, yoga) and ways of coping with the stress of the modern world, hypnosis experienced a rebirth. Researchers found new and potent uses for it in therapy, and the trance state began to be recognized as a highly effective tool for modifying behavior and for healing.

—Genevieve Slomski, Ph.D.

See also Alternative medicine; Anesthesia; Anesthesiology; Anxiety; Asthma; Bed-wetting; Brain; Meditation; Pain management; Psychiatry; Psychosomatic disorders; Stress; Stress reduction.

FOR FURTHER INFORMATION:

Brown, Peter. *The Hypnotic Brain: Hypnotherapy and Social Communication.* New Haven, Conn.: Yale University Press, 1994. This scholarly work examines how communication in human beings arose, the importance of nonverbal communication, the rise in oral cultures, and evidence for the common "everyday" trance.

Burrows, Graham D., Robb O. Stanley, and Peter B. Bloom, eds. *International Handbook of Clinical Hypnosis*. New York: Wiley, 2001. Takes a practical approach in explaining both the scientific and clinical aspects of hypnosis and providing information on a range of available psychological and physical treatments.

Forrest, Derek. *Hypnotism: A History*. New York: Penguin, 2000. This book offers a history of hypnotism and its predecessor, mesmerism. Traces the major figures of mesmerism, leading up through Sigmund Freud and hypnotism's influence in the twentieth century.

Hadley, Josie, and Carol Staudacher. *Hypnosis for Change*. 3d ed. New York: Ballantine Books, 2000. This popular account provides step-by-step details on the practice of self-hypnosis. It also offers a brief historical sketch of hypnosis, explores all facets of induction, and examines various aspects of hypnotic communication. Includes a bibliography.

Yapko, Michael D. *Trancework: An Introduction to the Practice of Clinical Hypnosis*. 3d ed. Washington, D.C.: Taylor & Francis, 2003. Describes what hypnosis is and why it works in a clinical setting, surveys a broad range of hypnotic methods and techniques, and provides several trance scripts.

Zahourek, Rothlyn P., ed. *Clinical Hypnosis and Therapeutic Suggestion in Patient Care*. New York: Brunner/Mazel, 1990. Representing a variety of disciplines, the contributors to this book argue that hypnosis is a natural, noninvasive tool that can be of use in patient care.

HYPOCHONDRIASIS

DISEASE/DISORDER

ALSO KNOWN AS: Hypochondriacal neurosis or hypochondriacal reaction

ANATOMY OR SYSTEM AFFECTED: Psychic-emotional system, all bodily systems

SPECIALTIES AND RELATED FIELDS: Psychiatry, psychology

DEFINITION: Unwarranted belief about or anxiety over having a serious disease which is based on one's subjective interpretation of physical symptoms or sensations; the belief or anxiety is main-

tained in spite of appropriate medical assurances that there is no serious disease.

KEY TERMS:

defense mechanisms: automatic, unconscious mental processes that become activated in the presence of emotional distress and anxiety; these processes work to maintain inner harmony by preventing mental awareness of that which would be otherwise too emotionally painful to endure

hypochondria: an earlier term for hypochondriasis; from classical Greek, it means the abdominal region of the body below the rib cage, from which black bile was believed to cause melancholy and yellow bile was believed to cause ill-temper

hypochondriacal neurosis: an earlier, but still-used, term for hypochondriasis; because experts have disagreed about what "neurosis" means precisely, the term is considered less descriptive than "hypochondriasis"

hypochondriacal reaction: another earlier term for hypochondriasis; experts who still prefer this term view hypochondriasis as a transient reaction to life stress and tend not to see it as a mental-emotional disorder in its own right

primary hypochondriasis: hypochondriasis as a disorder in its own right, and not accompanied by another psychiatric disorder such as generalized anxiety or panic

secondary hypochondriasis: the experience of hypochondriacal symptoms as part of an underlying, causal condition such as panic disorder, generalized anxiety disorder, schizophrenia, or major depression with psychotic features

somatization disorder: the somatoform disorder most similar to hypochondriasis; in somatization, the preoccupation is primarily with symptoms that one experiences and not with a disease that one is fearful of getting, an important distinction when these conditions are treated

somatoform disorders: the grouping of disorders that includes hypochondriasis; these disorders feature symptoms that suggest physical disease but that are actually caused by psychological upset

CAUSES AND SYMPTOMS

With hypochondriasis, the real problem is the patient's excessive worry and mental preoccupation with having or developing a disease, not the disease about which the patient is so worried. While concern about contracting a serious disease is common and normal, and may even make one more prudent, excessive worry, endless rumination, and obsessive interpretation of every symptom and sensation can disable and prevent effective functioning. A diagnosis of hypochondriasis is made when the patient's dread about the disease or diseases impairs normal activity and persists despite appropriate medical reassurances and evidence to the contrary. Even though hypochondriacs can acknowledge intellectually the possibility that their fears might be without rational foundation, the acknowledgment itself fails to bring any relief.

Researchers estimate that a low of 3 percent to a high of 14 percent of all medical (versus psychiatric) patients have hypochondriasis. Just how prevalent it is in the population as a whole is unknown. What is known is that the disorder shows up slightly more in men than in women, starts at any age but most often between twenty and thirty, shows up most often in physicians' offices with patients who are in their forties and fifties, and tends to run in families.

Most clinicians believe that hypochondriasis has a primary psychological cause or causes but that, in general, hypochondriacs have only a vague awareness that they are doing something that perpetuates and worsens their hypochondriacal symptoms. Hypochondriacs do not feign illness; they genuinely believe themselves to be sick, or about to become so.

Clinicians usually favor one of four hypotheses about how hypochondriasis starts. The hypotheses are based on anecdotal, clinical experience with patients who have gotten better when treated specifically for hypochondriasis. Researchers have rarely studied hypochondriasis using strict experimental methods. Nevertheless, the anecdotal evidence is important, because it gives clinicians a way to think about how to treat the condition.

The most popular view among mental health professionals sees hypochondriacs as essentially angry, but deep down inside. Because their life experience is of hurt, disappointment, rejection, and loss, they engage in a two-stage process to make up for their sad state of affairs. Though they believe themselves unlovable and unacceptable as they are, they solicit attention and caring by presenting themselves either as ill or as dangerously close to becoming ill. Their fundamental anger fosters their development of an interpersonal pattern in which they bite the emotional hands which seek to feed them. Endless worry and rumination soon render ineffective others' concern. No amount of reassurance al-

INFORMATION ON HYPOCHONDRIASIS
CAUSES: Psychological disorders
SYMPTOMS: Excessive worry, endless rumination, and obsessive interpretation of symptoms and sensations; impaired normal activity; chronic persistance despite appropriate medical reassurances and contrary evidence
DURATION: Chronic, although at times temporary
TREATMENTS: Psychotherapy, limited drug therapy

lays their preoccupation and anxiety. In this way, those moved to show concern tire, grow impatient, and finally give up their efforts to help, proving to the worried hypochondriacs that no one really does care about them after all. Meanwhile, the hypochondriacs remain sad and angry.

This view often assumes that hypochondriasis is actually a form of defense mechanism which transfers angry, hostile, and critical feelings felt toward others into physical symptoms and signs of disease. Because hypochondriacs find it too difficult to admit that they feel angry, isolated, and unloved, they hide from the emotional energy associated with these powerful feelings and transfer them into bodily symptoms. This process seems to occur most often when hypochondriacal people harbor feelings of reproach because they are bereaved and lonely. In effect, they are angry at being left alone and left uncared for, and they redirect the emotion inwardly as self-reproach manifested in physical complaints.

Others hypothesize that hypochondriasis enables those who either believe themselves to be basically bad and unworthy of happiness or feel guilty for being alive ("existential guilt") to atone for their wrongdoings and, thereby, undo the guilt that they are always fighting not to feel. The mental anguish, emotional sadness, and physical pain so prevalent in hypochondriasis make reparation for the patients' real, exaggerated, or imagined badness.

A third view is sociological in orientation. Health providers who endorse it see hypochondriasis as society's way of letting people who feel frightened and overwhelmed by life's challenges escape from having to face those challenges, even if temporarily. Hypochondriacs take on a "sick role" which removes societal expectations that they will face responsibilities. In presenting themselves to the world as too sick to function, they also present themselves as excused from doing so. A schoolchild's stomachache on the day of a big test provides a relatively common and potentially harmless example of this role at work. Non-physically disabled adults who seek refuge from life stress by staying in bed, and who find themselves with true physical paralysis years later, provide a more serious and regrettable example.

A fourth view utilizes some experimental data which suggest that hypochondriacal people may have lower thresholds for (and lower tolerances of) emotional and physical pain. The data suggest that hypochondriacs experience physical and/or emotional sensations that are a magnification of what is normal experience. Thus, a sensation that would be sinus pressure for most people would be experienced as severe sinus headache in the hypochondriac. Hypersensitivity (lower threshold) to bodily sensations keeps hypochondriacs ever on watch for these upsetting, intense sensations because of how amplified the physical and emotional experiences are. What seems to most people an exaggerated concern with symptoms is simply prudent, self-protective vigilance to hypochondriacs.

Regardless of why the disorder develops, the majority of hypochondriacs go to their physicians with concerns about stomach and intestinal problems or heart and blood circulation problems. These complaints are usually only part of broader concerns about other organ systems and other anatomical locations. The key clinical feature of the disorder of hypochondriasis, however, is not where and how many bodily complaints there are but the patients' belief that they are seriously sick, or are just about to become so, and that the disease has yet to be detected. Laboratory tests that reveal healthy organs, physician reassurances that they are well, and long periods in which the dreaded disease fails to manifest itself are not reassuring at all. In fact, before the hypochondriasis itself is treated psychologically, it seems that nothing can stop the frantic rumination and accompanying nervousness, even the patients' acknowledgment that they may be exaggerating their reaction to their heartbeat, headache, diarrhea, morning cough, or perspiration. Hypochondriacs seem genuinely unable not to worry.

Hypochondriacs typically present their medical history in great detail and at great length. Often, they have an elaborate, exotic, and complex pathophysiological theory to explain how they acquired the disease and what it is doing, or will soon do, to them. At times, they cite recent research and give great importance to other causes, tests, or treatments that they and their health providers have not yet tried. Because their actual problem is not, strictly speaking, medical (or not only medical) and because they usually frustrate professional caretakers such as physicians, as well as nonprofessional caretakers such as family and friends, breakdown in the helping process is common. Worried patients tax physicians' time and resources, while busy physicians feel increasingly drained for what they believe is no good reason. The hypochondriacal patients sense that their concerns are not respected or taken seriously; they start to sense resentment. Phone calls to physicians' offices go unreturned for longer and longer periods. The perceived lack of access to their health providers makes the hypochondriac worry even more frenetically. The physicians increasingly believe that these patients are unappreciative—that they are, in fact, healthy and that they are not cooperating with treatment goals. Instead, these hypochondriacal patients are seen as excessively demanding. Anger builds on both sides, relationships deteriorate, and the hypochondriacs begin to "doctor-shop," while the physicians lose them as patients.

Although hypochondriasis is usually chronic, with periods in which it is more and less severe, temporary hypochondriacal reactions are also commonly seen. Such reactions most often occur when patients have experienced a death or serious illness of someone close to them or some other major life stressor, including their own recovery from a life-threatening illness.

When these reactions persist for less than six months, the technical diagnosis is a condition called "somatoform disorder not otherwise specified," and not hypochondriasis. When external stressors cause the reaction, the hypochondriacal symptoms usually remit when the stressors dissipate or are resolved. The important exception to this rule occurs when family, friends, or health professionals inadvertently reinforce the worry and preoccupation through inappropriate amounts of attention. In effect, they reward hypochondriacal behavior and increase the likelihood that it will persist. A mother may never have received more support and help at home than following breast cancer surgery. A father may never have felt his children's affection as much as when he recuperated from having a heart attack. An employee may have never obtained special allowances on the job or received so many calls from coworkers as when recovering from herniated disk surgery. A student may never have gotten as special treatment or as many gifts from teammates as when treated for rheumatic fever. What began as a transient hypochondriacal reaction can become chronic, primary hypochondriasis.

The life of hypochondriacs is unhappy and unrewarding. Nervous tension, depression, hopelessness, and a general lack of interest in life mark the fabric of the hypochondriacs' daily routines. Actual clinical, depressive disorders can easily coexist with hypochondriasis, to the point that even antidepression medications will simultaneously alleviate hypochondriacal symptoms.

Hypochondriasis often accompanies physical illness in the elderly. As a group, the elderly have declining health, experience diminished physical capacities, and are at increased risk for contracting and developing disease. Sometimes, earlier tendencies toward hypochondriasis simply intensify with age. Sometimes, old age is simply when it first appears. Hypochondriasis is not, however, a typical or expected aspect of normal aging; most elderly people are not hypochondriacal. In those who are, however, hypochondriasis is most likely a symptom of depression, abandonment, or loneliness, and these are the conditions that should first be treated.

Treatment and Therapy

The most important aspect of treating hypochondriasis is assessing whether true organic disease exists. Many diseases in their early stages are diffuse and affect multiple organ systems. Neurologic diseases (such as multiple sclerosis), hormonal abnormalities (such as Graves' disease), and autoimmune/connective tissue diseases (such as systemic lupus) can all manifest themselves early in ways that are difficult to diagnose accurately. The frantic and obsessive reporting of hypochondriacal patients can just as easily be the worried and detailed reporting of patients with early parathyroid disease; both report symptoms that are multiple, vague, and diffuse. The danger of hypochondriasis lies in its being diagnosed in place of true organic disease, which is exactly the kind of event hypochondriacs fear will happen.

Of course, there is nothing to prevent someone with true hypochondriasis from getting or having true physical illness. Worrying about illness neither protects from nor prevents illness. Moreover, barring a sudden, lethal accident or event, every hypochondriac is bound to develop organic illness sooner or later. Physical illness can coexist with hypochondriasis—and does so when attitudes, symptoms, and mental and emotional states are extreme and disproportionate to the medical problem at hand.

The goal in treating hypochondriasis is care, not cure. These patients have ongoing mental illness or chronic maladaptation and seem to need physical symptoms to justify how they feel. Neither surgical nor medical interventions will ameliorate a psychological need for symptoms. The best treatments (when hypochondriasis cannot itself be the target of treatment, which is most of the time) are long term in orientation and seek to help patients tolerate and accommodate their symptoms while health providers learn to understand and adapt to these difficult-to-treat patients.

Medications have proved useful in treating hypochondriasis only when accompanied by pharmacotherapy-sensitive conditions such as major depression or generalized anxiety. When hypochondriasis coexists with either mental or physical disease, the latter must be treated in its own right. Secondary hypochondriasis means that the primary disorder warrants primary treatment.

The course of hypochondriasis is unclear. Clinicians' anecdotal experience tends to endorse the perception that these people are impossible as patients. Outcome studies, however, belie the pessimism. The research suggests that many who are treated get better, and the more the following conditions are present, the better the outcome is likely to be: coexisting anxiety or depressive disorder, rapid onset, onset at a younger age, higher socioeconomic status, absence of organic disease, and absence of a personality disorder.

A fifty-six-year-old married male, for example, recounted his history as never having been in really good health at any time in his life. He made many physician office visits and had, over the years, seen many physicians, though without ever feeling emotionally connected to them. Over the past several months, he felt increasingly concerned that he was having headaches "all over" his head and that they were caused by an undetected tumor in the middle of his brain, "where no X ray could detect it." He had read about magnetic resonance imaging (MRI) in a health letter to which he subscribed and said that he wanted this procedure performed "to catch the tumor early." Various prescribed medications for his headache usually brought no relief.

While productive at work and promoted several times, he had been passed over for his last promotion because, he believed, his superiors did not like him. He also stated that he believed that many on the job saw him as cynical and pessimistic but that no one appreciated the "pain and mental anxiety" he endured "day in and day out."

His spouse of thirty-two years had advanced significantly at a job she had begun ten years earlier, and she seemed to him to be closer to their three children than he was. She was increasingly involved with outside voluntary activities, which kept her quite busy. She reported that she often asked him to join her in at least some of her activities but he always said no. She said that when she arrived home late, he was often in a state of physical upset, but for which she could never seem to do the "right thing to help him." In their joint interview, each admitted often feeling angry at and frustrated with the other. She could never determine why he was sick so often and why her efforts to help only seemed to make his situation worse. He could not understand how she could leave him all alone feeling as physically bad as he did. He believed that she never seemed to worry that something might happen to him while she was out being "a community do-gooder." The husband was suffering from a classic case of hypochondriasis.

PERSPECTIVE AND PROSPECTS

Both the concept and term "hypochondriasis" have ancient origins and reflect a view that all persons are subject to their own humoral ebb and flow. Humors were once thought to be bodily fluids that maintained health, regulated physical functioning, and caused certain personality traits. In classical Greek, *hypochondria*, the plural of *hypochondrion*, referred to both a part of the anatomy and the condition known today as hypochondriasis. *Hypo* means "under," "below," or "beneath," and *chondrion* means literally "cartilage" but in this case refers specifically to the bottom tip of cartilage at the breastbone (the xiphoid or, more formally, xiphisternum). Here, below the breastbone but above the navel, two humors were thought to flow in excess in the hypochondriacal person. The liver, producing black bile, made people melancholic, depressed, and depressing; the spleen, producing yellow bile, made people bilious, cross, and cynical. This view, or a variant of it, persisted until the middle to late eighteenth century.

Sigmund Freud and other psychiatrists treated hypochondriacal symptoms with some success while approaching the disorder as a defense mechanism rather than as an excess of bodily fluids. Their treatment for the first time cast a psychological role for what had been seen as a physical problem. Mental health professionals whose theoretical orientation is psychoanalytic or psychodynamic continue to deal with hypochondriasis as they deal with other defense mechanisms.

In the 1970's, some researchers began to suggest that hypochondriasis was being incorrectly applied to describe a discrete disorder, when it was really only an adjective that described a cluster of nonspecific behaviors. They argued that hypochondriasis is not a real diagnosis. Other researchers disagreed and argued for differentiating between primary and secondary hypochondriasis. Their view has proved to have significant pragmatic utility in treating the wide range of patients who exhibit symptoms of hypochondriasis, and it remains the prevailing view.

Given the general unwillingness of patients with hypochondriasis to admit that they have a psychological problem and not some yet-to-be-found organic condition, the interpersonal difficulties that often arise between health providers and these patients, and the serious potential of concurrent organic disease, it is not surprising why hypochondriasis continues to challenge both persons afflicted with this disorder and those who treat them.

—Paul Moglia, Ph.D.

See also Anxiety; Bipolar disorders; Depression; Factitious disorders; Midlife crisis; Neurosis; Obsessive-compulsive disorder; Over-the-counter medications; Panic attacks; Phobias; Psychiatric disorders; Psychiatry; Psychiatry, child and adolescent; Psychiatry, geriatric; Psychosomatic disorders; Stress; Stress reduction.

FOR FURTHER INFORMATION:

Asmundson, Gordon J. G., et al., eds. *Health Anxiety: Clinical and Research Perspectives on Hypochondriasis and Related Conditions.* New York: Wiley, 2001. Assembles a wealth of information from the fields of medicine and psychology on the causes, assessment, and treatment of health anxiety related disorders.

Barsky, Arthur J. "Somatoform Disorders." In *Comprehensive Textbook of Psychiatry VI.* Vol. 1, edited by Harold I. Kaplan and Benjamin J. Sadock. 6th ed. Baltimore: Williams & Wilkins, 1995. While Kaplan and Sadock's book remains the standard psychiatric reference for psychiatrists and nonpsychiatric physicians alike, Barsky's chapter includes an excellent discussion of hypochondriasis that is readily intelligible to laypeople.

Ben-Tovim, David I., and Adrian Esterman. "Zero Progress with Hypochondriasis." *The Lancet* 352, no. 9143 (December 5, 1998): 1798-1799. Despite behavioral research on patients suffering from hypochondriasis, no acceptable treatment for this condition has been discovered. It is important for doctors to adequately examine these patients, however, because even hypochondriacal patients can fall ill.

De Jong, Peter J., Marie-Anne Haenen, Anton Schmidt, and Birgit Mayer. "Hypochondriasis: The Role of Fear-Confirming Reasoning." *Behaviour Research and Therapy* 36, no. 1 (January, 1998): 65-74. This article investigates whether hypochondriacal patients are prone to selectively search for danger-confirming information when asked to judge the validity of conditional rules in the context of general and health threats.

Hill, John. *Hypochondriasis: A Practical Treatise.* New York: AMS Press, 1992. Originally published in 1766, this well-regarded and readable work presents the world of hypochondriacs in ways that challenge stereotypical and biased views of them.

Starcevic, Vladen, and Don R. Lipsitt, eds. *Hypochondriasis: Modern Perspectives on an Ancient Malady.* New York: Oxford University Press, 2000. Provides an integrative overview of hypochondriasis as a mental disorder with diverse manifestations.

HYPOGLYCEMIA

DISEASE/DISORDER

ANATOMY OR SYSTEM AFFECTED: Blood, endocrine system, glands

SPECIALTIES AND RELATED FIELDS: Endocrinology, family medicine, hematology, internal medicine, serology

DEFINITION: The condition in which concentration of glucose in the blood is too low to meet the needs of key organs, especially the brain; this condition limits treatments for diabetes mellitus.

KEY TERMS:

fasting hypoglycemia: hypoglycemia that occurs when no food is available from the intestinal tract; usually caused by failure of the neural, hormonal, and/or enzymatic mechanisms that convert stored fuels (primarily glycogen) into glucose

glucagon: a pancreatic hormone which signals an elevated concentration of glucose in the circulation

gluconeogenesis: the synthesis of molecules of glucose from smaller carbohydrates and amino acids

glucose: a simple sugar, readily converted to metabolic energy by most cells of the body and essential for the welfare of brain cells

glycogen: a storage form of carbohydrate, composed of many molecules of glucose linked together; is found in many tissues of the body and serves as a major source of circulating glucose

glycogenolysis: the cleavage of glycogen into its constituent molecules of glucose

hypoglycemic unawareness: the occurrence of hypoglycemia without the warning symptoms of trembling, palpitations, hunger, or anxiety

hypoglycemic unresponsiveness: inadequate recovery of the circulating glucose concentration after an episode of hypoglycemia

insulin: a pancreatic hormone which signals a reduced concentration of glucose in the circulation

neuroglycopenia: abnormal function of the brain, caused by an inadequate supply of glucose from the circulation

reactive hypoglycemia: hypoglycemia that occurs within a few hours after ingestion of a meal

CAUSES AND SYMPTOMS

The condition known as hypoglycemia exists when the concentration of glucose in the bloodstream is too low to meet bodily needs for fuel, particularly those of the brain. Ordinarily, physiological compensatory mechanisms are called into play when the circulating concentration of glucose falls below about 3.5 millimoles. Activation of the sympathetic nervous system and the secretion of glucagon are especially important in promoting glycogenolysis and gluconeogenesis. Symptoms of sympathetic nervous activation normally become apparent with glucose concentrations that are less than about 3 millimoles. Brain function is usually demonstrably abnormal at glucose concentrations below about 2 millimoles; sustained hypoglycemia in this range can lead to permanent brain damage.

Some of the symptoms of hypoglycemia occur as by-products of activation of the sympathetic nervous system. These symptoms include trembling, pallor, palpitations and rapid heartbeat, sweating, abdominal discomfort, and feelings of anxiety and/or hunger. These symptoms are not dangerous in themselves; in fact, they may be considered to be beneficial, as they alert the individual to obtain food. Meanwhile, the sympathetic nervous system signals compensatory mechanisms. The manifestations of abnormal brain function during hypoglycemia include blunting of higher cognitive functions, disturbed mentation, confusion, loss of normal control of behavior, headache, lethargy, impaired vision, abnormal speech, paralysis, neurologic deficits, coma, and epileptic seizures. The individual is usually unaware of the appearance of these symptoms, which can present real danger. For example, episodes of hypoglycemia have occurred while individuals were driving motor vehicles, leading to serious injury and death. After recovery from hypoglycemia, the patient may have no memory of the episode.

There are two major categories of hypoglycemia: fasting and reactive. The most serious, fasting hypoglycemia, represents impairment of the mechanisms responsible for the production of glucose when food is not available. These mechanisms include the functions of cells in the liver and brain that monitor the availability of circulating glucose. Additionally, there is a coordinated hormonal response involving the secretion of glucagon, growth hormone, and other hormones and the inhibition of the secretion of insulin. The normal consequences of these processes include the addition of glucose to the circulation, primarily from glycogenolysis, as well as a slowing of the rate of utilization of circulating glucose by many tissues of the body, especially the liver, skeletal and cardiac muscle, and fat. Even after days without food, the body normally avoids hypoglycemia through breakdown of stored proteins and activation of gluconeogenesis. There is considerable redundancy in the systems that maintain glucose concentration, so that the occurrence of hypoglycemia often reflects the presence of defects in more than one of these mechanisms.

The other category of hypoglycemia, reactive hypoglycemia, includes disorders in which there is disproportionately prolonged and/or great activity of the physiologic systems that normally cause storage of the glucose derived from ingested foods. When a normal person eats a meal, the passage of food through the stomach and intestines elicits a complex and well-orchestrated neural and hormonal response, culminating in the secretion of insulin from the beta cells of the islets of Langerhans in the pancreas. The insulin signals the cells in muscle, adipose tissue, and the liver to stop producing glucose and to derive energy from glucose obtained from the circulation. Glucose in excess of the body's immediate needs for fuel is taken up and stored as glycogen is or utilized for the manufacture of proteins. Normally, the signals for the uptake and storage of glucose reach their peak of activity simultaneously with the entry into the circulation of glucose from the food undergoing digestion. As a result, the concentration of glucose in the circulation fluctuates only slightly. In individuals with reactive hypoglycemia, however, the entry of glucose from the digestive

---

INFORMATION ON HYPOGLYCEMIA

CAUSES: Endocrine disorder, malnutrition, advanced stages of cancer, inherited metabolic disorders, severe infections (including overwhelming bacterial infection and malaria), certain drugs

SYMPTOMS: Trembling, pallor, palpitations and rapid heartbeat, sweating, abdominal discomfort, feelings of anxiety and/or hunger, disturbed thoughts, confusion, loss of normal control of behavior, headache, lethargy, impaired vision, abnormal speech

DURATION: Temporary to long-term

TREATMENTS: Drugs inhibiting secretion of insulin, hormonal therapy

---

tract and the signals for its uptake and storage are not well synchronized. When signals for the cellular uptake of glucose persist after the intestinally derived glucose has dissipated, hypoglycemia can result. Although the degree of hypoglycemia may be severe and potentially dangerous, recovery can take place without assistance if the individual's general nutritional state is adequate and the systems for activation of glycogenolysis and gluconeogenesis are intact.

DIAGNOSIS AND TREATMENT

The diagnostic evaluation of an individual who is suspected of having hypoglycemia begins with verification of the condition. Evaluation of a patient's symptoms can be confusing. On one hand, the symptoms arising from the sympathetic nervous system and those of neuroglycopenia may occur in a variety of nonhypoglycemic conditions. On the other hand, persons with recurrent hypoglycemia may have few or no obvious symptoms. Therefore, it is most important to document the concentration of glucose in the blood.

To establish the diagnosis of fasting hypoglycemia, the patient is kept without food for periods of time up to seventy-two hours, with frequent monitoring of the blood glucose. Should hypoglycemia occur, blood is taken for measurements of the key regulatory neurosecretions and hormones, including insulin, glucagon, growth hormone, cortisol, and epinephrine, as well as general indices of the function of the liver and kidneys. If there is suspicion of an abnormality in an enzyme involved in glucose production, the diagnosis can be confirmed by measurement of the relevant enzymatic activity in circulating blood cells or, if necessary, in a biopsy specimen of the liver.

Fasting hypoglycemia may be caused by any condition that inhibits the production of glucose or that causes an inappropriately great utilization of circulating glucose when food is not available. Insulin produces hypoglycemia through both of these mechanisms. Excessive circulating insulin ranks as one of the most important causes of fasting hypoglycemia, most cases of which result from the treatment of diabetes mellitus with insulin or with an oral drug of the sulfonylurea class. If the patient is known to be taking insulin or a sulfonylurea drug for diabetes, the cause of hypoglycemia is obvious; appropriate modification of the treatment should be made. Hypoglycemia caused by oral sulfonylureas is particularly troublesome because of the prolonged retention of these drugs in the body. The passage of several days may be required for recovery, during which time the patient needs continuous intravenous infusion of glucose.

Excessive insulin secretion may also result from increased numbers of pancreatic beta cells; the abnormal beta cells may be so numerous that they form benign or malignant tumors, called insulinomas. The preferred treatment of an insulinoma is surgery, if feasible. When the tumor can be removed surgically, the operation is often curative. Unfortunately, insulinomas are sometimes difficult for the surgeon to find. Magnetic resonance imaging (MRI), computed tomography (CT) scanning, ultrasonography, or angiography may help localize the tumor. Some insulinomas are multiple and/or malignant, rendering total removal impossible. In these circumstances, hypoglycemia can be relieved by drugs that inhibit the secretion of insulin.

Malignant tumors arising from various tissues of the body may produce hormones that act like insulin with respect to their effects on glucose metabolism. In some cases, these hormones are members of the family of insulin-like growth factors, which resemble insulin structurally. Malnutrition probably has an important role in predisposing patients with malignancy to hypoglycemia, which tends to occur when the cancer is far advanced.

Fasting hypoglycemia can be caused by disorders affecting various parts of the endocrine system. One such disorder is adrenal insufficiency; continued secretion of cortisol by the adrenal cortex is required for maintenance of normal glycogen stores and of the enzymes of glycogenolysis and gluconeogenesis. Severe hypothyroidism also may lead to hypoglycemia. Impairment in the function of the anterior pituitary gland predisposes a patient to hypoglycemia through several mechanisms, including reduced function of the thyroid gland and adrenal cortices (which depend on pituitary secretions for normal activity) and reduced secretion of growth hormone. Growth hormone plays an important physiologic role in the prevention of fasting hypoglycemia by signaling metabolic changes that allow heart and skeletal muscles to derive energy from stored fats, thereby sparing glucose for the brain. Specific replacement therapies are available for deficiencies of thyroxine, cortisol, and growth hormone.

Hypoglycemia has occasionally been reported as a side effect of treatment with medications other than those intended for treatment of diabetes. Drugs which have been implicated include sulfonamides, used for treatment of bacterial infections; quinine, used for treatment of falciparum malaria; pentamidine isethionate, given by injection for treatment of pneumocystosis; ritodrine, used for inhibition of premature labor; and propranolol or disopyramide, both of which are used for treatment of cardiac arrhythmias. Malnourished patients seem to be especially susceptible to the hypoglycemic effects of these medications, and management should consist of nutritional repletion in addition to discontinuation of the drug responsible. In children, aspirin or other medicines containing salicylates may produce hypoglycemia.

Alcohol hypoglycemia occurs in persons with low bodily stores of glycogen when there is no food in the intestine. In this circumstance, the only potential source of glucose for the brain is gluconeogenesis. When such an individual drinks alcohol, its metabolism within the liver prevents the precursors of glucose from entering the pathways of gluconeogenesis. This variety of fasting hypoglycemia can occur in persons who are not chronic alcoholics: It requires the ingestion of only a moderate amount of alcohol, on the order of three mixed drinks. Treatment involves the nutritional repletion of glycogen stores and the limitation of alcohol intake.

Severe infections, including overwhelming bacterial infection and malaria, can produce hypoglycemia by mechanisms that are not well understood. Patients with very severe liver damage can develop fasting hypoglycemia, because the pathways of glycogenolysis and gluconeogenesis in the liver are by far the major sources of circulating glucose in the fasted state. In such cases, the occurrence of hypoglycemia usually marks a near-terminal stage of liver disease. Uremia, the syndrome produced by kidney failure, can also lead to fasting hypoglycemia.

Some types of fasting hypoglycemia occur predominantly in infants and children. Babies in the first year of life may have an inappropriately high secretion of insulin. This problem occurs especially in newborn infants whose mothers had increased circulating glucose during pregnancy. Children from two to ten years of age may develop ketotic hypoglycemia, which is probably related to insufficient gluconeogenesis. These disorders tend to improve with time. Fasting hypoglycemia is also an important manifestation of a variety of inherited disorders of metabolism characterized by the abnormality or absence of one of the necessary enzymes or cofactors of glycogenolysis and gluconeogenesis or of fat metabolism (which supplies the energy for gluconeogenesis). Most of these disorders become evident in infancy or childhood. If there is a hereditary or acquired deficiency of an enzyme of glucose production, the problem can be circumvented by provision of a continuous supply of glucose to the affected individual.

There are several other rare causes of fasting hypoglycemia. A few individuals have had circulating antibodies that caused hypoglycemia by interacting with the patient's own insulin, or with receptors for insulin on the patient's cells. Although the autonomic (involuntary) nervous system has an important role in signaling recovery from hypoglycemia, diseases affecting this branch of the nervous system do not usually produce hypoglycemia; presumably, hormonal mechanisms can substitute for the missing neural signals.

Reactive hypoglycemia can occur with an unusually rapid passage of foodstuffs through the upper intestinal tract, such as may occur after partial or total removal of the stomach. Persons predisposed to maturity-onset diabetes may also have reactive hypoglycemia, probably because of the delay in the secretion of insulin in response to a meal. Finally, reactive hypoglycemia need not indicate the presence of any identifiable disease and may occur in otherwise normal individuals.

Diagnosis of reactive hypoglycemia is made difficult by the variability of symptoms and of glucose concentrations from day to day. Adding to the diagnostic uncertainty, circulating glucose normally rises and falls after meals, especially those rich in carbohydrates. Consequently, entirely normal and asymptomatic individuals may sometimes have glucose concentrations at or below the levels found in persons with reactive hypoglycemia. Therefore, the glucose tolerance test, in which blood samples are taken at intervals for several hours after the patient drinks a solution containing 50 to 100 grams of glucose, is quite unreliable and should not be employed for the diagnosis of reactive hypoglycemia. Proper diagnosis of reactive hypoglycemia depends on careful correlation of the patient's symptoms with the circulating glucose level, preferably measured on several occasions after ingestion of ordinary meals. Some persons develop symptoms such as weakness, nausea, sweating, and tremulousness after meals, but without a significant reduction of circulating glucose. This symptom complex should not be confused with hypoglycemia.

When rapid passage of food through the stomach and upper intestine causes reactive hypoglycemia, the administration of drugs that slow intestinal transit may be helpful. When reactive hypoglycemia has no evident pathological cause, the patient is usually advised to take multiple small meals throughout the day instead of the usual three meals and to avoid concentrated sweets. These dietary modifications can help avoid hypoglycemia by reducing the stimulus to secrete insulin.

Two rare inherited disorders of metabolism can produce reactive hypoglycemia after the ingestion of certain foods. In hereditary fructose intolerance, the offending nutrient is fructose, a sugar found in fruits as well as ordinary table sugar. In galactosemia, the sugar responsible for hypoglycemia is galactose, a major component of milk products. Management of these conditions, which usually become apparent in infancy or childhood, consists of avoidance of the foods responsible.

PERSPECTIVE AND PROSPECTS

Fasting hypoglycemia is uncommon, except in the context of treatment of diabetes mellitus. The most serious public health problem associated with hypoglycemia is that it limits the therapeutic effectiveness of insulin and sulfonylurea drugs. Evidence suggests that elevation of the circulating glucose concentration (hyperglycemia) is responsible for much of the disability and premature death among patients with diabetes. In many of these patients, therapeutic regimens consisting of multiple daily injections of insulin or continuous infusion of insulin through a small needle placed under the skin can reduce the average circulating glucose to normal. Frequent serious hypoglycemia is the most important adverse consequence of such regimens. Persons with diabetes seem to be at especially high risk for dangerous hypoglycemia for two reasons. First, there is often a failure of the warning systems that ordinarily cause uncomfortable symptoms when the circulating glucose concentration declines, a situation termed hypoglycemic unawareness. As a consequence, when a patient with diabetes attempts to control his or her blood sugar with more frequent injections of insulin, there may occur unheralded episodes of hypoglycemia that can lead to serious alterations in mental activity or even loss of consciousness. Many patients with diabetes also have hypoglycemic unresponsiveness, an impaired ability to recover from episodes of hypoglycemia. Also, diabetes can interfere with the normal physiologic responses that cause the secretion of glucagon in response to a reduction of circulating glucose, thus eliminating one of the most important defenses against hypoglycemia. If both hypoglycemic unawareness and hypoglycemic unresponsiveness could be reversed, intensive treatment of diabetes would become safer and more widely applicable.

Reactive hypoglycemia, although seldom a clue to serious disease, has attracted public attention because of its peculiarly annoying symptoms. These symptoms, which reflect activation of the sympathetic nervous system, resemble those of fear and anxiety. The symptoms are not specific, and many patients with these complaints do not have hypoglycemia.

In summary, hypoglycemia indicates defective regulation of the supply of energy to the body. When severe or persistent, hypoglycemia can lead to serious behavioral disorder, obtunded consciousness, and even brain damage. Fasting hypoglycemia may be a clue to significant endocrine disease. Reactive hypoglycemia, while annoying, usually responds to simple dietary measures. The study of hypoglycemia has led to many important insights into the regulation of energy metabolism.

—Victor R. Lavis, M.D.

See also Blood and blood disorders; Diabetes mellitus; Endocrine disorders; Endocrinology; Endocrinology, pediatric; Hormones; Metabolism; Obesity; Pancreas; Pancreatitis; Vitamins and minerals.

For Further Information:

Chow, Cheryl, and James Chow. *Hypoglycemia for Dummies.* 2d ed. New York: Wiley, 2007. Part of the popular "Dummies" series, provides a wide range of expert information on diagnosis, risk factors, treatment options, diet and exercise regimens, advice on finding the right doctor, and setting up a support network.

Harmel, Anne Peters, and Ruchi Mathur. *Davidson's Diabetes Mellitus: Diagnosis and Treatment.* 5th ed. Philadelphia: W. B. Saunders, 2004. An important contribution to the study of diabetes and metabolism. Offers clear explanations of the physiological abnormalities in hypoglycemia and emphasizes the importance of fasting hypoglycemia as an index of serious illness.

Hypoglycemia Support Foundation. http://www.hypoglycemia.org/. Provides diet information, self-tests for the disease, and helpful Internet links.

Kahn, Ronald C., et al., eds. *Joslin's Diabetes Mellitus.* 14th ed. Philadelphia: Lippincott Williams & Wilkins, 2005. The definitive American textbook of diabetes. Covers all causes of hypoglycemia, not simply those related to diabetes.

Larsen, P. Reed, et al., eds. *Williams Textbook of Endocrinology.* 10th ed. Philadelphia: W. B. Saunders, 2003. Includes a comprehensive chapter called "Glucose Homeostasis and Hypoglycemia." Delineates especially well the coordination of the nervous and hormonal systems in physiologic defense against hypoglycemia, as well as the special problems of hypoglycemia in patients with diabetes mellitus.

Lincoln, Thomas A., and John A. Eaddy. *Beating the Blood Sugar Blues: Proven Methods and Wisdom for Controlling Hypoglycemia.* New York: McGraw-Hill, 2001. The authors, both type I diabetes patients, provide a thorough guide to understanding, preventing, and treating hypoglycemia, and intersperse the narrative with personal stories from doctors and patients.

Parker, James N., and Philip M. Parker, eds. *The 2002 Official Patient's Sourcebook on Hypoglycemia.* San Diego, Calif.: Icon Health, 2002. Draws from public, academic, government, and peer-reviewed research to provide a wide-ranging handbook for adult patients with hypoglycemia.

Hypoparathyroidism. *See* Hyperparathyroidism and hypoparathyroidism.

Hypospadias repair and urethroplasty
Procedure

Anatomy or system affected: Genitals, reproductive system

Specialties and related fields: General surgery, urology

Definition: Urethroplasty is any plastic surgery performed on the urethra; one of these procedures is the repair of hypospadias, the presence of an abnormal opening in the male urethra.

INDICATIONS AND PROCEDURES

Urethroplasty is performed to correct defects of the urethra, the tube leading from the bladder to the outside of the body through which urine exits the body. Hypospadias is a congenital defect of the distal end of the urethra in which it opens on the underside of the penis instead of at the tip. Less commonly, the opening can occur lower down on the underside of the penis or in the scrotum. Hypospadias is also associated with abnormalities in the kidneys.

The correction of hypospadias involves a technique known as a "flip-flap" repair: Two incisions on the undersurface of the glans and shaft of the penis are made, and skin from the glans is fashioned into an opening that is anatomically normal. The operation is usually done under general anesthesia.

The lines for both incisions are drawn and incisions carefully made to avoid damaging adjacent structures and erectile tissue. The prepuce is released from the body of the penis. A V-shaped flap is cut from the skin immediately below the hypospadias. The flap is rotated, and one side is sutured into one of the incisions made in the glans. The other side is similarly inserted into the other incision and sutured in place, forming a tube that extends the urethra. Excess skin from the prepuce is removed; the prepuce is sutured back into position on the shaft of the penis. The skin from the underside of the penis is brought together over the repaired urethra and sutured together. A catheter is frequently (but not universally) placed in the urethra and kept in place for up to three weeks. Some surgeons believe that the presence of a catheter helps to establish the new urethra. Others think that it only contributes to postoperative holes (fistulas) and do not use it, allowing the patient to urinate immediately through the newly constructed tube. The patient returns to the surgeon's office in a week for a postoperative check and the removal of sutures.

Another type of urethroplasty is the surgical repair of a discontinuity in the male urethra. Most commonly, this defect occurs on the underside of the penis and is attributable to the incomplete closure of the skin portions that normally fuse over the urethra during embryonic development. The technique is similar to that described above. Under general anesthesia, skin is removed from the prepuce of the penis and is sutured in place over the defect, closing the opening. A catheter may or may not be inserted. The patient returns to the surgeon's office in a week for a postoperative check and the removal of sutures.

USES AND COMPLICATIONS

The techniques associated with urethroplasty are used to repair congenital defects. Complications from these procedures are unusual, but they may include infection and stricture. Such problems can be avoided with careful attention to the finer details of the surgery.

The need for urethroplasty and hypospadias repair is unlikely to disappear. From a psychological standpoint, it benefits the patient to repair a hypospadias as early in life as possible, preferably before the age of three.

—*L. Fleming Fallon, Jr., M.D., Ph.D., M.P.H.*

See also Fistula repair; Genital disorders, male; Men's health; Neonatology; Pediatrics; Reproductive system; Surgery, pediatric; Urinary system; Urology; Urology, pediatric.

FOR FURTHER INFORMATION:

Baskin, Laurence S., ed. *Hypospadias and Genital Development*. New York: Kluwer Academic/Plenum, 2004.

Beers, Mark H., et al. *The Merck Manual of Diagnosis and Therapy*. 18th ed. Whitehouse Station, N.J.: Merck Research Laboratories, 2006.

Ferrari, Mario. *PDxMD Renal and Genitourinary Disorders*. New York: Elsevier, 2002.

Hadidi, Ahmed T., and Amir F. Azmy, eds. *Hypospadias Surgery: An Illustrated Guide*. New York: Springer, 2004.

Icon Health. *Hyperspadias: A Medical Dictionary, Bibliography, and Annotated Research Guide to Internet References*. San Diego, Calif.: Author, 2004.

Montague, Drogo K. *Disorders of Male Sexual Function*. Chicago: Year Book Medical, 1988.

Swanson, Janice M., and Katherine A. Forrest, eds. *Men's Reproductive Health*. New York: Springer, 1984.

HYPOTENSION

DISEASE/DISORDER

ALSO KNOWN AS: Low blood pressure

ANATOMY OR SYSTEM AFFECTED: Blood vessels, brain, circulatory system, heart, kidneys

SPECIALTIES AND RELATED FIELDS: Cardiology, critical care, emergency medicine, exercise physiology, geriatrics and general surgery, internal medicine, pharmacology

DEFINITION: Blood pressure that not only is low but also causes symptoms such as dizziness in the affected individual. It has multiple causes, including

INFORMATION ON HYPOTENSION

CAUSES: Blood loss, heart disease, heart attack, trauma, adverse drug reactions, infection, hormone-producing tumors, fever, dehydration, excessive heat, alcohol use, shock, burns

SYMPTOMS: Low blood pressure accompanied by rapid heartbeat, lightheadedness or dizziness, weakness, possibly fainting; sometimes kidney failure, strokes, heart attack

DURATION: Acute

TREATMENTS: Supportive measures such as fluids and oxygen therapy; treatment for underlying cause

blood loss, heart attack, trauma, reactions to medications, and overwhelming infection.

CAUSES AND SYMPTOMS

The body has a complex system for regulating blood pressure, which ensures adequate blood flow to each organ and tissue. The sympathetic and parasympathetic branches of the autonomic nervous system, various hormones produced by the adrenal and pituitary glands, the kidneys, the heart, and local mechanisms in all parts of the body control the amount of blood in the vessels, how much blood is squeezed out of the heart with each beat, and how much blood is available to any body system at a given time. A failure in any of these regulatory areas can cause the blood pressure to become too low for the person to function normally.

Normal blood pressure varies depending on the demands put on the body, how fit a person is, and the age of the individual. For most adults, 120/80 is considered normal; however, the top number (systolic pressure) can be as low as 90 and the bottom number (diastolic) as low as 60 and still be considered normal. When the blood pressure is lower than about 90/60 and the individual develops symptoms related to the low pressure, then that individual is diagnosed with hypotension. Low blood pressure by itself is not unhealthy, especially in athletic people, but when the flow of blood to the organs of the body is inadequate, symptoms develop. They include rapid heartbeat, lightheadedness or dizziness, weakness, and possibly fainting. Other symptoms vary with the cause of the low blood pressure.

Low blood pressure associated with insufficient blood flow to the body organs can cause kidney failure, strokes, and heart attacks. Orthostatic hypotension is low blood pressure and its associated symptoms that are most pronounced when a person goes from lying or sitting to standing.

Specific causes of hypotension include adverse drug reactions, diseases such as diabetes that damage the autonomic nervous system, hormone-producing tumors, fever, heart disease, dehydration, hemorrhage, excessive heat, alcohol use, heart attack, heart trauma, abnormal heart rhythms, overwhelming infection, anaphylaxis, burns, vomiting, and diarrhea.

TREATMENT AND THERAPY

The treatment of hypotension is primarily aimed at removing the underlying cause—for example, discontinuing a drug that causes blood vessels to dilate or wearing elastic stockings to improve blood flow back to the heart. If the low blood pressure is severe enough, then supportive treatment with fluids, oxygen, and other modalities may be required.

—*Rebecca Lovell Scott, Ph.D., PA-C*

See also Cardiology; Circulation; Dizziness and fainting; Heart; Hypertension; Kidneys; Nephrology; Nervous system; Neurology; Vascular medicine; Vascular system.

FOR FURTHER INFORMATION:

American Medical Association. *American Medical Association Family Medical Guide*. 4th rev. ed. Hoboken, N.J.: John Wiley & Sons, 2004.

Komaroff, Anthony, ed. *Harvard Medical School Family Health Guide*. New York: Free Press, 2005.

Stoppard, Miriam. *Family Health Guide*. New York: DK, 2004.

HYPOTHERMIA. *See* **HYPERTHERMIA AND HYPOTHERMIA.**

HYSTERECTOMY

PROCEDURE

ANATOMY OR SYSTEM AFFECTED: Reproductive system, uterus

SPECIALTIES AND RELATED FIELDS: Endocrinology, general surgery, gynecology, oncology

DEFINITION: The removal of the uterus and sometimes the ovaries and surrounding tissues, which is performed for a variety of indications, including uterine cancer and fibroids that cause symptoms.

KEY TERMS:

adenomyosis: a noncancerous disorder in which cells resembling the lining of the uterus are found within the muscle layer of the uterus, leading to abnormal vaginal bleeding and pain

estrogen: the female sex hormone produced by the ovaries and the adrenal gland that is responsible for the development of female secondary sex characteristics; the three types naturally produced by the body are estradiol, estrone, and estriol

Fallopian tubes: the structures located between the uterus and ovaries that are responsible for the transport of the egg; also called the oviducts

fibroid: a noncancerous tumor of the uterus, also known as leiomyoma; when large, these tumors can cause heavy menstrual bleeding leading to anemia or cause pressure symptoms in the pelvis

laparoscopy: a minimally invasive surgical procedure in which an instrument equipped with a small camera, called a laparoscope, is inserted through a small incision in the abdomen to visualize the pelvis or abdomen; surgical manipulation may be carried out during this procedure

menorrhagia: unusually heavy menstrual bleeding; when severe, it can lead to anemia

progesterone/progestin: a hormone produced in the ovaries that sustains pregnancy; birth control pills are composed primarily of progesterone, which works by suppressing ovulation

INDICATIONS AND PROCEDURES

The term "hysterectomy" comes from the Greek *hystera*, meaning "uterus," and *ektome*, meaning "to cut out." While hysterectomy refers to the removal of the uterus and, most commonly, the attached Fallopian tubes, there are several types of hysterectomies. Total hysterectomy, contrary to popular belief, does not mean that the ovaries are removed with the uterus. Rather, the term indicates the removal of the uterus and cervix. Subtotal, or partial, hysterectomy is the excision of the uterus above the cervix; the cervix is left in place. Either one or both ovaries may be removed with the uterus (unilateral oophorectomy or bilateral oophorectomy). Salpingo-oophorectomy refers to the removal of one of the Fallopian tubes along with the accompanying ovary, while bilateral salpingo-oophorectomy refers to the removal of both Fallopian tubes and ovaries.

Indications for hysterectomy can be divided into noncancerous and cancerous conditions. Within the noncancerous category, the most common indication for hysterectomy is symptomatic fibroids. Many women have fibroids, and the majority of fibroids do not cause symptoms and can be left alone. Symptomatic fibroids are those which are large enough to cause pressure symptoms in the pelvis, compress the bladder or rectum, or cause pain or discomfort during intercourse. Another type of symptomatic fibroids are those which cause excessively heavy menstrual bleeding and, when severe, anemia.

A hysterectomy is indicated in these situations if the patient fails to respond to less conservative therapy for symptomatic fibroids. Examples of conservative therapy for heavy bleeding include high-dose estrogen or birth control pills. A hysterectomy is usually performed only when childbearing is no longer desired, since removal of the uterus precludes pregnancy. Prior to hysterectomy, large fibroids may be shrunk with a course of a hormone called gonadotropin-releasing hormone. Unfortunately, this treatment results in menopausal symptoms, including hot flushes and bone density depletion, and therefore cannot be used for prolonged periods of time. More recently, treatments such as uterine artery embolization, in which the arteries feeding the uterus are blocked off using foreign particles such as gel foam, have been tried as an alternative to hysterectomy, in an attempt to preserve the uterus and avoid major surgery.

Another indication for hysterectomy is in patients who have had recurrent fibroids after myomectomy. A myomectomy is the surgical removal of isolated fibroids, rather than removal of the uterus itself. The benefit is that the uterus can be preserved, although the downside is that fibroids may regrow. Hysterectomy is the definitive treatment for uterine fibroids.

Another noncancerous indication for hysterectomy is adenomyosis, a painful condition whereby the cells of the uterine lining are abnormally embedded in the uterine muscle. No good treatments exist for this condition besides hysterectomy. Another indication for hysterectomy occurs in cases of abnormal uterine bleeding in which the bleeding is refractory to management with nonsurgical treatments, such as birth control pills or procedures that ablate the uterine lining. Other less common indications for hysterectomy are uterine prolapse (in which the uterus descends into the vaginal canal, causing discomfort or urinary incontinence), chronic pelvic pain (refractory to more conservative management), and large infections of the uterus and pelvis that are unresponsive to antibiotics. Hysterectomy may also be performed as part of a cesarean section if the surgeon encounters uncontrollable bleeding after delivery of the infant.

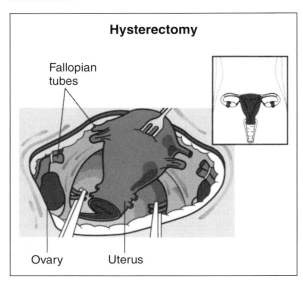

Hysterectomy

Fallopian tubes

Ovary   Uterus

The uterus, and sometimes such accompanying organs as the ovaries and Fallopian tubes, may be removed to treat disease conditions or as a contraceptive measure; the inset shows the location of the uterus.

Uterine cancer is a clear indication for hysterectomy. Often, the cancer causes abnormal uterine bleeding. Prior to hysterectomy, the cancer has usually been confirmed on biopsy of the uterine lining. If the cancer is small and localized to a small area of the uterus, then removal of the uterus alone may be curative. More often, however, uterine cancer may have spread more deeply into the uterine wall or even grown beyond the uterus. In these cases, hysterectomy may be accompanied by more extensive surgery that includes removing lymph nodes or other pelvic structures.

Most frequently, hysterectomy is accomplished through a 6- to 8-inch midline incision running either down from the navel or across the lower abdomen near or below the hairline (known as a "bikini incision"). This procedure is referred to as an abdominal hysterectomy. Vaginal hysterectomy is the removal of the uterus through the vaginal canal, rather than through a surgical opening in the abdomen. This procedure is most often performed to resolve prolapse (because the uterus has already descended into the vaginal canal) or when the uterus is not massively enlarged and can be pulled down and out through the vagina. If the hysterectomy is performed because of large fibroid tumors, then the abdominal approach is usually used. On rare occasions, a vaginal hysterectomy may be facilitated using laparoscopy. In these cases, laparoscopy enables visualization and manipulation of the uterus via small incisions in the abdomen to assist in removal of the uterus through the vaginal canal.

During the hysterectomy, the patient is almost always under general anesthesia. The patient lies on her back for abdominal hysterectomies. In vaginal hysterectomies, the patient's legs are placed in stirrups and the knees are spread apart to enable the gynecologist to gain access to the vaginal canal. The actual removal of the uterus involves clamping, transecting, and suture ligating the blood vessels that feed the uterus and the tissues that anchor the uterus in the pelvic cavity. Care is taken by the surgeon to avoid the ureters, the tubes carrying urine from the kidney to the bladder. The ureters are very close to the lower part of the uterus and can be damaged easily. If the entire uterus is removed, then the top end of the vagina, called the cuff, is sutured closed. If the cervix is left in place, then the top of the cervix is sutured closed.

After the surgery, the patient receives narcotic pain medication and antibiotics to prevent infection and is monitored carefully to confirm that vital signs are stable and recovery is appropriate. Laboratory tests may be performed to ensure that the patient is not unusually anemic and that important organs such as the kidneys are functioning properly. Until a patient is able to walk, a catheter (a rubber tube attached to a collecting bag) will be used to pass urine. Patients may initially take liquids by mouth. When they can tolerate liquids, indicating no apparent injury to the bowels, patients may begin to take solid food. A patient may be hospitalized for two to four days after the hysterectomy, although hospital stays in general have been shortening in length. On the whole, patients who receive vaginal hysterectomies have shorter hospital stays than patients receiving abdominal hysterectomies, assuming that no complications arise. Patients can usually resume normal sexual functioning six weeks after the surgery.

Uses and Complications

Hysterectomy can be used to provide relief from pressure, pain, and bleeding from the uterus. It may also be curative in the early stages of uterine cancer and can increase survival in later stages. For women who are finished with childbearing and whose lifestyles or responsibilities do not allow them to try more conservative treatments, many of which require several months to take effect, hysterectomy can provide definitive relief from symptoms within the defined time period needed to undergo scheduled surgery. In cases of life-threatening uterine hemorrhage, hysterectomy can save a woman's life.

The common complications of hysterectomy are those which are common to many major surgeries. One complication is excessive blood loss. The average blood loss during a hysterectomy is estimated at between 400 and 500 cubic centimeters (about a pint). When removal of the uterus is difficult, for instance because of the position of large fibroids, increased blood loss is likely to occur. When excessive blood loss is of concern, the patient's blood levels may be checked during the procedure. A patient who is significantly anemic may receive blood transfusions to avoid poor oxygenation of the major organs and to increase blood volume, and hence avoid shock. The number of transfusions depends on the amount of blood estimated to be lost. If a blood vessel continues to bleed after the patient leaves the operating room, then the patient may need to return to the operating room to have the bleeding vessel identified and sutured.

Another common complication of hysterectomy is infection. Even when aseptic techniques are followed, an infection may develop several days after the surgery. This is particularly true in vaginal hysterectomies, where the surgeon works through the vaginal canal, considered a clean but contaminated field. For this reason, patients are given antibiotics immediately prior to surgery in order to prevent infection. A patient who shows signs of infection after the surgery may be placed on an extended course of antibiotics. The source of these infections can range from the vaginal cuff site to the peritoneum (the lining of the pelvic and abdominal cavity) and the urinary tract.

The third major complication that can occur with hysterectomy is inadvertent damage to internal organs. The urinary tract and the bowels are particularly at risk during hysterectomy because of their proximity to the uterus. The ureters can be occluded inadvertently by the misplacement of a suture. If discovered early, this damage can be repaired. If the problem is not recognized, however, then a damaged ureter can result in kidney malfunction. For this reason, kidney function is carefully followed after the hysterectomy through blood tests. Since the bladder sits on the bottom half of the uterus, it is a common organ that can be damaged during a hysterectomy. If the bladder is accidentally entered using the scalpel during surgery, then it can usually be repaired during the procedure. Postsurgery, the patient may need prolonged catheterization of the bladder to enhance bladder recovery. The large and small intestines are another common site of surgical injury. They can be accidentally cut or sutured. Sometimes, this problem is not detected until after the patient has left the operating room, and the problem becomes apparent when normal bowel function does not return in a timely fashion postoperatively. The patient may experience nausea, vomiting, and abdominal distension and discomfort and may not be able to pass gas from the rectum.

Another complication that can occur after surgery is the formation of blood clots, particularly in the leg veins, as a result of the patient's immobility during and after surgery. These clots can be dangerous when they break off from their source and move into the lungs, a condition called pulmonary embolism. Large pulmonary emboli can be life-threatening. Pulmonary emboli can be prevented using warm compression stockings during and after surgery to promote blood flow. Early ambulation (walking) after surgery can also decrease the chances of developing leg vein clots and pulmonary emboli.

Long-term complications of hysterectomy also include scar formation in the pelvis, called adhesions, which can interfere with bowel function or cause pelvic pain. Some patients may experience the prolapse of the remaining pelvic organs (such as the bowels and bladder) into the space formerly occupied by the uterus. Procedures may be employed during the hysterectomy to anchor the vaginal cuff and close any spaces where prolapse might occur.

In rare cases, removal of the uterus can inadvertently decrease blood supply to any remaining ovaries, leading to ischemia and loss of ovarian function. In these cases, the patient may experience the symptoms of estrogen deficiency, also known as menopausal symptoms. They include hot flushes, vaginal dryness, and, when estrogen deficiency is prolonged, bone density loss. In women whose hysterectomies included removal of the ovaries, the hot flushes may become apparent a few days after surgery. In these cases, estrogen therapy or other medications may be of benefit.

The impact of a hysterectomy on a woman's psychological state varies from woman to woman. In women who have been suffering a great deal from their symptoms, be it pressure and pain or abnormal bleeding, a hysterectomy can be a relief and enable them to return to their activities of daily living. Hysterectomy can improve sexual function in many cases. In other women, a hysterectomy can trigger a sense of loss and represent the end of the woman's fertility, which is often associated with youth and vitality.

Perspective and Prospects

In ancient times, the complaints of women and the illnesses of the female organs were viewed as coming from an "unhappy uterus." It was believed that the uterus had the primary purpose of childbearing and that, when the uterus was not occupied with this function, it might show its wrath by abnormal bleeding and pain. These beliefs prevailed for centuries; early medical history indicates that women's gynecologic complaints were largely ignored. Moreover, no safe surgical procedures had been developed.

A noteworthy event in early American medical history was the operation attempted and documented by a frontier physician and surgeon, Ephraim McDowell. In 1809 in Danville, Kentucky, this daring young doctor carried out experimental surgery on a middle-aged woman to remove a huge ovarian tumor. Without the benefit of anesthesia and a sterile technique, he performed successful abdominal surgery on four out of five other patients.

Myomectomy, or removal of a fibroid tumor of the uterus, was the next procedure to be performed—first in France and later (about 1850) in Massachusetts by Washington Atlee. The first hysterectomy was successfully performed by Walter Burnham in the same decade, but he lost twelve of his next fifteen hysterectomy patients. In the text *Operative Gynecology* (1898), Howard A. Kelly of Baltimore describes one hundred hysterectomies that he performed in the late nineteenth century, all done because of pelvic infection. He lost only four patients, though convalescence for some survivors was prolonged.

Remarkable medical progress occurred in the nineteenth century in abdominal and vaginal surgical techniques. In the 1850's, Marion Sims of South Carolina was the first to perform vaginal surgery in the United States. He successfully repaired a vesicovaginal fistula, an abnormal opening between the bladder and the vagina through which urine escapes into the vagina. In the late nineteenth century, the "Manchester" operation for uterine prolapse was performed by A. Donald in Manchester, England. Prior to this procedure, uterine prolapse was treated with a pessary, a device inserted into the vagina to hold the uterus in place.

In the early part of the twentieth century, hysterectomy was considered a relatively dangerous procedure; many of the medical advances necessary for its success

(such as anesthesia, asepsis, antibiotics, and blood banks) were not yet available or were fraught with problems. Hysterectomy has now become one of the safer surgical procedures; mortality figures have dropped to between 0.2 and 0.5 percent, usually resulting from pulmonary embolism (a blood clot in the lungs), a complication common to almost all major surgeries.

In the 1930's, N. Sproat Heany of Chicago devised the present-day technique of vaginal hysterectomy. Vaginal (as opposed to abdominal) hysterectomy, it was believed, resulted in a less complicated procedure with shorter convalescence and more cosmetically pleasing results for most patients. For some time, vaginal hysterectomy was viewed as superior to abdominal hysterectomy. In the 1970's, between 25 and 40 percent of all hysterectomies were accomplished vaginally, depending on the age of the woman at the time of surgery. In 1981, however, a landmark study published by the U.S. Congress, weighing the costs, risks, and benefits of hysterectomy, stated that women undergoing vaginal hysterectomy are more likely to have postoperative fever and to receive antibiotic treatment. Moreover, vaginal hysterectomy patients may undergo further surgery at a rate as high as 5 to 10 percent.

By the late 1980's and early 1990's, the trend among many gynecologists had shifted away from hysterectomy to more conservative treatments, when possible. Physicians began to question whether hysterectomies were, in some or even in most cases, medically necessary. As more information became available to women regarding alternatives to hysterectomy (a major revenue-producing surgical procedure in the United States), many women became more apt to question their physicians when told that hysterectomy was the only possible solution to their gynecological problems.

—Genevieve Slomski, Ph.D.;
updated by Anne Lynn S. Chang, M.D.

See also Cancer; Cervical, ovarian, and uterine cancers; Contraception; Dysmenorrhea; Ectopic pregnancy; Endometriosis; Ethics; Genital disorders, female; Gynecology; Hormone replacement therapy (HRT); Hormones; Menorrhagia; Oncology; Reproductive system; Sex change surgery; Sterilization; Tubal ligation; Women's health.

For Further Information:

Clark, Jan. *Hysterectomy and the Alternatives: How to Ask the Right Questions and Explore Other Options.*

Rev. ed. London: Vermilion, 2000. Discusses the treatment of uterine fibroids and menstrual disorders and offers alternatives to radical hysterectomy.

Dennerstein, Lorraine, Carl Wood, and Ann Westmore. *Hysterectomy: New Options and Advances.* 2d ed. New York: Oxford University Press, 1995. This popular work on hysterectomy addresses all aspects of the procedure. Includes a bibliography and an index.

Doherty, Gerard M., and Lawrence W. Way, eds. *Current Surgical Diagnosis and Treatment.* 12th ed. New York: Lange Medical Books/McGraw-Hill, 2006. Provides concise summaries of gynecologic problems which could lead to hysterectomy.

Moore, Michele C., and Caroline M. de Costa. *Do You Really Need Surgery? A Sensible Guide to Hysterectomy and Other Procedures for Women.* New Brunswick, N.J.: Rutgers University Press, 2004. A guide for patients. Discusses anatomy, physiology, gynecological disorders, diagnosis, alternative treatments, and various surgeries.

Stenchever, Morton A., et al. *Comprehensive Gynecology.* 4th ed. St. Louis: Mosby, 2006. One of the definitive textbooks in the field of gynecology. It outlines in an objective and complete manner the indications for hysterectomy and the various types of hysterectomy. Also describes appropriate postoperative care and alternatives to hysterectomy.

IATROGENIC DISORDERS

DISEASE/DISORDER

ANATOMY OR SYSTEM AFFECTED: All
SPECIALTIES AND RELATED FIELDS: All
DEFINITION: Health problems caused by medical treatments.

CAUSES AND SYMPTOMS

Iatrogenic disorders may be attributable to inefficient or uncaring physicians or to the risks inherent in medical procedures that are necessary to prevent death or crippling disease. Such disorders are usually divided into those caused by medications, surgery, and medical misdiagnosis.

The average patient of any age expects physicians and the medical infrastructure to deliver perfect cures for all diseases. This is not possible because some diseases have no cure and because medical treatment always involves some potential risk to the persons being treated. In fact, a percentage—usually a small one—of the patients treated for any disease develop unexpected health problems (adverse reactions) which can be diseases themselves.

The term "iatrogenic disorder" is a catchall used to encompass the many different adverse reactions that accompany the practice of modern medicine. The number of such problems has grown as medical science has become more sophisticated. They are often blamed entirely on physicians and other medical staff involved in cases producing iatrogenic disorders.

This blame is correctly directed in instances where a physician and other staff involved are uncaring, inattentive, careless, or incompletely educated. However, iatrogenic disorders often result from the nature of modern medicine. Doctors frequently attempt therapeutic methods (such as surgery) that are innovative efforts which cure serious diseases but have some inherent risk of failure. They may also use therapeutic drugs that are powerful agents for cure of specific disease processes but that have side effects causing other health problems in some people who take them. In addition, doctors will very often utilize complicated overall therapy having adverse consequences that patients may not acknowledge despite physicians' attempts to explain them orally and with consent forms.

TREATMENT AND THERAPY

Despite careful efforts of most physicians—who are informed, caring, and efficient—iatrogenic disorders accompany many medical procedures. Public attention is, however, focused most on the effects of therapeutic agents, drugs and vaccines, because patients are often unaware that no therapeutic agent in use is ever perfectly safe. Even a clear physician description of the dos and don'ts associated with such therapy may be flawed by biological variation among patients, causing problems in one individual but not others. Furthermore, the explosion of new diseases and new versions of old diseases since the late 1980's has led to much more complex treatment regimens. Consequently, iatrogenic disorders occur much more often.

This has become particularly germane in treatment of the aged, acquired immunodeficiency syndrome (AIDS) patients, and the very young. Hence, several rules must be followed concerning therapeutic agents. First, wherever possible, these medications should be used only after other means fail and the benefits to be gained clearly outweigh the risks entailed. Second, therapy should begin with the lowest possible effective dose, and all dose increases should be accompanied by frequent symptom relief and toxicity monitoring. Third, patients and responsible family members must be made aware of all possible adverse symptoms, how to best counter them, and the foods or other medications to be avoided to diminish iatrogenic potential. Such problems, in the aged, are due to biochemical changes which alter their tolerance for many medications.

Many iatrogenic disorders are caused by the presence of bacterial contamination in wounds and the fact that surgical maintenance of sterility is not absolutely perfect. For example, iatrogenesis occurs after 30 percent of surgical procedures carried out at heavily contaminated surgical sites (such as emergency surgery of abdominal wounds). In addition, the use of antibiotics can be problematic. In many cases, the large doses of these therapeutic agents required to fight primary bacterial infection will cause superinfection by other microbes, such as fungi. Furthermore, wide antibiotic

---

INFORMATION ON IATROGENIC DISORDERS

CAUSES: Inherent medical risk, misdiagnosis, physician malpractice, medication error, surgical error

SYMPTOMS: Wide ranging

DURATION: Varies from acute to fatal

TREATMENTS: Depends on circumstances

use in hospitals has led to the creation of antibiotic-resistant bacteria.

For these reasons, treatment of surgical sites requires individualized attention. Clean wounds can be closed up immediately without high risk of infection, but deep wounds known to be contaminated prior to surgery are often best handled by closing up interior tissues and leaving skin and subcutaneous tissues open until it is clear that infection is under control. Many patients are frightened by such procedures and the pain involved, not understanding that it is in their best interest. Hence, they may resist treatment and accuse conscientious physicians of causing iatrogenic disorders. Such treatment is most crucial in the aged and in young children. In elderly patients the cause is diminution of body defenses against infection (for example, the immune system). It has been reported that the elderly experience a doubled or tripled chance of experiencing postoperative complications that may be seen as iatrogenic by their families. Young children are also more at risk than postpubertal individuals and "younger" adults, for reasons related to their incompletely developed immune systems.

Iatrogenesis resulting from misdiagnosis is too complicated an issue to be considered in depth here. In some cases, it is caused by physician inadequacy, but more often such problems are attributable to the great difficulty in diagnosing any disease absolutely.

It is essential for patients and physicians to communicate effectively. Such interaction lowers the occurrence of iatrogenic disorders because patients can decide to forgo treatment or to learn how to comply exactly with complex treatment protocols. Patients who do not receive adequate answers to questions posed to physicians should seek treatment elsewhere. Physicians should completely explain potential problems associated with therapeutic procedures by oral communication, informative consent forms, and well-educated counselors.

Because of the many iatrogenic disorders associated with medical therapy, physicians often believe that the best course of treatment—where a symptom is unclear and severe danger to patients is not imminent—is to allow nature to take its course so as to do no harm. This approach is often misunderstood by patients. To clarify the issue and to satisfy them, it should be explained—by the physician—that treatment can often be more dangerous than a perceived health problem.

It is hoped that the continued development of medical science, careful and complete therapy explanations by medical staffs, and better medical understanding and better treatment compliance by patients will decrease the incidence of iatrogenic disorders.

—Sanford S. Singer, Ph.D.

See also Antibiotics; Bacterial infections; Ethics; Hospitals; Law and medicine; Malpractice; Nausea and vomiting; Surgery, general; Surgical procedures; Wounds.

FOR FURTHER INFORMATION:

Apfel, Roberta J., and Susan M. Fisher. *To Do No Harm: DES and the Dilemmas of Modern Medicine.* New Haven, Conn.: Yale University Press, 1984. The book is well written and has a glossary of medical terms, twenty pages of footnotes, a bibliography of four hundred references, and an index, all of which enhance its usefulness.

Carroll, Paula. *Life Wish: One Woman's Struggle Against Medical Incompetence.* Alameda, Calif.: Medical Consumers, 1986. This personal narrative of a woman struggling to overcome breast cancer offers warnings of malpractice and surgical errors.

Farmer, Paul. *Infections and Inequalities: The Modern Plagues.* Berkeley: University of California Press, 2001. Physician-anthropologist Farmer examines why infectious diseases such as AIDS and tuberculosis target the poor. Uses public-health case studies of the pathogenic effects of poverty and other social conditions such as access to health care.

Levy, Stuart B. *The Antibiotic Paradox: How the Misuse of Antibiotics Destroys Their Curative Powers.* 2d ed. Cambridge, Mass.: Perseus, 2002. A leading researcher in molecular biology explores a modern-day massive evolutionary change in bacteria due to misuse of antibiotics. He argues that a buildup of new antibiotic-resistant bacteria in individuals and in the environment is leading medicine into a dangerous territory where "miracle" drugs may be obsolete.

Morath, Julianne M., and Joanne E. Turnbull. *To Do No Harm: Ensuring Patient Safety in Health Care Organizations.* San Francisco: Jossey-Bass, 2005. A manual on patient safety for health care personnel.

Preger, Leslie, ed. *Iatrogenic Diseases.* 2 vols. Boca Raton, Fla.: CRC Press, 1986. Offers helpful advice on diagnosing iatrogenic diseases. Includes bibliographical references and an index.

Sharpe, Virginia F., and Alan I. Faden. *Medical Harm: Historical, Conceptual, and Ethical Dimensions of Iatrogenic Illness.* New York: Cambridge University Press, 1998. Of the many seekers after a healthier life or of relief from suffering who rightfully expect benefit from the health care system, some are more harmed than helped. This book deals mostly with harmful medical events which happen in hospitals.

Vincent, Charles, Maeve Ennis, and Robert J. Audley, eds. *Medical Accidents*. New York: Oxford University Press, 1993. Covers such topics as diagnostic errors, iatrogenic disease, and medical malpractice. Also discusses liability insurance.

Wilson, Michael, Brian Henderson, and Rod McNab. *Bacterial Virulence Mechanisms*. New York: Cambridge University Press, 2002. Basing their discussion on research advances in microbiology, molecular biology, and cell biology, the authors describe the interactions that exist between bacteria and human cells both in health and during infection.

ILEOSTOMY AND COLOSTOMY

PROCEDURES

ANATOMY OR SYSTEM AFFECTED: Abdomen, gastrointestinal system, intestines

SPECIALTIES AND RELATED FIELDS: Gastroenterology

DEFINITION: Surgical procedures that reroute the intestines to a hole, or stoma, in the abdomen after the removal of all or part of the colon.

KEY TERMS:

anastomosis: the surgical connection of one tubular organ to another

appliance: any device for collecting or removing stool from a stoma

colon: the last section of the intestines, where most fluids are absorbed, located between the ileum and the rectum; also called the large bowel or intestine

ileum: the lower third of the small intestine, which joins with the colon

ostomy: a popular term for any operation that results in a stoma

rectum: the intestinal storage area for feces between the colon and anus

stoma: a surgically created passage between the intestines and the outer skin

stool: the waste matter of digestion excreted from the body through the anus or stoma

INDICATIONS AND PROCEDURES

Despite great advances in drugs and nonsurgical procedures, doctors can cure some disabling or life-threatening diseases of the intestines only on the operating ta-

ble. Common procedures of this type are the colostomy and ileostomy, both of which replace the anus with a stoma on the abdominal wall. Such surgery stresses patients considerably, and, in the aftermath, when they must entirely relearn the once-simple act of defecation, some drift into depression, despair, and withdrawal as their bowel functions consume their attention and disturb their social lives. Even for the large majority who adjust, and for whom the procedures are a life-lengthening boon, their postsurgical body, in most cases, requires a permanent, profound change in habits and a complete reliance on technology.

Colostomy and ileostomy are medical terms compounding *stoma* (from Greek, "mouth") and a prefix identifying the section of gut that ends in the newly created "mouth." If a portion of the colon is retained and ends in a stoma, the operation constructing it is called a colostomy. If the entire colon is removed and the lower section of the small bowel, or ileum, ends in a stoma, the operation constructing it is called an ileostomy. Nonmedical support groups for patients commonly use the back-formation "ostomy" to refer to any operation that creates a stoma (including a urostomy, in which a stoma is created for the excretion of urine) and to such patients as "ostomates," although neither term belongs to medical technical vocabulary.

Physicians determine that an ileostomy or a colostomy is necessary after inspecting the damaged intestinal segments by endoscopy, by imaging, or during surgery. In consultation with a surgeon, the patient agrees to undergo the procedure. The patient fasts before the surgery and receives laxatives and enemas (except in the case of obstructions or severe ulcerative colitis) to clean as much feces from the intestines as possible and thus reduce the chance of infection during surgery. The surgeon, often with the advice of an enterostomal therapist (ET), examines the patient's abdomen carefully, checking where the skin naturally folds and stretches when the patient assumes various common body positions, and a spot for the stoma is selected that is convenient for the patient and free of stress from muscles and skin tension. That place is marked. An area to the right and below the navel is the usual location for an ileostomy. The left side is commonly chosen for a colostomy.

In ileostomy, the surgeon makes the opening incision to the left of the navel, starting a few centimeters above it and continuing to the pelvic area. After the abdominal cavity is exposed, the tissues connecting the colon to surrounding structures are severed, starting at

The Results of Colostomy

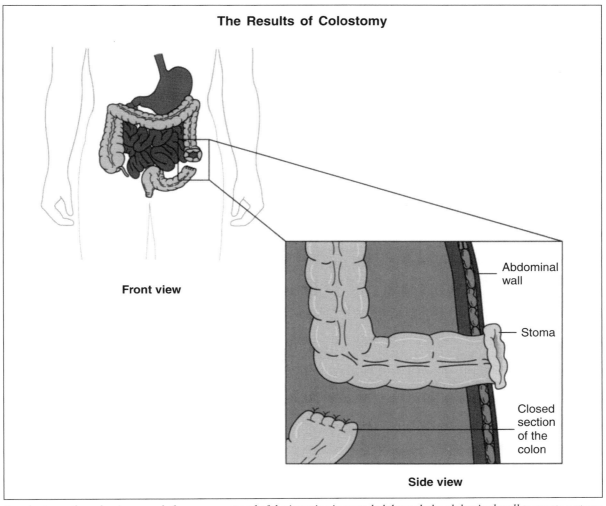

Front view

Abdominal wall

Stoma

Closed section of the colon

Side view

In colostomy, the colon is severed, the uppermost end of the intestine is extended through the abdominal wall to create a stoma through which fecal matter will be expelled, and the remaining section of the colon is closed off with sutures.

the cecum; the blood supply is cut and tied off; and clamps are placed over the ileum and rectum. Then the colon is cut free of the small intestine and rectum and is removed. If the operation is a "subtotal" procedure, the rectum is sutured shut and left in place or the open end is pulled through the abdominal wall as a "mucous stoma." (Such a second stoma is sometimes fashioned because the surgeon plans to connect the ileum and rectum in a later operation.) If the surgeon performs a proctocolectomy, the rectum is removed after the stoma is made and the anus is sutured shut.

The stoma is built by cutting a small round opening first in the skin and then in the abdominal wall and pulling the end of the ileum through the hole. The end sticks above the skin, is folded back over itself, and is sutured

to the edges of the hole, leaving the stoma protruding two to three centimeters. This basic ileostomy is called a Brooke ileostomy, after the English surgeon Bryan Brooke.

Variations on this basic procedure are employed depending on the wishes and health of the patient. A Kock pouch, named after its inventor, Nils Kock of Sweden, can be fashioned just behind the stoma in the abdominal cavity to act as an artificial rectum, collecting liquid waste until the ostomate wishes to void it; because this arrangement gives the patient control over defecation, it is called a continent ileostomy. The surgeon uses about 45 centimeters of ileum to form the pouch and adjusts the stoma so that it acts as a valve until a tube is inserted for drainage. In other procedures, the surgeon operates twice more on the ostomate, first detaching the ileum and closing the stoma and then reconnecting the bowel either to the rectum or to the anus.

If the ileum and rectum are joined, the procedure is called an ileorectal anastomosis. The rectum resumes its old job as a feces reservoir, and the patient defecates normally through the anus. This arrangement is seldom employed for ulcerative colitis patients, however, since the disease usually persists in the rectum. If the ileum is sutured directly to the anus, the procedure is called an ileoanal anastomosis. Because there is no rectum to collect feces, the surgeon must construct one. The pouch is made from loops of ileum that are slit along their length and stitched together. If not enough ileum remains from which to make a pouch, the surgeon pulls the end through the rectum and ties it directly to the anus, a procedure called an endorectal ileal pull-through. The anastomosis procedures require two operations—one for the temporary stoma and construction of the pouch, one to connect the pouch and the rectum, or anus—to give the artificial rectum a chance to heal properly and so prevent leaking.

Colostomies feature somewhat more variety of stoma placement than ileostomies, but since removal of the rectum, sigmoid colon, or both are the most common reasons for the creation of the stoma, it is usually placed on the lower left of the abdomen, near the hipbone. If more of the colon is removed, the stoma may be higher up toward the rib cage. The operation begins much as for an ileostomy, except that only the portion of the colon from the damaged or diseased area to the anus is removed; and the initial incision begins near that damaged section. The remaining, healthy colon is pulled through holes in the abdomen and skin, and its end is rolled back and fastened. The stoma protrudes out about two to three centimeters, so that an appliance for storing waste, if needed, can be attached.

There are three varieties of colostomy. The first, a single-barreled end colostomy, is the classical configuration. The rectum and anus are removed, and a single circular stoma, about 25 millimeters (1 inch) in diameter, is the permanent exit for stool. If, however, the surgeon believes that the colon and rectum can be rejoined, the rectum is left intact and closed. Either of two procedures can be used to give the colon a rest period between the removal of the diseased section and reconnection to the rectum. A double-barreled colostomy involves slicing through the colon and making side-by-side stomas from the ends. In a loop colostomy, the colon is not cut through; instead, a slit is made in one side, which is pulled through the skin and made into an oval stoma, usually larger than other stomas. In both cases, the upper colon discharges stool, and the lower length passes mucus.

USES AND COMPLICATIONS

Both colostomy and ileostomy are last-resort or emergency treatments. When a wound, such as one caused by a knife or gunshot, punctures the intestines, waste matter, full of bacteria, spills into the abdominal cavity. The severe infection that is sure to follow can kill a patient in days; thus, an emergency operation is required. The surgeon pulls healthy bowel through the abdominal wall and forms a temporary stoma (so that no more waste can leak out of the intestines), cleans out the spillage, and repairs the damaged bowel. In many cases, it is possible to reconnect the healthy bowel to the damaged portion after the wound has healed; at the same time, the stoma is closed, and the patient resumes defecation through the anus.

Emergency operations, however, account for only a small percentage of colostomies and ileostomies. About two-thirds of surgeries to form stomas are colostomies, most of which follow operations removing cancer (usually in the lower colon or rectum) or an obstruction. Diverticulitis, the inflammation of little pouches in the colon wall, may also require a colostomy; the diversion of wastes allows the inflammation to subside and the colon wall to heal, after which the stoma may be removed and the colon reconnected. Additionally, repair of some rare birth defects may entail a colostomy.

Ileostomies account for about one-quarter of stoma-creating procedures. Most are performed to eradicate ulcerative colitis, a chronic inflammation of the colon that begins in the rectum and may spread upward until the whole colon is involved. No drug or dietary treatment cures ulcerative colitis; when the condition becomes too unbearable for a patient to endure, an ileostomy removes the source of trouble: the colon itself. Long-standing ulcerative colitis is particularly likely to become cancerous, and the colon may be removed for that reason alone. Likewise, familial polyposis, a hereditary disease which dots the colon with toadstool-shaped lumps that are likely to become cancerous, may require removal of the colon and ileostomy.

Wounds, diverticulitis, familial polyposis, and birth defects, while not particularly rare, are the reasons for relatively few stomas. Together, colorectal cancer (particularly in the elderly) and ulcerative colitis (commonly disabling patients in their twenties) lead to hundreds of thousands of stoma operations yearly in the United States. As the average age of the population increases, so does the incidence of colon cancer and the need for ostomies.

Recovery from stoma surgery is prolonged. Surgery shocks the intestines, and several days pass before the gut resumes the wavelike contractions (called peristalsis) that enable digestion and push wastes toward the stoma. In the meantime, patients live on intravenous fluid nourishment. When bowel motion restarts and wastes begin coming through the stoma, the ileostomate must develop new habits to cope with the flow of wastes (which are always fluid because the ileum does not remove sufficient water to solidify the waste matter) by learning to attach and empty appliances and to keep the stoma clean. Colostomates, especially those who have lost only their sigmoid colon, can look forward to passing firm stools and may eventually be able to live without an appliance, but months of diarrhea occur before the bowel regains full operation.

Many complications can plague the new anatomy, some of which require surgical correction. The most serious include intestinal obstruction, scar adhesions that distort the shape of the bowel, retraction of the stoma, abscesses, prolapse (more of the bowel pushing out of the body), and kidney stones (which form because persistent diarrhea can dehydrate ostomates). Less threatening, but demanding attention, are offensive odors, diarrhea, skin irritation, and bowel inflammation. Steady advances in surgical technique have lowered the complication rates, and few patients die because of the surgery.

Ostomates often must live with the stoma for the rest of their lives. Feces exit through the stoma, rather than the anus, forcing patients to "toilet train" themselves all over again. Some stomas are continent; that is, they hold back wastes until the patient is ready to defecate by draining them with a tube. Many, however, are not, and stool and gas steadily seep through the opening, where the waste matter is collected in an appliance, usually a plastic bag that seals over the stoma.

Having a plastic bag of stool on the abdomen and needing to empty it periodically to prevent it from leaking, instead of defecating by sitting down on a toilet, proves a difficult adjustment for some patients, both physically and psychologically. Several aid resources help new ostomates adjust. Specially trained registered nurses called enterostomal therapists teach patients how to manage their new stomas and how to attach appliances or insert catheters to drain continent stomas;

they also help care for the stomas after the operation and periodically review their patients' progress. Gastroenterologists, physicians who specialize in the intestinal tract, can provide medical guidance and directly inspect the bowel wall behind the stoma through an endoscope, a flexible fiber-optic tube, should trouble develop. For those ostomates who feel isolated and depressed because of the stoma, the United Ostomy Association, a support group with branches throughout the United States, organizes social events and provides information and encouragement, often sending representatives to meet patients soon after surgery.

It is unfortunate that the widely felt repugnance for surgery involving the intestines and the social taboo against discussing defecation and excrement in polite conversation have obscured the triumph of stoma procedures. Much riskier and less rehabilitating surgeries, such as cardiac bypasses and organ transplantations, occupy the limelight, while ileostomies and colostomies, which prolong or improve more lives, receive scant popular attention. Medical journalists report that many patients, when told that they need a colostomy, know little or nothing of the procedure. After the doctor explains, they typically are dismayed and horrified. Nevertheless, few refuse the operation. On the other hand, potential ileostomates who suffer from ulcerative colitis are almost always better informed and look forward to the operation as the end to years of intense abdominal distress and fears about cancer.

Out of the hospital, ostomates literally face a new and different life. As well as learning to handle appliances or irrigate artificial rectums, they must face the fact that a major organ of their bodies is changed. The need for the stoma may anger or depress them, and this fixation on the change, if unalleviated, can evolve into loss of self-esteem and attendant social withdrawal. Many ostomates experience guilt in the belief that the disease and stoma, as well as the effects of the stoma on their families, are somehow their own fault.

These reactions require social and psychological therapy, extending care well beyond that afforded by the surgeon and the hospital. Support groups and the enterostomal therapist supply the majority of this care, but occasionally professional psychological help is required. The repulsion that patients feel for stomas and the consequent chance of morbid psychological reactions have encouraged surgeons to prefer anastomoses to stomas when possible, even though anastomoses are more difficult, have higher failure rates, and require a longer recovery period.

Moreover, the impression lingers, encouraged by popular accounts of research linking diet to disease, that most serious intestinal maladies (cancer in particular) result solely from poor eating habits. This type of reasoning sometimes leads to the insinuation that a stoma amounts to a kind of punishment for those habits, which is a hasty and erroneous conclusion that can worsen the guilt some ostomates feel. More often, factors over which people may have no control, such as genetic susceptibility and environmental toxins, contribute to the diseases that make stomas necessary.

Fortunately, the great majority of ostomates do adjust to their new lives; they seldom have any other alternative. Providing that the original need for surgery has been eliminated—the cancer has been removed, for example—they can look forward to an undiminished life span and few if any restrictions upon appetite, sexual function, or exercise. About 95 percent of ostomates recover completely, returning to their previous occupations after recovery, and of these the majority believe themselves to be in good or excellent health. Without the operations, all of them would have led drastically impaired lives, and many would have died. The high success rate places the ileostomy and colostomy procedures among the ranks of surgical interventions that rescue the seriously ill from otherwise incurable organic diseases.

PERSPECTIVE AND PROSPECTS

Although drastic techniques requiring much skill from surgeons and stamina from patients, ostomies did not originate with modern medicine and its sophisticated technology for sustaining patients during operations. Some colostomies date from the last quarter of the eighteenth century. In the nineteenth century, the number of operations creating a stoma—then called "artificial" or "preternatural" anus—increased, although without antiseptic conditions or anesthesia a patient's chances for survival were not good. Surgeons sometimes placed the stomas on the back instead of the abdomen. In 1908, William Ernest Miles conducted the first operation to remove a cancerous rectum; since the patient's intestines were still moving waste matter, which needed an exit, Miles created a stoma, thereby establishing one of the most common surgeries of the twentieth century.

Still, colostomies and ileostomies did not proliferate until after World War II. Since then, refinements in surgical techniques and postoperative care have steadily reduced the chance of complications and the length of the recovery period. At the same time, several variations of permanent and temporary stomas have been developed.

Like many other extreme surgical interventions, the ileostomy and colostomy testify to the limits of biomedical knowledge: Most of these surgeries are performed because other remedies fail. Until researchers discover the mechanisms causing cancer, ulcerative colitis, and other deadly lower bowel diseases and develop nonsurgical cures, ileostomies and colostomies will remain common, especially among the elderly.

—*Roger Smith, Ph.D.*

See also Bypass surgery; Cancer; Colitis; Colon and rectal surgery; Colon cancer; Crohn's disease; Digestion; Diverticulitis and diverticulosis; Gastrectomy; Gastroenterology; Gastroenterology, pediatric; Gastrointestinal disorders; Gastrointestinal system; Intestinal disorders; Intestines.

FOR FURTHER INFORMATION:

Adrouny, Richard. *Understanding Colon Cancer.* Jackson: University Press of Mississippi, 2002. An excellent lay guide to the disease, offering information on topics such as diagnosis, prognosis, treatment, demographics, high-risk conditions, the sequence from bowel polyps to cancer, the warning signs, the stages of the disease, and theories of how colon cancer spreads.

Brandt, Lawrence J., and Penny Steiner-Grossman, eds. *Treating IBD: A Patient's Guide to the Medical and Surgical Management of Inflammatory Bowel Disease.* Reprint. New York: Raven Press, 1996. Although devoted to inflammatory bowel disease (IBD) in general, this book contains a section on surgical cures for ulcerative colitis and Crohn's disease. Types of ileostomy and anastomosis are described thoroughly in lay terms, and drawings and photographs depict the bowel reconstructions.

Bub, David S., et al. *One Hundred Questions and Answers About Colorectal Cancer.* Sudbury, Mass.: Jones and Bartlett, 2003. Provides authoritative answers to questions about treatment options, posttreatment quality of life, and sources of support.

Doherty, Gerard M., and Lawrence W. Way, eds. *Current Surgical Diagnosis and Treatment.* 12th ed. New York: Lange Medical Books/McGraw-Hill, 2006. A reference work on general surgery for physicians, this tome is nevertheless comprehensible to laypersons familiar with medical terminology. Presents succinct overviews of the stoma procedures and their potential complications and contains finely detailed illustrations.

Fries, Colleen Farley. "Managing an Ostomy." *Nursing* 29, no. 8 (August, 1999): 26. Ostomies are used to assist patients with conditions like ulcerative colitis and bowel obstruction. The selection of an ostomy should be based on the patient's needs and is available in one- or two-piece devices and a number of sizes.

Kalibjian, Cliff. *Straight from the Gut: Living with Crohn's Disease and Ulcerative Colitis.* Cambridge, Mass.: O'Reilly and Associates, 2003. Shares numerous personal stories from those suffering from colitis and offers advice on all aspects of living with the disease.

Mullen, Barbara Dorr, and Kerry Anne McGinn. *The Ostomy Book: Living Comfortably with Colostomies, Ileostomies, and Urostomies.* Rev. ed. Palo Alto, Calif.: Bull, 1992. An amusingly written, inspirational account of the most typical of ostomy cases: a colostomy necessitated by rectal cancer. It is Mullen's own story, and she relates her emotional turmoil with candor, making her account invaluable reading for anyone who must undergo a colostomy.

Parker, James N., and Philip M. Parker, eds. *The 2002 Official Patient's Sourcebook on Ulcerative Colitis.* San Diego, Calif.: Icon Health, 2002. Draws from public, academic, government, and peer-reviewed research to provide a wide-ranging reference about the causes, treatments, and risk factors of colitis.

United Ostomy Association. http://www.uoa.org/. A support group for ostomy patients that stresses education, information, support, and advocacy.

IMAGING AND RADIOLOGY

PROCEDURE

ANATOMY OR SYSTEM AFFECTED: All

SPECIALTIES AND RELATED FIELDS: Nuclear medicine, radiology

DEFINITION: Medical imaging uses radiation that passes through the body to construct images of the insides of the body.

KEY TERMS:

computed tomography (CT): a scanning procedure using X rays

fluoroscope: a machine that uses a fluorescent screen instead of photographic film to display X-ray images

magnetic resonance imaging (MRI): an imaging method using radio waves

positron emission tomography (PET): a scanning procedure using gamma rays from injected radioactive pharmaceuticals

single photon emission computed tomography (SPECT): a scanning procedure using gamma rays from injected radioactive pharmaceuticals

tomography: a method to produce a three-dimensional image of the internal structure of the body by observing and recording radiation transmitted, reflected, or emitted by structures inside the body; observations are made of sections, or slices, of the body that are assembled to form the final image

ultrasound: an imaging method using high-frequency sound

INDICATIONS AND PROCEDURES

Before the advent of radiology, physicians were forced to rely on visual clues, palpation (examination by touch), and exploratory surgery to discover what lay beneath a patient's skin. X rays provided the first path around this limitation and allowed physicians to peer beneath the skin without surgery. X rays are electromagnetic radiation similar to visible light, but they have much higher energies than visible light, which makes them more penetrating.

Circumstances under which a doctor needs to "see" inside the body and might use X rays to do so include a patient who has fallen and now experiences localized pain and swelling in the leg (possible broken bone); a patient with severe pain in the lower back who passes blood in the urine (possible kidney stone); a patient who experiences intermittent and squeezing chest pain, nausea, and shortness of breath (possible constricted arteries in the heart); and a patient with a history of localized stomach pain and heartburn, also called acid reflux (possible inflamed esophagus, hiatal hernia, or ulcer).

All medical imaging devices require a source of radiation, a detector, and a way to position the patient. For X rays, the patient stands in front of a film holder or lies on a table over a film holder while X rays from an X-ray tube pass through the patient and cast the patient's shadow onto the film. The film must be as large as the body part being examined. Dense constituents such as bones show up as white on X-ray negatives, while various other body tissues show up as shades of gray depending upon the fraction of the X rays that they block.

X-ray film has been developed to have excellent resolution and contrast, and an X ray is a permanent record. It is not easy to take several X rays in quick suc-

An MRI allows physicians to visualize soft tissues inside the body, such as the brain and nasopharyngeal tissues. (Digital Stock)

cession, however, as might be done to examine the upper gastrointestinal tract. An alternative is to use fluoroscopy, in which a screen coated with special compounds is used in the place of film. These compounds fluoresce when struck by X rays. Advantages are that the image is immediate (no film to develop) and moving images can be viewed. The image can be made brighter by an image intensifier—a television camera-like device that amplifies the image—and a permanent record can be made by photographing this final image.

An ultrasound unit adapts sonar to medical purposes. The unit consists of a probe; electronics to generate, receive, and analyze signals; and a monitor to display the results. Such a device is relatively inexpensive compared with other types of scanners, and at the intensities used, ultrasound waves do not harm the body. The ultrasound probe contains a transducer, a crystal that can change electrical signals into sound waves and can also act as a receiver changing sound waves into electrical signals. During the examination, a gel is spread over the patient's skin in the area of interest. The gel provides good acoustical coupling between the probe and the patient's body tissue. In order to create an image of

structures as small as 1 millimeter, ultrasound frequencies between 3 and 7 megahertz are used. The crystal inside the probe emits sound waves while rapidly rocking back and forth, producing a wedge of sound pulses. The crystal then becomes a receiver and picks up sound echoes that form as the sound passes from one type of tissue into another. Distance can be determined from the time elapsed between sending a pulse and receiving the echo. Combining this distance information with the direction and intensity of the echo allows a computer to build an image of the structures inside the body.

This image is displayed on a monitor screen and can also be printed for a permanent record. The probe is moved around to provide the least obstructed view of the target. Since ultrasound waves pass easily through soft tissues such as the liver and fluid-filled organs such as the gallbladder or the uterus during pregnancy, ultrasound is particularly useful to examine these organs. Ultrasound does not penetrate bone or gas, and the latter property makes it difficult to examine the digestive tract with ultrasound.

Like ultrasound, magnetic resonance imaging (MRI), uses no potentially harmful radiation, but it is the most expensive of the imaging techniques. MRI uses a very large, superconducting magnet. Once the magnetic field is established, superconducting magnets require very little electrical power. In order to be superconducting, the magnet is wound with niobium-titanium wire and maintained at liquid helium temperature (about 4 Kelvins above absolute zero). The magnet itself is in the form of a very large, hollow cylinder into which the patient can be inserted. The magnetic field inside the cylinder is uniform and very strong, typically 0.5 to 2.0 tesla; for comparison, the strength of the earth's magnetic field is only about 0.00005 tesla near the surface. There are also three sets of much smaller (.0018 to .0027 of a tesla) "gradient" magnets, which are used to tweak the magnetic field at pinpoint locations during the scan. Hydrogen atoms are among the most abundant atoms in soft tissue. In a strong magnetic field, the spin axis of hydrogen nuclei (protons) precesses about magnetic field lines. The exact frequency with which it precesses depends on the proton's surroundings, or the type of tissue in which it is found.

The patient rests on a table that moves into the tunnel formed by the magnet. The magnetic field causes no noticeable sensation, but claustrophobic patients may become anxious. To combat this effect, newer machines have wider tunnels or have one side open. An insulated wire coil may be placed on the patient over the area to be examined, or coils mounted on the magnet may be used. A brief pulse of radiofrequency waves is broadcast from the coil at the same time that the gradient magnets adjust the magnetic field to the right value in a narrow slice of the patient. If the radiofrequency is at the precession frequency, then those protons with which it resonates will absorb energy. After the radiofrequency pulse, the protons produce an echo that radiates energy back to the coil. Analysis of this energy allows the identification of the type of tissue, which, along with location information from the gradient magnets, allows a computer to construct an image of the internal tissues of the patient. The image can be either two-dimensional or three-dimensional, as needed. Two-dimensional slices can be vertical, horizontal, or in any plane desired.

A scan of the brain and spinal column can detect areas of damage to the myelin (insulating sheath) surrounding nerve fibers that is the hallmark of multiple sclerosis. MRI scans are also used in diagnosing tumors, infections of the brain, strokes, torn ligaments, and many other conditions. As with X rays, contrast agents may be injected into the patient to make certain tissues or systems stand out. For example, the blood vessels in the heart may be examined in this fashion. Depending upon the size of the region to be scanned, the procedure takes from twenty to ninety minutes, and the patient must remain as still as possible during this time. Currents in the gradient magnets produce loud thumping sounds. These may be masked by providing the patient with music through earphones during the examination.

Physicians now depend so much on MRI investigations that more than 60 million are performed each year around the world. Underscoring this importance, the 2003 Nobel Prize in Medicine or Physiology was awarded to Paul C. Lauterbur and Sir Peter Mansfield for their work leading to the development of the MRI technique.

A nuclear medicine scan, also called nuclear radiology or isotope study, uses radioactive pharmaceuticals that have been injected into or ingested by the patient. The radiation dose to the patient is strictly controlled and is the least possible for the procedure to be effective. The radioactive isotopes used emit gamma rays—essentially high-energy X rays—which easily pass through the body and are observed by an array of gamma detectors. The patient lies on a table while the detector array is positioned near the target organ. In some applications, the array slowly scans a region. A computer receives information on the location and intensity of the detected gamma rays and constructs an image from this information. The image is fuzzy and lacks the fine detail that can be seen with X rays or ultrasound, but it shows directly how well the target organ functions.

To be useful for this purpose, radioactive isotopes must emit penetrating gamma rays, have a short half-life, and either be taken up by the target organ or be capable of being attached to a molecule that is taken up by the target organ. A short half-life is desirable to ensure that the isotope will cease to be radioactive not too long after it has served its purpose. Technetium-99m is frequently used because it is taken up by the thyroid and salivary glands (if those are the targets), it can be used to tag other biologically active molecules, and its half-life is only 6.01 hours.

For a thyroid study, the patient may be given a drink or a pill containing iodine-123 (13.1 hour half-life). About twenty-four hours later, the gamma emission from the thyroid is measured. This procedure shows how well the thyroid works in general. The patient may then be injected with technetium-99m and several scans made over the next hour. This provides another measure of the thyroid's functioning. It also allows a measure of the thyroid's size and shape. Any area of inactivity suggests a blockage or damage, while an unusual area of activity suggests an abnormally high tissue growth rate such as a tumor. In general, a region of rapidly growing tissue shows up as a hot spot on a nuclear medicine scan, which makes it possible to see a healing bone fracture that an X ray might miss.

A positron emission tomography (PET) scan is a special type of nuclear medicine scan that capitalizes on a property of the gamma rays emitted during positron annihilation. Positrons are positively charged and are the electron's antiparticle. Since they are oppositely charged, positrons and electrons are strongly attracted to each other, and as soon as they touch, they mutually annihilate, converting their energy into two gamma rays emitted at precisely 180 degrees to each other.

A gantry houses a large ring of gamma ray detectors arranged like a doughnut on its side. The patient rests on a movable table that carries the patient into, and perhaps through, the detector ring. Depending upon the purpose of the examination, one of several radioactive pharmaceuticals is administered. For example, fluorine-18 (half-life 109.8 minutes) is attached to glucose molecules and used to monitor the brain's metabolism. Since active areas of the brain draw the most glucose, a PET scan can watch the brain at work. When a fluorine nucleus emits a positron, the positron encounters an electron almost at once and is annihilated. The gamma ray detectors continually register hits from natural background radiation, but if two detectors located 180 degrees around the ring from each other record gamma rays of the right energy (0.511 million electron volts) and within a few nanoseconds of each other, it is virtually certain that they originated from a positron annihilation in the patient. A computer then draws a straight line between the two detectors and through the patient. Where two or more lines intersect is the location of the activity.

A single photon emission computed tomography (SPECT) scan is similar to a PET scan, but it detects only one photon at a time instead of a pair. In order to define the direction of a gamma ray photon, a collimator is placed in front of the detector array. The collimator is a slab of 5-centimeter-long lead straws pointing at the patient so that a gamma ray can reach the detector only by traveling up a straw. Such a collimator and detector array is called an Anger camera. A ring of cameras around the patient allows a computer to con-

struct a three-dimensional image of the target organ. SPECT combines the organ function information of nuclear medicine with some of the resolution of a computed tomography (CT) scan.

The CT apparatus consists of a movable table on which the patient rests and a gantry that houses the X-ray equipment. A doughnut hole in the gantry is large enough for the patient and table to pass through. An X-ray tube is mounted in the doughnut, and an array of X-ray detectors are mounted in the doughnut directly opposite from the X-ray source. As the doughnut rotates all the way around, the X-ray beam is sent through a narrow "slice" of the patient. Instead of the normal X-ray silhouette of the patient as illuminated from one direction, silhouettes from all directions are obtained, but only as numbers, not yet as images.

The information available consists of where the detector was when it picked up the signal and how strong the signal was. As the scan continues, the computer uses this information to construct an image of that slice of the patient. While the doughnut carries the X-ray tube and detectors around and around the patient, the table advances slowly and continuously until the whole body (or the desired segment) has been scanned. Blood clots and ruptured vessels in the brain are easily detected, as well as tumors in soft tissues such as the liver.

USES AND COMPLICATIONS

Bones, bone breaks, and some tumors show up well on an X ray, but soft tissue images may require additional techniques. For examination of the upper gastrointestinal tract, the patient is given a barium solution to drink while standing in front of the X-ray detector. Barium blocks X rays and coats the esophagus and stomach lining, thereby outlining them in detail on the X ray. In the "barium swallow," a quick series of X rays is taken to follow the progress of the barium into the stomach. Constrictions in the esophagus, the action of the stomach valve, and the presence of a hiatal hernia (the upper part of the stomach bulging through a weakened diaphragm) become visible. As the barium proceeds, a stomach ulcer may stand out in outline.

To check for kidney stones and to examine the kidneys, ureters, and urinary bladder, an intravenous pyelogram (IVP) is performed. First, a contrast solution (based on iodine, which blocks X rays) is injected into the patient's vein. The patient may feel a brief warm flush as the body reacts to the iodine, but this reaction passes quickly. The solution used soon passes through the patient's system: through the kidneys, through the ureters, and to the bladder. A series of X rays is then taken in which kidney stones may be revealed; any swelling of a kidney or blockage of a ureter will show up, if present.

The angiogram, a similar but more extensive procedure, is used to examine the blood vessels of the heart or other location. In this procedure, a catheter (fine plastic tube) is inserted into the femoral artery at the groin or into a blood vessel in the upper arm. The patient is given medication for pain and anxiety. Using a fluoroscope monitor, the physician maneuvers the catheter to the desired location and then injects the contrast solution through the catheter. Several X rays are taken from various angles, and any blockages or constrictions are generally apparent. The catheter is then withdrawn, and the patient is required to rest.

CT scanning represents a major step forward in X-ray technology. A patient might suffer a sudden loss of muscle control and feeling in part of the body (possible stroke). The doctor would like to X-ray the brain for signs of a ruptured or blocked blood vessel, but contrast agents are not useful for the brain. Without them, internal organs and tissues appear only as faint ghosts in an X ray. A CT scan uses computer technology to convert special X-ray images into clear views of the organs.

While prudence dictates that radiation exposure be kept to a minimum, the medical benefits of procedures using radiation generally outweigh the risks. Provided that a radiation dose is not overwhelmingly massive, the body has amazing recuperative properties and is able to repair most radiation damage. Everyone is exposed daily to background radiation from naturally occurring trace amounts of radioactive elements and from cosmic rays. The accompanying table lists the typical radiation doses received in several medical procedures, using the millisievert (mSv) as the unit of measurement, and provides the equivalent whole-body dose received from natural background radiation. None of these procedures generates radiation above allowable limits, but it should be noted that a medical procedure may expose the target organ to many times the average body dose.

A typical X-ray image shows different types of tissue as various shades of gray. Recent advances in medical imaging include digitizing any image and using powerful computer programs to enhance the subtle differences between different types of tissue, even coloring them so that they are immediately obvious to the physician. Three-dimensional images can be constructed and rotated so that they can be examined from every angle. A physician can see exactly what problems will be encountered in removing a tumor. Computers can scan X rays used to screen for breast cancer, called mammograms, and draw the radiologist's attention to any questionable regions. Finally, computers can merge images

COMPARISON OF RADIATION DOSES FOR VARIOUS PROCEDURES

Procedure	Typical Effective Dose	Natural Background Equivalent
Ultrasound scan	none	none
MRI	none	none
Chest X ray	0.1 mSv	10 days
Thyroid iodine uptake (whole-body dose)	2 mSv	8 months
Thyroid scan Tc-99m (whole-body dose)	5 mSv	1 year, 7 months
Whole-body PET scan with fluorine-tagged glucose	6 mSv	2 years
Chest CT scan	8 mSv	2 years, 8 months
Whole-body CT scan	10 mSv	3 years, 4 months

from complementary techniques such as PET (shows functionality of the organ) with MRI (shows high-resolution detail) to give a more complete view.

PERSPECTIVE AND PROSPECTS

November 8, 1895, was a Friday. That evening, Wilhelm Conrad Röntgen was quite late for dinner; he ate little and quickly returned to his laboratory. That afternoon, he had made an astounding and disquieting discovery. Many scientists of the day, including Röntgen, were studying cathode rays. The required apparatus was an evacuated glass tube with electrodes sealed inside at either end. When a high voltage was placed across the electrodes, cathode rays (electrons) streamed from the cathode, and where they struck the glass tube, the glass fluoresced.

Röntgen covered the tube with black paper and darkened the room, but still a fluorescent screen some distance away from the tube glowed whenever he operated the tube. Since cathode rays cannot travel far through air, Röntgen deduced that some unknown type of radiation must be coming from the tube. He called it X radiation (X for unknown). Placing bits of wood or metal between the tube and the screen cast shadows on the screen, some darker and some lighter. The key moment came when Röntgen held up a small lead disk. The expected shadow of the lead appeared, but holding the disk, Röntgen saw the shadows of his finger bones. He opened his hand, and the shadowy skeleton hand opened. Röntgen wondered if he could be hallucinating. In those days, some people believed that dreaming about or imagining seeing a skeleton was a premonition of one's impending death. Röntgen was concerned that others might think him crazy if he were to describe what he had seen, so he needed proof.

In the ensuing weeks, Röntgen made an intense study of the properties of X rays. Three days before Christmas, he placed photographic film in a black paper package and had his wife, Bertha, place her hand on it while he exposed it with X rays for fifteen minutes. The photograph showed the bones of Bertha Röntgen's hand, with a ring on her finger. Röntgen sent a copy of the photograph along with an explanation to a friend, but it soon found its way into newspapers all over the world. Only four months after the public announcement, Thomas Edison's company began marketing "complete outfits for x-ray work." While some considered looking at skeletons while people were still using them revoltingly indecent, the medical usefulness of X rays was immediately apparent. The first Nobel Prize in Physics ever awarded went to Röntgen in 1901 for his discovery of X rays.

In spite of the obvious medical advantages, relatively few doctors used X rays at first, but the public found them a source of entertainment. Edison built a fluoroscope for use at amusement parks. Looking through a hooded visor, spectators placed their hands between an X-ray tube and a fluorescent screen and watched their bones wiggle as they moved their hands. Casual exposure to X rays continued into the 1950's with the use of fluoroscopes by shoe stores to see how well shoes fit.

The widespread use of medical X rays was hampered by the lack of trained operators and proper equipment. This situation changed with World War I, when X-ray teams were trained and equipped by the hundreds. Marie Curie was a prime force in establishing such teams for the French and Belgian militaries. From this modest beginning, the various imaging techniques have evolved to provide the physician with "magic eyes" that can peer inside the body.

—*Charles W. Rogers, Ph.D.*

See also Angiography; Angioplasty; Computed tomography (CT) scanning; Echocardiography; Magnetic resonance imaging (MRI); Mammography; Neuroimaging; Noninvasive tests; Nuclear medicine; Nuclear radiology; Positron emission tomography (PET) scanning; Radiation sickness; Radiation therapy; Radiopharmaceuticals; Ultrasonography.

FOR FURTHER INFORMATION:

Giger, Maryellen L., and Charles A. Pelizzari. "Advances in Tumor Imaging." *Scientific American* 275, no. 3 (September, 1996): 110-112. Describes how combining images from complementary techniques such as MRI and PET is particularly helpful, as is forming three-dimensional color images. Computer-aided diagnosis provides an automatic second opinion.

Mould, Richard F. *A Century of X-Rays and Radioactivity in Medicine.* Philadelphia: Institute of Physics, 1993. A treasure trove of historical photographs and basic explanations outlining the development of X rays and nuclear medicine.

Raichle, Marcus E. "Visualizing the Mind." *Scientific American* 270, no. 4 (April, 1994): 58-64. Discusses how PET and CT scans are used to provide images of the brain in action.

Ter-Pogossian, Michel M., Marcus E. Raichle, and Burton E. Sobel. "Positron-Emission Tomography."

Scientific American 243, no. 4 (October, 1980): 170-181. A good basic explanation of the PET technique, including the equipment and how it is used.

Weissleder, Ralph, et al. *Primer of Diagnostic Imaging*. 4th ed. Philadelphia: Mosby, 2007. Contains information on chest, cardiac, gastrointestinal, genitourinary, musculoskeletal, neurologic, head and neck, vascular, breast, obstetric, pediatric, and nuclear imaging.

IMMUNE SYSTEM
BIOLOGY

ANATOMY OR SYSTEM AFFECTED: Blood, cells, circulatory system, glands, liver, lymphatic system, spleen

SPECIALTIES AND RELATED FIELDS: Cytology, hematology, immunology, microbiology, preventive medicine, serology

DEFINITION: A system—including the spleen, thymus, lymphatic system, and specialized cells—that protects the body from foreign substances.

KEY TERMS:

antibody: any of the proteins produced in the body during an immune response; recognizes and attacks foreign antigen substances

antigen: a substance within the human body recognized as foreign either by antibodies or by special immune cells; the cause behind the stimulation of the immune response

autoimmunity: an abnormal immune reaction against antigens

immunosuppression: a decrease in the effectiveness of the immune system

pathogen: any disease-causing organism, including a virus, bacterium, protozoan, mold or yeast, or other parasite

STRUCTURE AND FUNCTIONS

The immune system is capable of recognizing and identifying many different substances foreign to the human body. To function properly, this system must receive, interpret, and transmit large amounts of information about invaders from outside or within the body. These constant and ever-changing threats to the body must be met and destroyed by one complex system—namely, the human immune system. Many organs and parts of the body play a major role in maintaining resistance; some have more important roles than others, but all parts must work in unison. The circulatory and lym-

phatic systems, along with specific organs, are of primary importance in the overall workings of the immune system.

Blood. Besides the outer protective layer of the skin and mucous membranes, the first line of defense in the immune system includes the blood in the circulatory system. About 50 percent of human blood is made up of a fluid called plasma, which contains water, proteins, carbohydrates, vitamins, hormones, and cellular waste. The other half of blood is composed of white cells, red cells, and platelets. The red blood cells, called erythrocytes, are responsible for moving oxygen from the lungs to the other parts of the body. The special platelet cells, called thrombocytes, enable the blood to form clots, thus preventing severe bleeding. An unborn child produces red and white blood cells in the spleen and liver, while a newborn makes blood in the center of bones, called the marrow. After maturity, all red and most white blood cells are produced in the bone marrow. Although the red cells and platelets are vital, it is the white cells that play a major role in the immune system.

In a broad sense, white blood cells surround and engulf foreign matter and adjacent dying cells in a process called phagocytosis. The function is possible since the white blood cells can move, unlike red corpuscles, by pushing their bodies out and pulling forward. Red corpuscles move because of the flow of the blood within the circulatory system. White blood cells move in the lymph vessels, where they work to defend the body against disease, but are also transported through the blood. Bacteria and other foreign material can remain alive within a white corpuscle, but sometimes the corpuscle dies from the toxins produced by the bacteria. The resulting formation of pus is actually an accumulation of dead white blood cells. At other times, the white corpuscles win and the foreign matter is destroyed.

Three major types of white blood cells, known collectively as leukocytes, are involved in immune responses. All three—granulocytes, monocytes, and lymphocytes—arise from areas in either bone marrow, the spleen, or the liver.

The granulocytes, each of which is about twice the size of a red blood cell, originate from red bone marrow and live only about twelve hours. Under the classification of granulocytes, distinct cells have different structures, sizes, and shapes. These specialized granulocytes include the neutrophils, eosinophils, and basophils. None of these cells has a specific memory for future immune responses. The neutrophil granulocyte eats and digests small foreign matter with the help of special enzymes. Between 40 and 75 percent of the white blood cells in the human body are neutrophils. When these highly mobile neutrophil cells arrive at an injury site, they burst, releasing their enzymes and melting away the surrounding tissues. Eosinophils are similar to neutrophils but seem to be specialized in fighting infection caused by parasites, because of the seven toxic proteins that they use to fight. They are also effective against fungal, bacterial, viral, or protozoan infections. Basophils, which are smaller in size, move from the bone marrow through the body and act as a control by preventing overreactions during an immune response. Basophils prevent coagulation, but they cannot destroy foreign matter. These cells account for less than 1 percent of the white blood cells found in the blood.

The second group of leukocytes includes the monocytes, the largest cells found in the blood. Monocytes are two to three times as large as red cells, yet they are not very numerous, making up 3 to 9 percent of all the leukocytes in the blood. After only a few days in the blood, they move to areas between tissues. Over the course of months or years, the monocytes enlarge ten times in size in order to specialize in phagocytosis. After this growth, they are called macrophages. They are also referred to as terminal cells since they cannot divide, and thus do not reproduce.

The third type of leukocyte, and the most sophisticated of the white blood cells, are called lymphocytes because they come from the lymph system as well as bone marrow. The T lymphocytes, which are primarily responsible for immunity, can change into helper, killer, and suppressor cells. Besides being able to recognize foreign matter precisely, they can live freely in the blood, grow larger and divide, and then change back to their original form after working against the invader. Lymphocytes circulate throughout the body, moving from the bloodstream through the lymph fluid and back into the blood. The two major types of lymphocytes are T lymphocytes (also called T cells) and B lymphocytes (also called B cells). Both T and B cells can recognize foreign matter and hook onto it. Some of these special "memory" cells remain in the body for life, preventing a specific invader from causing illness when it is encountered again in the future. These specialized cells must have a way to travel through the body; one of these transport systems is the lymphatic system.

The lymphatic system. This system is a closed network of vessels that help in circulating fluids from the body and returning them to the bloodstream. The lymphatic system also defends against disease-causing foreign materials, known as antigens. The smallest components of the lymph system are the lymphatic capillaries that run parallel to the blood capillaries. The fluid inside these capillaries, which has come across the thin wall membrane from tissues all across the body, is called lymph. These capillaries merge into larger lymphatic vessels, which then merge into a type of collecting area called a lymph node. The lymph fluid is drained into trunks that join one of two collecting ducts. The larger left thoracic duct collects lymph from the upper arm, head, and neck of the left side of the body before emptying into a vein near the neck and shoulder. The right lymphatic duct does the same for the right side of the body. After leaving the collecting ducts, the lymph fluid becomes part of the blood plasma in the veins and returns to the right atrium of the heart. Lymph does not flow like blood in veins and arteries; instead, it is controlled by muscular activity.

The spleen. This largest lymphatic organ is located in the upper left part of the abdominal cavity, behind the stomach and under the diaphragm. The hollow spaces within the spleen are filled with blood, making it soft and elastic. The white blood cells in the lining of these hollow cavities engulf and destroy foreign materials, as well as damaged red blood cells that pass through the spleen.

The thymus. This gland is located between the lungs and above the heart, just behind the upper part of the breastbone. It contains large numbers of white cells; some are inactive, but others develop and leave the thymus to become functional in the immune system.

The liver. Located in the upper right part of the abdominal cavity below the diaphragm, the liver is well protected by the ribs. Since it is the largest gland in the body, it plays a major role in metabolism while also aiding the body's ability to clot blood. In addition, various liver cells, called macrophages, help in destroying damaged red blood cells. The liver's connection to the immune system is its ability to also destroy foreign substances through phagocytosis.

Bone marrow. Marrow is located in the center of bones. It can be divided into two types, red or yellow marrow. It is the red marrow that aids in the formation of white and red blood cells. The yellow marrow stores fat and is not involved in producing blood cells. Some white blood cells come from bone marrow cells. They are released into the blood and are carried to the thymus gland, where they undergo special processing that changes them into T lymphocytes (the letter *T* shows that they came from the thymus gland). The other lymphocytes that do not reach the thymus after leaving the bone marrow are named B lymphocytes (*B* because they came from bone marrow). These B lymphocytes are abundant in lymph nodes, the spleen, bone marrow, secretory glands, intestinal lining, and reticuloendothelial tissue.

THE RESPONSES OF THE IMMUNE SYSTEM

Failures of the immune system can lead to devastating diseases, either because the immune system attacks itself or because it fails to defend against outside foreign antigen matter. An antigen can be any substance that stimulates the body to fight, ranging from a bacterial infection to the virus that causes acquired immunodeficiency syndrome (AIDS).

When the body fights against an antigen, the immune system can produce two types of response, either a cellular immune response or a humoral immune response. The cellular response involves specific types of cells that recognize, attack, and destroy the invading antigen. The humoral immune response is actually the body's main defense against a bacterium, virus, or fungus in the blood or body fluids. This response involves various chemicals in the bloodstream that fight against the invaders.

Another way of looking at how the body fights to keep itself healthy is to separate the immune responses into either primary or secondary responses. The second time that a given antigen enters the body, the immune system attacks with what is called the secondary immune response stored in special immune memories, making it faster and more extensive than the primary response that occurred when the antigen was first encountered. This immune memory must be built for each antigen before the body becomes immune to the wide variety of diseases and conditions to which one is exposed on a daily basis.

The body begins to build this memory prior to birth by making an inventory of all the molecules within the body. Foreign substances not in this memory are considered to be antigens, which will activate an immune response. When an antigen is first encountered, the primary response occurs, producing lymphocytes that are sensitized to the invader. Many types of lymphocytes can respond in order to create the appropriate antibody molecules, which are then released into the lymph and transported to the blood. This process may last several weeks. During this primary immune response, the

B cells and T cells serve as memory cells. Because a memory for the antigen has been stored, if this antigen is encountered in the future the memory cells can react more quickly and effectively. In this secondary immune response, the antibodies are ready to react by attaching themselves to the surfaces of the antigens. There must be a specific type of antibody produced for every type of antigen. These new antibodies may survive only a few months, but the memory cells live much longer.

There are four main ways that an antibody can bind to an antigen. The antibody can pull together clusters of invading organisms to prevent the antigens from spreading. Another possibility is for this special component of the blood to punch a hole in the invader and destroy it. The antibody can also combine with the antigen, which makes it easier to destroy. In the case of a virus or a toxin, the antibody can neutralize the harmful activity by covering the outside of the antigen. With so many ways for an antibody to attach to an antigen, it is equally important for the antibody memory to be established. It is this special memory that leads to future immunity.

These memory cells are responsible for the four different types of immunity, two of which are acquired actively and two of which are acquired passively. The first type is naturally acquired active immunity, which results after the body is exposed to a live pathogen and develops the disease. The second type is artificially acquired active immunity, such as that gained after a vaccination. The immune response is triggered after an injection of weakened or dead pathogens is received, but the body does not suffer the severe symptoms of the disease. An example would be a smallpox vaccination. The third type of immunity is artificially acquired passive immunity, gained through an injection of prepared antibodies. This method is considered passive since the antibodies, called gamma globulin, were made by another person. This type of immunity usually does not last more than a few weeks, and the person will be susceptible to that pathogen in the future. Naturally acquired passive immunity occurs when the antibodies pass to the fetus from the mother, but it includes only those antibodies available in the blood of the mother. This process gives an infant certain short-term immunities for the first year of life.

These types of immunity are usually desirable, but there are occasions when an immune response is not wanted, such as after an organ transplant. When tissue or organs are transplanted from one person to another, the body may reject the foreign tissue, triggering an immune response and possibly destroying the new organ. Consequently, attempts are made to match the tissue between recipient and donor. In an effort to halt the immune response, immunosuppressive drugs are given to interfere with the recipient's ability to form antibodies, and drugs can be administered to destroy the lymphocytes that produce these antibodies. Unfortunately, the recipient is often left unprotected against infections, since the immune system is not functioning normally.

Perspective and Prospects

In the same way that the discovery of penicillin shocked the world, immunology has created endless possibilities in medicine. When surgeons found that they could transplant an organ from one person to another, the interest in immunology exploded.

This field of medicine has discovered that the immune system's power and effectiveness can be lessened because of several factors. Improper diet, stress, disease, and excessive physical activity levels can depress the immune system. Other factors that can modify immunity include age, genetics, and metabolic and environmental factors. The anatomical, physiological, and microbial factors are shown in the susceptibility of the young and the very old to infections. For the young, the system is immature, while the aged have suffered a lifetime of assaults from pathogens. The impact of psychological stress is difficult to measure, yet it holds the potential for negatively affecting the immune system.

Before immunology can be fully understood, more knowledge must be gained about how antibodies are made and how they develop memories. Lymphocytes must be examined to discover what role they play in the immune response. Studies must look at not only the whole picture of the immune system but also its smaller parts—the organs and how each participates. Such studies could lead to better success in transplanting these organs. Unanswered questions remain about how the immune system relates to other body systems. The relationships among the brain and nervous system, hormones, and the respiratory system leave many areas ripe for further study.

Recent research has identified the significant importance of Class I major histocompatibility proteins (I-MHCPs) in the cellular immune system. When disease-associated proteins occur in a cell, they are broken into pieces by the cell's proteolytic machinery. Cell proteins become attached to antigen fragments and transport them to the surface of the cell, where they are "presented" to the body's defense mechanisms. I-MHCPs are these transport molecules. The I-MHCPs holding an antigen fragment can attach to certain immature T cells. Once such a T cell and I-MHCP-antigen complex hook up, the T cell reproduces many times. This important link between the cellular immune system and I-MHCPs has been shown in recent times by the epidemic of diseases like AIDS, which kills T cells. Class II MHCPs (II-MHCPs) interact similarly in antibody production by the humoral immune system. Understanding of the genes used in production of the I-MHCPs and the II-MHCPs has led to great hope for methods to control their production, possibilities for eventual cure of AIDS, emerging cancer treatments, and better understanding of the production of antibodies.

Additional information is needed on defects in the system, as are explanations for its dysfunctions. With greater knowledge of immunology, it may be possible to conquer AIDS, allergies, and asthma and to develop birth control methods based on the immune response. Doctors may be able to cure cancer, diabetes, herpes, infertility, multiple sclerosis, and rheumatoid arthritis. The possibilities are endless and could also include perfecting transplants of organs and skin grafts and preventing birth defects and even obesity. Through human gene therapy, those at risk for genetic disorders could be diagnosed and those with existing genetic conditions could be treated. Genetically engineered drugs and gene replacement therapy could relieve the stress on the human immune system. Until these methods become feasible, however, individuals must protect the natural immunity supplied by their bodies.

—*Maxine M. Urton, Ph.D.*

See also Acquired immunodeficiency syndrome (AIDS); Allergies; Antioxidants; Autoimmune disorders; Blood and blood disorders; Bone marrow transplantation; Cells; Chemotherapy; Circulation; Cytology; Cytopathology; Dialysis; Endocrinology; Endocrinology, pediatric; Glands; Healing; Hematology; Hematology, pediatric; Histiocytosis; Homeopathy; Hormones; Host-defense mechanisms; Human immunodeficiency virus (HIV); Immunization and vaccination; Immunodeficiency disorders; Immunology; Immunopathology; Infection; Kawasaki disease; Liver; Lymphatic system; Multiple chemical sensitivity syndrome; Oncology; Preventive medicine; Serology; Severe combined immunodeficiency syndrome (SCID); Skin; Stress reduction; Systems and organs; Transfusion; Transplantation; Wiskott-Aldrich syndrome.

FOR FURTHER INFORMATION:

Adelman, Daniel C., et al., eds. *Manual of Allergy and Immunology*. 4th ed. Philadelphia: Lippincott Williams & Wilkins, 2002. Examines research developments and the clinical diagnosis and treatment of allergies and immune disorders. Topics include asthma, disorders of the eye, diseases of the lung, anaphylaxism, insect allergies, drug allergies, rheumatic diseases, transplantation immunology, and immunization.

Delves, Peter J., et al. *Roitt's Essential Immunology*. 11th ed. Malden, Mass.: Blackwell, 2006. Provides a fine description of immunology.

Frank, Steven A. *Immunology and Evolution of Infectious Disease*. Princeton, N.J.: Princeton University Press, 2002. Blends research from molecular biology, immunology, pathogen biology, and population dynamics to discuss how and why parasites vary to escape recognition by the immune system, vaccine design, and the control of epidemics.

Immune Web. http://www.immuneweb.org/. A mailing list and resource center for people with chronic fatigue syndrome, multiple chemical sensitivities, lupus, allergies, environmental illness, fibromyalgia, candida, and other immune system disorders.

Janeway, Charles A., Jr., et al. *Immunobiology: The Immune System in Health and Disease*. 6th ed. New York: Garland Science, 2005. An excellent text that provides a lucid and comprehensive examination of the immune system, covering such topics as immunobiology and innate immunity, the recognition of antigen, the development of mature lymphocyte receptor repertoires, the adaptive immune response, and the evolution of the immune system.

Kindt, Thomas J., Richard A. Goldsby, and Barbara A. Osborne. *Kuby Immunology*. 6th ed. New York: W. H. Freeman, 2007. Excellent text that gives an overview of the immune system and its role with cells and organs, and discusses such topics as the generation of B-cell and T-cell responses, immune effector mechanisms, and the immune system in health and disease.

Life, Death, and the Immune System. New York: W. H. Freeman, 1994. This comprehensive collection of articles from *Scientific American* provides basic information and research directions on AIDS, autoimmune disorders, and allergies, as well as an excellent discussion of the immune system in general.

Marieb, Elaine N. *Essentials of Human Anatomy and Physiology*. 8th ed. San Francisco: Pearson/ Benjamin Cummings, 2006. This introductory anatomy and physiology textbook, easily accessible to those with little science background, is richly illustrated with diagrams and photographs, which help to illuminate body systems and processes.

Tortora, Gerard J., and Bryan Derrickson. *Principles of Anatomy and Physiology*. 11th ed. Hoboken, N.J.: John Wiley & Sons, 2006. An outstanding textbook of human anatomy and physiology.

IMMUNIZATION AND VACCINATION

PROCEDURE

ANATOMY OR SYSTEM AFFECTED: Blood, cells, immune system

SPECIALTIES AND RELATED FIELDS: Immunology, microbiology, preventive medicine, public health

DEFINITION: Immunization is the process by which exposure to an infectious agent or chemical confers an organism with resistance to that agent; vaccination involves the injection of a killed or attenuated microorganism, with the intention of inducing immunity.

KEY TERMS:

active immunity: immunity resulting from antibody production following exposure to an antigen

antibody: a protein secreted by lymphocytes in response to antigen stimuli, such as bacteria or viruses; also referred to as immunoglobulin

antigen: any chemical substance that stimulates the production of antibodies

attenuation: the weakening or elimination of the pathogenic properties of a microorganism; ideally, the organism is rendered harmless

passive immunity: immunity resulting from the introduction of preformed antibodies

serotype: a subgroup member within a larger species that is similar, but not identical, to other members of the species

toxoid: a toxin that has been chemically treated to eliminate its toxic properties but that retains the same antigens as the original

vaccinia: a virus which causes a poxlike illness in cattle (cowpox) and serves as smallpox vaccine in humans because of its similarity to the smallpox virus

THE FUNDAMENTALS OF IMMUNIZATION

The major day-to-day function of the immune response is to protect the body from infection. Exposure to foreign antigens such as infectious agents results in the stimulation of either of two components of the immune

Immunization and the Action of Vaccines

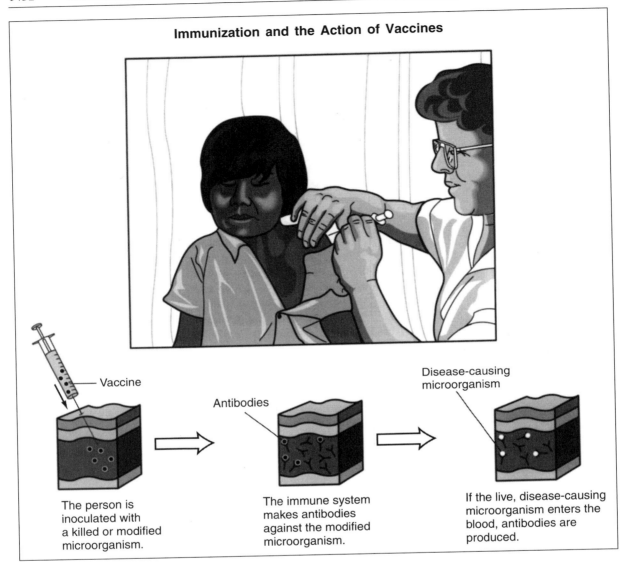

Vaccine

Antibodies

Disease-causing microorganism

The person is inoculated with a killed or modified microorganism.

The immune system makes antibodies against the modified microorganism.

If the live, disease-causing microorganism enters the blood, antibodies are produced.

system: the humoral (or antibody) immune response or the cellular immune response. Although no clear division exists between these two facets of the immune system, the antibody response deals primarily with organisms such as bacteria that live outside the cell. The cellular response deals primarily with microbes that live within a cell, such as intracellular bacteria or viral-infected cells.

A specialized class of white cells called B lymphocytes carries out the production of antibodies. Stimulation of these cells results from a complicated interaction between a variety of cells, including antigen-presenting cells (macrophage and dendritic cells) and both T and B lymphocytes. The response is specific in

that each type of T or B cell can interact with only a single antigen. The B cell that produces antibodies against a particular characteristic or shape on the surface of a bacterium reacts only with that particular determinant. In turn, the antibodies secreted by that B cell can interact only with specific determinants.

Antibodies secreted by B cells are themselves inert proteins. A variety of effects can result, however, when an antibody binds an antigen. The specific results depend on the nature of the antigen. For example, binding of an antibody to a toxin results in the neutralization of that substance. If the antigen is on the surface of a bacterial cell, the antibody can act as a flag that attracts other chemicals circulating in the blood. The technical term for an antibody bound to a bacterium is an opsonin. The antibody-bacterium complex becomes much more likely to be ingested and destroyed by a specialized cell called a phagocyte than if the antibody were not present. Likewise, if the antigen is an extracellular virus particle, binding of the antibody may inhibit the ability of the virus to infect a cell.

The cellular immune system also reacts in a specific manner. A subclass of T lymphocytes called cytotoxic T cells reacts with specific antigenic determinants on the surface of infected cells. When the T cells bind to a target, the result is the local release of toxic chemicals that ultimately kill the target.

The development of vaccines against specific infectious microbial agents resulted in the control or elimination of many diseases caused by these agents. The first formal vaccine developed for the prevention of

disease was that used by Edward Jenner against smallpox during the 1790's. Another century would pass before the molecular basis for vaccine function would begin to be understood.

Immunity to an antigen or disease may be induced using either of two methods. If preformed antibodies produced in another human or animal are inoculated into an individual, the result is passive immunity. Passive immunity can be advantageous in that the recipient achieves immunity in a short period of time. For example, if a person has been exposed to a toxin or has come into contact with an infectious agent, passive immunity can provide a rapid, short-term protection. Yet, since the individual does not generate the capacity to produce that antibody and the preformed antibodies are gradually removed from the body, no long-range protection is achieved.

Recommended Childhood Immunization Schedule, Ages 0-6 (2007)										
	Birth	1 mo.	2 mos.	4 mos.	6 mos.	12 mos.	15 mos.	18 mos.	19-23 mos.	4-6 yrs.
Hepatitis B	Dose 1	Dose 1	Dose 2		Dose 3	Dose 3	Dose 3			
Rotavirus			Doses 1, 2, 3	Doses 1, 2, 3	Doses 1, 2, 3					
Diphtheria, tetanus, pertussis (DTaP)			Doses 1, 2, 3	Doses 1, 2, 3	Doses 1, 2, 3		Dose 4	Dose 4		Dose 5
H. influenzae type B (HiB)			Doses 1, 2, 3	Doses 1, 2, 3	Doses 1, 2, 3	Dose 4	Dose 4			
Polio			Doses 1, 2	Doses 1, 2		Dose 3	Dose 3			Dose 4
Influenza					Yearly	Yearly	Yearly	Yearly	Yearly	Yearly
Measles, mumps, rubella (MMR)						Dose 1	Dose 1			Dose 2
Chickenpox (Varicella)						Dose 1	Dose 1			
Pneumococcal vaccine (PCV)			Doses 1, 2, 3	Doses 1, 2, 3	Doses 1, 2, 3	Dose 4	Dose 4			
Hepatitis A						Doses 1, 2	Doses 1, 2			

Approved by the Advisory Committee on Immunization Practices, the American Academy of Pediatrics, and the American Academy of Family Physicians.

The stimulation of antibody production through exposure to antigens, such as those found in a vaccine, results in active immunity. Development of effective active immunity requires a time span of several days to several weeks. The immunity is long-term, however, often lasting for the life span of the individual. Furthermore, each additional exposure to that same antigen, either through a vaccine booster or through natural exposure, results in a more rapid, greater response than those achieved previously. This increased rate of reaction is referred to as an anamnestic response.

The actual material utilized in a vaccine is variable, depending on the form of antigen. The earliest vaccine, that utilized by Jenner against smallpox, consisted of a virus that caused a disease in cattle called cowpox. The word "vaccination" is itself derived from this use; *vacca* is the Latin word for cow. While cowpox is distinct from the disease smallpox, the viruses that cause the two diseases contain similar antigenic determinants. Jenner made this observation. He exploited the fact that exposure to the cowpox virus results in active immunization against smallpox.

The use of attenuated strains of bacteria or viruses applies the same principle of cross-reaction. Attenuated organisms are mutants that have lost the ability to cause disease but that retain the antigenic character of the virulent strain. The most notable application of attenuation is the Sabin oral poliovirus vaccine (OPV). By testing hundreds of virus isolates for the ability to cause polio in monkeys, Albert Sabin was able to isolate certain strains that did not cause disease. These strains formed the basis for his vaccine. Similar testing resulted in the development of attenuated virus vaccines against a wide variety of agents, including those against measles, mumps, and rubella. Likewise, the Bacillus Calmette-Guérin (BCG) strain of *Mycobacterium tuberculosis* serves as a vaccine against the agent that causes tuberculosis. Unfortunately, the vaccine does not always result in immunity for the recipient. It is not used in the United States.

In some cases, the isolation of attenuated strains of microorganisms has proved difficult. For this reason, inactivated or killed microorganisms often serve as the basis for vaccine production. The Salk inactivated poliovirus vaccine represents the best-known example. By treating poliovirus with a solution of the chemical formalin, Jonas Salk was able to inactivate the organism. The virus retained its antigenic potential and served as an effective vaccine. A similar process has resulted in vaccines to protect against other bacterial diseases, such as bubonic plague, cholera, and pertussis (whooping cough), and against viral influenza.

In some cases, the vaccine is not directed against the etiological agent itself but against toxic materials produced by the agent. This is the case with diphtheria and tetanus. The vaccines are produced by treating the diphtheria and tetanus toxins secreted by these bacteria with formalin. The toxoids that result are antigenically similar to the actual toxins and so are able to induce immunity. They are incapable, however, of causing the deleterious effects of the respective diseases.

Only those determinants of a virus or bacterium that stimulate neutralizing antibodies are necessary in most vaccines. For this reason, the use of genetically engineered vaccines was begun in the 1980's. The first example put into use was the production of a vaccine against the hepatitis B virus (HBV). The gene that encodes the surface antigen of HBV was isolated and inserted into a piece of genetic material within the yeast *Saccharomyces*. The HBV antigen produced by the yeast was purified and subsequently found to be as effective in a vaccine as the whole virus. Since no live virus is involved, there is no danger of an attenuated strain reverting to its virulent parent. Recently, similar technology has been applied to produce vaccines that protect against chickenpox and hepatitis A virus.

HISTORY AND MAJOR SUCCESSES

Since the first use of vaccination by Edward Jenner in the 1790's for the prevention of smallpox, immunization techniques have been developed for protection against most major infectious illnesses. The term "vaccination" was originally applied to immunization against smallpox, but its definition has long been expanded to include most immunization techniques. "Vaccination" and "immunization" are used interchangeably, although there are technical differences in the definitions of the words.

The nineteenth century improvements in public health measures, combined with the passage of laws for compulsory vaccination, resulted in a steady decrease in the number of smallpox cases in the United States and most countries of Europe. Even as late as 1930, however, approximately 49,000 cases were reported in the United States. In the 1950's, large numbers of cases were still being reported in areas of Africa and Asia. At that time, the World Health Organization (WHO) of the United Nations decided on a plan for the elimination of smallpox based on the fact that humans served as the sole reservoir for the smallpox virus; animals are not naturally infected with smallpox. Through the use of mass immunization techniques, the plan was to isolate areas of infection into smaller and smaller pockets.

Ironically, the origins of the vaccine in use during the 1960's are unknown. The original strain of cowpox used by Jenner was lost sometime during the nineteenth century. The strain used in the vaccine during the twentieth century, called vaccinia virus, may have originated from an isolate obtained during the Franco-Prussian War in the 1870's.

The plan for the elimination of smallpox developed by WHO ultimately proved completely successful. There are actually two different forms of smallpox. The last known natural case of variola major was reported in Bangladesh in 1974. The last known case of variola minor was reported in Somalia in 1976. Although an outbreak of smallpox resulting from a laboratory accident was reported in Great Britain, there were no additional naturally caused cases of smallpox. In 1978, WHO declared the world to be free of smallpox.

Although vaccination was effective in immunizing most persons against smallpox, use of the vaccine itself was associated with some risk. Serious complications were rare but did occasionally occur. With the disappearance of the disease, the need for routine immunization lessened, and, in 1971, compulsory vaccination of children in the United States was discontinued. In 1976, the routine vaccination of hospital employees was also discontinued. By the 1990's, the only known sites of existence of smallpox virus were freezers in four laboratories. The September 11, 2001, terrorist attacks at the World Trade Center and the Pentagon introduced a new era in which the fear of terrorists' use of biological agents has prompted renewed discussions about the reintroduction of the smallpox vaccine.

The use of vaccines for the elimination of poliomyelitis represents another success story. Although sporadic outbreaks of polio occurred in earlier centuries and probably as long ago as the time of ancient Egypt, the first epidemics appeared in the late nineteenth century. Ironically, this increase in the incidence of polio was caused by improvements in public health. Poliovirus is easily transmitted through a fecal-oral route, but the majority of cases, particularly in young children, are without symptoms, or asymptomatic. With improvements in sanitation, the first exposure to polio was often delayed until later childhood or, as in the case of President Franklin Delano Roosevelt, in the adult years. Under these circumstances, the disease is often more severe.

In 1955, the inactivated poliovirus vaccine developed by Jonas Salk was introduced for general use; in 1961, Albert Sabin's oral poliovirus vaccine was licensed for use. By the 1990's, polio had been eliminated from the Western Hemisphere and from developed countries elsewhere. In 2003, the WHO developed the Global Polio Eradication Initiative, the purpose of which is both to monitor outbreaks of polio and to address the means of preventing its transmission. Despite setbacks in portions of Asia and Africa, the number of newly diagnosed cases of polio has been reduced to fewer than two thousand worldwide in 2006. Since eradication of polio is not complete, the American Academy of Pediatrics (AAP) recommends that children receive immunizations by their first birthday and boosters at eighteen months of age and again prior to starting school. Adults who plan to travel to areas of the world in which polio is found should also be immunized.

The most significant advancement in twentieth century health care in the United States has been the elimination of most major childhood diseases. In addition to poliovirus immunization, children routinely receive a variety of early immunizations. Measles, mumps, and rubella (MMR) vaccines are administered in a single preparation at fifteen months of age. All three contain live attenuated viruses. The measles vaccine was first introduced in 1966 and resulted in a decline in reported measles cases of nearly 99 percent by the 1980's. Beginning about 1986, however, increasing numbers of cases of measles were reported among young adults who had been previously immunized. For this reason, the AAP recommends that children receive boosters of measles vaccine prior to entering high school, at approximately eleven to twelve years of age. A series of the diphtheria, pertussis, and tetanus (DPT) vaccine is administered at two, four, six, and eighteen months, with tetanus and diphtheria boosters recommended at ten-year intervals throughout the remainder of life.

With the elimination of most other major childhood illnesses, *Hemophilus influenzae* type B infections moved into the dubious position of being among the most significant causes of illness and death among young children. In 1985, a vaccine developed from the outer coat of the bacterium was licensed for use. The vaccine worked poorly in children under the age of two, the major population at risk. Consequently, an improved vaccine was developed and licensed by 1987. The second vaccine consisted of a portion of the influenza coat joined to diphtheria toxoid. It was found to immunize children effectively at eighteen months of age; immunization with the vaccine is recommended by the age of fifteen months.

By 1991, a total of nineteen vaccines had been licensed in the United States by the Food and Drug Administration (FDA) for uses in either children or adults. Aside from the eight previously described vaccines for children, eleven vaccines (five viral and six bacterial) are recommended for special circumstances. For example, in 1986, a genetically engineered hepatitis B virus vaccine was developed and licensed. The gene that encodes the virus surface antigen was placed in a small piece of deoxyribonucleic acid (DNA), a plasmid, and inserted into the common baker's yeast *Saccharomyces cerevisiae*. The antigen that is produced is used in a three-dose series to immunize individuals at risk for the disease: health care workers, institutional staff persons, and anyone else who is likely to come into contact with the virus.

Although routine vaccination of children has virtually eliminated most health-threatening infectious disease from that population, immunization of adults against preventable diseases has not been as successful. It was estimated that, in the late twentieth century, 50,000 to 70,000 adults died yearly from diseases that were preventable through immunization, such as pneumococcal pneumonia, influenza, and hepatitis B.

Historically, pneumococcal pneumonia, caused by the bacterium *Streptococcus pneumonia*, has been a killer of adults. In the 1990's, an estimated 40,000 persons, primarily the elderly, died from this disease. The available vaccine is a polysaccharide vaccine, representing serotypes for twenty-three of the major strains of the bacterium. When administered by the age of fifty, the vaccine provides a significant degree of protection against the organism.

Between 1957 and 2005, yearly influenza outbreaks averaged between ten thousand to twenty-five thousand deaths from the disease in the United States alone. Two of the epidemics each resulted in more than 40,000 deaths. Most of these deaths were in elderly adults. Although the usefulness of vaccination among the elderly is limited, immunization against influenza will often lessen the severity of the disease, even if it fails to prevent infection. The appearance of a new outbreak of avian influenza in 2003, usually referred to simply as the "bird flu," raised new concerns about

In the News: Combination Vaccine Pediarix for Infants

In December, 2002, the U.S. Food and Drug Administration (FDA) approved a multicomponent vaccine containing diphtheria and tetanus toxoids, acellular pertussis adsorbed (DTaP), hepatitis B (HepB; recombinant), and inactivated poliovirus (IPV) components. This vaccine, manufactured by GlaxoSmithKline Biologicals in Belgium, is called DTaP-HepB-IPV combined vaccine, or Pediarix. It is intended to be given to infants in three injections, one each at two, four, and six months of age. Pediarix provides protection against diphtheria, tetanus, pertussis (whooping cough), hepatitis B, and poliomyelitis in a series of only three injections instead of the nine injections previously given to infants. Thus, for patients and practitioners alike, it provides benefits such as saved office visits and decreased costs. Most important, the shorter injection series makes it much easier for parents, increasing the likelihood that parents will have their children immunized against these serious diseases.

The Pediarix vaccine has been subjected to numerous worldwide clinical trials to evaluate its safety and immunogenicity, or impact on the immune system. Data indicate that the vaccine is both safe and effective, with no significant adverse effects being reported. In these trials, the immunogenicity of each of the components in the combined vaccine was not shown to differ significantly from the immunogenicity of the components administered separately. These studies, involving more than seven thousand infants, reported minor adverse affects, including injection-site soreness (pain, redness, or swelling), fever, and irritability. The Pediarix vaccine has been associated with a greater frequency of fever in comparison to the separately administered vaccine components. Infants who are hypersensitive to any component of the vaccine, including yeast, neomycin, and polymyxin B, should not be given the vaccine. The Advisory Committee on Immunization Practices (ACIP), the Committee on Infectious Diseases of the American Academy of Pediatrics, and the American Academy of Family Physicians all have recommended this vaccine for routine use.

—Steven A. Kuhl, Ph.D.

what appears to be a particularly virulent strain of influenza; by 2006, approximately 260 persons were reportedly diagnosed with the virus, of whom 150 died. A vaccine has not yet been developed against this strain.

Some specialized vaccines are recommended only for international travelers. Both killed and live attenuated oral vaccines against typhoid are licensed. The ease of administration of an oral vaccine has made this form the preferred choice. In addition, vaccines against cholera, dengue fever, plague, and yellow fever may be used in appropriate circumstances.

Although active immunization in most circumstances remains the preferred method of protection through vaccination, situations occur in which passive immunization may provide therapeutic treatment. Individuals may be immunosuppressed or lack a functional immune system. This condition may result from infection (acquired immunodeficiency syndrome, or AIDS), medical intervention (chemotherapy), or congenital reasons (severe combined immunodeficiency disease, or SCID). Whatever the cause, active immunization does not develop. In addition, there are circumstances in which the necessary time for the development of immunity through active immunization is not available, such as with exposure to tetanus toxin, the hepatitis virus, or rabies. For passive immunization or replacement therapy in immunodeficiency disorders, immunoglobulin is usually prepared from pools of plasma obtained from large numbers of blood donors. Specific immunoglobulins, directed against specific targets such as rabies or tetanus, are prepared from plasma containing high concentrations of these antibodies.

PERSPECTIVE AND PROSPECTS

The elimination of smallpox represents the classic example in which the efficacy of a vaccine resulted in the eradication of disease. Smallpox was an ancient disease, with origins as early as the twelfth century B.C.E. It appeared in the Middle East in the sixth century C.E., with subsequent dissemination into northern Africa and southern Europe as a result of the Arab invasions from the sixth to the eighth centuries. The disease spread throughout Europe with the return of the Crusaders during the eleventh and twelfth centuries and reached the Americas as a result of the African slave trade in the sixteenth century. It has been estimated that, at its peak during the eighteenth century, smallpox killed 400,000 persons each year and caused more than one-third of all cases of blindness. It has also been estimated that smallpox or other diseases killed approximately 85 percent of the American Indians who died during colonial periods, certainly far more than the number who died from bullet wounds.

The principle of immunization in prevention did not originate with Edward Jenner, the English physician credited with development of the smallpox vaccine in the 1790's. A practice called variolation was well known in China and parts of the Middle East for centuries prior to Jenner. Variolation consisted of the inhalation of dried crust prepared from the pocks obtained from individuals suffering from mild cases of smallpox. A variation involved removing small amounts of fluid from an active smallpox pustule and scratching the liquid into the skin of children. Lady Mary Wortley Montagu, wife of the British ambassador to the Ottoman Empire, introduced the practice of variolation into Great Britain during the early eighteenth century. Use of variolation was empirical: The practice was often successful. The possibility remained, however, that immunization might actually introduce the disease.

Born in 1749, Jenner first became aware of the protective effects of cowpox from the story of a local dairymaid who had been exposed to the disease. After years of study and observation, he became convinced of the story's validity. In 1796, he immunized an eight-year-old boy with material from a cowpox lesion. No ill effects were seen. Further immunizations supported the theory that cowpox protected against smallpox. Jenner called this material variolae vaccinae. Richard Dunning, a Plymouth physician, in an 1800 analysis of the procedure, was the first to use the term "vaccination."

Wider application of the principle of vaccination followed from Louis Pasteur's studies during the 1870's and 1880's. With his attenuation of the bacterium that caused chicken cholera, Pasteur demonstrated that one could manipulate the virulence of a microorganism. This practice soon led to his development of vaccines against both anthrax and rabies. It is ironic that no clinical trials have ever been conducted to test rabies vaccine.

The twentieth century saw the development of effective vaccines against most major childhood diseases. Use of the DPT toxoid became routine in the United States about 1945. Development of the oral Sabin vaccine and inactivated Salk vaccines during the 1950's resulted in the complete elimination of poliomyelitis from the Western Hemisphere by the 1990's. The use of genetic engineering, in which only the genes necessary to synthesize specific antigens are utilized, was first applied to the hepatitis B vaccine. It has recently been applied successfully to create vaccines against chickenpox and hepatitis A virus. A vaccine against hepatitis C virus is under development. This technology provides the potential for manufacturing vaccine "cocktails," or combinations of such genes from a variety of infectious agents in a single vaccine.

In 2000, the FDA approved conjugate pneumococcal vaccine (Prevnar) for use in children under the age of two years for the prevention of pneumococcal infections. The AAP recommended Prevnar for use in all children twenty-three months of age and younger. The AAP also recommended Prevnar for all immunocompromised children twenty-four to fifty-nine months of age who are at high risk for invasive pneumococcal infection. Prevnar may be administered in a series of four inoculations given at two, four, six, and twelve to fifteen months of age. Pneumococcal infections are a major cause of meningitis and septicemia in infants and children.

The most recent vaccine to be licensed is one directed against infection by certain strains of the human papillomavirus (HPV). HPV is most commonly associated with genital warts, and infection by some strains may also lead to the development of cervical cancer. HPV is not associated only with sexual transmission, as the virus may also be spread by hand, and the American Cancer Society estimates that more than six million persons are exposed to HPV each year. Approximately 9,700 women will develop cervical cancer, with some 3,700 deaths each year in the United States. In 2006, a vaccine called Gardasil, directed against the four most common types of HPV, was licensed. A three-dose regimen is recommended for girls and women in the nine to twenty-six age group.

Attempts to develop a vaccine against AIDS have proven largely unsuccessful. The mechanism that has been exploited by other vaccines, namely the stimulation of T cells to produce antibodies that protect a recipient, is nonfunctional in AIDS, and successful development of a vaccine against AIDS will require scientific ingenuity.

—Richard Adler, Ph.D.;
L. Fleming Fallon, Jr., M.D., Ph.D., M.P.H.;
updated by Richard Adler, Ph.D.

See also Acquired immunodeficiency syndrome (AIDS); Anthrax; Antibiotics; Bacterial infections; Bacteriology; Chickenpox; Childhood infectious diseases; Cholera; Diphtheria; Disease; Environmental health; Hepatitis; Host-defense mechanisms; Human papillomavirus (HPV); Immune system; Immunology; Influenza; Measles; Microbiology; Mumps; Pathology; Plague; Poliomyelitis; Preventive medicine; Rubella; Smallpox; Tuberculosis; Viral infections; Whooping cough; World Health Organization.

For Further Information:

Behbehani, Abbas. *The Smallpox Story in Words and Pictures.* Kansas City: University of Kansas Medical Center, 1988. The book includes the history of Edward Jenner and his use of cowpox in the first smallpox vaccine. The drawings and photographs are of particular interest.

Brock, Thomas D., ed. *Microorganisms: From Smallpox to Lyme Disease.* New York: W. H. Freeman, 1990. A collection of readings from *Scientific American* magazine. Included is a section on the role of vaccines in the prevention of disease, including their role in the elimination of smallpox. Also found are articles on synthetic vaccines and vaccination in Third World countries.

Delves, Peter J., et al. *Roitt's Essential Immunology.* 11th ed. Malden, Mass.: Blackwell, 2006. An excellent textbook on the subject of immunology. Much of the book is detailed and requires some background in biology. Nevertheless, the chapters which deal with infection and immunization are clear and contain much that will interest nonscientists. Numerous graphs illustrate material from the text.

Grandi, Guido, ed. *Genomics, Proteomics, and Vaccines.* Hoboken, N.J.: John Wiley & Sons, 2004. The authors begin with a history of vaccine development and proceed with both classical methods and a description of how new generations of vaccines have built upon biotechnology. Best appreciated by those with a science background.

Plotkin, Stanley A., and Walter A. Orenstein, eds. *Vaccines.* 4th ed. Philadelphia: Saunders, 2004. An excellent description of the role of vaccines in the prevention of disease. The book begins with a history of immunization practices. Each subsequent chapter deals with a specific disease and the role and history of vaccine production in its prevention. While enough detail is provided to interest someone in the field, the text is appropriate for nonscientists.

Rosario, Diane. *Immunization Resource Guide: Where to Find Answers to All Your Questions About Childhood Vaccinations.* Burlington, Iowa: Patter, 2001. Provides parents with information on all sides of the controversial vaccination issue and resources to make informed decisions. Includes reviews of over ninety books covering all aspects of childhood vaccinations and detailed listings of more than 130 vaccine and health organizations, periodicals, and publishers.

Vaccine Page, The. http://www.vaccines.com. Site provides access to current news about vaccines and an annotated database of vaccine resources on the Internet.

Immunodeficiency disorders

Disease/disorder

Anatomy or system affected: Immune system

Specialties and related fields: Genetics, immunology

Definition: Genetic or acquired disorders that result from disturbances in the normal functioning of the immune system.

Key terms:

antibody: protein immunoglobulin secreted by B lymphocytes; the production of antibodies is induced by specific foreign invaders, and they combine with and destroy only those invaders

B lymphocytes: also referred to as B cells; white cells of the immune system that produce antibodies; produced within the bone marrow

phagocytes: white cells of the immune system that destroy invading foreign bodies by engulfing and digesting them in a nonspecific immune response; includes macrophages and neutrophils

stem cells: multipotential precursor cells within the bone marrow that develop into white cell populations, including lymphocytes and phagocytic cells

T lymphocyte: a type of immune cell that kills host cells infected by bacteria or viruses and secretes chemicals (interleukins) that regulate the immune response

Causes and Symptoms

The defense of the body against foreign invaders is provided by the immune system. In nonspecific immunity, phagocytic cells engulf and destroy invading particles. Specific immunity consists of very specialized cell types that are synthesized in response to a particular type of foreign invader. Self-replicating stem cells within the bone marrow give rise to lymphocytes, which mediate specific immunity. Lymphocytes establish self-replacing colonies within the thymus, spleen, and lymph nodes. The various categories of T lympho-

cytes are derived from the thymus colonies, while B lymphocytes develop and mature within the bone marrow. B lymphocytes secrete highly specific antibodies that attack bacteria and some viruses.

T lymphocytes do not secrete antibodies. Cytotoxic T cells directly attack body cells that have been infected with a bacterium or virus, while helper T cells regulate the immune response, either by directly interacting with other lymphocytes or by secreting chemicals, called interleukins, which regulate those cells. In immunodeficiency disorders, some or all of these defenses are compromised, which can have life-threatening consequences. Immunodeficiency diseases are generally the result of genetic abnormalities and are present from birth; others may be acquired through infection or exposure to damaging drug or radiation treatments. Depending upon the specific defect, the result may range from limited defects involving a class of cells to an entire shutdown of the immune system; prognosis depends on the severity of the defect. Since these defects generally involve recessive traits, expression of immune deficiencies usually result from mutations on the X chromosome; sex-linked traits are generally observed only in males, since males carry a single X chromosome.

The most severe immunodeficiency disorder is attributable to the absence of stem cells, which results in a total lack of both B and T lymphocytes. This rare genetic condition is referred to as severe combined immunodeficiency syndrome (SCID). Affected infants show a failure to thrive from birth and can easily die from common bacterial or viral infections. The term SCID encompasses a variety of genetic deficiencies. Certain forms are sex-linked, while other types may be autosomal (non-sex-linked). The most common autosomal form is a deficiency in the enzyme adenosine deaminase, resulting in disruption of deoxyribonucleic acid (DNA) synthesis in the stem cells.

Major syndromes that involve defects specific to the T lymphocyte population are characterized by recurrent viral and fungal infections. DiGeorge syndrome results from improper development of the thymus, which in turn results in insufficient production of T lymphocytes, often accompanied by other structural abnormalities in the infant. In severe cases, death results in early childhood from overwhelming viral infections.

The most common disorders affecting B lymphocytes are forms of hypogammaglobulinemia. This condition is characterized by insufficient levels of antibody. The cause is generally associated with increased rates of antibody breakdown or loss in the urine secondary to kidney malfunction. Bruton's agammaglobulinemia is a rare, sex-linked form of the condition, in which B cells fail to mature properly. Severe bacterial infections are the most common symptom. When the disorder is left untreated, infants generally die of severe pneumonia prior to six months of age.

Several immunodeficiency disorders may be the result of partial defects in the production and/or function of B and T lymphocytes. Wiskott-Aldrich syndrome is a genetically inherited disease manifested by recurrent infections and an itchy, scaly inflammation of the skin. Certain classes of antibodies are absent or scarce. Chronic mucocutaneous candidiasis is characterized by chronic fungal infection of the skin and mucous membranes; reduced levels of T cells are responsible for this disfiguring disorder.

Immunodeficiency disorders may also be the result of defects in phagocytic cells; the underlying cause of most of these disorders is ill-defined but often involves deficiencies in hydrolytic enzymes. In chronic granulomatosis, an inherited enzyme deficiency prevents the immune system from destroying bacteria that have been phagocytized. Infants affected by this disorder develop severe infections and chronic inflammations of internal organs and bones. The bacteria responsible for these infections are generally common flora that are not considered pathogens in healthy individuals.

Immune disorders may involve defects in antibody production. However, certain forms of inherited disorders involve another group of proteins called complement. Complement actually represents a group of serum proteins which interact with each other in a series. The pathway may be activated either specifically from antibody-target interactions or nonspecifically by surface components of certain bacteria. Intermediates in the complement pathway attract or stimulate phagocytosis (opsonins), induce inflammation, and play roles in cell destruction. Some of the intermediates are enzymes that regulate the activation of complement components. The most important intermediate in the pathway is the C3 component. C3 is a protein that acts as an opsonin and at the same time is involved in activating later steps in the sequence. Defects in C3 result in increased susceptibility to infection. Similar immune problems may result from defects in other complement intermediates.

Most of the disorders that affect the immune system are not inherited but develop sometime during the person's life. They are either the result of an infection or a consequence of another disease or its treatment. The use of corticosteroids to treat inflammations, or the illicit use of them in muscle-building, can interfere with the proper production and function of T lymphocytes. Other immunosuppressive drugs used to diminish the possibilities of graft or transplant rejection, or in the treatment of autoimmune diseases, can severely depress antibody production. Chemotherapeutic agents used in the treatment of cancer can affect DNA replication and severely compromise the entire immune system. Whole-body radiation can damage or destroy bone marrow stem cells.

Acquired immunodeficiency syndrome (AIDS) is caused by the human immunodeficiency virus (HIV). HIV is transmitted primarily through unprotected sexual contact, sharing of needles for intravenous drug use, transfusion with contaminated blood products, or contact with contaminated body fluids. HIV specifically infects one type of regulatory T lymphocyte, the helper T cell, resulting in severe immune depression. The virus may be harbored in an inapparent form for years. Initial symptoms may be quite mild, but they generally progress so that the affected individual becomes susceptible to a host of opportunistic bacterial and fungal infections. A rare form of cancer called Kaposi's sarcoma is associated with infection by a particular human herpesvirus, HHV8, in persons with AIDS. AIDS also produces neurological damage in about one-third of infected individuals.

TREATMENT AND THERAPY

Most treatment of immunodeficient individuals is palliative. Infections are treated with antibiotics whenever possible. Individuals are counseled to avoid situations in which they may be exposed to contagious agents.

Treatment of immunodeficiency disorders may also target the source of the deficiency. For example, in DiGeorge syndrome, characterized by the congenital absence of the thymus, fetal thymus transplants may correct the problem, with improvement in lymphocyte levels seen within hours after the transplants. The use of thymus extracts has also been beneficial. Syndromes such as hypogammaglobulinemia can be managed by injection with mixtures of antibodies. Drug therapy to substitute for some absent immune components of Wiskott-Aldrich syndrome has been shown to have variable effects. The most effective treatment for chronic mucocutaneous candidiasis is aggressive antifungal medication to eradicate the causative organism; treatment must continue for several months because fungal infections are slow to respond to therapy and frequently recur. Chronic granulomatosis is notoriously difficult to treat, and the most effective therapy has been antibiotic and antifungal agents used aggressively during an overt infection.

Because of the magnitude of the defects, many inherited immunodeficiency disorders are difficult to treat successfully and are commonly fatal early in life. Chronic granulomatosis is usually fatal within the first few years of life, and only about 20 percent of patients reach the age of twenty. SCID is a serious disorder in which affected infants can die before a proper diagnosis is made. For individuals with these and other serious immunodeficiency disorders, maintenance in an environment free of bacteria, viruses, and fungi, such as a sterile "bubble," has been the best means to prevent life-threatening infections. Such an approach, however, precludes the possibility of a normal life. The most effective treatment for individuals with severely compromised immune systems is bone marrow transplantation. In this procedure, bone marrow from a compatible individual is introduced into the bone marrow of the patient. If the procedure works—and the success rate is high—in approximately one to six months the transplant recipient's immune system will be reconstituted and functional. Bone marrow transplantation is a permanent cure for these disorders, since the transplanted marrow will contain stem cells that produce all the cell types of the immune system. The difficulties in transplantation include finding a compatible donor and preventing infections during the period after the transplant.

Drug therapy for AIDS utilizes treatments that interfere with replication of the virus. The first drug to be approved for use was zidovudine (formerly AZT), a DNA analogue, but its success was somewhat limited, as it was associated with severe side effects and the creation of resistant virus. More recent treatments utilize drug "cocktails," combinations of drugs that act at different stages of viral replication. Vaccines and antibiotic therapy are used to prevent or treat the opportunistic illnesses that accompany AIDS. Various drugs may also help to ease symptoms of AIDS such as appetite disturbances, nausea, pain, insomnia, anxiety, depression, fever, and diarrhea. A combination of therapies has been shown to increase life expectancy in AIDS patients. Many patients choose to participate in clinical trials of experimental drugs not approved for general use in the hope that the new drug will be more effective at alleviating the disease. Others seek out alternative or nontraditional medical treatments that have a long history of use in Western cultures. These treatments include acupuncture, herbology, meditation, and homeopathy. An important aspect of therapy for AIDS patients is maintaining mental health through support groups and supportive caregivers.

Illicit use of corticosteroids can seriously compromise the immune system and may lead to permanent damage. The best therapy for this type of acquired immunodeficiency is prevention—that is, to not misuse the drugs. In their supervised use to control inflammation or other disease symptoms, normal immune function will return after treatment has been completed. A huge risk to cancer patients who are being treated with chemotherapy and/or radiation therapy is the depression of the immune system, which can lead to a host of infections being contracted and not easily fought off by the body's compromised immune system. These individuals should avoid exposure to infectious agents when possible and be attentive to lifestyle modifications that can strengthen the immune system and encourage its speedy recovery, including a nutritious diet, plenty of rest, and avoidance of stress. Close monitoring for any signs of infection facilitates rapid antibiotic therapy, which can prevent serious complications.

PERSPECTIVE AND PROSPECTS

Prior to the gains in scientific knowledge about the mechanics of the immune system, individuals with genetic immunodeficiency disorders would die of serious infections during their first few years of life. Even when it was finally realized that these individuals suffered from defects of the immune system, little could be done for most of the disorders, except to treat infections as they developed and to avoid contact with potential disease-causing organisms—a near impossibility if one is to lead a normal life. Housing persons with SCID in sterile bubbles was uncommon because of the expense and impracticality. During the 1970's, bone marrow transplants were first developed; by the 1990's they had progressed to a greater than 80 percent success rate. As a result of improved transplant-rejection drugs, transplants from donors with less-than-perfect tissue matches are now possible. Bone marrow transplantation has been a source of cure for many individuals with immune disorders.

Bone marrow transplantation is not suitable or possible in every case of immunodeficiency disorder, and scientists have long sought a means to cure the genetic defects themselves. In 1992, French Anderson of the National Institutes of Health conducted the first gene therapy trial on a young girl suffering from SCID. Some of the girl's bone marrow cells were removed from her body and exposed to an inactivated virus containing a normal gene for ADA, the defective enzyme. Some of the stem cells in the marrow incorporated the healthy gene, and the engineered cells were returned to her body. The cells lodged in her bone marrow, where they produced healthy immune cells. The procedure was repeated successfully in three other children shortly afterward.

Among the exciting applications of research into the molecular biology of immunodeficiencies has been the identification of specific genetic defects. Bone marrow stem cells can now be isolated and identified. In the future, such cells may be engineered such that the defective gene associated with the deficiency may be replaced by a normal copy. Since the cells are those from the same individual, transplantation problems can be avoided.

—Karen E. Kalumuck, Ph.D.;
updated by Richard Adler, Ph.D.

See also Acquired immunodeficiency syndrome (AIDS); Allergies; Arthritis; Asthma; Autoimmune disorders; Blood and blood disorders; Bone marrow transplantation; Cells; Cytology; Cytopathology; DiGeorge syndrome; Gene therapy; Hematology; Hematology, pediatric; Host-defense mechanisms; Human immunodeficiency virus (HIV); Immune system; Immunology; Immunopathology; Serology; Wiskott-Aldrich syndrome.

FOR FURTHER INFORMATION:

Abbas, Abul K., and Andrew K. Lichtman. *Basic Immunology: Functions and Disorders of the Immune System.* 2d ed. Philadelphia: Elsevier Saunders, 2006. Provides introductory text to the basics of immunology and describes the primary disorders that impair its function. Illustrations, case studies, review questions, key point summaries, and a glossary are included.

Bartlett, John G., and Ann K. Finkbeiner. *The Guide to Living with HIV Infection.* 5th ed. Baltimore: Johns Hopkins University Press, 2001. This informative book developed at The Johns Hopkins University AIDS Clinic is a great resource for information about the disease and a guide for patients and caregivers in living with the disease.

Delves, Peter J., et al. *Roitt's Essential Immunology.* 11th ed. Malden, Mass.: Blackwell, 2006. A thorough introduction to the science of immunology. Well illustrated. Includes an extensive section on immunodeficiency disorders.

Fehervari, Zoltan, and Shiman Sakaguchi. "Peacekeepers of the Immune System." *Scientific American*, October, 2006, 56-63. Discussion of new discoveries pertaining to understanding the role of regulatory T cells in maintaining the immune response. Particularly relevant to autoimmune diseases.

Frank, Steven A. *Immunology and Evolution of Infectious Disease.* Princeton, N.J.: Princeton University Press, 2002. Blends research from molecular biology, immunology, pathogen biology, and population dynamics to discuss how and why parasites vary to escape recognition by the immune system, vaccine design, and the control of epidemics.

Immune Web. http://immuneweb.org/. A site that offers good articles on several immunodeficiency disorders, "safe" product lists, and annotated links to other Internet sites, among other features.

Parker, James N., and Philip M. Parker, eds. *The Official Parent's Sourcebook on Primary Immunodeficiency.* San Diego, Calif.: Icon Health, 2002. Draws from public, academic, government, and peer-reviewed research to provide a wide-ranging handbook for parents whose children suffer from primary immunodeficiency.

Sticherling, Michael, and Enno Christophers, eds. *Treatment of Autoimmune Disorders.* New York: Springer-Verlag, 2003. Explores the basic mechanisms of autoimmune disorders; neurological, gastrointestinal, ophthalmological, and skin diseases; and current and future therapeutic options.

Stine, Gerald J. *AIDS Update: 2007*. Upper Saddle River, N.J.: Prentice Hall, 2007. An overview of AIDS, its cause, and methods of treating it. Included are sections outlining the immunodeficiency disorders that are sequelae to HIV infection.

IMMUNOLOGY

SPECIALTY

ANATOMY OR SYSTEM AFFECTED: Blood, cells, immune system

SPECIALTIES AND RELATED FIELDS: Cytology, hematology, microbiology, preventive medicine, serology

DEFINITION: The study of the immune system, its protection of the body from foreign agents, and its malfunction in autoimmune diseases, in which the body's defenses react against the body's own cells or tissues.

KEY TERMS:

antibody: a protein produced by lymphocytes in response to an antigen; binds only to a specific antigen

antigen: any substance perceived by immunological defenses to be foreign and against which antibody is produced; generally a protein

autoantibody: an antibody produced against tissue antigens within a host—that is, self-antigens

complement: a series of about twenty serum proteins that, when sequentially activated by immune complexes, may trigger cell damage

determinant: a region on the surface of an antigen capable of creating an immune response or of combining with an antibody produced by an immune response

Hashimoto's disease: thyroiditis; among the earliest characterized autoimmune diseases

systemic lupus erythematosus (SLE): commonly called lupus; a chronic inflammatory disease characterized by an arthritic condition and a rash

lymphocyte: a small white blood cell constituting about 25 percent of all blood cells; two basic types are B cells (antibody production) and T cells (cellular immunity)

tolerance: the state in which an organism does not normally react against its own tissue

SCIENCE AND PROFESSION

The field of immunology deals with the ability of the immune system to react against an enormous repertoire of stimulation by antigens. In most instances, these antigens are foreign infectious agents such as viruses or bacteria. Inherent in this process is the ability to react against nearly any known determinant, whether natural or artificially produced. The most reactive antigenic determinants are proteins, though to a lesser degree, other substances such as carbohydrates (sugars), lipids (fats), and nucleic acids may also stimulate a response.

In general, the body exhibits tolerance during the constant exposure to its own tissue. The precise reasons behind tolerance are vague, but the basis for the lack of response lies in two major mechanisms: the elimination during development of immunological cells capable of responding to the body's own tissue and the active prevention of existing reactive cells from responding to self-antigens. When this regulation fails, autoimmune disease may result.

There are two major types of immunological defense: humoral immunity and cell-mediated immunity. Humoral immunity refers to the soluble substances in blood serum, primarily antibody and complement, while cellular immunity refers to the portion of the immune response that is directly mediated by cells. Though these processes are sometimes categorized separately, they do in fact interact with and regulate each other.

Antibodies are produced by cells called B lymphocytes in response to foreign antigens. These proteins bind to the antigen in a specific manner, resulting in a complex that can be removed readily by phagocytic white blood cells. More important in the context of autoimmunity, antibody-antigen complexes also activate the complement pathway, a series of some twenty enzymes and serum proteins. The end result of activation is the lysis of the antigenic targets. In general, the targets are bacteria; in autoimmune disease, the target may be any cell in the body.

The cellular response utilizes any of several types of cytotoxic cells. These can include a specialized lymphocyte called the T cell (so named because of its development in the thymus) or another unusual type of large granular lymphocyte called the natural killer (NK) cell. NK and cytotoxic T cells function in a similar manner—by binding to the target and releasing toxic granules in apposition to its cell membrane.

Though autoimmune diseases differ in scope, they do tend to exhibit certain common factors. The pathologies associated with most of these illnesses result in part from the production of autoantibodies, which are antibodies produced against the body's own cells or tissues. If the antibody binds to tissue in a particular organ, complement is activated in the tissue, causing the destruction of those regions of the organ. For example, Goodpasture's syndrome is characterized by the deposition of autoantibodies directed against the membrane of the glomerulus in the kidneys. Complement activation can result in severe organ pathology and subsequent kidney failure.

If the autoantibody binds to soluble material in blood serum, the resultant antibody-antigen complexes are carried along in the circulation, and there is the possibility that they will lodge in various areas of the body. For example, systemic lupus erythematosus (SLE) results from the production of autoantibodies against soluble nucleoprotein, which is released from cells as they undergo normal death and lysis. The immune complexes frequently lodge in the kidney, where they can cause renal failure.

This is not to say that all autoimmune diseases result solely from autoantibody production. Though a precise role for either cytotoxic T cells or NK cells in human autoimmune disease has not been fully confirmed, several observations make such an association likely. First, large numbers of T cells are found in certain organ-specific diseases, including thyroiditis and pernicious anemia. Second, animal models of similar diseases show a specific role for such cells in the pathology of these diseases. Thus, it is likely that these cells do participate in the organ destruction.

Autoimmune disorders can be categorized in the form of a disease spectrum. At one end of the spectrum one can place organ-specific diseases. For example, Hashimoto's disease is an autoimmune thyroid disorder characterized by the production of autoantibodies against thyroid antigens. The extensive infiltration and proliferation of lymphocytes is observed (although, as described above, their roles are unproved), along with the subsequent destruction of follicular tissue.

Likewise, diabetes mellitus, Type I (formerly called juvenile-onset diabetes) may be an organ-specific autoimmune disease. In this case, however, autoantibodies are directed against the beta cells of the pancreas, which produce insulin. In pernicious (or megaloblastic) anemia, antibodies are produced against intrinsic factor, a molecule necessary for uptake of vitamin B_{12}. Subsequent pathology results from lack of absorption of the vitamin. Addison's disease, from which U.S. president John F. Kennedy suffered, is a potentially life-threatening condition resulting from antibody production against the adrenal cortex. Myasthenia gravis is characterized by severe heart or skeletal muscle weakness caused by antibodies directed against neurotransmitter receptors on the muscle. In fact, cells from any organ may be potential targets for production of an autoantibody.

Certain organ-specific autoimmune diseases in the spectrum are characterized not by antibodies directed against any specific organ, but by cellular infiltration triggered in some manner by less specific autoantibodies. For example, biliary cirrhosis, an inflammatory condition of the liver, is characterized by the obstruction of bile flow through the liver ductules. Though extensive cellular infiltration is observed, serum antibodies are directed against mitochondrial antigens, which are found within all cells. Certain types of chronic hepatitis also exhibit an analogous situation.

In some cases, antibodies may be directed against circulatory cells. Antibodies directed against red blood cells may cause subsequent lysis of the cells, leading to hemolytic anemia. Often, these are temporary conditions that have resulted from the binding of a pharmacologic chemical such as an antibiotic to the surface of the cell, which triggers an immune response. A more serious condition is hemolytic disease of the newborn (HDN), one example being erythroblastosis fetalis, or Rh disease. In this case, a mother lacking the Rh protein on her blood cells may produce an immune response against that protein, which is present in the blood of the fetus she is carrying during pregnancy. Prior to 1967, when an effective preventive measure became available, HDN was a serious problem for many pregnancies. Antibodies directed against blood platelets can cause a reduction in the number of those cells, resulting in thrombocytopenia purpura. An analogous situation can be seen with other cell types.

At the other end of the autoimmune spectrum are those diseases that are not cell- or organ-specific but result in widespread lesions in various parts of the body. Lupus received its name from the butterfly rash often seen on the faces of patients, which resembles a wolf-bite (lupus is Latin for "wolf"). Pathologic changes can be found at various sites in the body, however, including the kidneys, joints, and blood vessels. Likewise, rheumatoid arthritis is characterized by the production of rheumatoid factor, an antibody molecule directed against other antibodies in blood serum. The resultant immune complexes lodge in joints, causing the joint pain and destruction associated with severe arthritis.

In most cases, the specific reason for the production of autoantibodies is unknown. Genetic factors are certainly involved, since some autoimmune diseases run in families. Some may be triggered by bacterial or viral infections. Viral antigens may be expressed on the surfaces of certain cells or the virus itself may be attached to the cell. Heart muscle appears to express antigenic determinants in common with certain streptococcal bacteria. A mild "strep throat" may be followed several weeks later by severe rheumatic fever.

The binding of drugs to cell surfaces may trigger an immune response. For example, penicillin may bind to the surfaces of red blood cells, triggering a hemolytic anemia. Likewise, sedormid may bind to the membrane of platelets.

Most cases of autoimmune disease, however, are triggered by no apparent cause. They may "simply" involve a breakdown of the normal regulatory mechanisms associated with the immune response.

Diagnostic and Treatment Techniques

The regulation of self-reactive lymphocytes is necessary for the maintenance of tolerance by the immune system. When regulation breaks down or is otherwise defective, either humoral or cellular immunity is generated against the cells or tissues. The resultant pathology may be simply a painful nuisance or may have potentially fatal consequences. The difference relates to the extent of damage to particular organs, in the case of organ-specific autoimmune reactions, or to the level of tissue damage in systemic disease.

Despite differences in pathology, the mechanisms of tissue damage are similar in most autoimmune diseases. Most involve the formation of immune complexes. Either antibodies bind to cell surfaces or immune complexes form in the circulation. In either case, the result is complement activation. Components of the complement pathway, in turn, can either directly damage cell membranes or trigger the infiltration of a variety of cytotoxic cells.

Because the damage associated with most autoimmune diseases results from parallel processes, methods of treatment vary little in theory from one illness to another. Most involve the treatment of resultant symptoms; for example, the use of aspirin to reduce minor inflammation and, when necessary, the use of steroids to reduce the level of the immune response.

The treatment of autoimmune diseases does not eliminate the problem. The disease remains, but under ideal conditions, it is held under control. At the same time, there exists the danger of side effects of treatment. For example, most methods that reduce the level of the immune response are nonspecific; reducing the severity of the autoimmune disease may cause the patient to become more susceptible to infections by bacteria or viruses.

Certain approaches have been successful in the palliative treatment of some forms of autoimmune disease. For example, patients with myasthenia gravis (MG) exhibit significant muscle weakness. A myasthenia gravis patient may have difficulty breathing and may experience extreme fatigue, in severe cases being unable to open his or her mouth or eyelids. Associated with the disease are autoantibodies produced against the receptor for the neurotransmitter acetylcholine (ACh), the chemical utilized by nerves in regulating movement by the muscle. By blocking the ACh receptor, these antibodies inhibit the ability of nerves to control muscle movement. In effect, the patient loses control of the muscles.

Patients with myasthenia gravis often exhibit abnormalities of the thymus, the gland associated with T-cell production. In addition, there is evidence that the thymus contains ACh receptors that are particularly antigenic (perhaps exacerbating the illness). Removal of the thymus, even in adults, often aids in reducing the symptoms of the disease. The thymus, though not superfluous in adults, carries out its main functions during the early years of life, through adolescence. Thus, its removal generally has few major implications.

Often, MG will respond to more conventional forms of treatment. Steroid treatment will often reduce symptoms. Metabolic controls may also aid in reducing symptoms. For example, during normal nerve transmission of ACh, the enzyme cholinesterase is present to break down ACh, thereby regulating muscle movement. The use of anticholinesterase drugs to prolong the presence of ACh at the site of the receptor on the muscle has also been of benefit to some patients.

Systemic lupus erythematosus is among the most common of systemic autoimmune diseases. The disease usually strikes women in the prime of life, between the ages of twenty and forty. It is characterized by a butterfly rash over the facial region, weakness, fatigue, and often a fever. In many respects, the symptoms are those of severe arthritis. As the disease progresses, tissue or organ degradation may occur in the kidney or heart.

The specific cause of the symptomology is the formation of immune complexes, which consist of antibodies against cell components such as DNA or nucleoprotein. Complexes in the kidney have been large enough to observe with the electron microscope, particularly when the complexes contain cell nuclei. Similar complexes have been observed in regions of the skin characterized by inflammation and a rash. The immune complexes are sometimes ingested (phagocytized) by scavenger neutrophils, which make up the largest proportion (65 percent) of white blood cells. The presence of these so-called LE cells, white cells with ingested antibody-bound nuclei, was at one time used for the diagnosis of lupus.

As is true for many autoimmune diseases, the control of lupus often involves the use of steroids as immunosuppressive drugs. These have included drugs such as cyclosporin, which blocks T-cell function, and antimitotic drugs such as azathioprine or methotrexate, which block the proliferation of immune cells. Generalized immunosuppression as a side effect is a concern. Often, using combinations of steroids and immunosuppressives makes it possible to use lower concentrations of each, increasing the drugs' effectiveness and reducing the danger of toxicity.

Other palliative treatments of symptomology can increase patient comfort. For example, aspirin may be used to reduce inflammation or joint pain. Topical steroids can reduce the rash. Since lupus may significantly increase the photosensitivity of the skin, staying out of direct sunlight, or at least covering the surface of the skin, may reduce skin lesions. It should be emphasized again that these treatments deal only with symptoms; none will cure the disease.

Since some systemic diseases result from immune complex disorders, a reduction of the levels of such complexes has been found to be beneficial to some patients. Treatment involves a process called plasmapheresis. Plasma, the liquid portion of the blood, is removed from the patient (a small proportion at a time), after which the immune complexes are separated from the plasma. Though a temporary measure, since additional complexes continue to form, the process does prove useful.

Rheumatoid arthritis is another common autoimmune disorder. As is true of most autoimmune diseases, rheumatoid arthritis is primarily a disease of women. Symptomatology results from the lodging of immune complexes in joints, resulting in the inflammation of those joints. Many cases result from the formation of antibodies directed against other antibody molecules—a case of the immune system turning against itself. Pathology results both from complement activation and from the infiltration of a variety of cells into the joint; the result is damage to both cartilage and bone.

Medical treatment usually begins with the anti-inflammatory drug of choice: aspirin. Other common treatments are those that increase patient comfort: rest, proper exercise, and weight loss, if necessary. In severe cases, steroids may be prescribed.

In general, autoimmune diseases are characterized by alternating periods of symptomatology and remission. Treatments are generally similar in their approach of reducing inflammation as the first line of intervention, with the use of immunosuppression being the last resort. Since the precise origin of most of these disorders is unknown, prevention remains difficult.

PERSPECTIVE AND PROSPECTS

During the 1950's, F. Macfarlane Burnet published his theory of clonal selection. Burnet believed that antibody specificity was predetermined in the B cell as it underwent development and maturation. Selection of the cell by the appropriate antigen resulted in proliferation of that specific cell, a process of clonal selection.

Burnet also had to account for tolerance, however, the inability of immune cells to respond against their own antigens. Burnet theorized that during prenatal development, exposure to self-antigens, or determinants, resulted in the abortion of any self-reactive cells. Only those self-reactive immune cells that were directed against sequestered antigens survived.

Though Burnet's theories have reached the level of dogma in the field of immunology, they fail to account for certain autoimmune disorders. In the "correct" circumstances, the body does react against itself. Though they were not recognized at the time as such, autoimmune disorders were recognized as early as 1866. In that year, W. W. Gull demonstrated the link between chilling and a syndrome called paroxysmal hemoglobinuria. When external tissue such as skin is exposed to cold, large amounts of hemoglobin are discharged into the urine. In 1904, Karl Landsteiner established the autoimmune basis for the disease by demonstrating the role of complement in the lysis of red blood cells, causing the release of hemoglobin and the symptomatology of the disorder. Further, he demonstrated that one could cause the lysis of normal cells by mixing them with sera from hemoglobinurics.

Hashimoto's disease was among the first organ-specific autoimmune diseases to be described. The disease was first described in 1912 by Hakaru Hashimoto, a Japanese surgeon, and the immune basis for the disease was established independently by Ernest Witebsky and Noel Rose in the United States, and by Deborah Doniach and Ivan Roitt in Great Britain, in 1957.

Since the 1950's, dozens of autoimmune disorders have been described. Treatment of these disorders remains, for the most part, nonspecific. Research in the area, in addition to attempts to define the precise trigger for autoimmune disease, has attempted to develop ways to suppress specifically those immune reactions responsible for the symptomatology. Successes have been associated with vaccines directed against components involved with the reactions under investigation. For example, since the production of autoantibodies is the basis for some forms of disease, the generation of additional antibody molecules directed against determinants on the autoantibodies at fault could serve to neutralize the effects of those components. This procedure could be likened to a police department that arrests its own dishonest officers. There is a precedent for such an operation. Newborn children of mothers suffering from myasthenia gravis synthesize just such antibodies against the inappropriate MG antibodies that have crossed the placenta. Synthesis does seem to ameliorate the symptoms of the disease.

There is no question that autoimmune disorders represent an aberrant form of immune response. Nevertheless, an understanding of the underlying mechanism will shed light on exactly how the immune system is regulated. For example, it remains unclear how antibody production is controlled following a normal immune response. In the presence of an antigen, antibody levels increase for a period of days to weeks, reach a plateau, and then slowly decrease as additional production comes to a halt. The means by which the shutdown takes place remains nebulous.

Tolerance does not result solely from an absence of T or B cells that respond to antigens; it involves an active suppression of the process. A more detailed understanding of the process will lead to a more thorough understanding of the immune system in general.

—*Richard Adler, Ph.D.*

See also Acquired immunodeficiency syndrome (AIDS); Allergies; Autoimmune disorders; Blood and blood disorders; Bone marrow transplantation; Cells; Chemotherapy; Circulation; Cytology; Cytopathology; Dialysis; Endocrinology; Endocrinology, pediatric; Glands; Healing; Hematology; Hematology, pediatric; Histiocytosis; Homeopathy; Hormones; Host-defense mechanisms; Human immunodeficiency virus (HIV); Immune system; Immunization and vaccination; Immunodeficiency disorders; Immunopathology; Infection; Kawasaki disease; Liver; Lymphatic system; Multiple chemical sensitivity syndrome; Myasthenia gravis; Oncology; Serology; Severe combined immunodeficiency syndrome (SCID); Skin; Transfusion; Transplantation; Wiskott-Aldrich syndrome.

FOR FURTHER INFORMATION:

Delves, Peter J., et al. *Roitt's Essential Immunology.* 11th ed. Malden, Mass.: Blackwell, 2006. Several chapters deal specifically with immune disorders. Concise, with a large number of illustrations, but does require a basic knowledge of biology.

Fettner, Ann Giudici. *Viruses: Agents of Change.* New York: McGraw-Hill, 1990. Though argumentative in her approach, Fettner provides a simple discussion of the role of viruses in disease. Included are sections on autoimmunity and the possible roles played by viruses.

Frank, Steven A. *Immunology and Evolution of Infectious Disease.* Princeton, N.J.: Princeton University Press, 2002. Blends research from molecular biology, immunology, pathogen biology, and population dynamics to discuss how and why parasites vary to escape recognition by the immune system, vaccine design, and the control of epidemics.

Janeway, Charles A., Jr., et al. *Immunobiology: The Immune System in Health and Disease.* 6th ed. New York: Garland Science, 2005. An excellent text that provides a lucid and comprehensive examination of the immune system, covering such topics as immunobiology and innate immunity, the recognition of antigen, the development of mature lymphocyte receptor repertoires, the adaptive immune response, and the evolution of the immune system.

Kindt, Thomas J., Richard A. Goldsby, and Barbara A. Osborne. *Kuby Immunology.* 6th ed. New York: W. H. Freeman, 2007. Excellent text that gives an overview of the immune system and its role with cells and organs, and discusses such topics as the generation of B-cell and T-cell responses, immune effector mechanisms, and the immune system in health and disease.

Parkham, Peter. *The Immune System.* 2d ed. New York: Garland Science, 2005. A basic immunology text that details how cells and molecules work together in defending the body against invading microorganisms, describes situations in which the immune system cannot control disease, and examines what happens when the immune system overreacts.

Rose, Noel R., and Ian. R. Mackay, eds. *The Autoimmune Diseases*. 4th ed. St. Louis: Elsevier Academic Press, 2006. A well-written textbook containing thorough discussions of autoimmune disorders. Primarily for those with a background in immunology, but does provide much basic information.

IMMUNOPATHOLOGY

SPECIALTY

ANATOMY OR SYSTEM AFFECTED: All

SPECIALTIES AND RELATED FIELDS: Dermatology, genetics, hematology, immunology, pathology, serology

DEFINITION: The study of disease processes that have an immunological basis or pathogenesis involving either B cells (antibodies) and complement or T cells, including damage to tissues and cells caused by hypersensitivity reactions.

KEY TERMS:

antibody: a molecule of the immune system, produced by B cells and targeted toward eliminating a specific antigen

B cells: also known as B lymphocytes; the antibody-producing cells of the immune system

congenital: something that is present at birth.

hypersensitivity: reactions in which the immune system response is exaggerated

immunodeficiency: a state in which the immune system components that are meant to protect an individual are in a weakened state or absent altogether

T cells: also known as T lymphocytes; the immune system cells involved in cellular immunity and regulation of the immune response

SCIENCE AND PROFESSION

Immunopathology is the subdiscipline of immunology that deals with the four basic types of pathologies caused by the immune system: autoimmune disorders, congenital immunodeficiencies, acquired immunodeficiencies, and hypersensitivity reactions. Physicians who deal with such disorders are trained in immunology and/or pathology.

Autoimmune disorders are those in which the body fails to distinguish between self and nonself, leading to attack by the immune system on the tissues or organs of the body. There are many autoimmune disorders, and the symptoms are extremely varied, depending on the site and extent of the attack. Some disorders are tissue-specific, while others affect tissues and organs throughout the body. Examples of autoimmune disorders are multiple sclerosis (MS), systemic lupus erythematosus (SLE), and myasthenia gravis.

Congenital (primary) immunodeficiencies are those conditions in which there is an absence or a failure of the immune system at birth. Often they are the result of a failure of one or more components of the immune system to develop during the fetal stages. Most congenital deficiencies have a genetic basis. An example of a primary immunodeficiency disorder is DiGeorge syndrome, in which T cells are deficient as a result of a developmental problem of the thymus. The most severe of these disorders is severe combined immunodeficiency disorder (SCID), in which both B and T cells do not develop or function properly. Complement deficiencies fall into this category as well. Complement is a series of proteins that combine to generate an attack on invading cells, such as bacteria.

Acquired (secondary) immunodeficiencies are those that arise later in life, following a change in some environmental condition or exposure, such as accidents or surgery that damages or removes the spleen or lymph nodes, radiation exposure that damages the bone marrow, and cancers that attack or destroy parts of the immune system. Lymphocytic leukemias (malignancies of bone marrow precursors of B and T cells) are an example of acquired immune system diseases. Malnutrition or the use of certain drugs (especially opiates) may also affect the immune system responses in a negative way. Finally, viruses, such as human immunodeficiency virus (HIV), can attack and suppress the human immune system components, leading to a deficient ability to defend the body from daily attack by microorganisms.

In contrast to the immunodeficiency syndromes, hypersensitivity reactions are those in which the immune system overreacts in its attempt to keep the body healthy, and by doing so causes localized or systemic reactions that can range from annoying to life-threatening. Hypersensitivity reactions are classified according to their molecular mechanism of action and may overlap with other categories, such as autoimmune disorders. Type I reactions are those which most people would recognize as allergies. Here, a series of chemicals, including immunoglobulin E (IgE), are released into the bloodstream, triggering the effects commonly associated with allergies: runny nose, itchy eyes, and difficulty breathing. The most severe case is anaphylaxis, sometimes seen in individuals with allergies to bee or wasp venom or to certain food substances. Type II reactions are those in which existing antibodies in the bloodstream bind to antigens that are seen as foreign and begin the process of tissue destruction. Examples include transfusion reactions, in which the wrong blood type is given to an individual, and erythroblastosis fetalis (hemolytic disease of the newborn), in which maternal antibodies attack a developing fetus that has a different set of antigens. Type III disorders are those in which large immune complexes form and are deposited in the bloodstream or kidneys, leading to disorders such as vasculitis and glomerulonephritis. Type IV reactions are those involving T cell attack; they include contact dermatitis (such as poison ivy reactions) and transplant rejection.

Diagnostic and Treatment Techniques

Specialists who deal with immunopathologies may provide treatments that vary widely, as do the disorders themselves. The goal of all therapy is to restore the immune system to its normal balance so that it can continue to protect the body from the constant barrage of invading microorganisms. Individuals with immune system deficiencies are told to avoid contact with other individuals as much as possible, since most viruses and bacteria are spread through personal contact. Prophylactic regimens of antibiotics, antivirals, and antifungals are helpful in most of those with immunodeficiencies, but in those with more severe forms, bone marrow transplants are the treatment of choice. The use of passive immunization—transferring antibodies from healthy individuals into those with immunodeficiencies—is helpful in some cases. In acquired immunodeficiency syndrome (AIDS), drug combinations, or "cocktails," are aimed at suppressing replication of HIV, which attacks the T cells and keeps them from functioning.

Because most hypersensitivity reactions are temporary immunopathologies, their treatment involves short-term therapies to restore balance to the system. Antihistamines, for instance, help many allergy sufferers, as do air purifiers and lifestyle changes. Careful tissue and blood typing can eliminate or lower the instances of the other types of hypersensitivities.

Treatment for autoimmune disorders is also quite variable, because of the wide variety of manifestations and underlying causes. Treatments commonly include immunosuppressive drugs and replacement of hormones or other chemicals that the body is lacking.

Perspective and Prospects

Since immunology itself is a field that is still in its infancy, recognition of immune disorders and their treatments is relatively new. Autoimmunity was first described by Paul Ehrlich at the turn of the twentieth century, and he called the phenomenon "horror autotoxicus," a name that struck fear in patients and providers alike. Hypersensitivitiy reactions, especially allergies, were recognized hundreds of years ago, and various chemical prescriptions were used to control the symptoms, but it was not until the mid-twentieth century that the molecular basis of allergies began to be understood. Immunodeficiencies are still being described, and the understanding of their basis is quite incomplete.

Some immunodeficiencies, if detected early enough, may be candidates for future gene therapy. In those cases where a single gene defect can be identified, introduction of the functional gene into the developing tissue may be able to reverse the course of the disease, partially or completely. Other options include transplantation of the thymus or bone marrow in order to allow normal functioning of the immune system components.

One of the most exciting potential treatments for secondary immunodeficiencies is vaccination. The ability to block AIDS through early immunization looks promising, although still many years away from use.

—*Kerry L. Cheesman, Ph.D.*

See also Acquired immunodeficiency syndrome (AIDS); Allergies; Arthritis; Autoimmune disorders; Blood and blood disorders; Bone marrow transplantation; Cells; Chemotherapy; Cytology; Cytopathology; Endocrinology; Endocrinology, pediatric; Glands; Hematology; Hematology, pediatric; Hemolytic disease of the newborn; Host-defense mechanisms; Human immunodeficiency virus (HIV); Immune system; Immunization and vaccination; Immunology; Kawasaki disease; Leukemia; Lymphatic system; Multiple chemical sensitivity syndrome; Myasthenia gravis; Oncology; Rh factor; Serology; Severe combined immunodeficiency syndrome (SCID); Skin; Systemic lupus erythematosus (SLE); Transfusion; Transplantation; Wiskott-Aldrich syndrome.

For Further Information:

Abbas, Abul K., and Andrew K. Lichtman. *Basic Immunology: Functions and Disorders of the Immune System*. 2d ed. Philadelphia: Elsevier Saunders, 2006. An easy-to-read introduction to the human immune system. Includes excellent figures and a thorough glossary.

Fischer, A. M., et al. "Naturally Occurring Primary Deficiencies of the Immune System." *Annual Review of Immunology* 15 (1997): 93-124. A good, although somewhat technical, review of primary deficiencies and the literature in the field.

Janeway, Charles A., Jr., et al. *Immunobiology: The Immune System in Health and Disease.* 6th ed. New York: Garland Science, 2005. A classic undergraduate text on immunology, containing well-written and thorough chapters on failures of host defense mechanisms and allergy and hypersensitivity.

National Institutes of Health (NIH). http://www.nih .gov/. This Web site contains dozens of easy-to-read pamphlets that are useful for those needing basic information on immune system disorders, including *Understanding the Immune System*, *Something in the Air: Airborne Allergens*, and *Food Allergy: An Overview*.

IMPETIGO

DISEASE/DISORDER

ANATOMY OR SYSTEM AFFECTED: Immune system, skin

SPECIALTIES AND RELATED FIELDS: Bacteriology, dermatology, emergency medicine, family medicine, internal medicine, microbiology, pediatrics, sports medicine

DEFINITION: A superficial bacterial infection of the skin.

CAUSES AND SYMPTOMS

Impetigo is a superficial bacterial skin infection usually caused by group A streptococcus, *Staphylococcus aureus*, or a mixture of both. Group A streptococcus was originally the predominant pathogen, but recently *S. aureus* has become the most common strain. Impetigo caused by either of these bacteria are clinically identical.

Children are most commonly affected by impetigo, and infection is often preceded by minor trauma such as insect bites. Outbreaks predominantly occur during the summer months, when the climate is hot and humid. Impetigo is very contagious and easily spread in crowded conditions such as families, schools, the military, and athletics. Poverty and poor personal hygiene can also predispose individuals to infection.

A typical infection first develops as multiple vesico-pustules, which rupture and form a characteristic golden yellow crust. The lesions are painless but commonly pruritic (itchy), and scratching can serve to

---

> **INFORMATION ON IMPETIGO**
>
> **CAUSES:** Bacterial infection
> **SYMPTOMS:** Skin inflammation, blisters, itchiness, scabbing
> **DURATION:** Acute
> **TREATMENTS:** Injection of antibiotics (penicillin, erythromycin)

spread infection. Systemic symptoms are rare, but there can be local lymphadenopathy. The face, particularly the region around the mouth, is a common site of infection.

TREATMENT AND THERAPY

Topical and oral antibiotics have been used for the treatment of impetigo. Historically, the treatment of choice was penicillin or ampicillin. This has changed, however, as the most predominant bacteria is now *S. aureus* instead of group A streptococcus, which almost universally produces a beta-lactamase that makes them resistant to penicillin. It is now recommended to use a beta-lactamase-resistant penicillin such as dicloxacillin or a first-generation cephalosporin such as cephalexin. Erythromycin can be used if the patient is allergic to penicillin.

Topical antibiotics such as mupirocin and fucidic acid (not available in the United States) are very effective treatments. Mupirocin has been shown to be as effective as erythromycin. Topical antibiotics are usually used with mild or moderate cases and oral antibiotics reserved for more advanced cases. Topical antibiotics are as effective and have fewer side effects, which make them a better choice in less severe cases. A ten-day course is recommended whether oral or topical antibiotics are used.

Gentle cleansing of the area with soap and water can be helpful. Personal hygiene may be discussed with the patient to help prevent recurrence of infection. Frequent hand washing and not sharing bath linens can help prevent spread of the bacteria. The lesions usually heal without scarring.

—Jeffrey B. Roberts, M.D.,
and Jeffrey R. Bytomski, D.O.

See also Antibiotics; Bacterial infections; Blisters; Childhood infectious diseases; Dermatology; Dermatology, pediatric; Rashes; Skin; Skin disorders; Staphylococcal infections; Streptococcal infections.

FOR FURTHER INFORMATION:

Bhumbra, Nasreen A., and Sophia G. McCullough. "Skin and Subcutaneous Infections." In *Update on Infectious Diseases*, edited by Richard I. Haddy and Karen W. Krigger. Philadelphia: W. B. Saunders, 2003.

Swartz, Morton N., and Mark S. Pasternack. "Cellulitis and Subcutaneous Tissue Infection." In *Mandell, Douglas, and Bennett's Principles and Practice of Infectious Diseases*, edited by Gerald L. Mandell, John E. Bennett, and Raphael Dolin. 6th ed. New York: Elsevier/Churchill Livingstone, 2005.

Taylor, Julie Scott. "Interventions for Impetigo." *American Family Physician* 70, no. 9 (November 1, 2004).

IMPOTENCE. *See* SEXUAL DYSFUNCTION.

IN VITRO FERTILIZATION
PROCEDURE

ANATOMY OR SYSTEM AFFECTED: Cells, reproductive system, uterus

SPECIALTIES AND RELATED FIELDS: Embryology, genetics, gynecology

DEFINITION: A procedure whereby eggs and sperm are combined in the laboratory to achieve fertilization, usually followed by the introduction of the resulting embryos into the uterus.

KEY TERMS:

chromosome: a structure found in the cell nucleus that is composed of deoxyribonucleic acid (DNA) and associated proteins; chromosomes are responsible for carrying genetic information and can be observed under a microscope

clomiphene: a synthetic estrogenic substance used to induce ovulation in women who do not ovulate regularly; it is taken orally as a medication

endometriosis: a condition whereby cells of the uterine lining are found in abnormal locations, such as the pelvic cavity or ovary; endometriosis can lead to pelvic pain and the development of scars that can block the Fallopian tubes

Fallopian tube: one of two structures that conduct the egg, as it is released from the ovary, into the uterus

follicle: a spherical mass of cells and fluid within the ovary, from which the mature egg is produced

implantation: the process in which an embryo attaches and burrows into the lining of the uterus

in vitro: a Latin term used to indicate a process that has taken place outside of an organism, such as in a laboratory test tube or petri dish

ovulation: the process whereby the egg is released from the ovary and can be fertilized by sperm; this event occurs approximately at the middle portion of a woman's menstrual cycle

semen analysis: analysis of a recently ejaculated semen specimen, which includes a sperm count and an estimate of the percentage of motile sperm

zygote: the single cell formed after fertilization that is the result of the fusion of egg and sperm; it can develop into a new individual organism

INDICATIONS AND PROCEDURES

The purpose of fertilization is to create a new organism or individual that has the same number of chromosomes as the parent individuals but which has a unique mixing of genetic traits from both the mother and the father. In animals, this is accomplished by the fusion of egg and sperm cells. Both egg and sperm contain half the number of chromosomes needed to produce a healthy individual. The fusion of egg and sperm results in a zygote, or fertilized egg, which can develop into an individual organism.

Eggs and sperm are both gametes, cells that are specialized to carry out reproductive functions. The sperm cells are produced in the testicles of the male. Sperm production is continuous in the male, and millions of sperm are made within the testicles each day. Sperm cells contain genetic material within their head and are equipped with a flagellum, or whiplike tail, to enable them to swim within a liquid medium. The egg, or ovum, is about .01 millimeter in size and hundreds of times larger than the sperm. It is produced in the ovaries of females and contains cytoplasm, the cellular substance and specialized cell structures that are needed for the zygote to form and grow. In women, a single mature egg is usually made with each menstrual cycle and is released from the follicle contained in one of the ovaries. As women age, their ovaries become depleted of follicles, and eventually, at the menopause, ovulation no longer occurs. Therefore, a woman's age can contribute significantly to her ability to conceive. Other causes of ovarian failure that may lead to infertility include the use of chemotherapeutic agents and premature ovarian failure syndrome.

In natural, or in vivo, fertilization, sperm from the male are deposited in the vaginal canal of the female during sexual intercourse. The sperm are contained in nutritive fluid, called semen. The sperm are able to swim up the cervical canal (the lower part of the uterus) only during and around the time of female ovulation, as the cervical mucus becomes permeable to sperm at this time. Once within the uterine cavity, the sperm make their way up into the Fallopian tubes, where they can meet the egg and proceed with fertilization.

Several steps lead to fertilization. The egg is surrounded by a layer of cells called the corona radiata. This layer is loose and easily penetrated by sperm. The next layer is the zona pellucida, which is a critical barrier in fertilization. One of the sugarcoated proteins in the zona pellucida, ZP3, captures a sperm cell by binding to its head. This causes a structure on the head of the sperm, called an acrosome, to release enzymes. This process is called the acrosomal reaction. These enzymes then digest the coat on the head of the sperm cell and digest a path for the sperm through the zona pellucida. After this, the sperm reaches the membrane of the egg, and the sperm and egg cells fuse. The chromosomes of the sperm and egg join, thus completing the process of fertilization. Subsequently, the fertilized egg travels back into the uterus and implants into the lining of the uterus, where it continues to develop as an embryo and then as a fetus.

When the natural anatomy or physiology of the reproductive system is abnormal, infertility can result. For instance, endometriosis in women can cause severe scarring of the pelvic cavity, leading to occluded Fallopian tubes or ovaries that are completely encased in scar tissue. In these cases, the egg may have difficulty reaching the Fallopian tube canal and hence is unable to meet sperm to achieve fertilization. Another cause of pelvic scarring is pelvic inflammatory disease (PID), which can be caused by sexually transmitted diseases (STDs) or ruptures in the gastrointestinal tract.

In vitro fertilization (IVF) may be indicated when a couple experiences infertility. Infertility is defined as the lack of conception after one to two years of unprotected intercourse. There are many causes of infertility, which may be attributable to either the male or the female partner. Usually when an infertile couple seeks medical attention, they are asked to give a detailed history and receive physical examinations by the physician. Depending on the findings, the couple will be asked to undergo testing to better identify the cause of the infertility. Men will be asked to give a semen sample. The sample will be analyzed in the laboratory to ensure that adequate numbers of sperm are present and that they are able to move appropriately, a procedure called semen analysis. Women may be assessed for anatomic defects, such as whether the Fallopian tubes are blocked or large fibroid tumors in the uterus may prevent sperm from entering the Fallopian tubes. This assessment may be accomplished using a technique

The Process of In Vitro Fertilization

9 to 13 days: Woman undergoes ultrasound to monitor ripening of the eggs in her ovaries.

1 to 8 days: During the first eight days of menstrual cycle, woman is given fertility drugs to stimulate the ripening of several eggs.

16 to 17 days: Eggs are examined to see if they have been fertilized and have started to develop into embryos. If so, several two- or four-cell embryos are placed in the woman's uterus.

14 to 15 days (immediately before ovulation): Ripe eggs are removed by laparoscopy or by ultrasound-guided needle aspiration through the vagina or abdomen. Eggs are mixed with sperm in a dish, which is then incubated.

called a hysterosalpingogram, in which dye is introduced into the uterine cavity and an X-ray picture is taken. If a woman's Fallopian tubes are blocked, then no dye will spill into the pelvic cavity. If a woman's tubes are open, then dye will be seen spilling into the pelvic cavity. In addition, women may also undergo assessments regarding their ovarian function and ability to produce eggs. Blood tests may be drawn to assess for appropriate hormone levels.

If the cause of infertility is found to be blocked Fallopian tubes, then IVF may be indicated. Sometimes, women with irregular menstrual cycles who do not ovulate at predictable intervals may be treated with a medication called clomiphene, in order to induce ovulation. If a woman fails to achieve spontaneous conception after several months of clomiphene therapy, then the physician may proceed with in vitro fertilization as the next step in the attempt to achieve conception.

Another example of when IVF may be indicated is in cases where the sperm are defective. For instance, some men may have sperm that have difficulty swimming appropriately or penetrating the egg. In such cases, the sperm may need to be injected artificially into the egg to achieve fertilization, a procedure call intracytoplasmic sperm injection (ICSI). In order to perform this procedure, eggs must be harvested from the woman. The eggs are then placed in a petri dish, where they are injected with the sperm. Because fertilization is occurring outside the body in this situation, this procedure is also a type of in vitro fertilization. After the eggs have matured for a few days in the laboratory, the healthiest-looking zygotes are placed into the woman's uterus, a procedure called embryo transfer.

Another example in which intracytoplasmic sperm injection might be used is when the couple's infertility is caused by the man's inability to ejaculate sperm. This might occur, for instance, with a lack or occlusion of the vas deferens, the tubes that carry sperm from the testicles to the urethra where the sperm can exit the body. To obtain sperm for IVF in these cases, the male partner may undergo testicular sperm extraction, in which sperm are removed from the testicles. The sperm are then injected into the ova to achieve fertilization in vitro.

The procedures for IVF involve the induction of ovulation in the woman using hormones that stimulate the ovaries. These are usually hormones that are similar to endogenous follicle-stimulating hormone (FSH), which is responsible for follicle growth within the ovary. These exogenous hormones lead to the develop-

ment of multiple follicles within both ovaries. The size and number of these follicles is observed by ultrasound, and when the appropriate number and size is achieved, the ovum harvest is performed. This procedure involves taking the woman to the operating room, where she is given anesthesia and placed on her back with her legs in stirrups and knees apart. A needle attached to a vacuum device is carefully introduced into the vaginal canal with ultrasound guidance. With the ultrasound helping to locate the ovaries and follicles precisely, the needle is inserted into the follicle through the posterior vagina. The fluid within the follicle is aspirated, and the egg usually is suctioned out of the follicle along with the follicular fluid and placed into a test tube. The same procedure is repeated until a sufficient number of eggs have been harvested or the follicles have been depleted. The eggs are then taken to the laboratory, where they are examined under a microscope.

A sperm sample is then collected from the male partner, and the sample is washed and analyzed to ensure that the sperm appear healthy and able to fertilize the eggs. The sperm are then introduced to the eggs within a petri dish containing tissue culture fluid. If intracytoplasmic sperm injection is to be performed, then single sperm are taken up into a glass needle and injected into individual eggs at this time. The petri dish is placed in an incubator for a few days. Once the embryos have developed sufficiently, a few healthy ones are chosen to be introduced into the woman's uterus through embryo transfer. This involves picking up the embryos into a semiflexible tube. The tube is then inserted carefully through the cervical canal into the uterine cavity, where the embryos are released. Embryos that are not transferred into the woman's uterus can be frozen using cryopreservation for future use.

Uses and Complications

IVF enables couples who suffer from infertility to conceive and bear children. Specifically, IVF is most helpful for couples whose infertility is caused by blocked Fallopian tubes or the inability of sperm to reach and penetrate the egg. In couples where the woman is unable to produce her own eggs, donor eggs from another woman may be used in IVF. If a man is unable to produce his own sperm, then sperm donors may be used in IVF.

Recent technology has enabled early prenatal diagnosis for inheritable conditions using cells taken from the early embryo during the six-to-eight-cell stage, called blastomere biopsy. Inheritable diseases caused by single gene defects, such as cystic fibrosis, Duchenne's muscular dystrophy, sickle cell disease, hemophilia, and Tay-Sachs disease, have been detected using preimplantation diagnosis. This type of prenatal diagnosis is possible only through the IVF process, as the early embryo would not be accessible to the physician in cases of spontaneous conception. Procedures such as blastomere biopsy are far from common, however, given the technical difficulty and economic costs of such procedures.

The complications associated with the IVF process include a condition called ovarian hyperstimulation syndrome. This situation can occur when a woman receives hormones to stimulate ovulation. In these cases, the follicles within the ovary become excessively stimulated and grossly enlarge the ovary. When this condition is severe, the woman can suffer abdominal pain, fluid imbalances, electrolyte imbalances, abnormal kidney function, and an accumulation of fluid in the abdominal cavity or lungs. Her blood may have an abnormal tendency to form clots, and her blood pressure may become dangerously low. These patients are monitored carefully and require hospitalization, as severe ovarian hyperstimulation syndrome can be fatal.

Other complications of the IVF process can occur during the ovum harvest procedure. These include the risks of anesthesia and infection (because the needle is a foreign body introduced through the vagina, a nonsterile field). Another risk involves bleeding. Although the needle for harvesting the eggs is under ultrasound guidance, the risk of the needle inadvertently puncturing neighboring blood vessels still exists. In addition, the ovaries themselves may bleed when punctured, as they are highly vascular organs. Bleeding that is severe and life-threatening may require abdominal or pelvic surgery to identify the location of the bleeding and to stop the bleeding with sutures. If the patient becomes significantly anemic from the bleeding, she may require a blood transfusion.

Other risks of IVF are incurred during the embryo culture process. During this process, the petri dishes containing the embryos may become contaminated with microorganisms. In addition, problems with the tissue culture medium or with the incubation process may lead to poor embryo development and the lack of any viable embryos to transfer into the woman. Another risk is the fact that embryos transferred into the uterus may not implant themselves in the lining.

The rate of achieving pregnancy after IVF is directly related to the number of embryos transferred into the uterus. When multiple embryos are transferred back into the uterus, however, the woman is at risk for a multiple gestation pregnancy. Multiple gestation pregnancies lead to an increased risk of spontaneous abortion (miscarriage) and preterm birth, as well as other pregnancy complications such as low birth weight, growth restriction in utero, increased risk of congenital anomalies, placental abnormalities, preeclampsia (a hypertensive disease of pregnancy), umbilical cord accidents and malpresentations (when the fetus is not lying in the uterus with the head down, making vaginal birth difficult). More long-term risks of in vitro fertilization are the increased risk for complications during pregnancy. For instance, women whose pregnancies were a result of assisted reproductive technologies such as IVF are at increased risk for preterm birth, when compared to age-matched women whose pregnancies were a result of spontaneous conception.

In addition, the long-term outcomes of children conceived using IVF is unknown, as the first children born as a result of this technique are beginning to enter middle age. Whether they will live normal life spans is unknown. Whether they will have normal reproductive outcomes themselves remains unclear. Whether they are more prone to diseases such as cancer later in life is also unknown.

PERSPECTIVE AND PROSPECTS

The first baby conceived through in vitro fertilization was Louise Brown, who was born in 1978. The English team responsible for this important breakthrough consisted of Patrick Steptoe, a surgeon from Oldham Hospital, and Robert Edwards, a reproductive physiologist from Cambridge University. In the 1960's, animal breeding programs had successfully utilized in vitro fertilization. In 1965, Edwards reported that he had successfully induced maturation of a human egg in vitro. Edwards teamed up with Steptoe and another colleague, Jean Purdy. In 1970, they reported that they had achieved in vitro fertilization and cleavage (cell division) in human eggs. The first successful birth of an IVF baby in the United States occurred in 1981 in Norfolk, Virginia. The first successful use of a previously frozen human embryo occurred in Australia in 1984; two years later, a similar procedure was employed successfully in the United States.

A couple can undergo multiple cycles of IVF. A 1996 study reported data from large centers in three countries which showed that the cumulative pregnancy rate after six cycles of IVF was approximately 60 percent.

However, if a couple fails to achieve pregnancy after six cycles, then the chances of achieving pregnancy through IVF fall significantly. At that time, the infertile couple may be counseled to seek alternative means of becoming parents, such as adoption.

In vitro fertilization and its related procedures have provided opportunities to conceive for couples who would otherwise be childless. These opportunities have led to many ethical controversies as well. What should be done with frozen embryos that are not used? What are the rights of egg or sperm donors once the child is born? What are the rights of the child to know his or her parentage and family history of medical problems? What are the rights of surrogate mothers? How many embryos should be transferred back into the woman, given the fact that multiple gestations are at increased risk for poor outcomes such as premature delivery? Is there a certain age at which women should not attempt pregnancy? Some countries such as Australia, Norway, Spain, and the United Kingdom have responded to some of these questions by passing legislation regulating IVF. Other countries have been slower to respond, leaving decisions related to IVF to physicians, the patients themselves, and the court system.

As more couples delay childbearing, the prevalence of infertility and the desire for IVF and other assisted reproductive technologies is likely to increase. Human reproduction is not an efficient process, and the older the female partner becomes, the less likely it is that natural conception will occur. For instance, a 1986 survey in the United States reported that the percentage of married women who were infertile between the ages of twenty and twenty-four was only 7 percent. By the ages of forty to forty-four, this percentage became 28 percent. This statistic is partly attributable to the fact that the total length of time during which conception is possible is less in older women, as older women ovulate less frequently than do younger women.

—Anne Lynn S. Chang, M.D.

See also Assisted reproductive technologies; Conception; Embryology; Ethics; Gamete intrafallopian transfer (GIFT); Genetic engineering; Gynecology; Hormones; Infertility, female; Infertility, male; Multiple births; Obstetrics; Pregnancy and gestation; Reproductive system; Women's health.

FOR FURTHER INFORMATION:

Gardner, David K., ed. *In Vitro Fertilization: A Practical Approach*. New York: Informa Healthcare, 2007. Discusses established procedures and techniques, as well as current research. Explores the history of IVF.

Sher, Geoffrey, Virginia Marriage Davis, and Jean Stoess. *In Vitro Fertilization: The A.R.T. of Making Babies*. 3d ed. New York: Facts On File, 2005. Dr. Sher and his clinical associates describe for patients in words and line drawings the process of evaluating patients and the procedures involved in IVF. The book also includes a glossary and an index.

Speroff, Leon, and Marc A. Fritz. *Clinical Gynecologic Endocrinology and Infertility*. 7th ed. Philadelphia: Lippincott Williams & Wilkins, 2005. A comprehensive textbook that outlines the evaluation and treatment of infertility, including in vitro fertilization. Also discusses the biology behind reproductive processes.

Stenchever, Morton A., et al. *Comprehensive Gynecology*. 4th ed. St. Louis: Mosby, 2006. The definitive gynecologic textbook, it offers well-written chapters on prenatal diagnosis, reproductive endocrinology, and infertility.

Wisot, Arthur L., and David R. Meldrum. *Conceptions and Misconceptions: The Informed Consumer's Guide Through the Maze of In Vitro Fertilization and Other Assisted Reproduction Techniques*. 2d ed. Point Roberts, Wash.: Hartley & Marks, 2004. Written by two leading fertility experts, this book is an excellent guide through the maze of in vitro fertilization and other assisted reproductive techniques. Includes an excellent discussion of the basic physiology of conception and reproduction.

INCONTINENCE
DISEASE/DISORDER

ANATOMY OR SYSTEM AFFECTED: Abdomen, bladder, gastrointestinal system, urinary system

SPECIALTIES AND RELATED FIELDS: Family medicine, geriatrics and gerontology, gynecology, internal medicine, obstetrics, pediatrics, psychiatry, urology

DEFINITION: Involuntary loss of urine or feces, primarily a social and hygienic problem that particularly affects the older population.

KEY TERMS:

atonic bladder: a bladder characterized by weak muscles

enuresis: bed-wetting

frequency: urination at short intervals; a common problem accompanying incontinence

micturition: the act of urinating

nocturia: nighttime urination

sphincter: a ring-shaped muscle that surrounds a natural opening in the body and can open or close it by expanding or contracting

urge incontinence: a strong desire to urinate followed by leakage of urine

urgency: a strong desire to void urine immediately

CAUSES AND SYMPTOMS

Continence is a skill acquired in humans by the interaction of two processes: socialization of the infant and maturation of the central nervous system. Without society's expectation of continence, and without broadly accepted definitions of appropriate behavior, the concept of "incontinence" would be meaningless. There are many causes for urinary incontinence. Three broad (interrelated and often overlapping) categories are physiologic voiding dysfunction, factors directly influencing voiding function, and factors affecting the individual's capacity to manage voiding.

The causes of physiologic voiding dysfunction involve an abnormality in bladder or sphincter function, or both. The bladder and sphincter have only two functions: to store urine until the appropriate time for urination and then to empty it completely. Voiding dysfunction involves the failure of one or both of these mechanisms. Four basic types of voiding dysfunction can be distinguished: detrusor instability, genuine stress incontinence, outflow obstruction, and atonic bladder.

Detrusor instability is a condition characterized by involuntary bladder (detrusor muscle) contraction during filling. While all the causes of bladder instability are not fully understood, it can be associated with the following: neurologic disease (brain and spinal cord abnormalities), inflammation of the bladder wall, bladder outlet obstruction, stress urinary incontinence, and idiopathic (spontaneous or primary) dysfunction. Detrusor instability usually causes symptoms of frequency, urgency, and possibly nocturia or enuresis.

Genuine stress incontinence is caused by a failure to hold urine during bladder filling as a result of an incompetent urethral sphincter mechanism. If the closure mechanism of the bladder outlet fails to hold urine, incontinence will occur. This is usually manifested during physical exertion or abdominal stress (such as coughing or sneezing). It can occur in either sex, but it is more common in women because of their shorter urethra and the physical trauma of childbirth. Men can experience stress incontinence following traumatic or surgical damage to the sphincter.

INFORMATION ON INCONTINENCE

CAUSES: Neurological disease, bladder inflammation, obstruction, prostate gland enlargement, urinary tract infection, diuretics, endocrine disorders (*e.g.*, diabetes mellitus, thyroid disorders), aging, pregnancy and childbirth

SYMPTOMS: Frequent urination, straining to void, poor urinary stream, feeling of urgency with resulting leakage

DURATION: Ranges from acute to chronic

TREATMENTS: Drug therapy, surgery, bladder training

Obstruction of the outflow of urine during voiding can produce various symptoms, including frequency, straining to void, poor urinary stream, preurination and posturination dribbling, and a feeling of urgency with resulting leakage (urge incontinence). In severe cases, the bladder is never completely emptied and a volume of residual urine persists. Overflow incontinence can result. Common causes of bladder outlet obstruction are prostatic enlargement, bladder neck narrowing, or urethral obstruction. Functional obstruction occurs when a neurologic lesion prevents the coordinated relaxation of the sphincter during voiding. This phenomenon is termed detrusor-sphincter dyssynergia.

An atonic bladder—one with weak muscle walls—does not produce a sufficient contraction to empty completely. Emptying can be enhanced by abdominal straining or manual expression, but a large residual volume persists. The sensation of retaining urine might or might not be present. If sensation is present, frequency of urination is common because only a small portion of the bladder volume is emptied each time. Sensation is often diminished, and the residual urine volume can be considerable (100 to 1,000 milliliters). Overflow incontinence often occurs.

An acute urinary tract infection can cause transient incontinence, even in a fit, healthy young person who normally has no voiding dysfunction. Acute frequency and urgency with disturbed sensation and pain can result in the inability to reach a toilet in time or to detect when incontinence is occurring. If an underlying voiding dysfunction is also present, an acute urinary tract infection is likely to cause incontinence.

Many drugs can also disturb the delicate balance of normal functioning. The most obvious category consists of diuretics, those drugs which increase urinary discharge; a large, swift production of urine will give most people frequency and urgency. If the bladder is unstable, it might not be able to handle a sudden influx of urine, and urge incontinence can result. Sedation can affect voiding function directly (for example, diazepam can lower urethral resistance) or can make the individual less responsive to signals from the bladder and thus unable to maintain continence. Other commonly prescribed drugs have secondary actions on voiding function. Not all patients, however, will experience urinary side effects from these drugs.

Various endocrine disorders can upset normal voiding function. Diabetes can cause polydypsia (extreme thirst), requiring the storage of a large volume of urine. Glycosuria (sugar in the urine) might encourage urinary tract infection. Thyroid imbalances can aggravate an overactive or underactive bladder. Pituitary gland disorders can result in the production of excessive urine volumes because of an antidiuretic hormone deficiency. Estrogen deficiency in postmenopausal women causes atrophic changes in the vaginal and urethral tissues and will worsen stress incontinence and an unstable bladder.

Several bladder pathologies can also cause incontinence by disrupting normal functioning. A patient with a neoplasm (abnormal tissue growth), whether benign or malignant, or a stone in the bladder occasionally experiences incontinence as a symptom. These are infrequent causes of incontinence.

Often it takes something else in addition to the underlying problem to tip the balance and produce incontinence. This is especially true for elderly and disabled persons who are delicately balanced between continence and incontinence. For example, immobility—anything that impedes access—is likely to induce incontinence. Immobility can be the result of the gradual worsening of a chronic condition, such as arthritis, multiple sclerosis, or Parkinson's disease, until eventually the individual simply cannot reach a toilet in time. The condition may be acute—an accident or illness that suddenly renders a person immobile might be the start of failure to control the bladder.

In the case of children, most daytime wetting persists until the child reaches school age. It is less common than bed-wetting (enuresis), and the two often go together. One in ten five-year-old children, however, still wets the bed regularly. With no treatment, this figure gradually falls to 5 percent of ten-year-olds and to 2 percent of adults. It is twice as common in boys as in girls, has strong familial tendencies, and is associated with stressful events in the third or fourth year of life. A urinary tract infection is sometimes the cause.

Fecal, as opposed to urinary, incontinence is generally caused by underlying disorders of the colon, rectum, or anus; neurogenic disorders; or fecal impaction. Severe diarrhea increases the likelihood of having fecal incontinence. Some of the more common disorders that can cause diarrhea are ulcerative colitis, carcinoma, infection, radiation therapy, and the effect of drugs (for example, broad-spectrum antibiotics, laxative abuse, or iron supplements). Fecal incontinence tends to be a common, if seldom reported, accompaniment.

The pelvic floor muscles support the anal sphincter, and any weakness will cause a tendency to fecal stress incontinence. The vital flap valve formed by the anorectal angle can be lost if these muscles are weak. An increase in abdominal pressure would therefore tend to force the rectal contents down and out of the anal canal. This might be the result of congenital abnormalities or of later trauma (for example, childbirth, anal surgery, or direct trauma). A lifelong habit of straining at stool might also cause muscle weakness.

The medulla and higher cortical centers of the brain have a role in coordinating and controlling the defecation reflex. Therefore, any neurologic disorder that impairs the ability to detect or inhibit impending defecation will probably result in a tendency to incontinence, similar in causation to the uninhibited or unstable bladder. For example, the paraplegic can lose all direct sensation of and voluntary control over bowel activity. Neurologic disorders such as multiple sclerosis, cerebrovascular accident, and diffuse dementia can affect sensation or inhibition, or a combination of both. Incontinence occurs with some demented people because of a physical inability to inhibit defecation. With others, it occurs because the awareness that such behavior is inappropriate has been lost.

Severe constipation with impaction of feces is probably the most common cause of fecal incontinence, and it predominates as a cause among the elderly and those living in extended care facilities. Chronic constipation leads to impaction when the fluid content of the feces is progressively absorbed by the colon, leaving hard, rounded rocks in the bowel. This hard matter promotes mucus production and bacterial activity, which causes a foul-smelling brown fluid to accumulate. If the rectum is overdistended for any length of time, the internal and external sphincters become relaxed, allowing passage of this mucus as spurious diarrhea. The patient's symptoms usually include fairly continuous leakage of fluid stool without any awareness of control.

Most children are continent of feces by the age of four years, but 1 percent still have problems at seven years of age. More boys than girls are incontinent, suggesting that developmental factors can be relevant because boys mature more slowly. Fecal incontinence or conscious soiling in childhood (sometimes referred to as encopresis) has, like nocturnal enuresis, long been regarded as evidence of a psychiatric or psychologic disorder in the child. The evidence, however, does not support the claim that most fecally incontinent children are disturbed.

Such children usually have fastidious, overanxious parents who are intent on toilet training. The child is punished for soiling, so defecation tends to be inhibited, both in the underwear and in the toilet. When toilet training is attempted, the child may be repeatedly seated on the toilet in the absence of a full rectum and be unable to perform. The situation becomes fraught with anxiety, and bowel movements become associated with unpleasantness in the child's mind. The child therefore retains feces and becomes constipated. Defecation then becomes difficult and painful as well.

TREATMENT AND THERAPY

The two primary methods of treating urinary incontinence involve medical and surgical intervention (drug therapy and surgery) and bladder training.

Many drugs can be prescribed to help those with urinary incontinence. Often the results are disappointing, although some drugs can be useful for carefully selected and accurately diagnosed patients. Drugs are often used to control detrusor instability and urge incontinence by relaxing the detrusor muscle and inhibiting reflex contractions. This therapy is helpful in some patients. Sometimes when the drug is given in large enough doses to be effective, however, the side effects are so troublesome that the therapy must be abandoned. Drugs that reduce bladder contractions must be used cautiously in patients who have voiding difficulty, since urinary retention can be precipitated. Careful assessment must be made of residual urine. Drug therapy is also used with caution in patients with a residual volume greater than 100 milliliters. Some drugs are used in an attempt to prevent stress incontinence by increasing urethral tone. Phenylpropanolamine and ephedrine, those most often used, are thought to act on the alpha receptors in the urethra.

Drug therapy can also be used to relieve outflow ob-struction. Phenoxybenzamine is most commonly used, but this drug can have dangerous side effects, such as tachycardia (an abnormally fast heartbeat) or postural hypotension. If the bladder does not contract sufficiently to ensure complete emptying, drug therapy can be attempted to increase the force of the voiding contractions. Carbachol, bethanechol, and distigmine bromide have all been used with some success. Other drugs might be useful in treating factors affecting incontinence—for example, antibiotics to treat a urinary tract infection or laxatives to treat or prevent constipation.

Many drugs can exacerbate a tendency to incontinence. For those who are prone to incontinence, medications and dosage schedules are chosen that will have a minimal effect on bladder control. For example, a slow-acting diuretic, in a divided dose, can help someone with urgency and weak sphincter tone to avoid incontinence. An analgesic might be preferable to night sedation for those who need pain relief but who wet the bed at night if they are sedated.

Turning to surgical intervention, none of the several surgical approaches that have been used in an attempt to treat an unstable bladder has gained widespread use. Cystodistention (stretching the bladder under general anesthesia) and bladder transection, for example, are presumed to act by disturbing the neurologic pathways that control uninhibited contractions. Many vaginal and suprapubic procedures are available to help correct genuine stress incontinence in women. Surgery can also be used to relieve outflow obstruction—for example, to remove an enlarged prostate gland, divide a stricture, or widen a narrow urethra.

In cases of severe intractable incontinence, major surgery is an option. For those with a damaged urethra, a neourethra can be constructed. For those with a nonfunctioning sphincter, an artificial sphincter can be implanted. In some patients, a urinary diversion with a stoma (outlet) is the only and best alternative for continence. Although a drastic solution, a urostomy might be easier to cope with than an incontinent urethra, because an effective appliance will contain the urine.

Urinary incontinence is occasionally the result of surgery, usually urologic or gynecologic but sometimes a major pelvic or spinal procedure. Such iatrogenic incontinence can be caused by neurologic or sphincter damage, leading to various dysfunctional voiding patterns.

Several different types of bladder training or retraining are distinguishable and can be used in different circumstances. The most important element for success is that the correct regimen be selected for each patient and situation. A thorough assessment identifies those patients who will benefit from bladder training and determines the most appropriate method. Other factors that contribute to the incontinence should also be treated (for example, a urinary tract infection or constipation), because ignoring them will impair the success of a program.

Bladder training is most suitable for people with the symptoms of frequency, urgency, and urge incontinence (with or without an underlying unstable bladder) and for those with nonspecific incontinence. The elderly often have these symptoms. Patients with voiding dysfunction, other than an unstable bladder, are unlikely to benefit from bladder training.

The aim of bladder training is to restore the patient with frequency, urgency, and urge incontinence to a more normal and convenient voiding pattern. Ultimately, voiding should occur at intervals of three to four hours (or even longer) without any urgency or incontinence. Drug therapy is sometimes combined with bladder training for those with detrusor instability.

Bladder training aims to restore an individual's confidence in the bladder's ability to hold urine and to reestablish a more normal pattern. Initially, a patient keeps a baseline chart for three to seven days, recording how often urine is passed and when incontinence occurs. This chart is reviewed with the program supervisor, and an individual regimen is developed. The purpose is to extend the time between voiding gradually, encouraging the patient to practice delaying the need to void, rather than giving in to the feeling of urgency. Initially, the times chosen can be at set intervals throughout the day (for example, every one or two hours) or can be variable, according to the individual's pattern as indicated by the baseline chart. When the baseline chart reveals a definite pattern to the incontinence, it might be possible to set voiding times in accordance with and in anticipation of this pattern.

A pattern of voiding is set for patients throughout the day (timed voiding). Usually no pattern is set at night, even if nocturia or nocturnal enuresis is a problem. Patients are instructed to pass urine as necessary during the night. Sometimes the provision of a suitable pad or appliance helps to increase confidence and means that, if incontinence does occur, the results will not be disastrous. If urgency is experienced, patients are taught to sit or stand still and try to suppress the sensation rather than to rush immediately to the toilet. A

normal fluid intake is encouraged because the goal is to have the patient continent and able to drink fluids adequately.

As patients achieve the target intervals without having to urinate prematurely or leaking, the intervals can gradually be lengthened. The speed of progress depends on the individual and on other variables, such as the initial severity of symptoms, motivation, and the amount of professional support. Patients usually remain at one time interval for one to two weeks before it is increased by fifteen to thirty minutes for another two weeks. Once the target of three- to four-hour voiding without urgency has been achieved, it is useful to maintain the chart and set times for at least another month to prevent relapse.

Some people find that practicing pelvic muscle exercises helps to suppress urgency. Any weakness in the pelvic floor muscles will cause a tendency not only to urinary incontinence but also to fecal stress incontinence. Mild weakness can respond to pelvic muscle exercises similar to those used in alleviating the symptoms of stress incontinence, but with a concentration on the posterior rather than the anterior portion of the pelvic muscles. Rectal tone is assessed by digital examination, during which the patient is instructed to squeeze. Regular contractions on the posterior portion of the pelvic muscles are then practiced often for at least two months (usually in sets of twenty-five, three times a day).

In cases of fecal impaction, a course of disposable phosphate enemas—one or two daily for seven to ten days, or until no further return is obtained—is the treatment of choice. A single enema is seldom efficient, even if an apparently good result is obtained, because impaction is often extensive: The first enema merely clears the lowest portion of the bowel. If fecal incontinence persists once the bowel has been totally cleared (a plain abdominal X ray can be helpful in confirming this), the condition is assumed to be neurogenic in origin rather than caused by the impaction.

PERSPECTIVE AND PROSPECTS

Historically, most health professionals have been profoundly ignorant of the causes and management of incontinence. Incontinence was often regarded as a condition over which there was no control, rather than as a symptom of an underlying physiologic disorder or as a symptom of a patient with a unique combination of problems, needs, and potentials. The unfortunate result of such limited understanding was passive acceptance of the symptom of incontinence. Incontinence, often viewed as repulsive, is often a condition that is merely tolerated. As public recognition of the implications of incontinence has increased, however, the stigma associated with it has slowly decreased. It has become common knowledge that millions of Americans suffer from incontinence, and most pharmacies and supermarkets have a section for incontinence products.

At one time, incontinence was primarily regarded as a "nursing" problem, with nurses providing custodial care—keeping the patient as clean and comfortable as possible and preventing pressure ulcers from developing. Gradually, nurses were not alone in acknowledging that incontinence was a symptom requiring investigation and intervention; those in other health professions also began to realize this need. In the 1980's, research dollars began to be allocated for the study of incontinence. In 1988, U.S. Surgeon General C. Everett Koop estimated that 8 billion dollars was being spent by the federal government on incontinence in the United States annually.

As incontinence began to be recognized by the public as a health problem rather than as an inevitable part of aging, more people admitted having the symptoms of incontinence and sought medical attention. It has been estimated that, of all cases of incontinence, more than one-third can be cured, another one-third can be dramatically improved, and most of the remainder can be significantly improved.

—*Genevieve Slomski, Ph.D.*

See also Bed-wetting; Constipation; Diarrhea and dysentery; Digestion; Sphincterectomy; Stone removal; Stones; Urinary disorders; Urinary system; Urology; Urology, pediatric.

FOR FURTHER INFORMATION:

Dierich, Mary, and Felecia Froe. *Overcoming Incontinence: A Straightforward Guide to Your Options.* New York: John Wiley & Sons, 2000. The authors present no-nonsense, practical advice on incontinence. Readers will learn how the urinary system works and how and when to seek professional help.

Jeter, Katherine, Nancy Faller, and Christine Norton, eds. *Nursing for Continence.* Philadelphia: W. B. Saunders, 1990. This work, written by a group of nurses, addresses the diagnosis, treatment, and management of incontinence in all age groups and in special populations and circumstances in a practical, thorough, and sensitive manner.

Nathanson, Laura Walther. *The Portable Pediatrician: A Practicing Pediatrician's Guide to Your Child's Growth, Development, Health, and Behavior from Birth to Age Five.* 2d ed. New York: HarperCollins, 2002. An engaging, easy-to-read guide for parents to assess their child's development, medical symptoms, and behavioral problems, including bedwetting.

National Association for Continence. http://www.nafc .org/. A clearinghouse for information and services related to incontinence and assistive devices. Provides education, advocacy, and support on the causes, prevention, diagnosis, treatment, and management alternatives for persons with incontinence.

Newman, Diane Kaschack. *Managing and Treating Urinary Incontinence.* Baltimore: Health Professions Press, 2002. A comprehensive resource on incontinence, covering everything from the causes of incontinence to evaluation and therapy. Includes excellent practical information such as self-care practices that will minimize urinary symptoms, tools for health professionals that can be used to train staff and educate patients, and appendices on diet habits, bladder retraining, and mechanical devices used to reduce incontinence.

Parker, William, Amy Rosenman, and Rachel Parker. *The Incontinence Solution: Answers for Women of All Ages.* New York: Simon & Schuster, 2002. A consumer-oriented guide to incontinence with an accessible question-and-answer format. Covers causes and diagnosis, treatments, childbirth and incontinence, interstitial cystitis, and defining and diagnosing prolapse.

Vasavada, Sandip P., et al., eds. *Female Urology, Urogynecology, and Voiding Dysfunction.* New York: Marcel Dekker, 2005. The book begins with fundamentals of the female genitourinary tract, then analyzes the dynamics of continence mechanisms. Female urinary incontinence is treated as a multifaceted subject.

INDIGESTION

DISEASE/DISORDER

ALSO KNOWN AS: Functional dyspepsia

ANATOMY OR SYSTEM AFFECTED: Gastrointestinal system

SPECIALTIES AND RELATED FIELDS: Family medicine, gastroenterology, internal medicine

DEFINITION: Discomfort in the abdomen following meals.

CAUSES AND SYMPTOMS

Indigestion is a nonspecific term used to describe a variety of sensations. Burning, fullness, gaseousness, and gnawing sensation in the abdomen are all symptoms that patients may describe as indigestion. While some people who complain of indigestion have acid reflux disease or ulcers, these are by no means the only causes. Fullness or bloating following the ingestion of milk, cheese, or other dairy products may be symptoms of lactose intolerance. This is one of the few cases of indigestion that is truly a problem in the digestive process, namely in the breakdown of milk sugars. Abdominal discomfort associated with alternating bouts of diarrhea and constipation may signal irritable bowel syndrome (IBS). More rare causes of similar discomfort include diffuse esophageal spasm, in which the food pipe contracts abnormally, and inflammation in the gallbladder.

Since the term "indigestion" is so vague, care must be taken to distinguish it from cardiac pain (angina). Psychiatric causes of abdominal pain must also be considered, especially when other etiologies have been ruled out.

TREATMENT AND THERAPY

Since the causes of indigestion are so varied, it is useful to arrive at a more precise diagnosis before offering treatment. Prior to embarking on a lengthy workup, however, some simple measures should be attempted. If symptoms resolve entirely with these measures, then no further investigation or treatment is usually required. Any particular foods that appear to worsen symptoms should be eliminated from the diet. This is especially true for dairy products and wheat, which are offensive factors in lactose intolerance and celiac sprue, respectively. Patients should also try avoiding spicy foods for a period of time. Eating slowly and having frequent small meals are good habits for people with indigestion. Some people find relief with over-the-counter remedies such as magnesium or bismuth mixtures. Antacids can also be tried, especially if acid reflux is suspected.

If symptoms persist, or if they are accompanied by trouble swallowing, vomiting, weight loss, or a change in bowel movements, then more thorough investigation is needed. This is often done through blood tests, X rays, or endoscopy.

—*Ahmad Kamal, M.D.*

See also Abdomen; Abdominal disorders; Acid reflux disease; Appetite loss; Constipation; Crohn's dis-

---

INFORMATION ON INDIGESTION

CAUSES: Varies; may include acid reflux disease, ulcers, lactose intolerance, celiac sprue, irritable bowel syndrome (IBS)
SYMPTOMS: Burning, fullness, gaseousness, and gnawing sensation in abdomen
DURATION: Temporary, often recurrent
TREATMENTS: Avoidance of food triggers (*e.g.*, dairy products, wheat) or spicy foods; change in eating habits (slower eating, frequent small meals); over-the-counter drugs (magnesium, bismuth mixtures, antacids)

---

ease; Diarrhea and dysentery; Digestion; Gallbladder diseases; Gastroenterology; Gastroenterology, pediatric; Gastrointestinal disorders; Gastrointestinal system; Heartburn; Intestinal disorders; Nausea and vomiting; Nutrition; Stress; Ulcer surgery; Ulcers.

FOR FURTHER INFORMATION:

Beers, Mark H., et al. *The Merck Manual of Diagnosis and Therapy*. 18th ed. Whitehouse Station, N.J.: Merck Research Laboratories, 2006.

Kasper, Dennis L., et al., eds. *Harrison's Principles of Internal Medicine*. 16th ed. New York: McGraw-Hill, 2005.

Peikin, Steven R. *Gastrointestinal Health*. New York: HarperCollins, 1999.

Toews, Victoria Dolby. *User's Guide to Healthy Digestion: Learn How You Can Put an End to Heartburn, Indigestion, Constipation, and Other Digestive Problems*. North Bergen, N.J.: Basic Health, 2003.

INFARCTION, MYOCARDIAL. *See* HEART ATTACK.

INFECTION

DISEASE/DISORDER

ANATOMY OR SYSTEM AFFECTED: All
SPECIALTIES AND RELATED FIELDS: Bacteriology, family medicine, hematology, internal medicine, virology
DEFINITION: Invasion of the body by disease-causing organisms such as bacteria, viruses, fungi, and parasites; symptoms of infection may include pain, swelling, fever, and loss of normal function.

KEY TERMS:

antibiotic: a substance that destroys or inhibits the growth of microorganisms, such as bacteria

antibody: a small protein secreted from specialized white blood cells which binds to and aids in the destruction of pathogens

antigen: a substance found on pathogens to which the antibodies bind; also, any substance considered foreign by the body

bacteria: small microorganisms; some bacteria found normally in and on the body have helpful functions, while others that invade the body or disrupt the normal bacteria are harmful and often infectious

edema: an abnormal accumulation of fluid in the body tissues; tissue with edema is swollen in appearance

infectious: referring to a microorganism that is capable of causing disease, often with the ability to spread from one person to another

inflammation: a tissue reaction to injury which may or may not involve infection; pain, heat, redness, and edema are the usual signs of inflammation

pathogen: a microorganism or substance capable of producing a disease, such as a bacterium causing an infection

phagocytosis: the ingestion and destruction of a pathogen or abnormal tissue by specialized white blood cells known as phagocytes

virus: a very small organism which is dependent upon a host cell to meet its metabolic needs and to reproduce

PROCESS AND EFFECTS

Healthy people live with potential pathogens; that is, people have on and in their bodies non-disease-causing bacteria. They live in harmony with these organisms and in fact benefit from their presence. For example, some of the bacteria found in the intestinal tract supply vitamin K, which is important in blood-clotting reactions.

The human body has several features that prevent disease-causing organisms from inducing an infection. These features include anatomical barriers, such as unbroken skin, and the mucus in the nose, mouth, and lungs, which can trap pathogens. Another defense is the acid within the stomach, and even bacteria that are normally present in certain areas of the body can force out more harmful bacteria. The immune system is specially developed to ward off intruders.

Immune cells and factors secreted from these cells provide the next line of defense against invading organisms. Antibodies are secreted from specialized white blood cells known as plasma cells. These antibodies are very specific for the recognition of pathogens. For example, one antibody will recognize a particular strain of bacteria but not another. Antibodies attach themselves to the part of the bacterium called the antigen. Once bound to the antigen, they aid in the destruction of the pathogen. In addition to plasma cells, other white blood cells help in combating infections. These include the phagocytes called macrophages and neutrophils. Both of these types of immune cells have the ability to eat and digest pathogens such as bacteria in a process known as phagocytosis.

Microorganisms that cause disease must, in some way, overwhelm the body's natural defenses and immune system. Bacteria capable of causing infections may even be naturally occurring organisms that have left their normal environment and overcome the elements that normally hold them at bay. For example, some normal bacteria that reside in the mouth may cause pneumonia (inflammation of the lungs) if they gain access to the lungs.

Other infections can be caused by pathogens that do not normally reside in the body. One can "catch" a cold or the flu, or even a sexually transmitted disease. These kinds of infections are called communicable or transmissible infections. Similarly, a physician treating someone who has been bitten by a bat, skunk, or dog will want to know whether the animal has rabies. Rabies is a viral infection that is transmitted via a bite which breaks the skin and contaminates the wound with infectious saliva.

No matter what the route of infection, the body must mount a response to the intruding microorganism. Often the signs and symptoms one observes are not caused by the direct action of the infecting pathogen, but rather reflect the immune system's response to the infection. The most frequent signs and symptoms in-

---

INFORMATION ON INFECTION

CAUSES: Exposure to bacteria, viruses, fungi, or parasites

SYMPTOMS: Pain, swelling, fever, fatigue, loss of normal function

DURATION: Acute to chronic

TREATMENTS: Drug therapy (antibiotics, antiviral agents, antifungal agents, etc.)

clude inflammation and pain at the site of infection, as well as fever.

The inflammatory response is a nonspecific defense that is triggered whenever body tissues are injured, as in the case of infection. The goal of the inflammatory response is to prevent the spread of the infectious agent to nearby tissues, destroy the pathogens, remove the damaged tissues, and begin the healing process.

The signs of inflammation include redness, edema (tissue swelling), heat, pain, and loss of normal function. At first glance, these reactions do not appear to be beneficial to the body, but they do help fight the infection and aid in the healing process. The redness is attributable to an increase in blood flow to the area of infection. This increase in blood to the site of infection helps provide nutrients to the tissue, as well as removing some of the waste products that develop as the immune system fights the infection. With this increase in blood flow comes an increase in the temperature and the amount of blood that leaks out of blood vessels into the tissue spaces, causing edema at the site of infection. Some of the blood that leaks into the site of infection contains clotting proteins that help form a clot around the infected area, thereby reducing the chances that the pathogen could escape into the bloodstream or uninfected tissue nearby. Pain is present when the damaged tissue releases waste products and the pathogen releases toxins. The swelling of the injured area and the pain associated with infections keep the patient from using that area of the body and thus aid in healing. It is interesting to note that while some painkillers such as aspirin reduce the inflammatory reaction by stopping the production of some of the chemicals released during inflammation, the aspirin-like drugs do nothing to harm the pathogen, only the body's response to the microorganism.

Some of the same chemicals that are found in inflamed tissues also cause fever. This abnormally high body temperature represents the body's response to an invading microorganism. The body's thermostat, located in a region of the brain known as the hypothalamus, is set at about 37 degrees Celsius (98.6 degrees Fahrenheit). During an infection, the thermostat is reset to a higher level. Chemicals called pyrogens are released from white blood cells called macrophages. Once again, aspirin-like drugs can be used to reduce the fever by inhibiting the action of some of these chemicals in the hypothalamus.

The body responds to viral infections in a similar way. Virally infected cells, however, secrete interferon, exerting an antiviral action which may provide protection to uninfected neighboring cells. It appears that interferon acts to inhibit the virus from replicating. Therefore, cells that are already infected must be destroyed to rid the body of the remaining virus.

In addition to being part of the inflammatory response, certain white blood cells play an important role in attempting to remove the pathogen. Soon after inflammation begins, macrophages already present at the site of infection start to destroy the microorganism. At the same time, chemicals are being released from both the damaged tissue and the macrophages, which recruit other white blood cells such as neutrophils. The neutrophils, like the macrophages, are effective at attacking and destroying bacteria but, unlike the macrophages, they often die in the battle against infection. Dead neutrophils are seen as a white exudate called pus.

Other manifestations of infection include systemic (whole-body) effects in addition to changes at the site of infection. As noted, fever is a systemic effect mediated by chemicals from the site of infection. Some of these same factors have the ability to act on the bone marrow to increase the production of white blood cells. Physicians look for fever and an increase in white blood cell number as a sign of infection. If the infection is severe, the bone marrow may not be able to keep up with the demand and an overall decrease in white blood cell number is found.

COMPLICATIONS AND DISORDERS

Physicians and other health care workers must use patient history, signs and symptoms, and laboratory tests to determine the type of infection and the most appropriate treatment. Patient history can often tell the examiner how and when the infection started. For example, the patient may have cut himself or herself, been exposed to someone with an infectious disease, or had intimate contact with someone carrying a sexually transmitted disease. Signs of infection—edema, pain, fever—are usually rather easy to detect, but some symptoms may be rather vague, such as feeling tired and weak. These general signs and symptoms may indicate to a physician that the patient has an infection, but they will not provide information about the type of microorganism causing the infection. Nevertheless, some microorganisms do cause specific symptoms. For example, the varicella-zoster virus that causes chickenpox or the paramyxovirus that causes measles leave characteristic rashes.

When the microorganism does not have a characteristic sign, physicians must use laboratory tests to determine the pathogen involved. Diagnosis of the disease relies on identifying the causative pathogen by microscopic examination of a specimen of infected tissue or body fluid, by growing the microorganism using culture techniques, or by detecting antibodies in the blood that have developed against the pathogen.

Once the physician determines what type of microorganism has caused the infection, he or she will have to determine the best treatment to eradicate the disease. Drug therapy usually consists of antibiotics and other antimicrobial agents. The selection of the appropriate drug is important, as certain pathogens are susceptible only to certain antibiotics. Unfortunately, few effective antiviral drugs are available for many infectious viruses. In these cases, drugs can be used to treat symptoms such as fever, pain, diarrhea, and vomiting rather than to destroy the virus.

Anti-infective drugs are commonly used by physicians to treat infections. Agents that kill or inhibit the growth of bacteria are known as antibiotics and can be applied directly to the site of infection (topical), given by mouth (oral), or injected. The latter two modes of administration allow the drug to be carried throughout the body by way of the blood. Some antibiotic drugs are effective against only certain strains of infectious bacteria. Antibiotics that act against several types of bacteria are referred to as broad-spectrum antibiotics. Some bacteria develop resistance to a particular antibiotic and require that the physician switch agents or use a combination of antibiotics. Antibiotic therapy for the treatment of infections should be used when the body has been invaded by harmful bacteria, when the bacteria are reproducing at a more rapid rate than the immune system can handle, or to prevent infections in individuals with an impaired immune system.

Some serious common bacterial infections include gonorrhea, which is sexually transmitted and treatable with penicillin; bacterial meningitis, which causes inflammation of the coverings around the brain and is treatable with a variety of antibiotics; pertussis (or whooping cough), which is transmitted by water droplets in air and treatable with erythromycin; pneumonia, which causes shortness of breath, is transmitted via the air, and can be treated with antibiotics; tuberculosis, which infects the lungs and is treatable with various antibiotics; and salmonella (or typhoid fever), which is transmitted in food or water contaminated with fecal material, causes fever, headaches, and digestive problems, and is treated with antibiotics. It should be noted that antibiotics are not effective in viral infections; only bacterial infections are treated with antibiotics.

Antiviral drugs such as acyclovir, amantadine, and zidovudine (formerly known as azidothymide, or AZT) are used in the treatment of infection by a virus. These drugs have been difficult to develop. Most viruses live within the cells of the patient, and the drug must in some way kill the virus without harming the host cells. In fact, antiviral agents cannot completely cure an illness, and infected patients often experience recurrent disease. Nevertheless, they do reduce the severity of these infections.

There are several common viral infections. Human immunodeficiency virus (HIV) infection, which causes acquired immunodeficiency syndrome (AIDS), is transmitted by sexual contact or contaminated needles or blood products; it is often treated with zidovudine but remains lethal. Chickenpox (varicella-zoster virus), which is transmitted by airborne droplets or direct contact, is treated with acyclovir. The common cold is caused by numerous viruses that are transmitted by direct contact or air droplets and has no effective treatment other than drugs that reduce the symptoms. Hepatitis is transmitted by contaminated food, sexual contact, and blood; it causes flulike symptoms and jaundice (a yellow tinge to the skin caused by liver problems) and may be helped with the drug interferon. Influenza viruses ("the flu") are transmitted by airborne droplets; the only treatment for the flu is of its symptoms. Measles is transmitted by virus-containing water droplets and causes fever and a rash; treatment consists of alleviating the symptoms. Mononucleosis is transmitted via saliva and causes swollen lymph nodes, fever, a sore throat, and generalized tiredness; a patient with mononucleosis can only receive treatment for the symptoms, as no cure is available. Poliomyelitis (polio) is transmitted by fecally contaminated material or airborne droplets and can eventually cause paralysis; no treatment is available. Rabies is caused by a bite from an infected animal, as the virus is present in the saliva; the major symptoms include fever, tiredness, and spasms of the throat, and there is no effective treatment for rabies after these symptoms have appeared. Rubella is transmitted by virus-containing air droplets and is associated with a fever and rash; there is no treatment other than for the symptoms.

A major problem with infectious diseases is that there is almost always lag time between when the microorganism has entered the body and the onset of signs and symptoms. This gap may last from a few hours or days to several years. A patient without noticeable symptoms is likely to spread the pathogen. Thus a cycle is set up in which individuals unknowingly infect others who, in turn, pass on the disease-causing agent. Large numbers of people can quickly become infected.

One way to prevent the spread of infectious agents is to vaccinate patients. Diseases such as diphtheria, measles, mumps, rubella, poliomyelitis, and pertussis are rare in the United States because of an aggressive immunization program. When a patient is vaccinated, the vaccine usually contains a dead or inactive pathogen. After the vaccine is administered (usually by injection), the immune system responds by making antibodies against the antigens on the microorganism. Since the pathogen in the vaccine is unable to cause disease, the patient has no symptoms after immunization. The next time that the person is exposed to the infectious agent, his or her immune system is prepared to fight it before symptoms become evident.

In addition to immunization to prevent infection, individuals can largely avoid serious infectious diseases through good hygiene with respect to food and drink, frequent washing, the avoidance of contact with fecal material and urine, and the avoidance of contact with individuals who are infected and capable of transmitting the disease. When such avoidance is impractical, other protective measures can be taken.

Sexually transmitted diseases are usually preventable by using barrier contraceptives and practicing "safe sex." The most common of these diseases include chlamydial infections, trichomoniasis, genital herpes, and HIV infections. Prevention is particularly important in the viral infections of herpes and HIV, as there are no known cures.

Some infections can be acquired at birth, including gonorrhea, genital herpes, chlamydial infections, and salmonella. These microorganisms exist in the birth canal, and some infectious agents can even pass from the mother to the fetus via the placenta. The more serious infections transmitted in this manner are rubella, syphilis, toxoplasmosis, HIV, and the cytomegalovirus. The risk of transmitting these infections can be reduced by treating the mother before delivery or performing a cesarean section (surgical delivery from the uterus), thereby avoiding the birth canal.

PERSPECTIVE AND PROSPECTS

The ancient Egyptians were probably the first to recognize infection and the body's response to the introduction of a disease-causing microorganism: Some hiero-

glyphics appear to represent the inflammatory process. Sometime in the fifth century B.C.E., the Greeks noted that patients who had acquired an infectious disease and survived did not usually contract the same illness a second time.

More solid scientific evidence about infections was provided in the nineteenth century by Edward Jenner, an English physician and scientist. Jenner was able to document that milkmaids seemed to be protected against smallpox because of their exposure to cowpox. With this knowledge, he vaccinated a boy with material from a cowpox pustule. The boy had a typical inflammatory response, and he showed no symptoms of smallpox after being injected with the disease a few months later. His immune system protected him from the virus. Since that time, scientists have reached a much better understanding of how the body deals with infection.

Many scientists are focusing their attention on how pathogens are transmitted from the source of infection to susceptible individuals. Epidemiology is the study of the distribution and causes of diseases that are prevalent in humans. Since some infectious diseases are communicable (transmittable), epidemiologists gather data when an outbreak occurs in a population. These data include the source of infectious agents (the tissues involved), the microorganisms causing the disease, and the method by which the pathogens are transmitted from one person to another. Physicians and other health care workers help in the battle against infections by identifying susceptible individuals; developing and evaluating sources, methods, and ways to control the spread of the pathogens; and improving preventive measures, which usually include extensive educational efforts for the general population. With this knowledge, scientists and physicians attempt to eradicate the disease.

While scientists and physicians have made great advances in the understanding of infection, many problems remain. The spread of certain diseases, such as sexually transmitted diseases, is difficult to control except by modifying human behavior. The most difficult to treat are viral illnesses in which the drugs that are used are ineffective in completely eradicating the virus, and bacterial diseases in which the bacteria have developed drug resistance. Because these microorganisms evolve rapidly, new strains continually emerge. When a new infectious agent develops, it is often years before scientists can devise an effective drug or vaccine to treat the disease. In the meantime, large numbers of patients may become ill and even die. Perhaps the most effective way to combat infection is to use preventive measures whenever practical.

—*Matthew Berria, Ph.D.*

See also Bacterial infections; Bites and stings; Childhood infectious diseases; Disease; Ear infections and disorders; Eye infections and disorders; Fever; Fungal infections; Iatrogenic disorders; Inflammation; Insect-borne diseases; Lice, mites, and ticks; Parasitic diseases; Prion diseases; Staphylococcal infections; Streptococcal infections; Viral infections; Zoonoses; *specific diseases.*

FOR FURTHER INFORMATION:

Biddle, Wayne. *A Field Guide to Germs.* 2d ed. New York: Anchor Books, 2002. This comprehensive book is easily accessible to the nonspecialist and includes a discussion of nearly every virus, bacterium, and fungus known to cause human and nonhuman animal disease. The history of the microbe and the treatment of diseases are included.

Frank, Steven A. *Immunology and Evolution of Infectious Disease.* Princeton, N.J.: Princeton University Press, 2002. Blends research from molecular biology, immunology, pathogen biology, and population dynamics to discuss how and why parasites vary to escape recognition by the immune system, vaccine design, and the control of epidemics.

Gorbach, Sherwood L., John G. Bartlett, and Neil R. Blacklow, eds. *Infectious Diseases.* 3d ed. Philadelphia: W. B. Saunders, 2003. A thorough discussion of infectious diseases. Included is a brief history, an account of the mechanisms of disease and immunity, and a concise discussion of a broad range of infectious agents.

Leikin, Jerrold B., and Martin S. Lipsky, eds. *American Medical Association Complete Medical Encyclopedia.* New York: Random House Reference, 2003. Covers, in alphabetical order, medical terms, diseases, and medical procedures. Lists all major infectious illnesses, with their causes and treatments. Does an excellent job of explaining rather complex medical subjects for a nonprofessional audience.

Merrill, Ray M., and Thomas C. Timmreck. *Introduction to Epidemiology.* 4th ed. Sudbury, Mass.: Jones and Bartlett, 2006. A book in the Jones and Bartlett series in health sciences. Discusses epidemiological methods. Includes a bibliography and an index.

Shaw, Michael, ed. *Everything You Need to Know About Diseases.* Springhouse, Pa.: Springhouse Press, 1996. This well-illustrated consumer reference, compiled by more than one hundred doctors and medical experts, describes five hundred illnesses and conditions, their causes, symptoms, diagnosis, treatment, and prevention. A valuable reference book for everyone interested in health and disease. Of particular interest is chapter 19, "Infection."

Sompayrac, Lauren. *How Pathogenic Viruses Work.* Sudbury, Mass.: Jones and Bartlett, 2002. Engaging exploration of the basics of virology. The author uses twelve of the most common viral infections to demonstrate how viruses "devise" various solutions to stay alive.

Wilson, Michael, Brian Henderson, and Rod McNab. *Bacterial Virulence Mechanisms.* New York: Cambridge University Press, 2002. Basing their discussion on research advances in microbiology, molecular biology, and cell biology, the authors describe the interactions that exist between bacteria and human cells both in health and during infection.

INFERTILITY, FEMALE
DISEASE/DISORDER

ANATOMY OR SYSTEM AFFECTED: Genitals, reproductive system, uterus

SPECIALTIES AND RELATED FIELDS: Endocrinology, gynecology

DEFINITION: The inability to achieve a desired pregnancy as a result of dysfunction of female reproductive organs.

KEY TERMS:

cervix: the bottom portion of the uterus, protruding into the vagina; the cervical canal, an opening in the cervix, allows sperm to pass from the vagina into the uterus

endometriosis: a disease in which patches of the uterine lining, the endometrium, implant on or in other organs

follicles: spherical structures in the ovary that contain the maturing ova (eggs)

hormone: a chemical signal that serves to coordinate the functions of different body parts; the hormones important in female reproduction are produced by the brain, the pituitary, and the ovaries

implantation: the process in which the early embryo attaches to the uterine lining; a critical event in pregnancy

ovaries: the pair of structures in the female that produce ova (eggs) and hormones *oviducts:* the pair of tubes leading from the top of the uterus upward toward the ovaries; also called the Fallopian tubes

ovulation: the process in which an ovum is released from its follicle in the ovary; ovulation must occur for conception to be possible

pelvic inflammatory disease: a general term that refers to a state of inflammation and infection in the pelvic organs; may be caused by a sexually transmitted disease

uterus: the organ in which the embryo implants and grows

vagina: the tube-shaped organ that serves as the site for sperm deposition during intercourse

CAUSES AND SYMPTOMS

Infertility is defined as the failure of a couple to conceive a child despite regular sexual activity over a period of at least one year. Studies have estimated that in the United States 10 percent to 15 percent of couples are infertile. In about half of these couples, it is the woman who is affected.

The causes of female infertility are centered in the reproductive organs: the ovaries, oviducts, uterus, cervix, and vagina. The frequency of specific problems among infertile women is as follows: ovarian problems, 20 percent to 30 percent; damage to the oviducts, 30 percent to 50 percent; uterine problems, 5 percent to 10 percent; and cervical or vaginal abnormalities, 5 percent to 10 percent. Another 10 percent of women have unexplained infertility.

The ovaries have two important roles in conception: the production of ova, culminating in ovulation, and the production of hormones. Ovulation usually occurs halfway through a woman's four-week menstrual cycle. In the two weeks preceding ovulation, follicle-stimulating hormone (FSH) from the pituitary gland causes follicles in the ovaries to grow and the ova within them to mature. As the follicles grow, they produce increasing amounts of estrogen. Near the middle of the cycle, the estrogen causes the pituitary gland to release a surge of luteinizing hormone (LH), which causes ovulation of the largest follicle in the ovary.

Anovulation (lack of ovulation) can result either directly—from an inability to produce LH, FSH, or estrogen—or indirectly—because of the presence of other hormones that interfere with the signaling systems between the pituitary and ovaries. For example, the woman may have an excess production of androgen (testosterone-like) hormones, either in her ovaries or in her adrenal glands, or her pituitary may produce too much prolactin, a hormone that is normally secreted in large amounts only after the birth of a child.

Besides ovulation, the ovaries have another critical role in conception since they produce hormones that act on the uterus to allow it to support an embryo. In the first two weeks of the menstrual cycle, the uterine lining is prepared for a possible pregnancy by estrogen from the ovaries. Following ovulation, the uterus is maintained in a state that can support an embryo by progesterone, which is produced in the ovary by the follicle that just ovulated, now called a corpus luteum. Because of the effects of hormones from the corpus luteum on the uterus, the corpus luteum is essential to the survival of the embryo. If conception does not occur, the corpus luteum disintegrates and stops producing progesterone. As progesterone levels decline, the uterine lining can no longer be maintained and is shed as the menstrual flow.

Failure of the pregnancy can result from improper function of the corpus luteum, such as an inability to produce enough progesterone to sustain the uterine lining. The corpus luteum may also produce progesterone initially but then disintegrate too early. These problems in corpus luteum function, referred to as luteal phase insufficiency, may be caused by the same types of hormonal abnormalities that cause lack of ovulation.

Some cases of infertility may be associated with an abnormally shaped uterus or vagina. Such malformations of the reproductive organs are common in women whose mothers took diethylstilbestrol (DES) during pregnancy. DES was prescribed to many pregnant women from 1941 to about 1970 as a protection against miscarriage; infertility and other problems occurred in the offspring of these women.

INFORMATION ON FEMALE INFERTILITY

CAUSES: Endometriosis, cervical problems, anovulation, hormonal imbalance, abnormally shaped uterus or vagina, pelvic inflammatory disease

SYMPTOMS: Often asymptomatic; can include lack of menstrual periods, blocked Fallopian tubes, abdominal pain with endometriosis

DURATION: Short-term to chronic

TREATMENTS: Fertility drugs, surgery, fertility procedures (*e.g.*, in vitro fertilization)

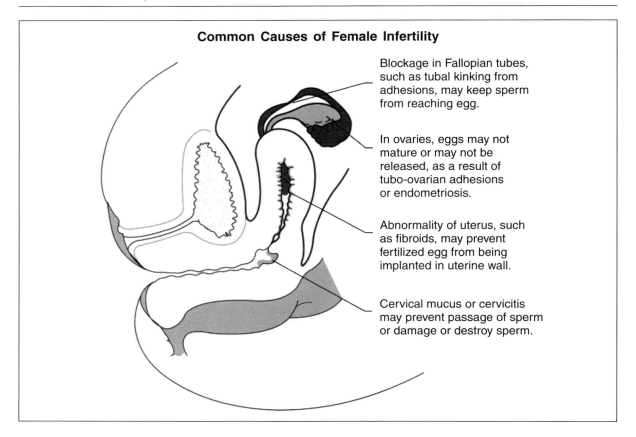

Common Causes of Female Infertility

Blockage in Fallopian tubes, such as tubal kinking from adhesions, may keep sperm from reaching egg.

In ovaries, eggs may not mature or may not be released, as a result of tubo-ovarian adhesions or endometriosis.

Abnormality of uterus, such as fibroids, may prevent fertilized egg from being implanted in uterine wall.

Cervical mucus or cervicitis may prevent passage of sperm or damage or destroy sperm.

Conception depends on normal function of the oviducts (or Fallopian tubes), thin tubes with an inner diameter of only a few millimeters; they are attached to the top of the uterus and curve upward toward the ovaries. The inner end of each tube, located near one of the ovaries, waves back and forth at the time of ovulation, drawing the mature ovum into the opening of the oviduct. Once in the oviduct, the ovum is propelled along by movements of the oviduct wall. Meanwhile, if intercourse has occurred recently, the man's sperm will be moving upward in the female system, swimming through the uterus and the oviducts. Fertilization, the union of the sperm and ovum, will occur in the oviduct, and then the fertilized ovum will pass down the oviduct and reach the uterus about three days after ovulation.

Infertility can result from scar tissue formation inside the oviduct, resulting in physical blockage and inability to transport the ovum, sperm, or both. The most common cause of scar tissue formation in the reproductive organs is pelvic inflammatory disease (PID), a condition characterized by inflammation that spreads throughout the female reproductive tract. PID may be initiated by a sexually transmitted disease such as gon-orrhea or chlamydia. Physicians in the United States have documented an increase in infertility attributable to tubal damage caused by sexually transmitted diseases.

Damage to the outside of the oviduct can also cause infertility, because such damage can interfere with the mobility of the oviduct, which is necessary to the capture of the ovum at the time of ovulation. External damage to the oviduct may occur as an aftermath of abdominal surgery, when adhesions induced by surgical cutting are likely to form. An adhesion is an abnormal scar tissue connection between adjacent structures.

Another possible cause of damage to the oviduct, resulting in infertility, is the presence of endometriosis. Endometriosis refers to a condition in which patches of the uterine lining implant in or on the surface of other organs. These patches are thought to arise during menstruation, when the uterine lining (endometrium) is normally shed from the body through the cervix and vagina; in a woman with endometriosis, for unknown reasons, the endometrium is carried to the interior of the pelvic cavity by passing up the oviducts. The endometrial patches can lodge in the oviduct itself, causing blockage, or can adhere to the outer surface of the oviducts, interfering with mobility.

Endometriosis can cause infertility by interfering with organs other than the oviducts. Endometrial patches on the outside of the uterus can cause distortions in the shape or placement of the uterus, interfering with embryonic implantation. Ovulation may be prevented by the presence of the endometrial tissues on the surface of the ovary. Yet the presence of endometriosis is not always associated with infertility. Thirty percent to forty percent of women with endometriosis cannot conceive, but the remainder appear to be fertile.

Another critical site in conception is the cervix. The cervix, the entryway to the uterus from the vagina, represents the first barrier through which sperm must pass on their way to the ovum. The cervix consists of a ring of strong, elastic tissue with a narrow canal. Glands in the cervix produce the mucus that fills the cervical canal and through which sperm swim en route to the ovum. The amount and quality of the cervical mucus change throughout the menstrual cycle, under the influence of hormones from the ovary. At ovulation, the mucus is in a state that is most easily penetrated by sperm; after ovulation, the mucus becomes almost impenetrable.

Cervical problems that can lead to infertility include production of a mucus that does not allow sperm passage at the time of ovulation (hostile mucus syndrome) and interference with sperm transport caused by narrowing of the cervical canal. Such narrowing may be the result of a developmental abnormality or the presence of an infection, possibly a sexually transmitted disease.

TREATMENT AND THERAPY

The diagnosis of the exact cause of a woman's infertility is crucial to successful treatment. A complete medical history should reveal any obvious problems of previous infection or menstrual cycle irregularity. Adequacy of ovulation and luteal phase function can be determined from records of menstrual cycle length and changes in body temperature (body temperature is higher after ovulation). Hormone levels can be measured with tests of blood or urine samples. If damage to the oviducts or uterus is suspected, hysterosalpingography will be performed. In this procedure, the injection of a special fluid into the uterus is followed by X-ray analysis of the fluid movement; the shape of the uterine cavity and the oviducts will be revealed. Cervical functioning can be assessed with the postcoital test,

in which the physician attempts to recover sperm from the woman's uterus some hours after she has had intercourse with her partner. If a uterine problem is suspected, the woman may have an endometrial biopsy, in which a small sample of the uterine lining is removed and examined for abnormalities. Sometimes, exploratory surgery is performed to pinpoint the location of scar tissue or the location of endometriosis patches.

Surgery may be used for treatment as well as diagnosis. Damage to the oviducts can sometimes be repaired surgically, and surgical removal of endometrial patches is a standard treatment for endometriosis. Often, however, surgery is a last resort, because of the likelihood of the development of postsurgical adhesions, which can further complicate the infertility. Newer forms of surgery using lasers and freezing offer better success because of a reduced risk of adhesions.

Some women with hormonal difficulties can be treated successfully with so-called fertility drugs. There are actually several different drugs and hormones that fall under this heading: Clomiphene citrate (Clomid), human menopausal gonadotropin (HMG), gonadotropin-releasing hormone (GnRH), bromocriptine mesylate (Parlodel), and menotropins (Pergonal) are commonly used, with the exact choice depending on the woman's particular problem. The pregnancy rate with fertility drug treatment varies from 20 percent to 70 percent. One problem with some of the drugs is the risk of multiple pregnancy (more than one fetus in the uterus). Hyperstimulation of the ovaries, a condition characterized by enlarged ovaries, can be fatal as a result of severe hormone imbalances. Other possible problems include nausea, dizziness, headache, and general malaise.

Artificial insemination is an old technique that is still useful in various types of infertility. A previously collected sperm sample is placed in the woman's vagina or uterus using a special tube. Artificial insemination is always performed at the time of ovulation, in order to maximize the chance of pregnancy. The ovulation date can be determined with body temperature records or by hormone measurements. In some cases, this procedure is combined with fertility drug treatment. Since the sperm can be placed directly in the uterus, it is useful in treating hostile mucus syndrome and certain types of male infertility. The sperm sample can be provided either by the woman's partner or by a donor. The pregnancy rate after artificial insemination is highly variable (14 percent to 68 percent), depending on the particular infertility problem in the couple. There is a slight risk of infection, and, if donated semen is used, there may be no guarantee that the semen is free from sexually transmitted diseases or that the donor does not carry some genetic defect.

Another infertility treatment is gamete intrafallopian transfer (GIFT), the surgical placement of ova and sperm directly into the woman's oviducts. In order to be a candidate for this procedure, the woman must have at least one partially undamaged oviduct and a functional uterus. Ova are collected surgically from the ovaries after stimulation with a fertility drug, and a semen sample is collected from the male. The ova and the sperm are introduced into the oviducts through the same abdominal incision used to collect the ova. This procedure is useful in certain types of male infertility, if the woman produces an impenetrable cervical mucus, or if the ovarian ends of the oviducts are damaged. The range of infertility problems that may be resolved with GIFT can be extended by using donated ova or sperm. The success rate is about 33 percent overall, but the rate varies with the type of infertility present.

In vitro fertilization is known colloquially as the "test-tube baby" technique. In this procedure, ova are collected surgically after stimulation with fertility drugs and then placed in a laboratory dish and combined with sperm from the man. The actual fertilization, when a sperm penetrates the ovum, will occur in the dish. The resulting embryo is allowed to remain in the dish for two days, during which time it will have acquired two to four cells. Then, the embryo is placed in the woman's uterine cavity using a flexible tube. In vitro fertilization can be used in women who are infertile because of endometriosis, damaged oviducts, impenetrable cervical mucus, or ovarian failure. As with GIFT, in vitro fertilization may utilize either donated ova or donated sperm, or extra embryos that have been produced by one couple may be implanted in a second woman. The pregnancy rate with this procedure varies from 15 percent to 25 percent.

Embryo freezing is a secondary procedure that can increase the chances of pregnancy for an infertile couple. When ova are collected for the in vitro fertilization procedure, doctors try to collect as many as possible. All these ova are then combined with sperm for fertilization. No more than three or four embryos are ever placed in the woman's uterus, however, because a pregnancy with a large number of fetuses carries significant health risks. The extra embryos can be frozen for later use, if the first ones implanted in the uterus do not survive. This spares the woman additional surgery to collect more ova if they are needed. The freezing technique does not appear to cause any defects in the embryo.

Some women may benefit from nonsurgical embryo transfer. In this procedure, a fertile woman is artificially inseminated at the time of her ovulation; five days later, her uterus is flushed with a sterile solution, washing out the resulting embryo before it implants in the uterus. The retrieved embryo is then transferred to the uterus of another woman, who will carry it to term. Typically, the sperm provider and the woman who receives the embryo are the infertile couple who wish to rear the child, but the technique can be used in other circumstances as well. Embryo transfer can be used if the woman has damaged oviducts or is unable to ovulate, or if she has a genetic disease that could be passed to her offspring, because in this case the baby is not genetically related to the woman who carries it.

Some infertile women who are unable to achieve a pregnancy themselves turn to the use of a surrogate, a woman who will agree to bear a child and then turn it over to the infertile woman to rear as her own. In the typical situation, the surrogate is artificially inseminated with the sperm of the infertile woman's husband. The surrogate then proceeds with pregnancy and delivery as normal, but relinquishes the child to the infertile couple after its birth.

In Western societies, couples are often advised to seek fertility treatment if one year of unprotected sexual intercourse has failed to produce a pregnancy. However, in 2002, the findings of a study conducted in Europe noted that even couples in their late thirties have a 91 percent chance of getting pregnant naturally within two years. This finding led some doctors to suggest healthy younger couples—women who do not experience menstrual abnormalities or men who have appropriate sperm counts, for example—wait two years before consulting fertility specialists.

PERSPECTIVE AND PROSPECTS

One of the biggest problems that infertile couples face is the emotional upheaval that comes with the diagnosis of the infertility. Bearing and rearing children is an experience that most women treasure. When a woman is told that she is infertile, she may feel that her femininity and self-worth are diminished. In addition to the emotional difficulty that may come with the recognition of infertility, more stress may be in store as the couple proceeds through treatment. The various treatments can cause embarrassment and sometimes physical pain, and fertility drugs themselves are known to cause emotional swings. For these reasons, a couple with an infertility problem is often advised to seek help from a private counselor or a support group.

Along with the emotional and physical trauma of infertility treatment, there is a considerable financial burden as well. Infertility treatments, in general, are very expensive, especially the more sophisticated procedures such as in vitro fertilization and GIFT. Since the chances of a single procedure resulting in a pregnancy are often low, the couple may be faced with submitting to multiple procedures repeated many times. The cost over several years of treatment—a realistic possibility—can be staggering. Many health insurance companies in the United States refuse to cover the costs of such treatment and are required to do so in only a few states.

Some of the treatments are accompanied by unresolved legal questions. In the case of nonsurgical embryo transfer, is the legal mother of the child the ovum donor or the woman who gives birth to the child? The same question of legal parentage arises in cases of surrogacy. Does a child born using donated ovum or sperm have a legal right to any information about the donor, such as medical history? How extensive should governmental regulation of infertility clinics be? For example, should there be standards for ensuring that donated sperm or ova are free from genetic defects? In the United States, some states have begun to address these issues, but no uniform policies have been set at the federal level.

The legal questions are largely unresolved because American society is still involved in religious and philosophical debates over the proprieties of various infertility treatments. Some religions hold that any interference in conception is unacceptable. To these denominations, even artificial insemination is wrong. Other groups approve of treatments confined to a husband and wife, but disapprove of a third party being involved as a donor or surrogate. Many people disapprove of any infertility treatment to help an individual who is not married. The basic problem underlying all these issues is that these technologies challenge the traditional definitions of parenthood.

—*Marcia Watson-Whitmyre, Ph.D.*

See also Assisted reproductive technologies; Conception; Contraception; Ectopic pregnancy; Endocrinology; Endometriosis; Gamete intrafallopian transfer (GIFT); Gynecology; Hormones; Hysterectomy; In vitro fertilization; Infertility, male; Menopause; Menstruation; Miscarriage; Obstetrics; Ovarian cysts; Pelvic inflammatory disease (PID); Pregnancy and gestation; Sexual dysfunction; Sperm banks; Sterilization; Stress; Tubal ligation; Women's health.

FOR FURTHER INFORMATION:

Berger, Gary S., Mark Fuerst, and Marc Goldstein. *The Couple's Guide to Fertility.* 3d ed. New York: Broadway Books, 2001. Surveys fertility treatment options, including hormone therapies, surgery, in vitro fertilization, sperm injection, egg and sperm donors, adoption, surrogate motherhood, and alternative therapies.

Harkness, Carla. *The Infertility Book: A Comprehensive Medical and Emotional Guide.* Rev. ed. Berkeley, Calif.: Celestial Arts, 1996. Written as a guide for the infertile couple, this book offers emotional support as well as medical information. The text is augmented by firsthand accounts of individuals' reactions to their infertility and the treatments.

InterNational Council on Infertility Information Dissemination. http://www.inciid.org/. INCIID's mission is to provide online resources of comprehensive, consumer-targeted infertility information that cover cutting-edge technologies and treatments. Provides fact sheets of treatments, an interactive area for member participation, library and glossary, and a comprehensive professional directory of clinics and doctors who specialize in infertility.

Phillips, Robert H., and Glenda Motta. *Coping with Endometriosis: A Practical Guide to Understanding, Treating and Living with Chronic Endometriosis.* New York: Putnam, 2000. Educates the reader on current research and addresses the psychological and emotional concerns brought on by a diagnosis.

Quilligan, Edward J., and Frederick P. Zuspan, eds. *Current Therapy in Obstetrics and Gynecology.* 5th ed. Philadelphia: Saunders, 2000. This excellent handbook provides detailed information on procedures for various infertility causes and treatments, arranged alphabetically amid other gynecological subjects.

Speroff, Leon, and Marc A. Fritz. *Clinical Gynecologic Endocrinology and Infertility.* 7th ed. Philadelphia: Lippincott Williams & Wilkins, 2005. A good basic textbook that can help the reader understand the normal functioning of the female reproductive system and the events associated with infertility.

Turkington, Carol, and Michael M. Alper. *Encyclopedia of Fertility and Infertility.* New York: Facts On

File, 2001. Offers a wide range of information on infertility for the general reader, including causes and remedies, treatment options, medical advances, and birth control techniques. Appendixes give resources for further information and support from organizations, periodicals and Web sites, and fertility clinics.

Weschler, Toni. *Taking Charge of Your Fertility.* Rev. ed. New York: HarperCollins, 2001. This book encourages women to become responsible consumers of their own reproductive health. Includes excellent discussions of infertility, natural birth control, and achieving pregnancy.

Wisot, Arthur L., and David R. Meldrum. *Conceptions and Misconceptions: The Informed Consumer's Guide Through the Maze of In Vitro Fertilization and Other Assisted Reproduction Techniques.* 2d ed. Point Roberts, Wash.: Hartley & Marks, 2004. Written by two leading fertility experts, this book is an excellent guide through the maze of in vitro fertilization and other assisted reproductive techniques. Includes an excellent discussion of the basic physiology of conception and reproduction.

Zouves, Christo. *Expecting Miracles: On the Path of Hope from Infertility to Parenthood.* New York: Berkley, 2003. Provides the human side of reproductive medicine by telling several personal stories and giving an in-depth look at the options, decisions, and unexpected twists, turns, and disappointments that infertile couples experience.

INFERTILITY, MALE
DISEASE/DISORDER

ANATOMY OR SYSTEM AFFECTED: Genitals, reproductive system

SPECIALTIES AND RELATED FIELDS: Endocrinology, urology

DEFINITION: The inability to achieve a desired pregnancy as a result of dysfunction of male reproductive organs.

KEY TERMS:

antibody: a chemical produced by lymphocytes (blood cells) that enables these cells to destroy foreign materials, such as bacteria

cryopreservation: a special process utilizing cryoprotectants that enables living cells to survive in a frozen state

cryoprotectant: one of several chemicals that enables living cells to survive in a frozen state; some cryoprotectants are made by animals that survive freezing

epididymis: an organ attached to the testis in which

INFORMATION ON MALE INFERTILITY

CAUSES: Low sperm count, infection, blockage of sperm ducts (from swollen tissue or tumor), premature release of sperm from epididymis, improper scrotal temperature, varicoceles

SYMPTOMS: Typically asymptomatic

DURATION: Short-term to chronic

TREATMENTS: Surgery, hormonal therapy, fertility procedures (*e.g.*, artificial insemination)

---

newly formed sperm reach maturity (that is, become capable of fertilizing an egg)

infertility: the inability to produce a normal pregnancy after one to two years of intercourse in the absence of any contraception; it may be caused by male and/or female factors

insemination: the placement of semen in the female reproductive tract, which may occur naturally as a result of sexual intercourse or artificially as a result of a medical procedure

testis: either of two male gonads that are suspended in the scrotum and produce sperm

varicocele: a swollen testicular vein in the scrotum occurring as a result of improper valvular function

CAUSES AND SYMPTOMS

To create a baby requires three things: normal sperm from a man, a normal egg from a woman, and a normal, mature uterus. Anything that blocks the availability of the sperm, egg, or uterus can cause infertility. Infertility can be thought of as an abnormal, unwanted form of contraception.

Many different factors may be responsible for infertility. In general, these factors may be infectious, chemical (from inside or outside the body, such as pharmaceuticals, toxins, or illegal drugs), or anatomical. Genetic factors may be responsible as well, since genes control the formation of body chemicals (such as hormones and antibodies) and body structures (one's anatomy). The way that these factors work is illustrated by male infertility.

The process by which sperm are made begins in a man's testis (or testicle). Because the transformation of testis cells into sperm is controlled by genes and hormones, abnormalities can cause infertility. Sperm released from the testis become mature in the epididymis. Sperm travel from the testis to the epididymis through ducts (tubes) in the male reproductive tract. A blockage of these ducts or premature release of sperm from the epididymis can cause infertility.

A blockage of reproductive ducts can occur as a result of a bodily enlargement, such as swollen tissue, a tumor, or cancer. An infection usually causes tissue swelling and can leave ducts permanently scarred, narrowed, or blocked. Infection can have a direct detrimental effect on the production of normal sperm. Cancer and the drugs or chemicals used to treat cancer can also damage a man's reproductive tract.

Another factor that may be important to male fertility is scrotal temperature. The temperature in the scrotum, the sac that holds the testes, is somewhat cooler than body temperature. The normal production of sperm seems to be dependent upon a cool testicular environment.

The leading cause of male infertility may be varicoceles, which occur when one-way valves fail in the veins that take blood away from the testicles. When these venous valves become leaky, blood flow becomes sluggish and causes the veins to swell. Many men with varicoceles are infertile, but the exact reason for this association is unknown. The reasons sometimes given are increased scrotal temperature and improper removal of materials (hormones) from the testis.

Mature sperm capable of fertilizing an egg are normally placed in the female reproductive tract by the ejaculation phase of sexual intercourse. The sperm are accompanied by fluid called seminal plasma; together, they form semen. A blockage of the ducts that transport the semen into the woman or toxic chemicals, including antibodies, in the semen can cause infertility.

For conception to take place—that is, for an egg to be fertilized after sperm enters the female tract—a normal egg must be present in the portion of the tract called the Fallopian tube, and sperm must move through the female tract to that egg. If the egg is absent or is abnormal, or if normal sperm cannot reach the egg, female infertility will result. The female factors that determine whether sperm fertilize an egg are the same as the male factors: anatomy, chemicals, infection, and genes.

In Western societies, couples are often advised to seek fertility treatment if one year of unprotected sexual intercourse has failed to produce a pregnancy. However, in 2002, the findings of a study conducted in Europe noted that even couples in their late thirties have a 91 percent chance of getting pregnant naturally within two years. This finding led some doctors to suggest healthy younger couples—women who do not ex-

perience menstrual abnormalities or men who have appropriate sperm counts, for example—wait two years before consulting fertility specialists.

For those that seek help with fertility issues, there are many methods available. Female infertility may be treated, depending upon the cause, by surgery, hormone therapy, or in vitro fertilization. Treatment of male infertility may be by surgery, hormone therapy, or therapeutic (artificial) insemination. Therapeutic insemination is often performed when the couple is composed of a fertile woman and an infertile man.

The first step for therapeutic insemination is for a physician to determine when an egg is ovulated or released into the Fallopian tube of the fertile woman. At the time of ovulation, semen is placed with medical instruments in the woman's reproductive tract, either on her cervix or in her uterus.

The semen used by the physician is obtained through masturbation by either the infertile man (the patient) or a fertile man (a donor), depending on the cause of the man's infertility. The freshly produced semen from either source usually undergoes laboratory testing and processing. Tests are used to evaluate the sperm quality. An effort may be made to enhance the sperm from an infertile patient and then to use these sperm for therapeutic insemination or in vitro fertilization. Other tests evaluate semen for transmissible diseases. During testing, which may require many days, the sperm can

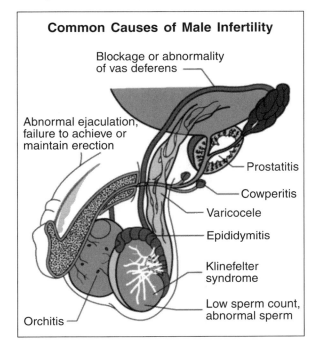

Common Causes of Male Infertility

Blockage or abnormality of vas deferens

Abnormal ejaculation; failure to achieve or maintain erection

Prostatitis

Cowperitis

Varicocele

Epididymitis

Klinefelter syndrome

Low sperm count, abnormal sperm

Orchitis

be kept alive by cryopreservation. Freshly ejaculated sperm remains fertile for only a few hours in the laboratory if it is not cryopreserved.

There are several processes that might enhance sperm from an infertile man. If the semen is infertile because it possesses too few normal sperm, an effort can be made to eliminate the abnormal sperm and to increase the concentration of normal sperm. Sperm may be abnormal in four basic ways: They may have abnormal structure, they may have abnormal movement, they may be incapable of fusing with an egg, or they may contain abnormal genes or chromosomes. Laboratory processes can often eliminate from semen those sperm with abnormal structure or abnormal movement. These processes usually involve replacing the seminal plasma with a culture medium. Removing the seminal plasma gets rid of substances that may be harmful to the sperm. After the plasma is removed, the normal sperm can be collected and concentrated. Pharmacologic agents can be added to the culture medium to increase sperm movement.

Testing for transmissible diseases is especially important if donor semen is used; these diseases may be genetic or infectious. There are many thousand genetic disorders. Most of these disorders are very rare and can be transmitted to offspring only if the sperm and the egg both have the same gene for the disorder. It is impossible, therefore, to test a donor for every possible genetic disorder; he is routinely tested only for a small group of troublesome disorders that are especially likely to occur in offspring. Tests for other disorders that the donor might transmit can be performed at the woman's request, usually based upon knowledge of genetic problems in her own family.

Much of the genetic information about a person is based on family history. Special laboratory procedures allow the genetic code inside individual cells to be interpreted. For this reason, it is important to store a sample of donor cells, not necessarily sperm, for many years after the procedure. These cells provide additional genetic information that might be important to the donor's offspring but not known at the time of insemination.

Semen can also be the source of infectious disease. Syphilis, gonorrhea, and acquired immunodeficiency syndrome (AIDS) are examples of venereal or sexually transmitted diseases (STDs). Tests for STDs can be done on blood and semen from a donor. These tests must be conducted in an approved manner, and the results must be negative before donor semen can be used

therapeutically. In some cases, a test must be repeated in order to verify that the semen is not infectious.

Cryopreservation of sperm is important to therapeutic insemination for two major reasons. First, it gives time to complete all necessary testing. Second, it allows an inventory of sperm from many different donors to be kept constantly available for selection and use by patients. Sperm properly cryopreserved for twenty years, when thawed and inseminated, can produce normal babies.

Cryopreservation involves treating freshly ejaculated sperm with a cryoprotectant pharmaceutical that enables the sperm to survive when frozen; the cryoprotectant for sperm is usually glycerol. Survival of frozen sperm is also dependent upon the rate of cooling, the storage temperature, and the rate of warming at the time of thawing. Sperm treated with a cryoprotectant have the best chance of survival if they are cooled about 1 degree Celsius per minute and stored at a temperature of −150 degrees Celsius or colder. An environment of liquid nitrogen is often used to attain these storage temperatures. The storage temperature must be kept constant to avoid the damaging effects of recrystallization. When sperm are to be thawed, survival is enhanced if they are warmed at 10 to 100 degrees Celsius per minute.

The cryopreservation procedure involves the actual formation of ice, although the ice is confined to the extracellular medium. Intracellular ice is lethal. Ice formation during cryopreservation causes the cells to lose water and to shrink. The cryoprotectant seems to replace intracellular water and thereby maintain cell volume.

An alternative process for low-temperature preservation of sperm is called vitrification. Vitrification uses temperatures as cold as cryopreservation, but it avoids ice formation altogether. Instead of using one cryoprotectant, vitrification uses a mixture of several. It employs a much slower cooling rate and a much faster warming rate. Technically, vitrification is more difficult to perform; therefore, it is seldom used by clinical sperm banks.

Human sperm can be shipped to almost any location for therapeutic insemination. Sperm is usually cryopreserved before shipment and thawed at the time of insemination.

Treatment and Therapy

The use of therapeutic insemination to treat two kinds of male infertility will be considered here. The first example is male infertility that cannot be treated by other means. The second example is a fertile man at high risk for becoming infertile because of his lifestyle or because he is receiving treatment for a life-threatening disease.

The first example might occur when a heterosexual couple, having used no contraception for a year or longer, has been unsuccessful in conceiving a baby. In 40 percent of infertility cases, the woman has the major, but not necessarily the only, problem preventing the pregnancy. In 40 percent of the cases, the man is the major factor. In 20 percent, each person makes a substantial contribution to the problem. Therefore, both partners must deal with the infertility and be involved in the treatment.

The solution to a couple's infertility involves evaluation and therapy. The couple will be evaluated in regard to their present sexual activity and history, such as whether either one has ever contributed to a pregnancy. The medical evaluation of both partners will include a physical examination, laboratory tests, and even imaging techniques such as X rays, ultrasonography, or magnetic resonance imaging (MRI). For the man, the physical examination will include a search for the presence of varicoceles, and the laboratory tests will include a semen analysis. About 15 to 30 percent of couples entering an infertility program achieve pregnancy during the evaluation phase of the program, before any therapy is begun.

Varicoceles are probably the most readily detected problem that may cause male infertility. They are three times more common in infertile men than in men with proved fertility. This association does not prove that varicoceles cause infertility, however, because surgery that corrects a varicocele does not always correct infertility.

If the medical evaluation determines that the female partner has a normal reproductive tract and is ovulating on a regular basis, and if it determines that the male partner has too few normal sperm to make a pregnancy likely, the couple may be asked to consider adopting a baby or undergoing therapeutic insemination. With therapeutic insemination, the woman actually becomes pregnant, and half of the baby's genes come from the mother. The other half of the genes come from the sperm donor, usually a person unknown to the couple. The physician performing therapeutic insemination may provide the couple with extensive information on several possible donors. Such information might include race, ethnic origin, blood type, physical characteristics, results of medical and genetic tests, and personal infor-

mation, but the donor usually remains anonymous. The semen from each donor has undergone laboratory testing and cryopreservation. The frozen semen is thawed at the time of insemination.

Although the idea of therapeutic insemination is simple, it usually involves some very complicated emotions. Although a couple may be very happy about all other aspects of their lives together, they are usually deeply disturbed to learn of the man's infertility. It may be extremely difficult for them to discuss his infertility with anyone else. Some people ridicule infertile men as being less virile or even being impotent. (This is not the case: The majority of infertile or sterile men have normal sex lives.) These feelings will influence the couple's selection of a sperm donor. Later, they must decide whether to tell the child about the circumstances of his or her birth. Sometimes, a child who originated through therapeutic insemination will try to learn the identity of the donor.

The donor must be considered as well. In a typical sperm bank, persons are subjected to a variety of tests before they are accepted as donors. Sperm donors are typically in their second decade of life, but some are older. These men are primarily, but not solely, motivated to be sperm donors by financial compensation. Payment effectively maintains donor cooperation for a period of several years. In addition to payment, the donor usually wants an assurance that he will not be held responsible, financially or legally, for the offspring produced by his semen. As a donor grows older, however, his attitude about his donation may change: He may wonder about the children he has helped to create.

Although male-factor infertility is the situation that benefits most from insemination and semen cryopreservation procedures, these procedures might be requested by a fertile couple that is at risk for male-factor infertility. Such couples may fear that the man's lifestyle, such as working with hazardous materials (solvents, toxins, radioisotopes, or explosives), may endanger his ability to produce sperm or may harm his genetic information. The man could be facing medical therapy that will cure a malignancy, such as Hodgkin's disease or a testicular tumor, but may render him sterile. A man facing such a situation may benefit from having some of his semen cryopreserved for his own future use, in the event that he actually becomes infertile.

Therapeutic insemination with a husband's semen is usually not as effective as with donor semen, especially when cryopreservation is involved. Although cryopreservation keeps cells alive in the frozen state, not all the cells survive. Men selected to be semen donors have sperm that survive freezing much better than the sperm of most men (although the reason for this ability is unknown). If a man undergoing medical treatment is already sick at the time that the decision is made to store his sperm, his concentration of functioning sperm may be less than normal.

There are ways to compensate for decreased semen quality. The semen may be processed in ways to increase the concentration of normal sperm. The processed semen may be placed directly into the woman's uterus (intrauterine insemination) rather than on her cervix, or in vitro fertilization may be used. In this procedure, the sperm and eggs are mixed in a laboratory and the resulting embryo is implanted in the woman. All these techniques have proved helpful to infertile couples wanting children.

PERSPECTIVE AND PROSPECTS

It has been estimated that infertility affects 8 to 15 percent of American marriages, which means that three to nine million American couples would like to, but cannot, have children without medical assistance. By the early 1990's, therapeutic insemination produced more than thirty thousand American babies yearly. This procedure advanced in the United States during the latter half of the twentieth century in large measure because of changes in attitudes, not because of new medical knowledge.

The medical knowledge to treat male infertility has been available for several centuries, even when the biological basis for pregnancy was not understood. The importance of sexual intercourse in reproduction was probably recognized by prehistoric humans. The Bible records stories of patriarchal families that knew the problem of infertility (Abraham and Sarah, Jacob and Rachel) and even indicates, in the story of Onan and Tamar (Genesis 38:9), that semen was understood to be important to reproduction. The possibility of therapeutic insemination was mentioned in the fifth century Talmud. Arabs used insemination in horse breeding as early as the fourteenth century, and Spaniards used it in human medicine during the fifteenth century.

The presence of sperm in semen was first observed by Antoni van Leeuwenhoek in the seventeenth century, but their importance and function in the fertilization process was not recognized until the nineteenth century. In 1824, Jean Louis Prévost and J. A. Dumas correctly guessed the role of sperm in fertilization, and in 1876, Oskar Hertwig and Hermann Fol proved that the union of sperm and egg was necessary to create an embryo.

Therapeutic insemination became an established but clandestine procedure in the late nineteenth century in the United States and England. Compassionate physicians pioneering therapeutic insemination encouraged secrecy to protect the self-esteem of the infertile man, his spouse, the offspring, and the donor. In an uncertain legal climate, the offspring might have been viewed as the illegitimate product of an adulterous act. Even by the beginning of the twenty-first century, many Americans continued to stigmatize masturbation and therapeutic insemination. Social attitudes, especially machismo, have limited the acceptability of therapeutic insemination to many infertile couples worldwide.

Cryopreservation of sperm became practical with the discovery of chemical cryoprotectants, reported in 1949 by Christopher Polge, Audrey Smith, and Alan Parkes of England. In 1953, American doctors R. G. Bunge and Jerome Sherman were the first to use this procedure to produce a human baby. Cryopreservation made possible the establishment of sperm banks; prior to this development, sperm donors had to provide the physician with semen immediately before insemination was to take place.

Recent research has shown a few promising new techniques: intracytoplasmic injection, which involves the placement of sperm into the ovum itself, and electroejaculation, which involves electrical stimulation of the penis to promote ejaculation. Intracytoplasmic injections are useful when the sperm are immotile or the woman's own immune system aggressively rejects the man's sperm. It is not always successful, however, and is affected by age and cycle. Electroejaculation has been successfully used in men with vascular compromise, as might be caused by diabetes mellitus, or with spinal cord injuries. It is also helpful in cases where men are unable to ejaculate for psychological reasons.

Researchers continue to theorize about new fertility-enhancing techniques using sperm. In 2003, scientists discovered that sperm has a type of chemical sensor that causes the sperm to swim vigorously toward concentrations of a chemical attractant. While researchers long have known that chemical signals are an important component of conception, the 2003 findings were the first to demonstrate that sperm will respond in a predictable and controllable way. The findings provided strong evidence that the egg signals its location to the sperm and the sperm responds by swimming toward the egg, a process which could prove promising for future contraception and infertility research. Scientists note that these findings might allow specific tests to be developed to determine if the egg is making the attractant or if the sperm has the receptor, thus helping in identifying those couples who are infertile because of poor signaling between the sperm and egg.

Therapeutic insemination and other alternative means of reproduction give rise to thorny issues of personal rights of various "parents" (social, birth, and genetic) and their offspring. In the United States, a few states have addressed these issues by enacting laws, usually to grant legitimacy to offspring of donor insemination. In the United Kingdom, Parliament established a central registry of sperm and egg donors. Offspring in the United Kingdom have access to nonidentifying donor information; these children are even able to learn whether they are genetically related to a prospective marriage partner.

—Armand M. Karow, Ph.D.;
updated by Paul Moglia, Ph.D.

See also Assisted reproductive technologies; Conception; Gamete intrafallopian transfer (GIFT); Genital disorders, male; In vitro fertilization; Infertility, female; Men's health; Pregnancy and gestation; Reproductive system; Sexual dysfunction; Sperm banks; Sterilization; Stress; Testicular surgery; Vasectomy.

FOR FURTHER INFORMATION:

Baran, Annette, and Reuben Pannor. *Lethal Secrets.* New York: Warner Books, 1993. The authors, medical social workers, discuss possible consequences of secrecy in donor insemination using a series of case histories.

Berger, Gary S., Mark Fuerst, and Marc Goldstein. *The Couple's Guide to Fertility.* 3d ed. New York: Broadway Books, 2001. Surveys fertility treatment options, including hormone therapies, surgery, in vitro fertilization, sperm injection, egg and sperm donors, adoption, surrogate motherhood, and alternative therapies.

Doherty, C. Maud, and Melanie M. Clark. *Fertility Handbook: A Guide to Getting Pregnant.* Omaha, Nebr.: Addicus Books, 2002. The authors, a reproductive endocrinologist and a former infertility patient, combine their experiences to explore current infertility options and treatments. Addresses the causes, getting diagnoses, choosing a fertility specialist, and utilizing new assisted reproductive technology.

Fisch, Harry, and Stephen Braun. *The Male Biological Clock: The Startling News About Aging, Sexuality, and Fertility in Men.* New York: Free Press, 2005. Discusses how testosterone levels decline with age. Also, examines the fertility industry.

Glover, Timothy D., and C. L. R. Barratt, eds. *Male Fertility and Infertility.* New York: Cambridge University Press, 1999. The editors have assembled a collection of essays by experts in the field. Includes bibliographical references and an index.

International Council on Infertility Information Dissemination. http://www.inciid.org/. INCIID's mission is to provide online resources of comprehensive, consumer-targeted infertility information that cover cutting-edge technologies and treatments. Provides fact sheets of treatments, an interactive area for member participation, library and glossary, and a comprehensive professional directory of clinics and doctors who specialize in infertility.

Schover, Leslie R., and Anthony J. Thomas. *Overcoming Male Infertility: Understanding Its Causes and Treatments.* New York: John Wiley & Sons, 2000. Clinical psychologist Schover has long worked with infertile couples, as urologist Thomas has with male infertility. Their combined skills and knowledge make this a valuable book. Patient-oriented, it conveys a vast amount of information understandably and maintains an underlying sense of humor.

Taguchi, Yosh, and Merrily Weisbord, eds. *Private Parts: An Owner's Guide to the Male Anatomy.* 3d ed. Toronto: McClelland & Stewart, 2003. A guide to male genital and sexual health, covering topics such as prostate trouble, erectile dysfunction, infertility, cancer, sexually transmitted diseases, vasectomies, and artificial insemination.

INFLAMMATION

DISEASE/DISORDER

ANATOMY OR SYSTEM AFFECTED: All

SPECIALTIES AND RELATED FIELDS: Family medicine, internal medicine, pathology, rheumatology

DEFINITION: The reaction of blood-filled living tissue to injury.

In inflammation, the following changes are seen locally: redness, swelling, heat, pain, and loss of function. These changes are chemically mediated. Inflammation may be caused by microbial infection; physical agents such as trauma, radiation, and burns; chemical

INFORMATION ON INFLAMMATION

CAUSES: Infection, injury, radiation, burns, chemical toxins, decomposing or necrotic tissue, immune system reactions
SYMPTOMS: Redness, swelling, heat, pain, loss of function
DURATION: Acute to chronic
TREATMENTS: Drug therapy (*e.g.*, antibiotics)

toxins; caustic substances such as strong acids or bases; decomposing or necrotic tissue; and reactions of the immune system. Acute inflammation is of relatively short duration (from a few minutes to a day or so), while chronic inflammation lasts longer. The local changes associated with inflammation include the outflow of fluid into the spaces between cells and the inflow or migration of white blood cells (leukocytes) to the area of injury. Chronic inflammation is characterized by the presence of leukocytes and macrophages, as well as by the proliferation of new blood vessels and connective tissue.

Inflammation is a protective mechanism for the body. Redness is attributable to increased blood flow to the injured area. Swelling is caused by the flow of fluid into the spaces between cells. Heat is produced by a combination of increased blood flow and chemical reactions in the local area. Pain results from the presence of two main chemicals found in the bloodstream: prostaglandins and bradykinin. Loss of function is a result of pain (the body limits movement to reduce discomfort) and swelling (interstitial fluid limits movement).

Acute inflammation. Many chemicals are involved in acute inflammation. Mediators of inflammation originate from blood plasma and from both damaged and normal cells. Vasoactive amines are a class of chemicals that increase the permeability of blood vessel and cell walls. The most well studied of these are histamine and serotonin. Histamine is stored in granules in mast cells that are found in both tissue and basophils, the latter being a type of cell found in the blood. Serotonin is found in mast cells and platelets; it is another type of cell found in the bloodstream. These substances cause vasodilation (expansion of the walls of blood vessels) and increased vascular permeability (leakage through the walls of small vessels, especially veins). Histamine and serotonin can be released by trauma or exposure to cold. Other chemicals that circulate in the blood can release histamine. Two of these are

part of the complement system; another is called interleukin-1. The effects of histamine diminish after approximately one hour.

Plasma proteases comprise three interrelated systems that explain much that is known about inflammation: the complement, kinin, and clotting systems. The complement system is composed of twenty different proteins involved in reactions against microbial agents that invade the body. The various chemicals act in a cascade, similar to falling dominoes: Each one sets off another in sequence. The result of these chemical actions is to increase vascular permeability, promote chemotaxis (the attraction of living cells to specific chemicals), engulf invading microorganisms, and destroy pathogens through a process called lysis.

The kinin system is responsible for releasing bradykinin, a chemical substance that causes contraction of smooth muscle tissue, dilation of blood vessels, and pain. The duration of action for bradykinin is brief because it is inactivated by the enzyme kininase. Bradykinin does not promote chemotaxis.

The clotting system is made up of a series of chemicals that result in the formation of a solid mass. The most commonly encountered example is the scab that forms at the site of a cut in the skin. Like the complement system, the clotting system is a cascade of thirteen different chemicals. In addition to producing a solid mass, the clotting system also increases vascular permeability and promotes chemotaxis for white blood cells.

Other substances are involved in acute inflammation. Among the most important of these is a class called prostaglandins. Several different prostaglandin molecules have been isolated; they are derived from the membranes of most cells. Prostaglandins cause pain, vasodilation, and fever. Aspirin counteracts the effects of prostaglandins, which explains the antipyretic (fever-reducing) and analgesic (pain-reducing) properties of the drug.

Another group of substances involved in acute inflammation are leukotrienes. The primary sources for these molecules are leukocytes, and some leukotrienes are found in mast cells. This group promotes vascular leakage but not chemotaxis. They also cause vasoconstriction (a decrease in the diameter of blood vessels) and bronchoconstriction (a decrease in the diameter of air passageways in the lungs). The effect of these leukotrienes is to slow blood flow and restrict air intake and outflow. A different type of leukotriene is found only in leukocytes. This type enhances chemotaxis but does not contribute to vascular leakage. In addition, leukotrienes cause white blood cells to stick to damaged tissues, speeding the removal of bacteria and promoting healing.

Other chemical substances are known to be involved with inflammation: platelet-activating factor, tumor necrosis factor, interleukin-1, cationic (positively charged) proteins, neutral proteases (enzymes that break down proteins), and oxygen metabolites (molecules resulting from reactions with oxygen). The sources of these are generally leukocytes, although some are derived from macrophages. They reinforce the effects of prostaglandins and leukotrienes.

There are four different outcomes for acute inflammation. There may be complete resolution in which the injured site is restored to normal; this outcome usually follows a mild injury or limited trauma where there has been only minor tissue destruction. Healing with scarring may occur, in which injured tissue is replaced with scar tissue that is rich in collagen, giving it strength but at the cost of normal function; this outcome follows more severe injury or extensive destruction of tissue. There may be the formation of an abscess, which is characterized by pus and which follows injuries that become infected with pyogenic (pus-forming) organisms. The fourth outcome is chronic inflammation.

Chronic inflammation. Acute inflammation may be followed by chronic inflammation. This reaction occurs when the organism, factor, or agent responsible for the acute inflammation is not removed or when the normal processes of healing fail to occur. Repeated episodes of acute inflammation may also lead to chronic inflammation, in which the stages of acute inflammation seem to remain for long periods of time. In addition, chronic inflammation may begin insidiously, such as with a low-grade infection that does not display the usual signs of acute inflammation; tuberculosis, rheumatoid arthritis, and chronic lung disease are examples of this third alternative.

Chronic inflammation typically occurs in one of the following conditions: prolonged exposure to potentially toxic substances such as asbestos, coal dust, and silica that are nondegradable; immune reactions against one's own tissue (autoimmune diseases such as lupus and rheumatoid arthritis); and persistent infection by an organism that is either resistant to drug therapy or insufficiently toxic to cause an immune reaction (such as viruses, tuberculosis, and leprosy). The characteristics of chronic inflammation are similar to those of acute inflammation but are less dramatic and more protracted.

—*L. Fleming Fallon, Jr., M.D., Ph.D., M.P.H.*

See also Abscess drainage; Abscesses; Anti-inflammatory drugs; Arthritis; Burns and scalds; Bursitis; Disease; Healing; Infection; Wounds; *specific diseases.*

FOR FURTHER INFORMATION:

Challem, Jack. *The Inflammation Syndrome: The Complete Nutritional Program to Prevent and Reverse Heart Disease, Arthritis, Diabetes, Allergies, and Asthma.* New York: Wiley, 2003. Explores the cumulative effect of low-grade inflammation that grows into chronic, debilitating diseases, including heart disease, diabetes, Syndrome X, obesity, arthritis, allergies, and asthma. Covers anti-inflammatory drugs and the impact of nutrition.

Gallin, John I., and Ralph Snyderman, eds. *Inflammation: Basic Principles and Clinical Correlates.* 3d ed. New York: Raven Press, 1999. This well-written book is for the reader who wants to know about inflammation in great detail.

Górski, Andrzej, Hubert Krotkiewski, and Michał Zimecki, eds. *Inflammation.* Boston: Kluwer, 2001. A series of papers review current understanding of inflammatory processes and responses, from allergies to life-threatening sepsis, and evaluate therapeutic strategies aimed at combating inflammatory diseases.

Kumar, Vinay, Abul K. Abbas, and Nelson Fausto, eds. *Robbins and Cotran Pathologic Basis of Disease.* 7th ed. Philadelphia: Elsevier Saunders, 2005. A widely used pathology text that contains a good discussion of inflammation. Written for health professionals, but the serious nonspecialist will find a wealth of material.

Meggs, William Joel, and Carol Svec. *The Inflammation Cure.* New York: McGraw-Hill, 2003. Examines recent research linkages between inflammation and heart disease, as well as diseases associated with aging including arthritis, Alzheimer's disease, osteoporosis, and some cancers. Covers causes, treatments, and lifestyle changes to promote wellness.

INFLUENZA
DISEASE/DISORDER

ANATOMY OR SYSTEM AFFECTED: Lungs, respiratory system

SPECIALTIES AND RELATED FIELDS: Epidemiology, family medicine, internal medicine, public health, virology

DEFINITION: Any one of a group of commonly experienced respiratory diseases caused by viruses, responsible for many major, worldwide epidemics.

KEY TERMS:

antibody: a protein substance produced by white blood cells (lymphocytes) in response to an antigen; combats bacterial, viral, chemical, or other invasive agents in the body

antigen: a chemical substance, often on a bacterial or viral surface, containing substances that activate the body's immune response

pneumonia: a respiratory tract infection that can be caused by bacteria or viruses; it is the major complication of influenza and the major cause of influenza deaths

ribonucleic acid (RNA): the material contained in the core of many viruses that is responsible for directing the replication of the virus inside the host cell

---

INFORMATION ON INFLUENZA

CAUSES: Viral infection

SYMPTOMS: Fever, malaise, headache, muscle pain (particularly in back and legs), coughing, nasal congestion, shivering, sore throat

DURATION: Acute

TREATMENTS: Typically alleviation of symptoms; sometimes antiviral drugs (*e.g.*, ribavirin)

CAUSES AND SYMPTOMS

Epidemics of what scientists believe was influenza have been reported in Europe and Asia for at least one thousand years. Epidemics of what could have been influenza were reported by ancient Greek and Roman historians. Influenza epidemics still occur, striking isolated societies, entire nations, or, as with pandemics, the entire world. Among the great plagues that have afflicted the world over the centuries, influenza is the one that remains active today. Smallpox has been conquered, and bubonic plague (the Black Death), yellow fever, and typhus no longer erupt every few years as they once did. Cholera still breaks out, but rarely as a major epidemic. Before acquired immunodeficiency syndrome (AIDS), influenza was called "the last of the great plagues."

The term "influenza" is from the Italian and refers to the fact that some early scientists thought that the disease was caused by the malevolent influence of the planets, stars, and other heavenly bodies. To others, this "influence" was a miasma or poisonous effluvium carried in the air—a theory that is closer to the truth.

In the eighteenth and nineteenth centuries, there were about twenty major epidemics of influenza in Europe and America. They were of varying severity—some mild, some harsh. In 1918, a pandemic of influenza became one of the worst afflictions ever endured by humankind. It came in three waves, the first in the spring of 1918. This wave was relatively mild and mortality rates were low, and it spread evenly through all age groups of the population. The second wave came in the fall, and it was the most devastating outbreak of disease seen since the great plagues of the Middle Ages. Up to 20 percent of its victims died, and about half the deaths were of people in the prime of life, twenty to forty years of age. The last wave came in the winter and was not as severe. By the time that the pandemic was over, more than 20 million people worldwide had died from it, with more than 500,000 deaths in the United States alone.

In 1918, scientists understood enough about microbiology to realize that a microorganism caused influenza, but they originally thought that it was a bacterium, *Haemophilus influenzae*, because this organism was isolated from some of the victims. *H. influenzae* causes many diseases, but influenza is not among them, as researchers found when infection from it failed to produce influenza symptoms in test subjects. It soon became apparent that the organism responsible for influenza was unlike any bacterium that science had yet encountered. Bacteria were easily seen in the microscope and could be collected in filters. Whatever it was that caused influenza was invisible to the microscope, and it could not be trapped in filters. So, scientists postulated that the influenza pathogen was far smaller than bacteria. They used the term "filtrable virus" to describe it—an interesting locution, because what they meant was that the organism could *not* be filtered by the devices that they were using. "Filter-passing virus," another term used at the time, is more accurate.

It was not until 1931, thirteen years after the great pandemic, that the first influenza virus was isolated. It was found in swine, and the methods used to discover it formed the basis for the techniques used to isolate the human influenza virus, a major event in microbiology that occurred in 1933. Recently, advances in molecular microbiology have allowed reconstruction of the 1918 influenza viral genome from pieces of viral RNA found in tissue samples from victims of the 1918 epidemic.

It was later found that there were not one but three kinds of human influenza virus: type A, which is the major cause of severe influenza outbreaks; type B, which also causes influenza epidemics but less often and which is usually less severe than type A; and the rarest, type C, which causes a mild, coldlike illness.

Further, it was discovered that there are different strains of virus within type A and type B, subtypes that are not identical to one another but that are related. Within each subtype there are variants. As these subtypes and variants began to appear, it became clear that the virus was capable of mutation. This was a critical discovery because it meant that influenza infection of one type would not necessarily immunize the victim against influenza of another type. This ability to mutate means that new influenza virus strains are constantly being developed—and are constantly threatening new waves of disease.

For example, in 1957, a new strain of influenza virus called the Asian flu came out of China and started a pandemic. Asian flu, or variants of it, caused the flu epidemics in the years from 1957 to 1968, but immunity to it spread so that the severity of the epidemics was gradually reduced. Then the Hong Kong flu, another new strain from the Far East, appeared. People had no immunity to it, so it caused another major pandemic. Hong Kong flu and its variants caused the epidemics that occurred in the next nine years. Then, in 1977, still another pandemic arose from a newer strain, also from Eastern Asia.

In 1976, another type, swine flu, appeared in the United States. This virus infects pigs and humans and is apparently a distant descendant of the virus that caused the 1918 pandemic. It was evidently not as hardy as the 1977 virus, because that one replaced it and swine flu disappeared, although some experts predict its return.

The reason that the influenza virus can mutate readily is related to its physiological structure. The virus is usually spherical, but the shape can vary. It is extremely small, about 0.0001 millimeter in diameter. Its surface is covered with spikes of protein, hemagglutinin and neuraminidase. They are the two major antigens that trigger the body's immune system to repel the virus and provide immunity against future infection. Hemagglutinin (H) causes red blood cells to agglutinate, or clump together. Neuraminidase (N) is an enzyme.

Inside the core of the virus are two additional antigens that trigger the production of antibodies, but these antibodies do not protect against future infection. Also in the core is a feature unique to influenza virus: Instead of a single strand of ribonucleic acid (RNA), there are eight individual strands, each one a single gene. Genes are said to be "encoded" to produce specific characteristics within an organism. When the virus invades a host cell, the RNA directs a process of replication in which components of the cell are used to make new viruses. The new viruses are then released to enter other cells and continue replicating.

The H and N antigens mutate gradually over the years because of changes in the RNA genes that encode for them. This process is called antigenic drift, and it refers to slight variations that appear in the influenza virus and account for minor and localized epidemics of the disease. When a particular strain of virus has been prevalent for some time, a "herd immunity" develops

An enlarged view of the influenza virus. (Digital Stock)

in the populations exposed to it, and incidence of disease from it declines. When the H or N antigen changes radically, the process is called antigenic shift. It creates a new subtype of the virus, one that can cause a major pandemic because there is no immunity to it. There are at least thirteen variants of H (labeled H1 to H13) and at least nine variants of N (labeled N1 to N9).

Before 1968, most influenza A viruses in circulation had H2N2 antigens on their surfaces. This type of virus was the Asian flu; it had been around for some years, so the world population had become relatively immune to it. Then, in 1968, a new virus appeared in Southeast Asia, with a combination of H3N2. The H antigen had changed completely, while the N antigen remained the same, but the combination was essentially a new virus; it gave rise to the worldwide epidemic of the Hong Kong flu.

It is known that influenza viruses from animals influence the structure of the human viruses and contribute the variations that become new strains capable of causing pandemics. There is an interesting theory of how the 1957, 1968, and 1977 pandemics that came out of China developed. The Chinese people not only eat an enormous amount of duck but also keep large flocks to eat insects that attack rice crops. Ducks carry a wide variety of influenza viruses in their intestines, and they live in close proximity to humans. This theory suggests that the influenza viruses from duck droppings modified the human influenza virus and created the new strains that caused the pandemics that emanated from China. Other animals, such as pigs, which gave the world swine flu, also harbor influenza viruses that can interact with the human influenza virus; however, most of the genetic intermingling and mutations of influenza viruses appear to occur in human hosts. Avian strains of influenza are currently of great concern because, while only a few people who have had close contact with sick birds or animals have been infected, these strains can cause severe, and often fatal, illness in people of all ages. These avian strains have thus far not acquired the ability to spread from person to person.

To cause disease, the virus must be inhaled, which is why the "influence" of poisonous effluvium carried in the air is a more correct attribution of the actual cause of the disease than the influence of heavenly bodies. Inside the upper respiratory tract, there is a layer of cilia-bearing cells (cells with small, hairlike filaments) that acts as a barrier against infection. Ordinarily, the tiny cilia spread a layer of mucus over respiratory tissues. The mucus collects infectious organisms and carries them to the stomach, where they are destroyed by stomach acids. The influenza virus causes the cilia-bearing cells to disintegrate, exposing a layer of cells beneath. The virus invades these and other host cells in the respiratory tract and begins replicating. Invasion and replication by the virus destroy the host cells. Destruction of the cells starts the inflammatory process that causes the symptoms of disease.

Influenza infection grows rapidly, and symptoms can appear in only a few hours, although the incubation period in most people is two days or so. Fever, malaise, headache, muscular pain (particularly in the back and legs), coughing, nasal congestion, shivering, and a sore throat are common symptoms. The disease can spread quickly among populations because the virus is airborne. There is good reason to believe that the virus can remain infective in the air for long periods of time. It has been reported that the crew members on a ship sailing past Cuba during an epidemic there were infected with the disease, presumably from virus-laden particles carried from shore by the wind.

The major complication of influenza is pneumonia, which can be caused by the influenza virus itself (primary influenza viral pneumonia), by infection from bacteria (secondary bacterial pneumonia), or by mixed viral and bacterial infection. Pneumonia is the major cause of death from influenza. In the severe pandemic of 1918, up to 20 percent of patients developed pneumonia and, of these, about half died.

Primary influenza viral pneumonia can come on suddenly, and it often progresses relentlessly with high fever, rapidly accumulating congestion in the lungs, and difficulty in breathing. Pneumonia caused by secondary bacterial infection can be caused by a large number of pathogens. In nonhospitalized patients, both children and adults, the common causes are pneumococci, streptococci, and *Haemophilus influenzae*. In older, infirm, or hospitalized patients, the common causes are pneumococci, staphylococci, and *Klebsiella pneumoniae*.

When influenza B is the pathogen, Reye's syndrome can develop, most often in children under eighteen. This disease, which causes brain and liver damage, is fatal in about 21 percent of cases.

TREATMENT AND THERAPY

There are two main goals of therapy for the patient with influenza: treatment and preventing the spread of the disease. The first aim of therapy is to keep the patient comfortable, address the symptoms of the disease that can be treated, and deal with any complications that may arise. Bed rest is recommended, particularly during the most severe stages of the disease. Exertion is to be avoided, in order to prevent excessive weakness that could encourage further infection. Aspirin, acetaminophen, and other drugs are given for fever, and painkillers are given to relieve aches and pains. Cough suppressants and expectorants can relieve the hacking coughs that develop. Drinking large amounts of liquids is advised to replace the fluids lost as a result of high fever and sweating.

Amantadine hydrochloride is sometimes given to patients with influenza A infection. It reduces fever and relieves respiratory symptoms. An analogue of amantadine, rimantadine, works similarly. In severe cases of influenza caused by either A or B virus, an antiviral drug called ribavirin can be administered as a mist to be breathed in by the patient. Ribavirin shortens the duration of fever and may alleviate primary influenza viral pneumonia.

Primary influenza viral pneumonia is usually treated in the intensive care unit of a hospital, where the patient is given oxygen and other procedures are used to give respiratory and hemodynamic support. Secondary bacterial pneumonia must be treated with appropriate antibiotics. Identifying the precise bacterium will help the physician decide which antibiotic to prescribe. This identification is not always feasible, however, in which case broad-spectrum antibiotics will be used. They are effective against the most common bacteria that cause these secondary infections: *Streptococcus pneumoniae*, *Staphylococcus aureus*, and *Haemophilus influenzae*.

In preventing the spread of influenza, the first line of defense is to isolate the patient from susceptible persons and to initiate a program of vaccination. Because the influenza virus is constantly mutating, vaccines are regularly reformulated to confer immunity to the current pathogens. For the most part, the differences are not great between one year's virus and the one causing the next year's disease. Current vaccines may confer immunity or may require adjustment. If a major antigenic mutation has occurred, however, immunity cannot be conferred unless a new vaccine is developed against the new strain. Because it can take months to develop a new vaccine, there is the danger that the epidemic will have run its course and infected entire populations by the time that the vaccine is ready. Fortunately, major pandemics of influenza usually start slowly, so researchers have the time to identify the new strain, create a vaccine, and disseminate it.

The usual recommendation is to vaccinate people who are at highest risk of complications from the disease. These people include those over sixty-five years of age; residents of nursing homes or other patients with chronic medical conditions; adults and children with chronic pulmonary or cardiovascular diseases, including children with asthma; adults and children who have been hospitalized during the previous year for metabolic disorders, such as diabetes mellitus, or for renal diseases, blood disorders, or immunosuppression; teenagers and children who are receiving long-term aspirin therapy (who may be at risk of developing Reye's syndrome as a result of influenza infection); and pregnant women whose third trimester occurs in winter.

When a family member brings influenza into the household, other members should be vaccinated. After vaccination, it usually takes about two weeks for immunity to develop. Amantadine may protect against influenza A in the meantime; it can be discontinued after immunity has been achieved. If, for any reason, a person cannot be vaccinated, amantadine should be given throughout the entire length of the epidemic, which may last six to eight weeks.

A history of influenza vaccine development beginning with the identification of the virus in 1933 illustrates how constant vigilance is required to combat the disease. Various influenza vaccines were developed from 1935 to 1942, but they were all unsatisfactory. Building on the work that had gone before them, Thomas Francis and Jonas Salk (who later developed the first polio vaccine) produced a vaccine in 1942 that conferred immunity against the current strains of both influenza A and influenza B. Intensive animal testing and human trials showed that the vaccine was effective for about a year.

In 1947, however, many people who had been vaccinated came down with the disease: A new strain of influenza A virus had surfaced. The old vaccine had no effect on it, and a new vaccine had to be developed. This pattern has been repeated constantly: The original vaccine of 1942 was effective until a new strain appeared and a new vaccine had to be developed. That one was satisfactory until the next new strain, the Asian flu, appeared in 1957, and the process had to be repeated to find a vaccine that would protect against it. Similarly, in 1968 and in 1977, new vaccines had to be developed, and these have had to be modified to match the changes in the virus.

In 1999, the Food and Drug Administration approved two new antivirals, zanamivir (Relenza) and oseltamivir (Tamiflu), for the prophylaxis and treatment of influenza A or B. These antivirals must be administered within the first forty-eight hours after the onset of symptoms to be effective, as is the case for amantadine or rimantadine. Strains of influenza may become resistant to amantadine and rimantadine, sometimes during a course of therapy. The efficacy of Relenza and Tamiflu for the treatment of either influenza A or B and the infrequent development of resistance have made these drugs the first choice for prophylaxis or treatment of influenza. Relenza must be administered by inhaler as an aerosolized power, and it can produce bronchospasm in asthmatics. Tamiflu is given orally as a capsule. Amantadine and rimantadine remain effective against strains of influenza A that have not developed resistance and may be chosen for prophylaxis or treatment of these strains as these older drugs are significantly less expensive.

In 2001, the FDA approved a nasally administered influenza vaccine for protection against influenza and the accompanying ear infections often seen as a complication. This nasal vaccine, called FluMist, is a vaccine composed of three live, attenuated strains of influenza virus, as recommended by the U.S. Public Health Service on an annual basis in the same manner as injectable influenza vaccine. This intranasal vaccine has been useful in children and adults. Because the virus in the intranasal vaccine is live, and not killed as in the injectable vaccine, however, it cannot be given to children under the age of five or adults over the age of fifty, or to a variety of other individuals who are unhealthy or who may have compromised immune systems.

The World Health Organization (WHO) maintains reference laboratories around the world to keep up with the mutations of the influenza viruses. Their vigilance discovers new varieties as they appear. The new variants are studied, and vaccines are prepared to immunize against those strains that seem likely to cause extensive epidemics. This activity blunts the force of new pandemics and saves millions of lives.

PERSPECTIVE AND PROSPECTS

Researchers are constantly working to prevent the recurrent epidemics and pandemics of influenza, or at least to make them less severe. The fact that vaccines have to be modified periodically, and new ones developed from time to time, will probably not change.

It is theoretically possible for a pandemic of the severity of 1918 to occur. If a new subtype of the influenza virus were to arise and its initial spread were rapid, it could rage around the globe before an effective vaccine could be developed and made available. Mass devastation and death could result.

Another major concern is the enormous number of influenza virus strains that are living in animals. Hundreds of different types of influenza virus have been isolated from birds alone. These strains have the potential of causing mutations in the human influenza virus, as the Chinese ducks did in causing the Asian flu, the Hong Kong flu viruses, and the virus that caused the pandemic of 1977. In 2004, infections spread by chickens in China resulted in a number of deaths and renewed concerns about mutations.

So far, medical science has been able to produce vaccines capable of protecting against the new mutant viruses as they arise. Even when a significant portion of any society is vaccinated, however, some people still become infected and there are no agents available that can kill the influenza virus. Furthermore, there are few therapeutic measures that can do any more than alleviate individual symptoms. Basically, the body's own immune system is the best therapy currently available.

Chemoprophylaxis (prevention of a disease by the use of a drug) with amantadine is effective in limiting the spread of disease caused by influenza A, but amantadine has some undesirable side effects, and the drug seems to have no effect on the virus itself. Rimantadine, a closely related compound, is equally effective as a chemoprophylactic agent and seems to be better tolerated. It is still considered an experimental drug, however, and it has not been licensed.

No chemotherapeutic agent (a drug capable of curing a disease) has yet been developed that will kill an influenza virus in the same way that an antibiotic destroys bacteria and other microorganisms. The search for antiviral agents is among the most urgent activities in medical science, and the problems are enormous. Yet the science is young. As researchers learn more about the structure, physiology, and activities of viruses, they will also develop means of controlling them.

When an agent is discovered that is safe and effective against influenza virus, it could be subject to the same limitations as the vaccines; that is, it may have to be modified periodically to remain effective against the new strains of influenza virus that are continually developing, and it may be necessary to develop new agents to deal with radically new mutants.

—C. Richard Falcon;
updated by H. Bradford Hawley, M.D.

See also Antibiotics; Avian influenza; Bacterial infections; Centers for Disease Control and Prevention (CDC); Epidemiology; Fever; Lungs; Microbiology; Nausea and vomiting; Noroviruses; Pneumonia; Pulmonary diseases; Pulmonary medicine; Pulmonary medicine, pediatric; Respiration; Reye's syndrome; Viral infections; World Health Organization; Zoonoses.

FOR FURTHER INFORMATION:

Biddle, Wayne. *A Field Guide to Germs*. 2d ed. New York: Henry Holt, 2002. This comprehensive book is easily accessible to the nonspecialist and includes a discussion of nearly every virus, bacterium, and fungus known to cause human and nonhuman animal disease. The history of the microbe and the treatment of diseases are included.

Giesecke, Johan. *Modern Infectious Disease Epidemiology*. 2d ed. New York: Oxford University Press, 2002. This book is divided into two sections. The first covers the tools and principles of epidemiology from an infectious disease perspective. The second covers the role of contact pattern from an assessment angle, exploring such topics as infectivity, incubation periods, seroepidemiology, and immunity.

Kimball, Chad. *Colds, Flu, and Other Common Ailments*. Detroit: Omnigraphics, 2002. A comprehensive guide for general readers covering treatment issues and controversies surrounding common ailments and injuries. Includes discussions on ailments of the nose, throat, lungs, ears, eyes, and head; common injuries; alternative therapies; choosing a doctor; and buying drugs and finding health information online.

Kiple, Kenneth F., ed. *The Cambridge World History of Human Disease*. New York: Cambridge University Press, 1993. The section on influenza gives a useful account of the epidemics and pandemics of influenza throughout the years.

Kolata, Gina. *Flu: The Story of the Great Influenza Pandemic of 1918 and the Search for the Virus That Caused It*. New York: Farrar, Straus and Giroux, 1999. Kolata's book vividly describes how the 1918 influenza outbreak, the most deadly pandemic the United States has ever faced, affected society. It not only offers an apocalyptic vision of the course of the disease but also details the ongoing efforts to track down its source.

Litin, Scott C., ed. *Mayo Clinic Family Health Book*. 3d ed. New York: HarperResource, 2003. A good general medical text for the layperson. The section on influenza is short but thorough.

Sahelian, Ray, and Victoria Dolby Toews. *The Common Cold Cure: Natural Remedies for Colds and Flu*. Garden City Park, N.Y.: Avery, 1999. The miseries of the common cold are many, and while a definitive medical cure remains elusive, its most annoying symptoms can certainly be addressed and, as Sahelian and Toews maintain, its duration shortened without the use of over-the-counter pharmaceuticals.

Tyrrell, David A., and Michael Fielder. *Cold Wars: The Fight Against the Common Cold*. New York: Oxford University Press, 2002. Traces the history of the common cold from ancient Egypt to the modern age and examines advances in its treatment.

Wagner, Edward K., and Martinez J. Hewlett. *Basic Virology*. 2d ed. Malden, Mass.: Blackwell Science, 2004. A very readable undergraduate text covering issues of virology and viral disease, properties of viruses and virus-cell interaction, working with viruses, and replication patterns of specific viruses.

INSECT-BORNE DISEASES
DISEASE/DISORDER

ANATOMY OR SYSTEM AFFECTED: All

SPECIALTIES AND RELATED FIELDS: Bacteriology, biochemistry, biotechnology, critical care, environmental health, epidemiology, microbiology, preventive medicine, public health

DEFINITION: Diseases transmitted by insects, which have a significant health and economic impact worldwide, causing illness, disability, and death.

KEY TERMS:

endemic: occurring naturally in a geographic area or population group

epidemic: any disease, injury, or health-related event occurring suddenly in numbers in excess of normal

mucous membranes: the inner lining of the mouth and nasal passages, as well as any membrane or lining containing mucus-secreting glands

parasite: an organism that obtains food and shelter from another organism or host

pathogen: a disease-producing microorganism such as bacteria, viruses, algae, and fungi

vector: an organism that transmits a disease from one host to another

CAUSES AND SYMPTOMS

Insects such as mosquitoes, blackflies, tsetse flies, eye flies, houseflies, fleas, and lice are responsible for

Dengue fever, also called breakbone fever, is rarely fatal, but it causes a high fever accompanied by severe pain and stiffness in the joints. In 2002, the World Health Organization (WHO) reported that every year 50 to 100 million people catch dengue, 500,000 are hospitalized for hemorrhagic fever, and at least 12,000 die. The disease is endemic in the tropics, where about 40 percent of the world's population lives. There is no vaccine or cure. Another form, hemorrhagic dengue, produces shock syndrome and follows a previous infection with dengue. The disease may infect people in as many as sixty-one countries.

West Nile virus was first reported in the United States in Queens, New York City, in 1999. In 2002, more than 4,000 human cases and 14,700 equine (horse) cases were documented. The virus causes high mortality in many species of birds and results in numer-

transmitting pathogens that inflict disease and illness on hundreds of millions of people each year. Mosquitoes and blackflies are the most medically and economically destructive of the bloodsucking insects. In 2002 alone, mosquito-borne diseases sickened 700 million people and killed more than 1.5 million. These diseases are generally one of three types. The first usually causes fever, rashes, joint pain, and occasional fatal infections. The second type is hemorrhagic, which causes bleeding from the mucous membranes and occasionally leads to fatal shock. The third type causes symptoms of encephalitis, an inflammation of the brain, and is identified with several epidemics.

The better-known mosquito-transmitted diseases include malaria, yellow fever, dengue fever, and West Nile virus. Malaria, responsible for the deaths of at least one million people in 2002, produces a high fever and chills and does not provide lasting immunity to a relapse. The disease is treated with quinine, but patients can still develop the deadly blackwater fever. Yellow fever is more deadly than malaria and is endemic in Central and South America, the West Indies, and Africa. There is no treatment for yellow fever, although at-risk individuals can be vaccinated to prevent infection. Patients with yellow fever may contract hepatitis and suffer renal (kidney) failure, hemorrhage (blood loss), shock, and death.

Mosquito-Borne Diseases

Mosquito	Habits	Features	Diseases
Aedes	Day biter, urban or rural	Head bent, body parallel to surface, black and white in color	Dengue, yellow fever, viral encephalitis
Anopheles	Night biter, mainly rural	Head and body in line, at angle to surface	Malaria, filariasis
Culex	Day biter, urban or rural	Shaped like *Aedes* but brown; whines in flight	Viral encephalitis, filariasis

INSECT-BORNE VIRAL DISEASES

Disease	Principal Vectors
Encephalitis, California	Mosquitoes: *Culex tarsalis, Aedes* species
Encephalitis, Eastern equine	Mosquitoes: *Aedes sollicitans, Culiseta melanura*
Encephalitis, St. Louis	Mosquitoes: *Culex pipiens pipiens, C. p. quinquefasciatus, C. tarsalis*
Encephalitis, Venezuelan	Mosquitoes: *Aedes serratus, Ae. scapularis, Ae. taeniorhynchus, Anopheles aquasalis, Culex vomifer, C. taeniopus, Haemogogus* species, *Mansonia titillans, Psorophora confinnis, P. ferox*
Encephalitis, Western equine	Mosquitoes: *Culex tarsalis* and others
Pappataci or sandfly fever	Sandfly: *Phlebotomus papatasii*
Rift Valley fever	Mosquitoes: *Eretmapodites chrysogaster, Aedes caballus, Ae. deboeri, Ae. circumluteolus, Ae. tarsalis, Culex theileri*
Yellow fever	Mosquitoes: *Aedes aegypti* (urban and jungle strains), *Ae. africanus, Ae. simpsoni, Ae. leucocelaenus, Sabethes chloroterus,* and others

ous horse deaths. Most infected people are symptom-free, with mild cases causing flulike symptoms such as fever, coughing, and weakness. Serious infections can progress to more severe headaches, high fevers, tremors, and partial paralysis, as well as encephalitis.

Biting blackflies are a nuisance that can affect tourism, agriculture, forestry, and recreation. For animals, these bites can cause weight loss, stress-related illnesses, and reduced egg, milk, and meat production. One of the most widespread of the blackfly diseases is onchocerciasis, or river blindness, a disease that can be transmitted to humans, cattle, and other large mammals. The serious effects can occur long after the initial fly bite and are caused by a worm that is transmitted to the host. The worm curls up in lumps on the body, causing coarsening of the skin, depigmentation (loss of color), and intense itching that can drive a person to suicide in severe cases. If the worm enters the eyes, then it can cause reduced peripheral vision, night blindness, and complete loss of vision. Blackfly fever, found in the New England area of the United States, is a severe reaction to bites that causes fever, nausea, headaches, and swollen lymph glands.

Tsetse flies, houseflies, and eye flies are responsible for numerous infections and diseases. The tsetse fly's bite can transmit parasites and cause sleeping sickness, a West African disease in humans. The parasite causes enlarged glands, loss of appetite, and extreme lethargy.

The patient eventually lapses into a coma, and the disease is fatal if not treated. A similar fatal disease called nagana occurs in animals, especially imported cattle and horses, cattle, goats, camels, and pigs.

Houseflies are nonbiting insects that can transfer pathogens from infected septic matter (feces) to human foodstuffs, sores, or mucous membranes. These pathogens can transmit cholera germs or cause diarrhea and eye infections. Eye flies drink fluid from eyes or blood from sores, ulcers, and small wounds on humans and animals. These very tiny black flies transmit bacteria, especially to children, and spread eye sores such as conjunctivitis (pinkeye) and other infections.

Biting midges are small flies that can transmit several diseases. Sandfly fever causes a short illness with fever in humans. Baronellosis, or Carrion's disease, occurs in South America in Peru, Ecuador, and Colombia in higher altitudes. Mild cases usually cause a slight fever, but severe cases can have an 80 percent mortality rate. After five to eight weeks, fever survivors develop large wartlike tumors all over the body, which cause pain and irritation. Leishmaniasis is a parasitic disease and ranges from a mild form with fevers and anemia to a disfiguring type with skin wounds to another form that can cause internal organ damage and death. Most forms infect animals and accidentally transfer to humans. In 2004, approximately twelve million people were infected worldwide. Other biting midges transmit diseases such as the Oropouche virus, which is found in tropical America. Severe flulike symptoms, with fever and vomiting, can last for up to two weeks but are usually not fatal.

Flea-borne murine (mice) typhus produces a typhuslike fever, eye rash, headache, chills, and general achiness. The most infamous disease transmitted by fleas, however, is the plague, which killed a quarter of the population of Europe in the fourteenth century. People become infected by receiving a flea bite, handling infected animals, or breathing infected respiratory droplets. The plague causes fever, chills, seizures, and severe headaches, followed by swollen lymph glands (or buboes) in the armpit, groin, or neck. Untreated septicemic plague is initially hard to diagnose because it invades the bloodstream directly, eventually spreading to the liver, kidney, spleen, lungs, eyes, and/or lining of the brain. This type of plague has a 40 percent mortality rate with treatment and a 100 percent fatality rate if untreated. Pneumonic plague, which is contracted by inhaling infected drops from another person or animal, causes severe, overwhelming pneumonia, shortness of breath, high fever, and blood in the phlegm. Life-threatening complications include shock, high fever, problems with blood clotting, and convulsions. Untreated pneumonic plague is almost always fatal, but a specific antibiotic treatment must be started fifteen to eighteen hours after symptoms appear in order to be effective.

Lice are responsible for several diseases, including louse-borne typhus, which comes from louse feces. Infection occurs through a scratch, contact with mucous membranes, or inhalation. Symptoms include fatigue, muscle aches, headache, coughing, rapid onset of fever, and a blotchy rash on the chest or abdomen. If untreated, the disease can cause delirium, low blood pressure, coma, and possibly death. Treatment with antibiotics usually provides a prompt cure. Brill-Zinsser disease is similar to a mild form of typhus and is a reoccurrence of louse-borne typhus, sometimes waiting as much as thirty years between outbreaks.

Symptoms of louse-borne relapsing fever include head and muscle aches, nausea, appetite loss, dizziness, coughing, vomiting, and the abrupt onset of fever. Severe infections cause the liver and spleen to swell and make breathing painful. Trench fever, or Wolhynian fever, occurred in Central Europe during World War I and World War II and is generally rare and seldom fatal. There may be no symptom or headaches, muscle aches, fever, and nausea.

Chagas' disease is found in South and Central America. Transmission of bacteria occurs through infected feces, and symptoms range from mild and flulike to severe chronic cardiac or digestive system disease. In 2004, an estimated twelve to eighteen million of more than ninety million people living where the disease is endemic were infected. Between 10 and 30 percent of infected people will develop chronic, life-threatening

INSECT-BORNE BACTERIAL AND RICKETTSIAL DISEASES

Disease	Disease Agent	Principal Vectors
Anthrax	*Bacillus anthracis*	Various horse flies by mechanical transmission
Carrion's disease	*Bartonella bacilliformis*	*Phlebotomus* sandflies
Food poisoning	*Shigella* and *Salmonella*	Various flies by mechanical transmission
Plague	*Yersinia pestis*	*Xenopsylla cheopis* and some other fleas
Trench fever	*Rickettsia quintana*	Human body louse *Pediculus humanus humanus*
Tularemia	*Francisella tularensis*	Deer flies and ticks
Typhus, louse-borne	*Rickettsia prowazekii*	Human body louse *Pediculus humanus humanus*
Typhus, murine	*Rickettsia mooseri*	Rat flea *Xenopsylla cheopis*; the rat louse *Polyplax spinulosa* is a zoonotic vector
Yaws	*Treponema pertenue*	*Hippelates* gnats

INSECT-BORNE PROTOZOAN DISEASES

Disease	Disease Agent	Principal Vectors
Chagas' disease	*Trypanosoma cruzi*	Assassin bugs: *Panstrongylus megistus* and many species of *Triatoma*
Kala-azar	*Leishmania donovani*	Sandflies: *Phlebotomus chinensis*, *P. major*, *P. argentipes*, *P. perniciosus*
Leishmaniasis, American mucocutaneous	*Leishmania braziliensis*	Sandflies: *Phlebotomus intermedius*, *P. longipalpus*, *P. pessoai*
Leishmaniasis, Mexican	*Leishmania mexicana*	Sandfly: *Phlebotomus flaviscutellatus*
Malaria, benign tertian	*Plasmodium vivax*	Mosquitoes: species of *Anopheles*
Malaria, malignant tertian	*Plasmodium falciparum*	Mosquitoes: *Anopheles stephensi*, *A. labranchiae*
Malaria, ovale tertian	*Plasmodium ovale*	Mosquitoes: *Anopheles gambiae*, *A. funestus*
Malaria, quartan	*Plasmodium malariae*	Mosquitoes: many species of *Anopheles*
Nagana (cattle, etc.)	*Trypanosoma brucei*	Tsetse fly: *Glossina morsitans*
Oriental sore	*Leishmania tropica*	Sandflies: *Phlebotomus papatasii* and *P. sergenti*
Sleeping sickness, East African	*Trypanosoma rhodesiense*	Tsetse flies: *Glossina morsitans* and *G. swynnertoni*
Sleeping sickness, West African	*Trypanosoma gambiense*	Tsetse flies: *Glossina tachinoides* and *G. palpalis*
Surra (camels, etc.)	*Trypanosoma evansi*	Horse flies in the family Tabanidae

symptoms or heart failure, and about will 50,000 die each year from infection. There is no vaccine or cure for Chagas' disease.

TREATMENT AND THERAPY

For most insect-borne diseases, treatment includes medical intervention such as antibiotics and vaccines to prevent transmission. As of 2007, vaccines for most of the diseases were still under development, and many of the diseases have no known cure. Educating people on how to avoid infection and treat the symptoms is essential.

Biological control involves reducing a target population by introducing a predator, pathogen, parasite, competitor, or toxin produced by a microorganism. This method of control was used as early as 1889 in California and became popular in early 1900's. Insecticides (or pesticides) replaced biological control and proved to be very successful in eliminating the insect vectors. Early pesticides were composed of natural botanicals (plant products) such as nicotine, rotenone, and pyrethrum mixed with chemicals such as lime sulfur, arsenic, mercuric chloride, and soaps. The scientific development of insecticides began as early as 1867, and the structures of botanical insecticides were known in the 1920's. In 1939, the insecticide properties of the first synthetic insecticide, DDT were discovered. DDT has provided a major benefit in the control of typhus, trench fever, and malaria, and it is still used in indoor insecticides for malaria control.

Pesticides may lose their effectiveness as the parasites become resistant to a specific toxin or insecticide. The focus in the early twenty-first century is on developing pesticides known as third-generation insecticides, mainly aimed at effecting mosquito development. Since these insecticides are developed for mosquitoes, they are less disruptive to the environment and less toxic to humans and other organisms.

Other preventive measures include insect growth regulators (IGRs), which are species-specific and prevents larvae from developing. Genetic control, which involves introducing sterile males to the population or the release of insects with only male-producing properties, results in so few females that the population declines. Genetic control methods also may involve population replacement in which the genetic structure is modified in a particular species of insect to prevent disease transmission. A gene can be inserted that would cause the insect to die after breeding and would be passed to offspring. A different gene insertion would kill the females, which are the bloodsuckers in most species, but not the males.

In addition to pesticides and insecticides, which may be applied over a large area, the elimination of insect breeding and gathering areas is very effective. General measures to prevent infection include using personal repellents on people and livestock, wearing light-colored clothing and long sleeves and pants during feeding times, stabling livestock during peak biting periods, managing sewage and fecal waste, using netting or fine mesh screening, reducing the number of strays and wild animals that can act as hosts, and keeping the air moving with fans.

PERSPECTIVE AND PROSPECTS

Insect-borne diseases have been infecting people throughout history. Malaria was noted in ancient times and written about prior to the first century C.E. Over time, some people speculated about a connection between insects and illness, but the scientific equipment and knowledge was not yet available to prove the existence of the pathogens. Initial observations led to improved hygiene and better housing, which greatly reduced plague and typhus. Malaria and yellow fever, however, did not respond to these developments.

In 1877, Sir Patrick Manson discovered that some mosquitoes can carry a parasite that infects people.

INSECT-BORNE WORM (HELMINTHIC) DISEASES

Contracted Through Ingesting Host

Disease	Parasite	Host
Dog tapeworm	*Dipylidium caninum*	Dog flea *Pulex irritans* and lice
Rodent tapeworm	*Hymenolepis diminuta*	Fleas including *Xenopsylla cheopis*; also roaches, moth and beetle larvae
Spiney-headed worm	*Macracanthorhynchus hirudinaceus*	Beetle larvae

Contracted from Blood-Sucking Flies

Disease	Parasite	Principal Vectors
Acanthocheilonemasis	*Acanthocheilonema perstans*	Biting midges: *Culicoides austeni* and *C. grahami*
Bancroft's filariasis	*Wuchereria bancrofti*	Mosquitoes: *Culex pipiens quinquefasciatus* and other *Culex*, *Aedes*, *Anopheles*, and *Mansonia* species
Brug's filariasis	*Brugia malayi*	Mosquitoes: *Mansonia, Anopheles, Aedes,* and *Armigeres* species
Dog heartworm	*Dirofilaria immitis*	Mosquitoes: *Culex pipiens, Aedes aegypti,* and others
Loiasis or African eyeworm	*Loa loa*	Mango flies: *Chrysops dimidiatus* and *C. silaceus*
Onchocerciasis	*Onchocerca volvulus*	Black flies: *Simulium damnosum, S. neavei, S. ochraceum,* and others
Ozzard's filariasis	*Mansonella ozzardi*	Biting midge: *Culicoides furens*

This discovery and subsequent work by many others stimulated the research into insect-borne diseases. The insect transmission of plague and typhus took ten to twelve years to understand, and others took decades. There were no specific drugs or vaccines for the diseases until 1925, except for quinine for malaria, which did not always work.

Research continues in an effort to find successful preventive and control measures, including the development of more effective pesticides, insecticides, and genetic controls. Attention must be paid to illnesses in humans and animals and the potential insect connection in order to fight existing diseases and recognize new or mutating ones. For example, some researchers speculate that bloodsucking stable flies may have caused the initial spread of human immunodeficiency virus (HIV) from chimpanzees to humans.

Although many insect-borne diseases were greatly reduced by 1970, they have since made a dramatic recovery in warm areas of the world, perhaps because of the evolution and adaptation of the pathogens. In addition, social problems such as poverty, famine, and war, which often result in overcrowded and unsanitary conditions, offer ideal breeding areas and easy transmission for numerous insect-borne illnesses and diseases.

—*Virginia L. Salmon*

See also Allergies; Bites and stings; Chagas' disease; Elephantiasis; Encephalitis; Epidemiology; Food poisoning; Leishmaniasis; Lice, mites, and ticks; Malaria; Parasitic diseases; Pinworms; Plague; Roundworms; Sleeping sickness; Tapeworms; Tropical medicine; Tularemia; Worms; Yellow fever; Zoonoses.

FOR FURTHER INFORMATION:

Busvine, James R. *Disease Transmission by Insects: Its Discovery and Ninety Years of Effort to Prevent It.* New York: Springer-Verlag, 1993. Describes the diseases and history of the discovery of the transmission, as well as a discussion of control measures and insecticides.

Harder, Ben. "Don't Let the Bugs Bite: Can Genetic Engineering Defeat Disease Spread by Insects?" *Science News* 166, no. 7 (August 14, 2004): 104. Discusses research on Chagas' disease and efforts to develop a genetic control.

Marquardt, William C., ed. *Biology of Disease Vectors.* 2d ed. New York: Elsevier Academic Press, 2005. This textbook is directed toward graduate students and researchers, but most of the information is accessible to the general reader.

O'Hanlon, Leslie Harris. "Tinkering with Genes to Fight Insect-Borne Disease: Researchers Create Genetically Modified Bugs to Fight Malaria, Chagas, and Other Diseases." *The Lancet* 363 (April 17, 2004): 1288. Discusses genetic engineering techniques and anticipated results.

Spielman, Andrew, and Michael D'Antonio. *Mosquito: A Natural History of Our Most Persistent and Deadly Foe.* New York: Hyperion, 2001. An account of the role that mosquitoes have played in human history.

Turkington, Carol A., and Rebecca J. Frey. "Malaria." In *The Gale Encyclopedia of Medicine*, edited by Jacqueline L. Longe. 3d ed. Farmington Hills, Mich.: Thomson Gale, 2006. A discussion of the history, causes, symptoms, diagnosis, treatment, prognosis, and prevention of malaria.

INSOMNIA. *See* SLEEP DISORDERS.

INSULIN RESISTANCE SYNDROME
DISEASE/DISORDER

ALSO KNOWN AS: Syndrome X, Deadly Quartet, metabolic syndrome

ANATOMY OR SYSTEM AFFECTED: All

SPECIALTIES AND RELATED FIELDS: Cardiology, endocrinology, internal medicine, nutrition

DEFINITION: A reduced sensitivity to the action of insulin, which brings glucose into body tissues to be used as a source of energy.

KEY TERMS:

glucose: blood sugar

insulin: a peptide hormone secreted by the pancreas; it helps the body by promoting glucose utilization, protein synthesis, and the formation and storage of neutral lipids by regulating the sugar metabolism

syndrome: a cluster of symptoms

CAUSES AND SYMPTOMS

Normally, after a meal, the body digests food, nutrients are absorbed into the blood, and the level of glucose (sugar) in the blood rises. Glucose is then quickly transported into cells for use, as glucose is the principal energy source in the human body. Most tissues, particularly skeletal muscle tissue, require insulin action to transport glucose into cells. Insulin, a hormone secreted by the pancreas, helps transport glucose into cells by binding with receptors on cells as a key would fit into a lock. Once the key—insulin—has fitted into the lock and unlocked the door, the cell allows the entry

**INFORMATION ON
INSULIN RESISTANCE SYNDROME**

CAUSES: Unclear, possibly genetic disorders; aggravated by obesity and physical inactivity
SYMPTOMS: Often asymptomatic; can include hypertension and obesity
DURATION: Typically long-term
TREATMENTS: Lifestyle changes (caloric restriction, weight loss, exercise); drug therapy (metformin, troglitazone)

of glucose, and the glucose can pass from the bloodstream into the cell. Inside cells, glucose is either used for energy or stored for future use in the form of glycogen in liver or muscle cells.

Insulin resistance occurs when the normal amount of insulin secreted by the pancreas is not able to unlock the door for glucose entering into cells. In some cases, the pancreas secretes additional insulin to maintain a normal blood glucose level. In other cases, when the body cells do not respond to even higher levels of insulin, glucose builds up in the blood, resulting in a high blood glucose (sugar) level, or Type II diabetes (non-insulin-dependent diabetes). Thus, the consequences of insulin resistance include decreased insulin function throughout the body, and hyperinsulinemia (a high insulin level in the blood).

However, insulin resistance does not occur alone. People with insulin resistance often have some other abnormalities, including an increased level of triglycerides (blood fat), a decreased level of high-density lipoprotein (HDL) cholesterol (good cholesterol), hypertension (high blood pressure), and obesity (overweight). This cluster of abnormalities, together with hyperinsulinemia and hyperglycemia (high blood glucose), is called insulin resistance syndrome, which is also known as Syndrome X or Deadly Quartet. The syndrome is a cluster of risk factors for heart disease, and insulin resistance may be the common factor linking other risk factors.

The cause of insulin resistance is still not clear as of today. Some scientists believe that a defect in specific genes may result in insulin resistance and Type II diabetes. What is currently known is that insulin resistance is aggravated by obesity and physical inactivity.

As a consequence of hyperinsulinemia, additional fat is stored in the body, because the body is trying to protect itself by turning excess insulin into triglyceride.

High insulin levels in the blood also contribute to high levels of low-density lipoprotein (LDL) cholesterol (so-called bad cholesterol), low levels of high-density lipoprotein (HDL) cholesterol, and hypertension. Obesity, associated with insulin resistance, often shows as upper body obesity.

Because insulin resistance syndrome does not have any outward physical signs, 20 to 25 percent of the "healthy" population may be insulin resistant but are not aware of it. Almost all individuals with Type II diabetes and many with hypertension, cardiovascular disease, and obesity are insulin resistant.

Anyone forty-five years or older should consider being tested for diabetes, and those who are also overweight are strongly recommended to do so. People should consider being tested if they are younger than forty-five, overweight, and have one or more of the following risk factors: a family history of diabetes, low HDL cholesterol and high triglycerides, high blood pressure, a history of gestational diabetes (diabetes during pregnancy) or having given birth to a baby weighing more than nine pounds, or a minority group background.

TREATMENT AND THERAPY

Insulin resistance often goes unrecognized until later in life when metabolic abnormalities develop. Thus, the first step of the treatment for this disorder is to identify those who may be at risk, including those who are overweight, have a parent or sibling with Type II diabetes, have low HDL and elevated triglycerides, and have high blood pressure. Women who had diabetes during pregnancy also have a higher risk for this disorder. Additionally, minority groups who are at higher risk for diabetes should be screened. They include African Americans, American Indians, Hispanic American/Latinos, and Asian American/Pacific Islanders.

Several tests can be used in screening for insulin resistance. The oral glucose tolerance test is a series of tests that measure blood glucose after fasting overnight and then two hours after ingesting a high-glucose concentrated drink. The fasting glucose test measures blood glucose after fasting overnight. Measuring fasting insulin levels is another means of screening for insulin resistance.

It is possible to reduce insulin resistance by caloric restriction, weight loss, exercise, and drug therapy. The multiple risk factor intervention treatment is usually recommended, aiming aggressively at reducing all cardiac risk factors that may exist. The key of this multiple risk factor intervention treatment is the modification of lifestyle. Lowering calorie intake can reduce insulin resistance within a few days. A diet low in saturated fat (less than 10 percent of total calories) and more moderate in total fat content (less than 40 percent of total calories) is beneficial. Concentrated sweets should be cut down. Weight loss, maintenance of ideal body weight, and regular exercise are essential. This kind of behavioral intervention is recommended for all those who have hypertension, high cholesterol, simple obesity, heart disease, diabetes, or insulin resistance syndrome.

If medical treatment is necessary, a variety of drugs are available, such as metformin and troglitazone. Metformin is a drug which enhances insulin sensitivity without affecting insulin secretion (not effective in the absence of insulin). It lowers glucose by decreasing glucose production in the liver. In addition, metformin decreases blood pressure, induces weight loss, and has a beneficial effect on lowering LDL cholesterol and triglyceride levels. Metformin has several gastrointestinal side effects, including diarrhea, nausea, and anorexia. These symptoms often improve with dosage reduction. Metformin also impairs absorption of vitamin B_{12} and folic acid but rarely causes clinical symptoms. In patients with kidney or heart disease, the use of metformin can increase the risk of lactic acidosis.

Troglitazone increases glucose transport. The treatment effect from troglitazone may not occur until two to three weeks after initiation of the drug. Troglitazone decreases the concentration of blood glucose and triglycerides, but increases HDL cholesterol. Some clinical trials have also shown that troglitazone decreases blood pressure. One important side effect of troglitazone is liver dysfunction. Thus, the liver function should be checked each month for the first six months of therapy, every two months for the next six months, and periodically thereafter. Often a combined therapy (using two or more drugs) plus behavioral intervention are used together for the treatment of insulin resistance.

Perspective and Prospects

No data are currently available to determine if long-term drug therapy aimed at reducing insulin resistance can prevent the development of diabetes and, consequently, heart disease. To investigate this issue, the Diabetes Prevention Program was recently initiated. This large randomized trial will compare four treatment groups—intensive lifestyle intervention, metformin, or troglitazone with standard diet and exercise, and a control group—to determine the effectiveness of these interventions on the prevention of Type II diabetes among high-risk people with insulin resistance. The United Kingdom Prospective Diabetes Study is a multicenter, prospective, randomized intervention trial, in which the combination effect of diet and drug therapy is being evaluated.

No drugs have been approved by the Food and Drug Administration (FDA) specifically for insulin resistance. Insulin resistance syndrome is more common in well-developed countries, such as the United States, where the population is becoming more sedentary and more obese. As both physical inactivity and obesity aggravate insulin resistance, more effective prevention and treatment of obesity should have a major impact on reducing the development of the Deadly Quartet.

—*Kimberly Y. Z. Forrest, Ph.D.; updated by Sharon W. Stark, R.N., A.P.R.N., D.N.Sc.*

See also Diabetes mellitus; Endocrine disorders; Endocrinology; Endocrinology, pediatric; Gestational diabetes; Hormones; Metabolic disorders; Metabolic syndrome; Obesity.

For Further Information:

Brook, Charles G. D., and Nicholas J. Marshall. *Essential Endocrinology.* 4th ed. Malden, Mass.: Blackwell Science, 2001. This text addresses the field of endocrinology, describing the physiology of the endocrine glands and the hormones that they produce. Includes an index.

Hansen, Barbara, and Eleazar Shafrir, eds. *Insulin Resistance and Insulin Resistance Syndrome.* New York: Taylor & Francis, 2002. Explores the cellular and whole body pathogenic mechanisms and phenotypic expressions in various models of insulin resistance.

Henry, Helen L., and Anthony W. Norman, eds. *Encyclopedia of Hormones.* 3 vols. San Diego, Calif.: Academic Press, 2003. A comprehensive overview of the role of hormones, the major physiological systems in which they operate, and the biological consequences of an excess or deficiency of a particular hormone.

Larsen, P. Reed, et al., eds. *Williams Textbook of Endocrinology.* 10th ed. Philadelphia: W. B. Saunders, 2003. Comprehensive information regarding endocrine diseases, pathophysiology, diagnoses, treatment, and prognoses.

National Institute of Diabetes and Digestive and Kidney Diseases. *Insulin Resistance and Pre-Diabetes.* http://diabetes.niddk.nih.gov/dm/pubs/insulin resistance/.

Reaven, Gerald M., Terry Kristen Strom, and Barry Fox. *Syndrome X, the Silent Killer: The New Heart Disease Risk.* New York: Simon & Schuster, 2001. Examines the diet-related causes of Syndrome X.

Romaine, Deborah S., and Jennifer B. Marks. *Syndrome X: Managing Insulin Resistance.* New York: HarperCollins, 2000. An accessible book that looks at causes, risk factors, treatments, and changes in lifestyle to promote wellness.

Wound Care Institute, Inc., for the Advancement of Wound Healing and Diabetic Foot Pathology. http://www.woundcare.org/. Users can search this site for a variety of articles on insulin resistance syndrome.

INTENSIVE CARE. *See* CRITICAL CARE; CRITICAL CARE, PEDIATRIC.

INTERNAL MEDICINE
SPECIALTY

ANATOMY OR SYSTEM AFFECTED: Abdomen, bladder, gallbladder, gastrointestinal system, glands, heart, intestines, kidneys, liver, lungs, pancreas, reproductive system, respiratory system, spleen, stomach, urinary system, uterus

SPECIALTIES AND RELATED FIELDS: Cardiology, endocrinology, gastroenterology, gynecology, nephrology, proctology, pulmonary medicine

DEFINITION: The field of medicine concerned with the diagnosis and treatment of disease of the body's inner organs and structures, usually including surgery on these organs.

KEY TERMS:

acute: referring to a short-term disease process

cellular biology: the study of the processes that take place within a cell

chronic: referring to a long-term disease process

inflammation: redness, pain, and heat resulting from trauma or infection; often the first step in the body's self-healing process

molecular biology: study of the interactions that occur among the molecules that make up living organisms

pathogen: any microorganism that can cause disease, including bacteria, viruses, fungi, yeasts, and parasites

trauma: physical injury to bodily tissue

SCIENCE AND PROFESSION

Internists, or practitioners of internal medicine, are skilled in the diagnosis and treatment of disease conditions that can occur virtually anywhere within the human body. They must be expert in human biology and anatomy and in pathophysiology (that is, the study of the processes that lead to disease conditions). By its nature, internal medicine embraces many other medical specialties, such as cardiology or gastroenterology. In fact, many internists become certified in related specialties.

The original model for the modern internist was Sir William Osler (1849-1919), a Canadian physician who practiced in the United States for much of his life. Osler was deeply beloved and respected for his compassion and humanity as well as his extraordinary skills in anatomy and diagnosis and in effecting cures for his patients. In his long career as physician and teacher of medicine, Osler formulated many of the guiding principles in the practice of internal medicine.

Knowledge of many scientific disciplines is required of internists. They must understand the physical and biological bases of disease. This involves knowledge of genetics, cellular biology, immunology, and the activities and nature of the various microorganisms that cause disease, such as bacteria, viruses, fungi, yeasts, and parasites.

Internists must understand the components and role of each type of cell in the human body and know how the cell functions. Human cells are not simple entities, but complex miniature organisms with many activities going on simultaneously, particularly metabolic processes. Just as important, internists must understand what happens within and outside of the cell in the disease process. For example, they must know how individual bacteria cause infection and how viruses invade cells, use them for their replication, and then destroy them. Internal medicine involves all the body's organ systems and structures, such as the heart and circulatory system, the gastrointestinal system, the genitourinary system, the respiratory system, the skin, the brain, and the skeletal system.

Internists must also be able to examine patients and diagnose the presence or absence of disease. This process involves a wide variety of techniques and procedures. It usually begins with an introductory interview, followed by physical examination of the patient. Pain is the most common symptom of disease, and manifestation of it is investigated thoroughly.

DIAGNOSTIC AND TREATMENT TECHNIQUES

Internists understand the intricate pathways of pain throughout the body and know that proper explanation of a pain will often lead directly or indirectly to a correct diagnosis of the underlying disorder. Much of the diagnostic skill of the internist, however, is in the understanding that pain may be ambiguous. Headache can point to the possibility of many disorders, ranging from sinusitis to severe pathologies within the brain. Pain in the chest can be caused by upper respiratory tract infection or heart disease. Pain in the limbs and/or joints may indicate physical trauma as a result of accidents or overexercising, or it may be attributable to arthritic or rheumatic disease or other causes. Abdominal pain can be present in literally dozens of different conditions. Similarly, back and neck pain can be caused simply by physical exertion or may point to a serious underlying disease.

Blood pressure and pulse are checked in the physical examination, and the doctor listens to heart and chest sounds through a stethoscope. The ears, mouth, and nose are examined. Body temperature is an important diagnostic consideration. Excess body heat or fever often accompanies infection and may also be present in other disease conditions. The doctor also checks for enlargement of lymph nodes and other signs that might suggest infection or other disorders.

Blood or urine samples are often taken for laboratory analysis. The internist will specify the tests he or she wants in the laboratory workup. These will include standard assays to give the internist a general picture of the patient's health and may include special tests for individual functions that the doctor may suspect are impaired.

Changes in the function of different body systems can lead the physician through the process of diagnosis. For example, such symptoms as dizziness; fainting; numbness; vision, speech, or hearing disturbances; or coma may be caused by dysfunction of the nervous system or may point to heart disease or other disorder. Abnormalities in respiratory function have specific meaning to the internist and may lead to a diagnosis ranging from a common cold to a more serious respiratory disease or a disease of other organs, such as the heart. Alterations in the skin may indicate a dermatological disorder or may suggest some internal condition.

Sometimes, a diagnosis is easy to make: The presenting symptoms are obvious signs of a specific disease. Sometimes, a group of symptoms, called a syndrome, may be ambiguous and could be related to any of a number of conditions. If the exact nature of a disease or its cause is uncertain, the internist will conduct a differential diagnosis in which possible causes of the disease are investigated in order to eliminate those that are not candidates and to pinpoint the actual cause.

Internists treat a wide variety of disorders. Among the most significant are the infectious diseases. They must study the pathogenesis (from *pathos*, meaning "disease" and *genesis*, meaning "origin" or "source") of infectious diseases in order to know how to diagnose and treat them. Harmful bacteria cause disease in different ways, but all damage and destroy body cells and tissue. Some cause infection at the point where they enter the body, such as at the site of a wound, or in the respiratory tract when they are breathed into the body. Sometimes, bacteria are carried from their site of entry to other parts of the body, where they colonize and cause infection.

The range of bacterial infections is enormous, but one thing that they often have in common is inflammation. Inflammation is the beginning of the immune process by which the body defends itself against invading pathogens. It starts when the body recognizes that the invading organism is a foreign entity by detecting foreign antigens (substances on the surfaces of invading organisms such as bacteria and viruses). The body then releases certain white blood cells, called leukocytes, that are specific for producing antibodies that can destroy the organism. Once the body has identified a foreign organism and created antibodies for it, the immune system will retain a memory of the organism and destroy it whenever it enters the body again.

When confronted with bacterial infection, internists may recognize the organism that causes it from the patient's symptoms, or they may have to take specimens from the site of inflammation and test them in order to identify the organism involved. Sometimes, the organism is identified by microscopic examination, often using a dye that stains certain bacteria. Sometimes, it is necessary to grow the organism in a culture medium in order to identify it. The organism may also be identified by its antigen or by the type of antibody that the immune system produces to fight it.

The signs of viral infection are often exactly the same as those of bacterial infection. The main difference is that the causative organism cannot be isolated and identified as easily. Unlike bacteria, viruses cannot be seen through a microscope or otherwise identified by many of the methods used for bacteria. They can be cultured, however, or antigens or antibodies may be detectable.

In addition to treating infectious diseases, internists are called on to treat dysfunction in all parts of the body. They treat many patients suffering from heart disease, the major killer of Americans. The heart is actually subject to a wide range of disorders, the most common and the most deadly of which is coronary artery disease. Internists have many means of diagnosing heart diseases and, often, predicting them. The patient's presenting symptoms and an analysis of the patient's lifestyle will often suggest the possibility of heart disease. Various in-office and laboratory procedures will inform the internist of the precise status of the patient's heart function and help direct the course of therapy.

Cancer, the second most common cause of mortality in the United States, is often seen by internists. Lung cancer is the leading cause of cancer death, followed by cancer of the colon or rectum, breast, prostate gland, urinary tract, and uterus. The lymph system, blood, mouth, pancreas, skin, stomach, and ovary are also common sites. The term "cancer" describes a large number of disorders. What all cancers have in common is that the cells of an organ multiply uncontrollably. As the cancer cells proliferate, they crowd out other cells and interfere with organ function. Sometimes cancer cells from one organ spread to neighboring organs or are carried to other parts of the body. This process is called metastasis, and it can indicate that the cancer has spread or is spreading throughout the body. Internists may be responsible for treating cancer patients throughout the disease process or may refer them to oncologists, or cancer specialists.

Diseases of the respiratory system are major concerns of the internist. In addition to bacterial and viral infections, there are many acute and chronic respiratory conditions. One major example is asthma. Its cause is unknown, but it is believed to be at least partially attributable to allergy. When an asthma attack occurs, airways in the lungs swell and constrict. Mucus builds up and airflow is restricted, causing the patient to wheeze and gasp for air. Many internists have become skilled in helping asthmatic patients, alleviating symptoms, and preventing attacks.

All parts of the body harbor the potential for disease, infectious and otherwise. They are all, to some degree, the province of internists. The kidneys and the urinary system, the gastrointestinal system, the immune system, the endocrine glands, the brain and the nervous system, and the skeletal system are all within the internist's broad purview. Often disorders in these various organs and systems can be treated fully by internists. When they believe that a patient needs a physician with greater knowledge in a particular area of medicine, however, internists will refer the patient to an appropriate specialist.

In addition to their diagnostic skills, internists must possess a wide knowledge of modern treatment modalities. Surgery is rarely among the procedures mastered by the internist, so surgical procedures are routinely referred to surgeons specializing in the particular techniques involved.

Primary among the internist's tools for fighting infectious diseases are the antibiotics. These are the mainstays of therapy for infections caused by bacteria and other nonviral microorganisms. Since the first antibiotics were developed in the 1930's and 1940's, literally hundreds more have been developed. Scores of these are in use, and new agents are constantly being introduced.

It is vital for internists to keep abreast of new antibiotics because disease-causing organisms are often able to develop resistance against antibiotic agents that have been in use for a long time. For example, many strains of bacteria that were susceptible to penicillin have developed the ability to counteract its antibiotic effect. Other agents had to be found to destroy these resistant strains. This phenomenon occurs across virtually the entire range of the available antibiotics: Prolonged use of a given agent often allows the target organism to develop resistance to it. Internists must also be skilled in the proper use of antibiotics. Knowing which agent or combination of agents to prescribe, in what amounts, and for how long are important considerations in developing the patient's treatment plan. Antibiotics are not useful for treating viral infections, but there are a limited number of antiviral agents available for treating certain diseases.

Immunization against infectious diseases can be an important concern of the internist. The most extensive immunization programs in the United States are directed toward the vaccination of children and thus are generally carried out by pediatricians and family practitioners. Internists are often responsible, however, for the immunization of adult patients. Immunization against influenza is recommended for the elderly, particularly when a new strain of influenza virus arises. It is also recommended that elderly hospitalized patients be vaccinated against pneumococcal pneumonia. Internists are a primary avenue of immunization against hepatitis B, particularly among high-risk target populations, such as medical personnel, intravenous drug abusers, and adult male homosexuals. Internists are also involved in immunizing patients who require special vaccinations because of exposure to disease or for travel to foreign countries.

Patients who require long-term or lifelong therapy for noninfectious diseases include individuals with heart diseases, high blood pressure, diabetes, cancer, respiratory disorders, and a host of other conditions. The challenge to the internist is to develop a regimen that is both efficacious and safe. Drug therapy is prominent in the internist's treatment armamentarium. In either short-term or long-term drug therapy, problems may arise. The patient may develop significant side effects or adverse reactions. The drug may lose its effectiveness after months or years of therapy. The condition may change and require dosage adjustments, additional medications, or a complete change of regimen.

Consistent monitoring of the patient's condition is an important part of therapy. The internist wants to ensure that the prescribed regimen is working and that the therapy is comfortable for the patient. For example, the earliest agents for high blood pressure, or hypertension, often had such disagreeable side effects that patients would stop taking them. Hypertension has virtually no symptoms. After the patient started taking medication, however, he or she could experience loss of energy, listlessness, impotence, dream disturbances, and many other unwelcome effects. Similarly, diabetes patients who are dependent on regular insulin injections sometimes neglect their therapy. They may balk against sticking themselves with needles three or four times a day, and they may not monitor their blood sugar adequately. Preventing the devastating and potentially fatal consequences of diabetes depends on rigorous compliance with all aspects of the diabetes regimen, including diet, insulin, and monitoring.

Thus, patient compliance with therapy becomes one of the major tasks of the internist and virtually any other physician: If the patient does not cooperate with the regimen that the doctor prescribes, the therapy is not likely to be effective. For this reason, many internists now make patient counseling part of their practice. The modern internist recognizes that patients must understand their therapeutic goals, why they are being given certain medicines, and what these drugs can be expected to accomplish. Further, many internists find that it is wise to alert their patients to possible adverse reactions, although they understand the necessity of not frightening the patient. Some internists find the time to discuss their therapeutic regimens thoroughly with their patients. Others use nursing staff or other health care workers to educate patients.

Treatment modalities change constantly, and internists are required to be aware of the latest advances in order to modify their therapy programs to take advantage of improvements in drugs or procedures. Not only are new drugs constantly being approved for use, but modern medical science is continually learning new facts about old diseases as well, and these new insights often radically alter the way a given disease is treated. A good example is a stomach ulcer. For years, it was thought that certain ulcers in the stomach were caused by erosion of the stomach wall by gastric juices. A group of investigators found, however, that a significant number of ulcer patients were also infected with the bacterium *Helicobacter pylori*. It has been suggested that infection may play a role in the development of these ulcers and that, therefore, therapy should be amended to include an antibacterial agent that is effective against *H. pylori*.

Furthermore, the internist's patient load is changing. Most internal medicine practices are treating increasing numbers of elderly patients, who have special needs. Internists must be aware of the constant advances in geriatric medicine in order to modify therapy for older patients.

PERSPECTIVE AND PROSPECTS

In the last decades of the twentieth century, internal medicine became somewhat fragmented as more and more physicians elected to practice in narrower specialties, such as cardiology, gastroenterology, hematology, or oncology, among many others. Specialties are still very much needed, but the practice of medicine seems to be headed back to the broader range of the internist.

As in the past, internists are at the forefront of progress in treatment. Recent generations have seen a far-reaching revolution in an understanding of the basic chemistry of life. As scientists elucidate the activities that occur at the molecular level of physical processes, insights are gained into exactly how the body works, as well as how antagonistic pathogens function. From this knowledge, new treatments have been devised for managing disease states.

A good example is the treatment of hypertension, one of the most common conditions seen by internists. Years ago, the only medications for high blood pressure were sedatives and diuretics. It was not fully understood exactly what occurred at the cellular and molecular level that caused vasoconstriction, which is the main physical characteristic of hypertension. Researchers discovered complex biochemical activities that contributed to vasoconstriction and other aspects of high blood pressure. They were then able to develop agents that could treat the condition more effectively than anything available before. Internists now have a wealth of antihypertensive agents with which to work. Some reduce blood pressure by reducing heart activity, some dilate blood vessels by direct action, and some interfere with the biochemical processes that cause vasoconstriction. In addition, most of the agents that internists and other physicians use for hypertension cause many fewer side effects and adverse reactions than their predecessors.

In the fight against infectious diseases, new research is combining genetics with molecular biology to elucidate the exact biochemical processes by which pathogenic organisms invade and damage body cells and tissues. This research is having an enormous impact on the understanding of bacteria and viruses: how they work, how they mutate, and, perhaps most important, in what ways they are vulnerable. With increased knowledge comes increased capability to design more efficient antibiotics and to find agents that will inhibit the pathogen's ability to develop resistant strains. Internists are among the leaders in the application of these technologies. Because they see such a wide range of disease conditions, internists often function as the main channel by which new medications and treatments reach the patient.

—C. Richard Falcon

See also Abdomen; Abdominal disorders; Angina; Arrhythmias; Arteriosclerosis; Bacterial infections; Beriberi; Bladder cancer; Bleeding; Bronchitis; Candidiasis; Cardiac arrest; Cardiology; Cardiology, pediatric; Cholecystitis; Cirrhosis; Colitis; Colonoscopy and sigmoidoscopy; Constipation; Coughing; Crohn's disease; Diabetes mellitus; Dialysis; Diarrhea and dysentery; Digestion; Diverticulitis and diverticulosis; *E. coli* infection; Emphysema; Endocarditis; Endoscopy; Gallbladder cancer; Gallbladder diseases; Gangrene; Gastroenterology; Gastroenterology, pediatric; Gastrointestinal disorders; Gastrointestinal system; Glands; Guillain-Barré syndrome; Gynecology; Heart; Heart attack; Heart disease; Heart failure; Heartburn; Hepatitis; Hernia; Incontinence; Indigestion; Influenza; Intestinal disorders; Intestines; Ischemia; Kidney cancer; Kidney disorders; Kidneys; Legionnaires' disease; Leprosy; Liver; Liver disorders; Lungs; Mitral valve prolapse; Multiple sclerosis; Nephritis; Nephrology; Nephrology, pediatric; Nonalcoholic steatohepatitis (NASH); Palpitations; Pancreas; Pancreatitis; Parasitic diseases; Peristalsis; Peritonitis; Pneumonia; Proctology; Pulmonary medicine; Pulmonary medicine, pediatric; Renal failure; Reproductive system; Reye's syndrome; Rheumatic fever; Rheumatoid arthritis; Roundworms; Scarlet fever; Schistosomiasis; Staphylococcal infections; Stone removal; Stones; Streptococcal infections; Tapeworms; Tumor removal; Tumors; Ulcer surgery; Ulcers; Urinary system; Urology; Urology, pediatric; Viral infections; Whooping cough; Worms.

FOR FURTHER INFORMATION:

Frank, Steven A. *Immunology and Evolution of Infectious Disease*. Princeton, N.J.: Princeton University Press, 2002. Blends research from molecular biology, immunology, pathogen biology, and population dynamics to discuss how and why parasites vary to escape recognition by the immune system, vaccine design, and the control of epidemics.

Kasper, Dennis L., et al., eds. *Harrison's Principles of Internal Medicine*. 16th ed. New York: McGraw-Hill, 2005. A standard text on internal medicine. Includes bibliographical references and an index.

Kiple, Kenneth, ed. *The Cambridge World History of Human Disease*. New York: Cambridge University Press, 1993. This text is useful for tracing the progress in medical practice through the years.

Litin, Scott C., ed. *Mayo Clinic Family Health Book*. 3d ed. New York: HarperResource, 2003. This text from the world-renowned medical facility was written for the layperson. Its coverage of medical practice in general and the diseases treated by the internist are clear and thorough.

Wagman, Richard J., ed. *The New Complete Medical and Health Encyclopedia*. 4 vols. Chicago: J. G. Ferguson, 2002. A good general medical reference work for the layperson. Its coverage of internal medicine is useful for clarifying the nature of the internist's practice and contrasting it with the subspecialties often practiced by internists.

INTERNET MEDICINE

SPECIALTY

ALSO KNOWN AS: E-medicine

ANATOMY OR SYSTEM AFFECTED: All

SPECIALTIES AND RELATED FIELDS: All

DEFINITION: The use of World Wide Web-based and other electronic long-distance communication technologies for health information, assessment, service delivery, training, and public health administration.

Key terms:

anonymous: of unknown authorship, unidentified by a singular identity

assessment: a thorough physical and/or psychiatric examination; a process of systematically collecting comprehensive information about health care behavior, physical and psychiatric conditions, and general well-being for the purpose of diagnosis or treatment planning

clinical trials: scientifically based research examinations of new treatment procedures, techniques, devices, or pharmaceuticals that are considered state of the art in the treatment of diseases and other medical disorders

confidential: a situation distinguished by the willing disclosure of intimate information because of assurances that the information will be protected from general distribution or unauthorized disclosure; information which, if disclosed, has the potential to be damaging or dangerous to the patient's reputation, status, or associates

diagnosis: a process of distinguishing knowledge about symptoms and problems that leads to the rendering of conclusions about physical and psychiatric illness; a label used to communicate specific health information among professionals, researchers, health systems, and insurance providers; a label which informs the process of treatment

Internet: a worldwide electronic system connecting individual computer users, computer networks, Web sites, and computer facilities for business, government, and organizational purposes

privacy: the state of being free from unwanted or unauthorized observation or other intrusion

professional licensing: state-granted privileges to health care and other professionals allowing them to deliver services or to participate in certain activities; a privilege that is revocable and subject to censure; a privilege usually granted only after thorough examination of the skill and practice of a person seeking licensure

profiling: the collection of data to summarily categorize and track the behavior of individual users or types of users, through electronic or other tracking systems, to learn more about their behavior, usually for the purpose of prediction, done either with or without the knowledge or consent of the user

screening: a triage process; a process of asking a few questions of an individual, as opposed to an assessment, in order to determine whether there is sufficient risk of a problematic condition being present to justify completing a detailed evaluation or, instead, to justify assigning that individual to a category of lesser or no risk

Web site: a location on the Internet that has an individual address and that presents information, usually in the form of individual pages, or Web pages, that the owner of the Web site wishes to make available to Internet users

Science and Profession

The Internet is a computer-based tool that is facilitating communication among vast numbers of individuals, groups, businesses, and governments. In addition to facilitating purely social and business-related ventures, the Internet is proving to be a valuable tool for improving the state of public health. This is because a new type of medical care and medical services has developed. These services, typically called telehealth, telemedicine, and e-medicine, use the Internet as a key tool in their dispensation, organization, and evaluation of health care services. Such services have taken the form of a variety of health care-related Web sites that provide services once available only through a face-to-face visit with a doctor or other health or social services professional. The Web sites are valuable in that they provide almost instantaneous information and other communications assistance to patients, their families, treatment professionals, trainers, trainees in the health care and social service professions, and medical researchers.

In terms of assisting patients, Internet-based medical approaches provide a variety of services to individual Internet users. First, they provide a wealth of information on different symptoms and medical conditions. They also allow for screening of such conditions to see if they warrant further attention from medical professionals and advice on how to handle minor health ailments and medical emergencies. They also help consumers to find medical advice, health care providers, self-help or support groups, and therapy over the Internet, all of which may or may not be supervised by medical professionals. Finally, they can give patients and their families information on different treatment options, including common procedures, the latest in alternative medicine, and even current clinical trials information.

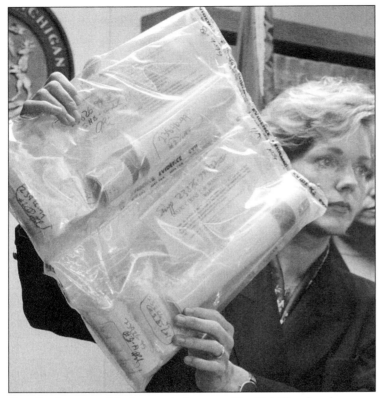

One disadvantage of the Internet is the ease with which illegal or dangerous substances, such as this home manufacturing kit for "date rape" drug gamma hydroxybutrate (GHB), can be distributed. (AP/Wide World Photos)

success or progress. Professionals may also use telemedicine in order to learn about new treatments and procedures, or to learn about new drugs and other pharmaceutical products. In addition, health care and social service providers may benefit their general practice by using the Internet to keep abreast of new clinical trials to test state-of-the-art treatments, changes in licensing laws affecting their practice, and the development of new health care databases for tracking, triage, and communication with insurance companies. Finally, some providers are actually using the Internet for health services delivery.

Health care providers in training and their trainers also benefit greatly from telemedicine. To trainees living in remote areas or those who might be highly mobile, such as those in the armed forces, the Internet provides immediate access to large online libraries, knowledgeable online teachers, and databases full of important medical information. Both long-established and new institutions interested in telemedicine increasingly are translating typical face-to-face training approaches into distance-based training programs utilizing the Internet. Encyclopedias, descriptions of techniques, pictures of what different conditions might look like both inside and outside the body, and even video of actual procedures are available online. Similarly, instruction in the use of such material is available online through training programs that lead to certificates of training and actual accredited degrees, ranging from bachelor's to doctoral degrees and postdoctoral training. In addition to helping individuals who are at remote locations, such material also can be used to reach a larger number of trainees than might typically be able to observe or attend such training. The increased ability to teach, show procedures, or give supervision at a distance using pictorial, written, oral, and video information greatly facilitates continuing education and improvement of general health care practice. It also helps to facilitate the evaluation of those practices and training sessions. Since all of the work takes place over the Internet, different aspects of the work can be monitored and evaluated electronically.

Internet medicine can also be very helpful for family members of individuals having medical problems. Often, family members do not know how best to help their significant others in times of medical need. To meet this need, Web sites may post a wide variety of information that can help people understand the conditions, the requirements of treatment, the limits of treatment, and things they can do to be helpful to the ill family member. Additionally, Web sites sometimes offer online support for family members through mechanisms such as e-mail and e-mail lists, also known as listservs, or other ongoing support groups in settings such as Internet chat rooms.

Health care and social service providers also find the Internet beneficial for their work. For some, it might be as simple as using the Internet to schedule appointments, or to communicate test results, reminder information about treatment procedures, or appointment reminders via e-mail with clients. For others, it might involve using special Web sites to conduct assessments of clients for the purpose of tracking their treatment

Much of the evaluation of this kind of information is done by researchers who are studying client, trainer, provider, or even health care system behavior and organization. This is done by evaluating information, also known as data, in individual sessions or visits to Web sites, as well as by examining data that is collected over time, across multiple visits. For instance, a person might first go to a Web site for information on a specific medical condition and then, at a later time or times, come back and look up different treatment approaches, or visit online discussion groups. What they do from time to time would be evaluated by researchers to see how individuals use the site, how long they stay on it, or what things they try searching for which may not yet be on the site. The process of watching behavior over time is called tracking. Tracking allows researchers to profile the users of Web sites to learn more about their behavior, usually for the purpose of predicting their behavior and response to treatment. By creating tracking databases of what happens with Web site users, the information gathered can be used to improve services and to decrease long-term health care service, training, and administration costs on a continuing basis.

Because of all the data being collected on how individuals are using different Web sites or other Internet-based services, there has been some concern over the individual's right to privacy and the protection of the information collected. For instance, some people have been concerned that if they are searching for information related to the human immunodeficiency virus (HIV) or substance use, they might be identified as being at risk for having that condition whether they do or not. Further, many individuals do not want that information linked to their identities or medical records. On one hand, they may be wishing to avoid solicitation of business from sellers of medical services or products because of their association with the condition; they do not want their personal information sold for that purpose to the providers of such products or services. On the other hand, they may also wish to maintain privacy and keep their information confidential so as to avoid having any threat to their future insurability or their ability to get health care coverage. As an example, if a health care provider such as a health maintenance organization (HMO) tracked users' information on a Web site and discovered, through the database, that someone who was now applying for coverage had certain medical conditions, that person might have a greater risk of being refused coverage if his or her time on the Web site was not completely anonymous. In sum, given these concerns, users of Internet medicine need to understand that there are differences between the terms privacy, confidentiality, and anonymity, as well as in the legal issues and protections one can exercise when using this type of medicine. Each Web site may be operating under different constraints, and so it is always important for users of these services to be sure they understand how the Web sites handle privacy. Finding out how a Web site protects or does not protect the privacy of its users is the only way users can determine how safe it is to reveal confidential information when they use a specific Web site.

DIAGNOSTIC AND TREATMENT TECHNIQUES

One of the biggest opportunities offered by Internet medicine is that of increasing the ability of individuals to do self-screening for medical conditions to see if they need medical assistance. Likewise, the ability of service providers to do screening and assessment for a larger number of people is increased relative to what can be done in person. This is because the assessments can be administered via the computer, saving valuable provider time. Additionally, assessments can be completed online and sent to providers in advance for immediate evaluation. While it may be some time before conclusive diagnoses can be offered via online technology, such advances are not far off; the differences between online and in-person assessments are being studied.

Intervention via the Internet is also much improved because large quantities of information can be dispensed electronically, printed out by clients or their families, or distributed to large numbers of individuals. Such informational interventions can be important for facilitating proper compliance with medical prescription regimens, helping clients to avoid bad drug interactions, or providing reminders about other things needed to facilitate wellness. Informational interventions can also be used for primary prevention, or preventing problems from happening in the first place. By providing suggestions for problem prevention, much suffering could be spared and many health care dollars can be saved. This is especially true for teenagers and college-age populations, who are often savvy Internet users.

Treatment also takes place on the Internet via simultaneous online interactions such as in chat rooms, communicating via videoconferencing as in a normal conversation but using video cameras, and simple asynchronous e-mail between the client and the provider. Generally this type of treatment is a complement to face-to-face treatment. For instance, some HMOs use online support groups as additional treatment for persons already receiving therapy. Others are using programs such as self-guided online courses that clients can work through to benefit their health. In general, practitioners are permitted to do this so long as they are properly licensed. This usually requires being licensed by the state in which they are practicing and/or where the client is receiving the services.

PERSPECTIVE AND PROSPECTS

The Internet continues to grow on a daily basis, with an increasing number of computer owners and Web sites taking advantage of its capabilities. Communications technologies are also improving constantly, allowing for almost instant individual communication of written, oral, and visual information at distances and speeds that were inconceivable in the past. As a result of these developments, as well as increases in health care costs and the potential economic and health benefits provided by Internet medicine, this specialty area is here to stay. Commitments by governments to examine such developments in health care underscore this likelihood. In 1998, for example, the Health Resources and Service Administration of the United States Department of Health and Human Services established the Office for the Advancement of Telehealth. This office is devoted to advancing the use of telehealth and Internet-based medicine to facilitate improvement in the state of public health and research on public health. The ability of such approaches to provide more services with streamlined administrative procedures and decreased costs holds much promise for improving the state of public health.

—*Nancy A. Piotrowski, Ph.D.*

See also Allied health; Alternative medicine; Clinical trials; Education, medical; Family medicine; Health maintenance organizations (HMOs); Herbal medicine; Noninvasive tests; Nursing; Pharmacology; Pharmacy; Physical examination; Screening; Self-medication; Telemedicine.

FOR FURTHER INFORMATION:

Armstrong, Myrna L., ed. *Telecommunications for Health Professionals: Providing Successful Distance Education and Telehealth.* New York: Springer, 1998. Provides strategies for using distance education and resources. Legal and ethical issues are discussed to inform patients, providers, students, and legislators.

Coiera, Enrico. *Guide to Health Informatics.* 2d ed. New York: Oxford University Press, 2003. The boundaries of appropriate communication of medical information via the Internet are outlined in this book tailored to the general reader, student, or trainer of health care provision.

Davis, James B., ed. *Health and Medicine on the Internet: A Comprehensive Guide to Medical Information on the World Wide Web.* 4th ed. Los Angeles: Practice Management Information, 2003. Provides an annual guide for individuals interested in Internet-based health care.

Goldstein, Douglas E. *E-Healthcare: Harness the Power of the Internet, e-Commerce, and e-Care.* Gaithersburg, Md.: Aspen, 2000. An easy to understand resource, for patients, service providers, and entrepreneurs interested in online health care, describing the types of services provided and important legal issues. Helpful CD-ROM included.

Kinsella, Audrey. *Home Telehealth in the Twenty-first Century: A Resource Book About Improved Care Services That Work.* Kensington, Md.: Information for Tomorrow, 2000. Provides an in-depth discussion of how telemedicine can help with chronic medical concerns.

McKenzie, Bruce C., ed. *Medicine and the Internet.* 3d ed. New York: Oxford University Press, 2002. Focuses on use of the Internet from a clinical point of view and discusses online medical advice. Intended for students and health care personnel.

Maheu, Marlene, Ace Allen, and Pamela Whitten. *E-Health, Telehealth, and Telemedicine: A Guide to Startup and Success.* San Francisco: Jossey-Bass, 2001. A resource guide for health organizations that want to use communication technologies to expand and transform their organizations. Covers topics such as program development, technical options, and ethical, legal, and regulatory issues.

Office for the Advancement of Telehealth. http://www.hrsa.gov/telehealth/. An organization devoted to advancing the use of telehealth and Internet-based medicine to facilitate improvement in the state of public health and research on public health.

Price, Joan. *Complete Idiot's Guide to Online Medical Resources.* Indianapolis: Que, 2000. Provides information on traditional and alternative medicine approaches, helping readers evaluate Internet-based information so as to avoid bad or unreliable advice or recommendations.

Interstitial pulmonary fibrosis (IPF)

Disease/disorder

Also known as: Idiopathic pulmonary fibrosis, cryptogenic fibrosing alveolitis

Anatomy or system affected: Heart, lungs

Specialties and related fields: Emergency medicine, internal medicine, pulmonary medicine

Definition: An inflammatory disease that results in the scarring and fibrosis of the lung alveolar tissue (air sacs).

Causes and Symptoms

Interstitial pulmonary fibrosis (IPF) is a chronic lung disease that causes scarring of the tissue between the air sacs (interstitium). It may be the result of a variety of causes, such as occupational exposure to silica or asbestos, drugs, radiation, and diseases such as sarcoidosis or connective tissue diseases (systemic lupus erythematosus, rheumatoid arthritis). When no known cause can be ascertained, the disease is known as idiopathic pulmonary fibrosis. It affects both sexes equally, with the highest incidence between the ages of forty and sixty.

The disease is characterized by an initial inflammation of the alveoli attributable to a known or unknown injury-causing agent, followed by healing by scarring and fibrosis of the interstitium. This results in a decreased transfer of oxygen to the blood, causing symptoms of increasing shortness of breath (dyspnea) and chest pain. The symptoms of the disease appear insidiously, with the patient noticing a dry cough and increasing shortness of breath, initially on exertion and eventually at rest. As the disease progresses, the patient is unable to perform daily activities and may require long-term oxygen therapy. Clubbing of the fingers and blueness of the extremities can be observed in these patients. Death is usually the result of respiratory failure, right-sided heart failure, a blood clot (embolism) in the lungs, stroke, or heart attack.

Diagnosis of IPF is made by correlating a chest X ray, a computed tomography (CT) chest scan, lung function tests, bronchoscopy, and a measurement of blood oxygen content. Lung biopsy and microscopic examination of the tissue is the only confirmatory test that would also show the extent of damage and help determine the prognosis of the disease.

Treatment and Therapy

Treatment must be initiated as soon as the diagnosis is made. Because of the chronic nature of the disease, most patients require lifelong treatment. Treatment modalities differ with age and the stage of the disease, but all aim at reducing the inflammation and stopping the fibrosis. Drugs are the mainstay of treatment, with prednisone (a corticosteroid) and cyclophosphamide being the most commonly used ones. Oxygen therapy improves the blood oxygen level in patients with severe breathlessness, and physical therapy and exercise also help in improving muscle strength and breathing. Patients with severe fibrosis require lung transplantation, the success rate of which is about 60 percent.

—*Rashmi Ramasubbaiah, M.D.,*
and Venkat Raghavan Tirumala, M.D., M.H.A.

See also Asbestos exposure; Lungs; Occupational health; Oxygen therapy; Pulmonary diseases; Pulmonary medicine; Respiration; Rheumatoid arthritis; Systemic lupus erythematosus (SLE).

For Further Information:

Kasper, Dennis L., et al., eds. *Harrison's Principles of Internal Medicine.* 16th ed. New York: McGraw-Hill, 2005.

Lynch, Joseph, ed. *Idiopathic Pulmonary Fibrosis.* New York: Marcel Dekker, 2004.

Parker, James N., and Philip M. Parker, eds. *The Official Patient's Sourcebook on Idiopathic Pulmonary Fibrosis.* San Diego, Calif.: Icon Health, 2002.

Rakel, Robert E., ed. *Textbook of Family Practice.* 6th ed. Philadelphia: W. B. Saunders, 2002.

Simpson, John, and Ann Millar. *Advances in Pulmonary Fibrosis.* Boca Raton, Fla.: CRC Press, 2004.

Information on Interstitial Pulmonary Fibrosis (IPF)

Causes: Various; may include occupational exposure to silica or asbestos, drugs, radiation, diseases (sarcoidosis, lupus erythematosus, rheumatoid arthritis)

Symptoms: Scarring of lung tissue, shortness of breath, chest pain, dry cough, clubbing of fingers, blue extremities; death may come from respiratory failure, heart failure, blood clot, stroke, heart attack

Duration: Progressive, eventually fatal

Treatments: Drugs (prednisone, cyclophosphamide); oxygen therapy; physical therapy and exercise; lung transplantation

INTESTINAL CANCER. *See* **STOMACH, INTESTINAL, AND PANCREATIC CANCERS.**

INTESTINAL DISORDERS
DISEASE/DISORDER
ANATOMY OR SYSTEM AFFECTED: Abdomen, anus, gastrointestinal system, intestines

SPECIALTIES AND RELATED FIELDS: Family medicine, gastroenterology, internal medicine

DEFINITION: Diseases or disorders of the small intestine, large intestine (or colon), liver, pancreas, and gallbladder.

KEY TERMS:
acute: the stage of a disease or presence of a symptom that begins abruptly, with marked intensity, and subsides after a short time

chronic: the stage of a disease or presence of a symptom that develops slowly and usually lasts for the lifetime of the individual

diarrhea: the passage of approximately six loose stools within a twenty-four-hour period caused by a variety of circumstances, such as infection, malabsorption, or irritable bowel

diverticulitis: inflammation or swelling of one or more diverticula, caused by the penetration of fecal material through thin-walled diverticula and the collection of bacteria or other irritating agents there

diverticulosis: the presence of diverticula in the colon, which may lead to diverticulitis

diverticulum: an outpouching through the muscular wall of a tubular organ, such as the stomach, small intestine, or colon

electrolytes: elements or compounds found in blood, interstitial fluid, and cell fluid that are critical for normal metabolism and function

peristalsis: the involuntary, coordinated, rhythmic contraction of the muscles of the gastrointestinal tract that forces partially digested food along its length

stricture: an abnormal narrowing of an organ because of pressure or inflammation

villi: folds within the small intestine that are important for the absorption of nutrients into the blood

PROCESS AND EFFECTS
Intestinal diseases and disorders are sometimes included with those of the digestive system. For the sake of clarity, this article makes the distinction between the structures of the digestive and intestinal tracts. The entire digestive tract, which includes the intestinal tract and is approximately 7.6 to 9.1 meters in length in adults, begins in the mouth and ends with the anus. It includes organs specific to digestion, such as the esophagus and stomach and their substructures. The intestinal tract, which constitutes the major part of the digestive tract, includes the small intestine, the large intestine (also known as the colon), and the organs that branch off these structures (the liver, pancreas, and gallbladder). The function of the small and large intestines is to break down food, absorb its nutrients into the bloodstream, and carry off waste products of digestion as feces.

The small intestine is approximately 6.1 meters long and 3.8 centimeters in diameter and is made up of the duodenum, the jejunum, and the ileum. It is where the process of digestion begins in full. The smaller products broken down by the stomach are received by the small intestine, where they are absorbed into the bloodstream through its lining by villi combined with bile (from the liver) and pancreatic juices.

Almost all food nutrients are absorbed in the small intestine. What passes into the large intestine is a mix of unabsorbed nutrients, water, fiber, and electrolytes. Most of the moisture from this process is removed as the mix passes through the large intestine, leaving solid waste products. Before excretion as feces, approximately 90 percent of the liquid that entered the large intestine has been reabsorbed. This reabsorption is necessary for health because the liquid contains sodium and water.

The large intestine is approximately 1.5 meters long and connected to the small intestine at the ileocecal valve. Waste products from the digestive process pass

---

INFORMATION ON INTESTINAL DISORDERS

CAUSES: Infection by bacteria or parasites, obstruction, cancer or tumor of rectum and colon, polyps

SYMPTOMS: Varies; can include persistent diarrhea, abdominal cramping or bloating, pain, swelling, fever, fatigue, constipation, nausea and vomiting, loss of appetite

DURATION: Acute or chronic

TREATMENTS: Surgery, anti-inflammatory and antidiarrheal medications, antibiotics, chemotherapy and/or radiation therapy through this valve into a large holding area of the large intestine called the cecum. The appendix is attached to this structure. The large intestine consists of the ascending colon (which begins on the right side of the abdomen and moves up toward the liver), the transverse colon (which crosses the abdomen), and the descending colon (which moves down the left side of the abdomen). The sigmoid colon is an S-shaped structure that connects to the descending colon and joins the rectum, a tube 12 to 20 centimeters long that leads to the anus. Small microorganisms in the large intestine break down waste products not broken down by the stomach and small intestines, resulting in gas (also known as flatus).

COMPLICATIONS AND DISORDERS

Diseases and disorders of the intestinal tract constitute a major health problem affecting many individuals at one point or another in their lives. The common diseases and disorders that affect the intestinal tract are those of acute inflammatory disorders (appendicitis), diverticular disorders (diverticulosis and diverticulitis), chronic inflammatory bowel disease (Crohn's disease and ulcerative colitis), intestinal infections (intestinal parasites and bacterial infections with *Salmonella*, *Shigella dysenteriae*, and *Escherichia coli*), intestinal obstructions, cancers or tumors of the rectum and colon, and polyps.

The most common acute inflammatory disorder is appendicitis. Its symptoms usually affect individuals between the ages of ten and thirty and include abdominal pain and tenderness, nausea and vomiting, loss of appetite, rapid heart rate, fever, and an elevated white blood cell count. Normally, the appendix, whose function is not clearly understood, fills and empties with food as regularly as does the cecum, of which it is a part. It sometimes becomes inflamed because of either kinking or obstruction, producing pressure and initiating symptoms. The most common major complication associated with appendicitis is perforation, which causes severe pain and an elevation of temperature. In these cases, a physician must be notified immediately. Treatment consists of surgical removal of the appendix.

Diverticular disorders include diverticulosis and diverticulitis. Diverticulosis is the presence of diverticula without any inflammation or symptoms. Diverticulitis is the result of an inflammation or infection of the intestine produced when food or bacteria are retained in a diverticulum. Signs of diverticulosis include cramplike pain in the left lower part of the abdomen, bowel irregu-

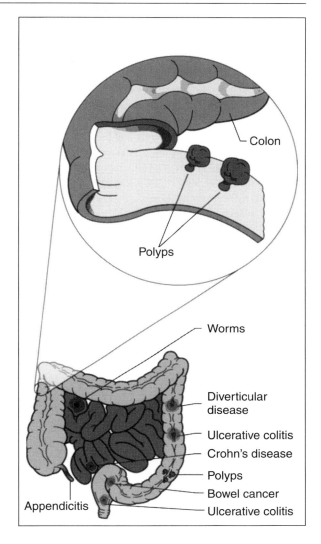

larity, diarrhea, constipation, and thin stools. There may be some intermittent rectal bleeding with diverticulitis.

Inflammatory bowel disease (IBD) of unknown cause is most common in whites (usually female) between the ages of fifteen and thirty-five, occurring most frequently in the American Jewish population. The two types of IBD are Crohn's disease, which is also known as regional enteritis, and ulcerative colitis. The disorders are considered to be separate diseases with similar characteristics.

Crohn's disease may affect any part of the intestinal tract but often affects the small intestine. The inflammation usually involves the entire thickness of the intestinal wall. Treatment for Crohn's disease depends on the presence or absence of symptoms. If there are no symptoms, treatment is not necessary. If there is evidence of inflammation, however, anti-inflammatory medication may be prescribed. Vitamin and mineral replacement may be given because of the problems of absorption associated with this disease. Surgery may be required at some point in the disease process because of its associated complications, such as obstruction.

Ulcerative colitis is characterized by tiny ulcers and abscesses in the inner lining of the colon, where it is usually confined. There is a tendency for these ulcerations to bleed, causing bloody diarrhea. The chronic nature of inflammatory bowel disease may cause a stricture, which can result in an obstruction requiring surgical intervention. As with Crohn's disease, the treatment for ulcerative colitis depends on the type of symptoms and may consist of medication, nutrition, or surgery. Anti-inflammatory drugs are used for flare-ups of the disease. Liquid food supplements may be given to compensate for nutrients lost in diarrhea. Intravenous therapy may be prescribed if the colon is considered too diseased to tolerate food.

There are many types of infections that affect the intestinal tract. The most common bacterial infections are caused by microorganisms such as *Salmonella* and *Shigella*. *Salmonella* bacteria are commonly found in meats, fruits (through contaminated fertilizer), poultry, eggs, dairy products, and contaminated marijuana. Pet turtles are also a source of this bacteria. The source of infections for *Shigella* bacteria is feces from an infected person, with the route of transmission being oral-fecal—for example, changing the soiled diaper of an infant, or having a bowel movement, and then eating or preparing food without properly washing the hands.

Intestinal parasites may also cause infection. The most common of these parasites, *Giardia lamblia*, is present where water supplies are contaminated by raw sewage. The primary treatment for these conditions consists of replacement of lost fluids and essential electrolytes. Although not normally used because they may interfere with the elimination of the causative agent, antidiarrheal medications may be prescribed.

Intestinal obstruction occurs when the normal flow of the intestine is partially or totally impeded because of an accumulation of contents, gas, or fluid. It may also be caused by the intestine's inability to propel contents along the intestinal tract in the process called peristalsis. Peristalsis may be obstructed by scars that bind together two normally separate anatomic surfaces (adhesions), hernias, or tumors. Another cause may be a paralytic ileus, a paralysis of the peristaltic movement of the intestinal tract caused by the effect of trauma or toxins on the nerve endings that regulate intestinal movement. Conservative treatment consists of decompression of the bowel using a nasogastric tube. Surgical treatment may be indicated if the bowel is completely obstructed.

While tumors of the small intestine are rare, tumors of the colon are common. Cancer of the colon and rectum is the second most common type of cancer in the United States (with lung cancer being the most common). The majority of intestinal tumors are benign (noncancerous) and discovered between the ages of forty and sixty. There are several types of benign tumors, which do not spread. They include lipomas, leiomyomas, angiomas, and adenomas. A small percentage of tumors of the small intestine is malignant (cancerous). The most common are adenocarcinomas, leiomyosarcomas, carcinoid tumors, and lymphomas. The symptoms of these tumors include weight loss, abdominal pain, nausea and vomiting, and bleeding. Treatment is dependent upon the stage and location of the tumor. Surgical removal of the tumor may be coupled with chemotherapy and/or radiation therapy.

Polyps are benign tumors of the large intestine and are common to individuals over the age of sixty. They arise from the lining of the colon and are usually found during tests to diagnose other conditions. Polyps include several different varieties, the most common of which is a hyperplastic polyp. Hyperplastic polyps are less than one-half of a centimeter in diameter and do not pose a health risk. Juvenile polyps can occur in childhood, and inflammatory polyps are believed to result from injury or inflammation, such as after an episode of ulcerative colitis. Neither of these conditions poses a health risk. There is a major category of polyps known as adenomas, however, which have the potential for malignancy. These types of polyps are generally removed to prevent the development of cancer.

Rectal cancer and colon cancer are two types of cancer common among both men and women. Factors that predispose an individual to these types of cancer include family history or a prior history of adenomatous colon polyps, colon cancer, or ulcerative colitis. The precise cause of these cancers is unknown, but diet is believed to play a significant role, specifically diets low in fiber and high in animal fat. One of the key symptoms of these conditions requiring immediate attention (especially for individuals over the age of forty) is rectal bleeding. Treatment consists of surgery to remove the affected part of the colon. The physician may prescribe additional treatment in the form of chemotherapy and/or radiation therapy.

PERSPECTIVE AND PROSPECTS

Problems associated with the intestinal tract are characterized by a variety of symptoms and treatments. These problems may be temporary in nature or may be manifestations of more serious underlying conditions interfering with the normal functions of absorption, fluid and electrolyte balance, and elimination. Symptoms are signs of malfunction and should not be ignored or go untreated.

Preventing problems associated with the intestinal tract may not always be possible because the causes of some intestinal diseases and disorders are unknown. Nevertheless, there has been substantial research related to intestinal diseases and disorders to support a strong correlation between nutrition and intestinal tract health. For example, there is evidence to support the relationship between the consumption of sugars, high amounts of animal protein and fat, and cholesterol and cancer-causing agents in the intestinal tract. Stress and its resulting influence on stomach acidity also contribute to intestinal ill health. Smoking and lack of regular exercise may also negatively influence normal peristalsis.

The prevention of these and other problems related to intestinal health are important not only to general health but also to work productivity. In the United States, for example, intestinal problems account for a large percentage of lost work time. Education about intestinal health and health issues beginning early in one's life will lower the incidence of some of the more common intestinal diseases and disorders.

—*John A. Bavaro, Ed.D., R.N.*

See also Abdomen; Abdominal disorders; Appendectomy; Appendicitis; Bacterial infections; Bariatric surgery; Bypass surgery; Celiac sprue; Cholecystitis; Colic; Colitis; Colon and rectal polyp removal; Colon and rectal surgery; Colon cancer; Colon therapy; Colonoscopy and sigmoidoscopy; Constipation; Crohn's disease; Diarrhea and dysentery; Digestion; Diverticulitis and diverticulosis; Enemas; Enterocolitis; Fistula repair; Food poisoning; Gastroenterology; Gastroenterology, pediatric; Gastrointestinal disorders; Gastrointestinal system; Hemorrhoid banding and removal; Hemorrhoids; Hernia; Hernia repair; Hirschsprung's disease; Ileostomy and colostomy; Indigestion; Internal medicine; Intestines; Irritable bowel syndrome (IBS); Lactose intolerance; Malabsorption; Malnutrition; Nutrition; Obesity; Obesity, childhood; Obstruction; Parasitic diseases; Peristalsis; Pinworms; Proctology; Roundworms; Soiling; Stomach, intestinal, and pancreatic cancers; Tapeworms; Tumor removal; Tumors; Worms.

FOR FURTHER INFORMATION:

Kapadia, Cyrus R., James M. Crawford, and Caroline Taylor. *An Atlas of Gastroenterology: A Guide to Diagnosis and Differential Diagnosis.* Boca Raton, Fla.: Pantheon, 2003. Provides a fully illustrated, nonspecialist understanding of myriad gastrointestinal diseases, including heartburn, dyspepsia, diarrhea, irritable bowel syndrome, and pancreatitis. Includes bibliographic references and index.

Leikin, Jerrold B., and Martin S. Lipsky, eds. *American Medical Association Complete Medical Encyclopedia.* New York: Random House Reference, 2003. Written in an encyclopedic format, this book is an authoritative guide to all aspects of medical and health topics. Contains many illustrations of various body systems and organs that are clearly presented and simple to understand.

Litin, Scott C., ed. *Mayo Clinic Family Health Book.* 3d ed. New York: HarperResource, 2003. This comprehensive medical guide was written for the general public by experts in the field of medicine. Intestinal disorders of the abdominal cavity are discussed in sections titled "Diseases and Disorders" and "Tests and Treatments."

Payne, Wayne A., and Dale B. Hahn, and Ellen Mauer. *Understanding Your Health.* 8th ed. New York: McGraw-Hill, 2004. An introductory textbook that is easy to read. Focuses on overall health and disease prevention. Each chapter offers a list of references and recommended readings related specifically to its content.

Peikin, Steven. *Gastrointestinal Health.* Rev. ed. New York: HarperCollins, 1999. Concerned almost wholly with the effect of nutrition on gastrointestinal (GI) maladies, the author offers a self-help guide for the afflicted. After explaining the GI tract's workings and describing common symptoms, Peikin specifies diets that he argues will relieve symptoms.

Tapley, Donald F., et al., eds. *The Columbia University College of Physicians and Surgeons Complete Home Medical Guide.* Rev. 3d ed. New York: Crown, 1995. An outstanding reference guide organized by each organ system and its function. Written in easily understandable terms and avoids the use of medical jargon. Part 3 provides in-depth information on how the body works and includes a full-color atlas showing major organ systems.

Tortora, Gerard J., and Bryan Derrickson. *Principles of Anatomy and Physiology*. 11th ed. Hoboken, N.J.: John Wiley & Sons, 2006. This highly readable text gives a clear and accurate description of the anatomy and physiology of the gastrointestinal system. The illustrations and diagrams are excellent. The authors include descriptions of major disorders and clinical applications.

INTESTINES

ANATOMY

ANATOMY OR SYSTEM INVOLVED: Abdomen, anus, gastrointestinal system

SPECIALTIES AND RELATED FIELDS: Gastroenterology, internal medicine

DEFINITION: The portion of the gastrointestinal tract from the lower end of the stomach to the anus, which consists of the small intestine and the colon (large intestine).

KEY TERMS:

amylase: the enzyme responsible for breaking down carbohydrates in the small intestine; amylase enters the intestinal tract from the salivary glands and the pancreas

colon: the large intestine, divided from the small intestine by the cecum (a controlled passageway) and ending at the sigmoid, which leads food waste into the rectum

fiber: food material derived from plant substances that retain the full structure of their cell walls despite the chemical effects of the digestive process

lipases: enzymes secreted by the pancreas into the small intestine; these serve to break down fatty materials (triglycerides) in the first intestinal stage of digestion

peristalsis: the muscular contraction in the walls of the intestines that propels food material forward through the bowels

STRUCTURE AND FUNCTIONS

After the initial process of digestion takes place in the stomach, food passes into the intestines, where the chemical action of several gastric juices separates out the nutritive content of fats, carbohydrates, and proteins. This nutritive material is then absorbed into the bloodstream through the walls of the intestines, while waste material is collected for excretion.

In adult humans, the small intestine and large intestine together represent a total length of about 9 meters (30 feet). Both small and large intestines are hoselike muscular organs; the former is much longer, but substantially narrower, than the latter. The two intestines are joined at the cecum, which is located in the right-lower abdominal cavity. The appendix, which is sometimes called a "blind pouch" because it is unessential to the main processes performed in the gastrointestinal tract, projects from the cecum.

The physical disposition and function of the large intestine, or colon, are distinct from those of the small intestine. As the large intestinal tube leaves the cecum, it assumes a specific shape, following horizontal and vertical lines within the abdominal cavity. This is not the case with the small intestine, whose extensive length (about 7 meters, or 23 feet) takes an intertwined "nesting" shape in the limited abdominal space available. By contrast, the colon, which is about 1.5 meters (5 feet) in length, has three easily identifiable sections: the ascending colon on the right side of the abdominal cavity, the transverse colon, and the descending colon on the left side of the abdomen. A final leftward bend in the colon at the sigmoid provides for its attachment to the rectum.

The two parts of the intestines carry out distinct functions in the overall digestive process. As food material passes from the lower end, or pylorus, of the stomach, only a part of the digestive process has occurred. Once partially digested food enters the small intestine, it is propelled through the intestine by means of a process of muscular contraction in the intestinal wall, which is called peristalsis.

As the food moves forward, different substances, some secreted from the lining of the intestine itself, and others—principally, bile and pancreatic fluid, which enter the upper intestine (duodenum) from the liver and pancreas—contribute to a further breaking down of food material.

Very small projections called villi are found along the interior surface of the small intestine. The villi absorb those portions of the food material that have been altered by the digestive process. From the villi, nutritive material is passed into the blood and lymphatic system for distribution to cells throughout the body. This process continues in the middle and end portions (jejunum and ileum, respectively) of the small intestine until, passing through the cecum, the remaining residue enters the large intestine.

The mixture of material contained in the large intestine, or colon, consists of indigestible food, bacteria, and substantial amounts of water. Most of the water is absorbed into the body through the walls of the colon, while the remaining waste material, or feces, is excreted through the rectum.

In order to understand how food materials are actually absorbed by the villi inside the small intestine and passed into the bloodstream, one must consider several chemical processes, according to the nature of the material in question.

For example, the triglyceride components of fat, chains of fatty acids attached to glycerol, are chemical compounds that do not dissolve in water (a major part of the main bloodstream). The pancreatic enzymes called lipases split the triglycerides into separate units of fatty acid. Once separated, these fatty acids become coated with bile salts secreted by the liver, a process that allows them to pass into the mucous cells lining the intestine. As this passage occurs, the coated fatty acids (micelles) resume their chainlike form as triglycerides. At this point, however, the triglycerides have assumed an altered chemical state. In this altered form, fats can be absorbed into the blood and carried throughout the body to be used as body "fuel" or, if unused, stored in fatty tissues.

Carbohydrates must be broken down into simple sugars (glucose, galactose, and fructose) before they can be absorbed by the cell linings of the small intestine. This process occurs when the more complex carbohydrates (both starches and sugars) are split by the chemical effects of the enzyme amylase, which enters the small intestine from the salivary glands and the pancreas.

Finally, proteins, which contain the amino acids so essential for the process of tissue formation in the body, must be split in several stages, the first of which occurs in the stomach itself. Here, proteins are partially broken down by the action of the gastric juices, mainly pepsin. Once protein material passes into the upper part of the small intestine, or duodenum, the process is accelerated by the influence of two main pancreatic enzymes: trypsin and chymotrypsin. These secretions cause the proteins to release amino acids in three forms: simple, dual, or triplicate bodies. It is not until these three forms are actually inside the cell walls of the small intestine that other enzymes split the dual and triplicate amino acids into their simplest single form, which can be absorbed into the veins that carry nourishment to the various organs of the body.

In the overall chemical process leading to the absorption of various body nutrients by the small and large intestines, there is a certain "absorptive specialization" in different zones of the gastrointestinal tract. Iron and calcium, for example, are absorbed in the duodenum, while proteins, fats, sugars, and all vitamins except vitamin B_{12} are absorbed in the jejunum. Finally, in the ileum, salt, vitamin B_{12}, and bile salts are processed.

DISORDERS AND DISEASES

Doctors have always known that the digestive processes of the intestines can be affected in either positive or negative ways by the nature of the food that is consumed. In the simplest terms, negative reactions are manifested by the obvious effects of indigestion and diarrhea. The control of such symptoms of improper or incomplete digestion may appear to the layperson to be a simple matter of using "over-the-counter" tablets such as laxatives or "antigas" pills. Treatment of the symptoms of indigestion, however, may provide only a superficial solution to a problem that is much more serious.

An area of important medical concern that goes beyond the general discomfort caused by imbalanced digestive functioning of the intestines involves peptic ulcers. A peptic ulcer is an open sore on the mucous membrane lining the gastrointestinal tract. The general label "peptic ulcer" was applied to this condition since the discovery, in the mid-1830's, of pepsin, the first clearly identified enzyme known to contribute to the chemical breakdown of ingested foods. Although later stages of research into the digestive process yielded much more extensive knowledge of the component elements of gastric juices, the specific name has remained attached to the general phenomenon of intestinal ulceration. The term "gastric ulcer" refers specifically to ulceration in the stomach lining.

Generally speaking, peptic ulcers occur when there is an imbalance between the task of digestion to be accomplished by the intestines and the amounts and levels of concentration of the gastric juices secreted into the gastrointestinal tract. When the amounts or concentrated strengths of gastric juices in the intestines exceed the level required for digestion (or flow into the intestine when no food has been ingested), these agents actually begin to digest the membranes of the intestine itself.

Various forms of treatment for intestinal ulcers have been developed, including both therapeutic drugs that have the capacity to counteract the corrosive effects of excessive gastric juices and, in the preventive vein, diets that contain natural combatants against intestinal disorders, especially high-fiber, unprocessed, or lightly processed foods.

In recent years, research into the causes of ulcers has extended into the field of gastrointestinal hormonal secretions originating not in the pancreas itself but in the intestine or stomach. These secretions reach the pancreas later through the bloodstream and stimulate its production of digestive juices. Such secretive processes may, if they fail to communicate properly balanced "codes" concerning the task of digestion that needs to take place in the intestines, cause an excessive supply (in volume or strength) of gastric juices, which can cause ulcerations to develop.

The most serious pathological condition that can affect the intestines is cancer of the colon. Thought to develop from a degenerative process originating in benign polyps (stem-based tumors that may develop in areas of the organism lined with mucous membrane, such as the nose, the colon, and, in females, the uterus), cancer of the colon has registered a survival rate that is statistically higher than those of cancers in other vital organs of the abdominal cavity (the liver and stomach, in particular). This is partly because—if the cancer is discovered in time—substantial areas of the colon that have been attacked by cancer can be removed surgically without endangering the continued essential functioning of the intestines.

Almost all questions relating to the pathology of the intestinal tract are somehow connected with the type of food that is eaten. Thus, medical science has turned increasingly to publicizing preventive dietary practices that can have a bearing on all functions of the intestines, from the simplest level of discomfort to the most serious level of chronic diseases.

As stated above, a relatively recent and valuable contribution to the knowledge of natural ways to aid in the absorptive work of both the small intestine and the colon—and to reduce the dangers of ulceration and/or intestinal cancer—involves the role of the fiber content of foods. Fiber is generally described as consisting of polysaccharides and lignin, two plant substances that, more than any other nutritive material, retain their natural forms as plant cell walls and are not broken down by human digestive enzymes. The plant food that is richest in these materials is wheat bran, which contains about 40 percent fiber. As fiber-rich foodstuffs such as bran pass through the gastrointestinal tract, the fiber material they contain is subject to fermentation by anaerobic bacteria in the colon. Two chemical results of

this complex process seem to be the removal of deoxycholic acid from the bile and the reduction of the cholesterol saturation level of the bile. Both effects are deemed beneficial, since the reduction of deoxycholic acid and cholesterol in intestinal bile tends, at the very least, to reduce the likelihood of developing gallstones. Fiber-rich diets in combination with the reduction of excess weight became standard symbols of preventive health care by the 1990's.

By the mid-twentieth century, typical personal diets in the Western world contained commercially refined foodstuffs that were rich in sugars and syrups, which are mainly fiber depleted. In addition to the specific disease-related factors mentioned above, medical science has noted that high consumption of fiber-depleted foods results in higher levels of energy intake (absorption of Calories) during the digestive process that occurs in the intestines. In simple terms, when Calorie intake exceeds the level required by the normally exercised body, the result is weight gain that may continue to the point of obesity.

PERSPECTIVE AND PROSPECTS

Medical science began to become aware of the various digestive functions of hormonal secretions only in the first decades of the twentieth century. Although the early nineteenth century American army surgeon William Beaumont was the first doctor to discover the presence of gastric juices in the intestines, his analysis of digestive fluids remained quite elementary. Beaumont could easily identify hydrochloric acid in stomach secretions. He also took samples of bile from the intestinal tract and performed laboratory experiments that proved the role of bile in breaking down fatty materials. What remained unsolved were the identity and origins of other components of gastric juice and an explanation for their controlled secretion from surrounding organs in the abdominal cavity into the intestines. Beaumont's view that mental concentration (including "negative mental concentration," or anxiety) induced the flow of gastric juices proved eventually to be only partially correct.

It was only in 1902 that the British doctors Ernest Henry Starling and Sir William Maddock Bayliss were able to show that, in addition to nerve "signals," certain chemical factors induced the flow of gastric juices, specifically from the pancreas into the intestinal tract. These doctors found that, in fact, the small intestine released into the bloodstream a "chemical transmitter" that, as it circulated to the other vital organs, stimulated the production and flow of the pancreatic juices necessary for digestion. They called this "chemical transmitter" secretin. To this initial agent would be added a whole category of secretions that are called "hormones," a term taken from the Greek word for "urging on."

A discovery was made in 1928 that helped to clarify the complex relationship of hormones, gastric juice secretion, and the carrying out of the digestive process by the small and large intestines. This was the discovery of pancreozymin, the second main "chemical transmitter" affecting the pancreas, by the American researcher Andrew Ivy. Pancreozymin was found to cause the release by the pancreas of an enzyme-rich fluid made up of three agents: trypsin, lipase, and amylase. Each agent proved to be an activator in the process of breaking down different nutrients (protein, fats, and carbohydrates, respectively).

Although the intestines are the ultimate destination of and seat of activity for the pancreatic juices released by command of this hormone (as well as of the last major digestion-linked hormone, gastrin, which was discovered in 1955), secretin alone has its origin in the intestines themselves. Both pancreozymin and gastrin are secreted from the stomach.

In time, researchers found that most gastrointestinal hormones are secreted by specialized cells that line the interior of the stomach. Such cells react at various levels according to the composition of the food that has been ingested, sending chemical signals, via the hormones they secrete, that determine the relative amounts and strengths of the several gastric juices that enter the intestines from the pancreas. A similar question of varied amounts and strengths of gastric juices was linked to the so-called vagus nerve function, which also activates pancreatic flow to the intestinal tract.

The functional relationship between these two activator agents—the one nervous and the other chemical—has become one of the primary interests of researchers who deal with the most common ailment attacking the intestinal organs: peptic ulceration.

—*Byron D. Cannon, Ph.D.*

See also Abdomen; Abdominal disorders; Bypass surgery; Colitis; Colon and rectal surgery; Colonoscopy and sigmoidoscopy; Digestion; Endoscopy; Enemas; Gastroenterology; Gastroenterology, pediatric; Gastrointestinal disorders; Gastrointestinal system; Hemorrhoids; Hernia; Internal medicine; Intestinal disorders; Laparoscopy; Malnutrition; Nutrition; Obstruction; Peristalsis; Proctology.

FOR FURTHER INFORMATION:

Feldman, Mark, Lawrence S. Friedman, and Lawrence J. Brandt, eds. *Sleisenger and Fordtran's Gastrointestinal and Liver Disease: Pathophysiology, Diagnosis, Management.* 8th ed. 2 vols. Philadelphia: W. B. Saunders, 2006. A comprehensive textbook.

Janowitz, Henry D. *Good Food for Bad Stomachs.* New York: Oxford University Press, 1997. A popular work on indigestion and diseases of the gastrointestinal system that suggests diet therapy. Includes an index.

_____. *Indigestion: Living Better with Upper Intestinal Problems from Heartburn to Ulcers and Gallstones.* New York: Oxford University Press, 1994. Uses a scientific and "commonsense" approach to address myriad gastrointestinal disorders.

Marieb, Elaine N., and Katja Hoehn. *Human Anatomy and Physiology.* 7th ed. San Francisco: Pearson Benjamin Cummings, 2007. This introductory anatomy and physiology textbook, easily accessible to those with little science background, is richly illustrated with diagrams and photographs, which help to illuminate body systems and processes.

Scanlon, Valerie, and Tina Sanders. *Essentials of Anatomy and Physiology.* 5th ed. Philadelphia: F. A. Davis, 2007. A text designed around three themes: the relationship between physiology and anatomy, the interrelations among the organ systems, and the relationship of each organ system to homeostasis.

Tortora, Gerard J., and Bryan Derrickson. *Principles of Anatomy and Physiology.* 11th ed. Hoboken, N.J.: John Wiley & Sons, 2006. An outstanding textbook of human anatomy and physiology, and a good first text to consult before reading more advanced gastroenterology texts and journal articles.

Wolfe, M. Michael, et al., eds. *Therapy of Digestive Disorders: A Companion to Sleisenger and Fordtran's Gastrointestinal and Liver Disease.* Philadelphia: W. B. Saunders, 2000. This resource is divided into sections that discuss such topics as esophageal, gastroduodenal, pancreaticobiliary, hepatic, intestinal, and miscellaneous disorders.

INTOXICATION

DISEASE/DISORDER

ALSO KNOWN AS: Inebriation

ANATOMY OR SYSTEM AFFECTED: Brain, heart, psychic-emotional, reproductive system, respiratory system

SPECIALTIES AND RELATED FIELDS: Cardiology, pathology, pharmacology, preventive medicine, psychiatry, public health, toxicology, vascular medicine

DEFINITION: a physical and mental state resulting from having consumed a psychoactive substance and characterized by maladaptive changes in physiological, psychological, mood, and/or cognitive processes.

CAUSES AND SYMPTOMS

Intoxication is a type of substance use disorder described in the *Diagnostic and Statistical Manual of Mental Disorders: DSM-IV-TR* (rev. 4th ed., 2000) by the American Psychiatric Association. Intoxication results from the consumption of substances such as alcohol, caffeine, marijuana, other illicit drugs, some mushrooms and other plants, and even over-the-counter and prescription drugs.

Intoxication is diagnosed via identification of the substance in the body system and the observation of characteristic symptoms in the person affected. Specific substances do certain things to the body and therefore create certain symptoms. Tests of breath and/or urine samples often are used to detect intoxication. Additionally, simply watching the individual for psychological and behavioral signs or asking the individual to perform certain tasks can help with detection. For instance, police officers suspecting alcohol intoxication may request individuals to try to walk a straight line or to close their eyes and try to stand up straight. Such tests allow the officers to observe the person's balance and body sway. Loss of balance or significant body sway can indicate intoxication.

Each substance has specific symptoms associated with its intoxication state. Therefore, when testing someone for intoxication, different tests may be needed to determine whether any individual substance has been used.

INFORMATION ON INTOXICATION

CAUSES: Overconsumption of substances such as alcohol, caffeine, marijuana, or other illicit drugs, prescription drugs

SYMPTOMS: Varies; with alcohol, may include slurred speech, coordination problems, unsteady gait, impairments in memory or attention, stupor, coma

DURATION: Temporary

TREATMENTS: Detoxification

Alcohol intoxication is marked by symptoms such as slurred speech, coordination problems, unsteady gait, nystagmus, impairments in memory or attention, and stupor. Nystagmus is an involuntary condition affecting the eyes in which they do not track the movement of objects smoothly. Stupor is a condition in which the person is in a daze and has numbed senses. With alcohol intoxication, stupor can escalate to coma. In addition to these symptoms, problematic behaviors may also manifest themselves, such as aggression, impaired judgment, mood problems, or problems interacting socially or at work.

TREATMENT AND THERAPY

Intoxication is short-lived; once a substance has been processed out of the body, the effects dissipate. Treatment usually consists of a process called detoxification, often shortened to detox. Typically, this usually is done in emergency rooms or inpatient units in hospitals. Sometimes, however, it may be done in community settings where nonmedical models of intervention are practiced. In all these settings, symptoms are monitored closely as the person withdraws from the substance, as withdrawal can be dangerous. Withdrawal varies from drug to drug. It also varies depending on how long the person has used the substance and how much has been used. Severe withdrawal from certain substances, such as alcohol, can be lethal.

PERSPECTIVE AND PROSPECTS

Intoxication for some substances is easier to identify than for others. Increasingly, methods are being developed to identify intoxication with greater ease via objective measures. For instance, technology to assess the iris of the eye to detect marijuana intoxication or the use of patches to detect substance use, such as with drugs that may be excreted in sweat, are two recent efforts.

—*Nancy A. Piotrowski, Ph.D.*

See also Addiction; Alcoholism; Caffeine; Club drugs; Coma; Marijuana; Poisoning; Toxicology.

FOR FURTHER INFORMATION:

American Psychiatric Association. *Diagnostic and Statistical Manual of Mental Disorders: DSM-IV-TR.* Rev. 4th ed. Washington, D.C.: Author, 2000.

Julien, Robert M. *A Primer of Drug Action: A Concise, Nontechnical Guide to the Actions, Uses, and Side Effects of Psychoactive Drugs.* 10th ed. New York: Worth, 2005.

Weil, Andrew, and Winifred Rosen. *From Chocolate to Morphine: Everything You Need to Know About Mind-Altering Drugs*. Rev. and updated ed. New York: Houghton Mifflin, 2004.

INTRAVENTRICULAR HEMORRHAGE
DISEASE/DISORDER

ANATOMY OR SYSTEM AFFECTED: Brain, nervous system

SPECIALTIES AND RELATED FIELDS: Neonatology, neurology

DEFINITION: Bleeding into or around the normal fluid spaces within the brain.

KEY TERMS:

cerebrospinal fluid (CSF): fluid produced within the ventricles of the brain that flows around the brain and spinal cord

cranial ultrasound: the use of sound waves to obtain a picture of the brain

hydrocephalus: a condition characterized by the abnormal accumulation of fluid within the cranial vault, often accompanied by enlargement of the head and damage to the brain

indomethacin: a nonsteroidal anti-inflammatory drug (NSAID) administered to preterm babies in an attempt to decrease the likelihood of developing intraventricular hemorrhage

ventricles: fluid-filled spaces within the brain

CAUSES AND SYMPTOMS

Intraventricular hemorrhage (IVH) occurs most commonly in premature babies, especially those weighing under 1,500 grams. IVHs have been seen as well in adults as a secondary complication of hemorrhagic stroke, leaving the individual with a poor prognosis.

IVH in premature babies is thought to occur when there is oxygen deprivation during delivery or complications following delivery. Since the blood vessels in the brain of the baby are fragile, they may rupture easily, resulting in excessive bleeding into (intraventricular) or around (periventricular) the ventricles. Generally, there are no outward symptoms. Some infants with IVH may suddenly develop seizures or anemia. IVH is usually diagnosed by cranial ultrasound routinely done on high-risk infants between three and ten days of life, since most cases occur by day three.

Intraventricular hemorrhages are categorized into four grades based on severity. Grade I involves bleeding confined to the small area where it began. Grade II involves blood extending into the ventricles, with no ventricular enlargement. Grade III involves more blood extending into the ventricles, with ventricular enlargement. Grade IV has blood collecting within the brain tissue (intraparenchymal hemorrhage), reflecting injury to the brain. Hydrocephalus is a common complication of Grade III or IV bleeds.

TREATMENT AND THERAPY

Premature babies are given intravenous indomethacin once daily for the first three days of life in order to decrease the likelihood of severe IVH. Steroids given to the mother prior to delivery have also decreased the frequency of severe IVH, as have improved monitoring and care of premature babies. No specific treatment exists for IVH, except to treat symptoms and underlying health problems. If hydrocephalus develops, it can be treated with frequent lumbar punctures or ventricular taps. If the condition persists, a shunt may be placed surgically to drain the extra CSF throughout life. In adults who suffer IVH secondary to hemorrhagic stroke, fibrolytic agents (so-called clot busters) are being evaluated as a mode of treatment.

PERSPECTIVE AND PROSPECTS

IVH has been reported in 35 to 50 percent of infants weighing under 1,500 grams. As gestational age increases, the likelihood of IVH decreases. Grade I IVHs rarely involve long-term problems. Those classified as Grade IV generally do result in long-term sequelae, in-

---

INFORMATION ON INTRAVENTRICULAR HEMORRHAGE

CAUSES: Unknown; possibly oxygen deprivation during premature delivery or subsequent complications, leading to rupture of blood vessels in brain

SYMPTOMS: Generally none, sometimes seizures or anemia; may result in hydrocephalus

DURATION: Acute, with possible long-term consequences if severe (motor problems, developmental delay, seizures, blindness, deafness)

TREATMENTS: Prevention through intravenous indomethacin during first three days of life, steroids given to mother prior to delivery; alleviation of symptoms; insertion of shunt for hydrocephalus cluding motor problems, developmental delay, seizures, blindness, and deafness.

—*Robin Kamienny Montvilo, R.N., Ph.D.*

See also Bleeding; Brain; Brain damage; Brain disorders; Hydrocephalus; Neonatology; Nervous system; Neurology; Neurology, pediatric; Perinatology; Premature birth; Shunts.

FOR FURTHER INFORMATION:

Klaus, Marshall H., and Avroy A. Fanaroff, eds. *Care of the High-Risk Neonate.* 5th ed. Philadelphia: W. B. Saunders, 2001.

Victor, Maurice, and Allan H. Ropper. *Adams and Victor's Principles of Neurology.* 7th ed. New York: McGraw-Hill, 2002.

Volpe, Joseph. *Neurology of the Newborn.* 4th ed. Philadelphia: W. B. Saunders, 2001.

INVASIVE TESTS

PROCEDURES

ANATOMY OR SYSTEM AFFECTED: All

SPECIALTIES AND RELATED FIELDS: All

DEFINITION: Tests that require the passage of an instrument through the body's protective barriers.

INDICATIONS AND PROCEDURES

Skin, sphincters, and gag and cough reflex systems are some of the defenses that can be penetrated to gather important diagnostic information. Invasive tests provide medical insights that are unattainable by noninvasive or laboratory tests. Invasive tests are typically performed last in a diagnostic protocol, however, because penetration of the body defenses is not without risk. An anesthetic agent is commonly used to minimize any discomfort or pain that may arise during the tests. Although invasive, these tests often circumvent the trauma of exploratory surgery.

In general, invasive tests may be classified as those that allow the physician to obtain samples of fluid, tissue, or tumors directly from their site of origin (through aspiration, lumbar puncture, and biopsy) or those that allow direct viewing of specific areas of the body through endoscopy. Some test procedures allow both direct viewing and sample collection; bronchoscopy is one such example.

One of the more familiar aspiration tests is amniocentesis. Amniocentesis involves removing 20 to 30 milliliters of fluid from the amniotic sac for analysis. This test is used in prenatal care at weeks fifteen to eighteen in order to assess the genetic makeup of the fetus or to detect developmental abnormalities.

Fluid from effusions can also be aspirated for analysis. Effusions are collections of an abnormally large quantity of fluid within a serous or synovial cavity. While a small amount of fluid is normal in these cavities, a large amount indicates a pathology that should be identified and treated. Once an effusion is tapped, the fluid is grossly examined for color and for clarity or turbidity. Microscopic investigations of the fluids are performed to assess the types of cells present (such as immune cells or malignant cells) and to identify microorganisms that may be present. Paracentesis is the removal of fluid from effusions within the abdominal, or peritoneal, cavity. If the effusion in this region is large, it is called ascites. Removal of fluid from the lung cavity, called thoracentesis, requires penetration of the chest wall between the ribs (intercostal spaces). Common causes of effusions include infections, congestive heart failure, kidney disease, and malignancy.

Synovial fluid is most commonly aspirated from the knee, but other joints can be investigated in this manner. Red blood cells, inflammatory cells, or crystals may be identified by microscopic evaluation of the aspirated fluid. Osteoarthritis, rheumatoid arthritis, and gout are some diseases that can be diagnosed through synovial fluid aspiration.

Cerebrospinal fluid (CSF) is housed within the bony cranium and spinal column. Fluid from this space is collected by lumbar puncture (spinal tap) and is drawn when a viral, bacterial, or fungal meningitis is suspected. Lumbar puncture may also be performed when a tumor or leukemia of the central nervous system is suspected, or to determine whether a subarachnoid hemorrhage is present.

Fine needle aspiration (FNA) is a specific kind of percutaneous (through-the-skin) needle biopsy. FNA can be used to collect a sample of cells from any palpable mass. By directly inserting a needle into the mass and then washing, or flushing, the region, some cells can be eroded from the tissue surface. These cells are set adrift in the fluid, which is sucked back into the flushing syringe. Microscopic evaluation of the cells can then be performed. Breast, neck, abdominal, and lymph nodes are some of the places where FNA is utilized.

Alternative biopsy techniques include gently scraping off a small surface, as in the Papanicolaou (Pap) smear of the cervix, or removing a deeper tissue sample, as in the punch biopsy of the cervix. Biopsy can sometimes require small surgical incisions to reach a certain organ, such as muscle, skin, breast, bone, or renal (kidney) biopsy.

Tissue biopsies may be taken directly from an organ without surgical incisions; one way to do this is with endoscopy. Typically, endoscopes are flexible probing instruments fitted with fiber-optic viewing devices. Often, a tool attachment allows the use of tiny cutting and sampling devices. Small pieces of tissue can be removed from some otherwise inaccessible areas of the body. Different kinds of endoscopes are used to accommodate the unique structural features of body regions, such as the bronchi, stomach, or colon. Sterile techniques are implemented in all cases.

Bronchoscopy is utilized in diagnosing pulmonary infections and lung cancers or in locating and removing foreign objects found in the airways. Esophagealgastroscopy is used to determine the source of upper gastrointestinal problems such as gastric or peptic ulcers, esophageal varices, esophageal reflux, or malignancy. Colonoscopy is similarly used to evaluate the origins of lower gastrointestinal problems. Colon polyps can be identified, and the mucosal lining of the colon can be evaluated for ulcerative colitis, diverticula, or adenocarcinomas.

Finally, arteriography (including angiography) and cardiac catheterization are important and frequently used invasive tests. These tests are used to evaluate the cardiovascular system. Angiography combines radiographic techniques with the injection of dyes into arteries. This combination allows the physician to determine whether an artery is blocked (occluded). Angiography is particularly useful in patients who have heart conditions, such as angina, and can be used to evaluate renal (kidney) arteries, aortic dissection, or cerebral aneurysms. The result of arteriography is a critical component in determining whether surgery or drug intervention is best for a given patient.

As a diagnostic tool, cardiac catheterization provides insight into the health of a heart. Pictures of the heart can be taken as the catheter is advanced into the right side and then the left side of the heart. A dye is injected into the heart so that the flow can be traced as the heart pumps. The heart chambers, valves, and blood vessels can be evaluated. Additionally, pressures within the heart chambers can be recorded.

USES AND COMPLICATIONS
The greatest health risk with any invasive test is infection. For this reason, sterile methods are used to keep infections and mortality caused by infections to a minimum. With proper care, the risks of invasive testing are surpassed by the benefits of the early and proper diagnosis that such tests provide.

—*Mary C. Fields, M.D.*

See also Amniocentesis; Angiography; Arthroscopy; Biopsy; Blood testing; Breast biopsy; Catheterization; Chorionic villus sampling; Colonoscopy and sigmoidoscopy; Cystoscopy; Endometrial biopsy; Endoscopy; Laparoscopy; Magnetic resonance imaging (MRI); Positron emission tomography (PET) scanning; Radiopharmaceuticals.

FOR FURTHER INFORMATION:
Cavanaugh, Bonita Morrow. *Nurse's Manual of Laboratory and Diagnostic Tests.* 4th ed. Philadelphia: F. A. Davis, 2003. Provides information on hundreds of laboratory and diagnostic tests, with each test presented in two distinct, cross-referenced sections: "Background Information" sections provide a complete description of each test and its purposes; "Clinical Application Data" sections focus on the information nurses most commonly need while caring for clients.

Classen, Meinhard, G. N. J. Tytgat, and C. J. Lightdale, eds. *Gastroenterological Endoscopy.* New York: Thieme Medical, 2002. Text that examines such topics as the impact of endoscopy, its history of use, diagnostic procedures and techniques, therapeutic procedures, descriptions of diseases involving the upper and lower intestine, endoscopic features of infectious diseases of the gastrointestinal tract, and pediatric endoscopy.

Dublin, Arthur B., ed. *Outpatient Invasive Radiologic Procedures: Diagnostic and Therapeutic.* Philadelphia: W. B. Saunders, 1989. Discusses such topics as radiography, radiotherapy, and diagnostic imaging. Also covers interventional radiography. Includes bibliographical references and an index.

Griffith, H. Winter. *Complete Guide to Symptoms, Illness, and Surgery.* Revised and updated by Stephen Moore and Kenneth Yoder. Rev. 4th ed. New York: Perigee, 2000. Covers more than five hundred diseases and disorders and includes information about causes and risk factors, preventive techniques, and diagnostic tests.

Pagana, Kathleen Deska, and Timothy J. Pagana. *Mosby's Diagnostic and Laboratory Test Reference.* 7th ed. St. Louis: Elsevier Mosby, 2005. A clinical handbook that gives alphabetically organized laboratory and diagnostic tests for easy reference. Each listing includes such things as alternate or abbreviated test names, type of test, normal findings, possible critical values, test explanation and related physiology, and potential complications.

Ravin, Carl E., ed. *Imaging and Invasive Radiology in the Intensive Care Unit*. New York: Churchill Livingstone, 1993. Discusses such topics as critical care medicine, diagnostic imaging, and interventional radiology. Includes bibliographical references and an index.

Sloan, John P. *Biopsy Pathology of the Breast*. 2d ed. New York: Oxford University Press, 2001. A practical guide to diagnosing breast pathology. Second edition examines the way in which advances in mammographic screening, more treatment options, greater involvement by pathologists in clinical management, and the expansion of molecular pathology have impacted the field.

Zaret, Barry L., ed. *Yale University School of Medicine Patient's Guide to Medical Tests*. Boston: Houghton Mifflin, 1997. Written and edited by Yale University School of Medicine faculty, this resource provides detailed information on types of diagnostic tests, how doctors use them, and what patients can do for themselves.

IRRITABLE BOWEL SYNDROME (IBS)
DISEASE/DISORDER

ALSO KNOWN AS: Irritable colon, mucous colitis, nervous colon, spastic colon or bowel

ANATOMY OR SYSTEM AFFECTED: Abdomen, anus, gastrointestinal system, intestines, nervous system

SPECIALTIES AND RELATED FIELDS: Alternative medicine, gastroenterology, nutrition

DEFINITION: A common intestinal disorder characterized by abdominal pain or discomfort and by altered bowel habits, consisting of diarrhea or constipation or alternating between diarrhea and constipation.

KEY TERMS:

biofeedback: the technique of making unconscious or involuntary bodily processes perceptible to the senses in order to manipulate them by conscious mental control

biopsychosocial: a model in medicine in which patients are assessed in terms of two important interconnected systems of the mind and the body; in simplest terms, the mind-body connection

colon: the large intestine

cognitive behavioral therapy: a type of psychotherapy that focuses on feelings and actions, especially on replacing negative thoughts with more positive thoughts, thereby resulting in more desirable outcomes

colonoscopy: the use of a small-diameter, flexible tube of optical fibers with an external light source to examine visually the interior of the body, specifically the colon

Crohn's disease: a disease characterized by inflammation of all layers (full thickness) of the intestines or any part of the digestive tract; early symptoms may resemble those of irritable bowel syndrome

defecation: passage of feces through the anus

feces: undigested food and other waste that is eliminated through the anus

gastroenterology: study of the function and diseases associated with the stomach, intestines, and other organs of the digestive tract such as the liver and pancreas

gut: the intestines

ileum: distal part of the small intestine, closest to the starting part of the colon; can be involved in ulcerative colitis

ischemic colitis: inadequate blood supply to the colon

lactose: a sugar found in milk and milk products; some people cannot digest lactose, causing lactose intolerance, which can produce symptoms that resemble those of irritable bowel syndrome

organic: arising from an organ

peristalsis: a series of muscular contractions that move food through the intestines during the process of digestion

physiological: pertaining to functioning; derived from physiology, the study of functions and of the biological, chemical, and physical factors and processes involved in a living organism and its parts

sigmoid: the distal part of the large colon, just before the rectum

sigmoidoscopy: similar to colonoscopy, with the tubular instrument with light instead inspecting only the anus, rectum, and sigmoid colon

somatic: pertaining to the body wall; in contrast to the viscera, which refers to the organs within body cavities

ulcerative colitis: an inflammatory disease that causes superficial ulcers in the ileum, colon, and rectum

CAUSES AND SYMPTOMS

Irritable bowel syndrome (IBS) is a gastrointestinal (GI) disorder characterized by abdominal pain or discomfort associated with diarrhea, constipation, or alternations between these two types of bowel motions. Other GI symptoms are related to this syndrome, including bloating, cramping, gas, heartburn, nausea, passage of mucus, an increased urge to defecate, and a feeling of incomplete defecation. Moreover, non-GI symptoms may accompany IBS, such as discomforts during menstruation, urination, and sexual activities. Although symptoms vary in intensity, they do not grow steadily worse over time but may wax and wane over the years.

IBS is sometimes referred to as a functional disorder. Several causes of IBS have been suggested, but there is no single organic cause that can explain this condition. IBS is understood as a disease with a common set of symptoms that are evaluated based either on the Manning criteria (established in 1978) or the Rome III criteria (updated in 2006) for standardized diagnosis of IBS and for distinguishing organic causes for the syndrome. The Manning criteria include the following: pain relief with defecation, sensation of incomplete defecation, passage of mucus, and frequent and looser stools associated with the onset of pain. The more symptoms are present, the higher the probability of IBS diagnosis. The Rome III criteria include recurrent abdominal pain or discomfort associated with two or more of the following: relief after defecation, frequency, and form (appearance) of stools associated with the onset of pain. The duration of these symptoms should at least be three days per month for the past three months or the onset of symptoms should at least be six months prior to diagnosis.

Three traditional physiological factors contribute to the symptoms of IBS: changes in GI motility, psychological aspects such as stress, and GI hypersensitivity. The GI motility responds to various stimuli such as

food, stress, and gut distention; the resulting changes in activity of the major part of the large intestine or colon can lead to IBS symptoms. Following food digestion by the stomach and the small intestine, the undigested material is propelled toward the rectum by peristalsis. When peristalsis becomes disrupted by IBS, the flow becomes too slow, causing constipation, or too fast, causing diarrhea.

Some foods and drinks appear more likely to trigger IBS attacks by disrupting peristalsis. Fatty foods, fried foods, milk products, chocolate, drinks with caffeine, and alcohol can exacerbate the symptoms of IBS, as well as some fruits or vegetables, such as cabbage, broccoli, cauliflower, or brussels sprouts. In some cases, however, no specific foods cause specific symptoms, as any food intake seems to worsen symptoms. Often, IBS-aggravating foods vary from person to person.

The nervous system processing between the brain and the intestines suggest that stress may be the culprit in IBS. Many IBS sufferers report symptoms following a meal when they experience stress. Psychologic stress has been shown to exacerbate GI symptoms in IBS. Stress may also be involved in some people who develop IBS following infection or inflammation of the bowel. In addition, psychiatric diseases are common among IBS patients, especially in those who are hospitalized.

A hypersensitive gut is characterized by enhanced perception of normal motility throughout the digestive tract. Recent studies have shown that specific parts of the brain show greater activation in IBS patients; these activated brain regions are associated with attention and response selection.

IBS is more commonly seen in women than in men, with up to 20 percent of the American population affected. Although it can occur at any time, IBS generally appears in the patient's teens and twenties, and it frequently is found in members of the same family. Americans and Europeans have similar frequencies of IBS.

TREATMENT AND THERAPY

Diagnosis of IBS is an involved process that is accomplished through a series of steps. A thorough history should be provided to the physician. A symptom-based criteria (Manning or Rome III) will be used to identify IBS. Moreover, alarming symptoms such as weight loss, unrelenting diarrhea, family history of colon cancer, and psychiatric aspects such as depression and suicidal thoughts will be ruled out. A physical examina-

IN THE NEWS:
A NOVEL APPROACH TO TREATING IBS SYMPTOMS

A new target for treatment of the symptoms of irritable bowel syndrome (IBS) is presented by the serotonin (5-HT) receptors that are present in nerves of the gastrointestinal (GI) tract and other organs. Receptors are proteins involved in the response of organs to various signals. Blocking these receptors can modify responses of the nerves in the GI tract. There are several types of 5-HT receptors; they are designated by numbers such as 5-HT3 and 5-HT4.

Alosetron (Lotronex) targets the 5-HT3 receptors in the GI tract. The desired effects of the drug include pain relief, normalization of bowel frequency, and decreased urgency for bowel movements in female patients with diarrhea-predominant IBS. The restrictive guidelines for alosetron were established because of its serious side effects: severe constipation and ischemic colitis that can potentially be fatal. Alosetron was withdrawn from the market but eventually reapproved by the Food and Drug Administration (FDA) with restrictive guidelines for its prescription.

A similar drug called cilansetron also targets the 5-HT3 receptors in the GI tract, and studies have shown that its effects on individuals with IBS are the same as for alosetron. It is the first 5-HT3 blocker specific for both male and female IBS patients suffering from diarrhea. In April, 2005, the FDA did not approve the product registration for cilansetron in the United States, even though the phase III registration trials were complete, and requested additional data from Solvay, the manufacturer. The FDA denial may be related to the challenges undergone by alosetron. By the end of 2005, Solvay suspended its product application in the United States, but it continues to discuss the introduction of cilansetron in the United Kingdom through the Medicines and Healthcare products Regulatory Agency (MHRA). The United Kingdom is the reference country for the introduction of cilansetron to the member countries of the European Union.

Tegaserod is a drug for treating constipation in IBS patients. It is marketed by Novartis as Zelnorm in the United States and Zelmac outside the United States. Tegaserod was approved by the FDA in 2002 for treatment of female patients suffering from constipation-predominant IBS. Tegaserod targets the 5-HT4 receptors in the GI tract. The desired effects of the drug include decreasing pain perception and reversing constipation through faster food transit in the GI tract. Tegaserod seems to be well tolerated by most patients, with most common side effects including headache, abdominal pain, and diarrhea. Evidence showed a link between the drug and an increased risk of heart attack and stroke, however, and it was withdrawn from the U.S. market in March, 2007.

More treatment options using the novel approach of targeting the serotonin (5-HT) receptors may be on the horizon as researchers learn more about the efficacy and safety of these new drugs in IBS patients.

—Miriam E. Schwartz, M.D., M.A., Ph.D., and
Colm A. Ó'Moráin, M.A., M.D., M.Sc., D.Sc.

tion will be performed on the first visit. Laboratory tests and a colonoscopy or sigmoidoscopy may be performed and a stool sample may be obtained—all of which will rule out serious diseases such as colon cancer, infection, and inflammatory diseases. Traditionally, IBS has been a diagnosis of exclusion.

Treatment options will include dietary and lifestyle changes, medications targeted toward the predominant symptoms, and psychological modalities. Generally, a low-fat, high-fiber diet lessens symptoms, although the tolerance of fiber as well as of all foods varies from person to person. Dietary changes vary according to the severity of the patient's symptoms. In mild cases of IBS, known aggravating foods should be identified and avoided. Symptoms may be eased by eating smaller meals. Since no diet has been found that controls all symptoms, a diary of symptoms and food intake is valuable in determining which foods are offensive. Establishment of fixed times for meals and bathroom visits helps regulate bowel habits as well.

In addition to dietary changes, medications are given to alleviate predominant IBS symptoms. Abdominal pain is treated with antispasmodic drugs such as dicyclomine, especially if the pain is associated with meals; these drugs relax the smooth muscles of the intestines. An antidiarrheal agent such as loperamide is used to reduce loose stools and to relieve abdominal pain. A newer medication called alosetron (Lotronex) is also used for diarrhea. Because alosetron has serious side effects, such as severe constipation and ischemic colitis, it was withdrawn from the market for a while; it is now available again, but with specific restrictions and only for severe IBS. Physicians must enroll in a special program with the manufacturer in order to prescribe alosetron. For constipation, bulk laxatives that supply increased dietary fiber such as psyllium (Metamucil, Fiberall, Konsyl, Colon Cleanse, and other similar products) are recommended. A new medication for constipation called tegaserod (Zelnorm) was made available in 2002 but was withdrawn in 2007 when evidence suggested that it raised the risk of heart attack and stroke.

Psychological treatments are imperative for IBS patients whose quality of life is severely impaired. Patients who have concomitant psychiatric conditions such as depression, history of sexual abuse, or any major life stress should be treated for their psychiatric ailments so that they can cope better with IBS.

Psychological counseling, cognitive behavioral therapy, hypnosis, biofeedback, and relaxation techniques are recommended to reduce anxiety and encourage learning to cope better with the pain of IBS. Severe pain from IBS can be treated with antidepressants such as tricyclics. Moderate exercise has also been shown to be beneficial.

In addition to dietary changes prescribed by doctors, alternative practitioners may advise herbal remedies to treat symptoms of IBS, such as Chinese herbal medicines, aloe vera, ginger, evening primrose, fennel, peppermint extract, chamomile, and rosemary. Aromatherapy, hydrotherapy, acupuncture, chiropractic, and osteopathy as alternative treatments may also be useful in some individuals.

PERSPECTIVE AND PROSPECTS

IBS was once believed to be a psychological disorder, but recent studies have shown that it is a true medical disorder with specific physiological characteristics and a significant impact on individuals who are afflicted with it. In addition, IBS has considerable effect on the society's health care burden. It has been reported that IBS is the second most common reason for seeing a physician (the first being the common cold) and accounts for 12 percent of visits to primary care and for the largest group seen by gastroenterologists. In terms of GI diseases, IBS is second only to gastroesophageal reflux disease (GERD) as most prevalent GI disorder in the United States. IBS affects 15.4 million people, and the economic costs (both direct and indirect) are in the billions of dollars. These costs are derived from work absenteeism, doctor visits, medical tests, and procedures, as well as other related expenses.

Although there is no cure for IBS, it is not a life-threatening condition. It has not been shown to cause intestinal bleeding or inflammation, as in Crohn's disease, ulcerative colitis, or cancer. Long-term management, though frustrating, involves commitment to therapy for six months or more to find the best combinations of medicine, diet, counseling, and support for control of IBS symptoms.

—Mary Hurd;
updated by Miriam E. Schwartz, M.D., M.A., Ph.D.,
and Colm A. Ó'Moráin, M.A., M.D., M.Sc., D.Sc.

See also Abdominal disorders; Colitis; Constipation; Crohn's disease; Diarrhea and dysentery; Gastroenterology; Gastrointestinal disorders; Gastrointestinal system; Intestinal disorders; Intestines; Lactose intolerance; Peristalsis.

FOR FURTHER INFORMATION:

"American Gastroenterological Association Technical Review on Irritable Bowel Syndrome." *Gastroenterology* 123, no. 6 (December, 2002): 2108-2131. An excellent and complete technical coverage of IBS. Available to the public on the American Gastroenterological Association Web site.

Chey, William D., et al. "Bacterial Overgrowth and IBS: Bridging the Gap." *Gastroenterology and Hepatology* 2, no. 8, supp. (August 9, 2006): 5-13. Provides excellent, up-to-date information about the diagnosis and treatment of IBS, especially the connection between bacterial infection and IBS.

Darnley, Simon, and Barbara Millar. *Understanding Irritable Bowel Syndrome.* New York: Wiley, 2003. A balanced overview of the different explanations of the disease available and the range of treatments to be found. Includes information about special diets, drugs, and alternative therapies, as well as personal stories of IBS patients.

Hadley, Susan K., and Stephen M. Gaarder. "Treatment of Irritable Bowel Syndrome." *American Family Physician* 72, no. 12 (December 15, 2005): 2501-2506. A review of different treatments available for IBS. The article is readily accessible and free to the public from the Web site of the American Academy of Family Physicians.

Irritable Bowel Syndrome Self Help and Support Group. http://www.ibsgroup.org/. Provides support to those who suffer from IBS or family members of an IBS patient and medical professionals who want to learn more about IBS. The IBS Support Group works to educate those who are living with IBS and to increase awareness about this and other functional gastrointestinal disorders.

Mertz, Howard R. "Irritable Bowel Syndrome." *New England Journal of Medicine* 349, no. 22 (November 27, 2003): 2136-2145. A medical review article on drug therapies available for IBS.

National Digestive Diseases Information Clearinghouse (NDDIC). *Irritable Bowel Syndrome.* http:// digestive.niddk.nih.gov/ddiseases/pubs/ibs/. A patient guide about IBS that can be read quickly. Covers basic topics of interest for those diagnosed with IBS.

ISCHEMIA
DISEASE/DISORDER

ANATOMY OR SYSTEM AFFECTED: Blood vessels, brain, circulatory system

SPECIALTIES AND RELATED FIELDS: Cardiology, critical care, neurology, vascular medicine

DEFINITION: The interruption or temporary restriction of blood flow to a particular area of the body, such as an organ.

CAUSES AND SYMPTOMS

When a localized area of the brain does not receive enough blood, neurons and supportive tissue such as glia are deprived of the essential oxygen and glucose that keeps them alive. If the brain does not receive sufficient blood for even a few minutes, the result is an ischemic stroke.

Although it is possible for ischemia to have no detectable symptoms, when it occurs to the internal carotid, middle cerebral, or vertebral-basilar arteries, symptoms such as confusion, impaired speech, double vision, or numbness on one side of the face can be experienced. In the majority of instances, these symptoms are temporary and do not result in permanent brain damage. If blood flow is restricted to the coronary artery of the heart (cardiac ischemia), then the heart muscle may suffer permanent damage. Symptoms of cardiac ischemia may include chest pain.

Ischemia is commonly caused by the formation of blood clots or by artherosclerosis, in which the walls of the arteries become narrowed as a result of the buildup of fat deposits.

INFORMATION ON ISCHEMIA

CAUSES: Blood clots, artherosclerosis

SYMPTOMS: Depends on location; may include confusion, impaired speech, double vision, numbness on one side of face, chest pain

DURATION: May be temporary or permanent

TREATMENTS: Drug therapy (*e.g.*, aspirin, nitroglycerin); surgery (*e.g.*, angioplasty)

TREATMENT AND THERAPY

Ischemic stroke can be assessed with high-resolution ultrasound equipment or magnetic resonance angiography (MRA) to detect blood flow. It is common to use computed tomography (CT) scanning or magnetic resonance imaging (MRI) to rule out the possibility that a blood vessel has burst, leading to a hemorrhage. Drug therapies such as administering aspirin or stronger blood-thinning agents help when ischemia is caused by clotting. Nitroglycerin can quickly open up coronary arteries and reduce the chest pain experienced when the heart is affected. Drugs that lower blood pressure are also helpful treatments.

Surgery might be needed to correct an obstruction that cannot be dissolved. Angioplasty can be used to expand affected arteries, particularly when the cause is atherosclerosis.

PERSPECTIVE AND PROSPECTS

Rudolf Virchow, a nineteenth century German physician, was the first to use the term "ischemia." Since the time that ischemia was originally identified, medical advances in diagnostics have been improved through the use of echocardiograms that send out sound waves to create an image of the heart's internal structures. When the affected organ is the brain, treatment improvements have included the administration of unique drugs that can mitigate damage to surrounding nerve cells indirectly affected by the lack of blood.

Much has been learned about the need for a balanced diet, regular exercise, and controlling hypertension as means to reduce the likelihood of suffering from an ischemic attack.

—*Bryan C. Auday, Ph.D.*

See also Angioplasty; Arteriosclerosis; Bypass surgery; Cardiology; Circulation; Claudication; Echocardiography; Heart; Heart attack; Heart disease; Heart failure; Hyperlipidemia; Hypertension; Strokes; Thrombosis and thrombus; Transient ischemic attacks (TIAs); Vascular medicine; Vascular system.

FOR FURTHER INFORMATION:

American Heart Association. *Heart Attack Treatment, Prevention, Recovery.* New York: Time Books, 1996.

Anagnostopoulos, Constantinos D., et al., eds. *Noninvasive Imaging of Myocardial Ischemia.* London: Springer, 2006.

Blumenfeld, Hal. *Neuroanatomy Through Clinical Cases.* Sunderland, Mass.: Sinauer Associates, 2002.

Kalat, James W. *Biological Psychology.* 9th ed. Belmont, Calif.: Thomson/Wadsworth, 2007.

Kolb, Bryan, and Ian Q. Whishaw. *Fundamentals of Human Neuropsychology.* 5th ed. New York: Worth, 2003.

Zillmer, Eric A., and Mary V. Spiers. *Principles of Neuropsychology.* Belmont, Calif.: Wadsworth, 2001.

ITCHING

DISEASE/DISORDER

ALSO KNOWN AS: Pruritus

ANATOMY OR SYSTEM AFFECTED: Skin

SPECIALTIES AND RELATED FIELDS: Dermatology, otorhinolaryngology, pharmacology, psychiatry

DEFINITION: An unpleasant sensation on or in the skin that causes a desire to scratch or rub the affected area.

CAUSES AND SYMPTOMS

Itching is elicited by the physical or chemical stimulation of nerve receptors in the skin. It can be caused by a wide variety of problems in a variety of different organ systems.

Nearly any skin lesion may itch; skin-related causes include such varied problems as eczema, psoriasis, contact dermatitis, insect bites, bacterial infections, fungal infections, sunburn, and exposure to wool. Viral infections such as chickenpox can cause intense itching. Itching of the eyes and nose are commonly associated with allergies. Itching without a skin rash may be caused by a number of internal problems. Various endocrine problems in children associated with itching include liver disease, kidney failure, thyroid disease, and diabetes. Some malignancies, particularly lymphomas, may cause itching. Hookworms and pinworms are both internal causes of itching, as are certain drugs. Finally, some women experience generalized itching during pregnancy.

Certain psychiatric problems are associated with

INFORMATION ON ITCHING

CAUSES: Eczema, psoriasis, contact dermatitis, insect bites, bacterial or viral infections, fungal infections, sunburn, exposure to wool, allergies, malignancies, parasites, reaction to certain drugs

SYMPTOMS: Varies; can include dry, red, or flaky skin; rashes; hives; pain and inflammation

DURATION: Acute to chronic

TREATMENTS: Hydration, moisturizing lotion, various medications (primarily antihistamines)

---

itching. Patients may scratch hard enough to create deep ulcers. The intensity of the itching seems to be related to the degree of nervous tension. In addition, patients who suffer from certain psychotic states or those who abuse drugs such as cocaine may experience a deep itching sensation that they describe as bugs crawling beneath the skin.

Itching may rarely be associated with neurologic disease in which changes in sensation are interpreted by the patient as itching. Occasionally, circulatory problems will cause itching, primarily on the legs. Both of these conditions are more common in older adults than in children or young adults.

TREATMENT AND THERAPY

Treatment should be directed toward the cause of the itching. Hydration (bathing followed by moisturizing lotion) may be helpful in providing relief. When itching is the result of an allergen such as poison ivy, however, a drying agent should be used. Various medications (primarily antihistamines) may relieve itching, but most also cause significant sleepiness.

—*Rebecca Lovell Scott, Ph.D., PA-C*

See also Allergies; Antihistamines; Athlete's foot; Bacterial infections; Bites and stings; Candidiasis; Chickenpox; Dermatitis; Dermatology; Dermatology, pediatric; Diabetes mellitus; Eczema; Endocrine system; Endocrinology; Endocrinology, pediatric; Fungal infections; Hemorrhoids; Hepatitis; Hives; Impetigo; Insect-borne diseases; Lice, mites, and ticks; Liver; Liver disorders; Parasitic diseases; Pinworms; Pityriasis rosea; Poisonous plants; Psoriasis; Rashes; Renal failure; Ringworm; Scabies; Sexually transmitted diseases (STDs); Skin; Skin disorders; Sunburn; Thyroid disorders; Viral infections; Worms.

FOR FURTHER INFORMATION:

Adelman, Daniel C., et al., eds. *Manual of Allergy and Immunology*. 4th ed. Philadelphia: Lippincott Williams & Wilkins, 2002.

Bernhard, Jeffrey D., ed. *Itch: Mechanisms and Management of Pruritus*. New York: McGraw-Hill, 1994.

Fleischer, Alan B., Jr. *The Clinical Management of Itching*. New York: Parthenon, 2000.

Litin, Scott C., ed. *Mayo Clinic Family Health Book*. 3d ed. New York: HarperResource, 2003.

Middlemiss, Prisca. *What's That Rash? How to Identify and Treat Childhood Rashes*. London: Hamlyn, 2002.

Turkington, Carol, and Jeffrey S. Dover. *The Encyclopedia of Skin and Skin Disorders*. New York: Facts On File, 2002.

Weedon, David. *Skin Pathology*. 2d ed. New York: Churchill Livingstone, 2002.

JAUNDICE

DISEASE/DISORDER

ANATOMY OR SYSTEM AFFECTED: Blood, liver, skin

SPECIALTIES AND RELATED FIELDS: Gastroenterology, hematology, internal medicine

DEFINITION: Yellow discoloration of skin resulting from increased levels of bilirubin in the blood.

CAUSES AND SYMPTOMS

Jaundice is not a disease per se, but rather a common sign of various disorders in the liver or the blood. Bilirubin is a pigment formed by the breakdown of hemoglobin, the oxygen-carrying molecule in red blood cells. Bilirubin is then transported to the liver, where it is processed into a water-soluble form. This process is known as conjugation. Conjugated bilirubin is secreted into the bile ducts and eventually excreted in feces. An increase in red blood cell breakdown, impairment in liver function, or blockage of the bile ducts can all result in the buildup of bilirubin. The first visible manifestation of this is often scleral icterus, a yellowing of the white part of the eyes. When levels of conjugated bilirubin are abnormally high, it may be seen in the urine as urobilinogen, which causes a darkening of the urine.

Once the bilirubin level in the blood exceeds 2.5 milligrams per deciliter, the yellow skin discoloration of jaundice can be seen. It is apparent first at the bottom of the tongue and later throughout the skin. Jaundice is sometimes associated with itching, presumably because of the deposition of bilirubin under the skin.

TREATMENT AND THERAPY

The treatment of jaundice depends on its cause. The first step is to determine whether there is an excess of conjugated bilirubin or unconjugated bilirubin. High levels of unconjugated bilirubin suggest an increase in red blood cell breakdown, known as hemolysis. This condition can be confirmed by examination of a peripheral blood smear and other laboratory studies. Most cases of hemolysis are the result of another underlying cause, such as infection or drugs. Hemolysis can also result from the body's immune system attacking its own red blood cells. Unconjugated bilirubin is also elevated in inherited disorders such as Gilbert's syndrome and Crigler-Najjar syndrome. These disorders are usually detected in early childhood.

Excess conjugated bilirubin, on the other hand, suggests a blockage in the biliary tree, which can be attributable to gallstones or, less commonly, a tumor. Gallstones can be confirmed with ultrasonography and may require surgery if they cause symptoms. Rarer causes of blockage in the biliary tree include strictures and sclerosing cholangitis. Disease of the liver itself can also result in high levels of conjugated bilirubin, but oftentimes both types of bilirubin are elevated. Such diseases include viral hepatitis (hepatitis A, B, or C), as well as alcohol and drug-induced hepatitis.

—Ahmad Kamal, M.D.

See also Cirrhosis; Gallbladder cancer; Gallbladder diseases; Hepatitis; Jaundice, neonatal; Liver; Liver disorders; Stones.

FOR FURTHER INFORMATION:

Arias, Irwin M., and James L. Boyer, eds. *The Liver: Biology and Pathobiology.* 4th ed. Philadelphia: Lippincott Williams & Wilkins, 2001.

Kasper, Dennis L., et al., eds. *Harrison's Principles of Internal Medicine.* 16th ed. New York: McGraw-Hill, 2005.

Palmer, Melissa. *Dr. Melissa Palmer's Guide to Hepatitis and Liver Disease.* Rev. ed. Garden City Park, N.Y.: Avery, 2004.

INFORMATION ON JAUNDICE

CAUSES: Excess of pigment bilirubin resulting from various liver or blood disorders, gallstones, tumors, infection (*e.g.*, hepatitis), or certain drugs

SYMPTOMS: Yellowing of skin and whites of eyes, dark urine, itchy skin

DURATION: Acute

TREATMENTS: Depends on cause; may include surgery to remove gallstones or tumors

---

JAUNDICE, NEONATAL

DISEASE/DISORDER

ANATOMY OR SYSTEM AFFECTED: Blood, bones, brain, liver, spleen

SPECIALTIES AND RELATED FIELDS: Hematology, neonatology, neurology

DEFINITION: A yellowish coloration visible on the skin that is the most frequent physical finding in newborn infants.

KEY TERMS:

bilirubin encephalopathy: damage to brain cells caused by excess bilirubin; also called kernicterus

---

**INFORMATION ON
NEONATAL JAUNDICE**

CAUSES: Excess of pigment bilirubin in newborns
SYMPTOMS: Typically yellowish skin; can include
sleepiness, lethargy, irritability, poor feeding,
vomiting, fever, high-pitched or shrill cry
DURATION: Acute
TREATMENTS: Phototherapy, exchange transfusion

---

exchange transfusion: the removal of an individual's
blood and its replacement with a donor's blood
hyperbilirubinemia: a condition in which the bilirubin
concentration in the blood reaches a level that is
higher than that generally found in umbilical cord
blood (1.5 milligrams per 100 milliliters)
hypertonia: an increase in muscle tone
hypotonia: a decrease in muscle tone
phototherapy: a treatment consisting of exposure to
light from a bank of fluorescent or other types of
lamps

CAUSES AND SYMPTOMS

Most jaundice found in children is neonatal nonhemolytic jaundice, a yellowish pigmentation of the skin
of some infants. The term "nonhemolytic" is used to
differentiate this condition from jaundice caused by
blood group incompatibilities (such as Rh or ABO
groups) or other enzyme abnormalities of the red blood
cells.

Neonatal nonhemolytic jaundice is the result of an
excess of the pigment bilirubin. Bilirubin is derived
from two major sources. One source is the normal destruction of circulating red blood cells (erythrocytes).
The normal life span of the erythrocytes varies from 80
to 120 days. Old erythrocytes are removed and destroyed in specific tissues in the spleen and liver, where
the hemoglobin of the red blood cells is broken down
and converted to bilirubin. This accounts for 75 percent
of the daily production of bilirubin, and 1 gram of hemoglobin yields 35 milligrams of bilirubin. The remaining 25 percent of bilirubin is derived from ineffective erythropoiesis (red blood cell formation) in the
bone marrow and other tissue heme or heme proteins
from the liver.

The bilirubin formed is transported in the plasma of
the blood and bound reversibly to albumin, a protein in

the blood and tissues. This bilirubin-albumin complex
is then transported to the liver, where it is converted
into a water-soluble compound (or conjugated) by the
enzyme glucuronyl transferase in the interior of the
liver cells. The conjugated bilirubin is excreted into
the bile capillaries and then into the intestine. Once in
the small intestine, the conjugated bilirubin is converted by bacteria in the colon into a colorless compound known as urobilinogen. In the newborn infant,
because of the lack of bacteria in the colon and the presence of the enzyme B-glucuronidase in the gut wall, a
significant amount of the conjugated bilirubin is de-
conjugated and reabsorbed back into the plasma pool, a
process known as the enterohepatic shunt.

Chemical hyperbilirubinemia can be defined as a serum concentration of bilirubin that exceeds 1.5 milligrams per 100 milliliters. Visible yellowing (icterus) of
the skin is caused by the combination of normal skin
color, bilirubin-albumin complexes located outside the
blood vessels, and precipitated bilirubin acid in the
membranes of the cell walls. It first becomes visible
when serum bilirubin reaches from 3 to 6 milligrams
per deciliter, depending on the infant's skin texture and
pigmentation and on the observer. In the neonate, jaundice is detected by blanching the skin over a bony structure with digital pressure, thus revealing the underlying
color of the skin and subcutaneous tissue. Jaundice is
first seen in the face and then progresses toward the
trunk and extremities.

In general, infants whose jaundice is restricted to the
face and trunk and does not extend below the umbilicus
have serum bilirubin levels of about 12 milligrams per
deciliter or less, while those whose hands and feet are
jaundiced have serum bilirubin levels in excess of 15
milligrams per deciliter. A more objective way to estimate the depth of jaundice in neonates is with the use of
an icterometer, a strip of transparent plastic with five
transverse yellow strips in different shades. The baby's
skin is blanched using pressure, and the resulting shade
of yellow is matched against a color scale. In recent
years, a transcutaneous bilirubinometer has been developed, which provides an electronic readout of an index that corresponds with a serum bilirubin concentration. A more precise way to judge jaundice is to draw a
small amount of blood (usually less than a tablespoon)
from the baby and to measure its serum concentration
in a laboratory.

A transient rise in serum bilirubin concentration is
almost universally seen in healthy newborns. This type
of jaundice, called physiologic jaundice, may be attrib-

utable to several factors. First, this condition may result from increased bilirubin load on liver cells caused by increased red blood cell volume, decreased red blood cell survival time, increased heme from muscles, or increased enterohepatic circulation of bilirubin. Second, the condition may result from decreased liver uptake of bilirubin from plasma caused by a decrease in specific proteins in liver cells (termed Y and Z proteins) for the transport of bilirubin. Third, it may result from defective bilirubin conjugation caused by decreased enzyme activity. Fourth, physiologic jaundice can result from defective bilirubin excretion.

The serum bilirubin level in newborns reaches its peak between forty-eight and seventy-two hours after birth and then decreases, so that the yellowish pigmentation may not be visible by the fifth to seventh day. The peak level of serum bilirubin in physiologic jaundice varies from a mean of 5 to 15 milligrams per 100 milliliters. A number of factors will confound the level of serum bilirubin present with this condition. They include maternal pregnancy history, complications, drugs, gestational age, early initiation of feeding, type of feeding (breast milk or formula), and ethnicity. The heterogeneity of the human population makes it difficult to apply a particular serum bilirubin level to the definition of physiologic jaundice. No jaundice should be dismissed as physiologic, however, without at least a review of maternal and neonatal history, an examination of the infant for signs of illness, and further laboratory investigation when indicated.

In some cases, excess bilirubin can cause neurotoxicity leading to brain damage known as bilirubin encephalopathy or kernicterus. This damage can result in either neonatal death or the development of long-term abnormal neurologic findings, such as cerebral palsy, a low intelligence quotient (IQ), lower school achievement, hyperactivity, and deafness. The identification of jaundiced newborn infants at risk for kernicterus is difficult. The data suggest that healthy infants with serum bilirubin levels as high as 25 to 30 milligrams per 100 milliliters may not have adverse neurologic effects, since the bilirubin is bound to adequate albumin and the blood-brain barrier formed by cerebral blood vessels is intact in these infants. Early hospital discharge policies practiced in many maternity centers, however, make it difficult to assess the evolution of physiologic as well as pathologic jaundice, or confounding factors such as infection. Clinicians, practitioners, and home health visitors need to pay special attention to the degree of jaundice and when it is associated with danger signs such as sleepiness, lethargy, irritability, poor feeding, vomiting, fever, high-pitched or shrill cry, hypertonia or hypotonia (depending on whether the infant is asleep or awake), neck and trunk arching, dark urine, or light stools.

TREATMENT AND THERAPY

The treatment of jaundice depends on the underlying pathology. For clinical purposes, the two major types need to be separated: jaundice resulting from hemolytic disease (Rh, ABO, and other blood group incompatibilities) and nonhemolytic jaundice. Nonhemolytic jaundice may be physiologic or an accentuation of physiologic jaundice, such as jaundice caused by polycythemia (an increased number of red blood cells), cephalhematoma (the collection of blood in the scalp between the bone and bone lining), bruising, cerebral or other hemorrhages, swallowed blood, increased enterohepatic shunting (because of breast-feeding, delayed passage of stools, or gastrointestinal tract obstruction), and infection or sepsis.

Although no general consensus exists concerning the management of nonhemolytic jaundice, infants with this condition are generally treated with phototherapy when the serum bilirubin level reaches between 15 and 18 milligrams per 100 milliliters, using the upper value for uncomplicated physiologic jaundice and the lower value when the jaundice has accentuating factors. Phototherapy consists of exposure of the baby's skin to light energy from a bank of fluorescent or other special lamps. The light converts the fat-soluble bilirubin, which cannot be excreted, into a water-soluble bilirubin, which can be easily excreted in the bile, thus lowering the serum concentration of bilirubin.

When the serum bilirubin level reaches between 20 and 25 milligrams per 100 milliliter—some clinicians advocate between 25 and 30 milligrams per 100 milliliters—exchange transfusion is generally recommended. In this method, all of the baby's bilirubin-containing blood is removed and exchanged with compatible blood, without bilirubin, from a donor. Both forms of treatment, phototherapy and exchange transfusion, aim to reduce or remove bilirubin from the baby's system, thereby preventing brain injury.

PERSPECTIVE AND PROSPECTS

Jaundice was identified as a major problem in newborn infants in the nineteenth century. Its association with brain injury was first described by German pathologist Johannes J. Orth in 1875. Fifty years later, brain damage was further identified with increased destruction of red blood cells because of hemolysis caused by Rh and ABO blood group incompatibilities.

It was also realized, however, that jaundice is encountered in normal newborn infants. The major problem has been to identify which infant is at risk for brain damage when bilirubin is at a particular level. Since there are multiple confounding factors, better means are being developed for identifying risks, such as laboratory methods to identify free (unbound) bilirubin and noninvasive clinical methods such as auditory evoked potential to measure brain waves in response to sound, the use of computers to analyze the shrillness of the baby's cry, and nuclear magnetic resonance (a form of X ray) to measure the energy metabolism of brain cells. In addition, methods to prevent the formation of bilirubin or to reduce its levels by decreasing the activity of the enzyme heme oxygenase are being studied.

—*Paul Y. K. Wu, M.D.*

See also Anemia; Blood and blood disorders; Cerebral palsy; Hematology, pediatric; Hemolytic disease of the newborn; Hepatitis; Jaundice; Light therapy; Liver; Liver disorders; Neonatalogy.

FOR FURTHER INFORMATION:

Appleby, Julie. "Jaundice-Caused Brain Damage Is on the Rise." *USA Today*, October 26, 2000, p. D10. Because babies are being sent home from the hospital earlier, many cases of jaundice are missed. There have been eighty-eight cases of jaundice-caused brain damage in the United States since 1984, the majority since 1990.

Behrman, Richard E., Robert M. Kliegman, and Hal B. Jenson, eds. *Nelson Textbook of Pediatrics*. 17th ed. Philadelphia: Saunders, 2004. Text covering all medical and surgical disorders in children with authoritative information on genetics, endocrinology, aetiology, epidemiology, pathology, pathophysiology, clinical manifestations, diagnosis, prevention, treatment, and prognosis.

Kirchner, Jeffrey T. "Clinical Assessment of Neonatal Jaundice." *American Family Physician* 62, no. 8 (October 15, 2000): 1880. Neonatal jaundice is a common condition, most often caused by normal physiologic mechanisms and not usually of significant concern. The decision to obtain a serum bilirubin level in a newborn usually is based on the child's appearance and the clinical judgment of the physician.

MacDonald, Mhairi G., Mary M. K. Seshia, and Martha D. Mullett, eds. *Avery's Neonatology: Pathophysiology and Management of the Newborn*. 6th ed. Philadelphia: Lippincott Williams & Wilkins, 2005. A standard textbook on the pathophysiology and management of the major disease processes affecting the neonate, first published in 1975. Two coeditors have joined Avery in bringing out this edition, now with sixty-one chapters.

Martin, Richard J., Avroy A. Fanaroff, and Michele C. Walsh, eds. *Fanaroff and Martin's Neonatal-Perinatal Medicine: Diseases of the Fetus and Infant*. 2 vols. 8th ed. Philadelphia: Mosby Elsevier, This classic reference work is one of the most comprehensive to date and features discussions on the diverse practice of neonatal-perinatal medicine, pregnancy disorders and their impact on the fetus, delivery room care, provisions for neonatal care, and the development and disorder of organ systems.

JAW WIRING

PROCEDURE

ANATOMY OR SYSTEM AFFECTED: Bones, gums, mouth, musculoskeletal system, teeth

SPECIALTIES AND RELATED FIELDS: Dentistry, emergency medicine, nutrition, orthodontics, plastic surgery, speech pathology

DEFINITION: A surgical procedure in which the upper and lower teeth are brought closely together and secured with wire in order to immobilize the jaw.

KEY TERMS:

arch bar: a pliable piece of metal with small hooked attachments; one is fitted along the upper teeth, another is fitted along the lower teeth, the two pieces are connected to the teeth with wires, and other wires are looped around the hooks and brought together to prevent jaw movement

facial edema: swelling of the facial tissue

intermaxillary fixation: the medical term for jaw wiring

mandible: the lower jawbone

maxilla: the upper jawbone

oral hygiene: care of the teeth and mouth

orthognathic surgery: jaw reconstruction

reduction: the restoration of a fractured bone to its normal position

zygoma: the cheekbone

INDICATIONS AND PROCEDURES

Jaw wiring is often necessary to repair fractures in the jaw. The principles of treatment for facial fractures, in which bones need to be lined up and held in position until healing takes place, are the same as for a fractured arm or leg. Whereas an arm or leg fracture is reduced and casted to hold the bones in proper alignment, however, this method cannot be used for fractures of the face. Instead, once the fractures have been reduced (the bones have been restored to their proper positions), the jaws are wired shut to prevent the displacement of bone or bone fragments until they have healed.

Fractures of the face can involve any of the facial bones. The lower jawbone (mandible) is the most commonly fractured facial bone. Nevertheless, the upper jawbone (maxilla), the cheekbone (zygoma), the nasal bones, or the orbits (formed from bones of the cranium and face around the eyes) may also suffer fractures. A fracture may involve an individual bone or a combination of bones. One of the most common causes of facial fractures is blunt trauma. A blow to the face, the impact from an automobile or motorcycle accident, and a gunshot wound to the face are some examples of such trauma.

When considering fractures of the face, more than simply the bony structures must be evaluated. The skeletal structure encapsulates and protects organs that are vital to the functions of seeing, breathing, eating, talking, and swallowing. Early identification and treatment of fractures of the face are necessary to maintain maximum function of these delicate organs. Therefore, even though facial fractures and related injuries to soft tissue are seldom fatal, they must be treated immediately, since improper care could result in disfigurement, permanent sensory impairment, and lifelong disabilities.

In addition to facial fractures, jaw wiring is sometimes performed to correct malformations of the facial bones, certain birth defects, and acquired disfigurements as a result of trauma or growth-related imperfections. At times, jaw wiring is performed to correct malformations that have caused headaches, chewing disorders, and breathing and speech impairments. This type of surgery is referred to as orthognathic or jaw reconstruction surgery, part of which may involve jaw wiring. This procedure may also be performed as a weight-loss treatment for obese persons.

When a patient is hospitalized for elective facial surgery involving jaw wiring, or intermaxillary fixation, ample time can be given to preparing the patient for the surgical procedure and both preoperative and postoperative care. For the patient who sustains facial trauma, however, the same opportunity for surgical preparation may not be possible.

Facial fractures can often be reduced and immobilized by jaw wiring on the day of the injury. When there is marked facial edema (swelling), when other serious injuries are present, or when the person has eaten within a certain period of time prior to the trauma, however, the surgery will need to be delayed until a general anesthetic can be administered safely and the patient's condition has stabilized to the point that the surgical procedure can be tolerated.

The purpose of jaw wiring is to reduce and stabilize the fracture in such a manner that proper alignment of the bone will be maintained until it has healed. If the surgery is for jaw reconstruction, then the bone is fractured and positioned by the surgeon. These surgical fractures also require stabilization so that they will heal in the intended position. Interosseous wiring (the wiring of one portion of bone to another) using stainless steel wire may be necessary to maintain proper bone alignment. Sometimes, compression plates are used to secure the bones together. At other times, a bite block splint is inserted between the teeth to provide stabilization. This splint resembles a denture plate. An appliance called an external fixation device may be needed to keep the bones in proper alignment until they are healed.

If the patient wears dentures, then the denture plates are wired to the bone, the lower plate to the mandible, and the upper plate to the maxilla, prior to the jaw-wiring procedure. If the patient has no teeth at all, a bite block splint must be wired to the mandible and the maxilla, similar to the way in which dentures would be wired into place.

Jaw wiring is accomplished by first attaching arch bars to the base of the teeth. Arch bars are pliable pieces of metal with small hooked attachments on one side. They come in precut lengths and can also be cut to fit the individual's mouth. One fits along the base of the lower dental arch, and the other fits along the base of the upper dental arch. Thin pieces of stainless-steel wire are passed around the base of each tooth and brought out, then hooked around the arch bar and twisted firmly into place to secure the arch bar itself. The wires are cut, and their edges are tucked down between the teeth to prevent them from poking into gum or cheek tissue. If the patient wears dentures, the arch bar is either wired or glued to the denture plate with a special glue before the plate is wired to the bone structure.

Once the arch bars are positioned and secured, then special rubber bands are drawn around the hooked attachments from the upper to the lower bar. These bands are what actually hold the jaw tightly together. They are usually replaced with thin wires a few days after surgery, when the danger of nausea and vomiting have passed. Wire cutters need to be kept within easy reach at all times, in the event of vomiting. Should this happen, only the wires that hold the teeth together are clipped, and they will need to be reapplied by the physician.

USES AND COMPLICATIONS

Until the 1970's, orthognathic surgery carried a purely cosmetic connotation among the general public. Gradually, with surgical practice, documentation, research, and reports of the results of orthognathic surgery, people have come to understand the importance of such surgery in terms of proper physical functioning, as well as psychological and social functioning. Surgical reconstruction of the face can produce amazing results, but it also comes with a price. The process sometimes takes several years and teamwork by dentists, orthodontists, oral and/or plastic surgeons, and sometimes even psychiatrists to achieve these results. It can also be very costly because some insurance companies still consider orthodontia and corrective surgery cosmetic rather than functional and do not accept claims for these services.

Whatever the reason for jaw wiring, this process involves much more than a simple surgical procedure. Patients are usually hospitalized. Many of them are young, and others have had little hospital experience and may be anxious about the outcome. Lack of family support or financial concerns may increase this anxiety. Other injuries may be present in addition to the facial ones, some of which could be life-threatening and need to be attended to first.

Since jaw wiring usually means that the jaws are tightly wired shut, careful immediate postoperative monitoring by a nurse is needed to ensure that respiratory functioning is adequate, nausea and vomiting are controlled, mouth care is performed, nutritional intake of an all-liquid diet is satisfactory, and facial swelling and pain are reported to the surgeon, if necessary.

Before being discharged from the hospital, patients need to be shown proper mouth care techniques. Primary among them is the use of an electrical appliance that delivers pulsating jets of water, saline, or a mouth care solution to areas between the teeth and under the gum line. It rinses out food debris and harmful bacteria from the mouth. Mouth care is very important during the period of time when the jaws are wired, so that healing is promoted and dental caries (cavities) are prevented.

Good nutritional habits are also important during this time. Since the patient's diet must be liquid in form, concerns about weight loss, adequate food variations, appropriate nutrients for healing, management of food preparation, and possible nutritional supplementation need to be addressed and resolved before a patient is discharged. Patients should have a written diet plan to use at home. Medications needed for pain and nausea, vitamins, and sometimes antibiotics will also need to be obtained in liquid form. Instructions regarding how to administer emergency care, when to call the doctor, and how to cut wires if vomiting occurs must be given.

Follow-up care with the physician will be needed to evaluate progress and to arrange for the clipping of wires and the removal of the arch bars. These procedures are usually done in the physician's office.

PERSPECTIVE AND PROSPECTS

It is likely that attempts were made to treat fractures of the face from the time of the cave dwellers, but no records of such attempts were kept. The earliest known records relating to the treatment of jaw fractures are found in the Smith Papyrus, which is thought to have been written about 25 to 30 centuries B.C.E. The author advises against the treatment of compound (open) fractures but recommends that the dislocation of the mandible be treated. Definite proof of the art of dentistry was found among the Etruscans, an ancient people living in what is now Tuscany and part of Umbria, in about 600 to 500 B.C.E.: Skeletal remains with the teeth bound with gold wire have been discovered.

In the time of Hippocrates (c. 460-c. 370 B.C.E.), the Greek physician known as the Father of Medicine, writings bear evidence that facial injuries or fractures were treated with some method of wiring. A section of the Corpus Hippocraticum reads:

If the jaw is broken right across, which rarely happens, one should adjust it in the manner described [one thumb inside the mouth and the fingers outside, for reduction]. After adjustment one should fasten the teeth together as was described above [with gold wire or, lacking that, with linen thread], for this will contribute greatly to immobility, especially if one joins them properly and fastens the ends as they should be.

The use of bandages to treat facial maladies was also practiced by some ancient cultures. Galen of Pergamum (129-c. 199 C.E.) and Soranus of Ephesus (98-138 C.E.) describe such methods. An ancient manuscript by Soranus of Ephesus illustrates the types of bandages used by the ancients to treat head and facial injuries.

Greek writings even suggested dietary practices in cases of jaw injury. When the mandible was fractured, liquid nourishment was recommended, and solid foods were withheld until bone healing was definite. Patients were also advised not to talk for a certain period of time.

In the thirteenth century, the Italian surgeon Guglielmo da Saliceto (c. 1210-c. 1277), also known as William of Saliceto, performed one of the first documented cases of jaw wiring, attaching the teeth of the lower jaw to the corresponding teeth of the upper jaw. He used linen and silk thread, twisting them together and then waxing the twist to keep it in place. In the next several centuries, however, the medieval literature lacks any references to the management of facial bone fractures. Whether the work of earlier surgeons was unknown or whether such surgical practices remained standard during these years, without notable progress, remains a mystery.

It was toward the end of the nineteenth century that the development of intermaxillary fixation by wiring was developed by an American physician and dentist, Thomas Lewis Gilmer (1849-1931). Gilmer carried out the jaw wiring procedure "by twisting wires around the necks of the teeth of the upper and lower jaws, by adjusting the lower teeth to the occlusion of the upper jaw, and by twisting together the connecting upper and lower wires for stabilization."

Many great names are associated with the twentieth century contributions to improved and refined methods of jaw wiring techniques and patient care during this process. Much was learned about the nature of facial fractures themselves from the work of French physician Rene LeFort. LeFort conducted a series of experiments in the early twentieth century to study facial fracture combinations. He subjected cadaver skulls to violent blows under many conditions and at various angles and then described the outcomes.

A survey of the progress made in jaw wiring would be incomplete without recognition of the impact that antibiotic therapy, advanced anesthetic techniques, and blood replacement therapy have had on this procedure and on medical science as a whole. These achievements paved the way for open surgical procedures and internal fixation, which have led to dramatic results and remarkable changes for individuals undergoing jaw wiring.

—*Karen A. Mattern*

See also Bones and the skeleton; Dentistry; Emergency medicine; Fracture and dislocation; Fracture repair; Hyperadiposis; Nutrition; Obesity; Orthodontics; Orthopedic surgery; Orthopedics; Orthopedics, pediatric; Plastic surgery.

FOR FURTHER INFORMATION:

Fonseca, Raymond J., et al., eds. *Oral and Maxillofacial Trauma*. 3d ed. St. Louis: Elsevier Saunders, 2005. This text discusses wounds and injuries to the face, mouth, and jaw, as well as therapies to treat them. Includes a bibliography and an index.

Niamtu, Joseph, III. "Cosmetic Oral and Maxillofacial Surgery Options." *The Journal of the American Dental Association* 131, no. 6 (June, 2000): 756-764. A global diagnosis and treatment plan that includes facial aesthetics can enhance cosmetic dentistry and serve to frame the work of the restorative dentist.

Proffit, William R., Raymond P. White, Jr., and David M. Sarver, eds. *Contemporary Treatment of Dentofacial Deformity*. St. Louis: Mosby, 2003. Explores the ways in which orthodontists, oral and maxillofacial surgeons, and facial plastic surgeons can work together to treat dentofacial deformities.

Reyneke, Johan P. *Essentials of Orthognathic Surgery*. Chicago: Quintessence, 2003. Discusses patients with dentofacial deformities, focusing on the surgical and orthodontic principles of orthognathic surgery rather than on research and treatment philosophies. Covers principles of clinical evaluation, treatment planning, and surgical procedures, and clinical cases are presented to demonstrate treatment outcomes.

Salter, Robert Bruce. *Textbook of Disorders and Injuries of the Musculoskeletal System*. 3d ed. Baltimore: Williams & Wilkins, 1999. Four sections of the book—"Basic Musculoskeletal Science and Its Applications," "Musculoskeletal Disorders: General and Specific," "Musculoskeletal Injuries," and "Research"—examine the diagnosis and treatment principles of disorders and trauma of the musculoskeletal system.

Watts, V., S. Madick, J. Pepperney, and C. Petras. "When Your Patient Has Jaw Surgery." *RN* 48 (October, 1985): 44-47. This article written for health care professionals focuses on jaw surgery as a result of facial deformities rather than fractures, describing some deformities. Also includes postoperative care of the patient.

Joint diseases. *See* **Arthritis.**

Joint replacement. *See* **Arthroplasty; Hip replacement.**

Juvenile rheumatoid arthritis
Disease/disorder

Anatomy or system affected: Back, circulatory system, eyes, heart, immune system, joints, musculoskeletal system

Specialties and related fields: Exercise physiology, family medicine, immunology, ophthalmology, orthopedics, pediatrics, psychology

Definition: A usually chronic autoimmune disease of unknown cause, characterized by joint swelling, pain, and sometimes the destruction of joints.

Key terms:

articular: of or relating to a joint or joints

autoimmune disease: a disease in which the body's immune system attacks itself

manifestation: an outward or visible expression

systemic: relating to the body as a whole, not limited to a particular part

Causes and Symptoms

Juvenile rheumatoid arthritis is an autoimmune disease of children that attacks the joints. It appears in three different subgroups that vary according to severity and type of extra-articular manifestation. Other significant variations within these subgroups include age at disease onset, the sex of affected children, genetic predisposition, and prognosis.

INFORMATION ON JUVENILE RHEUMATOID ARTHRITIS

Causes: Unknown

Symptoms: High, intermittent fevers; temporary red rash occurring during periods of fever; joint pain; occasionally polyarthritis

Duration: Acute and recurrent

Treatments: Alleviation of symptoms through medication (anti-inflammatory drugs), physical and occupational therapy, orthopedic treatment (*e.g.*, splinting)

The first major clinical pattern is systemic disease, which includes about 20 percent of children with juvenile rheumatoid arthritis. This type has the most dramatic onset and is the least common form of the illness. It affects boys more than girls and can begin at any age. The most characteristic manifestations are high, intermittent fevers and a temporary red rash occurring during periods of fever. Occasionally, more serious complications are involved. In some cases, systemic onset is marked by polyarthritis, which affects large and small multiple joints, and moves subsequently to disease of the knee or hip with no further involvement of other joints. The systemic complaints, which are often sudden and explosive in nature, may recur months or years later. Some children with systemic onset, however, never develop lasting arthritis.

Polyarticular juvenile rheumatoid arthritis, the second subgroup, includes children in whom five or more joints have been involved in the first six months of illness. It affects more girls than boys and can begin at any age. This subgroup includes about 25 percent of children with juvenile rheumatoid arthritis and is frequently mild. Within this subgroup exists a smaller subgroup, which includes about 5 percent of children with juvenile rheumatoid arthritis and rarely begins before the eighth birthday. The arthritis is often severe, with joint destruction occurring within the first year. Polyarthritis may involve swelling of the joints over a period of time, in which pain is not a prominent feature, or a sudden articular swelling, in which pain can be severe. Weight-bearing joints, usually knees and ankles, are often involved initially.

The third major subgroup is pauciarticular disease, which involves about 40 percent of all children with juvenile rheumatoid arthritis. In the initial episode of this type, only one joint is involved. More joints usually become involved within a few weeks or months, although occasionally involvement is restricted to one joint. Most often, the knee is the primary area, with the ankles and hips being the sites of minimal involvement.

Treatment and Therapy

The first step in treating juvenile rheumatoid arthritis is the identification of the child's problems and potential problems, which include active joint disease, disabilities, ocular disease, growth retardation, and psychosocial disability. Because the cause of chronic arthritis is not known, treatment suppresses the symptoms and does not cure the disease itself.

Drug therapy is used to relieve inflammatory pain and immobility. The major anti-inflammatory drug used for juvenile rheumatoid arthritis is aspirin. For children who cannot tolerate aspirin, a nonsteroidal anti-inflammatory drug (NSAID) may be substituted. Unfortunately, corticosteroids, the most effective anti-inflammatory drugs known, are of little benefit in treating juvenile rheumatoid arthritis because of their serious side effects. They can be used only in the treatment of severe, life-threatening systemic disease.

Physical and occupational therapy attempts to maintain strength and stamina and to preserve and increase the range of motion in the joints and in supporting muscles. All children with significant joint involvement should have a daily home program of activities and exercises directed toward the prevention and correction of disabilities which, after appropriate instruction, can be supervised by the parents. In addition to exercise, the program consists of the use of moist heat, adequate rest, and proper diet, which are aimed at maintaining strength. Children with severe disabilities may need hospitalization for intensive therapy.

Beyond physical therapy, orthopedic treatment for the joints may include splinting to preserve or repair joint motion. In the rehabilitation of older children who have suffered serious damage, the replacement of affected joints may provide good results.

Juvenile rheumatoid arthritis offers significant challenges for families. The family pediatrician or physician must act as teacher and adviser both to the patient and to family members. Other health care professionals who may be important to the care of children with juvenile rheumatoid arthritis are ophthalmologists, pediatric nurses, social workers, and psychiatrists, as well as the child's schoolteachers.

PERSPECTIVE AND PROSPECTS

Dr. George R. Still's finding in 1896 that juvenile rheumatoid arthritis includes at least three distinct joint afflictions first brought the subgroups to the attention of the medical profession and has fostered a greater understanding of the disease.

For most children with juvenile rheumatoid arthritis, early diagnosis and appropriate therapy point to a good prognosis. Of the children with systemic onset, at least 75 percent will enjoy a good outcome, whereas the rest may suffer severe arthritis, possibly resulting in disability. Between 80 and 90 percent of children with polyarthritis escape without permanent joint damage, although the disease itself may be chronic. The overall prospects for children with pauciarticular disease are not known.

Although most children suffering from juvenile rheumatoid arthritis eventually outgrow it, it is difficult for most parents to accept that accurate prediction for the ultimate outcome for their child is impossible. Nevertheless, a positive attitude, careful medical management, physical therapy, and psychologic support can improve the quality of life for all children with juvenile rheumatoid arthritis.

—Mary Hurd

See also Arthritis; Autoimmune disorders; Exercise; Massage; Musculoskeletal system; Orthopedics, pediatric.

FOR FURTHER INFORMATION:

Arthritis Foundation. http://www.arthritis.org/. Provides information on arthritis support groups, exercise classes, and other resources for persons with arthritis. Also offers information, education, and publications specific to juvenile arthritis.

Behrman, Richard E., Robert M. Kliegman, and Hal B. Jenson, eds. *Nelson Textbook of Pediatrics.* 17th ed. Philadelphia: Saunders, 2004. A great text for medical students rotating through pediatrics. It has thorough explanations of diseases and treatments.

Brewer, Earl J., and Kathy Cochran Angel. *The Arthritis Sourcebook.* 3d ed. New York: McGraw-Hill, 2000. A thorough guide to information on treatments, medications, and alternative therapies for the myriad forms of arthritis.

Brewer, Earl J., Edward H. Giannini, and Donald A. Person. *Juvenile Rheumatoid Arthritis.* 2d ed. Philadelphia: W. B. Saunders, 1982. A brief study of the condition of juvenile rheumatoid arthritis. Includes bibliographical references.

Kimball, Chad T. *Childhood Diseases and Disorders Sourcebook: Basic Consumer Health Information About Medical Problems Often Encountered in Preadolescent Children.* Detroit: Omnigraphics, 2002. Offers basic facts about cancer, sickle cell disease, diabetes, and other chronic conditions in children and discusses frequently used diagnostic tests, surgeries, and medications. Long-term care for seriously ill children is also presented.

Melvin, Jeanne L., and Virginia Wright, eds. *Pediatric Rheumatic Diseases.* Vol. 3. Bethesda, Md.: American Occupational Therapy Association, 2000. Covers essential information on team treatment for various disease groups, understanding pain in children, pediatric outcome assessment, the effects of arthritis and treatment on school achievement, surgical treatment, and detailed case studies, among other topics.

Merenstein, Gerald B., David W. Kaplan, and Adam A. Rosenberg. *Handbook of Pediatrics*. 18th ed. Stamford, Conn.: Appleton & Lange, 1997. This popular handbook provides comprehensive and easily accessible information on pediatrics. A reliable source of quick information on the care of children from infancy through adolescence, this edition has been completely revised, updated, and streamlined.

Parker, James N., and Philip M. Parker, eds. *Juvenile Rheumatoid Arthritis: The Official Patient's Sourcebook*. San Diego, Calif.: Icon Health, 2002. Draws from public, academic, government, and peer-reviewed research to provide a wide-ranging handbook for patients with juvenile arthritis.

KAPOSI'S SARCOMA

DISEASE/DISORDER

ANATOMY OR SYSTEM AFFECTED: Intestines, liver, lungs, skin

SPECIALTIES AND RELATED FIELDS: Internal medicine, oncology

DEFINITION: A disease in which cancer cells are found in tissues, causing lesions on the skin and/or mucous membranes and spreading to other organs in the body.

A Kaposi's sarcoma lesion on a patient with AIDS. (SIU School of Medicine)

CAUSES AND SYMPTOMS

It is uncertain whether Kaposi's sarcoma is actually cancer because, unlike cancer, it arises from several cell types. Although there is no accepted staging system for Kaposi's sarcoma, patients are grouped by the type that they have. The three types are classic, epidemic, and recurrent.

Classic Kaposi's sarcoma usually occurs in older men of Mediterranean heritage. It progresses slowly (over ten to fifteen years), with progression bringing lower limb swelling, impeded blood flow, possible spread to other organs, and other types of cancer in later life. Epidemic Kaposi's sarcoma, found in people with acquired immunodeficiency syndrome (AIDS), is a more virulent, fast-spreading, and fatal form, with symptoms of painless, either flat or raised, pink or purple plaques on the skin and mucosal surfaces. This type usually spreads to the lungs, liver, spleen, lymph nodes, digestive tract, and other internal organs. Recurrent Kaposi's sarcoma comes back after it has been treated in the original area where it started. Sometimes, it appears in another part of the body.

TREATMENT AND THERAPY

Four kinds of treatment are usually used: surgery (taking out the cancer), chemotherapy (using drugs to kill cancer cells), external beam radiation therapy (using high-dose X rays to kill cancer cells), and biological therapy (using the body's immune system to fight the cancer).

Classic Kaposi's sarcoma may be treated by radiation therapy, local excision (cutting out the lesion and some of the tissue around it), systemic chemotherapy (in which the drug enters the bloodstream, travels through the body, and kills cancer cells outside the original site), intralesional chemotherapy (in which the drug is injected into the lesion), or a combination of these treatments.

Epidemic Kaposi's sarcoma is treated by surgery, including electrodesiccation and curettage (burning the lesion and removing it with a sharp instrument) and cryotherapy (killing the tumor by freezing it). It

---

INFORMATION ON KAPOSI'S SARCOMA

CAUSES: Unknown; epidemic type found in patients with AIDS

SYMPTOMS: Flat or raised, pink or purple plaques on the skin and mucosal surfaces; lower limb swelling, impeded blood flow

DURATION: Ranges from acute to chronic with recurrent episodes

TREATMENTS: Surgery, chemotherapy, external beam radiation therapy, biological therapy can also be treated with chemotherapy or biological therapy.

PERSPECTIVE AND PROSPECTS

Until the early 1980's, Kaposi's sarcoma was found mainly in older male patients who had received organ transplants. The AIDS epidemic gave rise to cases in many other populations, such as homosexual men and African men. Recovery depends on the type of Kaposi's sarcoma, age, general health, and whether the condition is accompanied by AIDS.

—*Patricia A. Ainsa, M.P.H., Ph.D.*

See also Acquired immunodeficiency syndrome (AIDS); Biopsy; Cancer; Chemotherapy; Cryosurgery; Malignancy and metastasis; Oncology; Radiation therapy; Sarcoma.

FOR FURTHER INFORMATION:

Dollinger, Malin, et al. *Everyone's Guide to Cancer Therapy.* 4th rev. ed. Kansas City, Mo.: Andrews & McMeel, 2002.

Feigal, Ellen G., Alexandra M. Levine, and Robert J. Biggar. *AIDS-Related Cancers and Their Treatment.* New York: Marcel Dekker, 2000.

Gottlieb, Geoffrey J., and A. Bernard Ackerman. *Kaposi's Sarcoma: A Text and Atlas.* Philadelphia: Lea & Febiger, 1988.

Parker, James N., and Philip M. Parker, eds. *The Official Patient's Sourcebook on Kaposi's Sarcoma.* San Diego, Calif.: Icon Health, 2003.

Rutherford, George W., and James O. Kahn, eds. *The Epidemiology of AIDS-Related Kaposi's Sarcoma: A Symposium Sponsored by the San Francisco Center for AIDS Research, San Francisco, California, September 29, 1989.* New York: Raven Press, 1990.

Shepherd, Frances A. *Management of Kaposi's Sarcoma Associated with Human Immunodeficiency Virus Infection.* Ottawa: Health and Welfare Canada, 1991.

KARYOTYPING

PROCEDURE

ALSO KNOWN AS: Chromosome analysis

ANATOMY OR SYSTEM AFFECTED: Cells

SPECIALTIES AND RELATED FIELDS: Cytology, embryology, genetics, neonatology, obstetrics, oncology, pathology, perinatology

DEFINITION: The photographing of all the chromosomes of a single cell to identify extra, missing, or abnormal chromosomes.

KEY TERMS:

autosomes: all the chromosomes, except for the sex chromosomes

karyotype: a photograph of all the chromosomes in a single cell

mitosis: cell division

nondisjunction: a malfunction of mitosis, resulting in cells with an abnormal chromosome number

THE CELL AND CHROMOSOMES

Every cell in the human body—except for red blood cells—contains a nucleus with rod-shaped structures called chromosomes. The chromosomes, in turn, contain the genes, which are the units that transmit heredity from parents to offspring.

The forty-six individual chromosomes in a human cell exist as twenty-three pairs of so-called "homologues." Homologous chromosomes are similar in size and appearance. The first twenty-two pairs of homologues are referred to as autosomes, while pair number twenty-three contains two dissimilar chromosomes known as the X and Y or sex chromosomes, which determine gender. Sperm and eggs each have twenty-three chromosomes, or half the usual number. When a sperm fertilizes an egg, the normal chromosome number (forty-six) is reestablished in the first cell of life, the zygote.

Cells reproduce by mitosis, a process of simple division, the result being two identical daughter cells, each containing forty-six chromosomes. Since chromosomes contain the genetic information, it follows that mitosis must proceed with precision every time a cell divides. During the earliest stages of embryonic development, however, mistakes sometimes occur and the cells wind up with more or fewer chromosomes. This malfunction of mitosis is called nondisjunction, and the incorrect number of chromosomes is passed to all the cells in the developing embryo. This leads to a variety of abnormal conditions, all of which can be diagnosed with the procedure known as karyotyping.

PROCEDURE AND INTERPRETATION

A karyotype is a photograph of all the chromosomes in a single cell. The prefix "karyo-" refers to the nucleus, the part of the cell where chromosomes reside; the suffix "-type" means characterization. Thus, a karyotype is a characterization of a nucleus in terms of its chromosomes.

Karyotypes are performed on embryos to diagnose chromosomal abnormalities and on adults who suspect chromosomal aberrations that could be passed on to offspring. Although a karyotype can be constructed from almost any cell in the body that contains a nucleus, it is most often performed on white blood cells, which are easily harvested from a routine blood sample.

The procedure is simple. Once the blood is collected, the white cells are separated from the red. In the laboratory, the white blood cells are then stimulated to undergo mitosis. At the stage of mitosis when the chromosomes are most visible, the process is chemically halted. The chromosomes are then stained to make them more visible, after which they are photographed and the individual chromosomes cut out and rearranged as homologous pairs in descending order by size. Each pair of chromosomes is also given a number, the largest pair being designated number 1. Then another photograph is taken of the chromosomes in the rearranged format. The result is the karyotype. The entire process, from collecting the blood sample to growing the cells to preparing the karyotype, takes from one to three weeks.

Once the karyotype has been created, it is ready to be interpreted by a cytogeneticist, a person who is an expert in the study of chromosomes. The most common disorders visible with karyotyping are Down syndrome, an extra copy of chromosome number 21; Klinefelter syndrome, a male with an extra X chromosome, resulting in sterility and the development of some female features; and Turner syndrome, a female missing an X chromosome, resulting in sterility and a masculine body build.

PERSPECTIVE AND PROSPECTS
Karyotyping was first reported in the mid-1950's when chromosomes were examined in fetal cells collected from amniotic fluid. This was the beginning of the discipline of prenatal genetic diagnosis. At the time, there was no ultrasound to guide the needle through the amniotic membrane, which increased the risk of damaging the fetus. The karyotyping itself required four or five weeks of cell culture and was not always successful.

Today, karyotyping is commonly used to diagnose chromosomal abnormalities in both fetuses and already-born individuals. It is considered to be an absolutely safe procedure, the only risks being those inherent in penetrating the amniotic sac with a needle. Also, although the advent of ultrasound has greatly reduced the risk to the fetus, the possibility always exists of inadvertently collecting maternal cells when the mother's tissues are penetrated.

Karyotyping has been a fairly static procedure since its inception, having seen little innovation. Dyes are simply added to highlight the chromosomes for identification purposes. There is now, however, a new method called spectral karyotyping, which involves the use of fluorescent dyes that highlight specific regions of the chromosomes. A device called an interferometer is used to detect slight color variations invisible to the human eye and then assign visible colors to the homologous chromosomes. This method is superior to traditional karyotyping with chemical stains because it more clearly identifies chromosomes that are damaged or that contain fragments of other, nonhomologous chromosomes.

—*Robert T. Klose, Ph.D.*

See also Amniocentesis; Biopsy; Cells; Chorionic villus sampling; Cytology; DNA and RNA; Gene therapy; Genetic engineering; Genetics and inheritance; Laboratory tests.

FOR FURTHER INFORMATION:
Harris, Henry. *The Cells of the Body: A History of Somatic Cell Genetics.* Cold Spring Harbor, N.Y.: Cold Spring Harbor Laboratory Press, 1995.

Krogh, David. *Biology: A Guide to the Natural World.* 3d ed. Upper Saddle River, N.J.: Pearson Education, 2005

McGraw-Hill Concise Encyclopedia of Science and Technology. 5th ed. New York: McGraw-Hill, 2005.

Vogel, F., and A. G. Motulsky. *Human Genetics: Problems and Approaches.* 3d rev. ed. New York: Springer, 1997.

KAWASAKI DISEASE
DISEASE/DISORDER

ALSO KNOWN AS: Kawasaki syndrome, mucocutaneous lymph node syndrome (MLNS)

ANATOMY OR SYSTEM AFFECTED: Brain, blood vessels, circulatory system, heart, immune system, lymphatic system, mouth, skin

SPECIALTIES AND RELATED FIELDS: Cardiology, family medicine, immunology, pediatrics

DEFINITION: An inflammatory disease that affects numerous organs and systems in the body and typically occurs in children under the age of five.

CAUSES AND SYMPTOMS
The exact cause of Kawasaki disease is unknown. Approximately 80 percent of the victims are aged five and

---

INFORMATION ON KAWASAKI DISEASE

CAUSES: Unknown; possibly allergic reaction, viral or bacterial infection, or immune system response
SYMPTOMS: High fever; patchy rash; red lips, mouth, tongue, and throat; swollen lymph nodes in neck; swollen hands and feet; diarrhea; vomiting; stomach pain; joint pain; irritability; peeling skin on fingers and toes
DURATION: Two weeks to three months; long-term heart damage possible
TREATMENTS: Aspirin, gamma globulin

---

under. Some doctors believe that the disease may be an allergic reaction to certain types of infection. Others think that it is produced by a virus or bacterium. Some researchers believe that the source is an interaction of T cells, white blood cells that help regulate the immune system's response to infections, with toxins produced by bacteria.

Kawasaki disease begins rather abruptly with a fever that persists for five days or longer and can reach 104 degrees Fahrenheit. A red, patchy rash typically spreads over the chest and genital area and may cover the entire body. The lips, mouth, tongue, and throat become very red. The lymph nodes in the neck may be swollen, as well as the hands and feet. The hands, feet, eyes, and mucous membrane linings of the eyelids turn red. These symptoms may be accompanied by diarrhea, vomiting, stomach pain, joint pain, and irritability. As the fever subsides, there is a characteristic peeling of the skin from the fingers and toes. The symptoms associated with Kawasaki disease may last for two weeks up to three months.

TREATMENT AND THERAPY

Kawasaki disease should be treated as soon as it is diagnosed. A variety of prescribed medications may be used. Aspirin can reduce the fever, ease joint pain, and relieve the rash. Gamma globulin, purified antibodies found in blood, is administered intravenously to help fight infection and reduce the risk of the development of coronary artery abnormalities or damage to the heart muscle. If the disease is treated within ten days of its onset, then less than 20 percent of the patients experience any heart problems.

A doctor may order an electrocardiogram (ECG or EKG), chest radiograph, and echocardiogram in order to monitor heart functions. If liver or gallbladder mal-

function occurs, then ultrasonic imaging of those organs may be necessary.

PERSPECTIVE AND PROSPECTS

Tomisaku Kawasaki first identified Kawasaki disease in 1967 when he reported the symptoms in fifty children in cases occurring between the years of 1961 and 1967. In children under five, the disease has become the leading cause of acquired heart disease in the United States. About three thousand children are hospitalized with Kawasaki disease annually in the United States. Epidemics occurred in Japan in 1979, 1982, and 1985. Death from heart-related problems related to Kawasaki disease occurs in less than 2 percent of the victims. Less than 2 percent of children who experience Kawasaki disease have a reoccurrence.

—*Alvin K. Benson, Ph.D.*

See also Cardiology; Cardiology, pediatric; Childhood infectious diseases; Echocardiography; Electrocardiography (ECG or EKG); Epidemiology; Fever; Heart; Immune system; Immunology; Immunopathology; Lymphatic system; Rashes; Skin; Skin disorders.

FOR FURTHER INFORMATION:

Hawker, Jeremy, et al. *Communicable Disease Control Handbook.* 2d ed. Malden, Mass.: Blackwell, 2005.
Icon Health. *Kawasaki Disease: A Bibliography, Medical Dictionary, and Annotated Research Guide to Internet References.* San Diego, Calif.: Author, 2004.
Powell, Michael, and Oliver Fischer. *101 Diseases You Don't Want to Get.* New York: Thunder's Mouth Press, 2005.

KERATITIS

DISEASE/DISORDER

ANATOMY OR SYSTEM AFFECTED: Eyes
SPECIALTIES AND RELATED FIELDS: Family medicine, ophthalmology, optometry
DEFINITION: An inflammation of the cornea caused most often by the herpes simplex virus.

CAUSES AND SYMPTOMS

Keratitis produces an inflammation or irritation of the cornea, the outer transparent layer of the eye. It is generally caused when the cornea has been scratched, cut, or injured so that a pathway is established for the entry of infectious agents. The resulting infection may be superficial or may involve deeper layers of the cornea. The most common cause of keratitis is the herpes simplex virus, the same virus that produces cold sores. Initially, the virus causes inflammation of the conjunctiva, the membrane lining the eyelid. Typically, it then produces infection of the cornea with branchlike ulcerations. Less common causes of keratitis include adenoviruses, varicella zoster virus, bacteria, fungi, parasites, excessive exposure to ultraviolet light, vitamin A deficiency, rheumatic diseases, surgery on the cornea, adverse reaction to broad-spectrum antibiotics, trauma to the eye that leaves scar tissue, allergic reactions to eye makeup or other irritants, and congenital syphilis (often termed interstitial keratitis). Bacterial keratitis usually results from improper cleaning or care of contact lenses.

The symptoms of keratitis typically include one or more of the following: eye redness, tearing and itching of the eye, a sensation that foreign matter is in the eye, blurred vision or reduction of vision clarity, eyelids sticking together, pain, eye discharge, sensitivity to light, and cloudy appearance of the cornea. If keratitis is left untreated, then corneal tissue can be destroyed, scar tissue can form, and feeling in the cornea may eventually be lost. At the first sign of eye infection, proper treatment should be administered.

Treatment and Therapy

Medical treatment of keratitis varies according to the cause. Antiviral eyedrops are administered for viral keratitis. Oral or eyedrop antibiotics are used for other infections. Some ophthalmologists prefer to scrape diseased tissue from the cornea, apply anesthetic eyedrops, and cover the eye temporarily with a patch.

Information on Keratitis

Causes: Various; may include herpes or other viruses, congenital syphilis or other bacteria, fungi, parasites, excessive ultraviolet light, vitamin A deficiency, rheumatic diseases, eye surgery or other trauma, allergic reactions
Symptoms: Redness, tearing and itching, sensation of foreign matter, blurred or reduced vision, pain, discharge, light sensitivity, cloudy appearance of cornea
Duration: Acute
Treatments: Depends on cause; may include antiviral eyedrops, oral or eyedrop antibiotics, scraping away of diseased tissue, supplements for vitamin A deficiency

Later, the patient may wear a special type of contact lens to prevent a reoccurrence of the infection. For cases involving dry eyes, artificial tears are prescribed for lubrication. Contact lenses may need to be replaced. In the case of vitamin A deficiency, supplements and foods rich in vitamin A (such as carrots, mangoes, spinach, squash, and liver) are prescribed.

Perspective and Prospects

Approximately fifty thousand cases of keratitis are diagnosed worldwide each year. It is the most common cause of corneal blindness in the United States. If treatment for keratitis is started early, then it is typically very effective. In the treatment of keratitis caused by the herpes simplex virus, it is very important not to use topical corticosteroids, as they may worsen the infection and even lead to blindness. Because herpes simplex virus remains in the body after treatment, there is a 50 percent chance that keratitis may reoccur.

—*Alvin K. Benson, Ph.D.*

See also Blindness; Eye infections and disorders; Eyes; Herpes; Ophthalmology; Optometry; Optometry, pediatric; Viral infections; Vision disorders; Vitamins and minerals.

For Further Information:
Icon Health. *Keratitis: A Bibliography, Medical Dictionary, and Annotated Research Guide to Internet References.* San Diego, Calif.: Author, 2004.

Parker, James N., and Philip M. Parker, eds. *The Official Patient's Sourcebook on Keratitis.* San Diego, Calif.: Icon Health, 2002.

Wilhelmus, Kirk R., and Thomas J. Liesegang, eds. *Interstitial Keratitis.* Philadelphia: Saunders, 1994.

Keratoses. *See* Warts.

Kidney cancer
Disease/disorder
Also known as: Renal cancer, renal carcinoma
Anatomy or system affected: Kidneys, urinary system
Specialties and related fields: Nephrology, oncology, urology
Definition: A number of different malignant growths that occur in a kidney.
Key terms:
biological therapy: a type of medical treatment that stimulates the body's immune system or works with it to help it overcome disease

carcinoma: any cancer that begins in the skin or in tissues around body organs

chemotherapy: drug therapy for cancer, usually using multiple medications

embolization: a treatment that stops blood flow to a tumor by blocking small blood vessels

hematuria: blood in the urine, which may be visible (rust-colored or reddish urine) or microscopic (detectable only through laboratory tests)

kidney: one of a pair of abdominal organs which remove waste products from the blood and are involved in many regulatory processes of the body

malignant: cancerous; able to spread into and destroy nearby tissues and to spread to distant areas

metastasis: cancer that occurs at a distance from the primary location

magnetic resonance imaging (MRI): a radiologic technique that uses radio signals, magnets, and a computer to produce highly detailed images of tissues

nephrectomy: surgical removal of a kidney

radiation therapy: the use of high-energy rays to stop cancer cells from growing

renal: pertaining to the kidney

tumor suppressor gene: a gene that usually keeps tumors from growing

CAUSES AND SYMPTOMS

The most common type of kidney cancer is renal cell carcinoma (also known as hypernephroma or renal adenocarcinoma), which accounts for 90 to 95 percent of cases in adults. Renal cell carcinoma is about twice as common in men than in women and occurs most commonly between the ages of fifty and seventy.

The cause of kidney cancer is not known; however, various risk factors increase the chances of developing it. They include smoking, obesity, high blood pressure, chronic dialysis for kidney failure, and exposure to certain chemicals or industrial processes. Kidney cancer is also one part of a rare genetic disease called Von Hippel-Lindau syndrome.

The most common symptom of kidney cancer is hematuria, which occurs in about two-thirds of cases. The patient may notice a change in the color of the urine, or urinalysis may detect microscopic blood in normally colored urine. About one-third of patients have abdominal pain, and another third have a mass (lump) in the abdomen or flank. These three symptoms form the classic triad of findings that suggest kidney cancer. Other, less common symptoms include fever and weight loss. If the cancer has spread to the lungs or

> ### INFORMATION ON KIDNEY CANCER
>
> **CAUSES:** Unknown; risk factors include smoking, obesity, high blood pressure, dialysis, carcinogens
>
> **SYMPTOMS:** Hematuria, abdominal pain, mass in abdomen or flank; sometimes fever and weight loss
>
> **DURATION:** Chronic
>
> **TREATMENTS:** Depends on severity; may include kidney removal, chemotherapy, radiation therapy

bones, then the patient may cough or experience bone pain. On physical examination, a male patient may have a varicocele, a cluster of varicose veins in the scrotum. Laboratory studies may show elevated calcium in the blood, anemia, or, occasionally, an excess of red blood cells. Studies used to diagnose kidney cancer include intravenous pyelogram (IVP), an X ray of the kidneys and urinary tract using a special dye; computed tomography (CT) scan, a technique that generates detailed pictures from a series of X rays; and ultrasonography, the use of sound waves to create an image of the soft tissues of the body.

Less common types of adult kidney cancer include transitional cell cancer of renal pelvis, sarcoma, lymphoma, and metastases from other cancers such as melanoma (the deadliest form of skin cancer) and lung, breast, and stomach cancer. Kidney cancer itself may metastasize to the lungs, bones, liver, and the other kidney.

In children, the most common type of kidney cancer is Wilms tumor, which is caused by the loss of a tumor suppressor gene called WT1 found on chromosome 11. The most common finding is an abdominal mass. Other findings include abdominal pain, fever, hematuria, high blood pressure, or anemia. Unlike with adult kidney cancer, boys and girls have equal risk of developing Wilms tumor. This cancer occurs most commonly in young children (three to four years), although it may be found in younger and older children and in teens.

TREATMENT AND THERAPY

The treatment of kidney cancer depends on the age and health of the patient, the exact location and size of the tumor, and whether it has metastasized. Size, location, and metastasis are determined through the process of staging that includes extensive studies such as bone scans, CT scans, and MRIs.

The main treatment for adult kidney cancer is nephrectomy to remove the diseased kidney. Embolization or radiation therapy may be used to shrink the tumor before surgery, which makes it easier to remove. In cases where the cancer is too advanced for surgical treatment, these techniques may be used to relieve symptoms and make the patient more comfortable.

The treatment for Wilms tumor is a combination of surgery, chemotherapy, and radiation therapy. This has improved survival from about 60 percent in the 1950's to more than 90 percent in the early twenty-first century.

PERSPECTIVE AND PROSPECTS

Although chemotherapy has not been helpful in most adult kidney cancers, new drugs and new drug combination treatments are under investigation. Other new treatments include biological therapies with interferon alpha, interleukin-2, and other immune system modulators. Although the exact mechanism of these biological therapies is not entirely clear, they seem to slow, or even stop, the growth of cancer cells. They make it easier for the body's own immune system to destroy and remove cancer cells and appear to be particularly useful in treating metastatic disease.

Tumor vaccines and gene therapy are other biological treatments under development. The vaccines may prevent a cancer from starting, may treat a cancer that already exists, or may help rid the body of cancer cells that have not been eliminated by other forms of treatment. In the first decade of the twenty-first century, these vaccines are still being researched and available only to persons who enroll in experimental studies. Gene therapy actually changes the tiny genes that regulate cell growth and death. The goal is to improve the body's own ability to fight the cancer or to make the cancer more likely to respond to other forms of treatment. Researchers are also studying ablation (removal) of the cancer using radio frequencies or freezing.

—Rebecca Lovell Scott, Ph.D., PA-C

See also Cancer; Carcinoma; Chemotherapy; Dialysis; Gene therapy; Kidney disorders; Kidneys; Malignancy and metastasis; Nephrectomy; Nephrology; Nephrology, pediatric; Radiation therapy; Renal failure; Tumors; Urinary disorders; Urinary system; Urology; Urology, pediatric.

FOR FURTHER INFORMATION:

American Medical Association. *American Medical Association Family Medical Guide*. 4th rev. ed. Hoboken, N.J.: John Wiley & Sons, 2004.

Greenberg, Arthur, et al., eds. *Primer on Kidney Diseases*. 4th ed. Philadelphia: Elsevier Saunders, 2005.

Komaroff, Anthony, ed. *Harvard Medical School Family Health Guide*. New York: Free Press, 2005.

National Kidney Foundation. http://www.kidney.org/.

Schrier, Robert W., ed. *Diseases of the Kidney and Urinary Tract*. 8th ed. Philadelphia: Wolters Kluwer Health/Lippincott Williams & Wilkins, 2007.

Stoppard, Miriam. *Family Health Guide*. New York: DK, 2004.

KIDNEY DISORDERS

DISEASE/DISORDER

ANATOMY OR SYSTEM AFFECTED: Kidneys, urinary system

SPECIALTIES AND RELATED FIELDS: Internal medicine, nephrology, urology

DEFINITION: Disorders, from structural abnormalities to bacterial infections, that can affect the kidneys and may lead to renal failure.

KEY TERMS:

creatinine: the breakdown product of creatine, a nitrogenous compound found in muscle, blood, and urine

cystinosis: a congenital disease characterized by glucose and protein in the urine, as well as by cystine deposits in the liver and other organs, rickets, and growth retardation

hematuria: the abnormal presence of blood in the urine

hydronephrosis: the cessation of urine flow because of an obstruction of a ureter, allowing urine to build up in the pelvis of the kidney; can cause renal failure

oliguria: the diminished capacity to form and pass urine, so that metabolic products cannot be excreted efficiently

reflux: the abnormal backward flow of urine

toxemia: blood poisoning

uremia: the presence of excessive amounts of urea and other nitrogenous waste products in the blood

CAUSES AND SYMPTOMS

Disorders of the kidney can occur for a variety of reasons. The cause may be congenital (present from birth) or may develop very quickly and at any age. Many of these problems and disorders can be easily treated. The main areas of kidney disorders are classified as malformations in development of the kidney, part of the kid-

INFORMATION ON KIDNEY DISORDERS

CAUSES: Congenital defects, bacterial infections, trauma

SYMPTOMS: Varies; can include swelling, uremia, fever, rash, renal pain, body aches, nausea, fatigue, mental dullness

DURATION: Acute to chronic

TREATMENTS: Medications (diuretics, vasodilators, calcium antagonists, oral antibiotics); short-term dialysis; hemodialysis; catheterization; surgery such as transplantation

ney, or the ureter; glomerular disease; tubular and interstitial disease or disruption; vascular (other than glomerular) disease; and kidney dysfunction that occurs secondary to another disease.

The kidney frequently exhibits congenital anomalies, some of which occur during specific developmental stages. Agenesis occurs when the ureteric bud fails to develop normally. When the tissue does not develop, the ureter itself fails to form. If there is an obstruction where the ureter joins the pelvis of the kidney, there may be massive hydronephrosis (dilation). One or both kidneys may be unusually small, containing too few tubules. The kidneys may be displaced, too high or offset to one side or the other. They may even be fused. All these conditions could seriously affect the manufacture of urine, its excretion, or both.

Glomerulonephritis refers to a diverse group of conditions that share a common feature—primary involvement of the glomerulus. The significance of glomerulonephritis is that it is the most common cause of end-stage renal failure. Its features include urinary casts, high protein levels (proteinuria), hematuria, hypertension, edema (swelling), and uremia. The two forms of glomerulonephritis are primary and secondary. In the primary form, only the kidneys are affected, but in the secondary form, the lesion (affected area) is only one of a series of problems.

Nephrotic syndrome is usually defined as an abnormal condition of the kidney characterized by the presence of proteinuria together with edema and high fat and cholesterol levels. It occurs in glomerular disease, in thrombosis of a renal vein, and as a complication of many systemic diseases. Nephrotic syndrome occurs in a severe, primary form characterized by anorexia, weakness, proteinuria, and edema.

Interstitial nephritis is inflammation of the interstitial tissue of the kidney, including the kidneys. Acute interstitial nephritis is an immunologic, adverse reaction to certain drugs; drugs especially associated with it are nonsteroidal anti-inflammatory drugs (NSAIDs) and some antibiotics. Acute renal failure, fever, rash, and proteinuria are indicative signs of this condition. If the medication is stopped, normal kidney function returns. Chronic interstitial nephritis is defined as inflammation and structural changes associated with such conditions as ureteral obstruction, pyelonephritis, exposure of the kidney to a toxin, transplant rejection, or certain systemic diseases.

Kidney stones (calculi) are commonly manufactured from calcium oxalate and/or phosphate, triple phosphate, uric acid (urate), or a mixture of these. Calcium stones are not necessarily the result of high serum calcium, although they can be. Struvite calculi of magnesium ammonium (triple) phosphate mixed with calcium are bigger but softer than other types; they grow irregularly, filling much of the kidney pelvis. They arise from infection with urea-splitting organisms that cause alkaline urine. Urate stones are a complication of gout.

Those who have a tendency to develop stones may experience concomitant infection known as pyonephrosis. Pyonephrosis is a result of not only blockage at the junction of the ureter and kidney pelvis but also any constricture at this location. Bacteria from the bloodstream collect and cause an abscess to form. If the tube is completely blocked, the inflammation produces enough pus to rupture a portion of the kidney, and more of the abdominal cavity becomes involved.

Pyelonephritis is inflammation of the upper urinary tract. Acute pyelonephritis may be preceded by lower tract infection. The patient complains of lethargy, fever, and back pain. The major symptoms are fever, renal pain, and body aches accompanied by nausea and toxemia. Chronic pyelonephritis often affects the renal tubules and the small spaces within the kidney. Fibrous tissue may take over these areas and cause gradual shrinking of the functional kidney. The chronic form may also result from previous bacterial infection, reflux, obstruction, overuse of analgesics, X rays, and lead poisoning.

Obstruction may be caused by inadequate development of the renal tissue itself, closing off one or both ureters. Other malformations and certain calculi can also obstruct urine flow. Reflux may occur when the contraction of the bladder forces urine backward, up toward and into the kidney. Lesser degrees of reflux do not damage the kidney, but the greater the reflux, the more likely damage will occur. Bacterial infection is often attributable to *Escherichia coli*, but other bowel bacteria may also infect the area. They generally move upward from outside the body through the urinary organs, but they may move inward from the bloodstream.

Acute renal failure is defined as a sudden decline in normal renal function that leads to an increase in blood urea and creatinine. The onset may be fast (over days) or slow (over weeks) and is often reversible. It is characterized by oliguria and rapid accumulation of nitrogenous wastes in the blood, resulting in acidosis. Acute renal failure is caused by hemorrhage, trauma, burns, toxic injury to the kidney, acute pyelonephritis or glomerulonephritis, or lower urinary tract obstruction. Occasionally, it will progress into chronic renal failure.

Chronic renal failure may result from many other diseases. Its signs are sluggishness, fatigue, and mental dullness. Patients also display other systemic problems as a result of chronic renal failure. Almost all such patients are anemic; three-fourths of them develop hypertension. The skin becomes discolored; the muddy coloration is caused by anemia and the presence of excess melanin.

Renal symptoms suggestive of renal dysfunction include increases in frequency of urination, color changes in urine, areas of edema, and hypertension. The patient may experience only one symptom but is more likely to have a series of complaints. To determine the cause of renal disease, several diagnostic tools can be used to distinguish the type of pathogenic process affecting the kidney. The degree to which other body systems are involved determines whether the disease process is systemic or confined to the kidneys. Other valuable clues may be gathered from medical history, family history, and physical examination. The key factors, however, are renal size and renal histopathology.

Examination of the urine can reveal important data relative to renal health. Stick tests may show the abnormal presence of blood, glucose, and/or protein. Assaying the kind and amount of protein may pinpoint the cause of the disease. Urine contaminated with bacteria has always been used as an indication of some form of urinary tract infection. Microscopic examination of urine sediment may help diagnose acute renal failure. Blood tests may also indicate the source of a renal disorder. A series of blood tests might reveal rising urea and creatinine levels. The urea-to-creatinine ratio may

aid in determining if and which type of acute renal failure may be present. A high red cell count might suggest kidney stones, a tumor, or glomerular disease; a high white cell count would hint at inflammation and/or infection. Cells cast from the kidney tubules may indicate acute interstitial nephritis, while red cell breakdown products may mean glomerulonephritis. The diagnostician should also be diligent in tracking down possible septic causes. Repeated cultures of blood and urine should help ascertain if there is an abscess anywhere near the kidney.

X rays can provide useful information. An abdominal X ray may show urinary stones and abnormalities in the renal outline. Ultrasound will measure renal size, show scarring, and reveal dilation of the tract, perhaps as a result of an obstructive lesion. Abdominal ultrasound has become the investigation of choice because it can be performed at the patient's bedside.

Renal biopsy can give an accurate diagnosis of acute renal failure but may be more dangerous to the patient than the condition itself. The main indications for biopsy would be suspected acute glomerulonephritis and renal failure that has lasted six weeks.

TREATMENT AND THERAPY

If glomerulonephritis is suspected or diagnosed, its treatment seeks to avoid complications of the illness. The patient is monitored daily for fluid overload; as long as the patient is retaining fluid, blood tests that measure urea, creatinine, and salt balance are also run daily. The patient should stay in bed and restrict fluid as well as potassium intake. Medications may be prescribed: diuretics, vasodilators for hypertension, and calcium antagonists. If the cause is bacterial, a course of oral antibiotics may be given. If these measures are unsuccessful, short-term dialysis may be needed. Some urinary abnormalities may last for as long as a year.

The first measure undertaken to treat acute renal failure is to rebuild depressed fluid volumes: blood if the patient has hemorrhaged, plasma for burn patients, and electrolytes for a patient who is vomiting and has diarrhea. If infection is suspected as the underlying cause, an appropriate antibiotic should be administered when blood cultures confirm the presence of bacteria. After fluid volumes have been replenished, a diuretic may be necessary to reduce swelling of tissues within the kidney.

In chronic renal failure, the major undertaking is to relieve the obstruction of the urinary tract. If the blockage is within the bladder, simple catheterization may relieve it. If a stone or some similar obstacle is blocking a ureter, however, surgery to remove it may be necessary. A tube may be inserted to allow urine drainage, and the stone will pass or be removed.

In sufferers of recurrent stones, maintaining a high urine output is important, which requires the patient to drink fluids throughout the day and even at bedtime. Those enduring intense pain may need to be hospitalized. Analgesics for pain are administered, as well as forced fluid intake to increase urine output so that the stone might be passed. If these measures do not work, surgical intervention may be necessary.

Patients suffering from progressive, incurable renal failure need medical aid managing conservation of, substitution for, and eventual replacement of nephron function. Conservation attempts to prolong kidney function for as long as possible; renal function is aided by drug treatment. Substitution means the maintenance of kidney function by dialysis, especially hemodialysis. Replacement is the restoration of renal function by a kidney transplant. By this third stage of treatment, urine formation is independent of further drug treatment, and kidney function must be achieved by other means. Patients suffering from end-stage renal failure have two options: dialysis and transplantation. A patient may go from dialysis to transplantation. In fact, if a compatible donor (preferably a sibling) is available, a transplant is advisable. For those without a suitable donor, long-term hemodialysis is the first option.

Dialysis is defined as the diffusion of dissolved molecules through a semipermeable membrane. Several types of dialysis are available. Hemodialysis filters and cleans the blood as it passes through the semipermeable membranous tube in contact with a balanced salt solution (dialysate). Hemodialysis can be performed in a dialysis unit of a hospital or at home. It must usually be done two or three times a week, with each session lasting from three to six hours, depending on the type of membranes used and the size of the patient. Hemodialysis can lead to acute neurological changes. Lethargy, irritability, restlessness, headache, nausea, vomiting, and twitching may all occur. In some patients, neurological complications occur after dialysis is terminated. Convulsions are the most common of these consequences. In continuous abdominal peritoneal dialysis, a fresh amount of dialysate is introduced from a bag attached to a permanently implanted plastic tube. Wastes and water pass into the dialysate from the surrounding organs; then the fluid is collected four to eight hours later. Peritoneal dialysis is performed by the patient.

It is continuous, so the clearance rate of wastes is higher. The most important neurological complications of peritoneal dialysis are worsening of urea-induced brain abnormalities accompanied by twitching and, rarely, psychosis and convulsions.

Transplantation of a kidney is considered for patients with primary renal diseases as well as end-stage renal failure resulting from any number of systemic and metabolic diseases. Success rates are highest for those suffering from lupus nephritis, gout, and cystinosis. If a kidney is received from a close relative, there is a 97 percent one-year survival rate. Even if the organ transplant comes from a nonrelative, the survival rate is still 90 percent.

—Iona C. Baldridge

See also Dialysis; Edema; Genital disorders, male; Hemolytic uremic syndrome; Incontinence; Kidney cancer; Kidney transplantation; Kidneys; Lithotripsy; Nephrectomy; Nephritis; Nephrology; Nephrology, pediatric; Polycystic kidney disease; Pyelonephritis; Renal failure; Stone removal; Stones; Urethritis; Urinary disorders; Urinary system; Urology; Urology, pediatric.

For Further Information:

Cameron, J. Stewart. *History of the Treatment of Renal Failure by Dialysis.* New York: Oxford University Press, 2002. Traces the history of dialysis, including discussions of the concepts of diffusion and anticoagulation, early attempts of dialysis in animals and humans, and recent developments in the field.

Catto, Graeme R. D., and David A. Power, eds. *Nephrology in Clinical Practice.* London: Edward Arnold, 1988. This book addresses health care professionals in particular. Its goal is to educate practitioners in methods of recognition and diagnosis and of treatment.

Daugirdas, John T., Peter G. Blake, and Todd S. Ing, eds. *Handbook of Dialysis.* 3d ed. Philadelphia: Lippincott Williams & Wilkins, 2001. A practical guide that focuses primarily on the management of dialysis patients but also explores the physiologic basis for dialytic therapies and the pathophysiology of relevant disease states.

Dische, Frederick E. *Renal Pathology.* 2d ed. New York: Oxford University Press, 1995. For those in training for medical fields, this book describes renal anatomy and pathology. The terminology is somewhat simplified so that the descriptions are more understandable.

Greenberg, Arthur, et al., eds. *Primer on Kidney Diseases*. 4th ed. Philadelphia: Elsevier Saunders, 2005. A publication from the National Kidney Foundation that covers such topics as fluid and electrolyte disorders, hypertension, dialysis, and renal transplantation.

Morgan, Steven H., and Jean-Pierre Grunfeld, eds. *Inherited Disorders of the Kidney: Investigation and Management*. New York: Oxford University Press, 1999. Discusses a range of kidney disorders, including cystic diseases; glomerular, tubular, and metabolic disorders; hypertension; and carcinomas. Examines the role of genetics.

National Kidney Foundation. http://www.kidney.org/. Offers thorough information on myriad kidney problems and diseases; supports patient services such as transplantation, drug banks, and educational projects; and makes referrals to local agencies.

O'Callaghan, C. A., and Barry M. Brenner. *The Kidney at a Glance*. Malden, Mass.: Blackwell Science, 2000. Covers a range of topics related to the kidneys, presenting text on one page and accompanying illustrations on the facing page. Covers basic anatomy and physiology and the pathologies and presentations of renal and urinary tract disease.

Parker, James N., and Philip M. Parker, eds. *The 2002 Official Patient's Sourcebook on Kidney Failure*. San Diego, Calif.: Icon Health, 2002. Draws from public, academic, government, and peer-reviewed research to provide a wide-ranging reference about the causes, treatments, and risk factors of kidney disease and failure.

_____. *The Official Patient's Sourcebook on Urinary Tract Infection*. San Diego, Calif.: Icon Health, 2002. Draws from public, academic, government, and peer-reviewed research to provide a wide-ranging handbook for patients with recurring urinary tract infections.

Schrier, Robert W., ed. *Diseases of the Kidney and Urinary Tract*. 8th ed. Philadelphia: Wolters Kluwer Health/Lippincott Williams & Wilkins, 2007. Covers full range of the biochemical, structural, and functional correlations in the kidney, as well as hereditary diseases, urological diseases and neoplasms of the genitourinary tract, acute renal failure, and nutrition, drugs, and the kidney, among many additional topics.

Tierney, Lawrence M., Stephen J. McPhee, and Maxine A. Papadakis, eds. *Current Medical Diagnosis and Treatment 2007*. New York: McGraw-Hill Medical, 2006. This reference volume covers all aspects of internal medicine. It is readable and concisely describes more than one thousand diseases and disorders, as well as their medical management.

KIDNEY REMOVAL. *See* NEPHRECTOMY.

KIDNEY STONES. *See* KIDNEY DISORDERS; STONE REMOVAL; STONES.

KIDNEY TRANSPLANTATION
PROCEDURE

ANATOMY OR SYSTEM AFFECTED: Abdomen, kidneys, urinary system

SPECIALTIES AND RELATED FIELDS: General surgery, nephrology

DEFINITION: A surgical procedure that replaces the recipient's diseased, nonfunctioning kidney with a donated one.

KEY TERMS:

end-stage renal disease: the final phase of long-standing kidney disease, characterized by a nearly complete loss of function

hemodialysis: the use of an external apparatus to filter the blood of patients with end-stage renal disease

immunosuppression: the use of a variety of drugs to depress the immune system's response to foreign tissue; lowers the probability of rejection of transplanted organs

rejection: a cellular and chemical attack by the immune system on a transplanted organ, which is recognized as foreign to the body

renal: referring to the kidneys

INDICATIONS AND PROCEDURES

Transplantation of a human kidney from a donor to a recipient has been used since the middle of the twentieth century to improve the quality and length of life for people with renal failure. While hemodialysis—or the use of an artificial kidney machine, as it is commonly known—can be used satisfactorily for years, transplantation is often the ultimate goal because it can return the patient to a near-normal life.

The kidneys play a pivotal role in maintaining a stable internal environment by controlling fluid levels, excreting waste products, and regulating the blood concentration of acids and bases and of ions such as sodium and potassium. The kidneys are also responsible for regulating blood pressure by secreting substances that constrict the blood vessels. Clearly, the derangement of

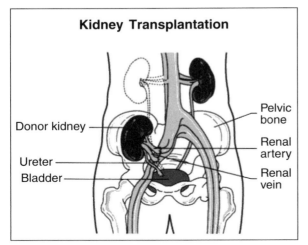

Kidney Transplantation

The donor kidney is usually attached in front of the pelvic bone, rather than in the location of the nonfunctioning kidney, which is not removed in some cases.

such complex functions, as occurs in renal disease, is life-threatening.

There are many reasons for renal failure, but the most frequent are inherited disorders, severe infections, toxic substances, allergic reactions, diabetes mellitus, and hypertension. The latter two, which are common illnesses in the United States, result in renal damage because of long-term injury to the blood vessels. The symptoms of minimally or nonfunctioning kidneys reflect an accumulation of toxic waste products and dramatic changes in the chemical composition of the blood. Every system is affected until coma and death ensue. The process of hemodialysis is used intermittently to cleanse the blood and maintain life. Transplantation in the otherwise healthy person, however, is preferred.

An extraordinary amount of cooperation and preparation is necessary for successful kidney transplantation. The donor organ may come from a living blood relative or from a cadaver within minutes of death. The organ is removed and maintained at low temperature in a special preservative solution for up to forty-eight hours. A suitable recipient is located through a national registry that can rapidly pair a cadaver organ to a waiting patient. The chosen candidate is immediately prepared for surgery, and through an abdominal incision, the kidney is placed in the abdomen and connected to the blood supply by its artery and vein. The ureter, the urine-collecting duct, is attached to the bladder. The recipient's own diseased kidneys may or may not be removed; their presence does not interfere with the trans-

planted organ. Within hours, the newly transplanted organ begins to form urine.

USES AND COMPLICATIONS

All transplanted organs and tissues face both immediate and long-term rejection by the recipient's immune system. Recognizing the donated kidney as foreign, or "nonself," the immune system attacks it both physically and chemically. The injury can be so severe as to result in the organ's death and the need for its surgical removal. In an attempt to prevent this reaction, certain steps are taken both before and after transplantation surgery.

Matching a donor and recipient involves careful selection that must minimize the physiological differences that exist between people. The blood types (the ABO and Rh systems) should be the same. Gene sequences on the sixth chromosome that code for immune system components are also matched as closely as possible in a process known as human leukocyte antigen (HLA) compatibility. Living, first-degree relatives, such as parents or siblings, often provide the best survival rates because of the genetic similarities between donor and recipient. The loss of one kidney in a healthy individual does not appear to affect the body.

The excellent success rates that have been achieved—nearly 80 percent—are attributable both to preoperative matching and to immunosuppression, which is begun shortly before surgery and continued for many months afterward. Potent drugs are used to inhibit the recipient's immune system, thereby protecting the new kidney from attack and significantly reducing rejection. Eventually, the drugs are tapered off and stopped, having allowed the body time to adjust to the foreign tissue and the kidney time to heal.

As can be expected in a procedure as difficult as kidney transplantation, the risks and complications are many. In the immediate postoperative period, hemorrhaging from the attached renal artery or vein, leakage from the ureter, organ malfunction, and immediate rejection can occur. Often, difficulties begin weeks or even months later, because of both rejection damage to the kidney and side effects related to severe immunosuppression. Immunosuppression leaves the body prey to bacterial, viral, and fungal infections, as well as cancer. Sometimes, a vicious cycle begins, in which life-threatening infections require the discontinuation of the immunosuppressive drugs, and the probability of organ rejection and irreparable kidney damage is heightened. Continual patient monitoring is absolutely essential to maintain the delicate balance between the risks and benefits involved in this procedure.

PERSPECTIVE AND PROSPECTS

Prior to 1962, when immunosuppressive drugs were unavailable and matching could only be based on blood type, kidney transplantation was an experimental procedure usually involving the organ of a living, first-degree relative. In the following decades, an extraordinary surge in information about the immune system and the genes that control the rejection response, as well as the discovery of powerful drugs, made transplantation a successful alternative for patients supported by hemodialysis. It also significantly increased the donor pool of organs by allowing unrelated cadaver kidneys to be used. It is in both areas, more precise matching and the development of less toxic postoperative drugs, that research continues. Contributions made in this field are readily used for research in all other organ transplantation as well.

—*Connie Rizzo, M.D., Ph.D.*

See also Circulation; Cysts; Dialysis; Hemolytic uremic syndrome; Internal medicine; Kidney cancer; Kidney disorders; Kidneys; Nephrectomy; Nephritis; Nephrology; Nephrology, pediatric; Polycystic kidney disease; Renal failure; Transplantation; Urinalysis; Urinary disorders; Urinary system; Urology; Urology, pediatric; Xenotransplantation.

FOR FURTHER INFORMATION:

American Kidney Fund. http://www.akfinc.org/. Provides financial assistance for individuals with chronic kidney failure.

Brezis, M., et al. "Renal Transplantation." In *Brenner and Rector's The Kidney*, edited by Barry M. Brenner and Floyd C. Rector, Jr. 6th ed. Philadelphia: W. B. Saunders, 1999. A chapter in a treatise which, at more than two thousand pages, is the most comprehensive and authoritative source on the normal and diseased human kidney.

Carpenter, C., and M. Lazarus. "Dialysis and Transplantation in Renal Failure." In *Harrison's Principles of Internal Medicine*, edited by Kurt Isselbacher et al. 14th ed. New York: McGraw-Hill, 1998. A chapter in a standard text on internal medicine. Includes bibliographical references and an index.

Danovitch, Gabriel, ed. *Handbook of Kidney Transplantation.* 4th ed. Philadelphia: Lippincott Williams & Wilkins, 2005. A clinical handbook that gives a practical overview of renal transplantation

and includes up-to-date coverage of topics such as immunosuppressive drugs, short- and long-term post-transplant management, complications, and ethical and legal issues.

National Kidney Foundation. http://www.kidney.org/. Offers thorough information on myriad kidney problems and diseases; supports patient services such as transplantation, drug banks, and educational projects; and makes referrals to local agencies.

Schrier, Robert W., ed. *Diseases of the Kidney and Urinary Tract.* 8th ed. Philadelphia: Wolters Kluwer Health/Lippincott Williams & Wilkins, 2007. Addresses the spectrum of systemic diseases and the kidney, covering malignancies, paraproteinemias, HIV, hepatitis, cryoglobulimea, sickle cell disease, sarcoidosis, and tropical diseases, in an atlas format.

KIDNEYS

ANATOMY

ANATOMY OR SYSTEM AFFECTED: Abdomen, circulatory system, urinary system

SPECIALTIES AND RELATED FIELDS: Hematology, nephrology, urology

DEFINITION: The organs that control the amount and composition of body water by separating the blood into waste products (which leave the body as urine) and nutrients (which are returned to the blood).

KEY TERMS:

Bowman's capsule: the group of renal cells that forms the cup of a nephron; fluids that seep from glomerular capillaries into the hollow wall of the capsule will be transformed into urine during their passage through the renal tubule leading from the capsule

glomerulus: a tuft or ball of capillaries contained within a Bowman's capsule

nephron: the almost-microscopic functional unit of the kidney, composed of special capillary blood vessels and of a Bowman's capsule connected to a renal tubule; each kidney has approximately 1.2 million nephrons

renal: of or relating to the kidneys

renal pelvis: the central pocket or sac of each kidney, which collects urine from all nephrons and channels it into the ureter

renal tubule: the tubular portion of a nephron that allows renal fluid to flow from the Bowman's capsule to the renal pelvis; these tubules, shaped like hairpins, are crucially important in the production of urine

ureter: the tube that transports urine from the renal pelvis to the urinary bladder

STRUCTURE AND FUNCTIONS

The normal human body has two kidneys, fist-sized organs located behind the abdomen and under the diaphragm. Each kidney, shaped like a bean, has a notch called the hilum, and the backbone separates the two kidneys. The kidneys make urine from blood. The renal artery transports blood into the kidney, while the renal vein transports blood out of the kidney. The blood vessels and the ureter connect with the kidney at its hilum.

The two kidneys are essentially identical in structure and function; consequently, kidney function can be discussed in the singular. The kidneys are a major functional unit of the circulatory system—unlike organs such as the brain, skin, or uterus, which are merely supported by that circulation. The kidney controls the environment of all cells of the body, an activity which is essential to life. That environment is salt water, and to understand the structure and function of the kidney, it is necessary to understand the nature of salt water in the body.

The human body is about 56 percent water, and the composition of this fluid is very important. One-third of this water is outside the cells; some of this extracellular fluid is between cells, and some of it is the liquid in blood vessels (blood is composed of liquid and cells). Two-thirds of the body's water is inside cells. The cell membrane surrounding each cell retains the intracellular fluid, but the water molecules move freely across the cell membrane. The size of each cell is determined by its water content. Cells swell or shrink based on the accumulation or loss of water molecules. The concentration of substances dissolved in the water determines whether water will accumulate inside or outside cells. Some of these dissolved substances are gases such as oxygen and carbon dioxide; some are minerals such as hydrogen, sodium, and calcium; some are sugars or proteins; and others are nutrients and waste products.

The amount and the composition of body water is controlled by the kidneys. Two other organs that aid in controlling the composition of body water are the lungs and the digestive tract; they can add or remove materials from the body water. The kidneys control the composition of body water primarily by removing materials from body water. Unlike the lungs and the digestive tract, however, the kidneys also regulate the amount of body water. The kidneys carry out both of these functions by acting on the blood. The kidney has three other important functions: It helps to control blood pressure, helps to control the manufacture of red blood cells, and participates in the manufacture of vitamin D. This article focuses on function of the normal kidney and what can make the kidney function abnormally.

Each kidney contains more than a million nephrons, its functional units, arranged in cones. A nephron is composed of blood vessels and a Bowman's capsule, a cup of renal cells containing the capillary tuft called a glomerulus and attached to a renal tubule.

A kidney has between eight and eighteen cones of nephrons. The base of each cone is near the surface of the kidney, and the peak of each cone is pointed at the renal pelvis, the central sac that collects and channels urine. Each nephron acts like a very sophisticated filtration system for the blood. Approximately 20 to 25 percent of all the blood in the body flows through the blood vessels of the kidneys every minute.

The action of the nephron actually begins with a porous filter, the glomerulus, that separates particles from a liquid. In this case, the liquid is blood plasma and the particles are blood cells and those protein molecules that are too large to pass through the glomerular pores. About 20 percent of the liquid in the blood seeps through the wall of glomeruli and into the inner space of Bowman's capsules. This liquid that crosses into a Bowman's capsule contains water, minerals, sugars, amino acids, and products of cell metabolism. The body needs to retain many of these substances, including water, so they must be recaptured by nephrons and returned to the blood.

The recapturing process occurs in the renal tubules.

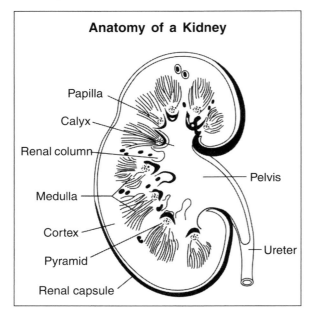

Anatomy of a Kidney

Papilla

Calyx

Renal column

Medulla

Cortex

Pyramid

Renal capsule

Pelvis

Ureter

This is the process in which the nephron differs from an ordinary filter. The tubules have special cells that are capable of selectively reabsorbing those materials that must be retained by the body. These materials are passed from the liquid inside the tubules, through the tubule cells, and into blood capillaries that are laced or braided around the outside wall of the tubules. About 99 percent of the water molecules that seep into the renal tubules from the glomeruli are returned to the blood. The substances that do not need to be retained by the body continue to flow through the tubules and eventually leave the kidney as urine.

The mechanism in the renal tubular cells that selectively reabsorbs substances from the tubular liquid is quite special. The membrane of each cell contains proteins that act as chemical pumps. These pump proteins pick up substances to be reabsorbed from the tubular liquid and pass those substances into and through the tubular cells, where they enter renal capillaries. The reabsorbed substances may be salts or electrolytes, such as sodium or bicarbonate, or they may be sugars or even amino acids. As these substances are reabsorbed, much of the tubular water is also reabsorbed.

The pump proteins can work in the opposite direction as well. They can move substances from the renal capillaries surrounding the tubules, through the wall of the tubules, and into the tubular liquid. This process is called tubular secretion. Substances that commonly undergo tubular secretion are potassium, ammonium, and acid.

The remarkable action of the pump proteins requires fuel—in this case, adenosine triphosphate (ATP). ATP is made by living cells from oxygen, sugar, fatty acids, and nucleic acids in the blood. Pump proteins stop working when cells are unable to make ATP.

The pressure of the blood flow through the glomeruli and the reabsorption process of the renal tubules are closely controlled. This control takes place directly in the kidney, which contains sensing mechanisms that respond to changes in fluid composition. The kidney makes a hormone, called renin, that increases blood pressure. Other sensors that respond to changes in fluid composition are located in the brain. When these sensors detect changes that require action, the brain, acting through the pituitary gland, releases hormones, such as antidiuretic hormone (ADH), that act on the kidney. Another important hormone that controls kidney function, aldosterone, comes from the adrenal gland. The actual means by which these hormones control kidney function, however, is only partially understood.

By other mechanisms, the kidney detects whether the blood contains sufficient red blood cells (erythrocytes). Red blood cells are responsible for carrying oxygen to all the other cells in the body. When more red blood cells are needed, the kidney makes a hormone called erythropoietin, which stimulates the bone marrow and causes it to make more red blood cells.

DISORDERS AND DISEASES

The advantage of having a pair of kidneys becomes obvious if renal function becomes impaired. A person does quite well with one kidney; in fact, half of one kidney is sufficient to keep an individual alive.

A kidney problem may be suspected if an individual experiences changes in urination, such as pain on urination, changes in frequency of urination (more often or less often than usual), or changes in the urine that is formed (such as in its amount, appearance, or odor). Puffiness of the skin all over the body, but especially of the hands, feet, ankles, and face, may indicate abnormal renal function. This puffiness signifies water retention. Kidney disease can also be manifested by severe pain in the lower back, side, abdomen, or sex organs. The pain may be long-lasting or may occur with startling suddenness.

A person can be born with abnormal kidneys; this is a form of kidney disease. Normal kidneys, however, can malfunction because of a problem in the kidney itself, a problem in the blood circulation, or a problem in the flow of urine from the kidneys. Examples of abnormal kidneys at birth, abnormal urinary flow (kidney stones), and kidney infection will be discussed.

The formation of the kidneys by a fetus is quite complex and is controlled by genes. The development of the kidneys, other parts of the urinary tract (the ureters, bladder, and urethra), and the sex organs are all closely related. There are many opportunities for the developmental process to go wrong. Sometimes no kidneys are formed, sometimes the two kidneys are fused together, and sometimes more than one pair of kidneys is formed.

One of the most common malformations of the kidney is polycystic kidney disease, a hereditary (genetic) disorder affecting about 2 in 1,000 people. In the United States, it is ten times more common than sickle cell disease and fifteen times more common than cystic fibrosis. In polycystic kidney disease, each kidney contains numerous fluid-filled sacs, or cysts, scattered throughout the organ. The cysts are of different sizes, some very small and some the size of a grape. Polycystic kidneys are noticeably enlarged.

The cysts are caused by a malformation of the renal tubules. A cyst is formed when a renal tubule develops a branch from the main tubule. Tubules are not supposed to form branches; if this occurs, however, then the branch may become sealed off from the original tubule so that it has no entrance or exit. These sealed-off tubules are the cysts. They are capable of secretory activity because their cells contain pump proteins. The cysts enlarge as they accumulate fluid, putting pressure on the blood vessels, their capillaries, and the nephrons. The flow of blood and of urine is hindered. Patients with polycystic kidney disease often develop high blood pressure, kidney stones, and kidney infections. The disease can begin before birth, but symptoms may not occur until childhood or early adulthood. The intensity or severity of the disease varies greatly, from symptomless to life-threatening. Treatment of mild polycystic kidney disease may consist of relieving the pain, curing the infection, and controlling the blood pressure. Treatment of severe or life-threatening polycystic renal disease requires dialysis or kidney transplantation.

Stones in the urinary tract are very common. About 1 in 100 Americans has stones, and 1 in 1,000 adults experiences such severe symptoms that hospitalization is required. Kidney stones are caused by a prolonged high concentration of certain minerals in the urine, usually calcium, oxalate, or urate. The stones usually consist of crystals bound together by proteins.

The size and shape of kidney stones vary greatly. They may be microscopic or the size of a pea or even larger; they may be smooth or jagged. The stones may be passed from the urinary tract during urination, but some require removal by a urologist. Microscopic stones may not cause any symptoms, while larger stones can be very painful and may produce blood in the urine. Because stones hinder the flow of urine, their presence can allow bacteria to grow in the urinary tract, producing an infection.

Kidney stones that produce symptoms and are not passed by the patient must be removed. Some stones may be removed with a ureteroscope while the patient is under general anesthesia. A ureteroscope is a urological instrument like a hollow tube. It is inserted into the urinary tract through the external opening of the urethra and passed through the bladder and into the ureter. The tube can actually be inserted into the renal pelvis. The optical system of the ureteroscope allows the physi-

cian to see inside the urinary tract. Through the ureteroscope, kidney stones may be broken up by applying ultrasonic, laser, or electrohydraulic (acoustic shock-wave) energy.

An alternative means of removing large kidney stones is extracorporeal shock-wave lithotripsy, or ESWL. ESWL is desirable because it uses shock waves to break up the stones, thus eliminating the need to insert medical instruments into the patient. In one method of ESWL, the anesthetized patient is placed in a tub of water. X-ray imaging locates and monitors the stones as shock waves crush them. The patient's tissues are not damaged, and the sandy remains of the stones are then passed with urine. The development of ESWL has offered a useful means of treating kidney stones, but it has not eliminated the need for surgical or ureteroscopic removal of these stones from some patients. Each patient and each stone is different; they require the professional evaluation of a urologist.

Urinary tract infections are common, affecting 10 to 20 percent of women at some point in their lives; they are less common in men. Pathogens usually infect the kidneys by ascending the urinary tract via the urethra, bladder, and ureters. The normal bladder is an effective barrier to these infections, but any obstruction to the flow of urine, such as enlarged prostate, renal cysts, pregnancy, or a urinary stone, will weaken this barrier. Sometimes, pathogens infect the kidneys through the blood. Most urinary tract infections can be effectively treated with antibiotics. It is important for the physician to choose an antibiotic that is effective against the causative pathogen. Each antibiotic is effective against only a few types of bacteria, and many different bacteria can cause urinary tract infections.

Infections involving the kidney are especially serious. Because the kidneys are essential to life, these infections must be treated promptly and completely. Some infections affect the kidney even after the infection is cured. The body reacts to pathogens by producing proteins called antibodies, which circulate in the bloodstream. Antibodies in the blood can coat and damage the glomerular filters in Bowman's capsules. This reduces the effectiveness of the filters, allowing blood and protein to enter the urine and causing the body to become puffy. The medical term for this serious kidney disease is glomerulonephritis. Treatment is available, but it is better to prevent the disease from occurring. If left untreated, the kidney damage may be so extensive that dialysis or transplantation is required to prevent death.

PERSPECTIVE AND PROSPECTS

The ancient Greeks seem to be the earliest people whose writings about the kidney have survived. They had no regard for the importance of this organ, mainly because their frame of reference consisted of four "humors." Even before 500 B.C.E., the Greeks were developing the doctrine of the four elements of the inanimate universe: air, fire, water, and earth. From this idea, Polybus, the son-in-law of Hippocrates, created the corollary of the four "humors" responsible for life: yellow bile (choler), blood, phlegm (pituita), and black bile (melancholia). The concept of humors dominated the thinking of Aristotle (384-322 B.C.E.) when he wrote about his study of the anatomy of kidneys in several animals, including humans. This approach delayed an understanding of even the basic concept that kidneys and urine are related, an idea finally proposed about 290 B.C.E. by Erasistratus of Ceos.

Knowledge of Erasistratus comes mainly from Galen (129-c. 199 C.E.). Galen, rather than applauding the advances of his forebears, ridiculed unfounded assertions. He conducted physiological experiments on living animals, such as observing the effect of cutting and tying one ureter while leaving the opposite one intact. His experiments yielded much information about renal physiology. The writings of Galen formed the foundation of medical knowledge for the next four hundred years. Students and teachers, rather than building upon the experimental process, accepted the proclamations of Galen as dogma.

The next great advance in renal knowledge came from the Italian anatomist Bartolommeo Eustachio (1520-1574), who, without the benefit of a microscope, discovered the renal tubules and their relationship to the renal vascular system. His descriptions and drawings of 1564 were lost in the Vatican library until 1714. In the meantime, another Italian, Lorenzo Bellini (1643-1704), independently discovered the renal tubules and discerned their function. A contemporary, Marcello Malpighi (1628-1694), discovered glomeruli and their relationship to tubules.

Subsequent advances had to wait until the nineteenth century, when knowledge of all aspects of human biology and medicine began a rapid advance. Many independent advances in the nineteenth and twentieth centuries—in surgery, pharmacology, and immunology—made the transplantation of kidneys and other major organs possible. General anesthesia was developed independently by two Americans: by Crawford Long in 1842 and by William T. G. Morton in 1846.

Antiseptic procedures were originated in 1867 by the Englishman Joseph Lister, and vascular surgical techniques were developed in 1902 by the French surgeon Alexis Carrel and the Hungarian surgeon Emerich Ullman. Anticoagulants were developed in 1914 and 1915, and systemic antibiotics were developed in the 1930's and 1940's. Blood typing was begun in Europe by Karl Landsteiner (1868-1943). Tissue immunology was first explained in 1953, and tissue typing was introduced in France and the United States in the 1960's. Immunosuppressive drugs were developed during this same period. Kidney transplantation is also possible because of extracorporeal support devices such as the dialysis machine, the heart-lung machine, and the organ perfusion machine.

The first transplant of a human kidney between identical twins was performed on December 23, 1954, by Joseph E. Murray. He later performed the first human kidney transplant between unrelated persons on April 5, 1962. By the 1990's, tens of thousands of kidney transplants were being performed in the United States every year. There are many more persons waiting for a transplant than there are kidneys available for transplantation. The solution to this problem is unclear. Transplants between living persons in the same family may be encouraged, and transplants from animals to humans may be perfected. It is even possible that a transplantable artificial kidney can be developed, but this task will be enormously difficult, considering all the functions of a natural kidney.

—*Armand M. Karow, Ph.D.*

See also Adrenalectomy; Blood and blood disorders; Circulation; Corticosteroids; Cysts; Dialysis; Hemolytic uremic syndrome; Internal medicine; Kidney cancer; Kidney disorders; Kidney transplantation; Laparoscopy; Lithotripsy; Nephrectomy; Nephritis; Nephrology; Nephrology, pediatric; Polycystic kidney disease; Pyelonephritis; Renal failure; Stone removal; Stones; Systems and organs; Transplantation; Urinalysis; Urinary disorders; Urinary system; Urology; Urology, pediatric.

FOR FURTHER INFORMATION:

Andreoli, Thomas E., et al., eds. *Cecil Essentials of Medicine.* 6th ed. Philadelphia: W. B. Saunders, 2004. This paperback book, written for physicians, describes diseases and their treatment in humans. Contains a good section on the kidneys.

Brenner, Barry M., and Samuel A. Levine, eds. *Brenner and Rector's The Kidney.* 7th ed. Philadelphia:

W. B. Saunders, 2004. This treatise, at more than two thousand pages, is the most comprehensive and authoritative source on the normal and diseased human kidney.

Eaton, Douglas C., and John D. Pooler. *Vander's Renal Physiology*. 6th ed. New York: Lange Medical Books/McGraw Hill, 2004. This paperback book, written for medical students, describes the anatomy and physiology of the normal human kidney. Provides extensive, exhaustive information in a comprehensible format. The text may be somewhat challenging for those who have not taken introductory college-level courses in chemistry and biology.

Gottschalk, Carl W., Robert W. Berliner, and Gerhard H. Giebisch, eds. *Renal Physiology: People and Ideas*. Bethesda, Md.: American Physiological Society, 1987. This collection of scholarly essays traces the historical development of renal physiology. While the work is exhaustive and comprehensive, emphasis is placed on the nineteenth and twentieth centuries.

Marieb, Elaine N. *Essentials of Human Anatomy and Physiology*. 8th ed. San Francisco: Pearson/Benjamin Cummings, 2006. This introductory anatomy and physiology textbook, easily accessible to those with little science background, is richly illustrated with diagrams and photographs, which help to illuminate body systems and processes.

O'Callaghan, C. A., and Barry M. Brenner. *The Kidney at a Glance*. Malden, Mass.: Blackwell Science, 2000. Covers a range of topics related to the kidneys, presenting text on one page and accompanying illustrations on the facing page. Covers basic anatomy and physiology and the pathologies and presentations of renal and urinary tract disease.

Voet, Donald, and Judith G. Voet. *Biochemistry*. 3d ed. Hoboken, N.J.: John Wiley & Sons, 2004. A good book to use for the description and explanation of the chemical processes taking place in the kidney and other areas of the body.

KINESIOLOGY
SPECIALTY

ANATOMY OR SYSTEM AFFECTED: Brain, cells, circulatory system, heart, lungs, muscles, musculoskeletal system, nervous system, psychic-emotional system, respiratory system, spine

SPECIALTIES AND RELATED FIELDS: Cardiology, exercise physiology, orthopedics, physical therapy, psychology, sports medicine

DEFINITION: The applied science of human movement, which combines the general areas of anatomy (the study of structure) and physiology (the study of function).

SCIENCE AND PROFESSION

In 1989, the American Academy of Physical Education endorsed the term "kinesiology" to describe the entire field traditionally known as physical education, which includes the following subdisciplines: exercise physiology, biomechanics, motor control and learning, sports nutrition, sports psychology, sports sociology, athletic training programs, pedagogy, adapted physical education, cardiac rehabilitation, and physical therapy.

Exercise physiology describes the body's muscular, cardiovascular, and respiratory functioning during both short-term and long-term exercise. Research has focused on muscle fiber typing, oxygen uptake assessment, lactic acid metabolism, thermoregulation, body composition, and muscle hypertrophy. Biomechanics applies Isaac Newton's laws of physics to improve the mechanical efficiency of muscle movement patterns; using high-speed video and computer analysis, flaws in joint and limb dynamics can be assessed and changed to optimize performance. Motor control and learning pinpoint the areas of the brain and spinal cord that are responsible for the acquisition and retention of motor skills. Understanding the neurological basis of reflex and voluntary muscle movements helps to refine teaching strategies and describe the mechanisms of fatigue.

Sports nutrition describes how the body stores, circulates, and converts nutrients for aerobic and anaerobic energy production through carbohydrate loading and other strategies. Sports psychology explores the workings of the mind before, during, and after exercise and competition. Sports sociology examines aspects such as cultural, ethnic, and gender differences; dynamics in small and large groups; and the role of sports in ethical and moral development. Athletic trainers work with sports physicians and surgeons to prevent and rehabilitate injuries caused by overuse, trauma, or disease. Physical therapists use clinical exercise therapy and other modalities in a variety of rehabilitation settings.

Allied health areas under the kinesiology umbrella include pedagogy (teaching progressions for movement skills), adapted physical education (activities for the physically and mentally challenged), and cardiac rehabilitation (recovery stages for those disabled by heart disease). Professional organizations in the field of kinesiology include the American College of Sports Medicine, the American Physical Therapy Association, the National Athletic Trainers Association, the National Strength and Conditioning Association, and the American Alliance for Health, Physical Education, Recreation, and Dance.

—*Daniel G. Graetzer, Ph.D.*

See also Allied health; Anatomy; Cardiac rehabilitation; Exercise physiology; Muscles; Nervous system; Neurology; Physical rehabilitation; Physiology; Respiration; Sports medicine.

FOR FURTHER INFORMATION:

Brooks, George A., and Thomas D. Fahey. *Fundamentals of Human Performance*. Mountain View, Calif.: Mayfield, 2000.

McArdle, William, Frank I. Katch, and Victor L. Katch. *Exercise Physiology: Energy, Nutrition, and Human Performance*. 6th ed. Philadelphia: Lippincott Williams & Wilkins, 2007.

Oatis, Carol A. *Kinesiology: The Mechanics and Pathomechanics of Human Movement*. Philadelphia: Lippincott Williams & Wilkins, 2004.

Plowman, Sharon A., and Denise L. Smith. *Exercise Physiology for Health, Fitness, and Performance*. San Francisco: Benjamin/Cummings, 2002.

Powers, Scott K., and Edward T. Howley. *Exercise Physiology: Theory and Application to Fitness and Performance*. 6th ed. New York: McGraw-Hill, 2007.

Sharkey, Brian J. *Fitness and Health*. 4th ed. Champaign, Ill.: Human Kinetics, 1997.

KLINEFELTER SYNDROME

DISEASE/DISORDER

ANATOMY OR SYSTEM AFFECTED: Breasts, endocrine system, genitals, hair, psychic-emotional system, reproductive system

SPECIALTIES AND RELATED FIELDS: Embryology, endocrinology, genetics, psychology

DEFINITION: A male chromosomal disorder causing infertility and significant femaleness.

CAUSES AND SYMPTOMS

Klinefelter syndrome is caused by a variation in the number of sex chromosomes. Normal males possess one X and one Y chromosome, while females have two X chromosomes. When an embryo has two X chromosomes and one Y chromosome (XXY), normal development and reproductive function are hampered and

---

> **INFORMATION ON KLINEFELTER SYNDROME**
>
> **CAUSES:** Genetic chromosomal disorder
> **SYMPTOMS:** Infertility, breast development, small testes that produce few, if any, sperm
> **DURATION:** Lifelong
> **TREATMENTS:** None; hormonal therapy for symptoms

the boy shows the symptoms of Klinefelter syndrome. These symptoms include breast development, incomplete maleness, and school or social difficulties. The major symptom is sterility or very reduced fertility. The testes remain small after puberty and produce few, if any, sperm.

In adolescence, breast tissue develops significantly in about 50 percent of all cases. In addition, normal facial and pubic hair may not develop in these boys. Although their average height is six feet, young men with Klinefelter syndrome are often unathletic and less physically strong or coordinated than their peers. Some affected individuals exhibit some degree of subnormal intelligence. Others appear passive and without self-confidence or experience difficulties learning language and speech.

TREATMENT AND THERAPY

Klinefelter syndrome is diagnosed using a karyotype, an analysis of the chromosomes from blood or cheek cells. It can determine the presence of forty-seven chromosomes, including one Y and two X. Although Klinefelter syndrome is genetic and cannot be cured, treatment in the form of a monthly injection of testosterone can be administered to supplement the usually insufficient amount produced by the boy's own testes. This therapy should enhance male physical development by increasing the size of the penis and causing pubic and facial hair growth and greater muscle bulk.

Hormone therapy cannot increase the size of the testes, however, nor can it cure sterility. It cannot reverse breast tissue development, which can only be treated by surgical removal. It may, however, increase self-esteem and a sense of maleness, thereby easing social interactions.

PERSPECTIVE AND PROSPECTS

Found in one or two of every thousand males born, Klinefelter syndrome is the most common human chromosomal variation. Described by Harry Klinefelter in 1942, its cause was discovered by Patricia Jacobs and John Strong in 1959. Affected males have normal erections and may suffer no major effects other than those mentioned above.

—*Grace D. Matzen*

See also Genetic diseases; Genetics and inheritance; Gynecomastia; Hermaphroditism and pseudohermaphroditism; Puberty and adolescence; Reproductive system; Sexual differentiation.

FOR FURTHER INFORMATION:

Bandmann, H.-J., and R. Breit, eds. *Klinefelter's Syndrome.* New York: Springer-Verlag, 1984.

Klinefelter Syndrome and Associates (KS&A). http://www.genetic.org/.

Larsen, P. Reed, et al., eds. *Williams Textbook of Endocrinology.* 10th ed. Philadelphia: W. B. Saunders, 2003.

Martin, Richard J., Avroy A. Fanaroff, and Michele C. Walsh, eds. *Fanaroff and Martin's Neonatal-Perinatal Medicine: Diseases of the Fetus and Infant.* 2 vols. 8th ed. Philadelphia: Mosby Elsevier, 2006.

Milunsky, Aubrey, ed. *Genetic Disorders of the Fetus: Diagnosis, Prevention, and Treatment.* 5th ed. Baltimore: Johns Hopkins University Press, 2004.

Morales, Ralph, Jr. *Out of the Darkness: An Autobiography of Living with Klinefelter Syndrome.* Louisville, Ky.: Chicago Spectrum Press, 2002.

Parker, James N., and Philip M. Parker, eds. *The Official Parent's Sourcebook on Klinefelter Syndrome.* San Diego, Calif.: Icon Health, 2002.

Sørensen, Kurt. *Klinefelter's Syndrome in Childhood, Adolescence, and Youth: A Genetic, Clinical, Developmental, Psychiatric, and Psychological Study.* Park Ridge, N.J.: Parthenon, 1988.

KLIPPEL-TRENAUNAY SYNDROME
DISEASE/DISORDER

ALSO KNOWN AS: Angio-osteohypertrophy, nevus vasculosus osteohypertrophicus syndrome, hemangiectasia hypertrophicans, Klippel-Trenaunay-Weber syndrome

ANATOMY OR SYSTEM AFFECTED: Blood vessels, circulatory system, gastrointestinal system, joints, lymphatic system

SPECIALTIES AND RELATED FIELDS: Genetics, internal medicine, pediatrics, vascular medicine

---

> ### INFORMATION ON KLIPPEL-TRENAUNAY SYNDROME
>
> **CAUSES:** Unknown, possibly genetic
> **SYMPTOMS:** Varicose veins, port-wine stains, limb or soft tissue hypertrophy, noticeable large vein running from lower leg into upper thigh, localized tumors, excessive bleeding
> **DURATION:** Lifelong
> **TREATMENTS:** Alleviation of symptoms, such as compression garments and leg elevation for varicose veins, surgery for limb hypertrophy, anticoagulants

---

DEFINITION: A rare congenital syndrome characterized by hemangiomas of the vascular system that can affect bone or soft tissue throughout the body.

CAUSES AND SYMPTOMS

Klippel-Trenaunay syndrome was first described in 1900 in patients exhibiting a combination of varicose veins, multiple vascular nevi (birthmarks on the skin sometimes called port-wine stains), and excessive growth or development (hypertrophy) of limbs or soft tissue. Increased vascularity is common. At birth, a large vein may be observed running from the lower leg into the upper thigh, referred to as the Klippel-Trenaunay vein.

The molecular basis for the disease is unclear, as most cases appear as simply random occurrences. Among those few cases which appear to be heritable, it is believed that an autosomal dominant gene may be at fault, possibly linked to chromosome numbers 5 or 11. Evidence suggests that, at the molecular level, deregulation of deoxyribonucleic acid (DNA) methylation of imprinted genes may play a role.

Whichever gene may be at fault, it is believed the mutation occurs early in embryonic development. The result is that the defect appears randomly among cells as they migrate and differentiate early during embryonic stages, resulting in the seemingly haphazard distribution of the trait as the fetus develops.

Diagnosis is based upon the triad of vascular or soft tissue defects, with venous or capillary malformations leading to localized, and often extensive, tumors. Preliminary diagnosis can be based upon any two of the characteristics. Another symptom may be excessive bleeding, especially from the rectum or detected in the urine.

Treatment and Therapy

If the disorder becomes apparent during the prenatal period, then the prognosis is generally poor. Treatment in the adult is generally symptomatic, although the possibility of internal organ involvement, as well as pulmonary embolisms, leaves the patient at risk even in the absence of symptoms.

Since varicose veins are generally apparent, the patient may wear compression garments, elevating the legs at intervals. Surgery may be necessary to correct limb hypertrophy. Because the formation of embolisms is a risk, the patient may utilize anticoagulants prophylactically, particularly prior to surgery. Corticosteroid use may help limit swelling in some cases. In the absence of significant malformations, the patient should simply be monitored on an annual basis.

Perspective and Prospects

The rare and sporadic nature of the disorder complicates routine screening. At best, proper prenatal care during pregnancy may result in diagnosis if the disorder does appear. Research into the molecular basis of the disorder may eventually determine its origins.

—*Richard Adler, Ph.D.*

See also Birthmarks; Skin; Skin disorders; Varicose veins; Vascular medicine; Vascular system.

For Further Information:

Baskerville, P. A., et al. "The Etiology of the Klippel-Trenaunay Syndrome." *Annals of Surgery* 202 (November, 1985): 624-627.

Evans, Jeff. "Klippel-Trenaunay Stains Predict Complications." *Skin and Allergy News* 34, no. 2 (February 1, 2003): 40.

Mulliken, John B., and Anthony E. Young, eds. *Vascular Birthmarks: Hemangiomas and Malformations.* Philadelphia: Saunders, 1988.

Telander, R. L., et al. "Prognosis and Management of Lesions of the Trunk in Children with Klippel-Trenaunay Syndrome." *Journal of Pediatric Surgery* 19 (1984): 417-422.

Kneecap removal

Procedure

Also known as: Patellectomy

Anatomy or system affected: Bones, joints, knees, legs, muscloskeletal system, tendons

Specialties and related fields: General surgery, orthopedics

Definition: The surgical removal of the kneecap.

Indications and Procedures

The kneecap, or patella, is the triangular bone at the front of the knee. It is held in position by the lower end of the quadriceps muscle, which surrounds the patella and is attached to the upper part of the tibia by the patellar tendon. The role of the kneecap is to protect the knee.

Kneecap removal surgery, or patellectomy, is performed as a result of fracture, frequent dislocation, or painful arthritis in the kneecap. Fracture is usually caused by a direct or sharp blow to the knee. Dislocation of the patella is often linked to a congenital abnormality, such as the underdevelopment of the lower end of the femur or excessive laxity of the ligaments that support the knee. Painful degenerative arthritic conditions, such as retropatellar arthritis and chondromalacia patellae, inflame and roughen the undersurface of the kneecap. Arthritic pain often worsens with the climbing of stairs or bending of the knee.

Before surgery begins, a clinical examination is conducted including blood and urine studies, and X rays of both knees. The knee is thoroughly cleansed with antiseptic soap. Anesthesia is administered either by local injection or spinal injection or by inhalation and injection (general anesthesia).

Surgery begins with an incision made around the kneecap. The skin is pulled back, exposing the muscle-covered kneecap. Surrounding muscle and connecting tendons attached to the kneecap are cut, and the kneecap is carefully removed. The remaining muscle is then sewn back together with strong suture material. Surgery is completed with the closing of the skin with sutures or clips. Full recovery takes about six weeks.

Uses and Complications

Following surgery, a scar will form along the incision. As the incision heals, the scar will recede gradually. Pain from the incision can be alleviated with heating pads. The affected leg should be elevated with pillows. Frequent movement of legs while resting in bed will decrease the likelihood of deep vein blood clots. General activity and returning to work is encouraged as soon as possible. Standing for prolonged periods of time, however, is not recommended during recovery. Following the approximate six-week recovery time, physical therapy is often used to restore strength to the knee.

Possible complications associated with kneecap removal include excessive bleeding and surgical wound infection. Additional complications can occur during recovery if general postoperative guidelines are not followed. Some loss of function can be expected.

—*Jason Georges*

See also Arthritis; Bones and the skeleton; Fracture and dislocation; Lower extremities; Orthopedic surgery; Orthopedics; Orthopedics, pediatric; Physical rehabilitation.

FOR FURTHER INFORMATION:

Doherty, Gerard M., and Lawrence W. Way, eds. *Current Surgical Diagnosis and Treatment*. 12th ed. New York: Lange Medical Books/McGraw-Hill, 2006.

Halpern, Brian. *The Knee Crisis Handbook: Understanding Pain, Preventing Trauma, Recovering from Knee Injury, and Building Healthy Knees for Life*. Emmaus, Pa.: Rodale Books, 2003.

Mulholland, Michael W., et al., eds. *Greenfield's Surgery: Scientific Principles and Practice*. 4th ed. Philadelphia: Lippincott Williams & Wilkins, 2006.

Tapley, Donald F., et al., eds. *The Columbia University College of Physicians and Surgeons Complete Home Medical Guide*. Rev. 3d ed. New York: Crown, 1995.

Tierney, Lawrence M., Stephen J. McPhee, and Maxine A. Papadakis, eds. *Current Medical Diagnosis and Treatment 2007*. New York: McGraw-Hill Medical, 2006.

KNOCK-KNEES

DISEASE/DISORDER

ALSO KNOWN AS: Genu valgum

ANATOMY OR SYSTEM AFFECTED: Bones, feet, hips, joints, knees, legs, ligaments, muscles

SPECIALTIES AND RELATED FIELDS: Orthopedics, pediatrics, physical therapy

DEFINITION: A deformity in which the knees are positioned close together or turn toward each other and the tibias and ankles are apart when the feet are placed in a normal standing position.

CAUSES AND SYMPTOMS

Knock-knees, affecting both knees or occasionally only one, are a normal condition as children mature. Infants' leg bones are slightly rotated because of uterine positioning. As toddlers' legs straighten after having bowlegs, their tibias and knees often temporarily rotate toward the body's axis, causing the feet to be several inches apart. When knock-knees are not representative of normal physical development, they occur because of health conditions such as infections, obesity, or fractured legs that disrupt knee growth. Knock-knees are sometimes a symptom of other conditions.

Mobility may be affected with knock-knees. Patients sometimes adjust leg and foot movement to compensate for altered knee positioning and imbalanced centers of gravity. Usually, children walk with their toes turned in for balance when they have knock-knees. Knock-kneed adults sometimes develop arthritis because of the strain on knee joints and ligaments. Knock-knees can also place stress on patients' backs and hips.

TREATMENT AND THERAPY

Medical professionals do not treat most knock-knees unless specific cases seem abnormal, cause pain, or impede movement. Growth usually corrects knee positioning. Physicians measure legs and the distance between ankles to assess the progress of natural correction. X rays are useful to detect bone problems that may exacerbate knock-knees. Photographs can document leg alignment.

Stretching the leg muscles can aid the natural resolution of knock-knees. Shoes designed with inserts can mitigate the stress on feet and manipulate patients to walk straight. Physical therapy can alleviate cartilage and joint pain associated with knock-knees.

If young patients do not outgrow knock-knees, ankle distances increase to 4 inches or more, or the condition worsens, particularly in one knee, then medical intervention often becomes necessary to ensure that patients are capable of normal movement. Physicians sometimes advise patients to wear a brace. If such efforts are unsuccessful, then the patient may undergo surgery to adjust leg bones and growth plates.

Treatment is essential for diseases or conditions in which knock-knees is a symptom. Some patients seek medical correction for aesthetic reasons.

INFORMATION ON KNOCK-KNEES

CAUSES: Normal condition in infants; infections, obesity, or fractures in older individuals

SYMPTOMS: Altered knee positioning, imbalanced center of gravity, sometimes arthritis

DURATION: Usually temporary

TREATMENTS: None, unless pain develops or movement is impeded; may include stretching, shoe inserts, physical therapy, orthopedic braces, surgery

PERSPECTIVE AND PROSPECTS

Beginning in the late nineteenth century, physicians routinely recommended therapeutic braces to treat knock-knees. During the 1950's, Soviet doctor Gavril Abramovich Ilizarov devised a fixator that encircles legs and uses tension to correct rotation problems associated with knock-knees. Italian doctor Antonio Bianchi-Maiocchi first used this device in Western countries in 1981. Dr. James Aronson brought the method to the United States in the 1980's. In that decade, Ukrainian doctor Veklich Vitaliy adapted Ilizarov's fixator for a procedure that is often used to correct severe knock-knees.

By the late twentieth century, however, physicians discouraged the use of braces to treat normal cases of knock-knees. Most advised patients to permit natural correction to occur, emphasizing that devices would not quicken that process.

—*Elizabeth D. Schafer, Ph.D.*

See also Bones and the skeleton; Growth; Lower extremities; Orthopedics; Orthopedics, pediatric.

FOR FURTHER INFORMATION:

Bianci-Maiocchi, Antonio, and James Aronson, eds. *Operative Principles of Ilizarov: Fracture Treatment, Nonunion, Osteomyelitis, Lengthening, Deformity Correction.* Baltimore: Williams & Wilkins, 1991.

England, Stephen P., ed. *Common Orthopedic Problems.* Philadelphia: W. B. Saunders, 1996.

Halpern, Brian. *The Knee Crisis Handbook: Understanding Pain, Preventing Trauma, Recovering from Knee Injury, and Building Healthy Knees for Life.* Emmaus, Pa.: Rodale Books, 2003.

Herring, John A., ed. *Tachdjian's Pediatric Orthopaedics.* 3d ed. 3 vols. Philadelphia: W. B. Saunders, 2002.

KWASHIORKOR

DISEASE/DISORDER

ALSO KNOWN AS: Malignant malnutrition, protein malnutrition, protein-calorie malnutrition, Mehl hrschaden

ANATOMY OR SYSTEM AFFECTED: Gastrointestinal system, muscles, skin

SPECIALTIES AND RELATED FIELDS: Family medicine, nutrition, pediatrics

DEFINITION: A form of malnutrition caused by inadequate protein intake.

INFORMATION ON KWASHIORKOR

CAUSES: Protein deprivation

SYMPTOMS: Fatigue, irritability, lethargy, poor growth, apathy, edema, decreased muscle mass, large belly, diarrhea, dermatitis, loss of skin pigmentation, changes in color and texture of hair, infections; may progress to shock, coma, and death

DURATION: Progressive if untreated

TREATMENTS: Depends on degree of malnutrition; may include treatment for shock and increased calorie intake (first as carbohydrates, simple sugars, and fats, then proteins)

CAUSES AND SYMPTOMS

Kwashiorkor occurs most commonly in areas of famine, limited food supply, and low levels of education, which can lead to inadequate knowledge of diet and appropriate dietary intakes. Early symptoms are general and include fatigue, irritability, and lethargy. As protein deprivation continues, symptoms include failure to gain weight and linear growth. Other progressed symptoms include apathy, decreased muscle mass, edema, a large protuberant belly (resulting from decreased albumin in the blood), diarrhea, and dermatitis. Skin may lose pigment where it has peeled away or darken where it has been irritated or traumatized. Hair may become thin and brittle and may change color, becoming lighter or reddish. As a result of immune system damage, patients may suffer from increased numbers of infections and increased severity of what normally might be mild infections. In the final stages, shock and/or coma usually precede death.

TREATMENT AND THERAPY

A physical examination may show an enlarged liver and generalized edema. Treatment varies depending on the degree of malnutrition. Patients in shock will require immediate treatment. Often, calories are given first in the form of carbohydrates, simple sugars, and fats. Proteins are started after other caloric sources have provided increased energy. Vitamin and mineral supplements are essential. Many children will have developed intolerance to milk lactose (sugar intolerance) and will need to be supplemented with lactase (an enzyme) if they are to benefit from milk products. Adequate diet with appropriate amounts of carbohydrates, fat, and protein will prevent kwashiorkor.

PERSPECTIVE AND PROSPECTS

Kwashiorkor means "deposed child" in one African dialect, referring to a child "deposed" from the mother's breast by a newborn sibling. Kwashiorkor is found largely in tropical and subtropical regions where the diet is high in starch (such as cereal grains or plantains) and low in protein. The incidence of kwashiorkor in children in the United States is extremely low, and only rare, isolated cases are seen. Treatment early in the course of kwashiorkor generally produces positive results. Treatment in later stages will improve a child's general health, but the child may be left with permanent physical ailments and intellectual disabilities. With delayed or no treatment, the condition is fatal.

—*Jason A. Hubbart, M.S.*

See also Edema; Food biochemistry; Malnutrition; Nutrition.

FOR FURTHER INFORMATION:

Champakam, S., S. G. Srikantia, and C. Gopalan. "Kwashiorkor and Mental Development." *American Journal of Clinical Nutrition* 21 (1968): 844.

Golden, M. H. N. "Severe Malnutrition." In *Oxford Textbook of Medicine*, edited by D. J. Weatherall, J. G. G. Ledingham, and D. A. Warrell. 3d ed. New York: Oxford University Press, 1996.

Kleinman, Ronald E., ed. *Pediatric Nutrition Handbook*. 5th ed. Elk Grove Village, Ill.: American Academy of Pediatrics, 2004.

KYPHOSIS

DISEASE/DISORDER

ALSO KNOWN AS: Dowager's hump

ANATOMY OR SYSTEM AFFECTED: Back, bones

SPECIALTIES AND RELATED FIELDS: Orthopedics

DEFINITION: A marked increase of the normal curvature of the thoracic vertebrae or upper back, sometimes referred to as dowager's hump because of its prevalence in elderly women.

CAUSES AND SYMPTOMS

Patients with kyphosis appear to be looking down with their shoulders markedly bent forward. They are unable to straighten their backs, their body height is reduced, and their arms therefore appear to be disproportionately long. The increased curvature of the thoracic vertebrae tilts the head forward, and the patient has to raise her head and hyperextend her neck in order to look forward. This posture increases the strain on the neck muscles and leads to discomfort in the neck, shoulders,

An elderly woman with kyphosis. (Custom Medical Stock Photo)

and upper back. It limits the field of vision and increases the patient's chances of tripping over an object not directly in the line of vision. It also shifts forward the body's center of gravity and increases the chances of falling.

In severe cases, kyphosis limits chest expansion during breathing. As a result, less air gets into the lungs, which become underventilated and prone to infections. Pneumonia is a common cause of death in these patients. In very severe cases, the curvature of the thoracic vertebrae is so pronounced that the lower ribs lie over the pelvic cavity. Patients with severe kyphosis are not able to lie flat on their backs, and many spend most of their time sitting up in a chair or in bed, propped by a number of pillows. Unless the patient changes positions frequently, the pressure exerted by the vertebrae on the skin and subcutaneous tissue may precipitate pressure sores (bed sores) on the upper back. Pressure sores may also develop on the buttocks. The sores often become infected, and the infection may spread to the blood, leading to septicemia and death.

INFORMATION ON KYPHOSIS

CAUSES: Osteoporosis, tumors, infection
SYMPTOMS: Inability to straighten one's back, reduced body height, appearance of disproportionately long arms, strain on neck muscles leading to discomfort, pain
DURATION: Chronic
TREATMENTS: Hormone therapy, drug therapy (*e.g.*, Fosamax, teriparatide)

The most common cause of kyphosis is osteoporosis, a disease in which the bone mass is reduced. As a result, the bones become mechanically weak and are unable to sustain the pressure of the body weight. The vertebrae gradually become wedged and partially collapsed, more so in the front (anteriorly) than in the back (posteriorly), thus increasing the forward curvature of the thoracic vertebrae. Sometimes, the compression of a vertebra is associated with sudden, very severe, and incapacitating pain that is usually relieved spontaneously after about four weeks. In most cases, however, the compression is a gradual process associated with slowly worsening back discomfort. The discomfort is caused by the strain imposed on the muscles on either side of the vertebrae. In rare instances, the nerves exiting the spinal cord become trapped by the wedged or collapsed vertebrae, and the patient experiences severe pain that tends to radiate to the area supplied by the entrapped nerve.

Less common causes of kyphosis include the compression of a vertebra as a result of tumors or infections. In these cases, the angulation of the thoracic curvature is very prominent.

TREATMENT AND THERAPY

The availability of medications to treat and prevent osteoporosis should reduce significantly the prevalence of both that disease and kyphosis.

—Ronald C. Hamdy, M.D.

See also Back pain; Bone disorders; Bones and the skeleton; Braces, orthopedic; Orthopedic surgery; Orthopedics; Orthopedics, pediatric; Osteoporosis; Pneumonia; Safety issues for the elderly; Spinal cord disorders; Spine, vertebrae, and disks.

FOR FURTHER INFORMATION:

Byyny, Richard L., and Leonard Speroff. *A Clinical Guide for the Care of Older Women.* 2d ed. Baltimore: Williams & Wilkins, 1996.

Currey, John D. *Bones: Structures and Mechanics.* Princeton, N.J.: Princeton University Press, 2002.

Heaney, Robert P. "Osteoporosis." In *Nutrition in Women's Health*, edited by Debra A. Krummel and Penny M. Kris-Etherton. Gaithersburg, Md.: Aspen, 1996.

Hodgson, Stephen F., ed. *Mayo Clinic on Osteoporosis: Keeping Bones Healthy and Strong and Reducing the Risk of Fractures.* Rochester, Minn.: Mayo Clinic, 2003.

Meredith, C. M. "Exercise in the Prevention of Osteoporosis." In *Nutrition of the Elderly*, edited by Hamish Munro and Gunter Schlierf. Nestle's Nutrition Workshop Series 29. New York: Raven Press, 1992.

Nelson, Miriam E., and Sarah Wernick. *Strong Women, Strong Bones: Everything You Need to Know to Prevent, Treat, and Beat Osteoporosis.* New York: G. P. Putnam, 2001.

Van De Graaff, Kent M. *Human Anatomy.* 6th ed. New York: McGraw Hill, 2002.

LABORATORY TESTS

PROCEDURES

ANATOMY OR SYSTEM AFFECTED: Blood, cells

SPECIALTIES AND RELATED FIELDS: Bacteriology, cytology, endocrinology, epidemiology, forensic medicine, genetics, hematology, histology, immunology, microbiology, oncology, pathology, pharmacology, serology, toxicology, virology

DEFINITION: The collection and analysis of body fluids such as blood and urine in order to establish a diagnosis or to monitor a treatment regimen.

KEY TERMS:

antibody: a protein produced in the body by the immune system that recognizes and binds selectively to foreign material (antigens) to facilitate their elimination; antibodies can be cultivated in animals or by artificial means in the laboratory and chemically altered for use as reagents in immunoassays

clinical chemistry: a chemistry specialty which deals with an analysis of the chemical components of body fluids

clinical laboratory: a general term for those areas of a medical facility where analyses of body fluids are performed

clinical microbiology: the scientific discipline involving the study of microscopic organisms (such as bacteria, fungi, and viruses) that cause disease

coagulation: the process of blood clotting, a very complicated process that can be affected by many disease states; the clotting process is inhibited for specimen collection purposes using substances called anticoagulants

hematology: the medical specialty dealing with the detection and diagnosis of blood-related diseases

immunoassay: the use of antibody-antigen recognition as the basis of a medically useful method of detecting and measuring a substance in body fluids

pathology: the medical specialty that deals with the structural and biochemical changes that are produced by disease

INDICATIONS AND PROCEDURES

Clinical laboratory testing is a vital element in diagnosis. After physical examination and the taking of the patient's medical history, the physician will often request that specific tests be performed on blood, urine, or other body fluids. Appropriate specimens are collected and forwarded to the laboratory for specimen processing.

Blood is the most common specimen submitted for testing in the clinical laboratory. In a hospital or large referral laboratory, there may be special personnel, called phlebotomists, employed to collect blood. In a small office laboratory, blood may be collected by the attending physician or nurse. Blood is collected in a syringe or in special tubes which may contain anticoagulants.

Urine is the next most common laboratory specimen and is collected as a result of a single void (random urine specimen) or for a time period of twenty-four hours or more. In the latter case, the collection container may also contain substances that act as a preservative. If a long-term urine specimen is necessary, it is very important for the patient to follow the directions regarding collection. Failure to follow these directions can lead to erroneous laboratory results.

Less commonly collected specimens include cerebrospinal fluid, gastric (stomach) fluid, and amniotic fluid. Cerebrospinal fluid is usually collected by a physician by direct sampling with a needle (lumbar puncture, or spinal tap). Gastric fluid is obtained by the insertion of a gastric collection tube. Amniotic fluid is collected by an obstetrician in the process called amniocentesis, in which a sample of the fluid surrounding the fetus is removed by the insertion of a needle through the mother's abdomen. Frequently, laboratory tests are also ordered on infectious material associated with a wound or surgical incision.

A major aspect of specimen collection is ensuring that the sample is correctly labeled and that no mix-up of specimens has occurred. Part of this process may involve checking identification armbands or asking patients or nursing staff to confirm identification. While this procedure may be exasperating to the patient or nursing personnel, it is a necessary part of detecting errors.

Immediately after the specimen is received in the laboratory, documentation of time of receipt and the tests requested is made, which is referred to as logging in the specimen. Each sample receives a special code called an accession number. The test performance and results are tracked with this number, since multiple specimens can be received on a single patient in a given day. This process is usually computerized and may utilize bar code labeling in a process very similar to that used for automatic cash-register pricing of grocery items.

In large hospital or referral laboratories, the processing center is responsible for distributing the sample to the laboratory sections, where various tests are performed. Since each test requires a specific amount of sample, specimen processing also involves determining that the correct amount of fluid has been collected and reserved for proper performance of the test.

For blood specimens, many laboratory determinations are made regarding plasma, or serum, which is the liquid component of blood that contains no cells. The whole blood specimen is separated into cellular and liquid components by centrifugation. The sample is spun rapidly so that the force of the spin sediments the cells, with the serum or plasma layer on top.

Once the specimen is distributed to the pertinent laboratory sections, testing is done using a variety of analytical techniques. The testing methodology is almost as varied as the types of analyses requested. A few general statements, however, are applicable. Automation is the guiding force behind laboratory test methodology development. Routinely ordered tests are done with instruments specifically designed to perform a group or panel of tests, rather than each test being performed individually by a technologist using manual chemistry methods. Automation coupled with computerization has greatly increased laboratory efficiency, decreased turnaround time (the time required for a test to be performed and results to be reported to the physician), eliminated human errors, and allowed more tests to be performed on smaller test sample material. The latter advantage is particularly important for pediatric specimens, in which sample size is usually an important consideration. Automation also eliminates much of the technologist's contact with the specimen, considerably reducing the risk of spreading infectious diseases.

Each section of the laboratory is responsible for a specific set of tests. The chemistry section performs chemical analyses of body fluids. Panels of tests related to kidney, heart, and liver function are also done. In addition, tests to measure amounts of therapeutic drugs,

IN THE NEWS: IN-HOME MEDICAL TESTING

In-home health testing has become increasingly popular as a result of its convenience, privacy, and affordability. Home tests can enable the consumer to determine the potential risk for developing a health problem even when no immediate signs or symptoms exist, or they can enable the consumer to follow a specific medical condition more accurately. Several home tests are available for over-the-counter purchase, including those that test for cholesterol levels, drugs of abuse, fecal occult blood, glucose levels, hepatitis C, human immunodeficiency virus (HIV), ovulation timing, pregnancy, prothrombin time screening, and vaginal pH. Home test kits should not be used as stand-alone measures to determine one's health care, but rather the results should be used in conjunction with proper medical advice in order to confirm the test results.

Most reports state that the test kits approved by the Food and Drug Administration (FDA) are either "about as accurate" or "fairly accurate," when compared to those that a doctor would use, provided that the instructions are carefully followed. The consumer should understand that no test is 100 percent accurate; test accuracy is improved when the consumer can read, understand, and follow the directions for test administration carefully. A home test kit will require accurate timing, specific collection materials, and typically a body fluid sample. Failure to comply with any of these factors could result in an inaccurate reading. If a product is not approved by the FDA, then the test's safety and efficacy is in question. Internet shopping for diagnostic test kits can be particularly misleading, since not all test kits available for purchase in this fashion are FDA-approved and some are illegal to sell over the Internet.

A search of the Clinical Laboratory Improvement Amendments (CLIA) database will inform the consumer if a home test has FDA approval. In order to use this search engine, the consumer must know if the test is considered a "test kit" (a consumer takes a sample, performs the test, and analyzes it, all on one's own) or a "collection kit" (a consumer takes a sample but sends it out to a laboratory for analysis). Collection kits are not currently listed on the CLIA database, although one can contact the FDA directly to find out if a kit is FDA-approved. The FDA maintains another database called Manufacturer and User Facility Device Experience (MAUDE), which lists reports on problems with kits and testing devices. The *Consumer Reports* magazine and Web site can also provide the consumer with additional product comparison information for a handful of home tests.

—*Bonita L. Marks, Ph.D.*

hormones, blood proteins, and cancer-related proteins are accomplished with immunoassay techniques. The development of antibody-related techniques has revolutionized testing in all areas of the clinical laboratory. The ability to customize antibody production and adapt it to specific analytical requirements has allowed the continual development of new tests and methodologies.

The hematology section is responsible for monitoring the level of blood cells and clotting factors. Other specialized tests to diagnose cancer of the blood cells may also be done. Blood typing and donor testing are technically hematology-related tests, but they are usually reserved for a separate section designated as blood bank or transfusion services. Transfusion service is a specialty in its own right and is almost always reserved for hospital-associated laboratories.

Microbiology is the section where body fluids are checked for infectious microorganisms. Once an organism is identified, the section can also determine which antibiotics may be useful for treatment by performing antibiotic susceptibility tests.

As the laboratory tests are performed, the results are recorded and reported to the physician. Computerization has permitted the transfer of patient results directly from the instrument performing the test to the patient's file, eliminating many tedious and error-prone clerical functions.

For hospital and reference laboratories, a laboratory director—either a physician (usually a pathologist) who specialized in laboratory medicine or a scientist with doctoral level training in a laboratory specialty—monitors the performance of the laboratory, helps physicians with the interpretation of ambiguous or complex laboratory results, and provides guidance on the introduction of new tests or instrumentation. Most laboratories also have a section supervisor or administrator who is an experienced medical technologist to oversee the daily laboratory routine.

In the United States, hospital and reference laboratories are inspected periodically by federal and state government agencies as well as professional medical societies to check the quality of the work performed. The most commonly used proficiency testing program is that administered by the College of American Pathology (CAP), which also sponsors a program of peer inspection of laboratories. Many state and federal agencies will accept CAP approval of a laboratory as a substitute for a detailed inspection by its own agency.

USES AND COMPLICATIONS

Because of the variety of laboratory testing, it is impractical to cover its applications in depth in a brief review. Instead, a few illustrative tests which are performed often or which are associated with familiar disorders will be presented. The most frequently ordered laboratory tests are serum glucose tests, serum electrolyte (salt) level measurements, and complete blood count (CBC) tests.

The maintenance of blood glucose (sugar) levels is essential for body activity and brain function. The laboratory measurement of blood glucose is one of the oldest known procedures performed in the clinical laboratory. It is part of the diagnostic procedures used to monitor and test for diabetes mellitus. Glucose and electrolyte testing are performed in the chemistry section of the laboratory, while a CBC takes place in hematology. Certain levels of electrolytes—sodium, chloride, potassium, and calcium—are needed for proper cardiac function. An abnormal level of these salts could also indicate possible hormonal or kidney malfunction. The CBC is a measure of the cell populations that carry oxygen (red blood cells), fight infection or invasion by foreign substances (white blood cells), and activate the blood-clotting mechanism (platelets). The white cell population is elevated in infections but also in cases of leukemia (malignant growth of a white cell population). More specialized testing is needed when leukemia is suspected. An instrument called a flow cytometer can be used to count and detect subtypes of white cells. These data, along with a pathologist's microscopic examination of a blood smear and the results of clinical examination, are used to arrive at a diagnosis of the specific type of leukemia present. The identification of the cell population causing the cancer is important for determining treatment and prognosis.

A deficiency of red cells or their oxygen-carrying hemoglobin molecule is called anemia. It can be caused by iron deficiency and other impairments of red cell production, chronic bleeding, or accelerated red cell destruction (hemolysis). Each of the causes must be either confirmed or ruled out through additional testing or by clinical examination.

Platelet deficiency is a major cause of clotting disorders, although many other causes of bleeding disorders exist. The specific defect can be determined by measuring the clotting time and by using special immunoassays to measure clotting substances in the blood.

Many hormonal (endocrine) disorders can be diagnosed through laboratory testing. For example, the thy-

Laboratory tests are vital in the diagnosis of disease. A scientist examines samples with a microscope. (PhotoDisc)

roid, the regulator gland for body metabolism, can produce a variety of symptoms when it is not functioning properly. Thyroid testing is the most common endocrine-related laboratory procedure requested by physicians. The blood levels of thyroid hormone and of the pituitary factor that stimulates the thyroid gland are measured in the laboratory using immunoassay methods. These types of assays can also be used to monitor other hormones involved in fertility, growth, and the function of the adrenal gland (the gland that helps maintain sugar metabolism and electrolyte balance).

Immunoassay methodology has also permitted the routine laboratory testing of therapeutic drugs as well as of drugs of abuse. In the past, the technology for analyzing drugs in biological fluids involved expensive, labor-intensive techniques that were impractical for routine laboratory use. With the introduction of immunologically based testing for drugs, however, it became possible to monitor patients on antibiotics, immunosuppressive agents, cardiac drugs, and antiseizure medication. Testing has been automated so that these drug levels can be performed as routine laboratory procedures. Assay results can be used to establish an individual dosage schedule so that dosage is main-

tained in the therapeutic range and does not exceed the concentration threshold, leading to toxic effects, or decline to values too low to achieve adequate treatment (subtherapeutic levels).

A continuing research effort is directed toward developing specific diagnostic cancer tests. These tests could be used to screen patients for tumors in order to detect them early, when therapy would be most effective. Substances that appear in body fluids coincident with the growth of tumors are referred to as tumor markers. The ideal tumor marker would appear only in patients afflicted with a specific type of cancer. Its concentration would reflect the size of the tumor as well as the presence of metastasis, in which tumor cells migrate from the initial cancer site to other sites in the body.

The ideal tumor marker has not yet been discovered. Most have not been specific or sensitive enough to use as a screening tool for detecting tumors, although they have been useful for monitoring the effects of therapy. One example of a useful marker is prostate-specific antigen (PSA). The level of this protein in serum is very low when the prostate gland is normal. When prostate cancer is present, however, the serum level, as measured by immunoassay, is elevated. The test can also be used for screening, provided that any positive result is confirmed by clinical examination. It is also used following prostate surgery or radiation therapy in order to determine the completeness of tumor removal. Continually high or rising levels of PSA in the serum following treatment indicate that residual tumor is still present.

In the microbiology department, the culturing of body fluids and antibiotic susceptibility studies allow the selection of the most appropriate antibiotic for treatment. The course and duration of treatment can then be followed in the chemistry laboratory using the therapeutic drug monitoring techniques discussed above. When an infection is suspected, body fluids are cultured or incubated with media selected to grow only specific microorganisms. Antibiotic susceptibility studies are performed by culturing the organism with various antibiotics until growth is arrested. Many strains of bacteria and other microorganisms will become resistant to an antibiotic which had proven effective previously, and patients who are allergic to some antibiotics may need to be treated with an alternative regimen.

The detection and identification of viruses has become a subspecialty in microbiology with distinctly different culturing techniques. Newer immunoassay methods and other biotechnologically based methods have made virus diagnosis easier. Acquired immunodeficiency syndrome (AIDS) testing is a prime example of the application of immunoassay techniques to virology testing. A detection technique which required growth of the human immunodeficiency virus (HIV) in the laboratory would be extraordinarily difficult and tedious. It would also be prohibitively expensive and time-consuming to screen large populations such as blood donors and high-risk groups. Instead, laboratory screening for HIV utilizes an automated immunoassay technique based on the detection of patient antibodies to virus-specific antigens. Although this test is very specific, the possibility of false positives is greatly minimized by confirming all positive screening results with another antibody test called a Western blot. In this test, a serum sample from a suspected HIV-positive patient is applied to a membrane impregnated with virus proteins. The virus proteins are localized at a characteristic position determined by their migration rate when the membrane coated with virus proteins is subjected to an electric field in a process called protein electrophoresis. After the membrane has been treated with patient serum and color development reagents, the presence in the patient sample of an antibody to one or more of these proteins is revealed as a colored stripe on the membrane. A combination of the two tests is a cost-efficient and extremely accurate procedure to confirm a suspected diagnosis of HIV infection.

PERSPECTIVE AND PROSPECTS

According to a study of the history of the clinical laboratory by J. Büttner, the concept of the modern hospital laboratory was first documented in 1791 when French physician and chemist Antoine-François de Fourcroy wrote that in hospitals "a chemical laboratory should be set up not far away from a ward having twenty or thirty beds." Büttner asserts that the two suppositions necessary for the creation of these laboratories were the idea that the results of laboratory examinations can be used as "chemical signs" in medical diagnosis and a new concept of disease which was the result of the "birth of the clinic" at the end of the eighteenth century.

During this phase of laboratory development, investigations were performed at patients' bedsides by physicians themselves. In the period from 1840 to 1855, clinical laboratories were established as operations distinct from hospitals and clinics. Most of these laboratories were developed in German-speaking countries and staffed by scientists who performed tests for the hospitals and taught medical students physiological chemistry. From 1855 onward, the concept of the clinical laboratory spread rapidly, with clinicians assuming directorship roles. The laboratory ultimately serving as a model for clinical laboratories in the United States was established by the renowned pathologist Rudolf Virchow at Berlin University. As the chair for pathological anatomy, he set up a "chemical department" within the institute for pathology in 1856. This laboratory represented a center of clinical chemistry research and established the clinical laboratory as integral to pathology.

Laboratories have evolved as essential but distinctly separate specialties of medical services. Although there is little or no participation in the analytical process by the physicians ordering the tests, a major part of a physician's diagnostic skill is knowing which tests to order as a supplement to examination and medical history. Laboratory tests cost money and time and may be useless in the diagnostic process if not ordered in a judicious fashion. The old medical admonishment to "treat the patient, not the laboratory result" is still an appropriate consideration. Moreover, responsibility for the correct interpretation of the results lies with the attending physician, who has access to all the pertinent patient data.

Laboratory results are usually interpreted with the help of a reference range. Reference ranges ideally represent laboratory values characteristic of a sample population which is free of known disease. If the results lie within this range, however, the laboratory result cannot always be assumed to rule out a specific diagnosis. Since considerable biological variation exists for most laboratory values, diseased individuals can sometimes yield test values in the normal range and, conversely, healthy individuals can occasionally have low or elevated values.

In order to verify a diagnosis, all laboratory results and clinical impressions should complement one another. The detection of blood-clotting deficiencies by the hematology department could be related to a poorly functioning liver, which will also be reflected in changes in enzymes and blood proteins measured in the chemistry laboratory. Cardiac disorders are diagnosed not only by examining an electrocardiograph (EKG or ECG) but also by measuring the levels of specific cardiac-related enzymes which rise to abnormally high levels when cardiac blood supply is diminished (such as with myocardial infarction, or heart attack). In summary, the clinical laboratory provides a valuable tool for physicians, but it should never displace clinical examination and medical history as methods of determining the final diagnosis.

—*David J. Wells, Jr., Ph.D.*

See also Amniocentesis; Bacteriology; Biopsy; Blood and blood disorders; Blood testing; Breast biopsy; Cells; Cytology; Cytopathology; DNA and RNA; Endometrial biopsy; Forensic pathology; Genetic engineering; Genetics and inheritance; Gram staining; Hematology; Hematology, pediatric; Histology; Hormones; Karyotyping; Microbiology; Microscopy; Pathology; Screening; Serology; Toxicology; Urinalysis.

FOR FURTHER INFORMATION:

Bennington, James L., ed. *Saunders Dictionary and Encyclopedia of Laboratory Medicine and Technology.* Philadelphia: W. B. Saunders, 1984. An excellent reference to laboratory vocabulary and terminology. Gives detailed information about complicated procedures and topics, rather than a simple dictionary definition.

Cavanaugh, Bonita Morrow. *Nurse's Manual of Laboratory and Diagnostic Tests.* 4th ed. Philadelphia: F. A. Davis, 2003. Provides information on hundreds of laboratory and diagnostic tests, with each test presented in two distinct, cross-referenced sections: "Background Information" sections provide a complete description of each test and its purposes; "Clinical Application Data" sections focus on the information nurses most commonly need while caring for clients.

Griffith, H. Winter. *Complete Guide to Symptoms, Illness, and Surgery.* Revised and updated by Stephen Moore and Kenneth Yoder. Rev. 4th ed. New York: Perigee, 2000. Covers more than five hundred diseases and disorders and includes information about causes and risk factors, preventive techniques, and diagnostic tests.

McPherson, Richard A., and Matthew R. Pincus, eds. *Henry's Clinical Diagnosis and Management by Laboratory Methods.* 21st ed. Philadelphia: Saunders Elsevier, 2007. The classic text on the clinical laboratory. Multiple authors cover all aspects of laboratory operations, including management and administration. The most recent edition should be consulted.

Pagana, Kathleen Deska, and Timothy J. Pagana. *Mosby's Diagnostic and Laboratory Test Reference.* 7th ed. St. Louis: Elsevier Mosby, 2005. A clinical handbook that gives alphabetically organized laboratory and diagnostic tests for easy reference. Each listing includes such things as alternate or abbreviated test names, type of test, normal findings, possible critical values, test explanation and related physiology, and potential complications.

Price, Christopher P., and David J. Newman, eds. *Principles and Practice of Immunoassay.* 2d ed. New York: Stockton Press, 1997. This work covers all aspects of immunoassays, including assay development, laboratory quality assurance, and test methodology.

Wu, Alan H. B., ed. *Tietz Clinical Guide to Laboratory Tests.* 4th ed. St. Louis: Saunders/Elsevier, 2006. A paperback condensation of the vital information needed for the interpretation of clinical laboratory tests. Tests are arranged alphabetically in tabular form for easy reference.

LACERATION REPAIR

PROCEDURE

ANATOMY OR SYSTEM AFFECTED: Skin

SPECIALTIES AND RELATED FIELDS: Emergency medicine, general surgery, plastic surgery

DEFINITION: The closure of an irregular skin wound.

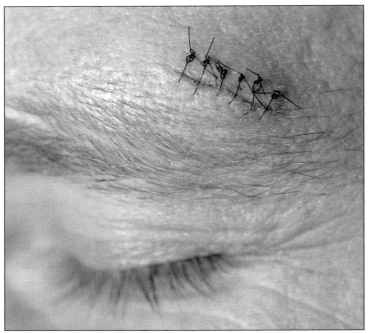

Stitches or sutures may be required to hold together the edges of lacerations that are large, deep, or ragged. (PhotoDisc)

INDICATIONS AND PROCEDURES

A laceration is a jagged, torn, mangled, or ragged wound. This type of wound is most commonly encountered in the skin, although any tissue may be lacerated. Lacerations are caused by sharp objects such as a piece of metal, glass, or a stick, or they may occur in accidents involving machinery or animals.

The first priority in laceration repair is to stop bleeding, thereby minimizing blood loss. This is usually accomplished by pressure either directly on the wound or on the injured blood vessel nearest the injury site.

The second priority with a laceration is to clean the wound, which involves the removal of any foreign material or debris. With penetrating injuries, this cleaning must be done carefully lest the removal of the object initiate bleeding. Tissue that has been destroyed beyond the body's ability to repair it must also be removed; this process is called debridement. Devitalized tissue is removed to prevent infection. The wound site is then cleaned through irrigation with saline and a disinfectant, usually a mild soap or a chemical.

Lacerations may then be treated for bacterial or other pathogenic contamination. Aqueous solutions containing an antibiotic are used with most wounds. If contamination with other pathogens is suspected, appropriate agents are used to rinse the wound. Antibiotic powders may be employed in field conditions, although this form of treatment is unusual in a hospital setting. Other than soap and water, there is no special treatment for viral contamination.

Closure of the wound is then completed. The edges are brought together and may be held in place with forceps. Sutures, or stitches, are inserted to hold the edges together while the tissue heals. On skin surfaces, these sutures are usually nonabsorbable and are later removed. The amount of time that sutures are kept in place varies with the location of the wound and the age of the patient: Mucous membranes heal more quickly than the palm, for example, and children's skin heals more rapidly than that of adults. Removable sutures are made of nylon or a similar material. Sutures that are used beneath the skin cannot be removed and are made of material that will break down within the body. Wound closure may also be accomplished with wire, staples, or adhesive tape. These materials have some advantages—durability (wire), ease of placement (staples), and minimal pain (tape)—and disadvantages—potential contamination (wire) and premature, accidental removal (tape). Lacerations should be rechecked by a physician when sutures or other means of wound closure are removed.

USES AND COMPLICATIONS

The techniques of laceration repair are used on all parts of the body where such wounds occur. Plastic surgery may be required to improve the appearance of the repaired tissue and to reduce scars when the patient believes that cosmetic results are an issue. In addition to scarring, other complications that may be associated with the repair of lacerations include infection and tetanus. All these problems can be minimized through good surgical techniques, the use of antibiotics, and careful postoperative care. The repair of lacerations to exposed facial skin is especially important. Careful technique minimizes scarring, as do some new methods of wound closure.

—*L. Fleming Fallon, Jr., M.D., Ph.D., M.P.H.*

See also Bleeding; Bruises; Emergency medicine; Grafts and grafting; Healing; Plastic surgery; Skin; Wounds.

FOR FURTHER INFORMATION:

American Academy of Orthopaedic Surgeons. *Emergency Care and Transportation of the Sick and Injured.* Edited by Benjamin Gulli, Les Chatelain, and Chris Stratford. 9th ed. Sudbury, Mass.: Jones and Bartlett, 2005.

Handal, Kathleen A. *The American Red Cross First Aid and Safety Handbook.* Boston: Little, Brown, 1992.

Mulholland, Michael W., et al., eds. *Greenfield's Surgery: Scientific Principles and Practice.* 4th ed. Philadelphia: Lippincott Williams & Wilkins, 2006.

Thygerson, Alton L. *First Aid and Emergency Care Workbook.* Boston: Jones and Bartlett, 1987.

Weedon, David. *Skin Pathology.* 2d ed. New York: Churchill Livingstone, 2002.

LACTOSE INTOLERANCE

DISEASE/DISORDER

ANATOMY OR SYSTEM AFFECTED: Gastrointestinal system, intestines, stomach

SPECIALTIES AND RELATED FIELDS: Gastroenterology, nutrition

DEFINITION: Lactose intolerance is an inability to break down and absorb milk sugar, known as lactose, resulting in stomach pain, gas, and diarrhea if lactose is consumed.

CAUSES AND SYMPTOMS

Lactose is a complex sugar commonly found in dairy products. It is composed of two simple sugars, glucose and galactose. In babies and young children, a gene produces an enzyme called lactase that breaks down lactose into its two component sugars, which are then absorbed into the bloodstream through the intestinal wall. In many people, sometime after early childhood, the lactase gene is "turned off." It no longer synthesizes lactase, which prevents the digestion and absorption of lactose.

INFORMATION ON LACTOSE INTOLERANCE

CAUSES: Insufficient lactase production

SYMPTOMS: Gas, cramping, and and diarrhea after consumption of lactose-containing food or drink

DURATION: One to two days

TREATMENTS: Avoidance of dairy produts, lactase pills

Normal bacterial inhabitants of the intestines synthesize lactase and break down the lactose molecules, producing large quantities of gas as a by-product. This can lead to cramping for the lactose-intolerant individual. The presence of lactose in the large intestine causes excessive amounts of water to move into the intestine, which can lead to diarrhea. Symptoms subside one to two days after the last lactose-containing food has been consumed.

TREATMENT AND THERAPY

Lactose intolerance can often be misdiagnosed as a host of gastrointestinal disorders, largely as a result of the commonness of its major symptoms, cramps and diarrhea. Typically, a dietary history must be kept. Patients with lactose intolerance will note an association between their symptoms and the consumption of milk products containing lactose. After elimination of these products from the diet, symptoms should not recur.

There is no treatment for lactose intolerance; prevention of symptoms is the general course of action. Avoidance of foods that contain lactose—including milk, ice cream, and cheese—is usually the best recourse. For those who wish to indulge in these products, over-the-counter lactase pills are available; their use usually prevents symptoms of the disorder.

PERSPECTIVE AND PROSPECTS

The vast majority of the world's population is lactose intolerant, yet this disorder was not recognized in the United States until the latter third of the twentieth century. Today, lactase supplements are available to help prevent symptoms for lactose-intolerant people who choose to consume dairy products. Alternatively, more and more dairy products are being manufactured as lactose-free; they can be consumed safely by the lactose-intolerant population.

—*Karen E. Kalumuck, Ph.D.*

See also Acid reflux disease; Diarrhea and dysentery; Digestion; Enzymes; Gastroenterology; Gastroenterology, pediatric; Gastrointestinal disorders; Gastrointestinal system; Irritable bowel syndrome (IBS); Metabolic disorders; Nutrition.

FOR FURTHER INFORMATION:

Dobler, Merri Lou. *Lactose Intolerance Nutrition Guide.* Chicago: American Dietetic Association, 2002.

Gracey, Michael, ed. *Diarrhea.* Boca Raton, Fla.: CRC Press, 1991.

Greenberger, Norton J. *Gastrointestinal Disorders: A Pathophysiologic Approach.* 4th ed. Chicago: Year Book Medical, 1989.

Icon Health. *Lactose Intolerance: A Medical Dictionary, Bibliography, and Annotated Research Guide to Internet References.* San Diego, Calif.: Author, 2004.

Janowitz, Henry D. *Your Gut Feelings: A Complete Guide to Living Better with Intestinal Problems.* Rev. ed. New York: Oxford University Press, 1994.

National Digestive Diseases Information Clearinghouse (NDDIC). National Institute of Diabetes and Digestive and Kidney Diseases (NIDDK). National Institutes of Health. *Lactose Intolerance.* http://digestive .niddk.nih.gov/ddiseases/pubs/lactoseintolerance/.

Peikin, Steven R. *Gastrointestinal Health.* Rev. ed. New York: HarperCollins, 1999.

LAMINECTOMY AND SPINAL FUSION
PROCEDURES

ANATOMY OR SYSTEM AFFECTED: Back, bones, spine

SPECIALTIES AND RELATED FIELDS: General surgery, orthopedics

DEFINITION: Surgical procedures that join two or more vertebrae, the arching bones that make up the spine.

INDICATIONS AND PROCEDURES

Laminectomies, which are designed to relieve pressure on the spinal cord, are often performed as the initial surgery in cases of extreme back pain caused by the compression of the spinal canal. An incision is made in the patient's back to expose the laminae, the flattened portions of the vertebral arch, and one or more adjacent laminae are chipped away. On occasion, several laminae are excised.

In such cases, spinal fusion, which involves the immobilization of the spine with steel rods or bone grafts, is indicated. Spinal fusion, like laminectomy a major surgery done under general anesthesia, is performed if X rays reveal unusual motion between adjacent vertebrae.

The causes of the severe back pain that usually precedes laminectomy or spinal fusion may be related to three conditions: osteoarthritis, which causes deterioration of the spinal joints; scoliosis caused by an injury or tumor that is destroying vertebrae; or spondylolisthesis, the dislocation of facet joints. In spinal fusion, when the damaged vertebrae are exposed, joint fusion is sometimes performed by using bone chips from the patient's pelvis. Following surgery, the vertebrae are held in place with plates or screws.

USES AND COMPLICATIONS

Both laminectomy and spinal fusion usually relieve the persistent back pain that has caused patients to seek treatment. Such surgery involves distinct risks, inasmuch as the spinal cord is exposed and there is often considerable blood loss. In the hands of a seasoned orthopedic surgeon, however, the risk is minimized.

Recovery from the surgery can be slow and often involves up to six weeks of confinement in bed. After this confinement, patients are usually required to wear a plaster cast until final vertebral fusion has occurred. This process can take half a year.

Fusion sometimes places an additional burden on the rest of the spinal column. In some cases, this pressure results in renewed back pain in other areas of the spine. Additional surgery may be indicated to control this pain.

—R. Baird Shuman, Ph.D.

See also Back pain; Bone grafting; Bones and the skeleton; Disk removal; Fracture and dislocation; Grafts and grafting; Orthopedic surgery; Orthopedics; Orthopedics, pediatric; Osteoarthritis; Scoliosis; Spinal cord disorders; Spine, vertebrae, and disks.

FOR FURTHER INFORMATION:

Boden, Scott D., ed. *Spinal Fusion.* Philadelphia: W. B. Saunders, 1998.

Devlin, Vincent J., ed. *Spine Secrets.* Philadelphia: Hanley & Belfus, 2003.

Frymoyer, John W., and Sam W. Wiesel, eds. *The Adult and Pediatric Spine: Principles, Practice, and Surgery.* 3d ed. Philadelphia: Lippincott Williams & Wilkins, 2004.

Hitchon, Patrick W., Setti Rengachary, and Vincent C. Traynelis, eds. *Techniques in Spinal Fusion and Stabilization.* New York: Thieme Medical, 1995.

Lewandrowski, Kai-Uwe, et al., eds. *Advances in Spinal Fusion: Molecular Science, Biomechanics, and Clinical Management.* New York: Marcel Dekker, 2004.

Nakamura, K., Y. Toyama, and Y. Hoshino, eds. *Cervical Laminoplasty.* New York: Springer, 2003.

Wetzel, F. Todd, and Edward Nathaniel Hanley, Jr. *Spine Surgery: A Practical Atlas.* New York: McGraw-Hill, 2002.

LAPAROSCOPY

PROCEDURE

ANATOMY OR SYSTEM AFFECTED: Abdomen, gallbladder, gastrointestinal system, intestines, kidneys, reproductive system, urinary system, uterus

SPECIALTIES AND RELATED FIELDS: Endocrinology, gastroenterology, general surgery, gynecology

DEFINITION: The examination of the abdominal organs with a laparoscope, a fiber-optic tube which can also be used to perform surgery to correct several disease conditions.

KEY TERMS:

abdomen: the area of the body between the diaphragm and the pelvis; it contains the visceral organs

cholecystectomy: the surgical removal of the gallbladder

ectopic pregnancy: the development of a fertilized egg in a Fallopian tube instead of the uterus; can be fatal to the mother unless it is corrected surgically

endometriosis: a female reproductive disease in which cells from the uterine lining (the endometrium) grow outside the uterus, causing severe pain and infertility and sometimes the need for hysterectomy

Fallopian tubes: the two tubes through which eggs pass on the way from the ovaries to the uterus

general anesthesia: anesthesia that induces unconsciousness

implant: a section of endometrial tissue found outside the uterus

local anesthesia: anesthesia that numbs the feeling in a body part, administered by injection or direct application to the skin

INDICATIONS AND PROCEDURES

Laparoscopy is a surgical technique for examining the abdominal organs and for treating surgically many diseases of these organs. The instrument used is called a laparoscope. It is a flexible tube that contains fiber optics for visualization purposes and a channel through which physicians can pass special surgical instruments into the abdominal cavity.

Upon insertion of a laparoscope into the abdomen through a small surgical incision (usually near the navel), physicians can observe the liver, kidneys, gallbladder, pancreas, spleen, and exterior aspects of the intestines in both sexes. Hence the technique is useful for detecting cirrhosis of the liver, the presence of stones and tumors, and many other diseases of the abdominal organs. The female reproductive organs can also be examined in this manner.

Before laparoscopy can be carried out, the patient must fast for at least twelve hours. The patient is given a local or general anesthetic, depending on the purpose of the procedure. In exploratory abdominal examinations, the instrument is inserted into the abdomen through a small incision in the abdominal wall after local anesthesia has numbed it. Often, especially when extensive surgery is anticipated, the procedure begins after general anesthesia produces unconsciousness. Upon the completion of exploration or surgery, the laparoscope is withdrawn and the incision is closed.

Laparoscopic abdominal examination is often used to detect endometriosis, the presence of endometrial cells outside the uterus. This procedure begins with the administration of local anesthesia when only exploration or biopsy is planned. General anesthesia is used when the removal of implants (endometrial tissue) is anticipated. The entry incision is made near the navel, and the laparoscope is inserted. The fiber-optics system is used to search the abdominal organs for implants. Visibility of the abdominal organs is usually enhanced by pumping in a harmless gas, such as carbon dioxide, to distend the abdomen. After the confirmation of endometriosis, surgical implant removal is carried out immediately, unless the decision is made to institute drug therapy instead. Full recovery from this surgery requires only a day of postoperative bed rest and a week of curtailing activities.

Laparoscopy can also be employed for female sterilization. The patient is given a general anesthetic. After laparoscopic visualization of the Fallopian tubes in the gas-distended abdomen is achieved, surgical instruments for tube cauterization or cutting are introduced and the sterilization is carried out. The entire procedure often requires only thirty minutes, which is one reason for its popularity. In addition, patients can go home in a few hours and have fully recovered after a day or two of bed rest and seven to ten days of curtailing activities.

USES AND COMPLICATIONS

Common laparoscopic surgeries are cholecystectomy (the removal of the gallbladder), the removal of gallstones and kidney stones, tumor resection, female sterilization by cutting or blocking the Fallopian tubes, the treatment of endometriosis through the removal of implants from abdominal organs, and the removal of biopsy samples from abdominal organs. Traditional uses of laparoscopy in female reproductive surgery are to identify and correct pelvic pain resulting from endometriosis, ectopic pregnancy, and pelvic tumors.

Laparoscopy has several advantages. There is rarely a need for patients on chronic drug therapy to discontinue medication before laparoscopy. In addition, the use of laparoscopy dramatically lowers surgical incision size, surgical trauma, length of hospital stay, and recovery time. Laparoscopy should be avoided, however, in cases of advanced abdominal wall cancer, severe respiratory or cardiovascular disease, or tuberculosis. Extreme obesity does not disqualify a patient from undergoing laparoscopy but makes the procedure much more difficult to perform.

As laparoscopic surgery has increased in scope, more procedures yield surgical tissues that are larger in size than the laparoscope channel (for example, the removal of gallbladders, gallstones, and ovaries). In many cases these organs and structures are cut into small pieces for removal. If potentially dangerous items are involved—such as malignancies that can spread on dissection—larger, more conventional incisions are often combined with laparoscopy.

PERSPECTIVE AND PROSPECTS

Since the 1970's, the uses of laparoscopy have constantly expanded. Once confined to the exploratory examination of the abdomen, the methodology has been applied to a large number of different types of surgery in addition to those already mentioned. Such versatility is attributable to the development of better laparoscopes, advanced instrumentation for diverse surgeries, and improved fiber-optic and video technologies.

As a consequence of these advances, many surgeons predict that most future abdominal surgery will be laparoscopic. The driving force for such innovation includes the public demand for quicker recovery times. In the United States, this desire is intensified by the requirements of insurance companies, employers, and the federal government for shorter hospital stays. Both changes are made possible by decreased severity of surgical trauma in laparoscopy when compared to traditional surgery, a result of the smaller incisions. The dramatic trend toward laparoscopy can be seen with cholecystectomies: Of those done in 1992, 70 percent were laparoscopic, compared to less than 1 percent in 1989.

—*Sanford S. Singer, Ph.D.*

See also Abdomen; Abdominal disorders; Appendectomy; Appendicitis; Biopsy; Cholecystectomy; Ectopic pregnancy; Endometriosis; Endoscopy; Gynecology; Internal medicine; Sterilization; Stone removal; Stones; Tubal ligation; Tumor removal; Tumors.

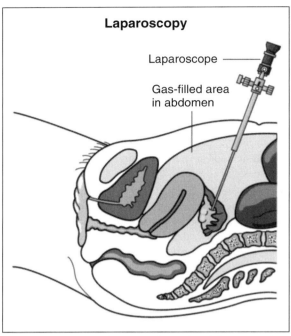

Laparoscopy

Laparoscope

Gas-filled area in abdomen

Many surgical procedures involving the abdomen, such as appendectomy or the removal of eggs from the ovaries for in vitro fertilization, can be performed using laparoscopy. Gas is pumped into the abdominal cavity, and a fiber-optic scope and instruments are inserted through a small hole in the skin.

FOR FURTHER INFORMATION:

Graber, John N., et al., eds. *Laparoscopic Abdominal Surgery.* New York: McGraw-Hill, 1993. A text for surgery residents and practicing surgeons wishing to gain an understanding of the theory and technique of laparoscopic surgery, written by experts in each area who were instrumental in the development of laparoscopic approaches. Abundantly illustrated with clear, detailed line drawings and color photographs.

Henderson, Lorraine, and Ros Wood. *Explaining Endometriosis.* 2d ed. St. Leonards, Australia: Allen and Unwin, 2001. Details possible causes, diagnosis, surgeries, and current treatment options for endometriosis.

Kapadia, Cyrus R., James M. Crawford, and Caroline Taylor. *An Atlas of Gastroenterology: A Guide to Diagnosis and Differential Diagnosis.* Boca Raton, Fla.: Pantheon, 2003. Provides a fully illustrated, nonspecialist understanding of myriad gastrointestinal diseases, including heartburn, dyspepsia, diarrhea, irritable bowel syndrome, and pancreatitis. Includes bibliographic references and index.

Reddick, Eddie Joe, ed. *An Atlas of Laparoscopic Surgery*. New York: Raven Press, 1993. Discusses such topics as cholecystectomy and peritoneoscopy. Includes an index.

Zollinger, Robert M., Jr., and Robert M. Zollinger, Sr. *Zollinger's Atlas of Surgical Operations*. 8th ed. New York: McGraw-Hill, 2003. A comprehensive examination of surgery. Covers basic surgical anatomy and vascular, gynecologic, gastrointestinal, and miscellaneous abdominal procedures.

Zucker, Karl A., ed. *Surgical Laparoscopy*. 2d ed. Philadelphia: Lippincott Williams & Wilkins, 2001. Discusses the gastrointestinal system, peritoneoscopy, and the methods of biliary tract surgery and endoscopic surgery.

LARYNGECTOMY

PROCEDURE

ANATOMY OR SYSTEM AFFECTED: Respiratory system, throat

SPECIALTIES AND RELATED FIELDS: General surgery, oncology, otorhinolaryngology

DEFINITION: The removal of all or part of the voice box, or larynx.

INDICATIONS AND PROCEDURES

Continued hoarseness and coughing can indicate laryngeal disorders. Polyps, which may be caused by excessive smoking or drinking, can form on the larynx. Children sometimes develop warts on it. Although these polyps and warts are generally benign, they should be removed and subjected to biopsy to preclude the presence of cancer.

Polyps, warts, and tumors are all detected quite easily with a laryngoscopic examination carried out by an otorhinolaryngologist with a mirror, an endoscope (a flexible fiber-optic tube), or a combination of the two. Such an examination, in addition to determining whether a growth is benign or cancerous, can detect signs of cancer in the lining of the larynx.

If cancer is detected early enough, radiation can usually control it. If the disease has advanced significantly, however, a laryngectomy may be necessary. In this surgical procedure, performed under general anesthesia, an incision is made in the neck and the larynx is removed. The windpipe directly below the larynx is then sewn to the skin around the surgical opening to form a permanent opening, or stoma, through which the patient breathes.

USES AND COMPLICATIONS

This surgery is used when cancer is sufficiently advanced that radiation therapy cannot destroy it. The major complication is that the patient's air supply is now taken through the stoma, meaning that swimming is precluded and that bathing must be undertaken with considerable caution.

A more apparent complication is that, with the loss of the larynx, one cannot speak. Through an extensive and painstaking course of speech therapy, however, esophageal speech can be achieved. This involves swallowing air and expelling it in such a way that it can be shaped by the palate, lips, and tongue into understandable words and sentences. An electronic larynx is also available. It makes a buzzing sound which, when pressed against the top of the throat, permits the patient to convert the sound into words.

—*R. Baird Shuman, Ph.D.*

See also Cancer; Endoscopy; Mouth and throat cancer; Otorhinolaryngology; Speech disorders; Tumors; Warts.

FOR FURTHER INFORMATION:

Blom, Eric D., Mark I. Singer, and Ronald C. Hamaker, eds. *Tracheoesophageal Voice Restoration Following Total Laryngectomy*. San Diego, Calif.: Singular, 1998.

Casper, Janina K., and Raymond H. Colton. *Clinical Manual for Laryngectomy and Head/Neck Cancer Rehabilitation*. 2d ed. San Diego, Calif.: Singular, 1998.

Edels, Yvonne, ed. *Laryngectomy: Diagnosis to Rehabilitation*. Rockville, Md.: Aspen Systems, 1983.

Ferrari, Mario. *PDxMD Ear, Nose, and Throat Disorders*. New York: Elsevier, 2002.

Griffith, H. Winter. *Complete Guide to Symptoms, Illness, and Surgery*. Revised and updated by Stephen Moore and Kenneth Yoder. Rev. 4th ed. New York: Perigee, 2000.

Montgomery, William W., ed. *Surgery of the Larynx, Trachea, Esophagus, and Neck*. Philadelphia: Saunders, 2002.

Zollinger, Robert M., Jr., and Robert M. Zollinger, Sr. *Zollinger's Atlas of Surgical Operations*. 8th ed. New York: McGraw-Hill, 2003.

Laryngitis

Disease/disorder

Anatomy or system affected: Throat

Specialties and related fields: Otorhinolaryngology, speech pathology

Definition: Inflammation of the larynx (voice box), often associated with common colds, bacterial infection, or straining the voice. The throat is dry, swallowing becomes difficult, and speech is a hoarse whisper.

Causes and Symptoms

The larynx, located directly above the windpipe (trachea), is the short, hollow tube containing the vocal cords, two heavily lined slits in a mucous membrane. Voiced sounds, such as vowels, result when air from the lungs induces vocal fold vibration. Laryngitis occurs when the folds are obstructed or do not vibrate properly; depending on the cause, laryngitis is classified as simple, chronic, diphtheritic, tuberculous, or syphilitic.

Simple laryngitis may be caused by bacterial infection (common cold, typhoid fever), a virus (influenza), or nonbacterial irritants (chemical fumes, dust, or tobacco smoke). The primary infection site is the mucous membrane lining the larynx. It becomes red and swollen, secreting a viscous discharge that impedes vocal fold vibration. In severe cases of viral infection, the larynx may become completely obstructed, causing suffocation.

Chronic laryngitis often results from excessive smoking, alcoholism, or consistent strain or abuse of the voice. It is an occupational hazard of auctioneers, orators, singers, and those who frequently shout for long periods, such as cheerleaders. Nondisease-induced chronic laryngitis may also be instigated by hysteria,

---

allergic reaction, remote disease of the nerves serving the voice, strong external pressure against the larynx, or irritation caused by tubes inserted down the throat to sustain breathing.

Diphtheritic laryngitis occurs when diphtheria afflicting the upper throat spreads to the larynx. The result may be a membrane of diseased cells infiltrating the mucous membrane and obstructing the vocal cords.

Tuberculous laryngitis is a secondary infection spread from the lungs. Tubular nodulelike growths are formed in larynx tissue, leaving ulcers on the surface. Starting at the vocal cords, this infection may spread over the entire larynx and eventually destroy the epiglottis and laryngeal cartilage.

Syphilitic laryngitis is one of the many complications of syphilis. Sores or mucous patches form in the larynx, eventually producing tissue destruction and scar formation. The mucous membrane becomes dry and covered with polyps (small bumps of tissue that project from the surface). These polyps distort the larynx, shorten the vocal cords, and produce persistent hoarseness.

Treatment and Therapy

Simple laryngitis is best treated by resting the voice. When it is absolutely necessary to speak, it should be with a soft, breathy voice, not a whisper. The throat should be kept well lubricated by frequent drinks of water and not cleared. Relative humidity in the recovery room should be maintained at 40 to 50 percent, and alcohol, tobacco, and decongestants should be avoided. Complete recovery usually occurs within several days.

A persistent hoarseness indicates a bacterial infection (usually curable by antibiotics) or polyps, cysts, or other fibrous growths on the vocal cords. These growths may become ulcerated and require surgical intervention. Although cancer of the larynx is not uncommon (2 percent of malignancies), it is usually completely curable if detected sufficiently early.

Systemic diseases not localized in the larynx, such as tuberculosis and syphilis, are best treated by antibiotics.

—George R. Plitnik, Ph.D.

See also Common cold; Laryngectomy; Multiple chemical sensitivity syndrome; Nasopharyngeal disorders; Otorhinolaryngology; Pharyngitis; Sore throat; Strep throat; Tonsillectomy and adenoid removal; Tonsillitis; Voice and vocal cord disorders.

> ## Information on Laryngitis
>
> **Causes:** Bacterial infection (common cold, typhoid fever, diphtheria, syphilis); viral infection (influenza); irritants (chemical fumes, dust, smoke, alcohol); consistent strain or abuse of voice
>
> **Symptoms:** Red and swollen larynx; discharge; obstruction that can cause suffocation if severe; polyps, cysts, or other fibrous growths on vocal cords
>
> **Duration:** Acute or chronic
>
> **Treatments:** Depends on cause; may include resting the voice, antibiotics, or surgery

FOR FURTHER INFORMATION:

Bellenir, Karen, and Peter D. Dresser, eds. *Contagious and Noncontagious Infectious Diseases Sourcebook*. Detroit: Omnigraphics, 1996.

Colton, Raymond H., Janina K. Casper, and Rebecca Leonard. *Understanding Voice Problems: A Physiological Perspective for Diagnosis and Treatment*. 3d ed. Philadelphia: Lippincott Williams & Wilkins, 2006.

Icon Health. *Laryngitis: A Medical Dictionary, Bibliography, and Annotated Research Guide to Internet References*. San Diego, Calif.: Author, 2004.

Ossoff, Robert H., et al., eds. *The Larynx*. Philadelphia: Lippincott Williams & Wilkins, 2003.

Sataloff, Robert T., ed. *Reflux Laryngitis and Related Disorders*. 3d ed. San Diego, Calif.: Plural, 2006.

Swartzberg, John Edward. *Wellness Self-Care Handbook: The Everyday Guide to Prevention and Home Remedies to Over 150 Common Ailments*. New York: Times Books, 1999.

LASER USE IN SURGERY

PROCEDURE

ANATOMY OR SYSTEM AFFECTED: Eyes, skin

SPECIALTIES AND RELATED FIELDS: Dermatology, oncology, ophthalmology, urology

DEFINITION: The application of laser technology to surgical procedures, such as the vaporization of blood clots or arterial plaque, the breaking up of kidney stones into small fragments, the removal of birthmarks, and the stoppage of hemorrhaging in the retina of the eye.

KEY TERMS:

ionization: a process in which a neutral atom loses one or more of its orbital electrons because of light, heat, or electrical collisions

laser: an acronym for light amplification by stimulated emission of radiation; a laser produces a very-high-intensity light beam at a single wavelength

optical fiber: a very thin thread made of high-purity glass, plastic, or quartz; used to transmit light from a laser into the body

photon: a particle of light whose energy depends on its wavelength (that is, its color); many billions of individual photons make up a light beam

pulsed laser: a laser technique used to deliver a light beam of high power for a very short time in order to localize the heating effect without damaging surrounding tissue

shock wave: a miniature explosion caused by intense local heating with a laser beam; used to fragment stones in the kidney or gallbladder

stimulated emission of radiation: the process in a laser whereby an avalanche of photons is created, all of which are synchronized in wavelength and direction of travel

wavelength: a property used to measure colors in the spectrum of light from infrared to ultraviolet; usually expressed in units of microns (one micron is equal to one-millionth of a meter)

THE FUNDAMENTALS OF LASER TECHNOLOGY

The first successful laser was built in 1960 by Theodore H. Maiman at the Hughes Aircraft Research Laboratory in Palo Alto, California. Since then, many applications have been developed for lasers. These include the compact disc player, telephone systems with fiber optics, guidance systems for military weapons, supermarket checkout scanners, quality control in industry, entertainment with laser light shows, and numerous medical applications.

Ordinary light sources such as flashlights, flames, and the sun do not emit laser light. The individual atoms emit their light waves in a random, uncoordinated manner, in the same way that water waves spread out at random when a handful of pebbles is thrown into a pool. In contrast, a laser beam consists of light waves that are all synchronized; they all have the same wavelength and remain in step as they travel in the same direction. Synchronizing the light emission from billions of atoms in a light source is the chief difficulty in building a laser.

The key idea for solving this problem had been proposed in an article on the general theory of light absorption and emission by atoms written by the famous physicist Albert Einstein in the 1920's. When an atom absorbs a burst of light energy (a photon), an electron in the atom is raised from a lower energy level to a higher one. A short time later, the electron spontaneously falls back down to the lower energy level, emitting a photon of light in the process. Einstein's contribution was to suggest a third mechanism in addition to ordinary absorption and emission. Based on theoretical arguments of symmetry and the conservation of energy, he proposed a new process called "stimulated emission of radiation." (The word "laser" is an acronym for light amplification by stimulated emission of radiation.)

To understand stimulated emission, consider an atom whose electron has been raised to a higher energy level, called an "excited state." This state is unstable, and the electron ordinarily will fall back down to the lower energy level in a short time. Suppose, however, that a photon of precisely the right energy strikes the atom while the electron is still in its temporary excited state. This photon cannot be absorbed because the electron is already in its excited state. Einstein reasoned that the incoming photon would cause the excited electron to fall to the lower energy level. A photon would then be emitted from the atom and would join the incoming photon. The two photons would be exactly synchronized in wavelength and direction.

If there were many atoms whose electrons had previously been raised to excited states, the process of stimulated emission would continue. The two photons could strike two other excited atoms and stimulate them to emit light energy, making a total of four photons. These four would trigger four more atoms, making eight photons, and so forth. Eventually, a so-called photon avalanche consisting of a huge number of synchronized light waves would be generated, which is the desired laser beam.

To make a successful laser, some additional requirements must be met. For one thing, a source of energy must be provided to raise most of the electrons to their excited states. For a gas laser, this energy is normally supplied by a high voltage. Examples of gas lasers are those using carbon dioxide, argon, or a mixture of helium and neon. A solid crystal, such as a clear ruby rod, would be excited by a bright burst of light from a device similar to a camera flash attachment. A solid-state diode laser is energized by a flow of electric current across a diode junction. In each case, it is necessary to "pump" the laser so that many atoms are in their excited state, ready and waiting to be triggered by an incoming photon to release their energy.

Another requirement for a successful laser is that the electrons must remain in their excited state for a longer-than-normal time. The problem with most materials is that electrons fall spontaneously to their lower energy level almost instantaneously, in less than one-millionth of a second. The photon avalanche effect requires that a substantial majority of the atoms be in their excited state. For very short-lived excited states, it is not possible to maintain this condition. Experimenters have no way to control the lifetime of excited states, so they must search for those atoms and molecules that already have the appropriate longer lifetime supplied by nature. It has not been possible to build a laser using hydrogen gas, for example, because hydrogen does not have any long-lived excited states. The spontaneous emission of

light takes place so quickly that there is no time for a photon avalanche to develop.

Another condition for laser action is to have two parallel mirrors at the ends of the laser material. The laser beam bounces back and forth many times between the mirrors at the speed of light, gaining or maintaining its energy from the excited atoms of the laser material. One of the mirrors is made slightly less than 100 percent reflecting, so that a small portion of the laser energy is allowed to exit in a narrow beam. For most medical applications, a thin optical fiber is joined directly to the end of the laser in order to transmit the beam to the desired location in the body.

Much research has been done to develop good optical fibers. The fiber should transmit a laser beam with very little loss of energy along the way. The technology of drawing thin glass fibers with few impurities or imperfections has become quite sophisticated. A fiber must be thin and uniform so that the laser beam will be forced to travel down its center, thus avoiding the loss of light energy through the walls.

For an ultraviolet laser, glass fibers cannot be used because of absorption. (The sun's ultraviolet radiation is absorbed by ordinary eyeglasses.) Special quartz fibers with low absorption have been developed for lasers in the ultraviolet region of the spectrum. In the infrared region of the spectrum, new optical materials are still under continuing investigation.

The wavelength (color) of a laser is determined entirely by the energy levels of the atoms or molecules being used. For example, a carbon dioxide laser always has a wavelength of 10.6 microns, which is infrared. The helium-neon gas laser always produces visible red light at a wavelength of 0.63 microns. A wide range of laser wavelengths has become available as a result of extensive research efforts by physicists and optical engineers. Since 1960, lasers have become much more rugged and dependable in construction. Some lasers operate with a continuous beam, while others produce very short pulses, depending on the desired application. Also, lasers can be designed to operate at a low power level for diagnostic purposes or a high power level for surgery.

Safety precautions must be followed when working with a laser. Not only the patient but also the surgical team must be protected from possible harmful radiation. The eyes must be protected from laser beam reflections from a shiny surface. Ultraviolet light is a special hazard because its high-energy photons can cause cell damage and genetic mutations. The great benefits

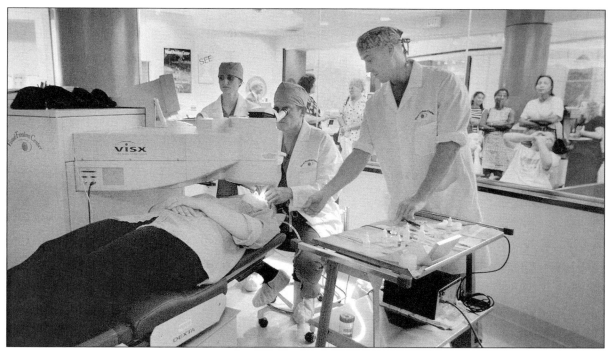

Lasers are taking a more prominent role in many procedures, especially eye surgery. Some worry that the popularity of laser vision correction—here a patient is treated at a shopping mall as spectators look on—has compromised safety. (AP/Wide World Photos)

of laser surgery can be negated by an inexperienced or careless surgeon.

USES AND COMPLICATIONS

The first medical use of a laser beam was for surgery on the retina of the eye, in 1963. Diabetic patients in particular frequently develop excessive blood vessels in the retina that give their eyes a typically reddish color. In advanced cases, the blood vessels can hemorrhage and eventually cause blindness. The green light of an argon laser will pass through the clear cornea and lens of the eye, but when it hits the dark brown melanin pigment of the retina, it will be absorbed and cause a tiny hot spot. The physician uses a series of laser pulses, carefully focused on affected areas of the retina, to burn away the extra blood vessels. The remarkable property of the laser beam in this procedure is that its energy penetrates to the rear of the eye, leaving the clear fluid unaffected.

In a greenhouse, light from the sun comes in through the glass but infrared radiation cannot get back out. This example illustrates that some materials, such as glass, are transparent for visible light but opaque for infrared light. Similarly, the front of the eye is transparent for visible light but absorbs infrared light. Therefore, an infrared laser such as the YAG (yttrium-aluminum-garnet) laser can be used for surgery near the front of the eye because its light energy is selectively absorbed there.

A particular problem following cataract surgery is that a secondary cataract may develop on the membrane behind the implanted artificial lens. About one-third of patients with such a lens implant require a second surgery to remove the secondary cataract. A YAG laser beam will pass through the cornea and artificial lens but can be focused to produce a hot spot at the site of the secondary cataract to destroy it. More than 200,000 such procedures are performed each year in the United States, and the result is a dramatic, almost instantaneous improvement of vision.

A third form of laser eye surgery, laser-assisted in situ keratomileusis (LASIK), became quite popular at the end of the twentieth century; it has, in fact, become the most commonly performed surgery in the country. In LASIK surgery, the cornea of the eyeball is reshaped to help patients overcome myopia (nearsightedness), hyperopia (farsightedness), or astigmatism. The procedure is done with a cool beam laser that can be used to remove thin layers of tissue from selected sites on the cornea to change its curvature. Success rates for the surgery are high: 90 to 95 percent of the patients get 20/40 vision, and 65 to 75 percent of the patients get 20/20 vision or better. The surgery is not without its problems, however. Because of its popularity and the large fee charged for a quick and fairly simple procedure, unqualified or less experienced physicians are oftentimes performing the delicate procedure; approximately 5 percent of patients receiving LASIK surgery receive less-than-satisfactory results. Two other corrective procedures for eyesight involving lasers are Kera-Vision Intacs (intrastomal corneal rings), which involves placing a lens in the cornea, and PRK (photorefractive keratectomy), where the cornea is scraped without LASIK's actual incision into the cornea.

Another dramatic medical application of the laser is the breaking up of stones in the kidney, ureter, or gallbladder. Such calcified, hard deposits previously could be removed only by surgery. It is now possible, for example, to insert an optical fiber of less than half a millimeter in diameter through the urethra and then transmit the laser beam to the site of the stone. High-power light pulses of very short duration (less than one-billionth of a second) create a shock wave that breaks the stone into small fragments that the body can eliminate.

Another promising application of laser surgery that has received much publicity is laser angioplasty, which is used to open up a blood vessel near the heart that is partially or wholly blocked by a deposit of plaque. The hope is that the laser procedure may be able to replace heart bypass surgery, but the results are still preliminary.

Laser angioplasty involves inserting a catheter that contains a fiberscope, an inflation cuff, and an optical fiber into the artery of the arm and advancing it into the coronary artery. The fiberscope enables the physician to see the blockage, the cuff is used to stop the blood flow temporarily, and the optical fiber transmits the laser energy that vaporizes the plaque. Sometimes, the laser method is used only to open up a small channel, after which balloon angioplasty is used to stretch the walls of the blood vessel.

The main risk in using the laser beam is that the alignment of the optical fiber inside the artery may be deflected and cause a puncture of the blood vessel wall. Improvements in the imaging system are needed. Also, further work must be done to see which light wavelengths are most effective in removing plaque and preventing recurrence of the obstruction.

The heating effect of a laser beam has been used by surgeons to control bleeding. For example, bleeding ulcers in the stomach, intestine, and colon have been successfully cauterized with laser light transmitted through an optical fiber. A similar procedure has been used to treat emphysema patients. An optical fiber is inserted through the wall of the chest, and the laser's heat is used to shrink the small blisters that are present on the surface of the lungs. Also, the heat from a laser has been used during internal surgery to seal the surrounding capillaries that contribute to bleeding.

For the preceding procedures, a carbon dioxide gas laser that emits infrared light is normally used. The reason is that water molecules in the tissue absorb the infrared wavelengths most efficiently. The optical fibers used to transmit infrared light are not as efficient and reliable as those used for visible or ultraviolet light, however, so further research on fiber materials is in progress.

One notable success of laser surgery has been the removal of birthmarks. Because of their typically reddish-purple coloration, birthmarks are commonly called port-wine stains. They can be quite unsightly, especially when located on the face of a person with an otherwise light complexion. To remove such a birthmark, the laser beam has to burn out the network of extra blood vessels under the skin. A similar procedure can be used to remove unwanted tattoos.

The color of the laser must be chosen so that its wavelength will be absorbed efficiently by the dark purple stain. What would happen if a purple laser beam were used? Its light would be reflected rather than absorbed by a purple object, and it would not produce the desired heating. Yellow or orange is most effectively absorbed by a purple object. The surgeon must be careful that the laser light is absorbed primarily by the purple birthmark without harming the normal, healthy tissue around it.

Experimental work is being done to determine whether laser surgery can be applied to cancer. Small malignant tumors in the lungs, bladder, and trachea have been treated with a technique called photodynamic therapy. The patient is injected with a colored dye that is preferentially absorbed in the tumor. Porphyrin, the reddish-brown pigment in blood, is one substance that has been known for many years to become concentrated in malignant tissue. The suspected site is irradiated with ultraviolet light from a krypton laser, causing it to glow like fluorescent paint, which allows the surgeon to determine the outline of the tumor. To perform the surgery, an intense red laser is focused on the tumor to kill the malignant tissue. Two separate optical fibers must be used for this procedure, one for the ultraviolet diagnosis and one for the red laser therapy.

The three traditional cancer treatments of surgery, chemotherapy, and radiation therapy all seek to limit damage to healthy tissue surrounding a tumor. Photodynamic surgery by laser must develop its methodology further to accomplish the same goal.

Much has already been accomplished in applying laser surgery to various body organs. Future developments are likely to emphasize microsurgery on smaller structures, such as individual cells or even genetic material in DNA molecules.

PERSPECTIVE AND PROSPECTS

Some inventions, such as the printing press, the steam engine, and the electric light bulb, were made by innovators who were trying to solve a particular practical problem of their time. Other inventions, such as the microscope, radio waves, and low-temperature superconductivity, initially were scientific curiosities arising from basic research, and their later applications were not at all anticipated. The laser belongs to this second category.

The first successful laser, built by Theodore Maiman, consisted of a small cylindrical ruby rod with shiny mirrored ends and a bright flash lamp to excite the atoms in the rod. His goal was to determine whether the separately excited atoms could be made to release their absorbed energy almost simultaneously in one coordinated burst of monochromatic (single wavelength) light.

No one could have foreseen the wide range of technological applications that resulted from Maiman's experiment. It is important to appreciate that he did not set out to improve telephone communication or eye surgery; those developments came about after the laser became available.

It is worthwhile here to summarize some of the general uses for lasers in modern technology. The tremendous advances in medical applications could not have happened without the concurrent development of new types of lasers, with a variety of wavelengths and power levels, needed for other industrial products.

Among laser applications are the following: the compact disc (CD) player, in which the laser beam replaces the LP record needle; optical fibers that can carry several thousand simultaneous telephone calls; supermarket check-out scanners, in which a laser beam reads the universal product code on each item; three-dimensional pictures, called holograms, that are displayed at many art museums; military applications, such as guided weapons and Star Wars technology; surveying, bridge building, and tunneling projects in which exact alignment is critical; and nuclear fusion research, in which high-power lasers can produce nuclear reactions that may become a future source of energy as coal and oil resources are depleted. Sophisticated advances in using lasers to control specific chemical reactions and to predict earthquakes are under development.

The future of laser technology in medicine will continue to advance as biologists, electrical and optical engineers, physicians, biophysicists, and people from related disciplines share this common interest.

—Hans G. Graetzer, Ph.D.;
updated by Cassandra Kircher, Ph.D.

See also Angioplasty; Astigmatism; Bionics and biotechnology; Bleeding; Blurred vision; Cataract surgery; Cataracts; Cervical procedures; Dermatology; Electrocauterization; Eye surgery; Eyes; Melanoma; Myopia; Neurosurgery; Ophthalmology; Refractive eye surgery; Skin; Skin disorders; Skin lesion removal; Stone removal; Stones; Tattoo removal; Ulcer surgery; Ulcers.

FOR FURTHER INFORMATION:

Alster, Tina S., and Lydia Preston. *Skin Savvy: The Essential Guide to Cosmetic Laser Surgery*. New York: Cadogan, 2002. A guide that provides an overview of current laser procedures in cosmetic surgery, information on the variety of lasers used for which procedures, and practical advice on whether or not certain surgeries would be right for specific conditions.

American Society for Laser Surgery and Medicine, Inc. http://www.aslms.org/. Site offers a database for referral to a laser practitioner, and links to the journal *Lasers in Surgery and Medicine*.

Azar, Dimitri T., and Douglas D. Koch, eds. *LASIK: Fundamentals, Surgical Techniques, and Complications*. New York: Marcel Dekker, 2003. A description of LASIK eye surgery and potential complications.

Buettner, Helmut, ed. *Mayo Clinic on Vision and Eye Health: Practical Answers on Glaucoma, Cataracts, Macular Degeneration, and Other Conditions*. Rochester, Minn.: Mayo Foundation for Medical Education and Research, 2002. A helpful handbook on all the medical, social, and emotional facets of vision impairment and the treatments available.

Goldman, Mitchel P., ed. *Cutaneous and Cosmetic Laser Surgery.* Philadelphia: Mosby Elsevier, 2006. Discusses methods of cosmetic surgery using lasers. Includes bibliographical references and an index.

IEEE Journal of Quantum Electronics 26, no. 12 (December, 1990). A special issue on lasers in biology and medicine. This journal is the professional publication of the Institute of Electrical and Electronic Engineers. The articles require some technical background on the part of the reader.

Narins, Rhoda S., and Paul Jarrod Frank. *Turn Back the Clock Without Losing Time: Everything You Need to Know About Simple Cosmetic Procedures.* New York: Three Rivers Press, 2002. A user-friendly guide to procedures that covers laser resurfacing and includes a "frequently asked questions" section for each treatment.

Sutton, Amy, ed. *Eye Care Sourcebook: Basic Consumer Health Information About Eye Care and Eye Disorders.* 2d ed. Detroit: Omnigraphics, 2003. A complete guide to eye care that includes such topics as eye anatomy, preventive vision care, refractive disorders and eye diseases, current research and clinical trials, and a list of organizations.

Victor, Steven, and Ina Yalof. *Ageless Beauty: A Dermatologist's Secrets for Looking Younger Without Surgery.* New York: Crown, 2003. Details several innovative approaches to skin care, including laser surgery.

LAW AND MEDICINE

ETHICS

DEFINITION: The use of medicine in legal contexts—to determine whether a person has been injured by the act of another, the extent of such an injury and its treatment, and whether a defendant was physically or emotionally capable of committing a crime or tort—and in related ethical and philosophical contexts—to determine when life begins (in the abortion debate) or how one evaluates "quality of life" (the euthanasia debate).

KEY TERMS:

compensable injury: an injury for which damages may be awarded

competency: the capacity to understand and act reasonably under given circumstances

diminished capacity: partial insanity; a legal determination that a defendant does not have the ability to achieve the state of mind required to commit a crime

DNA testing: a technique for identifying a person based on matching unique gene-bearing proteins (deoxyribonucleic acid, or DNA) from an organic sample taken from that person (such as hair, blood, or tissue) with another organic sample retrieved from the scene of a crime

emotional distress: damage to a plaintiff's emotional state caused by fear, anger, anxiety, stress, depression, or other negative emotions; such damage may be judged "compensable," or deserving of material compensation

euthanasia: the act of putting a person or other living being to death in order to end incurable pain or disease; popularly called "mercy killing"

forensic: having to do with a court of justice; forensic medicine and its various subspecialties apply medical science to the purposes of the law

insanity: a mental disease or defect that renders a person incapable of appreciating the wrongfulness of certain acts or of conforming to the requirements of the law

tort: a wrongful act for which civil courts, rather than criminal courts, are empowered to render justice

MEDICINE IN LEGAL AND ETHICAL DEBATES

Medicine as it relates to law is referred to as forensic medicine. Forensic medicine plays a part in three basic areas of the law. The first two involve the practical application of medicine in civil law and in criminal law. The third area involves the use of medical science to help in defining philosophical or ethical issues, such as when life begins and ends. Ethics in medicine, also called bioethics, refers to a set of moral standards and a code for behavior that govern people's interactions with one another and with society. Bioethics deals with moral issues and problems that have arisen as a result of modern medicine and research. Bioethical principles focus on autonomy (self-determination), beneficence (doing good), nonmaleficence (avoiding evil), and justice (the fair distribution of scarce resources).

In a civil case, a private party, the plaintiff, files a complaint in court against another party, the defendant, requesting that a judge or a jury settle a dispute between the two parties. A party to a civil suit can be an individual, a corporation, an association, a government organization, or any other group. A civil suit differs from a criminal case in that neither party is claiming that a crime (such as theft, kidnapping, or murder) was committed and that someone should be put in jail. Instead, the plaintiff in a civil suit is asking that the defendant pay some amount of money to the plaintiff to compensate for damages that the plaintiff has suffered because of something the defendant did.

In a criminal case, however, the state or federal government, on behalf of "the people," files a complaint with the court claiming that the defendant committed a crime, and the government seeks to have a judge or a jury determine the guilt or innocence of that defendant. If the defendant is determined to be guilty, the judge has the authority to punish the defendant, usually by imposing a fine, by requiring community service, by setting a jail sentence, or ultimately, in some states, by having the defendant put to death.

In both civil and criminal cases, medical science is called upon to provide evidence that can be used to prove or disprove a party's case. In a civil case, the parties will often resort to medical experts to determine the extent of a plaintiff's mental and physical injuries. These experts are doctors who act as witnesses in their areas of expertise and testify in a court of law. For example, a plaintiff in a civil suit might claim that he or she was born with birth defects as a result of drugs that the mother had taken during pregnancy and may present evidence of that injury and its cause by the testimony of doctors and medical research experts specializing in those related areas of medicine. Such testimony would be presented to the jury to show that the plaintiff's claim of birth defects being caused by such a drug is supported by medical research.

As medical science reveals more about the causes of disease, injuries, and the workings of the body, more distinct specialties have been created. This trend is reflected in the increasing number of expert witnesses: At the beginning of the twentieth century, a general practitioner was considered qualified to testify on most areas of medicine; today, the courts require expert witnesses to be specifically qualified in the area of medicine about which they testify.

The practice of using highly qualified and specialized doctors as expert witnesses has long been accepted by courts as an effective way to educate a jury regarding the extent, cause, and treatment of the injury in question, but there are some limitations on the use of such testimony. In order for the court to allow a medical expert to testify as to specific facts from which conclusions are to be drawn, the facts must be outside what is considered to be the general or common knowledge of a lay jury. For example, a court may not allow a party to use a medical expert to explain sprained ankles. The court would, however, allow a medical expert to explain toxic shock syndrome, because the existence, causes, and effects of that impairment are not common knowledge. The reasoning behind this limitation is that the jury members are supposed to form their own opinions when such opinions do not involve or require specialized knowledge. Only when it is necessary or helpful to the jury to be educated in a specialized area of knowledge is expert testimony usually allowed. In contrast to a lay witness, an expert witness is permitted to testify about the ultimate issue in the case. The medical expert in an accident case, for example, may testify about causation: whether the accident caused the injury that is the subject of plaintiff's lawsuit. Lay witnesses are not permitted to testify along these lines because they do not have the expertise to do so.

The court also recognizes a distinction between testimony from a medical expert and testimony from the plaintiff's treating doctor. Whereas the former educates the jury regarding an area of medicine that is relevant to the case, the latter does not. Instead, the treating doctor is called to testify to actual events or facts of the case that the doctor personally witnessed: that the plaintiff was examined on a certain date, the extent of his or her injuries, and so on. Thus, although an expert witness may not be allowed by the court to educate the jury on the subject of a sprained ankle or other topic of common knowledge, the fact that the plaintiff sustained a sprained ankle and was treated for it may be testified to by the treating doctor.

In a civil suit, the plaintiff must prove that he or she was injured by some act of the defendant. That injury can be economic (the loss of property or money), physical (such as a torn muscle or broken leg), or mental (stress or anxiety). Over the years, more and more types of injuries have become recognized as compensable injuries in civil cases. The term "pain and suffering" has been used to describe physical and emotional symptoms that a plaintiff may claim were caused by the defendant. Medical facts can help determine the existence and extent of all these types of injury.

Sometimes the expert will testify only hypothetically. In the hypothetical question, the expert may be asked to render an opinion based on certain assumptions concerning a hypothetical case that closely resembles the case at bar. The hypothetical question provides an opportunity for counsel to summarize his or her client's position. Sometimes, however, a medical expert will need to examine a plaintiff. It is not unusual for such examinations to take place years after the injury occurred, and the doctor will have to determine whether the injury exists, the extent of the injury, the cause of the injury, what (if any) limitations are caused by the injury, the treatment that is indicated, and the probable duration of the injury (perhaps based on the average rate of recovery for such an injury).

In the criminal justice system, medical experts may testify on a variety of scientific and medical issues. In the case of a murder, for example, it may be necessary to identify blood, tissue, bone, or some other human remains and to determine the source of those remains—namely, whether the remains belong to the alleged victim or perpetrator of the crime. Doctors who specialize in forensic medicine are often called upon to conduct special tests, such as DNA testing, to identify whose blood or tissue was found at the scene of a crime or on a murder weapon. Forensic experts can also determine the approximate time and cause of death. Testimony on these issues helps a jury determine the guilt or innocence of the accused.

Criminal cases occasionally also require the testimony of a forensic psychiatrist, who is an expert in mental and emotional disorders as they relate to legal principles. Testimony from such an expert assists in determining whether the defendant is "insane." According to section 4.01 of the Model Penal Code, a person is insane if he or she "lacks substantial capacity either to appreciate the criminality [wrongfulness] of his conduct or to conform his conduct to the requirements of the law." Not every state follows the Model Penal Code. Other variations of the insanity defense exist which deal with a person's ability to distinguish right from wrong. Psychiatric evaluations of the accused are performed to determine whether the defendant fit this definition at the time the crime was committed. Testimony regarding the defendant's insanity would significantly affect the case's outcome and sentencing.

A separate issue, unrelated to the defendant's mental condition at the time of the crime, is the defendant's "competency" to stand trial. According to Black's Law Dictionary (5th ed., 1979), a defendant "lacks competency to stand trial if he or she lacks capacity to understand the nature and object of the proceedings, to consult with counsel, and to assist in preparing his or her defense." The law ensures that an accused person's rights are protected by requiring that the defendant be capable of understanding these proceedings and their implications before he or she is allowed to stand trial. If either of the attorneys, or the judge, asserts that the defendant is not competent to stand trial, the court will hold a competency hearing to decide whether the defendant is "competent." In determining the competency of the defendant, the court will hear the testimony of psychiatric experts. If the defendant is determined to be incompetent at the time of the trial, the defendant will not be tried but may instead be sent to a mental institution until such time as he or she is competent to stand trial.

In addition to being used in civil cases and criminal cases, medical science is used to provide scientific information to support or disprove wholly nonscientific determinations. Such philosophical and ethical issues include abortion and euthanasia. In the long-running debate over the legality of abortion, for example, many issues and circumstances come into play, including rape and the possibility that pregnancy may endanger the woman's life. One central and hotly contested question, however, is "When does life begin?" This question may also involve an equally difficult and controversial one: "What is life?" The courts and various state legislatures have turned to medical science to address these profound, and possibly unanswerable, questions. Medical science has identified two key concepts to answer these questions: the concept of "viability" (that is, the ability of the fetus to survive outside the womb) and the distinction between the first, second, and third trimesters of a pregnancy. The distinction of trimesters was originally based on the concept of viability: A fetus generally could not survive outside the womb during the first trimester (that is, was not viable), while a fetus was generally considered viable during the third trimester. Thus, the courts and legislature would often use the concept of trimesters in determining a cutoff date after which an abortion could not be performed.

These concepts have been used as the basis for legislation to regulate and authorize abortions. Medical science is, however, a rapidly evolving field. Because it is now possible for a human egg, once fertilized, to become viable outside the womb, the legal foundation upon which abortions are based is becoming more unstable.

Another important area that has emerged from late twentieth and early twenty-first century technology concerns the use of human embryonic stem cells. Widely acknowledged as extremely valuable in assisting scientists in understanding basic mechanisms of embryo development and gene regulation, stem cell research holds the promise of enabling scientists to direct stem cells to grow into replacement organs and tissues to treat a wide variety of diseases. Embryos are valued in research for their ability to produce stem cells, which can be harvested to grow a variety of tissues for use in transplantation to treat serious illnesses such as cancer, heart disease, and diabetes.

THE APPLICATIONS OF MEDICAL TESTIMONY

Medical experts in almost every field of medicine have played a part in civil cases, criminal cases, and controversies involving philosophical and ethical issues. Sometimes, the interaction between medicine and the law has spawned new medical or legal subspecialties. In fact, medical expert testimony has become a field and an occupation in itself, supporting an entire group of medical professionals to the exclusion of medical practice. This phenomenon has in large part occurred in response to the greater acceptance by the courts of medical expert testimony and the increased reliability of recent medical testing.

Personal injury cases afford a good example of all the different types of testimony that come into play in civil suits. A physical injury case, as the name suggests, is based on a physical (or mental) injury, as opposed to a purely financial injury, suffered by the plaintiff. A physical injury case may involve an automobile accident and its resulting injuries. In such a case, doctors who are experts in the field of muscle damage, neurology (for head and nerve injuries), orthopedic surgery, and countless other areas could be called as experts, depending on the extent of the injuries.

Another type of case, called a product liability case, will often use expert medical testimony. A product liability case is one in which a person has been injured by a specific product on the market and sues the manufacturer, and often the seller, claiming that the product was defective. Famous examples of product liability cases include claims filed against manufacturers of asbestos products, certain tampons (for causing toxic shock syndrome), contraceptive devices such as the Dalkon Shield, and some generic or prescription drugs, such as thalidomide and Halcion. All these cases required medical experts in recently developed fields of medicine. Prior to the product liability suits filed against some tampon manufacturers, no one had heard of toxic shock syndrome. The testimony of medical experts was required to prove a link between an allegedly defective product and the resulting injury that was claimed. Without expert medical testimony in these cases, it would be impossible to prove that the defective products caused the injuries of which the defendants complained.

Another example of the medical profession developing to suit the law is in the area of workers' compensation. The California legislature, like the legislatures of many states, has established by statute (Labor Code section 3600 and following) a method by which to compensate any employee who has suffered a job-related injury. An employer is required by law to carry workers' compensation insurance, which will compensate an injured employee. If an employee is injured on the job in any manner, that employee is supposed to file a claim notifying his or her employer of the injury. The claim is then submitted to the workers' compensation insurance carrier. If the employer and the carrier accept liability, necessary treatment is provided to the employee. If the carrier denies further treatment or denies that an employee is disabled, the employee may file a claim with the Workers' Compensation Appeal Board. Once such a claim is filed, a judge will review all the medical reports of the injured worker. Additional medical evidence and testimony may be introduced to prove or disprove the employee's claim of injury or disability. The award of the Workers' Compensation Appeal Board is determined by the medical condition of the person claiming the injury. The growing popularity of workers' compensation has spawned an entire field of medicine, that of work-related injuries.

California courts routinely allow damages for "mental distress" in almost every type of tort action. Accordingly, psychiatrists and psychologists are routinely called upon to testify regarding whether a plaintiff has suffered such an injury. Emotional distress is not a specific medical condition, but rather a general emotional state, which may include anger, fear, frustration, anxiety, depression, and similar symptoms. Although psychiatric or psychological testimony is not required by the court for the plaintiff to recover damages for mental distress, it can be very effective in explaining to the jury the extent of the injuries and the effect of those injuries on the plaintiff's future life.

If a jury determines that the plaintiff suffered a physical or mental injury caused by the defendant, then, based on the medical testimony—of either the medical witness or the treating doctor—the jury may award any medical fees incurred, as well as anticipated medical fees and costs and compensation for the pain and suffering of the defendant. The jury may also award further damages not related to the medical condition of the plaintiff, if the case warrants such damages.

In criminal cases, particularly cases of homicide, forensic medicine often provides the key and fundamental evidence upon which the entire case is based. During the investigations of the assassination of President John F. Kennedy in the 1960's, the forensic evidence played a vital, although controversial, role. The testimony presented by the doctors who examined the president's body was used to reconstruct the crime. Forensic science was used to interpret the angle of entry of the bullets that killed Kennedy and thereby to extrapolate the source of the shots. Furthermore, forensic science was called upon to demonstrate how many shots were fired and the paths of the bullets upon entering the bodies of the president and Governor John Connally. Using medical evidence, along with other evidence, the Warren Commission concluded that the bullets all came from the book depository building behind the presidential caravan. Also using medical evidence and experts, critics of the Warren Commission's findings have alleged that the injuries suffered by the president could have been caused only by a bullet entering from the front of the president's neck and exiting the rear of the skull.

In another case, forensic evidence was able to reach a conclusive determination that certain bones were those of the Nazi war criminal Dr. Josef Mengele, known as the Angel of Death. In 1992, forensics experts discovered, using a method known as DNA testing, that some bones retrieved from a grave in Brazil were those of Mengele. In order to make this determination, doctors compared the DNA found in the blood of Mengele's son with DNA from the bones found in the grave. They found that the DNA from both sources was identical. Because DNA constitutes a "genetic fingerprint" that remains the same from parent to offspring, the doctors were able to conclude that the remains found in Brazil were those of Mengele.

DNA testing is now also commonly used in suits to determine the father of an infant. According to the Genetics Institute, DNA testing is at least 99.8 percent accurate. Medical science has so refined its ability to chart DNA "fingerprints" that the chance of coming upon two identical DNA patterns is approximately one in six billion. Prior to DNA testing, a blood testing method called human leukocyte antigen (HLA) typing was used to determine paternity, but this typing was only 95 percent accurate.

Some medical or scientific tests, while accepted by the courts, remain subject to much controversy. The Breathalyzer test, used to determine blood alcohol levels, is one such test. While the courts regularly accept the results of such tests to determine whether a suspect was intoxicated, the test is based on several assumptions and averages. Based on the alcohol content in the suspect's breath, the test extrapolates a probable amount of alcohol in the suspect's blood. The reliability of this test depends on the correct calibration of the equipment and the care of the person taking the readings. Since the tests are taken by nonmedical or nonscientific personnel in the field, mistaken readings are not uncommon. Furthermore, if the suspect used a spray breath freshener just before the test, the readings may be skewed, since such breath fresheners are usually alcohol-based.

PERSPECTIVE AND PROSPECTS

Medicine has always played some role in the outcome of court cases, but this relationship did not come into full flower until relatively recently. In the early twentieth century, courts placed strict limitations on the type and amount of medical testimony allowed into evidence. Often, certain types of medical evidence were not admissible because the science was not deemed reliable—there was too much room for error. The polygraph (lie detector), for example, could not be relied upon to reveal consistently whether a person was telling the truth, since it simply measured galvanic skin response, respiration rate, and other factors that only tend to be correlated with the subject's feelings of guilt. Most other evidence presented by medical experts concerned the likelihood of events or outcomes and therefore usually constituted opinion, rather than fact.

With the advent of new technologies in the later part of the twentieth century, medical science began to present "hard" (more precise) data that became more frequently accepted by the courts as reliable and relevant evidence. Even so, it took some time before medical scientists were able to present enough data to persuade the courts that the evidence of such methods as DNA "fingerprinting" was truly reliable. The acceptance of DNA testing, for example, was a long and hard-fought battle among legions of medical experts on both sides of the issue. Finally, DNA testing was accepted by the courts as a reliable source of evidence. As forensic medicine advances, no doubt its contribution to the law will also advance. The ability of the medical and other scientific professions to determine reliable conclusions relating to court cases is progressing rapidly with increases in scientific knowledge, methods, and technology.

In an ironic twist, however, this progress has clouded other areas of the law. In the early twentieth century, for example, no one could have dreamed of the technology that makes life support possible. With the advent of kidney dialysis machines, pacemakers, respirators, and other life support devices, medical science has achieved the ability to prolong an individual's bodily functioning. Whether this functioning alone is sufficient to define "life," however, remains a question that cannot be addressed by medical science alone but must be considered in the light of philosophical, ethical, and other values. Medicine is therefore becoming an area with which the law must contend. Issues that have challenged existing laws include abortion and the point at which life begins, euthanasia, the individual's right not to have life extended by extraordinary means if there is no hope of recovery, the right to reveal an individual's genetic predisposition toward disease, egg implantation, and genetic engineering. Medical science has propagated these dilemmas but may also be called upon to solve them.

—*Larry M. Roberts, J.D.;*
updated by Marcia J. Weiss, M.A., J.D.

See also Abortion; Animal rights vs. research; Assisted reproductive technologies; Autopsy; Blood testing; Cloning; Environmental health; Ethics; Euthanasia; Forensic pathology; Genetic engineering; In vitro fertilization; Malpractice; Occupational health; Screening.

FOR FURTHER INFORMATION:

Boumil, Marcia M., Clifford E. Elias, and Diane Bissonnette Moes. *Medical Liability in a Nutshell.* 2d ed. St. Paul, Minn.: Thomson/West, 2003. Succinctly discusses salient topics in medical liability: medical negligence, standard of care, intentional torts, informed consent and the right to refuse treatment, the duty of disclosure, causation and damages, and various defenses to liability.

Fremgen, Bonnie F. *Medical Law and Ethics.* 2d ed. Upper Saddle River, N.J.: Pearson Prentice-Hall, 2006. Essential legal and ethical principles for the health care provider. Contains case studies and legal citations.

Furrow, Barry R., et al. *Health Law: Cases, Materials, and Problems.* 5th ed. St. Paul, Minn.: West, 2004. Covers a range of issues related to health and the law, including cost control, prospective payment, health care antitrust, and federal and state regulation of health care delivery; legal and ethical issues created by reproductive technology and by the di-

lemmas of death and dying; and the core topics of professional liability and the physician-patient relationship.

Garner, Bryan A., ed. *Black's Law Dictionary.* 8th ed. St. Paul, Minn.: Thomson/West, 2004. The fundamental legal dictionary, containing definitions and examples of how the terms have been interpreted by courts.

James, Stuart H., and Jon J. Nordby, eds. *Forensic Science: An Introduction to Scientific and Investigative Techniques.* 2d ed. Boca Raton, Fla.: CRC Press, 2005. An introductory text that covers a range of topics, including trace evidence, forensic toxicology, DNA analysis, crime scene investigation, fingerprints, traumatic death, forensic anthropology, bloodstain patterns, and criminal profiling, among many others.

Jonsen, Albert R., Mark Siegler, and William J. Winslade. *Clinical Ethics: A Practical Approach to Ethical Decisions in Clinical Medicine.* 6th ed. New York: McGraw-Hill, 2006. Discusses the whole range of medical ethics, including legal issues, confidentiality, care of the dying patient, and euthanasia and assisted suicide.

Lewis, Marcia A., and Carol D. Tamparo. *Medical Law, Ethics, and Bioethics for Ambulatory Care.* 5th ed. Philadelphia: F. A. Davis, 2002. Directed to the general health care provider, the book covers practical topics such as management, guidelines and regulations for medical and allied health professionals, public duties, medical records, collection, allocation of scarce resources, genetic engineering, abortion, and life-and-death issues from the legal and ethical perspectives.

Munson, Ronald, comp. *Intervention and Reflection: Basic Issues in Medical Ethics.* 7th ed. New York: Wadsworth, 2004. An undergraduate text that combines social context, case studies, readings, and decision scenarios for topics that include abortion, advances in gene therapy, genetic discrimination, and health care rights.

Pence, Gregory E. *Classic Cases in Medical Ethics: Accounts of Cases That Have Shaped Medical Ethics, with Philosophical, Legal, and Historical Backgrounds.* 4th ed. Boston: McGraw-Hill, 2004. Surveys important cases that have defined and shaped the field of medical ethics. Each case is accompanied by careful discussion of pertinent philosophical theories and legal and ethical issues.

LEAD POISONING

DISEASE/DISORDER

ALSO KNOWN AS: Saturnism, plumbism, painter's colic

ANATOMY OR SYSTEM AFFECTED: Brain, circulatory system, endocrine system, musculoskeletal system, nervous system, reproductive system

SPECIALTIES AND RELATED FIELDS: Environmental health, pediatrics, preventive medicine, toxicology

DEFINITION: A condition caused by high levels of lead in the blood. This major preventable environmental health problem is found in both children and adults, but more frequently in children.

KEY TERMS:

arthralgia: severe joint pain, especially when inflammation is not present

chelation: the taking up or release of a metallic ion by an organic molecule

encephalopathy: any disease of the brain

lead: a limited naturally occurring element widely distributed throughout the environment by industrial uses and pollution

paresis: partial paralysis

paresthesia: an abnormal sensation, such as burning, tingling, tickling, or pricking

CAUSES AND SYMPTOMS

Lead poisoning is a major, preventable environmental health problem. Elevated lead levels in adults can increase blood pressure and cause fertility problems, nerve disorders, arthalgia, and problems with memory and concentration. Children under the age of six are at high risk for harm because their brains and nervous system are still maturing. Blood lead levels as low as 10 micrograms per deciliter are associated with harmful effects on children's ability to learn. Very high blood lead levels of 70 micrograms per deciliter can cause devastating health consequences, including seizures and other neurological symptoms, abdominal pain, developmental delays, attention deficit, hyperactivity, behavior disorders, hearing loss, anemia, coma, and death.

Children can be exposed to lead in many ways. Sources of exposure include automobile exhaust, lead-based paint, and environmental contaminants released by industrial processes that use or produce lead-containing materials. Contributors to childhood lead exposure also include lead-contaminated containers, food, dust, soil, air, and water; lead-containing ceramics and hobby supplies; substance abuse such as gaso-

line sniffing; parental transfer from lead-rich occupational environments; and traditional medicines such as azarcon and greta. Deteriorating lead-based paint in older homes is the most important source of lead exposure in children. Swallowing lead-based paint dust through normal hand-to-mouth activity or chewing directly on painted surfaces are major methods of lead ingestion. Children are often attracted to lead paint because of its sweet taste. Lead exposure in adults is usually a result of jobs in house painting, welding and smelting, the manufacturing of car batteries, and other occupations that expose them to lead.

Upon entering the human body, inorganic lead is not metabolized but is directly absorbed, distributed, and excreted. The rate at which lead is absorbed depends on its chemical and physical form and on the physiologic characteristics of the exposed person. Once in the blood, lead is distributed among three compartments: the blood; soft tissue zones such as the kidneys, bone marrow, liver, and brain; and mineralizing tissues such as bones and teeth. For lead poisoning to take place, major acute exposures to lead need not occur. The body accumulates lead and releases it slowly; therefore, even small doses over time can be toxic. It is the total body accumulation of lead that is related to the risk of adverse effects. Whether lead enters the body through inhalation or ingestion, the biologic effects are the same—interference with normal cell function and with certain physiologic processes.

By and large, children show a greater sensitivity to the effects of lead than do adults. Parents working in lead-related industries not only may inhale lead dust and lead oxide fumes but also may eat, drink, and smoke in or near contaminated areas, increasing the probability of lead ingestion and subsequent transfer to their children. Since lead readily crosses the placenta, the fetus is at risk. Fetal exposure can cause potentially

---

INFORMATION ON LEAD POISONING

CAUSES: Environmental exposure

SYMPTOMS: Varies; can include abdominal discomfort, fatigue, muscle pain, tremor, difficulty concentrating, headache, vomiting, weight loss, constipation, hearing loss, changes in consciousness

DURATION: Can be short-term or chronic

TREATMENTS: Chelation drug therapy

adverse neurological effects in utero and during post-natal development. The incomplete development of the blood-brain barrier in very young children, up to thirty-six months of age, increases the risk of the entry of lead into the developing nervous system, which can result in prolonged neurobehavioral disorders. Children absorb and retain more lead in proportion to their weight than do adults. Young children also show a greater prevalence of iron deficiency, a condition that can increase the gastrointestinal absorption of lead.

Symptoms of lead poisoning and lead intoxication vary because of differences in individual susceptibility, and the severity of symptoms increases with increased exposure. Symptoms of mild lead toxicity include abdominal discomfort, fatigue, muscle pain, or paresthesia. Moderate toxicity is indicated by arthralgia, tremor, fatigue, difficulty concentrating, headache, abdominal pain, vomiting, weight loss, and constipation. Severe toxicity symptoms include paresis or paralysis, encephalopathy, seizures, severe abdominal cramps, hearing loss, changes in consciousness, and coma.

TREATMENT AND THERAPY

If a child is suspected of having lead poisoning, laboratory tests are necessary to evaluate lead intoxication levels. Laboratory techniques defining lead toxicity include blood lead level screening, erythrocyte protoporphyrin (EP) and zinc protoporphyrin (ZPP) screening, creatinine, urinalysis, and hematocrit and hemoglobin tests with peripheral smear.

The physical examination for suspected lead poisoning cases includes special attention to hematologic, cardiovascular, gastrointestinal, and renal systems. Any neurological or behavioral changes are considered significant indicators. In addition, severe and prolonged lead poisoning may be indicated by a purplish line on the gums. A complete interview and medical evaluation of a suspected lead poisoning patient includes a full workup and medical history. Clues to potential exposure vectors can be obtained by discussing family and occupational history, use of traditional medicines, remodeling activities, hobbies, table and cookware, drinking water source, nutrition, proximity to industry or waste sites, and the physical condition and age of the patient's residence, school, and/or day care facility.

The treatment and management of lead poisoning first involves the separation of the patient from the source of lead. After a diagnosis of lead poisoning is made, local environmental health officials should be contacted to determine the lead source and what remediation action is necessary for its control. A diet high in calcium and iron may help to decrease the absorption of lead.

The Centers for Disease Control and Prevention recommends that children with blood lead levels of 45 micrograms per deciliter or greater should be referred for chelation therapy immediately. Several drugs are capable of binding or chelating lead, depleting both soft and hard (skeletal) tissues of lead and reducing its acute toxicity. All these drugs have potential side effects and must be used with caution. The most commonly used chelating agent is calcium disodium edetic acid, although several other agents are available.

—Randall L. Milstein, Ph.D.; updated by Sharon W. Stark, R.N., A.P.R.N., D.N.Sc.

See also Environmental diseases; Environmental health; Learning disabilities; Mental retardation; Occupational health; Poisoning; Safety issues for children; Screening; Toxicology.

FOR FURTHER INFORMATION:

Centers for Disease Control and Prevention. *Lead: Topic Home.* http://www.cdc.gov/lead/. This Web site provides a variety of information and sources related to lead, lead poisoning, statistics, treatment and prevention.

Goldstein, Inge F., and Martin Goldstein. *How Much Risk? A Guide to Understanding Environmental Health Hazards.* New York: Oxford University Press, 2002. A critical analysis of environmental health hazards and their threat to the public. Includes discussions of radiation from nuclear testing, radon in the home, the connection between electromagnetic fields and cancer, environmental factors and asthma, and pesticides and breast cancer.

Kessel, Irene, and John T. O'Connor. *Getting the Lead Out: The Complete Resource on How to Prevent and Cope with Lead Poisoning.* Rev. ed. Cambridge, Mass.: Perseus, 2001. A comprehensive resource for parents and homeowners describing the major sources of lead in the home and environment, as well as medical concerns, prevention strategies, and techniques for controlling lead hazards.

Morgan, Monroe T. *Environmental Health.* 3d ed. New York: Brooks Cole, 2002. Examines the links between environmental sciences and human population, focusing on the practices that support human life as well as the need to control factors that are harmful to human life.

National Safety Council. *Lead Poisoning.* http://www
.nsc.org/library/facts/lead.htm. This Web site provides an overview of lead poisoning, its sources, effects on health, treatment, and prevention.

Warren, Christian. *Brush with Death: A Social History
of Lead Poisoning.* Baltimore: Johns Hopkins University Press, 2000. Traces the history of lead poisoning from paint and gasoline in the United States.
Examines occupational, pediatric, and environmental exposure and the regulatory mechanisms, medical technologies, and epidemiological tools that arose
in response to lead poisoning.

LEARNING DISABILITIES
DISEASE/DISORDER

ANATOMY OR SYSTEM AFFECTED: Brain, nervous
system, psychic-emotional system

SPECIALTIES AND RELATED FIELDS: Neurology, pediatrics, psychology

DEFINITION: A variety of disorders involving the failure to learn an academic skill despite normal levels
of intelligence, maturation, and cultural and educational opportunity; estimates of the prevalence of
learning disabilities in the general population range
between 2 and 20 percent.

KEY TERMS:

achievement test: a measure of an individual's degree
of learning in an academic subject, such as reading,
mathematics, and written language

dyslexia: difficulty in reading, with an implied neurological cause

intelligence test: a psychological test designed to measure an individual's ability to think logically, act
purposefully, and react successfully to the environment; yields intelligence quotient (IQ) scores

neurological dysfunction: problems associated with
the way in which different sections and structures of
the brain perform tasks, such as verbal and spatial
reasoning and language production

neurology: the study of the central nervous system,
which is composed of the brain and spinal cord

perceptual deficits: problems in processing information from the environment, which may involve
distractibility, impulsivity, and figure-ground distortions (difficulty distinguishing foreground from
background)

standardized test: an instrument used to assess skill development in comparison to others of the same age
or grade

CAUSES AND SYMPTOMS

An understanding of learning disabilities must begin
with the knowledge that the definition, diagnosis, and
treatment of these disorders have historically generated
considerable disagreement and controversy. This is
primarily attributable to the fact that people with learning disabilities are a highly diverse group of individuals
with a wide variety of characteristics. Consequently,
differences of opinion among professionals remain to
such an extent that presenting a single universally accepted definition of learning disabilities is not possible.
Definitional differences most frequently center on the
relative emphases that alternative groups place on characteristics of these disorders. For example, experts in
medical fields typically describe these disorders from a
disease model and view them primarily as neurological
dysfunctions. Conversely, educators usually place
more emphasis on the academic problems that result
from learning disabilities. Despite these differences,
the most commonly accepted definitions, those developed by the United States Office of Education in 1977,
the Board of the Association for Children and Adults
with Learning Disabilities in 1985, and the National
Joint Committee for Learning Disabilities in 1981, do
include some areas of commonality.

Difficulty in academic functioning is included in the
three definitions, and virtually all descriptions of learning disabilities include this characteristic. Academic
deficits may be in one or more formal scholastic subjects, such as reading or mathematics. Often the deficits
will involve a component skill of the academic area,
such as problems with comprehension or word knowledge in reading or difficulty in calculating or applying
arithmetical reasoning in mathematics. The academic
difficulty may also be associated with more basic skills
of learning that influence functioning across academic
areas; these may involve deficits in listening, speaking,
and thinking. Dyslexia, a term for reading problems, is
the most common academic problem associated with
learning disabilities. Because reading skills are required in most academic activities to some degree,
many view dyslexia as the most serious form of learning disability.

The presumption of a neurological dysfunction as
the cause of these disorders is included, either directly
or indirectly, in each of the three definitions. Despite
this presumption, unless an individual has a known history of brain trauma, the neurological basis for learning
disabilities will not be identified in most cases because
current assessment technology does not allow for such

**INFORMATION ON
LEARNING DISABILITIES**

CAUSES: Unclear; possibly neurological deficits, genetic and hereditary influences, exposure to toxins during pregnancy or early childhood

SYMPTOMS: Difficulty in academic functioning (including deficits in listening, speaking, and thinking)

DURATION: Often chronic

TREATMENTS: Medication, patterning, teaching of specific reading skills and repeated language drills (imprinting)

precise diagnoses. Rather, at least minimal neurological dysfunction is simply assumed to be present in anyone who exhibits characteristics of a learning disorder.

The three definitions all state that individuals with learning disabilities experience learning problems despite possessing normal intelligence. This condition is referred to as a discrepancy between achievement and ability or potential.

Finally, each of the three definitions incorporates the idea that learning disabilities cannot be attributed to another handicapping condition such as mental retardation, vision or hearing problems, emotional or psychiatric disturbance, or social, cultural, or educational disadvantage. Consequently, these conditions must be excluded as primary contributors to academic difficulties.

Reports on the prevalence of learning disabilities differ according to the definitions and identification methods employed. Consequently, statistics on prevalence range between 2 and 20 percent of the population. Many of the higher reported percentages are actually estimates of prevalence that include individuals who are presumed to have a learning disorder but who have not been formally diagnosed. Males are believed to constitute the majority of individuals with learning disabilities, and estimated sex ratios range from 6:1 to 8:1. Some experts believe that this difference in incidence may reveal one of the causes of these disorders.

A number of causes of learning disabilities have been proposed, with none being universally accepted. Some of the most plausible causal theories include neurological deficits, genetic and hereditary influences, and exposure to toxins during fetal gestation or early childhood.

Evidence to support the assumption of a link between neurological dysfunction and learning disabilities has been provided by studies using sophisticated brain imaging techniques such as positron emission tomography (PET) and computed tomography (CT) scanning and magnetic resonance imaging (MRI). Studies using these techniques have, among other findings, indicated subtle abnormalities in the structure and electrical activity in the brains of individuals with learning disabilities. The use of such techniques has typically been confined to research; however, the continuing advancement of brain imaging technology holds promise not only in contributing greater understanding of the nature and causes of learning disabilities but also in treating the disorder.

Genetic and hereditary influences also have been proposed as causes. Supportive evidence comes from research indicating that identical twins are more likely to be concordant for learning disabilities than fraternal twins and that these disorders are more common in certain families.

A genetic cause of learning disabilities may be associated with extra X or Y chromosomes in certain individuals. The type and degree of impairment associated with these conditions vary according to many genetic and environmental factors, but they can involve problems with language development, visual perception, memory, and problem solving. Despite evidence to link chromosome abnormalities to those with learning disabilities, most experts agree that such genetic conditions account for only a portion of these individuals.

Exposure to toxins or poisons during fetal gestation and early childhood can also cause learning disabilities. During pregnancy nearly all substances the mother takes in are transferred to the fetus. Research has shown that mothers who smoke, drink alcohol, or use certain drugs or medications during pregnancy are more likely to have children with developmental problems, including learning disabilities. Yet not all children exposed to toxins during gestation will have such problems, and the consequences of exposure will vary according to the period when it occurred, the amount of toxin introduced, and the general health and nutrition of the mother and fetus.

Though not precisely involving toxins, two other conditions associated with gestation and childbirth have been linked to learning disabilities. The first, anoxia, or oxygen deprivation, occurring for a critical period of time during the birthing process has been tied to both mental retardation and learning disabilities. The second, and more speculative, involves exposure of the fetus to an abnormally large amount of testosterone during gestation. Differences in brain development are proposed to result from the exposure, causing learning disorders and other abnormalities. Known as the embryological theory, it may account for the large number of males with these disabilities, since they have greater amounts of testosterone than females.

The exposure of the immature brain during early childhood to insecticides, household cleaning fluids, alcohol, narcotics, and carbon monoxide, among other toxic substances, may also cause learning disabilities. Lead poisoning resulting from ingesting lead from paint, plaster, and other sources has been found in epidemic numbers in some sections of the country. Lead poisoning can damage the brain and cause learning disabilities, as well as a number of other serious problems.

The number and variety of proposed causes not only reflect differences in experts' training and consequent perspectives but also suggest the likelihood that these disorders can be caused by multiple conditions. This diversity of views also carries to methods for assessing and providing treatment and services to individuals with learning disabilities.

TREATMENT AND THERAPY

In 1975, the U.S. Congress adopted the Education for All Handicapped Children Act, which, along with other requirements, mandated that students with disabilities, including those with learning disabilities, be identified and provided appropriate educational services. Since that time, much effort has been devoted to developing adequate assessment practices for diagnosis and effective treatment strategies.

In the school setting, assessment of students suspected of having learning disabilities is conducted by a variety of professionals, including teachers specially trained in assessing learning disabilities, school nurses, classroom teachers, school psychologists, and school administrators. Collectively, these professionals are known as a multidisciplinary team. An additional requirement of this educational legislation is that parents must be given the opportunity to participate in the assessment process. Professionals outside the school setting, such as clinical psychologists and independent educational specialists, also conduct assessments to identify learning disabilities.

Because the definition of learning disabilities in the 1975 act includes a discrepancy between achievement and ability as a characteristic of the disorder, students suspected of having learning disabilities are usually administered a variety of formal and informal tests. Standardized tests of intelligence, such as the third edition of the Wechsler Intelligence Scale for Children, are administered to determine ability. Standardized tests of academic achievement, such as the Woodcock-Johnson Psychoeducational Battery and the Wide Range Achievement Test, also are administered to determine levels of academic skill.

Whether a discrepancy between ability and achievement exists to such a degree to warrant diagnosis of a learning disability is determined by various formulas comparing the scores derived from the intelligence and achievement tests. The precise methods and criteria used to determine a discrepancy vary according to differences among state regulations and school district practices. Consequently, a student diagnosed with a learning disability in one part of the United States may not be viewed as such in another area using different diagnostic criteria. This possibility has been raised in criticism of the use of the discrepancy criteria to identify these disorders. Other criticisms of the method include the use of intelligence quotient (IQ) scores (which are not as stable or accurate as many assume), the inconsistency of students' scores when using alternative achievement tests, and the lack of correspondence between what students are taught and what is tested on achievement tests.

In partial consequence of these and other problems with standardized tests, alternative informal assessment methods have been developed. One such method that is frequently employed is termed curriculum-based assessment (CBA). The CBA method uses materials and tasks taken directly from students' classroom curriculum. For example, in reading, CBA might involve determining the rate of words read per minute from a student's textbook. CBA has been demonstrated to be effective in distinguishing among some students with learning disabilities, those with other academic difficulties, and those without learning problems. Nevertheless, many professionals remain skeptical of CBA as a valid alternative to traditional standardized tests.

Other assessment techniques include vision and hearing tests, measures of language development, and tests examining motor coordination and sensory perception and processing. Observations and analyses of the classroom environment may also be conducted to determine how instructional practices and a student's behavior contribute to learning difficulties.

Based on the information gathered by the multidisciplinary team, a decision is made regarding the diagnosis of a learning disability. If a student is identified with one of these disorders, the team then develops an individual education plan to address identified educational needs. An important guideline in developing the plan is that students with these disorders should be educated to the greatest extent possible with their nonhandicapped peers, while still being provided with appropriate services. Considerable debate has occurred regarding how best to adhere to this guideline.

Programs for students with learning disabilities typically are implemented in self-contained classrooms, resource rooms, or regular classrooms. Self-contained classrooms usually contain ten to twenty students and one or more teachers specially trained to work with these disorders. Typically, these classrooms focus on teaching fundamental skills in basic academic subjects such as reading, writing, and mathematics. Depending on the teacher's training, efforts may also be directed toward developing perceptual, language, or social skills. Students in these programs usually spend some portion of their day with their peers in regular education meetings, but the majority of the day is spent in the self-contained classroom.

The popularity of self-contained classrooms has decreased significantly since the 1960's, when they were the primary setting in which students with learning disabilities were educated. This decrease is largely attributable to the stigmatizing effects of placing students in special settings and the lack of clear evidence to support the effectiveness of this approach.

Students receiving services in resource rooms typically spend a portion of their day in a class where they receive instruction and assistance from specially trained teachers. Students often spend one or two periods in the resource room with a small group of other students who may have similar learning problems or function at a comparable academic level. In the elementary grades, resource rooms usually focus on developing basic academic skills, whereas at the secondary level time is more typically spent in assisting students with their assignments from regular education classes.

Resource room programs are viewed as less restrictive than self-contained classrooms; however, they too have been criticized for segregating children with learning problems. Other criticisms center on scheduling difficulties inherent in the program and the potential for inconsistent instructional approaches and confusion over teaching responsibilities between the regular classroom and resource room teachers. Research on the effectiveness of resource room programs also has been mixed; nevertheless, they are found in most public schools across the United States.

Though they remain a minority, increasing numbers of students have their individual education plans implemented exclusively in a regular classroom. In most schools where such programs exist, teachers are given assistance by a consulting teacher with expertise in learning disabilities. Supporters of this approach point to the lack of stigma associated with segregating students and the absence of definitive research supporting other service models. Detractors are concerned about the potential for inadequate support for the classroom teacher, resulting in students receiving poor quality or insufficient services. The movement to provide services to educationally handicapped students in regular education settings, termed the Regular Education Initiative, has stirred much debate among professionals and parents. Resolution of the debate will greatly affect how individuals with learning disabilities are provided services.

No one specific method of teaching these students has been demonstrated to be superior to others. A variety of strategies have been developed, including perceptual training, multisensory teaching, modality matching, and direct instruction. Advocates of perceptual training believe that academic problems stem from underlying deficits in perceptual skills. They use various techniques aimed at developing perceptual abilities before trying to remedy or teach specific academic skills. Multisensory teaching involves presenting information to students through several senses. Instruction using this method may be conducted using tactile, auditory, visual, and kinesthetic exercises. Instruction involving modality matching begins with identifying the best learning style for a student, such as visual or auditory processing. Learning tasks are then presented via that mode. Direct instruction is based on the principles of behavioral psychology. The method involves developing precise educational goals, focusing on teaching the exact skill of concern, and providing frequent opportunities to perform the skill until it is mastered.

With the exception of direct instruction, research has generally failed to demonstrate that these strategies are uniquely effective with students with learning disabilities. Direct instruction, on the other hand, has been demonstrated effective but has also been criticized for focusing on isolated skills without dealing with the broader processing problems associated with these disorders. More promisingly, students with learning disabilities appear to benefit from teaching approaches that have been found effective with students without learning problems when instruction is geared to ability level and rate of learning.

Perspective and Prospects

Interest in disorders of learning can be identified throughout the history of medicine. The specific study of learning disabilities, however, can be traced to the efforts of a number of physicians working in the first quarter of the twentieth century who studied the brain and its associated pathology. One such researcher, Kurt Goldstein, identified a number of unusual characteristics, collectively termed perceptual deficits, which were associated with head injury.

Goldstein's work influenced a number of researchers affiliated with the Wayne County Training School, including Alfred Strauss, Laura Lehtinen, Newell Kephart, and William Cruickshank. These individuals worked with children with learning problems who exhibited many of the characteristics of brain injury identified by Goldstein. Consequently, they presumed that neurological dysfunction, whether it could specifically be identified or not, caused the learning difficulties. They also developed a set of instructional practices involving reduced environmental stimuli and exercises to develop perceptual skills. The work and writings of these individuals through the 1940's, 1950's, and 1960's were highly influential, and many programs for students with learning disabilities were based on their theoretical and instructional principles.

Samuel Orton, working in the 1920's and 1930's, also was influenced by research into brain injury in his conceptualization of children with reading problems. He observed that many of these children were left-handed or ambidextrous, reversed letters or words when reading or writing, and had coordination problems. Consequently, he proposed that reading disabilities resulted from abnormal brain development and an associated mixing of brain functions. Based on the work of Orton and his students, including Anna Gilmore and Bessie Stillman, a variety of teaching strategies were developed which focused on teaching phonics and using multisensory aids. In the 1960's, Elizabeth Slingerland applied Orton's concepts in the classroom setting, and they have been included in many programs for students with learning disabilities.

A number of other researchers have developed theories for the cause and treatment of learning disabilities. Some of the most influential include Helmer Mykelbust and Samuel Kirk, who emphasized gearing instruction to a student's strongest learning modality, and Norris Haring, Ogden Lindsley, and Joseph Jenkins, who applied principles of behavioral psychology to teaching.

The work of these and other researchers and educators raised professional and public awareness of learning disabilities and the special needs of individuals with the disorder. Consequently, the number of special education classrooms and programs increased dramatically in public schools across the United States in the 1960's and 1970's. Legislation on both state and federal levels, primarily resulting from litigation by parents to establish the educational rights of their children, also has had a profound impact on the availability of services for those with learning disabilities. The passage of the Education for All Handicapped Children Act in 1975 not only mandated appropriate educational services for students with learning disabilities but also generated funding, interest, and research in the field. The Regular Education Initiative has since prompted increased efforts to identify more effective assessment and treatment strategies and generated debates among professionals and the consumers of these services. Decisions resulting from these continuing debates will have a significant impact on future services for individuals with learning disabilities.

—*Paul F. Bell, Ph.D.*

See also Aphasia and dysphasia; Asperger's syndrome; Attention-deficit disorder; Autism; Brain; Brain disorders; Down syndrome; Dyslexia; Mental retardation; Neuralgia, neuritis, and neuropathy; Neurology; Neurology, pediatric; Psychiatry; Psychiatry, child and adolescent; Speech disorders.

For Further Information:

Bender, William N. *Learning Disabilities: Characteristics, Identification, and Teaching Strategies.* 5th ed. Boston: Pearson/Allyn & Bacon, 2004. A text with a pedagogical slant that examines the controversial issues of the changing definition of learning disabilities, theories, and medical aspects to assessment, placement, and instructional approaches.

Hallahan, Daniel P., et al. *Learning Disabilities: Foundations, Characteristics, and Effective Teaching.* 3d ed. Boston: Allyn & Bacon, 2004. This text addresses different learning disabilities and the education of the learning disabled. Includes a bibliography and indexes.

Jordan, Dale R. *Overcoming Dyslexia in Children, Adolescents, and Adults*. Austin, Tex.: Pro-Ed, 2002. Examines the role of genetics and brain development in relation to learning disabilities, and explains the perceptual and emotional nature of dyslexia. Eight "success stories," strategies for improving academic performance and social skills, and assessment checklists are included.

Learning Disabilities Association of America. http://www.ldanatl.org/. Information, publications, and referral service concerning learning disabilities. State and local groups provide services to families, including camps and recreation programs.

Levinson, Harold N. *Smart But Feeling Dumb: The Challenging New Research on Dyslexia—and How It May Help You*. Rev. ed. New York: Warner Books, 2003. Argues that the basis of dyslexia and other disorders is an inner ear dysfunction that can be cured with judicious application of the correct medications. Also discusses adults and families with dyslexia, speech disorders, and attention deficit disorders.

Lovitt, Thomas. *Introduction to Learning Disabilities*. Needham Heights, Mass.: Allyn & Bacon, 1989. This book is exceptionally well written and comprehensive in its review of topics associated with learning disabilities, including assessment and treatment issues, the history of these disorders, and recommendations for future efforts in the field.

Rief, Sandra F. *The ADHD Book of Lists: A Practical Guide for Helping Children and Teens with Attention Deficit Disorders*. San Francisco: Jossey-Bass, 2003. Designed for school personnel and parents, this resource book details recent research and strategies, supports, and interventions that help minimize the problems and optimize the success of children and teens with ADHD.

Swanson, H. Lee, Karen R. Harris, and Steve Graham, eds. *Handbook of Learning Disabilities*. New York: Guilford Press, 2003. A thorough text that synthesizes current understanding on the nature of learning disabilities, their causes, and how students with these difficulties can be identified and helped to succeed.

LEGIONNAIRES' DISEASE
DISEASE/DISORDER

ANATOMY OR SYSTEM AFFECTED: Chest, lungs, respiratory system

SPECIALTIES AND RELATED FIELDS: Bacteriology, environmental health, epidemiology, internal medicine, public health

DEFINITION: A rapidly progressing bacterial pneumonia caused by infection with an organism of the genus *Legionella* and characterized by influenza-like illness, with high fever, chills, headache, and muscle aches.

KEY TERMS:

alveolus: an outpouching of lung tissue in which gas exchange takes place between air in the lungs and blood capillaries

legionellosis: another name for any infection caused by a member of the genus *Legionella*; generally denotes Legionnaires' disease

macrophage: any of a variety of phagocytic cells; macrophages are found in highest numbers in tissue; alveolar macrophages are found in lungs and function to remove respiratory pathogens

phagocytes: white cells capable of ingesting and digesting microbes, a process referred to as phagocytosis; primarily refers to neutrophils and macrophages

Pontiac fever: a self-limiting, nonpneumonic disease caused by *Legionella* bacteria; clinically and epidemiologically distinct from Legionnaires' disease

virulence factor: a bacterial factor that enhances the pathogenic potential of the organism; includes products such as toxins and capsules

CAUSES AND SYMPTOMS

Legionnaires' disease, or legionellosis, is an acute bacterial pneumonia that was unknown prior to 1976. In July and August of that year, an outbreak of pneumonia occurred among persons who had either attended an American Legion convention in Philadelphia or had been in the vicinity of the Bellevue-Stratford Hotel in the downtown area. The likely source of the epidemic was a contaminated air-conditioning unit in the hotel. Though speculation among the media and general public suggested all sorts of causes for the epidemic, the specific etiological agent was isolated by January, 1977. It turned out to be a somewhat common bacterium, which was subsequently given the genus and species names *Legionella pneumophila*; the genus name reflected the first known victims, while the species name meant "lung-loving."

Within several years, additional strains of *Legionella* bacteria were isolated from patients suffering from bacterial pneumonia. Through 2005, forty-one species have been identified, of which eighteen have been associated with human disease. Most cases of Legionnaires' disease have been linked to infection by *L. pneumophila* or, to a lesser degree, *L. micdadei*.

Genetic evidence confirmed that *Legionella* was indeed a newly isolated bacterium. Several factors contributed to its previous invisibility. First, Legionnaires' disease is similar in its characteristics to other forms of nonbacterial pneumonia, such as that caused by viruses. Since no bacteria were readily isolated, there was no immediate reason to suspect a bacterium as the infectious agent. The second reason related to the initial difficulty of growing *Legionella* bacteria in the laboratory. Aspirates from pneumonia victims were inoculated onto routine laboratory media; most common bacteria grow quite readily on such media. No growth was observed, however, in the case of *Legionella*. Many nutrient supplements were tried. *Legionella* bacteria grew only on media that were supplemented with iron and the amino acid cysteine. Since the early 1980's, the medium of choice has been agar containing buffered charcoal yeast extract (BCYE). Nutrients such as amino acids, vitamins, and iron are included in the medium while the charcoal removes potentially toxic materials.

Legionellosis actually constitutes two separate clinical entities: Legionnaires' disease and Pontiac fever. Legionnaires' disease is potentially the more serious of the two. The victim is initially infected through a respiratory route. In general, the source of the infection is an aerosol generated by contaminated water supplies such as those found in the cooling units of building air-conditioning systems. Rarely, if at all, does the disease pass from person to person. Most infections are unapparent, with either mild disease or none at all. The estimate is that less than 5 percent of exposed individuals actually contract Legionnaires' disease. Certain factors seem to increase the chances that the infection will progress toward pneumonia. Often, the lungs of the victim have suffered from previous trauma, such as that caused by emphysema or smoking. The person is generally, though not always, middle-aged or older. These observations suggest that, in most instances, the person's immune system is quite capable of handling the infection.

The disease begins with a dry cough, muscle aches, and rising fever—symptoms that resemble the flu. The person may also suffer from vomiting and diarrhea. In

---

INFORMATION ON LEGIONNAIRES' DISEASE

CAUSES: Bacterial infection
SYMPTOMS: Dry cough, muscle aches, rising fever, possible vomiting and diarrhea
DURATION: Acute
TREATMENTS: Antibiotics (erythromycin, rifampin)

---

serious cases, the disease becomes progressively more severe over the next three to six days. The alveoli, or air sacs, of the lung become necrotized, increasing the difficulty in breathing. Small abscesses may also form in the lungs, as phagocytes infiltrate the area. The mortality rate has ranged from 15 to 60 percent in various outbreaks, although with early treatment, these numbers can be significantly lowered. Patients with other underlying lung problems, or who may be immunosuppressed, are at particular risk.

Pontiac fever is a much less serious form of disease. Named for the Michigan city in which a 1968 outbreak occurred in the Public Health Department building, the disease is self-limiting, nonpneumonic, and not life-threatening. Pontiac fever also seems to follow the inhalation of the etiological agent. Though the attack rate in exposed individuals appears to approach 100 percent, there is no infiltration of lung tissue and no abscess formation. A febrile period occurs one to two days following infection, with the individual progressing to recovery after several days. The difference between the two forms of disease remains obscure. There appears to be no obvious difference between the organisms associated with the two diseases, though strains associated with Pontiac fever may not replicate as readily inside human cells.

The mechanism by which infection by *Legionella* bacteria results in pneumonia is not altogether clear. Research into this area has centered on forms of virulence factors produced by the organism and their relationships to disease. Following their infiltration into the lung, *Legionella* bacteria are phagocytized by alveolar macrophages or other leukocytes (white blood cells). Unlike other ingested microbes, however, *Legionella* bacteria often survive the process and begin a process of intracellular replication. In this intracellular state, *Legionella* bacteria are shielded from many of the host's immune defenses.

Certain questions lend themselves to understanding

this approach in elucidating the mechanisms of Legionnaires' disease. First, are intracellular survival and multiplication necessary factors in the development of the disease? Second, if these factors are indeed relevant, exactly how does the organism manage to evade the killing mechanisms that exist inside the cell?

The first question has been dealt with by various animal studies. Guinea pigs were exposed to a *Legionella* aerosol, and lung aspirates were prepared after forty-eight hours. Large numbers of viable organisms were found inside alveolar macrophages. Few live *Legionella* bacteria, however, were observed outside cells. In addition, mutant *Legionella* bacteria that were incapable of intracellular growth showed reduced virulence in guinea pigs. Therefore, initial intracellular infection and multiplication does appear to be necessary to initiate the disease process.

The mechanism of intracellular survival is less clear. Macrophages are phagocytes that have a wide variety of means for killing ingested microorganisms. These mechanisms range from the production of reactive oxygen molecules to the synthesis of oxidizing agents such as peroxides. In addition, after a foreign microbe has been phagocytized within the membrane-bound vessel called a phagosome, a cell organelle, the lysosome, will fuse with the phagosome. Contained within the lysosome are large numbers of digestive enzymes that proceed to digest the target. Under normal circumstances, foreign microbes are ingested and digested, eliminating the threat of infection.

Somehow, *Legionella* bacteria evade these defense mechanisms. Different strains of *Legionella* bacteria appear to have evolved a variety of mechanisms for survival. In particular, there are two types of molecules, a phosphatase and a cytotoxin, whose presence is correlated with intracellular survival. Both appear to act by preventing the phagocytes from producing potentially lethal oxidation molecules such as hydrogen peroxide.

Another virulence factor that appears to be important for infectivity is a surface protein known as the macrophage infectivity potentiator, or MIP. The MIP proteins are apparently unique to *Legionella* bacteria; mutants that lack the MIP gene are significantly less virulent than wild-type strains. The MIP protein appears to be necessary for the internalization of *Legionella* bacteria by the macrophage, and for survival against the array of bacteriocidal activities.

A variety of other mechanisms may also exist that allow *Legionella* bacteria to escape the killing mechanisms of the macrophage. For example, in addition to the phosphatase, which removes phosphate molecules from host proteins or lipids, *Legionella* bacteria also produce protein kinases, which can add phosphate molecules to host cell proteins. In this manner, *Legionella* bacteria can potentially regulate the metabolism of the cells in which they find themselves by adding or subtracting phosphates from various sites or metabolic pathways.

Though a precise sequence of events that leads to the development of Legionnaires' disease remains to be worked out, certain steps appear to be necessary. Following the inhalation of a *Legionella* aerosol, probably from a contaminated water source, the organism lodges in the alveoli of the lung. Resident macrophages phagocytize the microbe, resulting in its internalization. Through a variety of virulence factors, *Legionella* survives, and multiplies within the macrophage. Death of the host cells along with the concomitant infiltration of other white cells results in the inflammation and lung damage recognized as Legionnaires' disease.

TREATMENT AND THERAPY

Despite the hysteria associated with the Philadelphia outbreak of Legionnaires' disease and the difficulty associated with the initial isolation of the etiological agent, there is nothing particularly unusual about the organism. The *Legionella* bacterium is a small, thin microbe some 2 to 10 micrometers in length, about the size of most average bacteria. Because of its characteristic staining pattern, it is classified as a gram-negative organism. This results from the molecular nature of its cell wall, which has a high lipopolysaccharide (LPS) content.

Since legionellosis can resemble other forms of pneumonia, improper diagnosis can be a problem. Though the prognosis of the disease is generally favorable with early intervention, improper or delayed treatment can prove fatal. In general, legionellosis is suspected in a patient with a progressive pneumonia for which other organisms do not appear to be a factor.

Legionnaires' disease pneumonia may be diagnosed microbiologically in a number of ways. The simplest, most rapid, and least costly test is the urinary antigen. The test is available only for *L. pneumophila* serogroup 1, but this organism is responsible for 80 percent of pneumonia cases. The antigen is detectable in the urine three days after symptoms begin and persists for several weeks. Expectorated sputum or secretions obtained through bronchoscopy may be stained and cultured. A special stain to visualize the bacteria through the microscope, called direct fluorescent antibody (DFA), is very specific but not very sensitive, because it requires large numbers of bacteria to be positive and such number are usually present only in the most severe cases. The definitive diagnostic method is culture using BCYE media. The bacteria grow slowly and colonies become visible only after three to five days of incubation. Lastly, blood (sera) may be collected as acute and convalescent specimens. A fourfold rise in the antibody titer is considered diagnostic. A single specimen of high titer (1:128 dilution or higher) is considered presumptive, but not definitive, evidence of infection. In the case of Pontiac fever, serologic testing is the usual method for diagnosis.

There are several aspects of the clinical significance of the gram-negative character of the organism, one of which is that this type of bacteria responds poorly to penicillin or penicillin derivatives. This serves to limit the type of antimicrobial therapy available for treatment of severe cases of legionellosis. Other antibiotics exist, of course, that exhibit antibacterial characteristics similar to those of penicillin—for example, the cephalosporins. And, indeed, penicillin derivatives have been used to treat at least some types of gram-negative infections. Legionellosis patients did not respond well, however, to treatment with any of these agents. It was subsequently found that the basis for the resistance by *Legionella* bacteria to these antibiotics lay in a type of extracellular enzyme produced by these bacteria—a beta-lactamase.

The lack of pharmacologic activity associated with the penicillins, the cephalosporins, and certain other antibiotics is thus easy to explain. The activity of these antibiotics is associated with the presence of a structure in the molecule called a beta-lactam ring. The beta-lactamase produced by the *Legionella* bacterium causes a break in the ring, rendering the antibiotic harmless to the microbe, and thus useless as a form of treatment. Such resistance has become increasingly common among bacteria, since the genes encoding the beta-lactamase are passed from organism to organism.

Fortunately, other antibiotics did prove to be useful in the treatment of legionellosis. To a certain extent, the determination of the antibiotics of choice was fortuitous. During the Philadelphia outbreak, the nature of the illness was unknown. The primary assumption was that an infectious agent was at fault, but determination of the nature of that agent lay months beyond the extent of the epidemic. Therefore, as would be true in the

treatment of any illness of unknown origin, various treatments were carried out. Two antibiotics in particular proved to be useful: erythromycin and rifampin. Erythromycin, which specifically inhibits bacterial protein synthesis, has continued to be useful. Though long-term use can result in liver damage and some individuals are hypersensitive to the drug, the intravenous administration of erythromycin remains the treatment of choice for legionellosis. Rifampin is used on occasion in association with other methods of treatment, but the high frequency of bacterial resistance to the drug precludes its use as a treatment of first choice.

Since the virulent properties of the *Legionella* bacterium depend on its intracellular presence in the macrophage, those antimicrobial agents that exhibit intracellular penetration would be expected to be most effective. Erythromycin fits this requirement, as do a number of other antibiotics. Newer antibiotics with intracellular activity have replaced erythromycin and rifampin as first choices for treatment of Legionnaires' disease pneumonia. Azithromycin, a macrolide antibiotic similar to erythromycin, yields higher intracellular levels than erythromycin and has proven to be more effective. Alternative monotherapy can be employed using one of the new respiratory fluoroquinolones such as levofloxacin or moxifloxacin. The quinolones are used for those who have undergone transplantation, as they do not interfere with the immunosuppressive drugs used in these patients.

Other aspects of treatment center on maintaining the comfort of the individual. This may include the use of analgesics for relief of pain. Pontiac fever is a self-limiting disease and requires only such symptomatic therapy.

Prevention of the disease is obviously preferable to dealing with the sequelae of infection. Epidemiological studies have demonstrated that the *Legionella* bacterium is a common soil organism that is often found in bodies of water contaminated by soil. The organism has been found in lakes and pond water, and it can survive for long periods in unchlorinated tap water. In fact, contaminated water appears to have been the source of infection for most outbreaks of the illness. Problems have often been associated with cooling towers, evaporative condensers, and other water supplies found with air-conditioning units of buildings. Infectious aerosols may be generated from these units, allowing for a respiratory route of infection. Though the disease is thus spread in an airborne manner, there is no evidence that it can be passed from person to person.

The epidemiological evidence for the disease supports an airborne hypothesis. Most outbreaks have occurred in regions of soil disruption, such as that occurring during construction. Subsequent isolation of *Legionella* bacteria from the cooling towers confirmed such contamination. Though the air-conditioning unit of the Bellevue-Stratford Hotel in Philadelphia was replaced prior to isolation of the organism, the assumption is that the unit was contaminated. The outbreaks of the disease during the summer, when air-conditioning use has peaked, are consistent with the role of air-conditioning units in the spread of *Legionella* bacteria.

The method by which the *Legionella* bacterium survives in the environment has not been completely determined. The organism is somewhat resistant both to chlorine treatment and to heat as high as 65 degrees Celsius. It appears to grow best in the presence of biological factors secreted by other microflora in the environment; growth stimulation may also be enhanced by the presence of physical factors such as sediment, silicone, and rubber compounds. Its ability to survive, and indeed be transmitted, may also be related to its tendency to penetrate and multiply intracellularly within environmental protozoa or amoeba.

Prevention of disease transmission must take into account these problems. Contamination of water supplies must be minimized. The resistance of the *Legionella* bacterium to standard methods of decontamination has made the process more difficult, and methods of choice remain controversial. Chlorination at relatively high levels remains the preferred method, with subsequent treatment at lower concentrations over the long term. The disadvantages of this method include the cost of constant treatment and the eventual corrosion of the units. Continuous or intermittent heating of the water has also proved effective in decontamination.

PERSPECTIVE AND PROSPECTS

Prior to August, 1976, Legionnaires' disease was unknown. From July 21 to 24 of that year, however, the Pennsylvania branch of the American Legion held its annual convention at the Bellevue-Stratford Hotel in Philadelphia. Some 4,000 delegates and their families attended the festivities. Following the convention, as delegates returned to their homes, a mysterious illness began to appear among the attendees. A total of 149 conventioneers and 72 others became ill. Characterized by a severe respiratory infection that progressed into pneumonia, and high fever, the illness proved fatal to 34 of the victims.

By August, it became clear to the Pennsylvania Department of Health that an epidemic was at hand. The cause of the outbreak was not clear, and rumors began to circulate. At various times, the news media explained the outbreak as a Communist plot against former military men, a Central Intelligence Agency test gone awry, and even an infectious agent arriving from space. The truth was less dramatic. By the beginning of 1977, David Fraser, Joseph McDade, and their colleagues from the Centers for Disease Control isolated the etiological agent: a bacterium subsequently named *Legionella pneumophila*.

With the isolation and identification of the organism, it became possible to explain earlier outbreaks of unusual illness. For example, during July and August of 1965, an outbreak of pneumonia at a chronic-care facility at St. Elizabeth's Hospital in Washington, D.C., resulted in 81 cases and 14 deaths. An outbreak among personnel at the Oakland County Health Department in Pontiac, Michigan, during July and August of 1968 of a disease that was subsequently called Pontiac fever was also traced to the same organism. In this case, however, though 144 persons were affected, none died. In fact, illness associated with the *Legionella* bacterium has been traced as far back as 1947. The 1976 outbreak was not new; it was merely the first time that medical personnel were able to isolate the organism that caused the disease.

The precise prevalence of the *Legionella* bacterium remains murky, but it is clearly more common than was at first realized. Despite the public's fear of the disease, in most instances it probably remains a mild respiratory infection, resembling nothing worse than a bad cold. Most cases remain undetected. A study of hospitalized community-acquired pneumonia patients conducted in Ohio showed that about 3 percent of cases were caused by *Legionella*. Estimates have suggested that as many as 25,000 persons in the United States develop infection. Based on seroconversions—the production of anti-*Legionella* antibody in the sera of persons—it has been estimated that more than 20 percent of the population of Michigan has been exposed to the organism. There is no reason to doubt that the same situation exists in many other states. In addition to sporadic cases, outbreaks continue to occur around the world. The most recent large outbreak was in Toronto. A colonized air-conditioning cooling tower atop the Seven Oaks Home for the Aged caused illness in 127 residents and workers, and 20 of the residents died.

The basis for the difference in severity between Legionnaires' disease and Pontiac fever is also unclear. There is no obvious difference between the two diseases that accounts for the differences in virulence. It also remains to be seen whether *Legionella* bacteria are associated with other illnesses.

The final lesson of Legionnaires' disease is as subtle as its initial appearance. Humans exist in an environment replete with infectious agents. Despite the battery of modern methods of treatment for illness, there always remains the potential for new outbreaks of previously unknown disease.

—*Richard Adler, Ph.D.;*
updated by H. Bradford Hawley, M.D.

See also Bacterial infections; Epidemiology; Lungs; Pneumonia; Pulmonary diseases; Pulmonary medicine; Pulmonary medicine, pediatric; Respiration.

FOR FURTHER INFORMATION:

Brock, Thomas D., ed. *Microorganisms: From Smallpox to Lyme Disease.* New York: W. H. Freeman, 1990. A collection of readings from *Scientific American.* The book includes a collection of accounts of the history of major infectious diseases. Divided into sections dealing with medical histories, methods of prevention, and means of transmission.

Dowling, John N., Asish K. Saha, and Robert H. Glew. "Virulence Factors of the Family *Legionellaceae.*" *Microbiological Reviews* 56 (March 1, 1992): 32. A thorough discussion of the roles played by various virulence factors related to intracellular survival of the bacterium. A review article for which basic knowledge of microbiology would be helpful. Nevertheless, the article contains a wealth of information on the subject.

Frank, Steven A. *Immunology and Evolution of Infectious Disease.* Princeton, N.J.: Princeton University Press, 2002. Blends research from molecular biology, immunology, pathogen biology, and population dynamics to discuss how and why parasites vary to escape recognition by the immune system, vaccine design, and the control of epidemics.

Gorbach, Sherwood L., John G. Bartlett, and Neil R. Blacklow, eds. *Infectious Diseases.* 3d ed. Philadelphia: W. B. Saunders, 2004. A thorough discussion of infectious diseases. Included is a brief history, an account of the mechanisms of disease and immunity, and a concise discussion of a broad range of infectious agents.

Hoebe, Christian J. P. A., and Jacob L. Kool. "Control of *Legionella* in Drinking-Water Systems." *The Lancet* 355, no. 9221 (June 17, 2000): 2093-2094. This article discusses the process of copper-silver ionization for the control of *Legionella.* This process has reduced *Legionella* counts when used simultaneously with continuous chlorine injection.

Kasper, Dennis L., et al., eds. *Harrison's Principles of Internal Medicine.* 16th ed. New York: McGraw-Hill, 2005. The standard textbook of internal medicine with an excellent chapter on Legionnaires' disease.

Ryan, Kenneth J., and C. George Ray, eds. *Sherris Medical Microbiology: An Introduction to Infectious Diseases.* 4th ed. New York: McGraw-Hill, 2004. A textbook dealing with major pathogenic organisms. The section on *Legionella* is a concise outline of what is known about the disease.

Springston, John. "*Legionella* Bacteria in Building Environments." *Occupational Hazards* 61, no. 8 (August, 1999): 51-56. *Legionella* bacteria tend to be unwanted occupants of the building environment. Their ability to contaminate domestic water systems, coupled with their potential to cause severe health complications, presents a very real concern to building owners and managers.

LEISHMANIASIS

DISEASE/DISORDER

ALSO KNOWN AS: Kala-azar

ANATOMY OR SYSTEM AFFECTED: Bones, immune system, lymphatic system, skin

SPECIALTIES AND RELATED FIELDS: Family medicine, public health

DEFINITION: A complex of diseases caused by protozoan parasites of the genus *Leishmania.*

CAUSES AND SYMPTOMS

Leishmaniasis, also known as kala-azar in its visceral form, is a parasitic disease that strikes nearly 2 million persons each year. At least 350 million persons, from eighty-eight subtropical and tropical countries around the world, are at risk of contracting the disease. Leishmaniasis has received more attention among United States' medical authorities because of the risk of contracting the disease faced by U.S. military personnel in Southwest Asia, including Iraq, and Central Asia, including Afghanistan. Leishmaniasis may be a contributor to the complex of illnesses called Gulf War syndrome reported from veterans of the first Persian Gulf War in 1991.

INFORMATION ON LEISHMANIASIS

CAUSES: Transmission of protozoa through sandflies

SYMPTOMS: Skin infection and ulcers; vomiting, fever, abdominal discomfort, diarrhea, weight loss, and cough in children; also fatigue, weakness, and appetite loss in adults; darkening, dry, and flaky skin; thinning hair; enlargement of spleen, liver, and lymph nodes

DURATION: Often chronic

TREATMENTS: Medications containing the mineral antimony (meglumine antimonite, stibogluconate) and sometimes amphotericin B, pentamidine, flagyl, and allopurinol; plastic surgery to correct disfigurement; removal of spleen

Leishmaniasis is caused by any of more than twenty species of the protozoan parasite *Leishmania*. They are transmitted by the bites of sandflies, small bloodsucking insects in the subfamily Phlebotominae. Humans are one of many mammalian hosts of these parasites. Infection can cause skin disease, called cutaneous leishmaniasis. *Leishmania* can also affect the mucous membranes, frequently resulting in ulcers, or cause systemic disease called visceral leishmaniasis, which is often fatal. Infection in children is usually sudden, with symptoms including vomiting, fever, abdominal discomfort, diarrhea, weight loss, and cough. Adults suffer from similar symptoms, but they may be accompanied by nonspecific symptoms such as fatigue, weakness, and loss of appetite. The skin may become darker, dry, and flaky, and the hair may begin to thin. Other signs include an enlarged spleen, liver, and lymph nodes.

Diagnosis is based on demonstration of the organism in spleen pulp, lymph nodes, liver, or peripheral blood. Species of *Leishmania* cannot be differentiated morphologically. They are distinguished on the basis of the disease produced, the host and its immune response, and geographical distribution.

TREATMENT AND THERAPY

Compounds containing the mineral antimony are the principal medications used to treat leishmaniasis. These compounds include meglumine antimonite and sodium stibogluconate. When these drugs are ineffective, other antiprotozoan medications may be utilized, including amphotericin B, pentamidine, flagyl, and allopurinol. With mucocutaneous leishmaniasis, plastic surgery may be needed to correct the disfigurement caused by destructive facial lesions. Removal of the spleen may be required in drug-resistant cases of visceral leishmaniasis. Relapse may occur and infection may persist despite treatment.

PERSPECTIVE AND PROSPECTS

Cases of infection by *Leishmania* have been reported on all the continents except Australia. In the Americas, *Leishmania* can be found from southern Mexico into the South American continent. The disease is widespread in the tropics. In the United States, cases have been reported in dogs, cats, and humans in Texas, Ohio, and Oklahoma.

The prognosis for leishmaniasis is quite variable and depends on the specific strain of infecting protozoan, as well as on the individual patient's immune system response to infection. Cure rates are high with antimony compounds. There are no preventive vaccines. Preventing sandfly bites is the most immediate form of protection. Insect repellent, appropriate clothing, screening of windows, and fine mesh netting will reduce exposure.

—Jason A. Hubbart, M.S.;
updated by David M. Lawrence

See also Bites and stings; Insect-borne diseases; Parasitic diseases; Protozoan diseases; Tropical medicine; Ulcers.

FOR FURTHER INFORMATION:

Chang, K.-P., and R. S. Bray, eds. *Leishmaniasis*. New York: Elsevier, 1985.

Hide, G., et al. *Trypanosomiasis and Leishmaniasis: Biology and Control*. Wallingford, Oxon, Eng.: CAB International, 1997.

Lane, R. P. "Sandflies (Phlebotominae)." In *Medical Insects and Arachnids*, edited by Richard P. Lane and Roger W. Crosskey. New York: Chapman & Hall, 1993.

Raghunath, D., and R. Nayak, eds. *Trends and Research in Leishmaniasis: With Particular Reference to Kala Azar*. New York: Tata/McGraw-Hill, 2005.

Ryan, Kenneth J., and C. George Ray, eds. *Sherris Medical Microbiology: An Introduction to Infectious Diseases*. 4th ed. New York: McGraw-Hill, 2004.

LEPROSY

DISEASE/DISORDER

ALSO KNOWN AS: Hansen's disease

ANATOMY OR SYSTEM AFFECTED: Immune system, nerves, nervous system, skin

SPECIALTIES AND RELATED FIELDS: Bacteriology, epidemiology, immunology, internal medicine, public health

DEFINITION: A bacterial infection that affects skin and nerves, causing symptoms ranging from mild numbness to gross disfiguration.

KEY TERMS:

acid-fast: the ability of a bacterium to retain a pink stain in the presence of a mixture of acid and alcohol

antibody: a protein found in the blood and produced by the immune system in response to bodily contact with an antigen

antigen: a foreign substance (such as a bacterium, toxin, or virus) to which the body makes an immune response

bacillus Calmette-Guérin (BCG): a vaccine for tuberculosis made from a harmless strain of *Mycobacterium bovis*

bacterium: microscopic single-celled organism that multiplies by simple division; bacteria are found everywhere; most are beneficial, but a few species cause disease

cellular immune response: the reaction of the body that produces active white blood cells that can destroy antigens associated with other body cells

humoral immune response: the reaction of the body that produces antibodies that can destroy antigens present in body fluids

hypersensitivity: an overreaction by the immune system to the presence of certain antigens; this overreaction often results in some damage to the person as well as the antigen

immune response: the working of the body's immune system to prevent or combat an infectious disease

CAUSES AND SYMPTOMS

Leprosy, also known as Hansen's disease, is caused by the bacterium *Mycobacterium leprae (M. leprae)*. Humans are the only natural host for this bacterium; it can be found only in leprosy victims. Most people who are exposed to this bacterium are unaffected by it; in the remainder, the bacterium grows inside skin and nerve cells, causing a wide range of symptoms that depend upon the person's immune response to the growth of the bacteria.

M. leprae is an obligate intracellular parasite, which means that it can grow only inside other cells. *M. leprae* has a unique waxy coating that helps to protect it while it is growing inside human skin and nerve cells. The bacterium grows very slowly, dividing once every twelve days, whereas the average bacterium will divide every twenty to sixty minutes. *M. leprae* grows best at temperatures slightly below body temperature (37 degrees Celsius). The leprosy bacterium is the only bacterium known to destroy peripheral nerve tissue (nerves that are not a part of the central nervous system) and will also destroy skin and mucous membranes. This bacterium is closely related to the bacterium that causes tuberculosis: *Mycobacterium tuberculosis*.

Leprosy is not very contagious. Several attempts to infect human volunteers with the bacteria have been unsuccessful. It is believed that acquiring leprosy from an infected person requires prolonged intimate contact with that person, such as living in the same house for a long time. Although the precise mode of transmission of *M. leprae* bacteria is unclear, it is highly probable that the bacteria are transferred from the nasal or respiratory secretions of the victim to the nasal passages or a skin wound of the recipient.

Once inside a person, *M. leprae* will grow and reproduce inside skin and nerve cells and destroy tissue. The exact mechanism of tissue destruction is not understood, but it probably results from a combination of nerve damage, massive accumulation of bacteria, and immunological reactions. Because the bacteria grow so slowly, the length of time from infection to appearance of the symptoms (the incubation period) is quite long. The average incubation period is two to seven years, but incubation can range from three months to forty years. Since the bacteria prefer temperatures slightly lower than normal body temperature, symptoms appear first in the cooler parts of the body, such as the hands, fingers, feet, face, nose, and earlobes. In severe cases, symptoms also appear in the eyes and the respiratory tract.

The symptoms associated with leprosy can range from very mild to quite severe, and the symptoms that a person gets depend heavily on that person's ability to mount a cellular immune response against the bacteria. In a normal infection, the human body is capable of defending itself through two processes of the immune system; the humoral immune response and the cellular immune response. The humoral response produces chemicals called antibodies that can attack and destroy infectious agents that are present in body fluids such as the blood. The cellular response produces white blood cells that can destroy infectious agents that are associated with cells. Since *M. leprae* hides and grows inside human cells, a cellular response is the only type of immune response that can be of any help in fighting the infection. The ability to generate a cellular immune response against *M. leprae* is dependent upon the genetic makeup and overall health of the victim, as well as the number of infecting bacteria and their ability to invade the body and cause disease. A quick and strong cellular response by a person infected with *M. leprae* will result in no symptoms or in the mild form of the disease: tuberculoid leprosy. A slow or weak cellular response by a person exposed to leprosy may result in the more severe form of the disease: lepromatous leprosy.

Only one in two hundred people exposed to leprosy will get some form of the disease. The earliest symptom is a slightly bleached, flat lesion several centimeters in diameter that is usually found on the upper body or on the arms or legs. About three-fourths of all patients with an early solitary lesion heal spontaneously; the rest progress to tuberculoid or lepromatous leprosy or to one of the many forms that fall between these two extremes.

Tuberculoid leprosy is characterized by flat skin lesions 5 to 20 centimeters in diameter. The lesions are lighter in color than the surrounding skin and are sometimes surrounded by nodules (lumps). The lesions contain only a few bacteria, and they, along with the surrounding tissue, are numb. These lesions are caused by a hypersensitive cellular immune response to the bacteria in the nerves and skin. In an attempt to destroy the bacteria, the immune system overreacts, and some of the surrounding nerve and skin tissue is damaged while the bacteria are being killed. This causes the areas of the skin to lose pigment as well as sensation. Often, tuberculoid leprosy patients can experience more extensive physical damage if the numbness around the lesions leads to accidental loss of digits, skin, and so forth. Leprosy victims may burn and cut themselves unknowingly, since they have no feeling in certain areas of their bodies.

INFORMATION ON LEPROSY

CAUSES: Bacterial infection
SYMPTOMS: Skin lesions, numbness, disfiguration
DURATION: Lifelong
TREATMENTS: Antibiotics

In lepromatous leprosy, the bacteria grow unchecked because of the weak cellular immune response. Often, there are more than 100 million bacterial cells present per square centimeter of tissue. These bacteria cause the formation of tumorlike growths called lepromas as well as tissue destruction of the skin and mucous membranes. Also, the presence of so many bacteria causes large numbers of antibacterial antibodies to be produced, but these antibodies are of no benefit in fighting off the infection. Instead, they can contribute to the formation of lesions and tissue damage both internally and on the skin through a process called immune complex hypersensitivity. This is a process whereby the large number of antibodies bind to the large number of bacteria in the body and form immune complexes. These complexes can be deposited in various parts of the body and trigger a chemical reaction that destroys the surrounding tissue. The large number of bacteria puts pressure on the nerves and destroys nerve tissue, which causes loss of sensation and tissue death.

The initial symptoms of lepromatous leprosy are skin lesions that can be spread out or nodular and are found on the cooler parts of the body, such as the inside of the nose, the front part of the eye, the face, the earlobes, the hands, and the feet. Often, the victim loses all facial features because the nodules enlarge the face, and the eyebrows and nose deteriorate, giving the victim a characteristic lionlike appearance. Severe lepromatous leprosy erodes bones; thus, fingers and toes become needlelike, pits form in the skull, nasal bones are destroyed, and teeth fall out. Also, the limbs become twisted and the hands become clawed. The destruction of the nerves leads to the inability to move the hands or feet, deformity of the feet, and chronic ulceration of the limbs. In addition, as is the case with tuberculoid leprosy, destruction of the small peripheral nerves leads to self-inflicted trauma and secondary infection (infection by another bacterium or virus). As the disease progresses, the growth of bacteria in the respiratory tract causes larynx problems and difficult breathing. Deterioration of the optic nerve leads to blindness. Bacteria can invade the bloodstream and spread infection throughout the whole body except the central nervous system. Death associated with leprosy usually results from respiratory obstruction, kidney failure, or secondary infection.

TREATMENT AND THERAPY

A physician can tell whether a person has leprosy by looking for characteristic symptoms (light-colored and numb lesions, nodules, and so forth) and by determining whether the patient may have been exposed to someone with leprosy. In addition, samples of scrapings from skin lesions, nasal secretions, fluid from nodules, or other tissue secretions can be examined for the presence of *M. leprae*. Samples are treated with a procedure called the acid-fast technique. Because of *M. leprae*'s waxy coating, these bacteria retain a pink stain after being washed in an acid-alcohol mixture, whereas all other bacteria lose the pink stain. Therefore, pink, rod-shaped bacteria observed in samples treated with the acid-fast technique indicate the presence of *M. leprae*. It is easy to find the acid-fast *M. leprae* in lepromatous leprosy patients because they have so many bacteria in their lesions, but the bacteria are more difficult to find in the lesions of tuberculoid leprosy patients. The lepromin test was originally developed to be used as a diagnostic tool for leprosy, in the same way that the tuberculin test is used as a diagnostic tool for tuberculosis. Lepromin, which is heat-killed *M. leprae* taken from nodules, is injected under the skin in the lepromin test. Two reactions are possible: an early reaction that appears twenty-four to forty-eight hours later and a late reaction that appears three to four weeks later. In both reactions, a hard red lump at the injection site indicates a positive lepromin test. This test is not specific for leprosy, however, because a person who has been exposed to *M. leprae*, *M. tuberculosis*, or the tuberculosis vaccine, Bacillus Calmette-Guérin (BCG), will show a positive early reaction. Even though this test is not useful as a diagnostic tool, it is useful in determining whether a patient has a strong or a weak cellular immune response to *M. leprae*. Tuberculoid leprosy patients show both the early and late reactions, while lepromatous leprosy patients show no reaction at all.

Leprosy can be treated with antibiotics. The antibiotic dapsone began to be used on a wide scale in the treatment of leprosy in 1950. Since that time, however, many dapsone-resistant strains of *M. leprae* have appeared. This means that, for some victims, this drug is no longer helpful in fighting the disease. In 1981, in response to the problem of dapsone-resistant strains, the World Health Organization (WHO) recommended a multidrug regimen for leprosy victims. For lepromatous leprosy patients, dapsone, rifampin, and clofazimine are recommended, whereas tuberculoid leprosy patients need take only dapsone and rifampin. Treatment is expected to continue until skin smears are free from acid-fast bacteria, which can last from two years up to the lifetime of the patient. Since 1989, the U.S. recommendations for tuberculoid leprosy are six months of rifampin and dapsone daily, then dapsone alone for three years. For lepromatous leprosy, the recommendation is to use rifampin and dapsone daily for three years, then dapsone only for the rest of the person's life. Often, antibiotics are given to family members of leprosy patients in order to prevent them from contracting the disease. Antibiotic therapy can make a leprosy victim noncontagious, stop the progress of the disease, and in some cases cause a reversal of some of the symptoms. Until treatment is complete, however, it is recommended that patients sleep in separate bedrooms, use their own linens and utensils, and not live in a house with children. Thus, leprosy victims can lead nearly normal lives without fear of infecting others in the community.

A man with leprosy receives a massage from a health care worker at a rehabilitation center in Thailand. (AP/Wide World Photos)

The best ways to keep from getting leprosy are to avoid exposure to leprosy bacteria and to receive antibiotic therapy following exposure. It should be possible to control and, eventually, eliminate leprosy. If every case of leprosy were treated, the disease could not spread and the bacteria would die out with the last leprosy victim. Progress in this direction is slow, however, because of ignorance, superstition, poverty, and overpopulation in areas with many leprosy cases. The first strategy in controlling leprosy is to treat all leprosy cases with antibiotics. As of 1991, about 50 percent of all leprosy victims were not receiving drug therapy. Second, the early detection and rigid isolation of lepromatous leprosy patients are important, as is preventive antibiotic therapy for individuals in close contact with those patients. Finally, even in the early twenty-first century, too many countries lack adequate basic health resources, and too many patients disabled by leprosy are not receiving adequate care. The development of a vaccine for leprosy would aid control efforts.

A global effort for the production of a vaccine for leprosy is being made under the auspices of WHO. The first problem with vaccine development is that, until recently, it was not possible to grow *M. leprae* bacteria outside of a leprosy victim; therefore, not much is known about the nature of the bacteria. Even though this bacterium was the first to be associated with a disease, it cannot be grown on an artificial laboratory medium, whereas nearly all other bacteria known can be grown artificially. It was not until 1960 that scientists at the Centers for Disease Control (CDC) discovered that the bacterium could be grown in the footpads of mice. Finally, in 1969, scientists at the National Hansen's Disease Center in Carville, Louisiana, found that the bacteria would grow in the tissues of the nine-banded armadillo. Several potential vaccines for leprosy have been tested since that time. One vaccine being tested is BCG, a live bacterial vaccine of the bacteria *Mycobacterium bovis*, which is a close relative of *M. leprae*. In four major trials with BCG, a range of 20 to 80 percent protection from leprosy was obtained. It is not known why there was such a wide variation in results. Recent strategies for vaccine development include making a modified BCG that contains *M. leprae* cell wall antigens. It is more advantageous to use BCG than *M. leprae* in a vaccine because BCG is much easier to grow. In addition, scientists are trying to find a way to grow *M. leprae* artificially so that larger quantities will be available to be used for a vaccine. In 1999, WHO set up a strategic plan titled "The Final Push Toward Leprosy Elimination: 2000-2005" and the Global Alliance for the Elimination of Leprosy was launched.

PERSPECTIVE AND PROSPECTS

Leprosy is one of the oldest known diseases. References to leprosy are contained in Indian writings that are more than three thousand years old. The Bible refers to leprosy and the isolation of lepers, although the term refers to other skin diseases as well. The examination of ancient skeletons has provided insights into how leprosy spread in past centuries. Early evidence suggests that the disease was highly contagious and that leprosy was widespread in Europe during the Middle Ages. Leprosy was so prevalent, in fact, that both governments and churches moved to deal with the problem. At that time, the cause of leprosy was unknown, and the disease was generally believed to be a punishment for some personal sin. Lepers were treated as outcasts and required to shout "unclean." They were required to wear gloves and distinctive clothes and carry a bell or clapper to warn people of their approach. They were forbidden to drink from public fountains, speak loudly, eat with healthy people, or attend church. Some lepers were even pronounced legally dead, burned at the stake, or buried alive. Later, they were isolated in asylums called leprosaria, and at one time about nineteen thousand leprosaria existed—mostly in France.

There was a sharp decrease in the number of leprosy cases in the sixteenth century. Several factors may have contributed to this decline, including the isolation of lepers, a better diet, warmer clothes, the plague epidemic, and the increase in tuberculosis, which may have provided resistance to leprosy. Leprosy is no longer as deadly or contagious as it once was, yet the stigma attached to this disease has remained. In an effort to alleviate the social stigma, the Fifth International Congress on Leprosy in 1948 banned the use of the word "leper" and encouraged the use of the term "Hansen's disease" instead of leprosy. *M. leprae*, the causative agent of leprosy, was first identified in the tissues of leprosy patients by the Norwegian physician Gerhard Armauer Hansen in 1873—hence the alternate name, Hansen's disease. Today, victims of leprosy are referred to as Hansenites or Hansenotic.

From the 1960's to the 1980's, estimates of the number of cases of leprosy worldwide ranged from 10 to 12 million. In 2001, at the Fifty-fourth World Health Assembly, it was announced that the global prevalence of leprosy had fallen to below 1 case per 10,000 by the end of 2000 and health experts believe that eliminating leprosy in all countries is an attainable goal by the year 2005. More than 600,000 new cases of leprosy were reported globally in 2002. A new combination of drugs known as multidrug therapy has been used to treat and completely cure patients. The drugs are donated free through foundations and since these donations began in 2000, more than 16 million of the "blister packs," each of which provides one month's treatment to one patient, have been shipped.

Leprosy is prevalent in tropical areas such as Africa, Southeast Asia, and South America. In the United States, most cases occur in Hawaii and small parts of Texas, California, Louisiana, and Florida. The number of new cases in the United States annually—mostly from foreign-born immigrants from leprosy-prone areas—has been very low in the last several decades.

—*Vicki J. Isola, Ph.D.*

See also Antibiotics; Bacterial infections; Immune system; Immunology; Nervous system; Numbness and tingling; Thalidomide; Tropical medicine; Tuberculosis; World Health Organization.

For Further Information:

Biddle, Wayne. *A Field Guide to Germs.* 2d ed. New York: Henry Holt, 2002. This comprehensive book is easily accessible to the nonspecialist and includes a discussion of nearly every virus, bacterium, and fungus known to cause human and nonhuman animal disease. The history of the microbe and the treatment of diseases are included.

Bloom, B. R. "Learning from Leprosy: A Perspective on Immunology and the Third World." *Journal of Immunology* 137 (July, 1986): i-x. This article discusses leprosy as a disease, the immune response to leprosy, possible leprosy vaccines, and the problems of administering vaccines in the Third World.

Donnelly, Karen J. *Leprosy (Hansen's Disease).* New York: Rosen, 2002. Traces the history of leprosy and discusses current and future directions in research. For young adults.

Frank, Steven A. *Immunology and Evolution of Infectious Disease.* Princeton, N.J.: Princeton University Press, 2002. Blends research from molecular biology, immunology, pathogen biology, and population dynamics to discuss how and why parasites vary to escape recognition by the immune system, vaccine design, and the control of epidemics.

Hastings, Robert C., ed. *Leprosy.* 2d ed. New York: Churchill Livingstone, 1994. This book contains a series of articles describing all aspects of leprosy, from the characteristics of the organism to the disease process to treatment.

Joklik, Wolfgang K., et al., eds. *Zinsser Microbiology.* 20th ed. Norwalk, Conn.: Appleton and Lange, 1992. An excellent textbook describing all infectious diseases. The information presented is thorough and logical, and it is supplemented by interesting diagrams, photographs, and charts. Discusses all diseases caused by species of mycobacteria, including leprosy and tuberculosis.

Mandell, Gerald L., John E. Bennett, and Raphael Dolin, eds. *Mandell, Douglas, and Bennett's Principles and Practice of Infectious Diseases.* 6th ed. New York: Elsevier/Churchill Livingstone, 2005. Describes leprosy, discussing the organism, epidemiology, symptoms, complications, and diagnosis; an expanded section on therapy is included.

Sehgal, Alfica. *Leprosy.* Philadelphia: Chelsea House, 2006. A book intended for young adults. Includes a historical overview and a scientific description.

Weedon, David. *Skin Pathology.* 2d ed. New York: Churchill Livingstone, 2002. Text with extensive photographs, covering tissue reaction patterns; the epidermis, dermis and subcutis; the skin in systemic and miscellaneous diseases; infections and infestations; and tumors, among other topics.

Leptin
Biology
Anatomy or system affected: All

Specialties and related fields: Biochemistry, cardiology, endocrinology, genetics, gynecology, nutrition

Definition: A protein hormone involved in regulation of food intake and obesity, with secondary effects on immunity, reproduction, and heart disease.

Structure and Functions

Leptin (from the Greek *leptos,* meaning "thin") is a protein hormone with important effects in regulating body weight, metabolism, and reproductive function. It is the product of the obese (ob) gene occurring on chromosome 7 in the human. Leptin is produced primarily by adipocytes (white fat cells). It is also produced by cells of the epithelium of the stomach and in the placenta. It appears that as adipocytes increase in size because of accumulation of triglycerides (fat molecules), they synthesize more and more leptin. However, the mechanism by which leptin production is controlled is largely unknown. It is likely that a number of hormones modulate leptin output, including corticosteroids and insulin.

DISORDERS AND DISEASES

At first leptin was assumed to be simply a signaling molecule involved in limiting food intake and increasing energy expenditure. Studies published as early as 1994 showed a remarkable difference in weight gain in mice deficient in leptin (mice with a nonfunctional ob gene). Daily injections of leptin into these animals resulted in a reduction of food intake within a few days and a 50 percent decrease in body weight within a month.

More recent studies in the human have not been as promising. It appears that leptin's effects on body weight are mediated through effects on hypothalamic (brain) centers that control feeding behavior and hunger, body temperature, and energy expenditure. If leptin levels are low, appetite is stimulated and use of energy limited. If leptin levels are high, appetite is reduced and energy use stimulated. The most likely target of leptin in the hypothalamus is inhibition of neuropeptide Y, a potent stimulator of food intake. However, this inhibition alone could not account for the effects seen, and studies looking at other hormones are under way.

Leptin also affects reproductive function in humans. It has long been known that very low body fat in human females is associated with cessation of menstrual cycles, and the onset of puberty is known to correlate with body composition (fat levels) as well as age. Several studies have suggested that leptin stimulates hypothalamic output of gonadotropin-releasing hormone, which in turn causes increases of luteinizing and follicle-stimulating hormones from the anterior pituitary gland. These hormones stimulate the onset of puberty. Prepubertal mice treated with leptin become thin and reach reproductive maturity earlier than control mice. One report has also indicated that humans with mutations in the ob gene that prevent them from producing leptin not only become obese but also fail to achieve puberty.

Leptin has been identified in placental tissues; newborn babies show higher levels than those found in their mothers. Leptin has also been found in human breast milk. Together, these findings suggest that leptin aids in intrauterine and neonatal growth and development, as well as in regulation of neonatal food intake.

Finally, leptin appears to have a role in immune system function. Studies have suggested a role for leptin in production of white blood cells and in the control of macrophage function. Mice that lack leptin have depressed immune systems, but the mechanisms for this remain unclear.

PERSPECTIVE AND PROSPECTS

Although early reports claimed that leptin could be useful in treating human obesity, clinical reports to date have not looked promising. It appears that deficiencies in leptin production are a rare cause of human obesity. However, since most obese individuals have plenty of leptin available, additional leptin will have no effect. In those individuals with a genetic deficiency of leptin, clinical use would require either daily injections of leptin or gene therapy. At this point neither of these options looks particularly promising.

—*Kerry L. Cheesman, Ph.D.*

See also Appetite loss; Endocrinology; Endocrinology, pediatric; Hormones; Immune system; Obesity; Obesity, childhood; Puberty and adolescence; Reproductive system; Weight loss and gain.

FOR FURTHER INFORMATION:

Barinaga, Marcia. "Obesity: Leptin Receptor Weighs In." *Science* 271 (January 5, 1996): 29. This article presents a summary of leptin receptor research accessible to the nonspecialist, as well as prospects for obesity drug research.

Brook, Charles G. D., and Nicholas J. Marshall. *Essential Endocrinology.* 4th ed. Malden, Mass.: Blackwell Science, 2001. This text addresses the field of endocrinology, describing the physiology of the endocrine glands and the hormones that they produce. Includes an index.

Castracane, V. Daniel, and Michael C. Henson, eds. *Leptin.* New York: Springer, 2006. Describes the discovery, history, roles, and regulation of leptin in all the major areas of physiology.

Goodman, H. Maurice. *Basic Medical Endocrinology.* 3d ed. Boston: Academic Press, 2003. Focuses on research advances in the understanding of hormones involved in regulating most aspects of bodily functions. Includes in-depth coverage of individual glands and regulatory principles.

Henry, Helen L., and Anthony W. Norman, eds. *Encyclopedia of Hormones.* 3 vols. San Diego, Calif.: Academic Press, 2003. A comprehensive overview of the role of hormones, the major physiological systems in which they operate, and the biological consequences of an excess or deficiency of a particular hormone.

Rink, Timothy J. "In Search of a Satiety Factor." *Nature* 372 (December 1, 1994): 372-373. A history of the research into weight regulation and how leptin supports prior theories is presented in a general news format. References are provided for further reading.

LEUKEMIA

DISEASE/DISORDER

ANATOMY OR SYSTEM AFFECTED: Blood

SPECIALTIES AND RELATED FIELDS: Hematology, internal medicine, serology, toxicology

DEFINITION: A family of cancers that affect the blood, characterized by an increase in the number of white blood cells.

KEY TERMS:

blast cell: an immature dividing cell

bone marrow: the tissue within bones that produces blood cells; in children, all bones have active marrow, but in adults, blood cell production occurs only in the trunk

bone marrow transplant: the removal of bone marrow from an immunologically matched individual for infusion into a patient whose bone marrow has been destroyed

chemotherapy: the use of drugs to kill rapidly growing cancer cells; this treatment will also kill some normal cells, producing undesirable side effects

granulocytes: white blood cells that generally help to fight bacterial infection; these cells are capable of passing from the blood capillaries into damaged tissues

hematopoiesis: the process by which blood cells develop in the bone marrow; this maturation is regulated by specific molecules called growth factors

immune system: the cells and organs of the body that fight infection; destruction of these cells leaves the body vulnerable to numerous diseases

lymphocytes: white blood cells that specifically target a foreign organism for destruction; the two classes of lymphocytes are B cells, which produce antibodies, and T cells, which kill infected cells

oncogenes: genes found in every cell which are capable of causing cancer if activated or mutated

CAUSES AND SYMPTOMS

The blood is essential for all the physiological processes of the body. It is composed of red cells called erythrocytes, white cells called leukocytes, and platelets, each of which has distinct functions. Erythrocytes, which contain hemoglobin, are essential for the trans-port of oxygen from the lungs to all the cells and organs of the body. Leukocytes are important for protecting the body against infection by bacteria, viruses, and other parasites. Platelets play a role in the formation of blood clots; therefore, these cells are critical in the process of wound healing. Blood cell development, or hematopoiesis, begins in the bone marrow with immature stem cells that can produce all three types of blood cells. Under the influence of special molecules called growth factors, these stem cells divide rapidly and form blast cells that become one of the three blood cell types. After several further divisions, these blast cells ultimately mature into fully functional erythrocytes, leukocytes, and platelets. In a healthy individual, the number of each type of blood cell remains relatively constant. Thus, the rate of new cell production is approximately equivalent to the rate of old cell destruction and removal.

Mature leukocytes are the key players in defending the body against infection. There are three types of leukocytes: monocytes, granulocytes, and lymphocytes. In leukemia, leukocytes multiply at an increased rate, resulting in an abnormally high number of white cells, a significant proportion of which are immature cells. All forms of leukemia are characterized by this abnormally regulated growth; therefore, leukemia is a cancer, even though tumor masses do not form. The cancerous cells live longer than the normal leukocytes and accumulate first in the bone marrow and then in the blood. Since these abnormal cells crowd the bone marrow, normal hematopoiesis cannot be maintained in a person with leukemia. The patient will usually become weak as a result of the lack of oxygen-carrying red cells and susceptible to bleeding because of a lack of platelets. The abnormal leukocytes do not function effectively in de-

---

INFORMATION ON LEUKEMIA

CAUSES: Unclear; possibly environmental and genetic factors

SYMPTOMS: Mild cold symptoms; fever; enlargement of lymph nodes, spleen, and liver; fatigue; paleness; weight loss; repeated infections; increased susceptibility to bleeding and bruising

DURATION: Acute or chronic with recurrent episodes

TREATMENTS: Chemotherapy, bone marrow transplantation

fending the body against infection, and they prevent normal leukocytes from developing; therefore, the patient is immunologically compromised. In addition, once the abnormal cells accumulate in the blood, they may hinder the functioning of other organs, such as the liver, kidney, lungs, and spleen.

It has become clear that leukemia, which was first recognized in 1845, is actually a pathology that comprises more than one disease. Leukemia has been divided into four main types, based on the type of leukocyte that is affected and the maturity of the leukocytes observed in the blood and the bone marrow. Both lymphocytes and granulocytes can be affected. When the cells are mainly immature blasts, the leukemia is termed acute, and when the cells are mostly mature, the leukemia is termed chronic. Therefore, the four types of leukemia are acute lymphocytic (ALL), acute granulocytic (AGL), chronic lymphocytic (CLL), and chronic granulocytic (CGL). The granulocytic leukemias are also known as myologenous leukemias (AML, CML) or nonlymphoid leukemias (ANLL, CNLL). These are the main types of leukemia, although there are additional rarer forms. These four forms of leukemia account for 5 percent of the cancer cases in the United States. The incidence of acute and chronic forms is approximately equivalent, but specific forms are more common at different stages of life. The major form in children is ALL; after puberty, there is a higher incidence of AGL. The chronic forms of leukemia occur in the adult population after the fourth or fifth decade of life, and men are twice as likely to be affected as women.

The causes of leukemia are still not completely understood, but scientists have put together many pieces of the puzzle. It is known that several environmental factors increase the risk of developing leukemia. Among these are exposure to radiation, chemicals such as chloramphenicol and benzene, and possibly viruses. In addition, there is a significant genetic component to this disease. Siblings of patients with leukemia have a higher risk of developing the disease, and chromosomal changes have been found in the cells of most patients, although they disappear when the patient is in remission. For example, the genetic basis of certain forms of CML is an exchange of information (translocation) between chromosome 22 and chromosome 9; the shortened chromosome 22 is referred to as the Philadelphia chromosome. These different "causes" can be linked by understanding how oncogenes function. Every person, as part of his or her genetic makeup, has

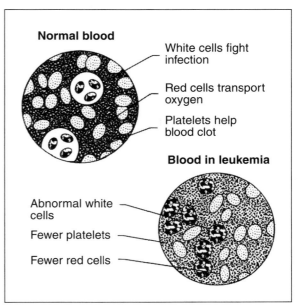

Leukemia is characterized by a high number of white blood cells and a reduced number of red blood cells and platelets; also, abnormal cells may be visible.

several oncogenes that are capable of causing cancer. In the healthy person, these oncogenes function in a carefully regulated manner to control cell growth. After exposure to an environmental or genetic influence that causes chromosome abnormalities, however, these oncogenes may become activated or deregulated so that uncontrolled cell growth occurs, resulting in the abnormally high number of cells seen in leukemia. The translocation associated with the Philadelphia chromosome results in abnormal expression of an oncogene encoding an enzyme that regulates cell division.

Leukemia is often difficult to diagnose in the early stages because the symptoms are similar to more common or less serious diseases. "Flulike" symptoms, sometimes accompanied by fever, may be the earliest evidence of acute leukemia; in children, the first symptoms may be less pronounced. The symptoms quickly become more pronounced as white cells accumulate in the lymph nodes, spleen, and liver, causing these organs to become enlarged. Fatigue, paleness, weight loss, repeated infections, and an increased susceptibility to bleeding and bruising are associated with leukemia. As the disease progresses, the fatigue and bleeding increase, various skin disorders develop, and the joints become painfully swollen. If untreated, the afflicted individual will die within a few months. Chronic leukemia has a more gradual progression and may be present for years before symptoms develop. When symptoms are present, they may be vague feelings of fatigue, fever, or loss of energy. There may be enlarged lymph nodes in the neck and armpits and a feeling of fullness in the abdomen because of an increase in the size of the spleen as much as tenfold. Loss of appetite and sweating at night may be initial symptoms. Often, chronic leukemia eventually leads to a syndrome resembling acute leukemia, which is ultimately fatal.

If these symptoms are present, a doctor will diagnose the presence of leukemia in two stages. First, blood will be drawn and a blood smear will be analyzed microscopically. This may indicate that there are fewer erythrocytes, leukocytes, and platelets than normal, and abnormal cells may be visible. A blood smear, however, may show only slight abnormalities, and the number of leukemic cells in the blood may not correspond to the extent of the disease in the bone marrow. This requires that the bone marrow itself be examined by means of a bone marrow biopsy. Bone marrow tissue can be obtained by inserting a needle into a bone such as the hip and aspirating a small sample of cells. This bone marrow biopsy, which is done under local anesthetic on an outpatient basis, is the definitive test for leukemia. Visual examination of the marrow usually reveals the presence of many abnormal cells, and this finding is often confirmed with biochemical and immunological tests. After a positive diagnosis, a doctor will also examine the cerebrospinal fluid to see if leukemic cells have invaded the central nervous system.

TREATMENT AND THERAPY

The treatment and life expectancy for leukemic patients varies significantly for each of the four types of leukemia. Treatment is designed to destroy all the abnormal cells and produce a complete remission, which is defined as the phase of recovery when the symptoms of the disease disappear and no abnormal cells can be observed in the blood or bone marrow. Unfortunately, a complete remission may be only temporary, since a small number of abnormal cells may still exist even though they are not observed under the microscope. These can, with time, multiply and repopulate the marrow, causing a relapse of the disease. With repeated relapses, the response to therapy becomes poorer and the durations of the remissions that follow become shorter. It is generally believed, however, that a remission that lasts five years in ALL, eight years in AGL, or twelve years in CGL may be permanent. Therefore, the goal of

leukemia research is to develop ways to prolong remission.

By the time acute leukemia has been diagnosed, abnormal cells have often spread throughout the bone marrow and into several organs; therefore, surgery and radiation are usually not effective. Treatment programs include chemotherapy or bone marrow transplants or both.

Chemotherapy is usually divided into several phases. In the first, or induction, phase, combinations of drugs are given to destroy all detectable abnormal cells and therefore induce a clinical remission. Vincristine, methotrexate, 6-mercaptopurine, L-asparaginase, daunorubicin, prednisone, and cytosine arabinoside are among the drugs that are used. Combinations that selectively kill more leukemic cells than they do normal cells are available for the treatment of ALL; however, in AGL no selective agents are available, resulting in the destruction of equal numbers of diseased and healthy cells. An alternative strategy does not rely on destroying the abnormal cells but instead seeks to induce immature leukemic cells to develop further. Once the cells are mature, they will no longer divide and will eventually die in the same way that a normal leukocyte does. Drugs such as cytarabine and retinoic acid have been tested, but the results are inconclusive.

Although the induction phase achieves clinical remission in more than 80 percent of patients, a second phase, called consolidation therapy, is essential to prevent relapse. Different combinations of anticancer drugs are used to kill any remaining cancer cells that were resistant to the drugs in the induction phase. Once the patient is in remission, higher doses of chemotherapy can be tolerated, and sometimes additional intensive treatments are given to reduce further the number of leukemic cells so that they will be unable to repopulate the tissues. During these phases of treatment, patients must be hospitalized. The destruction of their normal leukocytes along with the leukemic cells makes them very susceptible to infection. Their low numbers of surviving erythrocytes and platelets increase the probability of internal bleeding, and transfusions are often necessary. The dosages of chemotherapeutic agents must be carefully calculated to kill as many leukemic cells as possible without destroying so many normal cells that they cannot repopulate the marrow. In general, children handle intensive chemotherapy better than adults.

Following the induction and consolidation phases, maintenance therapy is sometimes used. In ALL, maintenance therapy is given for two to three years; however, its benefit in other forms of leukemia is a matter of controversy.

A second form of therapy is sometimes indicated for patients who have not responded to chemotherapy or are likely to relapse. Bone marrow transplantation has been increasingly used in leukemic patients to replace diseased marrow with normally functioning stem cells. In this procedure, the patient is treated with intensive chemotherapy and whole-body irradiation to destroy all leukemic and normal cells. Then a small amount of marrow from a normal donor is infused. The donor can be the patient himself, if the marrow was removed during a previous remission, or an immunologically matched donor, who is usually a sibling. If a sibling is not available, it may be possible to find a matched donor from the National Marrow Donor Program, which has on file approximately 350,000 people who have consented to be donors. Marrow is removed from the donor, broken up into small pieces, and given to the patient intravenously. The stem cells from the transplanted marrow circulate in the blood, enter the bones, and multiply. The first signs that the transplant is functioning normally occur in two to four weeks as the numbers of circulating granulocytes and platelets in the patient's blood increase. Eventually, in a successful transplant, the bone marrow cavity will be repopulated with normal cells.

Bone marrow transplantation is a dangerous procedure that requires highly trained caregivers. During this process, the patient is completely vulnerable to infection, since there is no functional immune system. The patient is placed in an isolation unit with special food-handling procedures. There is little chance that the patient will reject the transplanted marrow, because the immune system of the patient is suppressed. A larger problem remains, however, because it is possible for immune cells that existed in the donor's marrow to reject the tissues and organs of the patient. This graft-versus-host disease (GVHD) affects between 50 and 70 percent of bone marrow transplant patients. Even though the donor is immunologically matched, the match is not perfect, and the recently transplanted cells regard the cells in their new host as a "foreign" threat. Twenty percent of the patients who develop GVHD will die; therefore, drugs such as cyclophosphamide and cyclosporine, which suppress the immune system, are usually given to minimize this response. GVHD is not a problem if the donor is the patient. Since the availability of matching bone marrow cells is exceeded by

the need, recent studies have involved the testing of hematopoietic umbilical cord cells from unrelated donors. The incidence of relapse as well as GVHD was similar to that when using matched bone marrow cells, suggesting that cord blood cells have the potential to serve as an alternative to conventional transplants.

Aggressive chemotherapy and bone marrow transplantation have dramatically increased the number of long-lasting remissions. For those who survive the therapy, it appears that, in ALL, approximately 60 percent of children and 35 percent of adults may be cured of the leukemia. The outlook for permanent remission is 10 to 20 percent in AGL and 65 percent for CGL patients. Statistics for chronic lymphocytic leukemia have been difficult to predict, because individual cases that have been similarly treated have had very different outcomes. The average lifespan after a diagnosis of CLL is three to four years; however, some patients live longer than fifteen years.

Perspective and Prospects

As the number of deaths from infectious disease has decreased, cancer has become the second most common cause of disease-related death. It is estimated that one of three people in the United States will develop a form of cancer and that the disease will kill one of five people. The search for causes and treatments of various cancers is perhaps the most active area of biological research today. Multiple lines of experimentation are being pursued, and significant advances have been made.

Leukemia is one of the cancers that scientists understand fairly well, but many unanswered questions remain. Leukemia research can be divided into two broad approaches. In the first, the researcher seeks to modify and improve the current methods for treatment: chemotherapy and bone marrow transplantation. In the second, an effort is being made to understand more about the disease itself, with the hope that completely different strategies for treatment might present themselves.

The risks involved in current therapy for leukemia have been discussed in the previous section. Treatment schedules, individually designed for each patient, will add to the understanding of how other physiological characteristics affect treatment outcome. Significant advances in reducing the risk of GVHD are likely to come quickly. In marrow transplants in which the donor is the patient, research is in progress to improve ways to screen out abnormal cells, even if they are present at very low levels, before they are infused back into the patient. In addition, for transplants in which the donor is not the patient, techniques that remove the harmful components of the bone marrow are being developed. Bone marrow cells can be partially purified, resulting in an enriched population of stem cells. Administering these to the leukemic patient should greatly reduce the risk of GVHD. Since bone marrow can be stored easily, the day may come when healthy people will store a bone marrow stem cell sample in case they contract a disease that would require a transplant.

Basic research in leukemia focuses on a simple question, "Why are leukemic cells different from normal cells?" This question is asked from a variety of perspectives in the fields of immunology, cell biology, and genetics. Immunologists are looking for markers on the surfaces of leukemic cells that would distinguish them from their normal counterparts. If such markers are found, it should be possible to target leukemic cells for destruction by using monoclonal antibodies attached to drugs. These "smart drugs" would be able to home in on the diseased cells, leaving normal cells untouched or only slightly affected. This would be a great advance for leukemia treatment, since much of the risk for the leukemic patient following chemotherapy or bone marrow transplant involves susceptibility to infection because the normal immune cells have been destroyed. Similarly, it may be possible to "teach" the patient's immune system to destroy abnormal cells that it had previously ignored. Similar forms of immunotherapy have shown promise in treating forms of cancer such as melanoma.

Cell biologists are seeking to understand the normal hematopoietic process so that they can determine which steps of the process go awry in leukemia. Some of the growth factors involved in hematopoiesis have been identified, but it appears that the process is quite complex, and as yet scientists do not have a clear picture of normal hematopoiesis. When the understanding of the normal process becomes more complete, it may be possible to localize the defect in a leukemic patient and provide the missing growth factors. This might allow abnormal immature cells to complete the developmental process and relieve the symptoms of disease.

Geneticists are studying the chromosomal changes that underlie the onset of leukemia. As the oncogenes that are involved are identified, the reasons for their activation will also be determined. Once the effects of these genetic abnormalities are understood, it may be possible to intervene by genetically engineering stem cells so that they can develop normally.

These areas of research will likely converge to provide the leukemia treatments of the future. Leukemia is a cancer for which there is already a significant cure rate. It is not unreasonable to expect that this rate will approach 100 percent in the near future.

—Katherine B. Frederich, Ph.D.;
updated by Richard Adler, Ph.D.

See also Blood and blood disorders; Bone marrow transplantation; Cancer; Carcinogens; Chemotherapy; Malignancy and metastasis; Oncology; Radiation sickness.

FOR FURTHER INFORMATION:

Bellenir, Karen, ed. *Cancer Sourcebook: Basic Consumer Health Information About Major Forms and Stages of Cancer.* 5th ed. Detroit: Omnigraphics, 2007. This well-written volume provides the reader with a background against which to understand leukemia. Describes each of the four main types of leukemia in a straightforward and practical manner.

Dollinger, Malin, et al. *Everyone's Guide to Cancer Therapy.* 4th ed. Kansas City, Mo.: Andrews Mc-Meel, 2002. An excellent source of medical information about cancer, written for the general public. Various cancer sites in the body are described, and one essay focuses on sarcomas of the bone. A helpful glossary of medical terminology is provided.

Eyre, Harmon J., Dianne Partie Lange, and Lois B. Morris. *Informed Decisions: The Complete Book of Cancer Diagnosis, Treatment, and Recovery.* 2d ed. Atlanta: American Cancer Society, 2002. This text from the American Cancer Society is intended for the layperson. It is exemplary in its discussion of cancer.

Goldman, John, and Junia Melo. "Chronic Myeloid Leukemia: Advances in Biology and New Approaches to Treatment." *New England Journal of Medicine* 349, no. 15 (October 9, 2003): 1451-1464. Review of the causes and treatment for one form of leukemia, comparable to the research in general in that field.

Keene, Nancy. *Childhood Leukemia: A Guide for Families, Friends and Caregivers.* 3d ed. Cambridge, Mass.: O'Reilly and Associates, 2002. Keene uses the story of her daughter's battle with leukemia as a vehicle to explore the physical and emotional impacts of the disease. Offers guidance on coping with procedures, hospitalizations, school, and associated social, emotional, and financial problems.

Kimball, Chad T. *Childhood Diseases and Disorders Sourcebook: Basic Consumer Health Information*

About Medical Problems Often Encountered in Pre-adolescent Children. Detroit: Omnigraphics, 2002. Offers basic facts about cancer, sickle cell disease, diabetes, and other chronic conditions in children and discusses frequently used diagnostic tests, surgeries, and medications. Long-term care for seriously ill children is also presented.

Leukemia and Lymphoma Society of America. http://www.leukemia.org/. A group dedicated to funding blood cancer research, education, and patient services for patients with leukemia and other lymphatic diseases.

Rennie, Ed. *Beginning of the End of My Life.* Philadelphia: Xlibris, 2005. Diagnosed with leukemia, the author describes the impact on himself as well as his family. The nature of his treatment is presented.

Westcott, Patsy. *Living with Leukemia.* Austin, Tex.: Raintree-Steck-Vaughn, 1999. Designed for students in grades three through five, this book discusses a condition or disease through the stories of children experiencing it. Includes clear and easy-to-understand diagrams and full-color photographs.

LEUKODYSTROPHY

DISEASE/DISORDER

ANATOMY OR SYSTEM AFFECTED: Brain, ears, eyes, muscles, nerves

SPECIALTIES AND RELATED FIELDS: Biochemistry, family medicine, genetics, neurology, nutrition, occupational health, pediatrics, physical therapy

DEFINITION: A group of genetic disorders characterized by progressive deterioration of the white matter (myelin sheath) of the brain.

> ### INFORMATION ON LEUKODYSTROPHY
>
> **CAUSES:** Enzyme defect resulting in degeneration of the myelin sheath
> **SYMPTOMS:** Uncontrolled muscle stiffness, paralysis, speech difficulties, memory failures, personality changes, impaired reasoning, urinary incontinence, vision loss, hearing loss
> **DURATION:** Lifelong
> **TREATMENTS:** Medications (Lorenzo's oil or Lovastatin), dietary supplements, exercise, and occupational and speech therapy

---

CAUSES AND SYMPTOMS

Leukodystrophy is caused by a breakdown in the enzyme systems that metabolize fats (lipids) in the nerve cells. As a result, the body can no longer break down very long chain fatty acids (VLCFA), which then accumulate. This causes the substance around nerve fibers, known as the myelin sheath, to degenerate. The myelin sheath protects and insulates the axons of nerve cells, allowing them to transmit impulses between the nerve cells in the brain and other parts of the body. Loss of the myelin sheath around nerve cells short-circuits nerve impulses. As a result, the victim can experience uncontrolled muscle stiffness, paralysis, speech difficulties, memory failures, personality changes, impaired reasoning, urinary incontinence, loss of vision, and loss of hearing. These symptoms may be difficult to recognize during the early stages of the disease. Leukodystrophy usually begins in the back of the brain, eventually spreading throughout the white matter of the cerebral hemispheres and often into the spinal cord. Leukodystrophy is typically diagnosed with a blood test that is used to determine the amount of VLCFA in the body.

The myelin sheath is a complex chemical substance made from a variety of lipids. Different types of leukodystrophy affect one of the particular constituents of myelin. Specific leukodystrophies include adrenoleukodystrophy (ALD), metachromatic leukodystrophy (MLD), Zellweger's syndrome, and Alexander's disease. Having one type of leukodystrophy does not increase the risk of having another type.

TREATMENT AND THERAPY

The effects of leukodystrophy may be tempered through the use of various medications, dietary supplements, exercise programs, and occupational and speech therapies. For ALD, the most common form of leukodystrophy, Lorenzo's oil helps the body bring VLCFA levels back to normal. To be effective, Lorenzo's oil should be coupled with a very-low-fat diet. Lovastatin, an anticholesterol drug, does the same thing as Lorenzo's oil without the patient needing to be on a low-fat diet.

For some types of leukodystrophy, particularly MLD, bone marrow transplants have shown promise in slowing down the disease. Gene therapy is being investigated. The hope is to deliver genes to the patient that will stimulate the oligodendrocyte cells in the brain to produce myelin once again.

PERSPECTIVE AND PROSPECTS

Leukodystrophy is genetically inherited. Most types show up in early childhood, although there are some late childhood forms. Public awareness of the disease was greatly enhanced by the 1992 film *Lorenzo's Oil*, the true story of Augusto and Michaela Odone seeking a cure for ALD for their five-year-old son Lorenzo. They founded the Myelin Project, a research effort that continues to seek ways for victims of leukodystrophy to produce myelin that will insulate their nerve cells.

—Alvin K. Benson, Ph.D.

See also Brain; Brain damage; Brain disorders; Multiple sclerosis; Nervous system; Neuralgia, neuritis, and neuropathy; Neuroimaging; Neurology; Neurology, pediatric.

FOR FURTHER INFORMATION:

Icon Health. *Leukodystrophy: A Medical Dictionary, Bibliography, and Annotated Research Guide to Internet References*. San Diego, Calif.: Author, 2004.

Kimball, Chad T. *Childhood Diseases and Disorders Sourcebook: Basic Consumer Health Information About Medical Problems Often Encountered in Preadolescent Children*. Detroit: Omnigraphics, 2002.

Lazzarini, Robert A. *Myelin Biology and Disorders*. San Diego, Calif.: Elsevier Academic Press, 2004.

Salvati, S., ed. *A Multidisciplinary Approach to Myelin Diseases II*. New York: Plenum Press, 1994.

LICE, MITES, AND TICKS
DISEASE/DISORDER

ANATOMY OR SYSTEM AFFECTED: Ears, genitals, hair, skin

SPECIALTIES AND RELATED FIELDS: Dermatology, pediatrics, public health

DEFINITION: Parasites that live on the human body, causing severe itching, skin rashes, and sometimes more serious diseases.

KEY TERMS:

*louse (*pl. *lice):* a wingless insect that sucks blood and that can be involved in transmitting diseases

mite: a very small spider that is parasitic to humans and can carry disease

molt: to shed all or part of the skin or outer covering

parasite: an organism that lives off of another organism while contributing nothing to the survival of the host

tick: a wingless insect that sucks blood and can spread disease

CAUSES AND SYMPTOMS

Lice, mites, and ticks are parasites that live on human beings. Two species of lice survive on human blood:

INFORMATION ON LICE, MITES, AND TICKS

CAUSES: Bites or exposure to diseases through parasites

SYMPTOMS: Severe itching, rashes, development of diseases

DURATION: Acute to chronic

TREATMENTS: Insecticidal shampoos, medications, lotions

---

body lice and crab lice. Body lice are divided into two subspecies, the head louse (*Pediculus humanus capitis*) and the body louse (*Pediculus humanus corporis*). Head lice live on the scalp among the hairs of the head. Body lice actually live in and on clothing. They move off clothes and attach themselves to human skin to feed on blood frequently during the day. It is very difficult to tell the difference between these types of lice. They are both flat, wingless, grayish in color, and very small. The body louse is about .08 to .16 inch long, slightly larger than the head louse, which measures only .04 to .08 inch. Body lice are a slightly lighter shade of gray than are head lice.

Both subspecies of body lice live by sucking blood from their victims. These insects of the order *Anoplura* have three pointed tubes on their bodies called stylets that can jab into the skin and draw out blood. When not in use, the stylets are tucked away in a pouch. Body lice begin their lives as eggs dropped into the folds of clothing by mature adult females. Head lice eggs are glued to the base of a strand of hair on top of the head. The eggs, called nits, are about one-fourth the size of a mature female. After about seven to ten days, the nits hatch into young nymphs. Because hair grows about 0.3 millimeter a day, the nits hatch about 3 millimeters away from the scalp. After the nymph emerges, it leaves behind an empty egg shell still tightly cemented to the hair. Nymphs begin sucking blood as soon as they hatch. Within nine days, the nymph molts three times before a full adult louse is formed. Adults then live about two weeks, with females laying about ten eggs every day.

Lice are passed from head to head only by direct contact. This usually happens at school, often on the playground or in the gym. Head lice have different effects on different people. Some experience only slight itching, while others are terribly irritated and develop a swollen and inflamed scalp. An itching scalp is the most obvious symptom of head lice. Nits are visible upon inspection of hair near the scalp. On girls, they are usually found behind the ears, while on boys, they are most likely to be found attached near the top of the head. Parents should be very careful in treating head lice; they too can be infected. Head lice can be the transmitters of several dangerous infectious diseases, such as epidemic typhus, relapsing fever, and trench fever.

Body lice are less often found on children than are head lice. They thrive in clothing and bodies that are unclean for long periods of time. Body lice are especially troublesome and numerous on homeless people, prisoners of war, and others living in dirty conditions. (Cleanliness, however, is not a factor with head lice; they can thrive in clean or dirty hair.) Body lice have helped spread a number of contagious diseases, the most deadly of which is typhus. This disease starts with flulike symptoms, followed by a high fever and rash. During World War II, more than three million Russian prisoners of war died from louse-spread typhus. In recent years, however, typhus has been rare.

Crab lice (*Phthirus pubis*) are usually found living in pubic hair and are most likely to infect adults. Like all lice, they are very small, .083 inch in length when fully grown, but they cause great discomfort. As adults, they firmly grab pubic hair with their crablike legs (six per louse), insert their barbed tongue into the skin, and suck blood. The female lays its eggs about .08 inch from the skin. When the eggs hatch, the nymphs begin to feed and stop only while molting. Feeding causes intense itching and a rash. Rarely, but occasionally, the lice spread to the chest, eyebrows, or armpits. They can be passed on only by human carriers through direct contact. Crab lice cannot live on any other species except humans, and about 3 percent of people have them. Crab lice do not carry sexually transmitted diseases but are often associated with them.

Ticks are members of a blood-sucking family of insects called Ixodidae. Several different species suck blood from warm-blooded vertebrates, such as human beings, cows, and dogs. Common species in the United States and Canada include hard ticks and the American dog tick. Ticks have a hard, shieldlike plate on their backs called a scutum that makes them very difficult to crush. A female tick can

swell up to the size of a pea when ingesting blood and can lay from four thousand to six thousand eggs within four to ten days.

The eggs hatch after about a month, and six-legged larvae, called seed ticks, emerge. A seed tick waits on the tip of a leaf of grass or other low-growing plant until a suitable animal walks by. The seed tick grabs onto its meal and, after sucking enough blood, molts into its next stage, an eight-legged nymph called a yearling tick. It finds another host, sucks more blood, and then molts one more time into an adult. After another week of feeding, adults mate, the female produces its eggs, and the three-stage cycle begins all over again.

Ticks are very good survivors: Eight-legged nymphs can live more than a year without food, while adults can go without a meal of blood for more than two years.

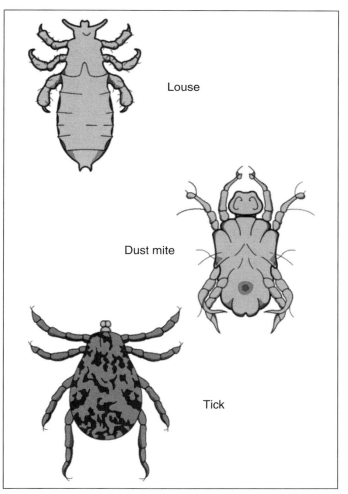

Louse

Dust mite

Tick

Magnified representations of a louse, a mite (normally microscopic), and a tick.

VIRAL DISEASES SPREAD BY TICKS

Disease	Principal Vector
Colorado tick fever	*Dermacentor andersoni*
Encephalitis, Far East Russian	*Ixodes persulcatus*
Louping ill	*Isodes ricinus*

Ticks carry many dangerous diseases, including Rocky Mountain spotted fever, Colorado tick fever, tularemia, anaplasmosis, and Lyme disease.

Mites are actually related to spiders, rather than insects. Dust mites (*Dermatophagiodes pteronyssinus*), the chief living forms found in house dust, are among the most numerous inhabitants of human environments. One study of 150 houses in Holland found mites in every one of them. Dust mites measure about .01 inch in diameter. They have eight legs, like all spiders, and are closely related to ear mites found in dogs and cats and scab mites found in sheep. House dust mites spend all of their life stages, from birth to death, in dust. There can be as many as five hundred mites in every gram of house dust. This measures out to about fourteen thousand mites per ounce of dust. They survive by eating human skin that is shed daily, scabs that fall off, and dandruff, which is about 10 percent fat and which they digest with the help of a fungus also found in house dust. Dust mites are responsible for some allergies and asthma attacks. They can also invade the skin and cause allergic reactions such as dermatitis. Although dust mites cannot penetrate the surface of the skin, they can live in ulcers, fungal infections, scabs, and other skin openings.

The scabies mite (*Sarcoptes scabei*) does burrow into the skin in search of its preferred food, skin cells and intestinal fluids. Female scabies mites are about .016 inch long, while males are only about half as big. The female lays its eggs only a few hours after mating and can lay two to three eggs a day for up to four weeks. The eggs hatch after only three to four days. The larvae often move about on the skin surface until they find a suitable space, usually between the fingers or at the bend in the knee, elbow, or wrist. The underarms, breasts, and genitals can also be invaded by these travelers. Frequently, they travel all the way down to the ankles or between the toes. Sometimes it takes up to six weeks before the pests are noticed by the person acting as their host.

Children are especially sensitive to the feces and eggs of scabies mites, which can cause an agonizing itch that is particularly irritating at night. Scabies mites are most active in the fall and winter, but they are transmissible at any time. They can be spread by shaking hands, by touching the infected areas of another person, and even by having contact with the clothes or bedsheets of the infected individual. Scabies mites do not carry any major diseases, but they do cause a good deal of itching and discomfort.

TREATMENT AND THERAPY

Treatments for lice, mites, and ticks vary according to the type and severity of infestation. The only way to protect a child against head lice is through regular inspection of the head. The hair should be combed and brushed every night; this will injure the lice, which will not be able to survive. Treatment involves an insecticidal shampoo such as Proderm, which contains malathion, or Kwell, which contains lindane or gamma benzene hexachlorine. These shampoos kill both the lice and the nits. Removing lice by hand or crushing them is a difficult and usually impossible task. The force required to remove a nit from a hair is greater than most parents can provide. Crushing a louse requires direct pressure of about five hundred thousand times the weight of a louse. The crushed body of a louse can also cause infection. The best treatment for body lice is washing clothes and infected areas with soap. Soap and hot water usually kill body lice. If an infection of either head or body lice is discovered, all members of a family should be checked, and a doctor should be consulted. If a child has head lice, his or her school should always be notified. If crab lice are discovered, a physician should be contacted immediately. Pubic lice can be treated with insecticides such as pyrethrin pediculicide. Pyrethrins are available over the counter in drugstores. Stronger treatments require a prescription. Crab lice can be controlled by washing clothing and bedding and drying them in a very hot dryer.

Ticks are very difficult to remove from the body. A tick should not be pulled or yanked out because its head, filled with jagged teeth, can remain in the wound and cause an infection. Ticks have to be removed so that their mouthparts do not break off. Unattached ticks can be brushed off with a hand, but an attached tick should not be removed with bare fingers. To remove a tick, the hands should be covered with a tissue or gloves. Then, the tick is grabbed with a pair of tweezers as close to its head as possible. Gentle, steady pressure is applied until the tick comes out. The tick should not be twisted or crushed until it is fully out. Body fluids from the tick can carry Lyme disease organisms, which can enter the body through broken skin. The safest way to kill the tick is to drown it in soapy water or crush it with the tweezers, avoiding contact with the hands. The site of the bite should be washed and checked carefully to see if any part of the head is still embedded. Anything that remains should be removed with tweezers, which will help prevent infection. If all parts cannot be removed, the spot should be rubbed with an antiseptic. A doctor should be consulted if the site becomes inflamed or filled with pus.

Scabies mites can be controlled by insecticidal lotions containing lindane or sulfur. The pesticide lindane is the one most commonly used for scabies mites, but it has been linked to cancer in some tests. Sulfur is preferred by most physicians because it is safer and more widely available. Sulfur requires three applications over three days, however, and frequently leaves stains on bedding and clothes. The fastest-acting miticide is permethrim. It usually requires only one application to be effective, but it is more toxic than sulfur.

Scabies mites can be controlled by washing the clothing, bedding, and towels used by the infected person. If scabies mites are found, other people with whom the child has had contact should be told so that they can seek treatment, even though they might not have started to itch. Scabies mites cannot live long if detached from their hosts, usually no more than two to three days. Sealing infected clothes in a plastic bag for a week or so will also kill most of the mites.

Dust mites can be controlled by reducing their sources of food. This can be accomplished by covering mattresses in plastic, keeping pets away from beds and sleeping areas, reducing humidity in the house, and vacuuming once a week. Killing dust mites requires vacuuming with a water vacuum or one with special dust filters, washing sheets and pillowcases in hot soapy water, freezing or heating blankets, or using pesticides such as mosquito repellents containing diethyl-m-toluamide (DEET) or products containing boric acid.

PERSPECTIVE AND PROSPECTS

New chemicals have proven very effective in the treatment of diseases spread by lice, mites, and ticks. Louse-spread typhus, once responsible for millions of deaths,

BACTERIAL AND RICKETTSIAL DISEASES SPREAD BY LICE, MITES, AND TICKS

Disease	Disease Agent	Principal Vectors
Boutonneuse fever	*Rickettsia conori*	Ticks: *Rhipicephalus sanguineus*, *R. secundus*, and species of *Haemaphysalis*, *Hyalomma*, *Amblyomma*, *Boophilis*, *Dermacentor*, and *Ixodes*
Q fever	*Coxiella burneti*	Ixodid ticks
Relapsing fever	*Borrelia*	*Ornithodoros* ticks
Rickettsialpox	*Rickettsia akari*	Mite: *Liponyssoides sanguineus*
Rocky Mountain spotted fever	*Rickettsia rickettsi*	Ticks: *Dermacentor andersoni*, *D. variabilis*, *Amblyomma americanus*, *Haemaphysalis leporispalustris* (rabbit-to-rabbit transmission)
Trench fever	*Rickettsia quintana*	Human body louse *Pediculus humanus humanus*
Tularemia	*Francisella tularensis*	Deer flies and ticks
Typhus, louse-borne	*Rickettsia prowazekii*	Human body louse *Pediculus humanus humanus*
Typhus, murine	*Rickettsia mooseri*	The rat louse *Polyplax spinulosa* and the tropical rat mite *Ornthonssus bacoti* are zoonotic vectors
Typhus, scrub	*Rickettsia tsutsugamushi*	Mites: *Leptotrombidium akamushi* and *L. deliensis*

is no longer a great danger. Improved standards of cleanliness have done much to eliminate the problem of body lice in all but the poorest populations in the United States. Unfortunately, head lice cannot be controlled simply by keeping things clean, so they continue to cause itching and scratching when contracted even by the cleanest children. Lice, mites, and ticks will always be with humans, but the diseases that these parasites spread, with a few exceptions such as Rocky Mountain spotted fever and Lyme disease, are now much less deadly because of new medicines and drug treatments.

—*Leslie V. Tischauser, Ph.D.*

See also Allergies; Asthma; Bites and stings; Dermatitis; Dermatology; Dermatology, pediatric; Insect-borne diseases; Itching; Lyme disease; Parasitic diseases; Rashes; Scabies; Skin; Skin disorders; Typhus.

FOR FURTHER INFORMATION:

Ashford, R. W., and W. Crewe. *The Parasites of "Homo sapiens": An Annotated Checklist of the Protozoa, Helminths, and Arthropods for Which We Are Home.* 2d ed. New York: Taylor & Francis, 2003. A comprehensive checklist of all the animals naturally parasitic in or on the human body. Each parasite includes a complete summary of characteristics.

Berenbaum, May R. *Ninety-nine Gnats, Nits, and Nibblers.* Urbana: University of Illinois Press, 1989. A scientist describes how insects affect human lives. Offers an informative description of the life cycles and habits of lice, mites, ticks, and other troublemakers.

Goddard, Jerome. *Physician's Guide to Arthropods of Medical Importance.* 4th ed. Boca Raton, Fla.: CRC Press, 2002. Nontechnical description of a wide variety of arthropods and conditions related to their stings or bites. Topics include allergy to venoms and the signs and symptoms of arthropod-borne diseases.

Olkowski, William, Sheila Daar, and Helga Olkowski. *Common-Sense Pest Control.* Newton, Conn.: Taunton Press, 1996. A very useful book by a biologist that describes the best methods of dealing with all kinds of insect problems, including lice, mites, and ticks. Offers detailed descriptions of how to remove these pests from your children and the environment safely.

Robinson, William H. *Urban Entomology: Insect and Mite Pests in the Human Environment.* London: Chapman & Hall, 1996. Discusses household pests in urban areas, including how to control them. Provides a bibliography and an index.

Service, M. W., ed. *Encyclopedia of Arthropod-Transmitted Infections of Man and Domesticated Animals.* New York: CAB International, 2001. Offers basic information related to the transmission, symptoms, treatment, and control of infections transmitted by biting midges, ticks, lice, and related organisms.

Sheorey, Harsha, John Walker, and Beverley-Ann Biggs. *Clinical Parasitology.* Melbourne: University of Melbourne Press, 2003. Reviews global parasitic diseases and includes information regarding classification and geographical distribution of parasites, details of diagnostic tests, availability and treatment regimens of drugs, and means of obtaining uncommon drugs.

Vanderhoof-Forschner, Karen. *Everything You Need to Know About Lyme Disease and Other Tick-Borne Disorders.* 2d ed. New York: John Wiley & Sons, 2003. A consumer guide that aims to provide basic knowledge and useful insights into the prevention and management of disease.

Weedon, David. *Skin Pathology.* 2d ed. New York: Churchill Livingstone, 2002. Text with extensive photographs, covering tissue reaction patterns; the epidermis, dermis and subcutis; the skin in systemic and miscellaneous diseases; infections and infestations; and tumors, among other topics.

LIGHT THERAPY

TREATMENT

ANATOMY OR SYSTEM AFFECTED: Brain, nervous system, psychic-emotional system, skin

SPECIALTIES AND RELATED FIELDS: Dermatology, gerontology, oncology, ophthalmology, psychiatry, psychology

DEFINITION: A noninvasive procedure using exposure to light as the mechanism for clinical treatment.

INDICATIONS AND PROCEDURES

Light therapy, or phototherapy, treats a variety of disorders. By exposing individuals to different kinds of light (for example, monochromatic, polychromatic, ultraviolet), symptoms can often be delayed, reduced, and eradicated. Immunological, neurotransmitter, and neuroendocrine systems play key roles in response to this type of treatment.

Best known in psychiatry, light therapy serves as a treatment for treat seasonal affective disorder (SAD), or winter depression; bulimia nervosa; sleep disorders; and "sundowner's syndrome," the late afternoon confusion and agitation sometimes accompanying Alzheimer's disease. Shift workers can also experience difficulties related to light exposure, and light therapies may provide some relief. Reduced environmental light is a factor in the etiology, onset, or maintenance of these problems. Thus, treatment involves exposing individuals to bright, full-spectrum light for specific time-periods. Duration of exposure and light intensity vary by the disorder and individual treated.

In dermatology and oncology, light therapy treats psoriasis, skin ulcers, tumors, and esophageal cancers. The type of light and the intensities used, however, vary considerably from those applied for the treatment of psychiatric disorders.

Uses and Complications

The side effects of light therapy are best documented in psychiatry: Insomnia, mania, and (less frequently) morning hot flashes have been noted. Persons with other sensitivity to light, such as those prone to migraines, may also need to exercise caution with light therapy in order to avoid undesirable effects. Careful monitoring by medical providers of the patient's response to treatment is necessary. Additionally, professionals advise morning administrations of light therapy.

Users of light therapy must also be cautioned to adhere closely to recommended doses and intensity of exposure to light. Use of light outside of prescribed parameters may be damaging to the eyes.

Light therapy is not effective universally; some patients may experience no improvement. For seasonal affective disorder, evidence suggests that younger individuals whose depression involves weight gain and increased sleep may be most likely to respond to treatment. For psoriasis, complementary treatments, such as psychotherapy, may facilitate a response to treatment.

Perspective and Prospects

Light and dark cycles are a biological reality; thus, it is no surprise that light affects physical, emotional, and mental well-being. As the interest in noninvasive interventions increases, the attention given to environmental treatments such as light therapy is likely to increase as well. Recent developments in the use of light therapy for sleep and behavioral disorders are fueling clinical, research, consumer, and other business interests in this procedure. Experimentation with different frequencies or colors of light, doses, intensities, and sites on the body for application of light are ongoing and likely to increase the diversity of uses for this type of treatment. Additionally applications of light-based interventions in the workplace and elsewhere may prove useful in preventing disorders related to light deprivation and in helping to affect productivity, directly and indirectly.

—*Nancy A. Piotrowski, Ph.D.*

See also Alternative medicine; Alzheimer's disease; Bulimia; Chronobiology; Depression; Dermatology; Psoriasis; Psychiatry; Seasonal affective disorder; Skin disorders; Sleep; Sleep disorders.

For Further Information:

Goldberg, Burton, comp. *Alternative Medicine: The Definitive Guide.* 2d ed. Portland, Oreg.: Ten Speed Press, 2002.

Hyman, Jane Wegscheider. *Light Book: How Natural and Artificial Light Affects Our Health, Mood, and Behavior.* New York: Putnam, 1990.

Jacobs, Jennifer, ed. *The Encyclopedia of Alternative Medicine: A Complete Family Guide to Complementary Therapies.* Rev. ed. Boston: Journey Edition, 1997.

Kastner, Mark, and Hugh Burroughs. *Alternative Healing: The Complete A-Z Guide to over 160 Different Alternative Therapies.* New York: Henry Holt, 1996.

Marshall, Fiona, and Peter Cheevers. *Positive Options for Seasonal Affective Disorder.* New York: Hunter House, 2003.

Palmer, John D. *The Living Clock: The Orchestrator of Biological Rhythms.* New York: Oxford University Press, 2002.

Lipids

Biology

Anatomy or system affected: Cells, gastrointestinal system

Specialties and related fields: Biochemistry, cytology, nutrition, vascular medicine

Definition: Organic compounds found in the tissues of plants and animals that serve as energy-storage molecules, function as solvents for water-insoluble vitamins, provide insulation against the loss of body heat, act as a protective cushion for vital organs, and are structural components of cell membranes.

Key terms:

alcohol: an organic compound containing a hydroxyl (–OH) group attached to a carbon atom *carboxylic acid:* an organic compound that contains the carboxyl (–CO2H) group

ester: the relatively non-water-soluble compound formed when an alcohol reacts with a carboxylic acid

fatty acid: an organic compound that is composed of a long hydrocarbon chain with a carboxyl group at one end

glycerol: a three-carbon alcohol that has one hydroxyl compound on each carbon atom

hydrocarbon: an organic compound composed of only hydrogen and carbon atoms that does not dissolve in water (water-insoluble)

hydrophilic: "water-loving" or "water-attracting"; a term given to molecules or regions of molecules that interact favorably with water

hydrophobic: "water-hating" or "water-repelling"; a term given to molecules or regions of molecules that do not interact favorably with water

saponification: a reaction in which a strong basic solution splits a molecule into a carboxylic acid unit and an alcohol unit

STRUCTURE AND FUNCTIONS

Lipids are a class of bio-organic compounds that are typically insoluble in water and relatively soluble in organic solvents such as alcohols, ethers, and hydrocarbons. Unlike the other classes of organic molecules found in biological systems (carbohydrates, proteins, and nucleic acids), lipids possess a unifying physical property—solubility behavior—rather than a unifying structural feature. Fats, oils, some vitamins and hormones, and most of the nonprotein components of cell membranes are lipids.

There are two categories of lipids—those that undergo saponification and those that are nonsaponifiable. The saponifiable lipids can be divided into simple and complex lipids. Simple lipids, which are composed of carbon, hydrogen, and oxygen, yield fatty acids and an alcohol upon saponification. Complex lipids contain one or more additional elements, such as phosphorus, nitrogen, and sulfur, yielding fatty acids, alcohol, and other compounds on saponification.

The fatty acid building blocks of saponifiable lipids may be either saturated, which means that as many hydrogen atoms as possible are attached to the carbon chain, or unsaturated, which means that at least two hydrogen atoms are missing. Saturated fatty acids are white solids at room temperature, while unsaturated ones are liquids at room temperature, because of a geo-

metrical difference in the long carbon chains. The carbon atoms of a saturated fatty acid are arranged in a zigzag or accordion configuration. These chains are stacked on top of one another in a very orderly and efficient fashion, making it difficult to separate the chains from one another. When carbons in the chain are missing hydrogen atoms, the regular zigzag of the chain is disrupted, leading to less efficient packing, which allows the chains to be separated more easily. Saturated fatty acids have a higher melting temperature because they require more energy to separate their chains than do unsaturated fatty acids. Unsaturated fatty acids can be converted into saturated ones by adding hydrogen atoms through a process called hydrogenation.

Simple lipids can be divided into triglycerides and waxes. Waxes such as beeswax, lanolin (from lamb's wool), and carnauba wax (from a palm tree) are esters formed from an alcohol with a long carbon chain and a fatty acid. These compounds, which are solids at room temperature, serve as protective coatings. Most plant leaves are coated with a wax film to prevent attack by microorganisms and loss of water through evaporation. Animal fur and bird feathers have a wax coating. For example, the wax coating on their feathers is what allows ducks to stay afloat.

Edible fats and oils such as lard (pig fat), tallow (beef fat), corn oil, and butter are triglycerides. Triglyceride molecules are fatty acid esters in which three fatty acids (all saturated, all unsaturated, or mixed) combine with one molecule of the alcohol glycerol. Oils are triglycerides that are liquid at room temperature, while fats are solid at room temperature. The fluidity of a triglyceride is dependent on the nature of its fatty acid chains; the more unsaturated the triglyceride, the more fluid its structure. The triglycerides found in animals tend to have more saturated fatty acids than do those found in plants. Vegetable oils and fish oils are frequently polyunsaturated.

Complex lipids are classified as phospholipids or glycolipids. Structurally, phospholipids are composed of fatty acids and a phosphate group. Glycerol-based lipids called phosphoglycerides contain glycerol, two fatty acids, and a phosphate group. The phosphoglyceride structure contains a hydrophilic (polar) head, the phosphate unit, and two hydrophobic (nonpolar) fatty acid tails. The polar head can interact strongly with water, while the nonpolar tails interact strongly with organic solvents and avoid water. Egg yolks contain a large amount of the phosphoglyceride phosphatidylcholine (also called lecithin). This lipid is used to form the emulsion mayonnaise from oil and vinegar. Normally, oil and water do not mix. The hydrophobic oil forms a separate layer on top of the water. Since lecithin's structure contains both a hydrophobic and a hydrophilic region, it can attach to the water with its polar head and the oil with its nonpolar tail, preventing the two materials from separating. Lipids derived from the alcohol sphingosine are called sphingolipids. They contain one fatty acid, one long hydrocarbon chain and a phosphate group. Like the phosphoglycerides, sphingolipids have a head-and-two-tail structure. Sphingolipids are important components in the protective and insulating coating that surrounds nerves.

Glycolipids differ from phospholipids in that they possess a sugar group in place of the phosphate group. Their structure is again the polar head and dual tail arrangement in which the sugar is the hydrophilic unit. Cerebrosides, which are sphingosine-based glycolipids containing a simple sugar such as galactose or glucose, are found in large amounts in the white matter of the brain and in the myelin sheath. Gangliosides, which are found in the gray matter of the brain, in neural tissue, and in the receptor sites for neurotransmitters, contain a more complex sugar component.

Nonsaponifiable lipids do not contain esters of fatty acids as their basic structural feature. Steroids are an important class of nonsaponifiable lipids. All steroids possess an identical four-ring framework called the steroid nucleus, but they differ in the groups that are attached to their ring systems. Examples of steroids are sterols such as cholesterol, the bile acids secreted by the liver, the sex hormones, corticosteroids secreted by the adrenal cortex, and digitoxin from the digitalis plant, which is used to treat heart disease.

Lipids constitute about 50 percent of the mass of most animal cell membranes. Biological membranes control the chemical environment of the space they enclose. They are selective filters controlling what substances enter and exit the cell, since they constitute a relatively impermeable barrier against most water-soluble molecules. The three types of lipids involved are phospholipids (most abundant), glycolipids, and cholesterol. Phospholipids, when surrounded by an aqueous environment, tend to organize into a double layer of lipid molecules, a bilayer, allowing their hydrophobic tails to be buried internally and their hydrophilic heads to be exposed to the water. These phospholipids have one saturated and one unsaturated tail. Differences in tail length and saturation influence the packing efficiency of the molecules and affect the flu-

idity of the membrane. Short, unsaturated tails increase the fluidity of the membrane. Cholesterol is important in maintaining the mechanical stability of the lipid bilayer, thereby preventing a change from the fluid state to a rigid crystalline state. It also decreases the permeability of small water-soluble molecules.

The lipid bilayer provides the basic structure of the membrane and serves as a two-dimensional solvent for protein molecules. Protein molecules are responsible for most membrane functions; for example, they can provide receptor sites, catalyze reactions, or transport molecules across the membrane. These proteins may extend across the bilayer (transmembrane proteins) or be associated with only one face of the bilayer. Cell membranes also have carbohydrates attached to the outer face of the bilayer. These carbohydrates are bound to membrane proteins or part of a glycolipid. Typically, 2 to 10 percent of a membrane's total weight is carbohydrate. Evidence exists that cell-surface carbohydrates are used as recognition sites for chemical processes.

Lipids play an important role in health and well-being. The body acquires lipids directly from dietary lipids and indirectly by converting other nutrients into lipids. There are two fatty acids, linoleic and linolenic acids, which are called essential fatty acids. Since these fatty acids cannot be synthesized in the body in sufficient amounts, their supply must come directly from dietary sources. Fortunately, these acids are widely found in foodstuffs, so deficiency is rarely observed in adults.

About 95 percent of the lipids in foods are triglycerides, which provide 30 to 50 percent of the calories in an average diet. Triglycerides produce 4,000 calories of energy per pound, compared to the 1,800 calories per pound produced by carbohydrates or proteins. Since the triglyceride is such an efficient energy source, the body converts carbohydrates and proteins into adipose (reserve fatty) tissue for storage to be used when extra fuel is required.

While carbohydrates and proteins undergo major degradation in the stomach, triglycerides remain intact, forming large globules that float to the top of the mixture. Fats spend a longer time than other nutrients in the stomach, slowing molecular activity before continuing into the intestines. Thus, a fat-laden meal gives longer satiety than a low-fat one.

In the small intestine, bile salts split fat globules into smaller droplets, allowing enzymes called lipases to saponify the triglycerides. In some instances, the fatty acids at the two ends are removed, leaving one attached as a monoglyceride. About 97 percent of dietary triglycerides are absorbed into the bloodstream; the remainder are excreted. Although glycerol and fatty acids with short carbon chains are water-soluble enough to dissolve in the blood, the long-chain fatty acids and monoglycerides are not. These insoluble materials recombine to form new triglycerides. Since these hydrophobic triglycerides would form large globules if they were dumped directly into the blood, small triglyceride droplets are surrounded with a protective protein coat that can dissolve in water, taking the encapsulated triglyceride with it. This structure is an example of a lipoprotein.

Cholesterol is found in relatively small (milligram) quantities in foods, compared to triglycerides. Cholesterol supplies raw materials for the production of bile salts and to be used as a structural constituent of brain and nerve tissue. Since these functions are important to animals but serve no purpose in plants, cholesterol is found only in animals. Only about 50 percent of dietary cholesterol is absorbed into the blood; the rest is excreted. Much of the body's supply of cholesterol is produced in the liver. For most individuals, the amount of cholesterol synthesized in the body is larger than the amount absorbed directly from the diet.

Digested lipids released from the intestine and those synthesized in the liver compose the lipid content of the blood. The fatty acids required by the liver are obtained directly from the bloodstream or by synthesis from sources such as glucose, amino acids, and alcohol. Liver-synthesized triglycerides are incorporated into lipoprotein packages before entering the bloodstream. There are three types of lipoprotein packages that transport lipids to and from the liver. Very-low-density lipoproteins (VLDLs) transport triglycerides to tissues; low-density lipoproteins (LDLs) transport the cholesterol from the liver to other cells; and high-density lipoproteins (HDLs) transport cholesterol from other tissues to the liver for destruction.

DISORDERS AND DISEASES

Lipid consumption is an important dietary concern. Lipid deficiency is rarely observed in adults but can occur in infants who are fed nonfat formulas. Since fatty acids are essential for growth, lipid consumption should not be restricted in individuals under two years of age. Excess lipid consumption is associated with health problems such as obesity and cardiovascular disease. Although excess calories from any dietary source can lead to obesity, the body must expend less energy to store dietary fat than to store dietary carbohydrate as body fat. Thus, high-fat diets produce more body fat than do high-carbohydrate, low-fat diets.

Atherosclerosis, or "hardening of the arteries," is the leading cause of cardiovascular disease. A strong correlation exists between diets high in saturated fats and the incidence of atherosclerosis. In this condition, deposits called plaques, which have a high cholesterol content, form on artery walls. Over time, these deposits narrow the artery and decrease its elasticity, resulting in reduced blood flow. Blockages can occur, resulting in heart attack or stroke. High serum cholesterol levels (total blood cholesterol content) often result in increased plaque formation. Since dietary cholesterol is not efficiently absorbed into the bloodstream and the serum cholesterol level is largely determined by the amount of cholesterol synthesized in the liver, high serum cholesterol levels are frequently related to high saturated fat intake.

Since the measurement of the serum cholesterol level gives the total cholesterol concentration of the blood, it can be a somewhat misleading predictor of atherosclerosis risk; cholesterol is not free in blood, but is encapsulated in lipoproteins. Since the cholesterol packaged in the LDL, cholesterol that can be deposited in plaques ("bad" cholesterol), has a very different fate from that in the HDL, which is transporting cholesterol for destruction ("good" cholesterol), measuring the ratio of LDL cholesterol to HDL cholesterol has been found to be a better indicator of atherosclerosis risk. Decreasing dietary intake of cholesterol and saturated fats, increasing water-soluble fibers in the diet, removing excess body weight, and increasing the amount of aerobic exercise will all serve to improve the LDL-C/HDL-C ratio.

A number of hereditary diseases are known that result from abnormal accumulation of the complex lipids utilized in membranes. These diseases are called lipid (or lysosomal) storage diseases, or lipidoses. In normal individuals, the amount of each complex lipid present in the body is relatively constant; in other words, the rate of formation equals the rate of destruction. The lipids are broken down by enzymes that attack specific bonds in the lipid structure. Lipid storage diseases occur when a lipid-degrading enzyme is defective or absent. In these cases, the lipid synthesis proceeds normally, but the degradation is impaired, causing the lipid or a partial degradation product to accumulate, with consequences such as an enlarged liver and spleen, mental retardation, blindness, and death.

Niemann-Pick, Gaucher's, and Tay-Sachs diseases are examples of lipidoses. Niemann-Pick disease is caused by a defect in an enzyme that breaks down sphingomyelin. The disease becomes apparent in infancy, causing mental retardation and death normally by age four. Gaucher's disease, a more common disease involving the accumulation of a glycolipid, produces two different syndromes. The acute cerebral form affects infants, causing severe nervous system abnormalities, retardation, and death before age one. The chronic form, which may become evident at any age, causes enlargement of the spleen, anemia, and erosion of the bones. In Tay-Sachs disease, a partially degraded lipid accumulates in the tissues of the central nervous system. Symptoms include progressive loss of vision, paralysis, and death at three or four years of age. Although Tay-Sachs disease is relatively rare (1 in 300,000 births), it has a high incidence in individuals of Eastern European Jewish descent (1 in 3,600 births). This defect is a recessive genetic trait that is found in one of every twenty-eight members of this population. For two parents who are both carriers of this trait, there is a one in four chance that their child will develop Tay-Sachs disease. Tests have been developed to detect the presence of the defective gene in the parent, and the amniotic fluid of a developing fetus can be sampled using a technique called amniocentesis to detect Tay-Sachs disease. Lipid storage diseases have no known cures; however, they can be prevented through genetic counseling.

PERSPECTIVE AND PROSPECTS

The ability of a cell to discriminate in its chemical exchanges with the environment is fundamental to life. How the cell membrane accomplishes this feat has been an intense subject of biochemical research since the beginning of the twentieth century.

In 1895, C. Overton observed that substances that are lipid-soluble enter cells more quickly than those that are lipid-insoluble. He reasoned that the membrane must be composed of lipids. About twenty years later, chemical analysis showed that membranes also contain proteins. Irwin Langmuir prepared the first artificial membrane in 1917 by mixing a phospholipid-containing hydrocarbon solution with water. Evaporation of the hydrocarbon left a phospholipid film on the surface of the water, which showed that only the hydrophilic heads contacted the water. When the Dutch biologists E. Gorter and F. Grendel deposited the lipids from red blood cell membranes on a water surface and decreased

the occupied surface area with a movable barrier, a continuous film resulted that occupied an area approximately twice the surface area of the original red blood cells. In 1935, all these observations, along with the fact that the surfaces of artificial membranes containing only phospholipids are less water-absorbent than the surfaces of true biological membranes, were combined by H. Davison and J. Danielli into a membrane model in which a phospholipid bilayer was sandwiched between two water-absorbent protein layers.

The technological advances of the 1950's in X-ray diffraction and electron microscopy allowed the structures of membranes to be probed directly. Such studies revealed that membranes are indeed composed of two parallel orderly arrays of lipids; although many of the proteins are attached to one of the faces of the bilayer, however, the Danielli-Davison model was too simplistic. The freeze-fracture technique of preparing cells for electron microscopy has provided the most information about the nature of membrane proteins. In this technique, the two layers are separated so that the inner topography can be studied. Instead of the smooth surface predicted by the Danielli-Davison model, a cobblestone-like surface was observed that resulted from proteins penetrating into the interior of the membrane. All experimental evidence supports the fluid mosaic model for biological membranes, in which proteins are dispersed and embedded in a phospholipid bilayer that is in a fluid state. How membranes function was the next question to be considered.

Although most of the small molecules needed by cells cross the barrier via protein channels, some essential nutrients, such as cholesterol in its LDL package, are too large to pass through a small channel. In 1986, Michael Brown and Joseph Goldstein received the Nobel Prize for their discovery of specific protein receptors on the membranes of liver cells to which LDL molecules attach. These receptors move across the surface until they encounter a shallow indentation or pit. As the pit deepens, the membrane closes behind the LDL, forming a coating allowing transport across the hydrophobic membrane interior. The presence of insufficient numbers of these receptors causes abnormal LDL-cholesterol buildup in the blood.

Many questions remain unanswered concerning the roles of proteins and glycolipids in membranes. Membranes are involved in the movement, growth, and development of cells. How the membrane is involved in the uncontrolled multiplication and migration in cancer is one medically important question. Experiments that will answer questions about how membrane structure affects functioning should lead to the development of new medical treatments.

—*Arlene R. Courtney, Ph.D.*

See also Arteriosclerosis; Cholesterol; Digestion; Fluids and electrolytes; Food biochemistry; Gaucher's disease; Heart disease; Hypercholesterolemia; Hyperlipidemia; Insulin resistance syndrome; Metabolic disorders; Metabolism; Niemann-Pick disease; Nonalcoholic steatohepatitis (NASH); Obesity; Obesity, childhood; Steroids; Tay-Sachs disease.

FOR FURTHER INFORMATION:

Bettleheim, F. A., et al. *Introduction to General, Organic, and Biochemistry.* 8th ed. New York: Brooks Cole, 2006. A text designed for students with little previous chemistry background. Chapter 17 discusses the structure and function of lipids, chapter 21 discusses the conversion of biological molecules into energy, and chapter 22 gives details of the synthesis of lipids in the body.

Bloomfield, Molly M., and Lawrence J. Stephens. *Chemistry and the Living Organism.* 6th ed. New York: John Wiley & Sons, 1996. A text written for allied health students that has a well-written chapter on lipids. Other chapters provide good elementary coverage on organic compounds such as alcohols, carboxylic acids, and esters.

Brown, Michael S., and Joseph L. Goldstein. "How LDL Receptors Influence Cholesterol and Atherosclerosis." *Scientific American* 251 (November, 1984): 58-66. An article in which the Nobel laureates describe their work on LDL membrane receptors. This article is of an intermediate technical nature.

Christian, Janet L., and Janet L. Greger. *Nutrition for Living.* 4th ed. Redwood City, Calif.: Benjamin/ Cummings, 1994. A human nutrition text written at a level requiring little or no technical knowledge. This book provides an elementary discussion of the nutritional aspects of fats and cholesterol.

Cornatzer, W. E. *Role of Nutrition in Health and Disease.* Springfield, Ill.: Charles C Thomas, 1989. Gives a comprehensive description of medical conditions in which lipids are involved.

Sikorski, Zdzisław E., and Anna Kołakowska, eds. *Chemical and Functional Properties of Food Lipids.* Boca Raton, Fla.: CRC Press, 2002. In seventeen chapters by international specialists, this book examines the nature, technological properties, reactiv-
ity, and health-related concerns and benefits of food lipids.

Vance, Dennis E., and Jean E. Vance, eds. *Biochemistry of Lipids, Lipoproteins, and Membranes.* 4th ed. Boston: Elsevier, 2002. First published in 1985, this edition details the startling advances made in lipid biochemistry and covers all aspects of lipids research.

LIPOSUCTION
PROCEDURE

ANATOMY OR SYSTEM AFFECTED: Abdomen, arms, hips, knees, legs

SPECIALTIES AND RELATED FIELDS: General surgery, plastic surgery

DEFINITION: The removal of fat deposits with a cannula and a suction pump in order to recontour body areas.

KEY TERMS:

abdomen: the area of the body between the diaphragm and the pelvis; it contains the visceral organs

adipose tissue: the tissue that stores fat

cannula: a tube used to drain body fluids or to administer medications

general anesthesia: anesthesia that induces unconsciousness

local anesthesia: anesthesia that numbs the feeling in a body part; administered by injection or direct application to the skin

subcutaneous: under the skin

INDICATIONS AND PROCEDURES

The fat contained in adipose tissue makes up 15 to 20 percent of the body weights of most healthy individuals. Much adipose tissue is found inside the abdominal cavity, but significant amounts are located under the skin of the abdomen, arms, breasts, hips, knees, legs, and throat. The quantity of this subcutaneous fat at any such site is based on individual heredity, age, and eating habits. When excessive eating greatly elevates body fat, a patient becomes obese, a condition that can be life-threatening. Until recently, the sole means for decreasing fat content resulting from obesity was time-consuming dieting, which requires much patience and will power. In addition, the positive consequences of long diets can be easily obliterated if dieters begin to overeat again. Recurrent overeating is common and often followed by the rapid regaining of the fat.

Persons who have undesired, unattractive fat deposits as a result of age, heredity, or obesity may undergo cosmetic surgery, such as so-called tummy tucks, to remove them. Such major procedures, however, often remove muscle along with fat and cause considerable scarring. Liposuction is a relatively easy way to lose unattractive body fat; it also is seen as a fast way to reverse obesity and is touted as more permanent than dieting. A cannula connected to a suction pump is inserted under the skin in the desired area. Then a chosen amount of fat is sucked out, the cannula is withdrawn, and the incision is closed. The result is a recontouring of the body part. Hence, liposuction has become a very popular cosmetic surgery procedure for the abdomen, arms, breasts, hips, knees, legs, and throat; many pounds can be removed from large areas such as the abdomen.

Liposuction begins with the administration of antibiotics and the anesthesia of the area to be recontoured. Local anesthesia is safer, but general anesthesia is used when necessary. The process usually begins after a 1.3-centimeter (0.5-inch) incision is made in a fold of the treated body region, so that the scar will not be noticeable after healing. At this time, a sterile cannula is introduced under the skin of the treatment area. Next, the surgeon uses suction through the cannula to remove the fat deposits. Liposuction produces temporary tunnels in adipose tissue. Upon completion of the procedure, the incision is closed and the surgical area is wrapped with tight bandages or covered with support garments. This final stage of recontouring helps the tissue to col-

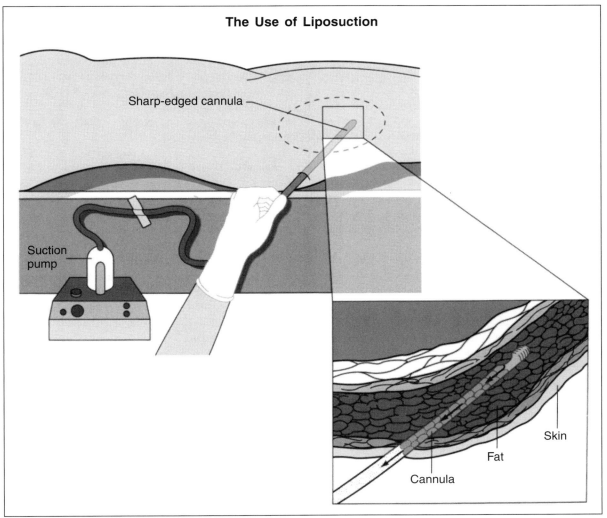

The Use of Liposuction

Sharp-edged cannula

Suction pump

Skin

Fat

Cannula

When unwanted areas of fat seem resistant to dieting and exercise, some patients turn to liposuction, the physical removal of fat deposits with a tube and a suction pump. The cosmetic results of this procedure may vary considerably.

lapse back into the desired shape during healing. In most patients, the skin around the area soon shrinks into the new contours. When this does not happen easily, because of old age or other factors, liposuction is accompanied by surgical skin removal.

USES AND COMPLICATIONS

Liposuction can be used for body recontouring only when undesired contours are attributable to fat deposits; those attributable to anatomical features such as bone structure cannot be treated in this manner.

A major principle on which liposuction is based is the supposition that the body contains a fixed number of fat cells and that, as people become fatter, the cells fill with droplets of fat and expand. The removal of fat cells by liposuction is deemed to decrease the future ability of the treated body part to become fat because fewer cells are available to be filled. Dieting and exercise are less successful than liposuction because they do not diminish the number of fat cells in adipose tissue, only decreasing fat cell size. Hence, when dieters return to eating excess food again or exercise stops, the fat cells expand again.

Another aspect of liposuction which is becoming popular is the ability to remove undesired fat from some body sites and insert it where the fat is wanted for recontouring. Most often, this transfer involves enlarging women's breasts or correcting cases in which the two breasts are of markedly different size. Liposuction also can be used to repair asymmetry in other body parts as a result of accidents.

Liposuction, as with any other surgery, has associated risks and complications. According to reputable practitioners, however, they are temporary and relatively minor, such as black-and-blue marks and the accumulation of blood and serum under the skin of treated areas. These complications are minimized by fluid removal during surgery and by the application of tight bandages or garments after the operation. Another related complication is that subcutaneous fat removal leads to fluid loss from the body. When large amounts of fat are removed, shock occurs if the fluid is not replaced quickly. Therefore, another component of successful liposuction is timely fluid replacement.

The more extensive and complex the liposuction procedure attempted, the more likely it is to cause complications. Particularly prone to problems are liposuction procedures in which major skin removal is required. Hence, surgeons who perform liposuction suggest that potential patients be realistic about the goals of the surgery. It is also recommended that patients choose reputable practitioners.

PERSPECTIVE AND PROSPECTS

Liposuction, currently viewed as relatively safe cosmetic surgery, originated in Europe in the late 1960's. In 1982, it reached the United States. Since that time, its use has burgeoned, and about a half million liposuction surgeries are carried out yearly. Although its first use was as a purely cosmetic procedure, liposuction is now done for noncosmetic reasons, including repairing injuries sustained in accidents. Women were once the sole liposuction patients. Now, men make up about one-quarter of treated individuals.

In the United States, liposuction is not presently accepted by insurance companies or considered tax deductible. This situation may change because several studies have found that obese people have a greater chance of developing cardiovascular disease and cancer. It must be noted, however, that liposuction offers only temporary relief from body fat. Although it does decrease fat deposition in a treated region, lack of proper calorie intake and exercise will deposit fat elsewhere in the body.

—*Sanford S. Singer, Ph.D.*

See also Bariatric surgery; Dermatology; Lipids; Nutrition; Obesity; Obesity, childhood; Plastic surgery; Skin; Weight loss and gain.

FOR FURTHER INFORMATION:

Schein, Jeffery R. "The Truth About Liposuction." *Consumers Digest* 30 (January/February, 1991): 71-74. Liposuction is the most popular type of cosmetic surgery, and that means that many people are assuming that liposuction can do more than it really can. Some facts about liposuction and physicians' certification are given.

Shelton, Ron M., and Terry Malloy. *Liposuction.* New York: Berkley, 2004. A consumer guide to liposuction that reviews the pros and cons and answers common questions.

Shiffman, Melvin A., and Alberto Di Giuseppe, eds. *Liposuction: Principles and Practice.* New York: Springer, 2006. A comprehensive book on the latest state-of-the-art methods.

Wilkinson, Tolbert S. *Atlas of Liposuction.* Philadelphia: Elsevier Saunders, 2005. A helpful atlas covering liposuction. Includes bibliographical references and an index.

Zollinger, Robert M., Jr., and Robert M. Zollinger, Sr.

Zollinger's Atlas of Surgical Operations. 8th ed. New York: McGraw-Hill, 2003. A comprehensive examination of surgery. Covers basic surgical anatomy and vascular, gynecologic, gastrointestinal, and miscellaneous abdominal procedures.

LISPING

DISEASE/DISORDER

ANATOMY OR SYSTEM AFFECTED: Mouth, teeth

SPECIALTIES AND RELATED FIELDS: Dentistry, speech pathology

DEFINITION: The defective pronunciation of the sibilants "s" and "z," usually substituted with a "th" sound.

CAUSES AND SYMPTOMS

A central or frontal lisp is caused by a child pushing the tongue past the teeth while speaking, which tends to occur in cases of an open bite. This produces the familiar lisp in which "s" and "z" sounds are pronounced like "th." Sometimes, the child tries to correct the protrusion of the tongue by pulling it in, but lisping still occurs because the correct position of the tongue has not been learned.

A lateral lisp involves the escape of air on both sides of the tongue, yielding an unpleasant "blubbering" sound. A possible cause is missing teeth, particularly the two upper front teeth.

A recessive lisp is caused by holding the tongue too far back in the mouth. The "s" and "z" sounds come out sounding more like "sh." This mild lisp is often associated in the popular media with the speech of an intoxicated person.

TREATMENT AND THERAPY

Speech therapists work with lisping children in two ways. In the phonetic placement method, the child is asked to pronounce the "t" sound and then prolong it. Once this is learned, the bite is closed and the child then practices moving the lips in a slightly protracted position; the tongue is moved back and forth until the "s" sound is achieved. This same process is used in learning to pronounce "z"; the "d" sound, however, is used in practice instead of a "t." In some cases, asking the child to pronounce "sh" first and then move the tongue forward along the roof of the mouth will produce an "s" sound.

In the auditory stimulation method, the speech therapist pronounces the correct sound repeatedly and com-

---

> ### INFORMATION ON LISPING
>
> **CAUSES:** Physiological defects, dental problems, missing teeth
> **SYMPTOMS:** Mispronunciation of sibilants *s* and *z*
> **DURATION:** Typically short-term but may be chronic
> **TREATMENTS:** Speech therapy

pares it to the incorrect articulation. This method is very successful in young children with lisps.

After a sound has been practiced by itself, the child attaches it to nonsense syllables and practices pronouncing them. Gradually, the sound is introduced in familiar words, followed by sentences. The final test is the use of the newly acquired sound in spontaneous conversation.

—Rose Secrest

See also Developmental stages; Motor skill development; Speech disorders; Stuttering; Voice and vocal cord disorders.

FOR FURTHER INFORMATION:

Bleile, Ken M. *Manual of Articulation and Phonological Disorders: Infancy Through Adulthood.* 2d ed. Clifton Park, N.Y.: Thomson Delmar Learning, 2004.

Gordon-Brannan, Mary E., and Curtis E. Weiss. *Clinical Management of Articulatory and Phonologic Disorders.* 3d ed. Philadelphia: Lippincott Williams & Wilkins, 2007.

Hamaguchi, Patricia McAleer. *Childhood Speech, Language, and Listening Problems: What Every Parent Should Know.* 2d ed. New York: Wiley, 2001.

Williams, A. Lynn. *Speech Disorders Resource Guide for Preschool Children.* Clifton Park, N.Y.: Thomson/Delmar Learning, 2003.

LITHOTRIPSY

PROCEDURE

ANATOMY OR SYSTEM AFFECTED: Abdomen, bladder, kidneys, urinary system

SPECIALTIES AND RELATED FIELDS: Nephrology, urology

DEFINITION: A method of breaking up stones in the kidneys, ureters, and urinary bladder using shock waves or high-frequency sound waves.

INDICATIONS AND PROCEDURES

Stone fragmentation using shock waves or ultrasonic waves is less invasive, less painful, and less time consuming than conventional open surgery to remove stones or the organs that contain them. With lithotripsy, blood loss is minimal and recovery is quick, with a low morbidity (injury rate).

In extracorporeal shock-wave lithotripsy (ESWL), the patient is given either local or general anesthesia. A machine called a lithotripter is placed on the abdomen over the site of the stones. An emitter in the lithotripter sends out shock waves that break the stones into fine fragments that can pass through the urinary tract without harm to the patient, who is encouraged to drink copious amounts of fluid following the procedure.

In ultrasonic lithotripsy, an incision is made in the skin. The stone is approached and visualized with an endoscope, a hollow instrument with a telescope at one end for visualization. The other end of the instrument is introduced via the urethra into the bladder or ureter or via a small skin hole into the kidney. For kidney stones, a small needle is introduced into the kidney through the back under X-ray control, and a nephrostomy tract is established between the skin and the kidney. The ultrasonographic lithotripsy probe is introduced through the endoscope and brought in contact with the stone.

A piezoceramic crystal is electrically stimulated, which generates ultrasonic waves that will fragment the stone. The design of the probe allows it to suction out the broken stone particles simultaneously. Larger stones can be fragmented into smaller pieces, which can then be grasped with forceps and pulled out. When a ureteral stone is treated by this method, a plastic tube (a double-J stent) is left in the ureter to prevent postoperative blockage and future scar formation. When a kidney stone is treated by this method, a large-caliber tube is left in the kidney (a nephrostomy tube) to drain the kidney and secure a tract for future X-ray studies and reinspection of the kidney for possible residual stone fragments.

USES AND COMPLICATIONS

The main morbidity associated with this procedure occurs during the establishment of the nephrostomy tract to gain access to the kidney, which can lead to bleeding, or during the introduction of the endoscope into the ureter, which can lead to perforation and future scarring. During stone fragmentation, it is imperative that the probe be in direct contact with the stone at all times, or it may cause ureteral perforation and bleeding. Overall, however, ultrasonographic lithotripsy is a safe and effective method of stone treatment, with few injuries and a quick recovery.

As with ultrasonic lithotripsy, few serious complications are associated with shock-wave lithotripsy. The presence of blood in the urine (hematuria) may be noted but is usually only temporary, as the stone fragments pass through the ureters, bladder, and urethra. Abdominal bruising may also occur, but this complication is minor in comparison to more invasive techniques. Severe pain that is unresponsive to medication may rarely signal perirenal hematoma. Other rare complications include pancreatitis and nerve palsy. Research is ongoing regarding the possibility of an association of ESWL with the development of hypertension in some patients.

—*Saeed Akhter, M.D.;*
updated by Victoria Price, Ph.D.

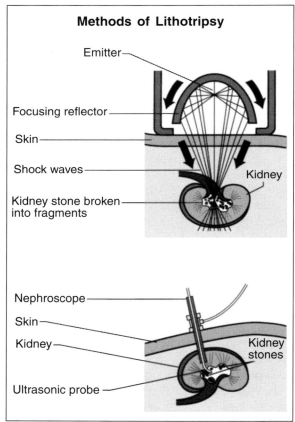

Methods of Lithotripsy

Emitter

Focusing reflector

Skin

Shock waves

Kidney

Kidney stone broken into fragments

Nephroscope

Skin

Kidney

Kidney stones

Ultrasonic probe

Kidney stones can be removed or broken into fragments using lithotripsy. In extracorporeal shock-wave lithotripsy (top), an emitter sends shock waves into tissues above the kidney stones, breaking the stones into very small fragments that can then be passed through the urine. In percutaneous lithotripsy (bottom), a nephroscope is inserted through the skin and into the kidney, where an ultrasonic probe breaks up and removes the stones.

See also Cholecystectomy; Gallbladder diseases; Kidney disorders; Kidneys; Nephrology; Stone removal; Stones; Ultrasonography; Urinary disorders; Urinary system; Urology.

FOR FURTHER INFORMATION:

Alexander, Ivy L., ed. *Urinary Tract And Kidney Diseases And Disorders Sourcebook: Basic Consumer Health Information About the Urinary System.* 2d ed. Detroit: Omnigraphics, 2005.

Leikin, Jerrold B., and Martin S. Lipsky, eds. *American Medical Association Complete Medical Encyclopedia.* New York: Random House Reference, 2003.

Parker, James N., and Philip M. Parker, eds. *The 2002 Official Patient's Sourcebook on Kidney Stones.* San Diego, Calif.: Icon Health, 2002.

Tanagho, Emil A., and Jack W. McAninich, eds. *Smith's General Urology.* 16th ed. New York: Lange Medical Books/McGraw-Hill, 2004.

Tierney, Lawrence M., Stephen J. McPhee, and Maxine A. Papadakis, eds. *Current Medical Diagnosis and Treatment 2007.* New York: McGraw-Hill Medical, 2006.

Walsh, Patrick C., and Darracott Vaughan. *Campbell's Urology.* 8th ed. New York: Elsevier, 2002.

LIVER

ANATOMY

ANATOMY OR SYSTEM AFFECTED: Abdomen, blood, circulatory system, endocrine system, gastrointestinal system, glands

SPECIALTIES AND RELATED FIELDS: Endocrinology, gastroenterology, hematology, internal medicine, toxicology

DEFINITION: A vital organ that controls blood sugar levels; metabolizes carbohydrates, lipids, and proteins; stores blood, iron, and some vitamins; degrades steroid hormones; and inactivates and/or excretes certain drugs and toxins.

KEY TERMS:

cirrhosis: a condition of the liver in which injured or dead cells are replaced with scar tissue

endoplasmic reticulum: a component of cells which in the liver is responsible for, among other things, the metabolism of xenobiotics

hepatitis: an infectious disease of the liver that is caused by a virus; at least three different types of hepatitis exist

hepatocyte: the functional cell of the liver; the liver contains only one type of functional cell

plasma proteins: any proteins found in the plasma of blood, which include those proteins necessary for blood clotting and some necessary for the transport of other molecules; most are produced by the liver

subclinical: referring to an infection in which the patient has no symptoms of disease; the infection is detected by other indicators, such as the presence of antibodies

virus: a subcellular particle that enters cells and causes cellular damage; it uses the cells' mechanisms to reproduce itself

xenobiotic: a nonbiological chemical that can enter a biological system; it could be a prescribed drug, a pollutant, or another substance

STRUCTURE AND FUNCTIONS

The liver, an accessory gland of the digestive system, is the largest organ in the human body. Located in the upper-right quadrant of the abdominal cavity, it abuts the diaphragm on the anterior surface. The liver is composed of two lobes of unequal size, with the large right lobe further divided into two smaller lobes. The organ is protected by the ribs, which cover nearly the entire surface. The liver contains only one type of functional cell, known as a hepatocyte. Closely associated with the organ is the gallbladder, a saclike structure which holds bile, a product of the hepatocytes. Bile is continually produced by the hepatocytes but is stored in the gallbladder until it is required for digestive products.

The liver is unique in that it receives blood from two different sources. The hepatic artery delivers blood to the liver from the systemic circulation. The liver also receives blood via the portal vein, which collects blood that has previously passed through the small intestine and has absorbed nutrients from the digestive system. As the blood enters the liver, it flows into dilated capillaries called sinusoids. Blood flow through sinusoids is much slower than through capillaries, and the exchange of materials between hepatocytes and the bloodstream is accomplished with little difficulty. This slower process also allows the liver to serve as a storage organ for blood, which gives the organ its characteristic dark red appearance.

The liver is essential to the normal functioning of the body. Its activities are many and varied: It regulates the metabolism of carbohydrates, lipids, and proteins; synthesizes proteins, particularly those of blood plasma that control clotting; serves as a storage site for some vitamins and iron; degrades steroid hormones; and inactivates and/or excretes certain drugs and toxins.

The liver plays a major role in carbohydrate metabolism. As carbohydrates are absorbed from the small intestine, they are transported to the liver through the portal vein. The liver regulates blood sugar levels by removing excess quantities. If the diet includes too much glucose, this substance is stored in the liver or skeletal muscle as glycogen. If the blood sugar levels are low, the glycogen is broken down into glucose and released to the bloodstream. The liver is also capable of converting amino acids, lipids, or simple carbohydrates into glucose.

The principal functions of the liver in lipid metabolism are twofold. First, it is responsible for the breakdown of large fat molecules into small compounds that can be used for energy. Second, it synthesizes triglycerides, cholesterol, and phospholipids from other fats. All three of these compounds play important roles in cellular function.

The synthesis of proteins by the liver is of major importance for the body. The liver is capable of synthesizing not only a variety of proteins but also the nonessential amino acids that are the building blocks of proteins. Many of the proteins that the liver synthesizes are found in blood plasma, including those factors responsible for blood clotting. In order to protect the body against deficiencies in these substances, the liver stores vitamins A, D, and B_{12}. It is also capable of storing iron, the mineral necessary for the production of hemoglobin.

Located in the smooth endoplasmic reticulum of hepatocytes are nonspecific enzymes called the mixed-function oxidases. They are capable of metabolizing a wide variety of hormones, including some polypeptide hormones and the steroid hormones, such as cortisol, estrogen, and testosterone. These same enzymes are responsible for the degradation of many foreign substances that enter the body, such as prescription medications, illegal drugs, and toxins. Most of the materials metabolized are made more water-soluble, and therefore more easily excreted, by the kidney. Others are removed from the hepatocytes in the bile that the cells produce.

Production of bile by the hepatocytes is of utmost importance to the digestive system. Bile is composed of lecithin, cholesterol, bile pigments, proteins, and bile acids, along with an isotonic solution similar to blood plasma. Bile is produced continually and stored in the gallbladder. Several minutes after a meal begins, the gallbladder releases bile to the duodenum of the small intestine. The highest rate of bile release occurs

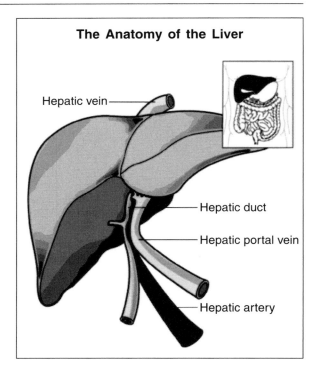

The Anatomy of the Liver

Hepatic vein

Hepatic duct

Hepatic portal vein

Hepatic artery

during the duodenal digestion of food and is controlled by the hormone cholecystokinin. In the duodenum, bile acts as an emulsifier of fat in the diet. It breaks large lipid droplets into many small lipid droplets, which can more easily be digested by enzymes in the small intestine. About 95 percent of the bile is reabsorbed and returned to the liver, and the other 5 percent is excreted with the feces. This provides one mechanism for the body to use the digestive system for the removal of waste products. One important product that is excreted in this manner is bilirubin, a by-product of the normal destruction of old red blood cells.

DISORDERS AND DISEASES

The liver is unique among body organs because it has the ability to regenerate in cases of injury or disease. It is estimated that in a young, healthy individual a liver which has suffered a physical injury could regenerate as much as 80 percent of the total organ. Many important organs are paired, such as the lungs and kidneys. Though the liver is a single organ, its ability to regenerate ensures normal function even in cases of severe injury.

The presence of liver disease is detectable in many ways. With some diseases, the liver becomes enlarged and can be felt below the ribs. This swelling may be associated with localized discomfort or pain in the region. In more severe cases of liver disease, the organ may actually shrink and recede further under the ribs, a condition easily detected by a physician.

The pathophysiology of the liver is characterized by certain physiologic events that occur regardless of the underlying cause. Within the liver, disease may result in portal hypertension, blockage of bile ducts, and cellular injury or death. Cellular injury may be manifest by fatty infiltration and by interference with cellular functions, including the synthesis of proteins necessary for blood clotting, the metabolism of drugs or toxins, the regulation of glucose, and the production of bile. Any or all of these physiologic changes can lead to effects in other parts of the body.

Disease of the liver is often detectable by routine blood tests that include liver function tests. The patient may show decreased levels in the blood serum of proteins that are normally produced by the liver, an increased blood-clotting time, or increased serum levels of enzymes that are normally found only in the liver. A yellow skin tone known as jaundice has been associated with liver disease. This discoloration of skin and the cornea of the eye is a result of excessively high levels of bilirubin in the blood. Bilirubin is a by-product of the breakdown of red blood cells that are near the end of their 120-day life cycle.

The injury or death of liver cells may present a pathology unique to the liver, the disease cirrhosis. When hepatocytes are injured or diseased, they begin to accumulate lipids in vacuoles, giving the liver a whitish appearance. Associated with the development of a fatty liver, the cells may divide to produce more cells that will ensure normal function. Sometimes, however, this stimulation of cell division leads to an excess of hepatocytes, a condition that may result in abnormal patterns of blood flow through the liver. In addition, this phenomenon may include the production of large nodules of connective tissue to replace dead or dying cells, a condition comparable to scarring. The development of scars may cause increased blood pressure in the portal veins and may block bile ducts. Cirrhosis may be caused by a variety of conditions, including alcoholism, exposure to toxic substances, or infection. It is irreversible and ultimately causes the death of the patient.

Diseases of the liver can be classified according to the following scheme: congenital liver disorders, viral and nonviral infections, drug-induced and toxin-induced disease, vascular disorders, metabolic disorders, iron accumulation, alcoholic liver disease, and tumors.

The most common types of congenital diseases of the liver involve abnormalities of the bile ducts or of the portal vein, which may be associated with portal hypertension. More important, however, are those diseases that lead to the formation of cysts, such as polycystic liver disease or hepatic fibrosis. Jaundice of the newborn, a discoloration of the skin at birth, usually clears within a week or so with no long-term effects.

Viral infections of the liver may be associated with the hepatitis viruses or other viruses less specific for the liver. The four most common hepatitis viruses are hepatitis A, hepatitis B, hepatitis C, and hepatitis D. Hepatitis can also be associated with yellow fever, infectious mononucleosis, cytomegalovirus infection, and herpes simplex.

Hepatitis A is also known as infectious hepatitis. It is generally transmitted via fecal contamination of milk, water, or seafood. It is most common in the areas of the world where untreated sewage may come into contact with the water supply or food sources. It has a short incubation period and is usually not fatal; it does not lead to chronic hepatitis. Hepatitis B, also known as serum hepatitis, is transmitted from persons with an active form of the disease or from carriers via contaminated blood or blood products. It is particularly prevalent among drug users who share needles. The threat of contraction of hepatitis B from a transfusion has been greatly reduced by the screening of blood products. Hepatitis B has a long incubation period, up to six months. The severity of the disease varies greatly from subclinical hepatitis (showing no symptoms) to chronic hepatitis and in some cases may result in death. The course of hepatitis C disease resembles that of hepatitis B and may lead to chronic hepatitis. Hepatitis D is believed to be a defective virus that is found only in the presence of hepatitis B. It is transmitted via the same route and can result in chronic hepatitis. It occurs more commonly in Europe than in the United States.

Hepatitis from any cause may show subclinical or mild, influenza-like symptoms. Acute hepatitis may cause loss of appetite, vomiting, fever, jaundice, and enlargement of the liver. The viruses that cause hepatitis replicate within the liver cells, which could be the cause of the injury to these cells. Hepatocyte injury could also be a result of the immune system's attempt to fight the virus, which may injure the cells of the liver in the process. In either case, the damaged cells swell before they die. The liver can also be infected by bacterial cells, which usually reach the liver as a result of a systemic infection.

Many toxins or drugs can injure the liver, in a general pattern that is similar to the effects of infectious agents. The assault on the cell often leads to fatty infiltration, followed by swelling and finally by the death of the hepatocyte. Even in less severe cases of injury, those that do not lead to death of the hepatocyte, there is often impairment of the metabolic activities of the liver that can lead to diverse systemic effects. One of these effects is the ability to metabolize foreign compounds or naturally occurring steroids; the accumulation of these compounds throughout the body can have wide-ranging consequences.

The liver is adversely affected by the constant intake of excessive quantities of ethyl alcohol. In the early stages of alcoholism, the physiologic changes may be a result of improper nutrition or of vitamin deficiencies. During the more advanced stages of alcoholism, the patient is likely to suffer from a fatty liver and, ultimately, from cirrhosis. While those who stop drinking may slow down the advancement of cirrhosis, the disease appears to be irreversible.

There are more than five thousand metabolic enzymes in the liver, each of which is controlled genetically. Important in the treatment of metabolic disease is early diagnosis, which may prevent damage to other organs or to the liver. Dietary control may be used to minimize the effects of such conditions, leading to a near-normal life. Examples of treatable metabolic diseases are galactosemia, a condition which prevents the conversion of galactose to glucose; fructosemia, a condition that leads to the accumulation of fructose-1-phosphate; and Wilson's disease, an accumulation of copper in vital organs as a result of a defect in copper metabolism. In each case, the accumulation of a certain substance can lead to cellular damage, but dietary control of the substance can minimize the effects. Hemochromatosis is a similar disease which leads to accumulation of iron in the liver. As with Wilson's disease, the deposition of this element is not limited to the liver and can accumulate in other vital tissues of the body as well.

Cancer of the liver is usually caused by its spread from another site. Primary liver cancers are rare and usually do not occur until late in life. Risk factors may include exposure to hepatotoxins, chronic liver disease, or hepatitis B. There are two types of primary carcinomas of the liver: hepatocellular carcinoma, which develops in hepatocytes, and cholangiocellular carcinoma, which develops in bile ducts.

PERSPECTIVE AND PROSPECTS

The liver is a vital organ that plays a major role in the homeostasis of the body. Any condition that adversely influences the liver will have wide-ranging effects on other organs and the patient as a whole.

Because one of its functions is the metabolism of pollutants, drugs (including alcohol), and hormones, the liver is often exposed to substances that are toxic to its hepatocytes. When these compounds are encountered, the liver efficiently alters them for excretion. Sometimes, however, these substances may do damage to the cells before the liver can metabolize them.

When a liver cell is injured, the end result may be the death of the cell. Fortunately, liver cells are efficient at cell division and can replace those cells that have been injured or that have died. With continued damage to liver cells, however, the body can no longer replace them, and the resulting decrease in liver function leads to extensive complications throughout the body. A decrease in liver function will not only have an effect on the digestive system but will have wide-ranging effects on glucose and lipid metabolism (normal functions of the blood whose proteins are synthesized by the liver) and on the ability to remove certain foreign substances or toxins from the blood. For example, if the ability to metabolize medication is impaired by liver disease, the patient's body may accumulate high, even toxic, levels of drugs. These substances can have pronounced effects, particularly on the nervous system. With liver injury, the once-simple act of determining a medication dosage can become a critical problem.

Because there is only one liver and because the liver cells are genetically programmed to divide a limited number of times, any liver injury or disease can have permanent effects. There is little that medicine can do to cure liver disease. For example, there is no treatment for the hepatitis viruses; the body's own defense mechanisms must ultimately rid itself of the disease. The medical community can treat the symptoms of hepatitis.

Cancer of the liver is also difficult to treat. Because it is not easily detected, the diagnosis is rarely early. Unless the cancer is restricted to one lobe that can be removed, surgery is rarely the answer. Treatment is further complicated by the fact that the liver cells are particularly sensitive to radiation and that the doses needed to treat the cancer would be deadly to hepatocytes. Chemotherapy remains the primary hope for a cure.

With the discovery of immunosuppressive drugs, liver transplantation has become a positive procedure in the treatment of liver disease, and the results are promising. The availability of healthy livers for transplant, however, makes this an option limited to a small percentage of patients.

—Annette O'Connor, Ph.D.

See also Abdomen; Abdominal disorders; Alcoholism; Anatomy; Blood and blood disorders; Circulation; Cirrhosis; Gastroenterology; Gastroenterology, pediatric; Gastrointestinal disorders; Gastrointestinal system; Hematology; Hematology, pediatric; Hepatitis; Internal medicine; Jaundice; Liver cancer; Liver disorders; Liver transplantation; Metabolism; Nonalcoholic steatohepatitis (NASH); Systems and organs; Transplantation; Wilson's disease.

FOR FURTHER INFORMATION:

Chandrasoma, Parakrama, and Clive R. Taylor. *Concise Pathology*. 3d ed. Stamford, Conn.: Appleton & Lange, 1998. A pathology book written for health care personnel. It is well designed, and most laypeople will be able to understand the clearly organized and simple explanations that are presented.

Dollinger, Malin, et al. *Everyone's Guide to Cancer Therapy*. 4th ed. Kansas City, Mo.: Andrews McMeel, 2002. A well-organized book on therapy for various cancers, including a special section on liver cancers. Clearly describes the methods of treatment that are available and the treatment of choice. Written for the layperson and easily understood.

Feldman, Mark, Lawrence S. Friedman, and Lawrence J. Brandt, eds. *Sleisenger and Fordtran's Gastrointestinal and Liver Disease: Pathophysiology, Diagnosis, Management*. 8th ed. 2 vols. Philadelphia: W. B. Saunders, 2006. A clinical text that covers basic liver anatomy; disorders of the gastrointestinal tract, biliary tree, pancreas, and liver; and related topics of nutrition and peritoneal diseases.

Guyton, Arthur C., and John E. Hall. *Textbook of Medical Physiology*. 11th ed. Philadelphia: Elsevier Saunders, 2006. Although this is a text for medical students, the material is presented so well and with such a useful background that general readers will be able to understand the information that it contains. Offers good illustrations and tables that help to put everything in context.

McCance, Kathryn L., and Sue M. Huether. *Pathophysiology: The Biologic Basis for Disease in Adults and Children*. 5th ed. St. Louis: Elsevier Mosby, 2006. A very well written book on pathophysiology which not only presents the facts regarding certain diseases but also explains their physiological bases. Designed for student nurses, but its description of the physiology of the organ provides an extensive background for the less informed reader.

Scanlon, Valerie, and Tina Sanders. *Essentials of Anatomy and Physiology*. 5th ed. Philadelphia: F. A. Davis, 2007. A text designed around three themes: the relationship between physiology and anatomy, the interrelations among the organ systems, and the relationship of each organ system to homeostasis.

LIVER CANCER

DISEASE/DISORDER

ANATOMY OR SYSTEM AFFECTED: Liver

SPECIALTIES AND RELATED FIELDS: Gastroenterology, immunology, oncology, radiology

DEFINITION: Malignancies of the liver, which may be primary (arising in the organ itself) but are more likely to be secondary (metastasizing from another site).

CAUSES AND SYMPTOMS

The liver filters the blood supply, removing and breaking down (metabolizing) toxins and delivering them through the biliary tract to the intestines for elimination with other wastes. Because of the large volume of blood flowing through the liver (about a quarter of the body's supply), blood-borne toxins or cancer cells migrating from tumors elsewhere (the process called metastasis) pose a constant threat. In fact, in the United States most liver cancers are metastatic; only about 1 percent actually originate in the liver. In Southeast Asia and sub-Saharan Africa, primary liver cancer is the most common type, accounting for as much as 30 percent of all cancers.

Two major types of cancer affect the liver: those involving liver cells (hepatocellular carcinomas) and those involving the bile ducts (cholangiocarcinomas). The first is by far the more common, although tumors may contain a mixture of both, and their development is similar. Tumors may arise in one location, forming a large mass; arise in several locations, forming nodes; or spread throughout the liver in a diffuse form. Liver cancers occur in men about four to eight times more frequently than in women and in blacks slightly more than in whites, although the proportions vary widely among different regions of the world. In the United States, most cancers arise in people fifty years old or older; in other areas, people older than forty are at risk.

Primary liver cancer has so much regional and gender variation because causative agents are more or less common in different areas and men are more often exposed. A leading risk factor in the United States and Europe is cirrhosis, a scarring of liver tissue following destruction by viruses, toxins, or interrupted blood flow. In the United States, long-term alcohol consumption is the most common cause of cirrhosis, and men have long been more likely than women to become alcoholics. Likewise, hemochromatosis, a hereditary disease leading to the toxic buildup of iron, is a cancer precursor and more common in men than in women. In Africa and Southeast Asia, the hepatitis B and C viruses are leading precancer diseases because hepatitis has long been endemic in those areas, whereas in the United States it is not widespread (although the number of infected people began to rise in the 1980's).

Diet and medical therapies have also been implicated as liver carcinogens. Food toxins, especially aflatoxin from mold growing on peanuts (which are a staple in parts of Africa and Asia); oral contraceptives; anabolic steroids; and the high levels of sex hormones used in some treatments are thought to increase the likelihood of hepatobiliary tumors. Genetic factors, radiation, and occupational exposure to volatile chemicals may also play a minor role.

Although researchers generally agree about which agents are liver cancer precursors, the exact mechanism leading to tumor development is not thoroughly understood. Nevertheless, one factor may be universal. Viruses and toxins injure or destroy liver and bile duct cells; the body reacts to repair the damage with inflammation and an increased rate of new cell growth, a condition called regenerative hyperplasia. If the toxin damage continues, triggering ever more hyperplasia, as is the case with hepatitis and alcoholic cirrhosis, formation of a tumor becomes almost inevitable.

Like lymph nodes, the liver collects migrating cancer cells, so the cancers that physicians detect there often are metastases from cancers arising elsewhere in the body. In fact, liver involvement may be found before the primary cancer has been recognized. Colorectal cancer is especially given to metastasizing to the liver, since the digestive tract's blood supply is directly linked to the liver through the portal vein; similarly, lung and breast cancer may spread to the liver. Such metastases indicate advanced cancers that do not bode well for the patient's survival.

Symptoms may be ambiguous. Two common symptoms are jaundice and enlargement of the liver, with accompanying tenderness. Jaundice, a yellowing of the skin and eyes, is caused by an accumulation of bilirubin. Bilirubin builds up because a tumor has blocked the bile duct that normally empties it into the small intestine. (Both symptoms may also occur as a result of either gallstones or cirrhosis.) Patients with liver cancer may also have a fever and retain fluid in the abdominal cavities.

TREATMENT AND THERAPY

Doctors suspecting liver cancer conduct tests designed to distinguish this disease from other disorders. Palpation of the liver may reveal that the organ is enlarged or contains an unusual tissue mass, which is likely to be a tumor. A rubbing sound heard through the stethoscope may also come from a tumor. Hepatocellular carcinoma often elevates the alpha-fetoprotein level in blood. Abdominal ultrasound or computed tomography (CT) scans can provide good evidence of a tumor in the liver, and a biopsy will supply a tissue sample capable of proving the presence of cancer, especially if the biopsy is done with CT scan or ultrasound guidance. A tumor can also disrupt normal biochemical action in the body, which doctors may detect in blood tests. Liver function blood tests may be abnormal with both primary and secondary liver cancer.

Under even the most favorable circumstances, the outlook for patients with liver cancer is still not good. If a primary cancer is found while still fairly small, surgical removal is the surest and fastest treatment, although it is a difficult, risky procedure because of the liver's complex, delicate structure. Radiation and chemotherapy have not succeeded in shrinking tumors effectively. Because symptoms usually appear late in the development of primary liver cancer, it seldom is found early enough for surgical cure; patients usually live only one to two months after detection. Those found with small, removable cancers live an average of twenty-nine months. Most liver cancers are metastases,

---

INFORMATION ON LIVER CANCER

CAUSES: Metastasized tumors, genetic factors, radiation, occupational exposure to chemicals, dietary toxins, medical therapies, cirrhosis
SYMPTOMS: Ambiguous; typically includes jaundice and liver enlargement and tenderness
DURATION: One to twenty-nine months; often fatal
TREATMENTS: Chemotherapy, surgery

Liver Cancer

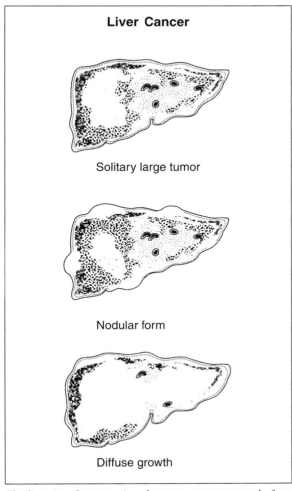

Solitary large tumor

Nodular form

Diffuse growth

The liver is a frequent site of cancer, most commonly from malignancies that have spread from their original site. The particular form the cancer takes depends on several factors, notably the primary source and its possible cause.

however, and removal of the liver tumor will not rid the patient of cancer. In general, hepatobiliary cancer patients have a 5 percent chance of living five years after diagnosis.

Liver cancer screening tests can locate tumors while they are still treatable, although routine physical examinations in Western nations seldom include such tests. Usually only patients with cirrhosis or chronic hepatitis are screened. The best ways to ward off liver cancer are to avoid viral infection and to abstain from alcohol. For those at risk for infection, such as health care workers, the most effective primary prevention is vaccination for hepatitis B.

—Roger Smith, Ph.D.

See also Alcoholism; Cancer; Carcinogens; Chemotherapy; Cirrhosis; Hepatitis; Jaundice; Liver; Liver disorders; Liver transplantation; Malignancy and metastasis; Oncology; Radiation therapy; Tumor removal; Tumors.

FOR FURTHER INFORMATION:

Curley, Steven A., ed. *Liver Cancer*. New York: Springer, 1998. Provides the general surgeon, surgical oncologist, radiation oncologist, and medical oncologist with current information regarding diagnosis and multimodality treatment approaches for patients with primary or metastatic hepatobiliary cancer.

Dollinger, Malin, et al. *Everyone's Guide to Cancer Therapy*. 4th ed. Kansas City, Mo.: Andrews McMeel, 2002. A well-organized book on therapy for various cancers, including a special section on liver cancers. Clearly describes the methods of treatment that are available and the treatment of choice. Written for the layperson and easily understood.

Eyre, Harmon J., Dianne Partie Lange, and Lois B. Morris. *Informed Decisions: The Complete Book of Cancer Diagnosis, Treatment, and Recovery*. 2d ed. Atlanta: American Cancer Society, 2002. The American Cancer Society endorses this excellent book, which provides a complete consumer reference for cancer diagnosis, treatment, and recovery.

Liver Cancer Network. http://www.livercancer.com/. A group founded through and supported by Pittsburgh's Allegheny General Hospital. The group's mission is to provide liver cancer patients and their families with the basic knowledge needed to better communicate with their physicians and to give patients and families hope for the future. Gives excellent information about the liver's anatomy, and the disease's diagnosis and treatment.

Parker, James N., and Philip M. Parker, eds. *The Official Patient's Sourcebook on Adult Primary Liver Cancer*. San Diego, Calif.: Icon Health, 2002. Guides patients in using the Internet to educate themselves about the disease and draws from public, academic, government, and peer-reviewed research to provide information on virtually all topics related to adult primary liver cancer, from the essentials to the most advanced areas of research.

Sachar, David B., Jerome D. Waye, and Blair S. Lewis. *Pocket Guide to Gastroenterology*. Rev. ed. Baltimore: Williams & Wilkins, 1991. Discusses such topics as gastroenterology, the digestive organs, and digestive system diseases. Includes bibliographical references and an index.

Shannon, Joyce Brennfleck. *Liver Disorders Sourcebook*. Detroit: Omnigraphics, 2000. This book includes basic consumer health information about the liver and how it works; liver diseases, including cancer, cirrhosis, hepatitis, and toxic and drug-related diseases; tips for maintaining a healthy liver; laboratory tests; radiology tests and facts about liver transplantation; and a section on support groups, a glossary, and resources listing.

Steen, R. Grant. *A Conspiracy of Cells: The Basic Science of Cancer*. New York: Plenum Press, 1993. Thorough, lucid explanations of all physiological aspects of cancer make this book instructive for readers willing to slog through the subject's complexity and terminology.

LIVER DISORDERS

DISEASE/DISORDER

ANATOMY OR SYSTEM AFFECTED: Liver

SPECIALTIES AND RELATED FIELDS: Gastroenterology, internal medicine

DEFINITION: As one of the most complex organs in the body, the liver is the target of a wide variety of toxins, infectious agents, and cancers that lead to hepatitis, cirrhosis, abscesses, and liver failure.

KEY TERMS:

abscess: a localized collection of pus and infectious microorganisms

ascites: the presence of free fluid in the abdominal cavity

bilirubin: a major component of bile, derived from the breakdown products of red blood cells

cirrhosis: the fibrous scar tissue that replaces the normally soft liver after repeated damage by viruses, chemicals, and/or alcohol

hepatitis: inflammation of the liver, such as that caused by viruses or toxins

jaundice: a yellow discoloration of the skin, eyes, and membranes caused by excess bilirubin in the blood

portal hypertension: elevated pressures in the portal veins caused by resistance to blood flow through a diseased liver; produces many regional problems, including ascites

portal system: a system of veins, unique to the liver, that carry nutrient-rich blood from the digestive organs to the liver

CAUSES AND SYMPTOMS

The liver is the largest internal organ, lying in the upper-right abdominal cavity. Intricately attached to it by a system of ducts on its lower surface is the pear-shaped gallbladder. Unique to the liver is a blood supply that derives from two separate sources: the hepatic artery, carrying freshly oxygenated blood from the heart, and the portal vein, carrying blood rich in the products of digestion from the digestive organs. The liver cells, or hepatocytes, are arranged in thin sheets that are separated by large pores, blood vessels, and ducts. The result is a very soft, spongy organ filled with a large volume of blood.

The liver performs a wide variety of complex and diverse functions, more so than any other organ. Most commonly known is the production of bile, which is formed from the breakdown of red blood cells, cholesterol, and salts; stored in the gallbladder; and used in the small intestine to digest fats. The liver also serves the all-important purpose of detoxification by chemically altering harmful substances such as alcohol, drugs, and ammonia from protein digestion. Additionally, the liver is involved in the formation of such essential materials as blood proteins, blood-clotting factors, and sugar and fat storage compounds.

Because of the liver's many responsibilities and unique position as an intermediary between the digestive process and the blood (via the portal vein), it easily falls prey to many disease-causing agents. Chemicals, illegal drugs, alcohol, viruses, parasites, hormones, and even medical drugs can damage the liver and have widespread effects on the rest of the body. The liver is also the most frequent target of cancer cells that have spread beyond their primary site. In the United States and other industrialized countries, liver disease is usually related to alcoholism and cancer, while in Third World countries it is often the result of infectious contamination by viruses and parasites.

There are two simplified methods of classifying liver disorders. The first is based on cause: infections (viruses and parasites), injury (alcohol and other toxins), inheritance (inability to perform certain functions), infiltration (iron and copper deposits), and tumors (both benign and malignant). The second method of classification is based on the result: hepatitis (inflammation), cirrhosis (permanent injury from alcohol or other toxins), and cancer, for example.

Each of these liver diseases produces a particular set of signs and symptoms depending on the length of time and the specific disruption of structure and function.

Pain and swelling rarely occur alone and are usually associated with one or more of the following: nausea and vomiting, jaundice, ascites, blood-clotting defects, and encephalopathy. Indeed, in some cases liver failure ensues, leading to coma and death.

Jaundice, a yellow discoloration of the skin and whites (sclera) of the eyes, is caused by the secretion of bile precursors (bilirubin) from the damaged liver cells directly into the blood rather than into the ducts leading to the gallbladder. Consequently, bilirubin accumulates in the body's tissues, including the skin and eyes. Ascites, the collection of fluid beneath the liver in the abdomen, is an important sign of liver disease. This fluid comes primarily from the portal vein system, which lies between the liver and the digestive organs. As the liver becomes congested and enlarged in response to injury or infection, blood flow becomes difficult and pressure begins to build, causing liquid to leak from the blood vessels into the abdominal cavity. Easy bruising, excessive bleeding, and other problems with blood clotting are important signs that reflect the failure of the liver to produce essential blood proteins. Neuropsychiatric symptoms such as a flapping hand tremor and encephalopathy (a state of mental confusion and disorientation that can quickly progress to coma) are not well understood, but it is likely that they result from an accumulation of toxic substances that would normally be cleared from the blood by the liver. Several other problems, such as the enlargement of male breasts, atrophy of the testicles, and other sexual changes, derive from the inability of the liver to clear the blood of hormones.

Hepatitis, an inflammation of the liver generally caused by viruses, is one of the most common diseases in the world. Hepatitis A, B, and C; Epstein-Barr virus (the causative agent of mononucleosis); and herpes are a few of the organisms that can infect the liver. Hepatitis A, transmitted through contaminated food, water, and shellfish, is usually a self-limited disease that resolves itself. Hepatitis B, transmitted through contact with infected blood and body secretions, is much more serious, with a carrier state, progressive organ damage, cancer, and death as possible sequelae. Hepatitis C is transmitted by intravenous drug use or blood transfusion. Infection most often causes no symptoms initially but leads to chronic infection in about 80 percent of individuals. Chronic infection progresses to cirrhosis in 20 to 30 percent of cases and may lead to liver cancer. Noninfectious causes of hepatitis in susceptible people include such frequently used substances as acetaminophen (Tylenol), halothane (general anesthesia), and oral contraceptives. Nonalcoholic steatohepatitis (NASH) is a disease that causes chronic inflammation and, upon biopsy, resembles alcoholic hepatitis. It is diagnosed in patients with persistent abnormal liver function tests, no evidence of hepatitis B or C, and consumption of less than 40 grams of ethanol per week. NASH is most often found in patients with obesity, Type II diabetes, and hyperlipidemia.

Cirrhosis is the result of continuous toxic exposure that injures the liver beyond repair. Fibrous scar tissue replaces the normally soft, spongy organ, making it small and firm, with few hepatocytes capable of functioning normally. Chronic alcohol abuse is by far the most frequent factor in the development of cirrhosis. Severe ascites, bleeding disorders, encephalopathy, and sex organ changes often herald imminent liver failure and death from this disease.

Liver cancer is most often secondary to malignancies that have spread from other sites. In Asia and Africa, primary tumors of the liver itself are much more common, in part because of several factors: a high incidence of hepatitis B infection, food toxins, and parasite infestation. Chronic injury appears to play the critical role in liver cancer; hence the risk factors that have been established are cirrhosis, hepatitis B and C, and long-term exposure to a variety of chemicals, hormones, and drugs. Benign tumors may occur in young women who use oral contraceptives, but they are relatively infrequent.

Several other hepatic diseases warrant mention. Liver abscesses, encapsulated areas filled with infectious material, can be caused by bacteria, fungi, and parasites. These organisms enter the bloodstream through ingestion, skin puncture, or even intestinal rupture (as occurs in appendicitis and diverticulitis), and

---

INFORMATION ON LIVER DISORDERS

CAUSES: Cirrhosis, infection, disease, abscess, liver failure, injury, genetic factors, tumors

SYMPTOMS: Varies; can include pain, swelling, nausea and vomiting, jaundice, easy bruising, excessive bleeding, blood clotting problems

DURATION: Acute to chronic

TREATMENTS: Drug therapy, surgery, transplant; most often symptomatic relief and supportive care

Signs and Symptoms of Liver Disease

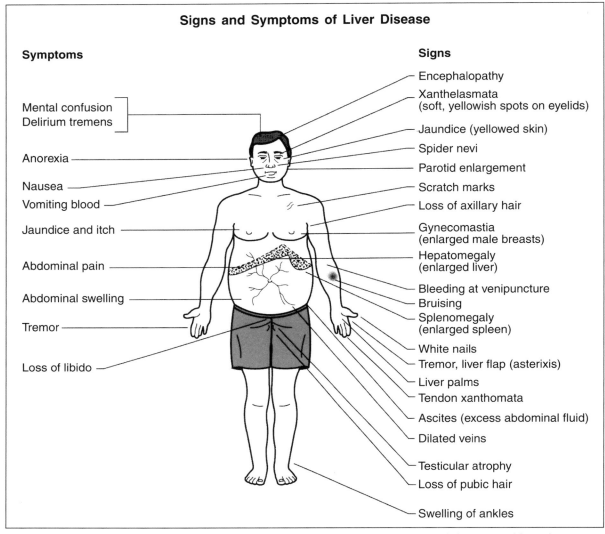

Symptoms

Mental confusion
Delirium tremens

Anorexia

Nausea

Vomiting blood

Jaundice and itch

Abdominal pain

Abdominal swelling

Tremor

Loss of libido

Signs

Encephalopathy

Xanthelasmata
(soft, yellowish spots on eyelids)

Jaundice (yellowed skin)

Spider nevi

Parotid enlargement

Scratch marks

Loss of axillary hair

Gynecomastia
(enlarged male breasts)

Hepatomegaly
(enlarged liver)

Bleeding at venipuncture

Bruising

Splenomegaly
(enlarged spleen)

White nails

Tremor, liver flap (asterixis)

Liver palms

Tendon xanthomata

Ascites (excess abdominal fluid)

Dilated veins

Testicular atrophy

Loss of pubic hair

Swelling of ankles

Particular combinations of these factors can provide clues to both the diagnosis and the extent of liver damage.

travel to the liver. Two unusual but notable disorders of iron and copper metabolism—hemochromatosis and Wilson's disease, respectively—have prominent liver involvement. While the disease mechanisms are not well understood, these essential metals are retained in excess and deposited in body tissues in toxic levels, causing damage. Finally, several genetic disorders of bile production run the gamut from mere nuisances to death in infancy. Disruption in bilirubin metabolism, the handling of red blood cell waste products by incorporation into bile, is affected to varying degrees. Severe jaundice reflects the accumulation of toxic levels of bilirubin in all body tissues, including the brain.

TREATMENT AND THERAPY

The diagnosis of a patient with suspected liver disease occurs in an orderly process that begins with a thorough history and physical examination, supported by a number of valuable blood tests and imaging techniques. Liver biopsy, the obtaining of a tissue sample for microscopic analysis, is often a final and definitive procedure if the disorder remains ambiguous. Both the cause and the chronology or state of the disease (whether of recent onset or advanced) determine treatment and outcome. While many signs and symptoms are nonspecific—nausea, vomiting, pain, hepatic enlargement, and jaundice—others such as ascites, encephalopathy, blood-clotting defects, and sex organ changes reflect significant organ damage and an advanced stage of disease. Careful questioning of the recent and past history of a patient can elicit facts that point to a diagnosis: exposure to known liver toxins such as alcohol, anesthetics, certain medications, and occupational chemicals; travel to countries with known contaminated water supplies (hepatitis A); blood transfusions, kidney dialysis, sexual promiscuity, or intravenous drug abuse (hepatitis B and C); weight loss that is unexplained (cancer); or even a history of gallstones (blocked bile ducts between the liver and gallbladder). Armed with suspicions from the history, the physician uses the physical examination to note signs that confirm or reject the possibilities. A small and firm liver with ascites, tremor, enlarged male breasts, and small, shrunken testicles all point to an advanced stage of cirrhosis, for example. An enlarged painful liver, with vomiting, jaundice, fever, and recent raw shellfish ingestion, would likely suggest hepatitis A.

Blood tests play the second critical role in evaluating liver disease. An elevated bilirubin level would correlate with the severity of jaundice. Blood protein levels (albumin) and blood-clotting factors (prothrombin) may be dangerously low, revealing a near inability of the hepatocytes to synthesize these vital substances. Special chemicals that exist primarily in liver cells (hepatic enzymes and the aminotransferases) may be quite high, because the cells die and release their contents into the blood. Finally, elevated white blood cell counts and special tests for individual infections (viruses, bacteria, fungi, and parasites) can positively establish the diagnosis.

Depending on the suspected disease, confirmation may be needed from various imaging techniques, chosen specifically for a particular diagnosis. Plain X rays do little to visualize the liver, although they can reveal air in the abdomen, a consequence of a perforated intestine, appendix, or ulcer. A much more advanced method, the computed tomography (CT) scan, combines computer-generated views of multiple cross-sectional X rays, providing a highly detailed examination of the liver and thereby establishing a diagnosis in the majority of cases. Two other techniques that have more specific uses are ultrasound, which uses sound wave transmission, and magnetic resonance imaging (MRI), which uses magnetic fields to create an image. Ultrasound can readily distinguish solid masses from those that are fluid-filled (tumors versus abscesses) and can view the bile ducts. MRI is quite helpful in determining blood flow problems such as portal hypertension.

Finally, if a precise diagnosis remains ambiguous, a biopsy is performed. A sample of liver tissue is obtained using a large needle inserted through the skin, under the guidance of an ultrasound image. The sample is then viewed microscopically, and both the cause and the extent of liver damage are readily apparent. Treatment options for the majority of liver diseases are improving. If drug toxicity is suspected, especially from alcohol, immediate withdrawal of the agent can prevent further damage, as has been shown in cirrhosis. Obstructing gallstones can be surgically removed to relieve pressure in the bile ducts. Combinations of surgery, radiation, and chemotherapy are used in liver cancer, but the prognosis is poor. Little can be done for the inherited diseases of bilirubin metabolism, while some success has been achieved in treating the iron and copper storage diseases.

Infections of viral origin have specific treatment regimens. Prevention of hepatitis A and B is possible if pooled serum immunoglobulin is given immediately after exposure. This substance is a concentrated form of antibodies obtained from infected individuals whose diseases have completely resolved; essentially, it is a method of giving passive immunity. Chronic hepatitis B may be effectively treated with several antiviral medications or interferon. Chronic hepatitis C is treated

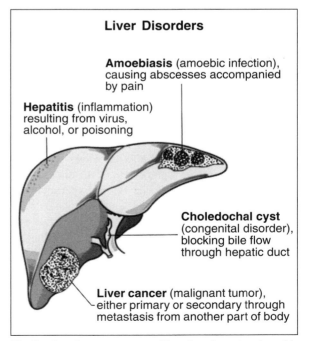

The liver's unique structure and functions leave it vulnerable to a wide range of diseases.

with a combination of an antiviral medication (Ribavirin) plus interferon. Response rates to therapy depend upon the viral load, the genotype of the virus, and compliance with treatment and range between 50 and 80 percent. There are no specific therapies proven effective for treatment of NASH. Treatment is recommended for associated medical conditions, including weight loss, reduction of lipids (cholesterol and triglycerides), and control of diabetes. One area in which effective treatment does exist is in bacterial, fungal, and parasitic infections and abscesses. Appropriate antibiotics and surgical drainage yield dramatic improvement in most cases.

In many cases of liver disease, symptom relief and nutritional support, often carried out in the hospital, are the only options. Pain relief and the administration of intravenous fluid and nutrients to counteract vomiting and dehydration are the first steps. Ascites is relieved through bed rest, salt restriction, diuretics, and paracentesis, a procedure that uses ultrasound to guide a needle into the abdomen and withdraw fluid. Attempts to correct encephalopathy by removing toxins such as ammonia from the blood are generally ineffective, and mental changes, along with other intractable symptoms, often herald complete liver failure and imminent death.

Clearly, preventive measures are the most important factor in liver disease. One effective measure that is widely available is the hepatitis B vaccine, which is recommended during childhood in a three-injection series. Hepatitis A vaccine is available and recommended in children older than one year. Hepatitis A and B vaccines are recommended to any non-immune adult with chronic liver disease.

PERSPECTIVE AND PROSPECTS

Liver transplantation offers approximately four thousand patients per year replacement of the diseased organ with a normal, donated one. Begun experimentally in the early 1960's after decades of low success rates (less than 20 percent), it has finally been accepted as a lifesaving operation, with survival rates exceeding 70 percent at five years. Technical improvements, especially intraoperative blood circulation and cadaver organ preservation, have been combined with advances in immunosuppressive therapy that counteract rejection and refined patient selection and timing. The result is that liver transplantation has become the method of choice for patients whose liver disease is life-threatening, progressive, and unresponsive to other treatments.

Specific guidelines exist for both children and adults to be considered candidates for the procedure. It is imperative that the person is otherwise healthy and that the heart, lungs, kidneys, and brain are functioning well. Malignancy, human immunodeficiency virus (HIV) infection, incorrectable congenital defects, and continuing drug or alcohol abuse are obvious contraindications. However, infants with inherited, inevitably fatal liver disorders are good candidates, as are adults with end-stage liver failure from chronic hepatitis, for example. Controversial indications, requiring case-by-case evaluation, include advanced viral hepatitis (as recurrent infection in the donated organ often occurs) and alcohol-induced cirrhosis (because of the likelihood of damage to other organs and the high relapse rate after surgery). Relapse is also very common if the transplantation is done for a primary liver cancer.

Careful donor selection is equally important. The principal source of cadaver organs is victims of head trauma who are declared brain-dead. Organs are accepted from those sixty years of age or younger who had no viral, bacterial, or fungal infections and who were otherwise healthy up to the time of death. In the United States, recipient-donor matches are made through a nationwide organ transplantation registry, with highest priority going to those most critically ill. Only twelve to eighteen hours can elapse between organ retrieval and implantation—beyond that, liver tissue begins to degenerate.

The use of immunosuppressive therapy, drugs that keep the recipient's immune system in check, has contributed significantly to success and survival. Rejection of the transplanted organ remains one of the most feared postoperative complications, along with hemorrhaging. Because the body recognizes the organ as foreign tissue, the immune system's white blood cells attack and damage the implanted donor liver. The use of drugs to counteract this process allows the new liver to heal and the body to adapt to the presence of foreign tissue. Despite the use of these potent drugs, which themselves have serious side effects, rejection continues to be a problem. Nevertheless, one-year survival rates are 87 percent, and at five years, 73 percent of transplant patients are alive.

—Connie Rizzo, M.D., Ph.D.
updated by James P. McKenna, M.D.

See also Abdomen; Abdominal disorders; Alcoholism; Cirrhosis; Hepatitis; Jaundice; Liver; Liver cancer; Liver transplantation; Nonalcoholic steatohepatitis (NASH); Wilson's disease.

FOR FURTHER INFORMATION:

American Liver Foundation. http://www.liverfoundation.org/. Provides physician referrals and information on support groups for persons with liver disease and their families.

Blumberg, Baruch S. *Hepatitis B: The Hunt for a Killer Virus*. Princeton, N.J.: Princeton University Press, 2003. A scientific memoir, the book traces the research and investigative twists and turns that led to the hepatitis B antigen, the elusive virus itself, and, finally, the vaccine.

Chopra, Sanjiv. *The Liver Book: A Comprehensive Guide to Diagnosis, Treatment, and Recovery*. New York: Simon & Schuster, 2002. Covers myriad information about liver disorders including how doctors diagnose liver ailments, what to expect from tests and screening, hepatitis B and hepatitis C, liver transplants, and the role of alternative treatments.

Feldman, Mark, Lawrence S. Friedman, and Lawrence J. Brandt, eds. *Sleisenger and Fordtran's Gastrointestinal and Liver Disease: Pathophysiology, Diagnosis, Management*. 8th ed. 2 vols. Philadelphia: W. B. Saunders, 2006. A clinical text that covers basic liver anatomy; disorders of the gastrointestinal tract, biliary tree, pancreas, and liver; and related topics of nutrition and peritoneal diseases.

Fishman, Mark, et al. *Medicine*. 5th ed. Philadelphia: J. B. Lippincott, 2004. This excellent soft cover text is the perfect place to start. Used by medical students and other health professionals, it is clear and understandable, exploring normal biology and the process of disease.

Goldman, Lee, and Dennis Ausiello, eds. *Cecil Textbook of Medicine*. 22d ed. Philadelphia: W. B. Saunders, 2004. This bible of internal medicine has a superb section on liver diseases that is somewhat difficult but so well written and thorough that it is worth the effort. The text is well supplemented with diagrams and photographs.

Yamada, Todataka, et al., eds. *Textbook of Gastroenterology*. 4th ed. Philadelphia: J. B. Lippincott, 2003. The reference text used by specialists in the field, covering all aspects of the digestive system. A large section is devoted to the liver and gallbladder.

LIVER TRANSPLANTATION

PROCEDURE

ANATOMY OR SYSTEM AFFECTED: Abdomen, gallbladder, liver

SPECIALTIES AND RELATED FIELDS: Gastroenterology, general surgery

DEFINITION: Surgery performed to replace a diseased, nonfunctional liver with one that is healthy and capable of carrying out normal liver functions.

KEY TERMS:

bile: fluid produced by the liver and stored in the gallbladder to be secreted into the intestine; contains salts, bile pigments (bilirubin), cholesterol, and other waste products

cirrhosis: a severe degenerative condition in which healthy liver tissue is replaced with nonfunctional scar tissue; alcohol and drug abuse are the most common causes

hepatic: of or referring to the liver

hepatitis: inflammation of the liver

jaundice: a yellowish coloration of the skin and mucous membranes caused by high levels of bilirubin in the blood; the result of liver malfunction

INDICATIONS AND PROCEDURES

Liver transplantation is performed on individuals whose livers are severely diseased and unable to carry out normal liver functions. The most common cause of liver failure in adults is cirrhosis, which results from alcohol and/or drug abuse. In this condition, the liver becomes filled with tough, nonfunctional scar tissue. Symptoms of cirrhosis, as well as other liver diseases, include abnormal levels of liver enzymes in the blood, jaundice, a lack of blood-clotting factors, the inability to dispose of bile, and the failure to detoxify metabolic by-products and other poisons, which can lead to coma and death. Other conditions that can lead to liver disease include hepatic cancer, long-term hepatitis B infection, and obstruction of the bile passages in the liver.

The donor liver may be obtained from a recently deceased individual, or a section of the liver can be obtained from a living donor. In either case, the donated organ must be a close immunological match to reduce the chance of transplant rejection. A preoperative injection is given to the recipient to dry up internal fluids and promote drowsiness. A vertical incision is made from just below the breastbone to the navel. Muscles are moved aside, and a second incision is made through the outer membranous lining of the body cavity, revealing the internal organs. Bypass tubes are inserted into the hepatic veins and connected to veins in the arm to divert the flow of blood from the liver. When this is completed, the hepatic veins are cut, and the liver and gallbladder are removed from the body cavity. The veins of the donor liver are connected to the recipient veins, and the bypass tubes are removed. The new liver is then connected to the intestine, and the incisions are closed.

USES AND COMPLICATIONS

Liver transplantation is performed only when the individual has no other chance for survival. Typically, there is a long waiting list for available organs. Certain factors such as blood type and protein markers on cell surfaces must be matched as closely as possible in order to avoid rejection by the recipient's immune system. A liver from a recently deceased donor may be kept functioning only for five hours with specific cooling fluid, thus limiting its ability to be transported long distances. Because of the lack of available transplant organs and the necessity of compatibility, many people die before an appropriate organ becomes available. It is possible to transplant a segment of liver from a close relative; the liver can grow considerably and regenerate itself. This is a preferable situation and eliminates the pressure of transporting a donor liver between hospitals while attempting to keep it functioning.

After liver transplantation, the patient is kept in an intensive care unit for several days and in bed for at least a week. Pain from the incisions is alleviated with drugs. Rejection is the major danger, even with closely matched donor organs. Drugs such as cyclosporine are administered to suppress the immune system and, in most cases, must be taken for life. These immunosuppressive drugs inhibit the normal functioning of the immune system, thus making the individual much more susceptible to frequent—and more severe—infections, including bacterial, fungal, and viral infections. Other possible complications of the long-term use of immunosuppressive drugs include cataracts, impaired wound healing, peptic ulcers, and steroid-induced diabetes mellitus. About 20 percent of patients suffer graft rejection, obstruction of the arteries, or infection. In the case of serious complications, another transplantation may be the patient's only hope for survival. In successful surgeries, patients are able to return to normal, active lives within a few weeks of the surgery.

PERSPECTIVE AND PROSPECTS

The first successful liver transplantation procedure was performed in 1967. Nevertheless, this surgery was considered an experimental procedure until 1983, when a National Institutes of Health (NIH) conference on liver transplantation accepted it as a routine procedure. In 1984, more than 250 liver transplantations were performed in the United States. Within five years, that number increased dramatically, to 2,188 transplantation procedures performed in 1989, and by 2002, the number had climbed to more than 5,300 transplants. Long-term results are steadily improving; currently, more than half of recipients survive for five years or more. Improvements in survival rates are attributable to improved methods of preserving donor livers, the advent of living donor transplantation, better methods to prevent graft rejection, more suitable selection of recipients (for example, hepatic cancer patients typically have a high rate of recurrence of the disease in their transplanted liver), and improved surgical techniques.

Future prospects include further improvements in surgical techniques and advanced drug therapy to prevent graft rejection but not totally compromise the disease-fighting ability of the patient's immune system. Efforts at public education regarding the need for donor organs may cause more individuals to contact donor organ societies, family, and friends regarding their wishes to donate organs in the event of untimely death. In addition, improved treatments for the diseases that lead to liver failure may help to decrease the need for this surgical procedure.

—*Karen E. Kalumuck, Ph.D.*

See also Abdomen; Abdominal disorders; Alcoholism; Circulation; Cirrhosis; Gastroenterology; Gastroenterology, pediatric; Gastrointestinal disorders; Gastrointestinal system; Hepatitis; Internal medicine; Jaundice; Liver; Liver disorders; Nonalcoholic steatohepatitis (NASH); Transplantation.

FOR FURTHER INFORMATION:

Ahmed, Moustafa. *Surviving Liver Diseases: Life with a Liver Transplant*. London: MegaZette, 1999. Designed for the layperson, this resource offers guidance on the prevention of liver disease and offers personal narrative regarding liver transplantation.

Belzer, Folkert O., and Hans W. Sollinger. "Immunology and Transplantation." In *Basic Surgery*, edited by Hiram C. Polk, Jr., H. Harlan Stone, and Bernard Gardner. 5th ed. St. Louis: Quality Medical, 1995. A chapter in a text discussing such topics as operative and diagnostical surgery.

Griffith, H. Winter. *Complete Guide to Symptoms, Ill-*

ness, and Surgery. Revised and updated by Stephen Moore and Kenneth Yoder. Rev. 4th ed. New York: Perigee, 2000. Covers more than five hundred diseases and disorders and includes information about causes and risk factors, preventive techniques, and diagnostic tests.

Mulholland, Michael W., et al., eds. *Greenfield's Surgery: Scientific Principles and Practice*. 4th ed. Philadelphia: Lippincott Williams & Wilkins, 2006. Covers the scope and practice of surgery and includes reviews of wound biology, immunology, the management of trauma and transplantation, surgical practice according to anatomic region and specialty, and musculoskeletal, neurologic, genitourinary, and reconstructive surgery.

United Network for Organ Sharing. http://www.unos .org/. A site that provides detailed information for patients and family members about the procedure, living with a transplant, current transplant research, and how to donate organs.

Youngson, Robert M. *The Surgery Book: An Illustrated Guide to Seventy-three of the Most Common Operations*. New York: St. Martin's Press, 1997. In a clear, easy-to-follow format, this dependable, comprehensive sourcebook answers questions about and gives information on a wealth of operations, including mastectomy, vasectomy, prostatectomy, cesarean section, hernia repair, hip replacement, heart bypass, and dozens more.

Zollinger, Robert M., Jr., and Robert M. Zollinger, Sr. *Zollinger's Atlas of Surgical Operations*. 8th ed. New York: McGraw-Hill, 2003. A comprehensive examination of surgery. Covers basic surgical anatomy and vascular, gynecologic, gastrointestinal, and miscellaneous abdominal procedures.

LOCKJAW. *See* TETANUS.

LOU GEHRIG'S DISEASE. *See* AMYOTROPHIC LATERAL SCLEROSIS.

LOWER EXTREMITIES
ANATOMY

ANATOMY OR SYSTEM AFFECTED: Bones, feet, hips, knees, legs, lymphatic system, musculoskeletal system, nerves, nervous system, skin

SPECIALTIES AND RELATED FIELDS: Neurology, orthopedics, physical therapy, podiatry

DEFINITION: The thighs, lower legs, and feet; the lower extremities are attached to the pelvis at the hip joint and consist of muscles, bones, blood vessels, lymph vessels, nerves, skin, and toenails.

KEY TERMS:

distal: farther away from the base or attached end

femur: the thigh bone

fibula: the smaller of the two bones in the lower leg, on the lateral side

knee: the joint between the thigh and the lower leg

lateral: on the outer side; toward the little toe when in reference to the leg

leg: the lower extremity, excluding the foot; the lower leg runs from the knee to the ankle

medial: on the side toward the midline; toward the big toe when in reference to the leg

proximal: closer to the base or attached end

tarsus: the ankle

thigh: the upper segment of the leg, from the hip joint to the knee

tibia: the larger of the two bones in the lower leg, on the medial side

STRUCTURE AND FUNCTIONS

The lower extremities consist of the thighs, lower legs, and feet. Each extremity attaches to the pelvis (innominate bone) at the hip joint. The lower extremity is made mostly of bones and muscles, but it also contains blood vessels, lymphatics, nerves, skin, toenails, and other structures. Important directional terms for the lower extremity include proximal (closer to the base or attached end), distal (further from the base or attached end), medial (on the same side as the tibia and big toe), and lateral (on the same side as the fibula and little toe). Along the foot, the lower surface is called plantar; the upper surface is called dorsal. The lower extremity is clothed in skin (or integument). The sole or plantar surface of the foot is unusual, along with the palm of the hand, in being completely hairless; it also contains the thickest outer skin layer (the stratum corneum) of any part of the body. Each toe has a hardened toenail on its dorsal surface.

The pelvic girdle that supports the lower extremity develops as three separate bones: the ilium, ischium, and pubis. All three help form the acetabulum, a socket into which the femur fits. Below the acetabulum, the ischium and pubis surround a large opening called the obturator foramen. The right and left pubis meet to form a pubic symphysis. The bones of the lower extremity include the femur, tibia, fibula, tarsals, metatarsals, and phalanges. The femur (thigh bone) is the largest bone in the body. Its rounded upper end, or head, fits into the acetabulum and is attached by a short neck. A rough-surfaced greater trochanter lies just beyond this neck and serves for the attachment of many muscles. The lesser trochanter, also for muscle attachments, lies just below the neck. The knee joint is covered and protected by the kneecap, or patella, the largest of the sesamoid bones formed within tendons at points of stress. The lower leg, from the knee to the ankle, contains two bones: the tibia on the medial side and the more slender fibula on the lateral side. The tarsus, or ankle, includes the talus, calcaneus, and five smaller bones. The talus (or astragalus) has a pulleylike facet for the tibia and other curved surfaces for articulation with the calcaneus and navicular. The calcaneus, or heel bone, is vertically enlarged in humans; the Achilles tendon attaches to its roughened lower tuberosity. Smaller tarsal bones include the navicular, the medial (or inner) cuneiform, the intermediate cuneiform, the lateral (or outer) cuneiform, and the cuboid. Beyond the tarsal bones, the foot is supported by five metatarsal bones. The big toe, or hallux, contains two phalanges; each of the remaining toes contains three phalanges.

The muscles of the lower extremity include extensors, which straighten joints, and flexors, which bend joints. Abductor muscles move the limbs sideways, away from the midline, while adductors pull the limbs back, toward the midline. The muscles of the iliac region attach the lower extremity to the body. The psoas major runs from the lumbar vertebrae to the lesser trochanter of the femur. The iliacus runs from the ilium and part of the sacrum to the femur, including the lesser trochanter. The anterior muscles of the thigh include the sartorius, the quadriceps femoris, and the articularis genus. The sartorius, the longest muscle in the body, flexes both hip and knee joints. It runs obliquely from the anterior border of the ilium across the front of the thigh to insert onto the medial side of the knee at the upper end of the tibia. The quadriceps femoris consists of the rectus femoris and the three vastus muscles; all four are strong extensors of the knee. The rectus femoris originates from the region surrounding the acetabulum. The vastus lateralis, vastus medialis, and vastus intermedius muscles all originate along the shaft of the femur. All four quadriceps muscles insert onto a common tendon which runs over the knee and inserts onto the top of the tibia. The patella is a sesamoid bone enclosed within this tendon where it runs over the front of the knee. The smaller articularis genus muscle originates on the anterior side of the shaft of the femur; it inserts onto the kneecap.

The extensor muscles of the hip and thigh help to maintain upright posture. The gluteus maximus, the largest of these muscles, originates from the posterior portion of the ilium and inserts high on the femur, especially onto the greater trochanter. The gluteus medius and gluteus minimis both originate from the outer surface of the ilium and insert onto the greater trochanter. The tensor fasciae latae originates along the iliac crest; it inserts onto a broad, sheetlike tendon (the fascia lata) which covers much of the lateral surface of the thigh. The piriformis runs from the sacrum to the greater trochanter of the femur. The obturator internus runs from the inner surface of the pelvis through the obturator foramen to the greater trochanter of the femur. The gemellus superior and the gemellus inferior originate from the rear margin of the ischium; they both insert onto the greater trochanter. The quadratus femoris originates from the lateral surface of the ischium; it inserts between the greater and lesser trochanters of the femur. The obturator externus originates along the outer surface of the pelvis below the obturator foramen and inserts near the greater trochanter.

The muscles on the medial (or inner) side of the thigh are all abductors of the thigh. The gracilis is a long, thin muscle that originates from the pubis, runs along the medial side of the thigh, and inserts high on the tibia. The pectineus originates anteriorly on the pubis and inserts onto the shaft of the femur below the lesser trochanter. The adductor longus originates from the pubis and inserts onto the posterior edge of the femur. The adductor brevis originates from the pubis and inserts onto the posterior edge of the femur. The adductor magnus is a large, triangular muscle that originates from the lower portion of the ischium and pubis; it expands to a long, thin insertion along the posterior edge of the femur.

The hamstring muscles run along the posterior side of the femur; they flex the knee and extend the hip joint. The biceps femoris originates from the posterior portion (the tuberosity) of the ischium and separately from the posterior edge of the femur. Both portions converge onto a common tendon which inserts primarily onto the top of the fibula. The semitendinosus originates from the posterior end of the ischium; it inserts by a long tendon onto the medial side of the tibia. The semimembranosus runs from the ischium to the posterior surface of the tibia.

The muscles on the front (anterior) side of the lower leg raise the foot by flexing it dorsally. At the ankle, their tendons are all held in place by two transverse bands, the extensor retinacula. The tibialis anterior originates along the anterior edge of the tibia; it inserts by a tendon onto the medial cuneiform and the base of the first metatarsal. The extensor hallucis longus originates from the anterior surface of the fibula; its tendon passes beneath the extensor retinacula to insert onto the distal phalanx of the big toe. The extensor digitorum longus originates near the top of the tibia and along the anterior side of the fibula. Its tendon passes beneath the extensor retinacula and splits into four tendons, inserted onto the second and third phalanges of the second through fifth digits. The peroneus tertius originates along the anterior edge of the fibula and runs alongside the extensor digitorum longus. It inserts onto the base of the fifth metatarsal bone.

The muscles on the posterior surface of the lower leg are mostly extensors of the foot; some also flex the knee. The gastrocnemius originates in two heads from opposite sides of the femur. It inserts onto the Achilles tendon, which attaches to the calcaneus. The soleus originates from the posterior surface of the fibula; it inserts onto the Achilles tendon. The plantaris originates from the posterior surface of the femur and inserts onto the posterior portion of the calcaneus. The popliteus runs from the lateral side of the femur across the back of the knee to insert onto the tibia. The flexor hallucis longus originates along the posterior surface of the fibula; its tendon runs around to the medial side of the ankle and inserts onto the base of the big toe. The flexor digitorum longus originates from the posterior surface of the tibia; its tendon crosses the sole of the foot obliquely and divides into four tendons which insert onto the distal phalanges of the second through fifth toes. The tibialis posterior originates from the posterior surfaces of the tibia, the fibula, and the interosseous membrane that joins them; its tendon passes around to insert onto the navicular bone. The peroneus longus originates along the lateral surface of the fibula; its tendon runs along a groove on the bottom of the cuboid to insert obliquely onto the base of the first metatarsal. The peroneus brevis originates along the lateral margin of the fibula; its tendon inserts onto the fifth metatarsal. The extensor digitorum brevis originates from the calcaneus and runs obliquely across the dorsal side of the foot, dividing into four tendons. One tendon inserts onto the base of the big toe; the remaining tendons insert onto the tendons of the extensor digitorum longus.

Several flexor muscles of the foot are attached to the plantar aponeurosis, a flat ligament which runs from the calcaneus along the sole of the foot to the bases of the toes and to several flexor tendons. The abductor hallucis originates from the calcaneus and the plantar aponeurosis; it inserts onto the base of the big toe. The flexor digitorum brevis originates from the plantar aponeurosis and the calcaneus; it divides into four portions, each of which gives rise to a tendon. These tendons run into the second through fifth toes, each splitting in half to insert onto opposite sides of the second phalanx, separated by the tendons of the flexor digitorum longus, which emerge between them. The abductor digiti quinti originates from the calcaneus and the plantar aponeurosis; it inserts onto the base of the fifth toe. The quadratus plantae originates from the calcaneus and inserts onto the tendons of the flexor digitorum longus. The four small lumbricals run from the tendons of the flexor digitorum longus to the corresponding tendons of the extensor digitorum longus. The flexor hallucis brevis originates from the cuboid and lateral cuneiform bones; its two portions insert onto the big toe from opposite sides. The adductor hallucis originates from the second through fourth metatarsals and also from the bases of the third through fifth toes. Its tendon inserts onto the base of the big toe. The flexor digiti quinti originates from the base of the fifth metatarsal and inserts onto the base of the fifth toe. The four dorsal interossei originate from the bases of the metatarsal bones; they insert onto the bases of the second through fourth toes. The three plantar interossei originate from the third through fifth metatarsals and run beneath these bones to insert onto the bases of the corresponding toes.

Blood vessels of the lower extremity include both arteries and veins. The common iliac arteries arise from the dorsal aorta; each divides into an internal and an external iliac. The internal iliac artery supplies many muscles of the thigh region and pelvis. The external iliac artery branches into an inferior epigastric artery and a deep iliac circumflex artery; it then continues along the femur as the femoral artery. The femoral artery gives rise to a deep femoral artery running to the medial and posterior regions of the thigh; the base of this artery also gives rise to two circumflex arteries that send branches upward into many thigh muscles. Near the knee, the femoral artery branches into a descending geniculate artery to the knee, then continues as the popliteal artery, forming several branches to the thigh muscles and other small branches to the knee before splitting into anterior and posterior tibial arteries.

The anterior tibial artery descends along the front of the tibia, forming several small branches. It then continues into the foot as the dorsalis pedis artery, giving rise to a lateral tarsal artery and an arcuate artery, both of which form arches by joining with branches of the peroneal artery. The deep plantar artery and hallucis dorsalis artery also branch from the dorsalis pedis artery, while individual arteries to the second through fourth metatarsals arise from the arcuate artery. Arterial branches to all the toes arise from the individual metatarsal arteries, including the hallucis dorsalis, forming a system of collateral circulation in which multiple alternate routes permit blood flow even if one of the routes is temporarily blocked.

The posterior tibial artery gives rise to a peroneal artery; the two arteries then run down the posterior side of the lower leg, forming small branches to the muscles of the lower leg and nutrient arteries to the tibia and fibula. The posterior tibial artery branches to the calcaneus before it splits into a medial plantar artery, which runs along the medial margin of the foot into the big toe, and a much larger lateral plantar artery. The lateral plantar artery runs across the foot obliquely to the lateral side, then turns and runs obliquely in the other direction to the base of the big toe, where it runs into the deep plantar artery to form a loop. From this loop arise a series of plantar metatarsal arteries to all five toes. Blood can reach each toe from either side, and the arch that supplies this blood can receive its blood either by way of the posterior tibial and lateral plantar arteries or by way of the anterior tibial and deep plantar arteries, providing another example of collateral circulation.

There are several important veins draining the lower extremity. The deep veins originate from a series of plantar digital veins draining the individual toes into a deep plantar venous arch. This arch is drained to either direction by a lateral plantar vein and a medial plantar vein, which later unite to form a posterior tibial vein; this vein and the peroneal vein run parallel to the corresponding arteries along the posterior side of the lower leg. An anterior tibial vein drains the anterior side of the lower leg and the dorsal side of the foot. Near the knee, the peroneal vein and the anterior and posterior tibial veins unite to form the popliteal vein, which continues into the thigh as the femoral vein. The femoral vein receives the deep femoral vein as a tributary, then the saphenous vein. The femoral vein then continues as the external iliac vein.

The lower extremity is also covered with a network of superficial veins that lie just beneath the skin. The vessels of this network are drained along the medial side of the lower leg and thigh by the great saphenous vein, which runs into the femoral vein just below the groin. The lateral side of the foot and the posterior surface of the lower leg are drained by the small saphenous vein, which drains into the popliteal vein.

The nerves to the lower extremity arise from two series of complex branchings, the lumbar plexus and sacral plexus. The largest nerve formed from the lumbar plexus is the femoral nerve, supplying muscles on the anterior side of the thigh and part of the lower leg. Other branches to the muscles include the obturator nerve to the adductor muscles and separate muscular branches to the psoas and iliacus muscles. Cutaneous sensory nerves to the skin include the lateral femoral cutaneous nerve to the lateral side of the thigh, the anterior cutaneous branches of the femoral nerve to the medial side of the thigh, and the saphenous nerve, a branch of the femoral nerve to the medial side of the lower leg.

The sacral plexus gives rise to the very large sciatic nerve and to several smaller nerves, including the superior gluteal and inferior gluteal nerves to the gluteal muscles, and separate muscular branches to the piriformis, quadratus femoris, obturator internus, and gemelli. Cutaneous branches such as the posterior femoral cutaneous nerve supply sensory fibers to the skin on the posterior surface of the thigh. The sciatic nerve, the largest nerve in the body, branches off to the hamstring muscles before splitting into tibial and peroneal nerves. The tibial nerve supplies the muscles on the posterior side of the lower leg and then runs onto the sole of the foot, where it splits into the medial and lateral plantar nerves, which together supply both cutaneous sensation and muscular innervation to the sole of the foot. The peroneal nerve divides into deep and superficial portions. The deep peroneal nerve supplies the muscles on the anterior side of the lower leg and the dorsal surface of the foot. The superficial peroneal nerve supplies cutaneous sensation to the lateral surface of the lower leg and the dorsal surface of the foot.

DISORDERS AND DISEASES

Many medical conditions and disorders affect the lower extremity; these include animal bites (including snakebites), injuries, fungus infections such as athlete's foot, contact dermatitis (including poison ivy), and an assortment of neuromuscular disorders, including nerve paralyses, muscular atrophies, and muscular dystrophies. Nerve paralyses of the lower extremities usually arise from traumatic injury.

Muscular atrophies are diseases in which muscle tissues become progressively weaker and smaller, usually beginning after the age of forty. Spastic movements sometimes occur. The small muscles of the hands and feet are usually affected sooner and more severely in comparison to the larger muscles of the legs and thighs. Amyotrophic lateral sclerosis (ALS), commonly known as Lou Gehrig's disease, is one such disease that usually begins with weakness and deterioration of the distal muscles. The disease proceeds to affect the rest of the extremities, then other parts of the body; it is usually fatal within three to five years after onset. A more rare type of atrophy, myelopathic muscular atrophy (or Aran-Duchenne atrophy), affects both upper and lower extremities and eventually spreads to the trunk. A degenerative lesion of the gray matter in the cervical region of the spinal cord is usually responsible.

Muscular dystrophy is a series of inherited diseases that begin in early childhood, affecting males more often than females. The most common type, Duchenne muscular dystrophy, is caused by a sex-linked recessive trait which impairs the body's ability to synthesize a large protein called dystrophin. Muscular dystrophy primarily affects the large muscles of the thigh and lower leg, impairing the ability to stand unassisted or to walk. The affected muscles become very weak but remain approximately normal in size and may even increase as muscle tissue is replaced by fatty and fibrous tissue. Progressive weakening makes walking and similar motor functions impossible, but, with proper care, patients can live for decades.

Sports injuries often occur in the lower extremities and are generally treated by orthopedic specialists. Fractured bones are generally set in casts and kept immobile until they heal. Injured or ruptured ligaments often require surgical treatment. Snakebites and other animal bites occur more often to the lower extremities than to other parts of the body. The bites of poisonous snakes must be treated quickly, before the venom reaches the heart. The patient must be kept calm and quiet, and experienced medical attention should be sought as soon as possible.

PERSPECTIVE AND PROSPECTS

The major muscles and bones of the lower extremities were studied in ancient societies by such individuals as Galen (or Caius Galenus), the physician to the Roman army in the second century. Ironically, the science of anatomy took many great strides because of the efforts of artists, who studied the human body in order to create realistic sculptures and paintings. During the Renaissance, Leonardo da Vinci (1452-1519) and Michelangelo (1475-1564) dissected human corpses illegally in their quest for this knowledge. Andreas Vesalius (1514-1564) produced the first well-illustrated anatomical texts, containing information that corrected many of the errors made by Galen.

Injuries to the leg are generally treated surgically. Whenever possible, broken bones are set in place, immobilized in a cast, and then allowed to heal. Muscles (or their tendons) must be sewn together. Nerve endings must be matched with their former locations if they are to grow back correctly. Gangrene, or tissue death from lack of circulation, occurs more often in the lower extremities than in the upper extremities. When the lower extremity is gangrenous or is injured beyond repair, an amputation is often performed. Artificial legs or partial legs are sometimes attached to the lower extremity.

—Eli C. Minkoff, Ph.D.

See also Amputation; Arthritis; Arthroplasty; Arthroscopy; Bone cancer; Bone disorders; Bone grafting; Bones and the skeleton; Bowlegs; Braces, orthopedic; Bunions; Bursitis; Feet; Flat feet; Foot disorders; Fracture and dislocation; Fracture repair; Frostbite; Grafts and grafting; Hammertoe correction; Hammertoes; Heel spur removal; Hemiplegia; Hip fracture repair; Hip replacement; Kneecap removal; Knock-knees; Liposuction; Motor skill development; Muscle sprains, spasms, and disorders; Muscles; Nail removal; Nails; Orthopedic surgery; Orthopedics; Orthopedics, pediatric; Osgood-Schlatter disease; Osteoarthritis; Osteochondritis juvenilis; Osteogenesis imperfecta; Osteopathic medicine; Paralysis; Paraplegia; Physical rehabilitation; Pigeon toes; Podiatry; Poliomyelitis; Prostheses; Quadriplegia; Rheumatoid arthritis; Rheumatology; Rickets; Tendon disorders; Tendon repair; Upper extremities; Varicose vein removal.

FOR FURTHER INFORMATION:

Agur, Anne M. R., and Arthur F. Dalley. *Grant's Atlas of Anatomy.* 11th ed. Philadelphia: Lippincott Williams & Wilkins, 2005. Excellent, detailed illustrations can be found in this standard reference work.

Crouch, James E. *Functional Human Anatomy.* 4th ed. Philadelphia: Lea & Febiger, 1985. A good beginning reference for an introduction to anatomy. This easy-to-read book provides clear explanations.

Currey, John D. *Bones: Structures and Mechanics.* Princeton, N.J.: Princeton University Press, 2002.

Very accessible overview of a range of information related to whole bones, bone tissue, and dentin and enamel. Topics include stiffness, strength, viscoelasticity, fatigue, fracture mechanics properties, buckling, impact fracture, and properties of cancellous bone.

Marieb, Elaine N. *Essentials of Human Anatomy and Physiology*. 8th ed. San Francisco: Pearson/Benjamin Cummings, 2006. This text discusses the functional significance of various anatomical structures, including the foot. Readers will enjoy the excellent pictures and diagrams of the foot and associated body parts.

Rosse, Cornelius, and Penelope Gaddum-Rosse. *Hollinshead's Textbook of Anatomy*. 5th ed. Philadelphia: Lippincott-Raven, 1997. Helpful descriptions and illustrations mark this thorough, detailed reference source.

Standring, Susan, et al., eds. *Gray's Anatomy*. 39th ed. New York: Elsevier Churchill Livingstone, 2005. This work stands as a classic in the field of anatomy. Thorough descriptions and excellent color illustrations are provided.

Van De Graaff, Kent M. *Human Anatomy*. 6th ed. New York: McGraw Hill, 2002. Chapters 8 through 11 present a first-rate introduction to bones, the skeleton, and joints. The many clear illustrations, photographs, clinical commentaries, and X rays, as well as a pronunciation guide, a complete index, and a glossary, make this a very accessible book for the nonspecialist reader.

LUMBAR PUNCTURE

PROCEDURE

ALSO KNOWN AS: Spinal tap

ANATOMY OR SYSTEM AFFECTED: Brain, nerves, nervous system, spine

SPECIALTIES AND RELATED FIELDS: Anesthesiology, biochemistry, critical care, general surgery, neurology, oncology, pathology

DEFINITION: A process in which the physician places a hollow needle into the lower part of the spinal canal, either to harvest cerebrospinal fluid for diagnosis or to inject substances into the spinal canal.

KEY TERMS:

aneurysm: ballooning within an artery or vein that protrudes through a weak spot

angiogram: film on which images of blood vessels treated with a medium that is opaque to X rays become visible

cerebrospinal fluid (CSF): watery fluid that surrounds the brain and the spinal cord

meningeal irritation: inflammation of the meninges, or membranes surrounding the brain and spinal cord

meningitis: inflammation of the membranes of the brain or spinal cord

myelography: X-ray examination of the spinal cord, tissues, and nerves within the spinal canal

subarachnoid hemorrhage: a condition in which blood from a ruptured cranial blood vessel invades the surface of the brain

vertebrae: pieces of bone or cartilage of which the backbone or spine is composed

xanthochromic spinal fluid: yellowish CSF, indicating either an abnormally high protein level or a brain hemorrhage

INDICATIONS AND PROCEDURES

A lumbar puncture, often referred to as a spinal tap, is indicated for the diagnosis of meningitis because it is the best method for detecting meningeal irritation. A laboratory examination of the cerebrospinal fluid (CSF) harvested through a lumbar puncture can detect problems relating to the brain and spinal cord. Meningitis cannot be diagnosed through imaging methods such as computed tomography (CT) scanning.

Some subarachnoid (brain) hemorrhages involve the loss of so little blood that they are not detectable radiologically. When this is the case, the CSF may contain small amounts of blood that continues to be present in successive testing. If diagnosis is delayed, then the blood from a subarachnoid hemorrhage may have dissipated, making the CSF yellowish. This indicates that the blood in it is being metabolized. When this is the case, an immediate angiogram is indicated.

CSF withdrawn through a lumbar puncture should be examined immediately by a pathologist or hematologist to detect the presence of blood or, if it is xanthochromic or yellowish, to indicate either that the protein level is abnormally high or that a subarachnoid hemorrhage exists and blood is spreading over the surface of the brain. Such leakage may indicate an aneurysm and generally requires prompt surgery.

Although lumbar puncture is essentially a diagnostic tool, it is sometimes indicated when CSF has built up to dangerous levels in the spinal canal and the patient is hydrocephalic. In such instances, excess CSF can be withdrawn from the spinal canal, but an immediate determination of the cause of the buildup is essential and treatment to eliminate the cause imperative.

Lumbar Puncture

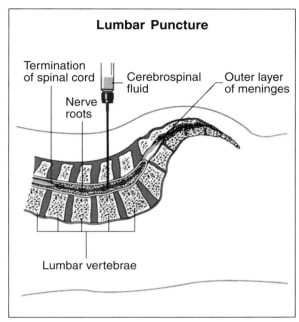

Termination of spinal cord

Nerve roots

Cerebrospinal fluid

Outer layer of meninges

Lumbar vertebrae

A lumbar puncture, commonly known as a spinal tap, is a diagnostic procedure in which cerebrospinal fluid is extracted from the meninges of the spine and analyzed for the presence of infection.

Patients undergoing lumbar punctures lie sideways, chin down and knees drawn up to separate the vertebrae. Local anesthetic is used to numb the area surrounding the lower vertebrae. A hollow needle inserted between two lower vertebrae is pushed into the spinal canal. The entire procedure, involving minimal discomfort, takes about twenty minutes. The puncture wound left by the needle is covered with a sterile bandage. Patients may experience a headache following the procedure, but it usually disappears quickly.

USES AND COMPLICATIONS

Lumbar puncture is used to inject dyes into the spinal canal to serve as a contrast medium in diagnostic procedures involving X rays, particularly myelography. It is also used to introduce medications into the CSF for the treatment of certain types of cancer. This use, often appropriate in cases of leukemia and carcinomas of the nervous system, is frequently employed in pediatric care.

Some surgical procedures require that patients be awake during surgery. In such cases, local anesthetics are introduced into the spinal canal through lumbar puncture, rendering patients still conscious but insensate.

As with any invasive procedure, there is risk of infection, but it is minimal. The procedure is performed under sterile conditions. One danger, in the case of a subarachnoid hemorrhage, is blood loss. Bleeding, in rare cases, may become uncontrollable and result in death. One cautionary note is that lumbar puncture should never be performed in cases where a brain abscess is suspected unless reliable CT scans or other tests have failed to reveal a mass or reveal only a small mass.

Lumbar puncture in and of itself is not a high-risk procedure, although the conditions that require its use often involve high risks for the patient. It is advisable in most cases for the procedure to be performed where immediate surgery can be carried out if the patient's condition deteriorates suddenly.

PERSPECTIVE AND PROSPECTS

The earliest use of CSF in diagnosis was in the nineteenth century, when such primitive tools as sharpened bird quills were used to penetrate the lumbar region. The technique came into its own in the mid-twentieth century, when most problems of the central nervous system were diagnosed through an examination of the CSF.

Because of the importance of CSF in diagnosing meningitis, cerebral hemorrhages, and other dangerous conditions, considerable progress and sophistication have accompanied the development of lumbar puncture. The imaging tools currently available to surgeons, neurologists, hematologists, and pathologists are so advanced and accurate, however, that lumbar puncture is used as a diagnostic tool somewhat less than in the past.

—*R. Baird Shuman, Ph.D.*

See also Anesthesia; Anesthesiology; Bacterial infections; Bacteriology; Biopsy; Bleeding; Fluids and electrolytes; Infection; Invasive tests; Meningitis; Nervous system; Neuroimaging; Neurology; Neurology, pediatric; Neurosurgery; Spine, vertebrae, and disks; Viral infections.

FOR FURTHER INFORMATION:

Bowden, Vicky R., and Cindy Smith Greenberg. *Pediatric Nursing Procedures.* Philadelphia: Lippincott Williams & Wilkins, 2003.

Colyar, Margaret R. *Well-Child Assessment for Primary Care Providers.* Philadelphia: F. A. Davis, 2003.

Doherty, Gerard M., and Lawrence W. Way, eds. *Current Surgical Diagnosis and Treatment.* 12th ed. New York: Lange Medical Books/McGraw-Hill, 2006.

Dougherty, Lisa, and Sara E. Lister, eds. *The Royal Marsden Hospital Manual of Clinical Nursing Procedures.* 6th ed. Malden, Mass.: Blackwell, 2004.

McAllister, Leslie D., et al. *Practical Neuro-oncology: A Guide to Patient Care.* Boston: Butterworth-Heinemann, 2002.

Lumpectomy. *See* **Mastectomy and lumpectomy.**

Lumps, breast. *See* **Breast cancer; Breast disorders; Breasts, female.**

Lung cancer
Disease/disorder

Anatomy or system affected: Chest, lungs, lymphatic system, respiratory system

Specialties and related fields: Environmental health, immunology, occupational health, oncology, pulmonary medicine, radiology

Definition: The appearance of malignant tumors in the lungs, which is usually associated with cigarette smoking.

Causes and Symptoms

Most forms of lung cancer fall within one of four categories: squamous cell (or epidermoid) carcinomas and adenocarcinomas (each of which accounts for approximately 30 percent of all pulmonary cancers), small or oat cell carcinomas (accounting for about 25 percent of lung cancers), and large cell carcinomas (which represent about 15 percent of lung cancers). Each of these forms can be further categorized on the basis of cell differentiation within the tumor: either well differentiated (resembling the original cell type) or moderately or poorly differentiated. Upon biopsy, stage groupings are also determined on the basis of size, invasiveness, and possible extent of metastasis.

Oat or small cell carcinomas usually consist of small, tightly packed, spindle-shaped cells, with a high nucleus-to-cytoplasm ratio within the cell. Oat cell carcinomas tend to metastasize early and widely, often to the bone marrow or brain. As a result, by the time that symptoms become apparent, the disease is generally widely disseminated within the body. Coupled with a resistance to most common forms of radiation and chemotherapy, oat cell carcinomas present a particularly poor prognosis. In general, patients diagnosed with this form of cancer have a survival period measured, at most, in months.

Adenocarcinomas are tumors of glandlike structure, presenting as nodules within peripheral tissue such as the bronchioles. Often these forms of tumors may arise from previously damaged or scarred tissue, such as has occurred among smokers. The development of adenocarcinoma of the lung is not as dependent upon smoke inhalation, however, as are other forms of lung cancer.

Squamous cell, also called epidermoid, carcinomas tend to be slower-growing malignancies which form among the flat epithelial cells on the surface of a variety of tissues, including the bladder, cervix, or skin, in addition to the lung. The cells are often polygonal in shape, with keratin nodes on the surface of lesions. Squamous cell carcinomas tend to metastasize less frequently than other forms of lung cancer, allowing for a more optimistic prognosis.

Large cell carcinomas are actually a more general form of cancer in which the cells are relatively large in size, with the cell nucleus being particularly enlarged. Often these carcinomas have arisen as either squamous cell carcinomas or adenocarcinomas. Metastasis, when it occurs, is frequently within the gastrointestinal tract.

There is no question that the single leading cause or factor resulting in lung cancer is smoking. Persons who do not smoke, and indeed even smokers who smoke fewer than five cigarettes per day, are at relatively low risk of developing any form of lung cancer. Those who smoke more than five cigarettes per day run an increased risk of developing lung cancer at rates approaching two hundred times that of the nonsmoker. This risk is greatest for oat cell carcinomas and least for adenocarcinomas (but still approximately a tenfold risk over that for nonsmokers). The relative risk is related to

---

Information on Lung Cancer

Causes: Smoking, exposure to other environmental toxins (asbestos, hydrocarbon products, nickel, vinyl chloride, uranium, pitchblende)

Symptoms: Persistent cough (sometimes accompanied by blood), difficulty breathing, chest pain, repeated and long-lasting attacks of bronchitis or pneumonia

Duration: Progressive and usually fatal

Treatments: Depends on stage; may include alleviation of symptoms, surgery, chemotherapy, radiation therapy the number of cigarettes smoked: The more cigarettes, the greater the risk. In addition, though other environmental hazards can be related to the development of lung cancers, the risk associated with those hazards is without exception amplified by cigarette smoke.

Exposure to other specific environmental factors has also been associated with the formation of certain forms of pulmonary cancers. Individuals chronically exposed to materials such as asbestos, hydrocarbon products (coal tars or roofing materials), nickel, vinyl chloride, or radiochemicals (uranium and pitchblende) are at increased risk. Chronically damaged lungs, for whatever reason, are at significantly increased risk for development of cancer.

The symptoms of lung cancer may represent the damage caused by the primary tumor or may be the result of metastasis to other organs. The most common symptom is a persistent cough, sometimes accompanied by blood in the sputum or difficulty breathing. Chest pain may be present, especially upon inhalation. There may also be repeated attacks of bronchitis or pneumonia that tend to persist for abnormal periods of time.

Treatment and Therapy

Diagnosis of a tumor in the lung generally includes a chest X ray, along with use of a variety of diagnostic tests: bronchography (X-ray observation of the bronchioles following application of an opaque material), tomography (cross-sectional observation of tissue), and cytologic examination of sputum or bronchiole washings. Confirmation of the diagnosis, in addition to determination of the specific type of tumor and its clinical stage, generally requires a needle biopsy of material from the lung.

The treatment of the tumor is dependent on the form of the disease and on the extent of its spread. Surgery remains the preferred method of treat-

In the News: Lack of Lung Cancer Symptoms in Some Women

In 2006, media stories reporting the death from lung cancer of Dana Reeve, widow of actor Christopher Reeve, focused on nonsmoking women who developed that disease. Reports concentrated on risk factors, including studies addressing the possible connection of estrogen with lung cancer, in order to educate women regarding screening. News accounts stressed that because lung cancer was often asymptomatic in women, female patients should not rely solely on symptoms to seek medical help, noting the work of researchers striving to develop effective methods to locate early-stage lung cancer. Articles noted the limitations of chest X rays, which do not detect most early-stage lung cancer tumors.

During 2005, the media had reported development of a potentially accurate lung cancer test in which dentists, physicians, or patients scraped samples of cheek cells inside the mouth to submit to medical laboratories for automated quantitative cytometry (AQC) evaluation. Researchers emphasized the low cost of this test, which did not need special equipment to take samples.

In the spring of 2006, the media reported on findings published in *Chest* journal that indicated tests for chronic obstructive pulmonary disease (COPD) might not reveal women had lung cancer because their lungs seemed to function normally during those tests and no symptoms were apparent. Researchers emphasized women at risk of having lung cancer should undergo other types of tests and that physicians should consider patients' age, smoking history, and environment when screening for that disease.

The media discussed the October, 2006, issue of *The New England Journal of Medicine*, which printed information regarding a New York-Presbyterian Hospital/Weill Cornell Medical College study evaluating the benefits of computed tomography (CT) scanning to detect lung cancer in asymptomatic subjects who smoked or were exposed to risk factors. This method, using low radiation dosages, alerted researchers to cancerous lung tumors in 484 of the 31,567 subjects scanned, enabling surgical removal before the cancer spread. Reports noted that because physicians could focus on small tumors, healthy lung tissue could be preserved during surgery.

Critics expressed concerns that the study lacked a control group to evaluate whether CT scans helped extend patients' life spans. They criticized the approach for resulting in unnecessary biopsies and surgeries for scan-detected tumors which later were determined to be benign, stressing that additional studies examining the role of CT scanning for lung cancer should be considered. The Lung Cancer Alliance, however, endorsed CT scans.

—*Elizabeth D. Schafer, Ph.D.*

A microscopic view of lung cancer cells. (PhotoDisc)

ment, but because of the nature of the disease, less than half the cases are operable at the time of diagnosis. Of these, a large proportion are beyond the point at which the surgical removal of the cancer and resection of remaining tissue are possible. A variety of chemotherapeutic measures are available and along with the use of radiation therapy can be used to produce a small number of cures or at least temporary alleviation of symptoms. Nevertheless, only a small proportion of lung cancers, perhaps 10 percent, respond with a permanent remission or cure.

Lung cancer represents the leading cause of cancer deaths among American men and women. In 2000, 164,000 new cases of lung cancer were reported, with 157,000 deaths reported. The prognosis for most forms of lung cancer remains poor.

—Richard Adler, Ph.D.

See also Addiction; Asbestos exposure; Bronchitis; Cancer; Carcinogens; Carcinoma; Chemotherapy; Lungs; Malignancy and metastasis; National Cancer Institute (NCI); Nicotine; Occupational health; Oncology; Pneumonia; Pulmonary diseases; Pulmonary medicine; Radiation therapy; Respiration; Smoking; Tumor removal; Tumors; Wheezing.

FOR FURTHER INFORMATION:

Dollinger, Malin, et al. *Everyone's Guide to Cancer Therapy.* 4th ed. Kansas City, Mo.: Andrews McMeel, 2002. A well-organized book on therapy for various cancers. Clearly describes the methods of treatment that are available and the treatment of choice. Written for the layperson and easily understood.

Eyre, Harmon J., Dianne Partie Lange, and Lois B. Morris. *Informed Decisions: The Complete Book of Cancer Diagnosis, Treatment, and Recovery.* 2d ed. Atlanta: American Cancer Society, 2002. This text from the American Cancer Society is intended for the layperson. It is exemplary in its discussion of cancer.

Henschke, Claudia I. *Lung Cancer: Myths, Facts, Choices—and Hope.* New York: W. W. Norton, 2003. An award-winning book that describes how the lungs work and how cancer develops. Reviews why early detection is so critical, provides questionnaires to pinpoint risk factors, and addresses practical concerns such as dealing with insurance issues.

Lung Cancer Online Foundation. http://www.lung canceronline.org/. A Web site that strives to improve the quality of care and quality of life for people with lung cancer by funding lung cancer research and providing information to patients and families.

Parles, Karen, and Joan H. Schiller. *One Hundred Questions and Answers About Lung Cancer.* Sudbury, Mass.: Jones and Bartlett, 2002. A patient-oriented guide that covers a range of topics related to lung cancer, including risk factors and causes; methods of prevention, screening, and diagnosis; available treatments and how to choose among them; and ways of coping with common emotional and physical difficulties associated with the diagnosis and treatment.

Pass, Harvey I., et al., eds. *Lung Cancer: Principles and Practice.* 3d ed. Philadelphia: Lippincott Williams & Wilkins, 2005. This illustrated text addresses neoplasms of the lungs. Includes a bibliography and an index.

Steen, R. Grant. *A Conspiracy of Cells: The Basic Science of Cancer.* New York: Plenum Press, 1993. Provides a fine discussion of a variety of factors which cause cancers to develop.

LUNG DISEASES. *See* PULMONARY DISEASES.

LUNG SURGERY

PROCEDURE

ANATOMY OR SYSTEM AFFECTED: Lungs, respiratory system

SPECIALTIES AND RELATED FIELDS: Emergency medicine, general surgery, pulmonary medicine

DEFINITION: The correction and treatment of such lung problems as bronchiectasis, cancer, emphysema, and pneumothorax.

KEY TERMS:

catheter: a flexible tube inserted into a body cavity to distend it or maintain an opening

diaphragm: the muscular partition that separates the abdomen and the thorax

expiration: the act of breathing out, which partly collapses the lungs

inspiration: the act of breathing in, which expands the lungs

trachea: a cartilaginous, air-carrying tube that runs from the larynx to the bronchi of the lungs

INDICATIONS AND PROCEDURES

Located in the chest (or thoracic) cavity, the lungs rest on the diaphragm. Each lung is connected to the trachea, which brings air in on inspiration and carries it away on expiration. Prior to its entry into the lungs, the trachea forms two bronchi. Each enters a lung near its middle and subdivides into smaller and smaller passages called bronchioles. The smallest tubes open into tiny air sacs called alveoli. Each alveolus contains blood vessels called capillaries which take up oxygen and release carbon dioxide into the lungs to be expelled as waste. Alveoli are arranged into lobules, which are united into lung lobes. The left lung contains two such lobes, and there are three in the larger right lung. Appropriate alveolar function is essential to life. To optimize their action, the lungs are surrounded by a double membrane, the pleura, and supplied by nerves that control expansion on inspiration and contraction on expiration. This size change, accomplished by muscular action, normally occurs eighteen times per minute throughout life. It slows during sleep and accelerates during exercise.

Good health requires adequate lung operation, which can be compromised in many ways. The best-known lung disorders are abscesses, asthma, bronchiectasis, bronchitis, cancer, emphysema, pneumonia, pneumothorax, and tuberculosis. Of these, lung cancer, abscesses, bronchiectasis, and pneumothorax can be corrected surgically.

Lung cancer is a leading cause of cancer death among both men and women. The disease has been attributed primarily to smoking, although causative agents such as asbestos, radioactive substances, and other air pollutants also have been implicated. The development of lung cancer is slow until severe symptoms appear. An early warning is a persistent cough unassociated with asthma or emphysema, chest pain, shortness of breath, fatigue, and general listlessness. The detection of lung cancer in its beginning stages requires regular chest X rays. Early detection greatly enhances long-term survival.

Lung cancer is best treated by surgery. This requires the removal of a small wedge of lung tissue, a lobectomy (lobe removal), or a pneumonectomy (lung removal), depending on the stage of the cancer. During surgery, general anesthesia is followed by an incision around the rib cage on the affected side, along a lower rib. The rib is then detached to produce a gap, and the tumor and/or section of the lung is removed. Postsurgical patients are kept in an intensive care unit for several days, where they are fed and given therapeutic drugs intravenously. Chest drainage tubes are used to drain the incision site. Convalescence takes several months after leaving the hospital. Complications can include infection at the site of the incision and lung collapse.

Lung abscesses most often result from the inhalation of food or tooth fragments. The symptoms are chills, fever, chest pain, and a severe cough that brings up phlegm containing blood and pus. Abscesses are often located using X rays. In many cases, antibiotics are curative. Severe and/or large lung abscesses, however, require surgical drainage or—in extreme cases—the surgical removal of affected lung tissue. For lung abscesses to require surgery, the affected tissue must be thick-walled and antibiotic-resistant. The simplest such cases involve the placement of a catheter in the abscess to act as a drain. In very severe cases, the affected lung portion (usually a wedge) is removed surgically, as with lung cancer.

Bronchiectasis, the distortion of air tubes, is often the result of childhood lung infections and takes years to develop. In most cases, it causes the production of large amounts of foul-smelling phlegm and predisposes the patient to repeated severe lung infections following colds. Diagnosis is by X ray, and treatment is often the use of antibiotics at the first sign of any cold. In some cases, the problem is severe enough to require lung surgery. Bronchiectasis that is severe enough to cause recurrent pneumonia in the same lung segment is treated by surgery when the air tube involved can be removed as well. The potential dangers of this procedure are infection and lung collapse, but they are uncommon.

Pneumothorax occurs when air enters the space between the pleura layers around a lung, causing the afflicted lung parts to collapse. It may be attributable to chest injury (such as knife wounds) or to air from ruptured blisters on the surface of the lungs. The symptoms of pneumothorax are breathlessness, chest pain, and chest tightness. Minor pneumothorax often cures itself, but severe pneumothorax can be fatal if left untreated. Surgery to correct major pneumothorax, although rare, must be carried out quickly. Minor pneumothorax cases that require surgical intervention usually involve the insertion of a catheter to remove the intrapleural air. Patients are then monitored for several days to ensure proper healing. In cases in which the leakage of air persists or a pleural tear is responsible for the pneumothorax, surgical repair of the pleura is required.

USES AND COMPLICATIONS

Lung surgery is straightforward but potentially dangerous because it can lead to death as a result of respiratory failure. After major operations, it is important for patients to convalesce slowly and to comply with the physician's instructions. It is particularly important for the patient to ensure that infection does not occur, to report pain and other danger signs, and to convalesce carefully. The resumption of work and physical activity should be as directed by a physician.

Major advances in treating problems associated with lung surgery include better diagnosis of their extent via computed tomography (CT) scanning and magnetic resonance imaging (MRI). Furthermore, the use of cytotoxic drugs and radiotherapy to treat cancer, including lung cancer, seems to minimize the severity of the surgical treatment of these lesions.

—*Sanford S. Singer, Ph.D.*

See also Abscess drainage; Abscesses; Cancer; Chest; Edema; Embolism; Heart transplantation; Internal medicine; Lung cancer; Lungs; Pleurisy; Pulmonary diseases; Pulmonary medicine; Pulmonary medicine, pediatric; Respiration; Resuscitation; Thoracic surgery; Thrombosis and thrombus; Transplantation; Tumor removal; Tumors.

FOR FURTHER INFORMATION:

Beers, Mark H., et al. *The Merck Manual of Diagnosis and Therapy*. 18th ed. Whitehouse Station, N.J.: Merck Research Laboratories, 2006. Contains a useful exposition of the characteristics, etiology, diagnosis, and treatment of lung disease. Designed for physicians, the material is also useful for less specialized readers.

Griffith, H. Winter. *Complete Guide to Symptoms, Illness, and Surgery*. Revised and updated by Stephen Moore and Kenneth Yoder. Rev. 4th ed. New York: Perigee, 2000. Covers more than five hundred diseases and disorders and includes information about causes and risk factors, preventive techniques, and diagnostic tests.

Matthews, Dawn D. *Lung Disorders Sourcebook*. Detroit: Omnigraphics, 2002. A comprehensive overview of lung anatomy, physiology, and dysfunctions culled from government agencies, the American Academy of Family Physicians, the American Lung Association, and the Mayo Foundation. Discusses thirty-five lung disorders in depth.

Professional Guide to Diseases. 8th ed. Ambler, Pa.: Lippincott Williams & Wilkins, 2005. A comprehensive yet concise medical reference covering more than six hundred disorders, this book includes information about the latest AIDS treatments, new parameters for defining diabetes, current information on cancers, updates on Alzheimer's disease, and more.

Tierney, Lawrence M., Stephen J. McPhee, and Maxine A. Papadakis, eds. *Current Medical Diagnosis and Treatment 2007*. New York: McGraw-Hill Medical, 2006. This text, updated yearly, is the point of reference for physicians and other health care practitioners. It incorporates each year's biomedical research discoveries that have immediate, relevant, and applicable use for the patient.

Lungs

ANATOMY

ANATOMY OR SYSTEM AFFECTED: Chest, respiratory system

SPECIALTIES AND RELATED FIELDS: Environmental health, exercise physiology, oncology, pulmonary medicine, vascular medicine

DEFINITION: Vital organs that allow gas exchange between an organism and its environment.

KEY TERMS:

aerobic respiration: the chemical reactions that use oxygen to produce energy; some small organisms do not use oxygen and are called anaerobic

alveoli: small, thin-walled sacs at the end of the airways; most gas exchange with the blood occurs here

cellular respiration: the chemical reactions that produce energy in the cell; these reactions can be aerobic or anaerobic

cilia: hairlike structures on cells that sweep mucus containing bacteria and foreign particles out of the airways

diffusion: the constant motion of molecules that tends to spread them from places of high concentration to those of lower concentration; gases move across the alveoli by diffusion

gas exchange: the movement of oxygen and carbon dioxide across the membrane of the lungs; other gases, such as nitrogen, may also cross the membrane

mucus: a thick, clear, slimy fluid produced in many parts of the body; in the lungs, mucus catches foreign material and provides lubrication to allow smooth airflow

respiration: the exchange of gases in breathing or the cellular chemistry that involves the same gases in the cell and produces energy

STRUCTURE AND FUNCTIONS

Efficient gas exchange with the environment is critical for larger organisms because oxygen is required for the last step in a series of cellular chemical reactions which processes nutrients from food. These reactions, called aerobic respiration, provide most of the energy that maintains life. Furthermore, as these reactions proceed, parts of larger carbon molecules are removed. Carbon dioxide is produced as a by-product and must be removed from the body. Hence, oxygen and carbon dioxide must be exchanged.

Small aerobic organisms can simply absorb the oxygen from air or water across their moist membranes or skins. The oxygen travels from where it is more concentrated to where it is less concentrated, a process called diffusion. The carbon dioxide inside the cells also diffuses across the membrane in the opposite direction to the environment. Larger organisms, however, have relatively less outside surface area and require special structures for their gas exchange. Various types of gills, swim bladders, and lungs are all examples of ways to absorb more oxygen and release more carbon dioxide.

This article focuses on one of these specialized structures: the lung. The lung is found in air-breathing land creatures. It allows oxygen to enter the blood and carbon dioxide to be removed. Form reflects function: The lung provides large amounts of moist surface area, close to many small blood vessels for gas exchange. Humans have a joined pair of lungs suspended in the chest cavity. The two lungs are somewhat different in size: The left lung is divided into two lobes, while the right has three lobes. This difference reflects the fact that the left side of the chest cavity has less room because of the position and shape of the heart.

The pathway to the lungs begins with the nose. The air entering each nostril is temporarily divided among three pathways (nasal conchae) and then warmed and moisturized by contact with a mucous membrane containing many blood vessels. Bacteria and particles get caught on the sticky mucus on this membrane. If objects pass this point they can be trapped by mucus lower in the tract and be swept out by waving cilia, hairlike fibers extending from cells of the airway that move in unison to push particles backward. Large particles that irritate the mucous membranes can cause a sneeze, which may eject the offending particle at speeds up to 169 kilometers per hour.

The air then continues to the pharynx (throat), where the nasal passageways and the mouth meet, and moves into the larynx, the organ that produces the voice. Swallowing pulls the larynx upward, allowing the epiglottis to flip over the opening and prevent food from entering this part of the airway. This movement of the larynx during swallowing can be felt by light touch with the fingers.

The trachea, or windpipe, follows. It is 11 centimeters long and made rigid by rings of cartilage. The inside of the trachea has cilia and also produces mucus. As the trachea approaches the lungs, it branches into two bronchi, which enter sides of the lungs at a midpoint between top and bottom. The walls of the bronchi contain cartilage rings and smooth muscles. Irritation in the larynx, the trachea, or the bronchi may cause coughing. Coughing is a reflex, like sneezing, that attempts to cast out impurities.

The bronchi continue to branch until they contain only smooth muscle; at this point, they are called bronchioles. The smooth muscle can contract or relax to allow the diameter of the bronchioles to adjust. Hence, the airflow can be changed according to the needs of the body. The pathways inside the lungs resemble an upside-down tree. Millions of cilia line the bronchial "tree" and constantly beat to remove particles. Each bronchial tube branches into several alveolar ducts. Each duct ends with a grapelike cluster of sacs called alveoli. The irregular branching that has led to this point ranges from eight to twenty-five divisions, with an average of twenty-three. Each alveolus has walls that are only one cell thick. Because of the large number of these air sacs, the lungs are very light in weight.

Gas exchange occurs in the alveoli. These structures are closely associated with the body's smallest blood vessels, the capillaries. Oxygen dissolves into the moisture on the vast surface of the alveoli. It then crosses the thin tissue of the lungs and moves into the capillaries to enter the blood. Carbon dioxide moves in the other direction to the lungs. Direction is maintained by the principle of diffusion: Flow is always from a higher to a lower concentration. The surface tension of the watery film inside the alveoli can cause a problem in gas exchange. Water molecules have a strong attraction for one another and can cause the alveoli to collapse to a smaller volume, reducing the surface area available for gas exchange. Fortunately, among the regular cells of the lining of the alveoli is found a second type of cell, called the type II cell. Type II cells produce surfactant, a mixture of chemicals that lowers the overall surface tension in the alveoli by separating the water molecules. Therefore, the alveoli stay fully inflated.

Roaming white blood cells called macrophages are a final defense against foreign objects at the alveolar level. Macrophages protect the lungs by attacking and eating bacteria and particles. They can be found elsewhere in the body performing the same function.

The pleural membrane is a double covering, one layer lining the outside of the lungs and the other lining the inside of the chest cavity. These two layers, which are really the same membrane, move over each other as breathing occurs, reducing friction. If air enters the space between the double membrane, however, the lung will collapse, a condition known as pneumothorax.

Air enters the entire airway by expansion of the chest cavity, or thorax. The cavity can be thought of as a box in which the top cannot be moved upward but the bottom and the sides may move outward. The arched diaphragm muscle at the base of the cavity contracts to lower the bottom of the box. Muscles between the ribs, called intercostals, contract to elevate the chest. The ribs, which slant downward when relaxed, move outward. This expansion pushes the walls out, increases the volume of the chest cavity, and lowers its internal pressure, causing air to be pushed into the lungs. Exhalation results when the muscles relax and allow the natural recoil of the lungs to expel the air.

Young children breathe differently than do older children or adults. Babies and toddlers have ribs that are nearly horizontal. They depend mainly on the descent of the diaphragm muscle for breathing. By two years of age, the ribs have moved to the adult position and rib muscles increase in importance. In addition, a sexual difference in breathing has been observed. Females tend to rely mainly on rib movement, while males tend to use both rib and diaphragm movement, with an emphasis on the diaphragm.

The rate of breathing is controlled by the medulla of the brain, which checks the carbon dioxide content of the blood. Activity produces more carbon dioxide and affects the rate. The normal relaxed breathing rate is about twelve times a minute. A person resting in bed may inhale 8 liters of air per minute, while a runner may reach 50 liters per minute. If a person relaxes and falls into a very shallow rhythm, a yawn attempts to break the pattern. A yawn is a deeper breath that causes more gas exchange.

DISORDERS AND DISEASES

The lungs are the only major internal organs exposed to the outside environment, and they tend to show the effects of both age and type of use. A child's lungs are pink, but with age this color becomes darker and mottled because of particles that are trapped inside the macrophages of the lung. The lungs of city dwellers and coal miners show the greatest effects because of the poor quality of the air being inhaled. Understanding the pathologies of the lungs is linked to understanding the function of the lung itself.

For example, smoking and air pollution are known to cause chronic bronchitis. The repeated irritation of the bronchi by pollutants causes the linings of the air tubules to thicken, closing down the airways. Muscles contract, and the secretion of mucus increases. Poor drainage may lead to pneumonia. Smoking tobacco can also lead to cancer of the lung, mouth, pharynx, and esophagus. Tobacco smoke may contain as many as forty-three carcinogenic (cancer-causing) chemicals. Lung cancer usually begins with changes in the lining of the bronchi among the cells with cilia and those that produce mucus. The long-term irritation of smoking eventually destroys these cells faster than the bronchi can replace them. Abnormal cells, without cilia or the ability to produce mucus, begin to take their place. These cells offer less protection and, as irritation and replacement continues, may become cancerous. In the United States, lung cancer is the leading cause of cancer deaths in both men and women, and evidence has revealed the danger of inhaling smoke from someone else's cigarette. Smoking also leads to greater risk of various other lung diseases.

Pneumonia is a general term for any inflammation that produces a fluid buildup in the lungs. The excess fluid makes breathing difficult by blocking the alveoli. The cause of the inflammation can be bacterial, viral, fungal, or chemical. For example, Legionnaires' disease is a type of pneumonia caused by a bacterium that lives in air conditioners, humidifiers, and other water-storage devices. Because it causes a lack of oxygen in the body, pneumonia can be fatal if it is not controlled: More than 70,000 deaths attributed to pneumonia occur in the United States each year. The very young and the very old are in the most danger, especially if they have already been weakened by other illnesses. Since the discovery of antibiotics, however, the majority of those infected recover.

Bronchitis is an inflammation of the mucous membrane of the bronchi that often follows a cold. A telltale symptom is a deep cough that eventually brings up gray or greenish phlegm. Bronchitis may be viral or bacterial; if the cause is bacterial, antibiotics can help in recovery. Chronic bronchitis can result from repeated attacks of bronchitis and is aggravated by smoking and air pollution.

Another lung disease is emphysema, which is usually caused by smoking. This condition is often seen in advanced cases of chronic bronchitis. In emphysema, the alveoli overinflate and break. Nearby alveoli are damaged and merge into larger units, leaving less surface area for gas exchange. Therefore, less of the air coming into the lungs comes into contact with the membrane. The increase in dead air space requires deeper breaths to obtain oxygen, and the lungs suffer further damage. Because the air sacs are permanently broken down, the damage is irreversible.

Tuberculosis is a highly contagious bacterial infection that damages the lungs and can spread to the kidneys and the bones. Immunization, screening for exposure, and antibiotics have controlled the number of cases found in countries with modern medical care systems. Worldwide, however, tuberculosis remains a major danger, and millions of lives are still lost to this disease every year.

According to the Mayo Clinic, cases of asthma appear to be increasing in the United States population. Asthma involves a hyperactive response of the airways. During an attack, the smooth muscles of the bronchi and bronchioles contract, and excess mucus is produced. In other cases, the airways may become inflamed and swollen. The cause may be allergies or other stimuli. Asthma is rarely fatal but interferes with normal functioning, as breathing becomes difficult. The blockage of breathing can be reversed with proper medications. Asthma does not lead to emphysema.

Respiratory distress syndrome occurs in about 50,000 premature infants every year. These infants have not yet developed the ability to produce sufficient surfactant in their alveoli to prevent collapse. The importance of surfactant can be illustrated by the difficulty of a baby's first breath. To inflate the alveoli requires up to twenty times the force of a normal breath. Without surfactant, the alveoli would collapse again and the next breath would be just as difficult. In 1990, a surfactant treatment derived from calf lungs became available. Treatment of premature babies with this surfactant before symptoms develop has resulted in an 88 percent survival rate.

Cystic fibrosis is a severe genetic problem in which the mucus produced in the airways (and the gastrointestinal tract) is abnormally thick. This thick mucus interferes with gas exchange, causing the heart to work harder and the valves to be damaged. As a result, the lung may collapse. Serious infections are more likely to occur. While about 50 percent of those with cystic fibrosis live only until their late teens and twenties, an increasing number of children and young adults with this disease are living into adult life. Progress on curing cystic fibrosis is being made: Researchers working in this area have located the gene that causes the condition.

If air is allowed to enter between the pleural membrane, the lungs will instantly collapse. The two lungs are independent enough so that one lung can be collapsed for healing while the other performs the gas exchange for the body. Furthermore, each lung subdivides into its lobes and then into ten bronchopulmonary segments. Each of these segments is a structural unit that can be removed surgically if diseased.

PERSPECTIVE AND PROSPECTS

The ancient Greeks established the first understandings of lung function. They rightly accepted that life depended on air but overgeneralized that air carried all disease. Empedocles of Agrigentum (c. 500-430 B.C.E.) demonstrated that air was a real substance by filling a wineskin with it. Empedocles erred, however, in explaining the mechanism of breathing. He compared the body to a pipe and thought that the movement of air in and out of the lungs caused vital air to move in and out of pores in the body's skin.

The writings of Galen of Pergamum (129-c. 199 C.E.) came to dominate Western medicine until the Renaissance. In his physiology, Galen attempted to connect the function of the lungs with the blood. He believed, however, that the liver produced a "vegetative" blood which traveled to the vena cava and then took different pathways. Some then flowed to other veins to nourish the whole body for growth. The rest entered the right side of the heart. Some of this substance entered the pulmonary artery into the lungs to allow impurities to be exhaled. The rest filtered to the left side of the heart through imagined pores in the septum.

In Galen's complicated scheme, the lungs were not only for exhaust: Vital air was inhaled there to be modified. The heart then pumped the modified air through the pulmonary vein to its left side. Here the air joined the blood to become "vital spirit," which traveled by arteries to warm the whole body. The brain converted this vital spirit into "animal spirit," distributing it by the nerves to cause movement and sensation. Galen did not know that blood traveled from one side of the heart to the other by moving through the lungs. He believed that the lungs acted as a reservoir of air for the heart. Galen also thought that breathing cooled the heart.

William Harvey (1578-1657) studied the position of valves in the veins and realized that Galen's vegetative blood traveled backward. Harvey then argued for a single blood that must go through the lungs to reach the other side of the heart. Blood travels in a circle, he bravely suggested. He was supported when the new microscopes discovered the necessary small vessels that connect arteries to veins.

Antoine-Laurent Lavoisier (1743-1794) noted that the lungs take in oxygen and that carbon dioxide is exhaled. He concluded that a slow combustion must occur in the lungs to warm the blood, while opponents noted that the lungs are not warmer than other parts of the body. By the 1790's, the idea was accepted that the lungs exchange Lavoisier's gases with the blood. Many believed that blood was the essence of life. In the 1850's, however, Georg Liebig and Hermann von Helmholtz showed that muscle tissue uses oxygen and releases carbon dioxide and heat. It was finally realized that the cells are the location of Lavoisier's slow fire of respiration and that the blood is the carrier of gases between the cells and the lungs.

—Paul R. Boehlke, Ph.D.

See also Abscess drainage; Abscesses; Allergies; Altitude sickness; Anatomy; Apnea; Asbestos exposure; Aspergillosis; Asphyxiation; Asthma; Avian influenza; Bacterial infections; Bronchiolitis; Bronchitis; Cancer; Chest; Childhood infectious diseases; Choking; Chronic obstructive pulmonary disease (COPD); Common cold; Coughing; Croup; Cyanosis; Cystic fibrosis; Diphtheria; Edema; Embolism; Emphysema; Environmental diseases; Environmental health; Exercise physiology; Heart transplantation; Hyperventilation; Influenza; Internal medicine; Interstitial pulmonary fibrosis (IPF); Kinesiology; Legionnaires' disease; Lung cancer; Lung surgery; Measles; Multiple chemical sensitivity syndrome; Nicotine; Occupational health; Oxygen therapy; Physiology; Plague; Pleurisy; Pneumonia; Pulmonary diseases; Pulmonary hypertension; Pulmonary medicine; Pulmonary medicine, pediatric; Respiration; Respiratory distress syndrome; Resuscitation; Smoking; Systems and organs; Thoracic surgery; Thrombolytic therapy and TPA; Thrombosis and thrombus; Toxoplasmosis; Transplantation; Tuberculosis; Tumor removal; Tumors; Wheezing; Whooping cough.

FOR FURTHER INFORMATION:

Corrin, Bryan, and Andrew G. Nicholson. *Pathology of the Lungs.* 2d ed. Edinburgh: Churchill Livingstone/

Elsevier, 2006. This volume discusses such topics as lung development, infectious diseases, vascular disease, tumors, and transplantation.

Levitzky, Michael G. *Pulmonary Physiology.* 7th ed. New York: McGraw-Hill Medical, 2007. A clinical text that describes the structure and function of the respiratory system. Covers topics such as the physical process of respiration from the interrelationship of basic lung mechanics, the microscopic changes at the alveolar level of gas exchange, the "nonrespiratory" functions of the lungs, and how the lungs respond to stress.

Mason, Robert J., et al., eds. *Murray and Nadel's Textbook of Respiratory Medicine.* 4th ed. Philadelphia: Elsevier Saunders, 2005. Details basic anatomy, physiology, pharmacology, pathology, and immunology of the lungs.

Sarosi, George A., and Scott F. Davies, eds. *Fungal Diseases of the Lung.* 3d ed. Philadelphia: Lippincott Williams & Wilkins, 2000. This resource covers a wide range of topics, including blastomycosis, coccidioidomycosis, cryptococcosis, and sporotrichosis.

Tapley, Donald F., et al., eds. *The Columbia University College of Physicians and Surgeons Complete Home Medical Guide.* Rev. 3d ed. New York: Crown, 1995. A comprehensive, practical health guide explaining all aspects of illness and treatment in common language. The section on respiratory diseases and lung health covers both the causes and the prevention of various diseases and problems.

West, John B. *Pulmonary Pathophysiology: The Essentials.* 6th ed. Baltimore: Lippincott Williams & Wilkins, 2003. Examines lungs afflicted with obstructive, restrictive, vascular, and environmental diseases. Bronchoactive drugs, the causes of hypoventilation, and the pathogenesis of asthma and pulmonary edema are new topics covered in this edition.

LUPUS. *See* SYSTEMIC LUPUS ERYTHEMATOSUS (SLE).

LYME DISEASE

DISEASE/DISORDER

ALSO KNOWN AS: Lyme borreliosis

ANATOMY OR SYSTEM AFFECTED: Eyes, heart, joints, knees, nerves, nervous system, skin

SPECIALTIES AND RELATED FIELDS: Bacteriology, cardiology, dermatology, epidemiology, neurology, ophthalmology, rheumatology

DEFINITION: Lyme disease is caused by bacteria transmitted by ticks. Initial symptoms include a spreading rash at the site of the tick bite; later, the central nervous system, heart, or joints may be affected.

KEY TERMS:

ectoparasite: an external parasite

seronegative Lyme disease: Lyme disease in which serum lacks a reaction with antibodies

spirochete: a long, helically coiled bacterial cell

CAUSES AND SYMPTOMS

Lyme disease is the most common tick-borne disease in the United States and Europe. It is caused by spirochete bacteria of the species complex *Borrelia burgdorferi sensu lato.* (This name refers to all bacteria causing Lyme disease.) *Borrelia burgdorferi sensu stricto* is the predominant cause of Lyme disease in the United States, while *Borrelia afzelii* and *Borrelia garinii* more often cause Lyme disease in Europe. The hard-bodied (Ixodes) tick transmits *Borrelia burgdorferi* to humans. Lyme disease is endemic in parts of New England, the upper Midwest, and Northern California. The tick species *Ixodes scapularis* (the black-legged tick or deer tick) transmits Lyme disease in the East and Midwest, while *Ixodes pacificus* (the Western black-legged tick) is the vector for Lyme disease in the West. In Europe, *Ixodes ricinus* (the sheep tick) is the vector.

Ticks are arachnid, obligate, blood-feeding ectoparasites with mouth parts that pierce the host skin. The tick saliva contains analgesics, anti-inflammatories, antihistamines, and anticoagulants that make it less likely that the tick bite will be detected. A tick takes three blood meals—as a larva, a nymph, and an adult—typically from different host species. The spirochete does not pass from adult tick into the tick eggs. When a tick larva feeds on a host infected with *Borrelia burgdorferi,* that larva becomes infected, molts to the nymph stage, and passes on the spirochete when it takes its next blood meal. In the eastern United States, the hosts infected with *Borrelia burgdorferi* on which the tick feeds are white-footed mice (the reservoirs of infection) and deer. There is a receptor that binds an outer membrane protein of the bacterium to maintain the bacteria in the tick gut. When the tick begins feeding on another host, a bacterial protein is produced that aids in detaching the bacteria from the receptor, and bacteria begin multiplying. The bacteria then go to the salivary glands and via saliva go to the host skin. Initially, there is little or no transmission of bacteria to the host. It

INFORMATION ON LYME DISEASE

CAUSES: Bacterial infection from bite of infected ticks

SYMPTOMS: Fatigue, malaise, chills and fever, headache, muscle and joint pain, swollen lymph nodes, rash, arthritis, nervous system abnormalities

DURATION: Acute

TREATMENTS: Oral antibiotics

takes at least twelve hours and perhaps as long as three days before the efficient transfer of bacteria. Even though the adult tick is twice as likely as the nymph to be infected with the Lyme spirochete, most cases of Lyme disease are noted in the late spring and summer, when nymphs seek blood meals from hosts. This may be because the smaller nymph is more difficult to notice.

Within a month after *Borrelia burgdorferi* bacteria enter the skin, a bull's-eye-shaped, rapidly expanding rash may form at the bite site. Bacteria travel through the bloodstream to other organs. Viral infection-like symptoms may develop, such as fatigue, headache, and neck pain. Respiratory symptoms, such as coughing, and vomiting or diarrhea do not occur. Not all who have the viral infection-like symptoms develop the rash or note a tick bite. About 60 percent of those who had the skin rash and were not treated develop arthritis, usually of the knee. About 10 percent develop neurological problems, usually facial nerve palsy. About 5 percent develop a cardiac complication as a result of atrioventricular block. The eyes may also be affected.

Lyme disease experts disagree about other possible effects. In some individuals, months after initial infection and treatment, symptoms such as muscle pain and fatigue seem to develop. Bacteria in some parts of the body may be resistant to antibiotic treatment, causing a persistent infection. Such infections would benefit from additional antibiotic treatment. A Lyme infection may be more severe because of coinfection from the tick with other pathogens, such as the rickettsial infection human granulocytic anaplasmosis and the protozoan disease babesiosis.

TREATMENT AND THERAPY

To prevent Lyme disease, avoiding exposure to ticks is key. In a tick-infected area, one should wear protective clothing, use tick repellent such as DEET, check daily for ticks, and promptly remove any ticks. To reduce the population of ticks around a house, the lawn should be kept mowed and brush cleared.

The rash of Lyme disease is treated with antibiotics such as doxycycline, amoxicillin, or cefuroxime axetil. For those under eight years of age and pregnant women, however, doxycycline is not recommended.

In the late 1990's, a vaccine against Lyme disease was available. This vaccine induced the production of antibodies to a *Borrelia burgdorferi* outer cell membrane surface lipoprotein. In 2002, the manufacturers of the vaccine withdrew it from the market because of problems involving postvaccination fatigue.

PERSPECTIVE AND PROSPECTS

The clinical symptoms of Lyme disease have been documented in European medical literature as early as the 1880's, but each clinical sign was considered a separate illness. In the 1970's, an outbreak of apparent juvenile rheumatoid arthritis, in some cases preceded by a rash, occurred in Old Lyme and Lyme, Connecticut. In 1975, this range of different symptoms was recognized as a single illness. *Borrelia burgdorferi* was identified in 1982 by Willy Burgdorfer, a tick-borne disease expert from the Rocky Mountain Labs in Montana.

In 2006, the Infectious Diseases Society of America (IDSA) released updated diagnosis and treatment guidelines for Lyme disease. These guidelines recommend a bull's-eye, or erythema migrans (EM), rash or positive laboratory tests to diagnose Lyme disease. The IDSA guidelines do not recognize a chronic form of Lyme disease, nor do they recognize seronegative Lyme disease except in early infections. This stance has generated a great deal of controversy. Both the International Lyme and Associated Disease Society (ILADS), a professional medical society, and the Lyme Disease Association, an all-volunteer association, have expressed concern about the stricter guidelines. They worry that patients with chronic Lyme disease will continue to suffer. There is much more to learn about the Lyme bacteria in order to aid patients.

—Susan J. Karcher, Ph.D.

See also Antibiotics; Arthritis; Bacterial infections; Bites and stings; Epidemiology; Lice, mites, and ticks.

FOR FURTHER INFORMATION:

American Lyme Disease Foundation. http://www.aldf .com/.

Edlow, Jonathan A. *Bull's-Eye: Unraveling the Medical Mystery of Lyme Disease*. 2d ed. New Haven, Conn.: Yale University Press, 2004.

International Lyme and Associated Disease Society (ILADS). http://www.ilads.org/.

Lyme Disease Association. http://www.lymedisease association.org/.

Stricker, Raphael B., Andrew Lautin, and Joseph J. Burrascano. "Lyme Disease: The Quest for Magic Bullets." *Chemotherapy* 52 (2006): 53-59.

Wormser, Gary P., et al. "The Clinical Assessment, Treatment, and Prevention of Lyme Disease, Human Granulocytic Anaplasmosis, and Babesiosis: Clinical Practice Guidelines by the Infectious Diseases Society of America." *Clinical Infectious Diseases* 43, no. 9 (2006): 1089-1134.

LYMPHADENOPATHY AND LYMPHOMA

DISEASE/DISORDER

ANATOMY OR SYSTEM AFFECTED: Lymphatic system

SPECIALTIES AND RELATED FIELDS: Hematology, internal medicine, oncology, vascular medicine

DEFINITION: Lymphadenopathy, or enlarged lymph nodes, refers to any disorder related to the lymphatic vessels of lymph nodes; lymphoma is a group of cancers consisting of unchecked multiplication of lymphatic tissue cells.

KEY TERMS:

B lymphocyte: a blood and lymphatic cell that plays a role in the secretion of antibodies

Hodgkin's disease: a malignant disorder of lymphoid tissue, generally first appearing in cervical lymph nodes, which is characterized by the presence of the Reed-Sternberg cell

lymphoma staging: a classification of lymphomas based upon the stage of the disease; used in the determination of treatment

non-Hodgkin's lymphoma: any malignant lymphoproliferative disorder other than Hodgkin's disease

Reed-Sternberg cell: a large atypical macrophage with multiple nuclei; found in patients with Hodgkin's disease

T lymphocyte: a blood and lymphatic cell that functions in cell-mediated immunity, which involves the direct attack of diseased tissues; subclasses of T cells aid B lymphocytes in the production of antibodies

CAUSES AND SYMPTOMS

The lymphatic system consists of a large complex of lymph vessels and groups of lymph nodes ("lymph glands"). The lymph vessels include a vast number of capillaries that collect fluid and dissolved proteins, carbohydrates, and fats from tissue fluids. The lacteals of the intestinal villi are lymph vessels that serve to absorb fats from the intestine and transport them to the bloodstream.

Lymph nodes are found throughout the body but are concentrated most heavily in regions of the head, neck, armpits, abdomen, and groin. Nodes function to filter out foreign materials, such as bacteria or viruses, which make their way into lymphatic vessels.

The sizes of lymph nodes vary: Some are as small as a pinhead, some as large as a bean. In general, they are shaped much like kidney beans, with an outer covering. Internally, they consist of a compartmentalized mass of tissue that contains large numbers of B and T lymphocytes as well as antigen-presenting cells (APC). The lymphatic circulation into the lymph nodes consists of a series of entering, or afferent, vessels, which empty into internal spaces, or sinuses. A network of connective tissue, the reticulum, regulates the lymph flow and serves as a site of attachment for lymphocytes and macrophages. The lymphatic circulation leaves the node through efferent, or exiting, vessels in the lower portion of the organ, the hilum.

Among the functions of lymph nodes are those of the immune response. B and T lymphocytes tend to congregate in specialized areas of the lymph nodes: B cells in the outer region, or cortex, and T cells in the underlying paracortex. When antigen is presented by an APC, T- and B-cell interaction triggers B-cell maturation and proliferation within the germinal centers of the cortex. The result may be a significant enlargement of the germinal centers and subsequently of the lymph node itself.

Lymphadenopathy, or enlarged lymph nodes, may signify a lymphoma, or cancer of the lymphatic system. More commonly, however, the enlarged node is sec-

---

INFORMATION ON LYMPHADENOPATHY AND LYMPHOMA

CAUSES: Disease, allergies, infection, viruses, genetic factors

SYMPTOMS: Enlarged lymph nodes, fatigue, mild fever, night sweats, weight loss

DURATION: Varies from acute to long-term

TREATMENTS: Varies; may include antibiotics, radiation therapy, chemotherapy, bone marrow transplantation

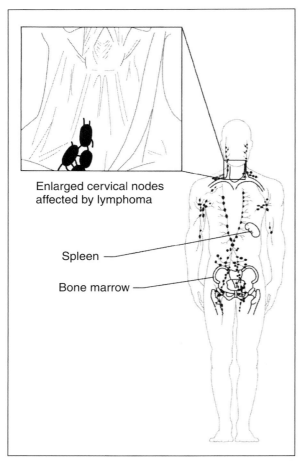

Enlarged cervical nodes
affected by lymphoma

Spleen

Bone marrow

Anatomy of the lymphatic system, showing major lymph nodes; enlarged lymph nodes may occur for a wide variety of reasons, including but not limited to lymphoma (cancer).

ondary to other phenomena, usually local infections. For example, an ear infection may result in the entrance of bacteria into local lymphatic vessels. These vessels drain into regional nodes of the neck. The result is an enlargement of the nodes in this area, as an immune response is carried out.

Enlarged nodes caused by infections can, in general, be easily differentiated from those caused by malignancies. Infectious nodes are generally smaller than 2 centimeters in diameter, soft, and tender. They usually occur in areas where common infections occur, such as the ears or the throat. Malignant lymph nodes are often large and occur in groups. They are generally firm and hard, and they often appear in unusual areas of the body (for example, along the diaphragm). In order to confirm a malignancy, a biopsy of material may be necessary.

Infectious nodes can also be caused by diseases such

as infectious mononucleosis, tuberculosis, and acquired immunodeficiency syndrome (AIDS). Lymphadenopathy syndrome (LAS), a generalized enlargement of the lymph nodes, is a common feature of the prodromal AIDS-related complex (ARC).

Since lymphadenopathy can be caused by any immune proliferation in the germinal centers, allergy-related illnesses may also cause enlargement of the lymph nodes. Consequently, immune disorders such as rheumatoid arthritis, systemic lupus erythematosus, and even hay fever allergies may show enlarged nodes as part of their syndromes.

As is the case for any cell in the body, cells constituting the lymphatic system may undergo a malignant transformation. The broadest definition of these lymphoproliferative diseases, or lymphomas, can include both Hodgkin's disease and Hodgkin's lymphomas, in addition to acute and chronic lymphocytic leukemias (ALL and CLL). With the understanding of, and ability to detect, specific cell markers, it is possible to classify many of these lymphomas on the basis of their cellular origin. Such is the case for ALL, CLL, Burkitt's lymphoma, and many other forms of non-Hodgkin's lymphomas. The cell type that ultimately forms the basis for Hodgkin's disease remains uncertain.

Hodgkin's disease is a malignant lymphoma that first presents itself as a painless enlargement of lymphoid tissue. Often, this is initially observed in the form of swollen lymph nodes in the neck or cervical region. Occasionally, the victim may exhibit a mild fever, night sweats, and weight loss. Untreated, the disease spreads from one lymphatic region to another, resulting in diffuse adenopathy. An enlarged spleen (splenomegaly) is a common result. As the disease spreads, other organs such as the liver, lungs, and bone marrow may be involved.

The disease is characterized by the presence of a characteristic cell type—the Reed-Sternberg cell. Reed-Sternberg cells appear to be of macrophage origin, with multilobed nuclei or multiple nuclei. They may also be present in other lymphatic disorders, but their presence is considered to be indicative of all cases of Hodgkin's disease. The precise relationship of the cell to the lymphoma is unclear, but some researchers in the field believe that the Reed-Sternberg cell is the actual malignant cell of the disease. The other infiltrative cells present in the node, including many B and T lymphocytes, may simply represent the reaction to the neoplasm. This interpretation, however, has been disputed.

Lymphoma staging is a system of classifying lymphomas according to the stage of development of the disease. Staging is important in that the prognosis and basis for treatment are in part determined by the stage of disease. Characterizing the form of Hodgkin's disease, therefore, involves two forms of classification. The first is a four-part classification based on the histology or cell type (Rye Conference classification). This scheme is based upon the proportion of Reed-Sternberg cells, ranging from their being "hard to find" to their being the predominant type. The prognosis becomes less favorable as the proportion of these cells increases.

Clinical staging, like that based on histology, is a four-part classification scheme (it is actually six parts, since stage III can be divided into subclasses). In this system, classification is based upon the extent of spread or extralymphatic involvement. For example, stage I features the involvement of a single lymph node region or a single extralymphatic site. Stage IV involves multiple disseminated foci. Early-stage disease is more easily treated and has a better prognosis than late-stage disease.

Non-Hodgkin's lymphomas (NHLs) represent a multitude of malignant disorders. Unlike Hodgkin's disease, they frequently arise in lymphatic tissue that is not easily observed; for example, in the gastrointestinal tract, tonsils, bone, and central nervous system. They have a tendency to spread rapidly, with malignant cells being released into the bloodstream early in the disease. Consequently, by the time diagnosis of NHL is made, the disease has often spread and the prognosis may be poor.

Though the etiology of most forms of NHL remains unknown, certain characteristics are evident in some forms of these diseases. For example, a portion of chromosome 14 is elongated in about 60 percent of NHL patients. Nearly one-third of patients with NHLs of B-cell origin demonstrate a chromosomal translocation, often involving a piece of chromosome 14 being translocated to chromosome 18. Though the relationship of these changes to disease is unclear, one can surmise that chromosomal defects play at least some role in the development of some forms of these disorders.

At least two forms of NHL are either caused by viruses or related to their presence: Burkitt's lymphoma and adult T-cell lymphoma/leukemia. Burkitt's lymphoma, which was first described by Denis Burkitt in central Africa, is a B-cell tumor that occurs primarily in children. It is generally presented as a large tumor of the jaw. This type of lymphoma is associated with early infection by the Epstein-Barr virus, or EBV (also the etiological agent of infectious mononucleosis). The relationship of the disorder to the virus remains unclear, and EBV may be either a specific cause or a necessary cofactor.

Specific chromosomal abnormalities are also associated with Burkitt's lymphoma. In 75 percent of cases, a translocation from chromosome 8 to chromosome 14 is evident, while in most other cases, a portion of chromosome 8 is translocated to either chromosome 2 or chromosome 22. Each of these translocations involves the transfer of the same gene from chromosome 8, the c-myc gene. The site to which the c-myc is translocated is in each instance a region that encodes protein chains for antibody production, proteins that are produced in large quantities. The c-myc gene product normally plays a role in committing a cell to divide. By being translocated into these specific regions, the c-myc gene product is overproduced, and the B cell undergoes continual replication.

Approximately 80 percent of NHL tumors are of B-cell origin; the remainder are primarily of T-cell origin. Those lymphomas that arise within the thymus, the organ of T-cell maturation, are called lymphoblastic lymphomas. Those that originate as more differentiated and mature T cells outside the thymus include a heterogeneous group of diseases (for example, peripheral T-cell lymphomas and Sézary syndrome). Often, by the time of diagnosis, these disorders have spread beyond the early stage of classification and have become difficult to treat.

TREATMENT AND THERAPY

Treatment and other means of dealing with lymphadenopathy depend on the specific cause. In the case of lymph node enlargement that is secondary to infections, treatment of the primary cause is sufficient to restore the normal appearance of the node. For example, in a situation in which nodes in the neck region are enlarged as the result of a throat infection, antibiotic treatment of the primary cause—that is, the bacterial infection—is sufficient. The nodes will resume their normal size after a short time.

Dealing with lymph node enlargement caused by lymphoma requires a much more aggressive form of treatment. There are many kinds of lymphomas, which differ in type of cell involvement and stage of differentiation of the involved cells. The manifestations of most lymphomas, however, are similar. In general, these disorders first present themselves as painless, enlarged nodes. Often, this occurs in the neck region, but in many forms of NHL, the lymphadenopathy may manifest itself elsewhere in the lymphatic system. As the disease progresses, splenomegaly (enlarged spleen) and hepatomegaly (enlarged liver) may manifest themselves. Frequently, the bone marrow becomes involved. If the enlarged node compresses a vital organ or vessel in the body, immediate surgery may be necessary. For example, if one of the veins of the heart is compressed, the patient may be in immediate, life-threatening danger. Treatment generally includes radiation therapy and/or chemotherapy.

As is true for lymphomas in general, Hodgkin's disease is found more commonly in males than in females. In the United States, it occurs at a rate of 2 per 100,000 population per year, resulting in more than 6,000 cases being diagnosed each year. Approximately 1,500 persons die of the disease each year. The cause of the disease is unknown, though attempts have been made to assign the Epstein-Barr virus to this role.

Hodgkin's disease has an unusual age incidence. The age-specific incidence exhibits a bimodal curve. The disease shows an initial peak among young adults between 15 and 30 years of age. The incidence drops after age 30, only to show an additional increase in frequency after age 50. This is in contrast to NHL, which shows a sharp increase in incidence only after age 45. The reasons for this are unknown.

As noted earlier, the staging of Hodgkin's disease is important in determining methods of treatment; the earlier the stage, the better the prognosis. Patients in stage I (single node or site of involvement) or stage II (two or more nodes on the same side of the diaphragm involved, or limited extralymphatic involvement) have a much better prognosis than patients in stages III and IV (splenic or disseminated disease). Prior to the mid-1960's, a diagnosis of Hodgkin's disease was almost a death sentence. The development of radiation therapy and chemotherapy has dramatically increased the chances for survival; long-term remission can be achieved in nearly 70 percent of patients, and the "cure" rate may be higher than 90 percent with early detection. In part, this has been the result of understanding the progression of the disease (reflected in the process of staging) and utilizing a therapeutic approach to eradicate the disease both at its current site and at likely sites of spreading.

Radiation therapy is the treatment of choice for patients in stages I and II; spreading beyond local nodes is still unlikely in these stages. The body is divided into three regions to which radiation may be delivered: The mantle field covers the upper chest and armpits, the para-aortic field is the region of the diaphragm and spleen, and the third field is the pelvic area. For example, a patient presenting lymphadenopathy in a single node in the neck region may undergo only "mantle" irradiation. As noted above, with early detection, such treatment is effective 90 percent of the time (based on five-year disease-free survival).

Beyond stage II, a combination of radiation therapy and chemotherapy treatment is warranted. A variety of chemotherapy programs have been developed, the most common of which is known by the acronym MOPP (nitrogen mustard/Oncovin/procarbazine/prednisone). With combined radiation therapy and chemotherapy, even stage III disease may go into remission 60 to 70 percent of the time, while 40 to 50 percent of stage IV patients may enter remission. In general, therapy takes six to twelve months.

Non-Hodgkin's lymphomas represent a heterogeneous group of malignancies. Eighty percent are of B-lymphocyte origin. The wide variety of types has made classification difficult. The most useful method of classification for clinical purposes is based on the relative aggressiveness of the disease, low-grade being the slowest growing, followed by intermediate-grade and high-grade, which is the most aggressive.

NHLs often arise in lymphoid areas outside the mainstream. For example, the first sign of disease may be an abdominal mass or pain. Fever and night sweats are uncommon, at least in the early stages. Consequently, once the disease is presented, it is often deep and widespread. Because the disorder is no longer localized by this stage, radiation therapy by itself is of limited use. For comparison, nearly half of Hodgkin's disease patients are in stage I at presentation; not quite 15 percent of NHL patients are in stages I and II. Consequently, treatment almost always involves extensive chemotherapy.

A variety of aggressive forms of chemotherapy may be applied. These may include either single drugs such as alkaloids (vincristine sulfate) and alkylating agents (chlorambucil) or combination programs such as that of MOPP. Low-grade types of NHL are frequently slow growing and respond well to less aggressive forms of therapy. Low-grade NHL patients often enter remission for years. Unfortunately, the disorder often recurs with time and may become resistant to treatment; remission may occur in 50 percent of the patients, but only about 10 percent survive disease-free after ten years. High-grade lymphomas are rapidly growing, and the prognosis for most patients in the short term is not good. Those patients who do achieve remission with aggressive therapy, however, often show no recurrence of disease. As many as 50 percent of these persons may be "cured." The difference in prognosis between low-grade and high-grade disease may relate to the characteristics of the malignant cell. A rapidly growing cancer cell may be more susceptible to aggressive therapy than a slow-growing cancer and more likely to die as a result. Thus, if a patient enters remission following therapy, there is greater likelihood that the cancer has been eradicated.

PERSPECTIVE AND PROSPECTS

What was likely Hodgkin's disease was first described in 1666 as an illness in which lymphoid tissues and the spleen had the appearance of a "cluster of grapes." The disorder was invariably fatal. In 1832, Thomas Hodgkin published a thorough description of the disease, including its progression from the cervical region of the body to other lymphatic regions and organs. The unusual histological appearance of the cellular mixture characteristic of Hodgkin's disease was noted during the nineteenth century. It was early in the twentieth century, however, that Dorothy Reed and Karl Sternberg described the cell that is characteristic of the disorder: the Reed-Sternberg cell. As noted earlier, the number and proportion of such cells are the bases for the classification of the disease.

Two forms of non-Hodgkin's lymphoma are known to be associated with specific viruses: Burkitt's lymphoma (BL) and adult T-cell leukemia (ATL). BL was described by Denis Burkitt, who studied the pattern of certain forms of lymphomas among Ugandan children during the late 1950's. He noted that nearly all cases were found in children between the ages of 2 and 14, and noted that most cases in Africa were found in the malarial belt. Burkitt suspected that a mosquito might be involved in the transmissions of BL. Though no link has been found with arthropod transmission, the idea that BL might be associated with a viral agent bore fruit. In 1964, Michael Epstein and Yvonne Barr reported the presence of a particle in BL tissue that resembled the herpes virus. The Epstein-Barr virus was eventually linked to BL, though the specific role played by the virus remains elusive.

Adult T-cell leukemia was first noted in Japan during the 1970's. Japanese scientists observed that the majority of NHLs there were of T-cell origin and ex-

hibited a similar clinical spectrum. The disease was later observed in the Caribbean basin, the southeastern United States, South America, and central Africa. In 1980, Robert Gallo isolated the etiological agent, the human T-cell lymphotrophic type I virus (HTLV-I).

The treatment of Hodgkin's disease represents one of the few success stories in dealing with cancers. In addition, some forms of NHL—notably, Burkitt's lymphoma—respond well to treatment. The prognosis for most patients with NHL, however, is less than optimal. In addition, the specific causes of most NHL syndromes are not known. Those with which a virus is linked may, in theory, be prevented by means of vaccination. The etiological agents or factors associated with the development of other forms of lymphomas remain elusive.

—*Richard Adler, Ph.D.*

See also Burkitt's lymphoma; Cancer; Carcinogens; Chemotherapy; Epstein-Barr virus; Hodgkin's disease; Infection; Lymphatic system; Malignancy and metastasis; Oncology; Radiation therapy.

FOR FURTHER INFORMATION:

Cerroni, Lorenzo, Helmut Kerl, and Kevin Gatter. *An Illustrated Guide to Skin Lymphoma*. 2d ed. Malden, Mass.: Blackwell, 2004. This book is an extremely practical guide to diagnosis that will help any pathologist spot skin lymphoma. It combines stunning pictures of histopathology (tissue specimens) with the clinical features, making it attractive and useful to pathologists and clinicians.

Delves, Peter J., et al. *Roitt's Essential Immunology*. 11th ed. Malden, Mass.: Blackwell, 2006. An outstanding textbook on immunology. The early chapters on the lymphatic system, lymph nodes, and the immune response provide an excellent background for the subject.

Greer, John, et al., eds. *Wintrobe's Clinical Hematology*. 11th ed. Philadelphia: Lippincott Williams & Wilkins, 2004. A textbook of hematologic disorders, with an excellent review of lymphatic diseases including Hodgkin's disease. Written for clinicians and students of medicine.

Holman, Peter. *One Hundred Questions and Answers About Lymphoma*. 2d ed. Sudbury, Mass.: Jones and Bartlett, 2007. A patient-oriented guide that covers a range of topics related to lymphatic diseases, including risk factors and causes; methods of prevention, screening, and diagnosis; available treatments and how to choose among them; and ways of coping with common emotional and physical difficulties associated with the diagnosis and treatment.

Jandl, James H. *Blood: Textbook of Hematology.* 2d ed. Boston: Little, Brown, 1996. A textbook on hematology. The book is quite detailed but is recommended for anyone who is seriously interested in the subject. Though the lymphatic system is not specifically covered, blood and lymphatic cells are extensively covered.

Knowles, Margaret A., and Peter J. Selby. *Introduction to the Cellular and Molecular Biology of Cancer.* 4th ed. New York: Oxford University Press, 2005. A general description of cancer and areas of research. The text discusses features of cancer and its possible origins. The possible role of oncogenes in the disease is also included. Though not intended for the layperson, the book does present a good overview of the subject.

Leukemia and Lymphoma Society. http://www.leukemia.org/. A group dedicated to funding blood cancer research, education, and patient services for patients with leukemia and other lymphatic diseases.

Lymphoma Information Network. http://www.lymphomainfo.net/. Offers information on the diagnosis and treatment options for adult and childhood Hodgkin's disease and resources for further research.

National Cancer Institute. *What You Need to Know About Non-Hodgkin's Lymphoma.* Rev. ed. Bethesda, Md.: U.S. Department of Health and Human Services, Public Health Service, National Institutes of Health, 1999. Aimed at the patient who has been diagnosed with non-Hodgkin's lymphoma, this publication offers the latest advice.

LYMPHATIC DISORDERS. *See* LYMPHADENOPATHY AND LYMPHOMA.

LYMPHATIC SYSTEM
ANATOMY
ANATOMY OR SYSTEM AFFECTED: Circulatory system, immune system, spleen

SPECIALTIES AND RELATED FIELDS: Hematology, immunology, vascular medicine

DEFINITION: A network of vessels, paralleling those of the circulatory system, and nodules that collects extravascular materials and fluids from tissue in order to return them to the bloodstream.

KEY TERMS:

antigen-presenting cell (APC): a type of macrophage or interstitial cell that initiates the immune response by "presenting" processed antigen to B and T lymphocytes

edema: an abnormal accumulation of fluids around tissues

lacteals: lymphatic capillaries in the villi of the small intestine that absorb fat, producing a milky substance called chyle

lymph: the straw-colored fluid of the lymphatic system; as much as 1 to 2 liters is collected from tissue each day and returned to the bloodstream

lymph node: a small, oval structure that filters tissue fluids; lymph nodes are found in areas such as the armpits, groin, mouth, and neck, and serve as sites of immune response

lymphocytes: cells of the lymphatic system; B lymphocytes function in antibody production, while T lymphocytes function in cellular immunity

Peyer's patches: lymphatic nodules in the ileum of the intestine; Peyer's patches are one kind of mucosal associated lymphoid tissue (MALT), which, unlike lymph nodes, are not enclosed by tissue capsules

spleen: a lymphatic organ found between the stomach and the diaphragm; destroys old blood cells and filters foreign material from the blood

thoracic duct: the largest lymphatic vessel, which collects lymphatic fluid and returns it to the bloodstream at the left subclavian vein in the region of the neck

thymus: the lymphatic gland in which T lymphocytes mature; located in humans just below the thyroid

STRUCTURE AND FUNCTIONS
The lymphatic system is a complex of capillaries, ducts, nodes, and organs that filters and maintains interstitial fluid—that is, fluid from body tissues. Fluid is collected from body tissues and returned to the bloodstream. In addition, the system functions as a site of the immune response, primarily in the spleen and the lymph nodes, and transports fat and protein to the bloodstream.

The organs of the lymphatic system are divided into primary lymphoid organs and secondary organs. The primary organs include the thymus and the bone marrow, which are sites where lymphocytes are produced and mature. Secondary lymphoid organs are those in which the immune response is carried out. These include both encapsulated organs such as the spleen and lymph nodes and unencapsulated organs such as the mucosal associated lymphoid tissue, which includes Peyer's patches in the intestine and Waldemeyer's ring in the throat (the tonsils and adenoids), which encircles the pharnyx. Lymph nodes are found throughout the body, but they occur in large numbers in the head, neck, armpits (the axial nodes), and abdomen and groin (the inguinal nodes).

The lymphatic vessels essentially parallel those of the bloodstream. The system originates in peripheral tissue as small openings, or sinuses, within the tissue. Fluid that drains from the tissue collects in these sinuses and forms lymph. In addition, a significant amount of liquid (1 to 2 liters) that is lost from blood capillaries each day also collects in the interstitial fluid. The lymph is physiologically similar to blood plasma in that it is a balanced solution of electrolytes containing some carbohydrates, lipids, and proteins. In general, the protein level is about half that found in blood, since most blood proteins are too large to pass through the endothelial walls of blood capillaries. Arguably, the major function of the lymphatic system is the return of this fluid, and its constituent materials, to the blood. The buildup of abnormal amounts of fluid in tissue results in swelling, or edema. Approximately 60 percent of lost fluid is returned to the blood through the lymphatics, and the remainder is collected directly into small blood capillaries.

Generally speaking, the peripheral portion of the lymphatic system is completely separate from that of the blood. Once the interstitial fluid is collected, it begins to move toward the thoracic duct. Since the duct is found in the neck region, this movement is primarily in an upward direction. The fluid moves through regional lymph nodes, such as those found in the groin or armpits, and gradually collects in the larger ducts of the major lymphatics. Though an extensive system of valves is found in the lymphatic system to prevent the movement of lymph in the wrong direction, no internal pumping mechanism analogous to the heart exists. The movement of the lymph is mediated by the musculature of the body: respiratory pressure, muscular movement, and the pulsing or motion of nearby organs. Lymphatic fluids from all portions of the body, except for the upper-right quadrant, eventually collect in the thoracic duct. Lymph from the upper-right quadrant of the body collects in the right lymphatic duct. The endothelia of these major lymphatic ducts are contiguous with those of the veins in the neck, and it is here that the fluid is returned to the bloodstream. Valves present in the lymphatic ducts serve to prevent the backup of blood from the bloodstream into the lymphatic system.

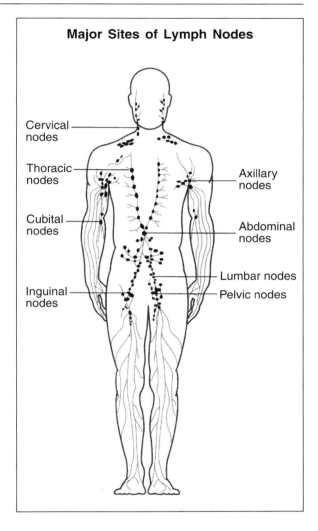

Major Sites of Lymph Nodes

Cervical nodes

Thoracic nodes

Cubital nodes

Inguinal nodes

Axillary nodes

Abdominal nodes

Lumbar nodes

Pelvic nodes

In addition to the electrolytes and proteins that collect in lymph, foreign materials such as infectious agents may also penetrate the skin or internal surfaces of the body. These materials pass into tissue fluids and also collect in the lymphatic system. From here, they travel to regional lymph nodes, where they are filtered out by phagocytic cells such as macrophages. In addition, antigen-collecting cells in the skin, including dendritic cells, may transport foreign materials such as bacteria to these regional nodes. These cells may intercalate, or interdigitate, among the lymphocytes of the lymph nodes and, along with the macrophages, "present" antigen to B and T cells. In this manner, the immune response is initiated.

An analogous situation exists in the blood system. In this case, however, it is the macrophages of the spleen that serve to filter foreign material, such as infectious agents, from the blood. Damaged or old red blood cells are removed in a similar manner. The macrophages then degrade the foreign material and "present" it to B and T lymphocytes in the spleen.

Most of the immune response occurs in the lymph nodes and the spleen. Once the interaction has occurred between the APCs and the lymphocytes, differentiation of the B and T cells begins. The B cells develop into plasma cells, which are essentially antibody-producing factories, while T cells may undergo proliferation. Within the nodes, B and T cells are generally confined to specific areas: the outer cortex for B cells and the underlying paracortex for T cells. Embedded within the cortex are collections of primary nodules, which consist primarily of B cells. Once antigenic stimulation occurs, the cells within the nodules enlarge and proliferate, forming secondary follicles that surround germinal centers. These germinal centers enlarge as B lymphocytes mature and proliferate, and they account for the enlargement of regional lymph nodes in the event of infection. In addition, blood vessels within the node may become enlarged, increasing blood flow. Though some of the activated lymphocytes eventually find their way to the bloodstream, most remain within the lymphatic system. Antibodies produced in response to an infection, however, are transported to the blood.

Since lymph nodes serve as regions of drainage for local tissue, they also represent a route through the body for cancer cells that break away from a tumor. For example, cells from a breast cancer may lodge in regional lymph nodes of the neck or armpit and travel from there to other areas of the body. Although specialized types of lymphocytes capable of killing tumor cells are found in the nodes, some cancer cells may survive. It is for this reason that, during the removal of tumors, localized nodes are examined for evidence of metastasis. If no cancer cells are observed in the nodes, the chances are high that the cancer has not spread.

Mucosal associated lymphatic tissue (MALT) is found along mucosal membranes in regions of the intestines (Peyer's patches and the appendix) and the throat (tonsils). The tonsils actually consist of a network of three groups of tissues that are located at the base of the tongue, at the back of the throat, and at the roof of the nasopharynx (adenoids). Like the spleen and the lymph nodes, MALT tissues may be sites of germinal centers. Unlike the spleen and lymph nodes, however, these tissues are not enclosed by defined capsules of connective tissue. They may be loosely organized, like the mucosa of the intestinal villi, or they may form organized regions like those of the tonsils and adenoids.

MALT appears to function to protect the body against respiratory or gastrointestinal agents. For example, agents such as bacteria or viruses that enter through the oral or respiratory route may stimulate an immune response by the tonsils. The swelling of the tonsils, tonsillitis, is the result of a localized immune response much like that found in the spleen or the lymph nodes. Germinal centers within the tissue represent areas of B cell maturation and proliferation. In the same way, the Peyer's patches consist of approximately thirty to forty nodules along the wall of the intestines. Gastrointestinal antigens that penetrate the intestinal wall stimulate germinal centers in these regions.

Digestion products of carbohydrates and proteins are actively transported into the villi of the small intestine and enter the bloodstream directly. Fats, however, enter the blood in a more roundabout way through the lymphatic system. Fats are digested in the small intestine and diffuse into underlying cells. There they are assembled into triglycerides and, along with cholesterol, are enclosed in protein envelopes; the resulting bodies are called chylomicrons. Once these bodies pass into the lacteals of the lymphatic system, the whitish fluid, chyle, is transported to a region at the beginning of the thoracic duct called the cisterna chyli. It is here that the fat enters the bloodstream.

DISORDERS AND DISEASES

If the interstitial fluid—that is, the fluid in the tissues—increases beyond the capacity of the lymphatic system to handle the situation, an abnormal accumulation of fluid will build up in the tissue. This creates a situation known as edema. A variety of etiological factors can cause edema. For example, burns, inflammation, and certain allergic reactions may increase the level of capillary permeability. This is particularly true if a large amount of protein is lost as the result of a serious burn.

An increase in capillary hydrostatic pressure may also increase the rate of fluid buildup in the tissues. This may be a by-product of several conditions: congestive heart failure, renal failure, or the use of a variety of drugs (estrogen, phenylbutazone). For example, an increase in the sodium concentration of the blood caused by retention resulting from renal failure or simply an excess of salt in the diet may cause water retention and increased blood volume. The sequelae include increased fluid leakage and edema. It is for this reason that a reduction in sodium intake is often recommended for those who suffer from this problem. Diuretics may be prescribed to promote the excretion of sodium and water. Similarly, venous obstruction as serious as phlebitis or as minor as the pressure from a tight bandage or clothing may increase hydrostatic pressure and lead to edema.

A buildup of fluid in the lungs, or pulmonary edema, may occur as a result of congestive heart failure. Hydrostatic pressure in the capillaries of the lungs is relatively low when compared with that of the circulation elsewhere. As a result, the "wetness" of lung tissue is minimal. In patients with serious congestive heart disease, capillary fluid is backed up into the lung (and, indeed, in tissues of the extremities). The result is fluid leakage into the alveoli and bronchioles. Though the lymphatics are capable of removing small amounts of excess fluids, at some point the leakage of plasma and dissolved proteins exceeds the capacity of the lymphatic system to handle the problem. The result is a vicious circle. Since less oxygen is taken up through the lungs, capillary permeability increases. More fluid and protein are then lost. Unless intervention is carried out, the patient may eventually drown in his or her own fluids.

Intervention for pulmonary edema generally involves elevating the head and knees of the patient (Fowler's position) and the administration of diuretics. A low-sodium diet, allowing for decreased fluid retention, may also relieve some of the stress on the lymphatic system. With time, the number of lymphatic vessels in the lungs may increase, allowing for a greater capacity to remove fluids.

A variety of disorders may directly involve the lymphatic system itself. Lymphedema, or the accumulation of lymph in tissue with subsequent swelling, may result from the absence of lymphatic vessels or from obstructions within the vessels. The symptoms of lymphedema, particularly in the lower extremities, include mild swelling that becomes increasingly severe with time. The problem may be exacerbated by menstruation or pregnancy. In some instances, lymphatic vessels may be absent, either congenitally or because of surgical removal. Diagnosis of the problem often requires the use of lymphangiography (lymphography). In this procedure, a contrast medium is injected, and the lymphatic vessels are examined by means of X rays.

The etiologic factors associated with lymphatic obstruction may either be congenital or have external causes. Milroy's disease is a hereditary lymphedema characterized by chronic obstructions. The obstruction of lymphatic vessels may also be caused by the presence of tumor cells or the infiltration of parasites. For example, elephantiasis is caused by an infestation of a parasitic worm that obstructs the flow of fluid. The affected limb or region of the body may swell to an astounding degree.

The treatment of most of these disorders is essentially symptomatic. An obstruction may be treated or removed. Often, lymphedema may be treated by having the patient sleep with the feet elevated. A low-salt diet or diuretics may be indicated, and a light massage in the direction of lymph flow may also be helpful.

As is true for all tissues in the body, the cells and organs of the lymphatic system may also undergo malignant transformation. Any neoplasm of lymphoid tissue is referred to as a lymphoma. In general, these are malignant. Though lymphomas may be of different forms and involve different types of cells, they are characterized by enlarged lymph nodes (generally in the neck), fever, and weight loss. Among the more common forms of lymphomas are Hodgkin's disease and non-Hodgkin's lymphomas, a mixed collection of malignant solid tumors originating among the secondary lymphoid tissues of the lymph nodes. Hodgkin's disease generally appears first among the cervical or axillary lymph nodes. Its manner of presentation usually allows for early diagnosis and treatment. As a result, the prognosis with early intervention has significantly improved since the 1960's.

Non-Hodgkin's lymphomas often develop in less obvious areas of the lymphatic system, such as the gastrointestinal tract, the central nervous system, and the oral and nasal pharynx. The result is that diagnosis is often delayed until the disease has spread, and therefore the prognosis is less optimistic. More than 80 percent of non-Hodgkin's lymphomas are of B-lymphocyte origin, and they often arise within the follicles of the lymph node. There is some evidence that neoplastic transformation may be related to antigen exposure. In some instances, molecular defects of the cell DNA may result in the neoplastic event. Non-Hodgkin's lymphomas may also be of T-lymphocyte or, less commonly, macrophage origin. Most treatments of lymphomas include both radiation therapy and chemotherapy.

PERSPECTIVE AND PROSPECTS

The first description of the lymphatic system was made by the Italian anatomist Gasparo Aselli in 1622. Aselli observed the lacteals in the intestinal walls of dogs that he had dissected, and he included diagrams of the lacteals in his text *De Lactibus* (1627), the first anatomical medical text with color plates.

The role of the lymphatic system in maintaining the fluid dynamics of the body was understood by the beginning of the twentieth century. Much of this knowledge resulted from the early work of the British physiologist Ernest Henry Starling.

Beginning about 1900, Starling's research centered on the secretion and circulation of lymph. It was known that the lymphatic system as a parallel to blood circulation was found only among the higher vertebrates. This indicated that it had developed relatively late during the course of evolution. There occurred, along with the increasing development of the body's circulatory system as organisms evolved, an increase in the hydrostatic pressure within the system—that is, as the circulatory system became more complex, blood vessels branched into smaller and thinner capillaries. The pressure within those capillaries became higher. Starling pointed out the significance of the hydrostatic pressures within the capillaries: Fluids and dissolved materials leak out of the capillaries into the tissues.

Starling did not believe, however, that protein was able to leak through the capillary walls. In the 1930's, Cecil Drinker demonstrated that protein is a major constituent of dissolved material in lymph and suggested that an important role of the lymphatic system is the return of this protein to the bloodstream. Drinker was unable to prove definitively that the protein in lymph originated with the blood, and it remained for H. S. Mayerson to confirm this point in the 1940's.

Lymphocytes had been observed in the blood as early as the nineteenth century. Their role in the immune process was not readily apparent, however, and various functions were assigned to them. In 1948, Astrid Fagraeus demonstrated that lymphocytes mature into antibody-producing plasma cells. It remained unclear whether this was the sole purpose of these cells.

In 1956, Bruce Glick and Timothy Chang, working with chickens, discovered that an organ called the bursa, found near the cloaca in the region of the tail, was the site of the production of antibody-producing cells. Their discovery, along with those of Robert Good and Jacques Miller some years later, showed that lymphocytes are not all identical; at least two distinct populations exist. It remained for Henry Claman and his coworkers, in 1966, to demonstrate that these two populations of lymphocytes act cooperatively in the production of antibodies.

In 1969, Ivan Roitt called those lymphocytes that mature in the thymus gland T cells. The lymphocytes that mature in the bursa, an organ found only in birds, were called B cells. Since mammals lack the bursa, B cells in these organisms mature within the bone marrow (considered a bursa equivalent). Once the cells are released from the marrow, they migrate into both the lymphatic system and the bloodstream.

—Richard Adler, Ph.D.

See also Angiography; Bacterial infections; Bladder cancer; Blood and blood disorders; Breast cancer; Breast disorders; Burkitt's lymphoma; Cancer; Cervical, ovarian, and uterine cancers; Chemotherapy; Circulation; Colon cancer; DiGeorge syndrome; Edema; Elephantiasis; Epstein-Barr virus; Gallbladder cancer; Histology; Hodgkin's disease; Immune system; Immunology; Immunopathology; Kawasaki disease; Kidney cancer; Liver cancer; Lower extremities; Lung cancer; Lymphadenopathy and lymphoma; Malignancy and metastasis; Mononucleosis; Mouth and throat cancer; Oncology; Prostate cancer; Skin cancer; Sleeping sickness; Splenectomy; Stomach, intestinal, and pancreatic cancers; Systems and organs; Testicular cancer; Tonsillectomy and adenoid removal; Tonsillitis; Tumors; Upper extremities; Vascular medicine; Vascular system.

For Further Information:

Delves, Peter J., et al. *Roitt's Essential Immunology.* 11th ed. Malden, Mass.: Blackwell, 2006. A standard immunology text. Though the lymphatic system is not singled out in any particular section of the book, its role in the immune response is an underlying theme throughout the text.

Dwyer, John M. *The Body at War: The Story of Our Immune System.* 2d ed. London: J. M. Dent, 1993. Provides a good general description of the immune system. The immune function of the lymphatic system, the roles of lymph nodes in the immune response, and the functions of lymphatic cells are described in a basic manner for the nonscientist.

Eales, Lesley-Jane. *Immunology for Life Scientists.* Hoboken, N.J.: John Wiley & Sons, 2003. A highly readable text for the nonspecialist that covers such topics as antigens, hypersensitivity, autoimmunity, reproductive immunity, and immunodeficiency.

Janeway, Charles A., Jr., et al. *Immunobiology: The Immune System in Health and Disease.* 6th ed. New York: Garland Science, 2005. An excellent text that provides a lucid and comprehensive examination of the immune system, covering such topics as immunobiology and innate immunity, the recognition of antigen, the development of mature lymphocyte receptor repertoires, the adaptive immune response, and the evolution of the immune system.

Kindt, Thomas J., Richard A. Goldsby, and Barbara A. Osborne. *Kuby Immunology.* 6th ed. New York: W. H. Freeman, 2007. An excellent textbook on the subject of immunology. The section on the cells and organs of the immune system is well organized and includes the latest information on lymphatic circulation. The immune function of the lymphatic system is the major emphasis.

LYMPHOMA. *See* **LYMPHADENOPATHY AND LYMPHOMA.**

MACULAR DEGENERATION

DISEASE/DISORDER

ANATOMY OR SYSTEM AFFECTED: Eyes

SPECIALTIES AND RELATED FIELDS: Ophthalmology

DEFINITION: A degenerative disease of the central portion of the retina that results primarily in loss of central vision.

CAUSES AND SYMPTOMS

The macula is located in the center of the retina, the light-sensitive tissue at the back of the eye. The retina instantly converts light, or an image, into electrical impulses. The retina then sends these impulses, or nerve signals, to the brain. One of the earliest signs of age-related macular degeneration (ARMD) seen by physicians during a dilated eye examination is deposits of tiny, bright yellow material called drusen, which is harder as a result of aging or softer and larger if associated with ARMD and vision loss. As parts of the eye in the retina and choroid become thinner or lose tissue, central vision and/or peripheral vision is affected, depending on the area of damage. Central vision is needed to see clearly and to perform everyday activities such as reading, writing, driving, and recognizing people and things. Peripheral vision, needed for walking, is much less commonly affected.

There are two forms of ARMD: early and advanced. About 90 percent of cases are early ARMD, although the advanced type affects 7 percent of those seventy-five years or older. Advanced ARMD is further categorized into two distinct types based on their clinical features: dry and wet. The dry form involves thinning of the macular tissues and disturbances in its pigmentation. About 70 percent of patients have the dry form. The remaining 30 percent have the wet form, which can involve bleeding within and beneath the retina, opaque deposits, and eventually scar tissue. The wet form accounts for 90 percent of all cases of legal blindness in macular degeneration patients.

Neither dry nor wet macular degeneration causes pain. The most common early sign of dry macular degeneration is blurring vision that prevents people from seeing details clearly that are in front of them, such as faces or words in a book. In the early stages of wet macular degeneration, straight lines appear wavy or crooked. This is the result of fluid leaking from blood vessels and lifting the macula, distorting vision.

A number of risk factors can affect the initial development of ARMD: age, smoking, genetic predisposition, and ethnicity. Two risk factors have also been studied and suggested in causing a progression of ARMD: nutrition and high blood pressure. Age is the most important risk factor for macular degeneration: The older the patient, the higher the risk. Studies have shown that having a family with a history of macular degeneration raises the risk factor. Because macular degeneration affects most patients later in life, however, it has proven difficult to study cases in successive generations of a family. Heavy smoking, at least a pack of cigarettes a day, can double a person's risk of developing ARMD. The more a person smokes, the higher the risk of macular degeneration. Moreover, the adverse effects of smoking persist, even fifteen to twenty years after quitting. Those with a family history of ARMD are more likely to develop the disease due to a genetic mutation of part of a gene called the complement factor H gene. With a family history of the disease, the risk is greater for developing the wet type than the dry type of ARMD. Studies have shown that non-Hispanic Caucasians have a greater risk of developing ARMD than do African Americans or Hispanics.

Poor dietary habits contribute to ARMD as well. A diet high in saturated fats may clog the vessels leading to the eyes, thus reducing the flow of nutrient-rich blood. Excess fat may deposit itself directly in the membrane behind the retina. In this case, nutrients might not be able to reach the cells that nourish the retina. High blood pressure has also been shown to increase the risk of developing ARMD in the second eye in those having ARMD in one eye.

An effective test to determine if a person has wet macular degeneration is fluorescent angiography. A special dye is injected into a vein in the patient's arm and then flows to the blood vessels in the eye. Photographs are taken of the retina. The dye highlights any problems in the blood vessels and allows the doctor to determine if they can be treated. Annual eye examinations that include dilation of the pupils are also useful in early detection. Early detection is important because a person destined to develop macular degeneration can sometimes be treated before symptoms appear, which may delay or reduce the severity of the disease. Anyone who notices a change in vision should contact an ophthalmologist immediately.

TREATMENT AND THERAPY

New and exciting treatments are in development for ARMD as extensive research is being done. Currently, there is no cure, and no treatment recommendations exist for those with dry type ARMD, the type that is much less threatening to vision. Some treatments, however, can slow the progression of wet type ARMD. Research has shown that stopping smoking is the most effective preventive measure in regard to developing ARMD and slowing its progression.

Antioxidants have proved promising in recent studies which show that they can lower the risk of progression to more advanced ARMD in those who have moderate or advanced disease. In a major clinical trial called the Age-Related Disease Study (AREDS), it was shown that patients with moderate or severe ARMD taking antioxidants vitamin C, vitamin E, and beta carotene plus zinc and copper had a lower risk of progression among both nonsmokers and smokers. Since the group of smokers who took zinc alone had the same lowered risk of progression as those smokers taking antioxidants plus zinc and copper, it was recommended that smokers with ARMD take zinc alone, as some antioxidants have shown to increase the risk of lung cancer and coronary heart disease when used at high doses.

Although no treatments can reverse the actual pathologic process of the disease of wet type ARMD, some treatments used by ophthalmologists are aimed at containing the damaged vessels that cause the loss of vision. They include laser photocoagulation, photodynamic therapy, intravitreous injections, and, as a last resort, macular translocation surgery.

Laser photocoagulation involves using a high-intensity thermal laser to burn off the blood supply to abnormal choroidal membranes. The benefits of this treatment are that it is done in the outpatient setting using only topic anesthetic drops and that it prevents the formation of new abnormal vessels associated with ARMD for two or three years. It is limited, however, to only those patients with well-defined abnormal areas (only about 15 percent of patients with ARMD). It cannot restore lost vision and may actually destroy normal retinal tissue along with the neovascular formation that is targeted.

Photodynamic therapy involves the injection of a dye called verteporfin which, when activated by a photo laser, forms substances that destroy the abnormal newly formed vessels associated with wet type ARMD. Thus, by the use of this dye and laser combination, the normal vessels are protected and the abnormal vessels are destroyed. It has also been shown that this treatment can be repeated safely.

The vascular endothelial growth factor (VEGF) inhibitors are a class of agents that block a factor involved in the disease process of ARMD. VEGF is essential for the formation of the new abnormal vessels that cause the loss of vision and the anatomic destruction associated with ARMD. The VEGF inhibitors block this factor, thereby limiting those destructive effects. Studies involving these agents have shown that a majority of patients showed improvement in their vision and marked anatomic improvement of their retinas.

Macular translocation surgery involves surgically removing the macula from a diseased area and attaching it to a healthier area of the retina. Although currently an experimental therapy and not well studied, it can be used for those patients in which no other treatment options are left. If performed successfully, macular translocation surgery can improve central vision and allow a majority of patients to read. Great risks are associated with this type of treatment, however, including detachment of the retina and the development of double vision. In addition, use of a steroid injection into the vitreous and/or the posterior sub-Tenon's space has shown short-term improvement in vision.

Many visual aids have been developed for patients with ARMD to make the most of their remaining vision, including magnifying glasses, powerful special lenses, and large-print books and reading materials. Voice synthesizers in electronic devices such as calculators, clocks, and phones are also very helpful. Maximizing room lighting by the use of stronger lights, opening windows, and painting walls brighter colors can help patients see better at home.

INFORMATION ON MACULAR DEGENERATION

CAUSES: Unclear; possibly aging, genetic factors, nutrition, smoking, sunlight exposure

SYMPTOMS: Dependent on form; can include blurred or distorted central vision, bleeding within and beneath retina, development of scar tissue, eventual blindness

DURATION: Typically long-term

TREATMENTS: Vision aids (*e.g.*, magnifying glasses, special lenses, electronic systems); laser photocoagulation; surgery; low-level radiation; injection of photosensitive chemicals into bloodstream

PERSPECTIVE AND PROSPECTS

Blindness or low vision affects 3.3 million Americans aged forty and over, or one in twenty-eight, according to the Eye Disease Prevalence Research Group study, sponsored by the National Eye Institute. This figure is projected to reach 5.5 million by the year 2020. The study reports that low vision and blindness increase significantly with age, particularly in people over age sixty-five. People eighty years of age and older currently make up 8 percent of the population but account for 69 percent of blindness. ARMD affects about 15 percent of the U.S. population by age fifty-five and more than 30 percent by age seventy-five. It is the most common cause of legal blindness in people over the age of sixty-five.

Although there is no cure for ARMD, many treatments are available to curtail progression of the disease. As extensive research continues in this area, advances in the diagnosis and treatment of this debilitating condition are anticipated by many in the field of ophthalmology. Currently, the National Eye Institute is studying the possibility of transplanting healthy cells into a diseased retina, evaluating families with a history of ARMD to understand genetic and hereditary factors that may cause the disease , and looking at certain anti-inflammatory treatments for the wet form of ARMD.

—Kenneth Dill, M.D.

See also Aging; Blindness; Blurred vision; Cataracts; Eye infections and disorders; Eye surgery; Eyes; Laser use in surgery; Myopia; Ophthalmology; Smoking; Vision disorders.

FOR FURTHER INFORMATION:

American Macular Degeneration Foundation. http://www.macular.org/. Provides information to clinicians and patients regarding the latest in research regarding ARMD. Offers an award-winning video for helping patients with ARMD cope with this debilitating illness.

D'Amato, Robert, and Joan Snyder. *Macular Degeneration: The Latest Scientific Discoveries and Treatments for Preserving Your Sight.* New York: Walker, 2000. Ophthalmologist and noted researcher D'Amato teams up with macular degeneration patient Snyder to write a reassuring, hopeful, and informative book providing the facts that sufferers need in order to understand the disorder, handle treatment options, and live successfully with low vision.

Kansai, Jack. *Diseases of the Macula.* New York: Elsevier, 2002. A clinical text that covers diseases that primarily affect the macula, such as age-related macular degeneration, together with secondary diseases that might have an indirect effect on macular

function, such as vascular and inflammatory disorders.

Macular Degeneration Foundation. http://www.eyesight.org/. Describes this charitable educational and research foundation dedicated to discovering the cause of and developing cures for macular degeneration.

MayoClinic.com. *Macular Degeneration.* http://www.mayoclinic.com/health/macular-degeneration/DS00284. Provides a comprehensive overview of the risk factors, symptoms, and treatment of ARMD.

Sardegna, Jill, et al. *Encyclopedia of Blindness and Vision Impairment.* 2d ed. New York: Facts On File, 2002. All aspects of vision impairment are covered in five hundred entries, including health and social issues, surgery and medications, adaptive aids, education, and helpful organizations. Twelve appendixes provide myriad resources for research, support, and services.

Sutton, Amy L., ed. *Eye Care Sourcebook: Basic Consumer Health Information About Eye Care and Eye Disorders.* 2d ed. Detroit: Omnigraphics, 2003. A complete guide to eye care that includes such topics as eye anatomy, preventive vision care, refractive disorders and eye diseases, current research and clinical trials, and a list of organizations.

MAGNETIC FIELD THERAPY
TREATMENT

ANATOMY OR SYSTEM AFFECTED: Cells, immune system

SPECIALTIES AND RELATED FIELDS: Alternative medicine

DEFINITION: A practical and inexpensive modality that uses magnets to relieve chronic and acute pain incurred through overuse or trauma.

INDICATIONS AND PROCEDURES

In this treatment method, which is based on physics principles called the Hall effect and Faraday's law, magnetic pads are placed on or near the site of injury or soreness in order to stimulate local circulation by attracting positive and negatively charged ions in the blood and lymph. This biomagnetic attraction of electrolytes utilizes an alternating pattern of polarities that penetrate 5 to 20 centimeters into the body's tissues, depending on field strength (which is normally between 300 and 950 gauss). A common magnet will not produce this effect because only the ions and fluid in vessels that are precisely in line with the north-south poles will be attracted. Many advocates claim that magnetic therapy works faster than diathermies such as ultrasound. A warm tingling sensation is often felt minutes after application because of the increase of microcirculation, which brings more oxygen, nutrients, white blood cells, and antibodies to the damaged tissues and which removes metabolic waste products.

USES AND COMPLICATIONS

Several forms of magnetic field therapy (including pulsed electromagnetic therapy) have been used for years in Japan, Germany, and other countries, and double-blind studies are being conducted in the United States to determine the validity of numerous testimonials. Disorders that are regularly treated with magnetic therapy in other countries include carpal tunnel syndrome, osteoarthritis, tendinitis, bursitis, migraine headaches, and energy problems such as chronic fatigue syndrome and malaise. Magnetic deficiency syndrome is now documented in Japanese medical literature, and many American physicians agree that proper magnetic balance in the tissues is an overlooked ingredient of health.

Magnetic pads come in several sizes and shapes to allow for comfortable attachment to any area of the body, including silver-dollar-sized pads that are one-eighth of an inch thick, for concentrated force, and 5-by-7-inch pads for larger areas such as the back. Magnetic massage balls, mattress pads, pillows, seat cushions, and orthotic insoles are also sold. The magnets are permanently charged and have no harmful side effects, although they are not recommended for pregnant women or patients wearing pacemakers. In 2005 and 2006, some respected medical journals reported positive treatment outcomes for the healing of surgical wounds. Because this result defies conventional medical wisdom, however, the use of magnetic field therapy in mainstream medicine remains controversial.

—Daniel G. Graetzer, Ph.D.;
updated by LeAnna DeAngelo, Ph.D.

See also Alternative medicine; Bursitis; Carpal tunnel syndrome; Chronic fatigue syndrome; Circulation; Fatigue; Migraine headaches; Osteoarthritis; Pain management; Tendon disorders.

FOR FURTHER INFORMATION:

Burroughs, Hugh, and Mark Kastner. *Alternative Healing: The Complete A-Z Guide to Over 160 Different Alternative Therapies*. La Mesa, Calif.: Halcyon, 1996.

Jacobs, Jennifer, ed. *The Encyclopedia of Alternative Medicine: A Complete Family Guide to Complementary Therapies*. Rev. ed. Boston: Journey Edition, 1997.

Null, Gary. *Healing with Magnets*. New York: Carroll & Graf, 2006.

Pelletier, Kenneth. *Best Alternative Medicine*. New York: Simon & Schuster, 2002.

Trivieri, Larry, Jr., and John W. Anderson, eds. *Alternative Medicine: The Definitive Guide*. 2d ed. Berkeley, Calif.: Ten Speed Press, 2002.

Vegari, G. *Magnetic Therapy*. Christchurch, New Zealand: Caxton, 2004.

White, R., K. Cutting, and P. Beldon. "Magnet Therapy: Opening the Debate." *Journal of Wound Care* 15, no. 5 (May, 2006): 208-209.

MAGNETIC RESONANCE IMAGING (MRI)

PROCEDURE

ANATOMY OR SYSTEM AFFECTED: All

SPECIALTIES AND RELATED FIELDS: Biotechnology, nuclear medicine, radiology

DEFINITION: A noninvasive, nonradiological method of obtaining detailed information concerning normal and diseased tissue.

KEY TERMS:

electromagnetic waves: a convenient way of understanding energy as a wave; visible light, X rays, and radiowaves, which have the longest wavelength and lowest energy, are the most familiar examples

Fourier transform: a mathematical method which allows MRI to utilize one radio frequency pulse and thereby examine all wavelengths, as opposed to examining each wavelength individually with a continuous wave

nucleus: the dense, positively charged, central core of an atom, containing its massive protons and neutrons

zeugmatography: a name applied to MRI characterizing the close relationship of nuclear magnetic forces and electromagnetic waves (from the Greek *zeugma,* meaning "to yoke together")

INDICATIONS AND PROCEDURES

In 1901, Wilhelm Conrad Röntgen won the first Nobel Prize in Physics for his discovery of X rays. Twentieth century applications of this radiation have produced medical miracles. Magnetic resonance imaging (MRI), often called nuclear magnetic resonance (NMR or nmr) imaging, differs in fundamental ways from X rays and other imaging methods. It is capable of producing a far richer array of three-dimensional images without the dangers attendant on ionizing radiation or the introduction of radioactive chemicals. MRI allows both safe diagnosis and study in healthy subjects. Furthermore, the method can be used to examine flowing matter, such as in the circulatory system.

The nuclei of hydrogen atoms behave like tiny magnets when they are placed in a magnetic field. When radio waves are superimposed on the magnetic waves, hydrogen atoms can be made to change their alignment with the magnetic field. The time required for the atoms to return to their original orientation, after the radio waves cease, varies with the nature of the tissue in which the hydrogen atoms reside. This combination of natural circumstances together with the marvels of modern electronics have made it possible to obtain detailed images of brain tumors, spinal fluid, and blood vessels.

The discovery, in the mid-1940's, by Edward M. Purcell and Felix Bloch of the basic techniques of nuclear magnetic resonance won for them the 1952 Nobel Prize in Physics. Their innovation changed dramatically the practice of chemistry, biochemistry, and biology. Following new theoretical and practical contributions, diagnostic medicine is participating fully in this revolution.

MRI Scanning

Magnet

Radio-wave source

Scanning plane

Radio-wave detector

This diagnostic imaging technique employs a powerful magnet to generate a magnetic field that is capable of aligning the protons in the body's hydrogen atoms, which are then knocked out of alignment by radio-wave pulses; as the protons realign, they emit radio signals that can be detected and used to create a cross-sectional image of the body.

Both permanent magnets and electromagnets are used, and each has advantages, but the superconducting magnet is rapidly becoming the standard. The essential factors in producing detailed images are constant field strength and a highly uniform field. A transmitter, connected to a radio frequency transmitter-receiver, is used to broadcast the signal and to receive the signal returned from the patient. A short but intense pulse of radio frequency power is required, and its duration is critical to control electronic noise, which obscures the signal required to form the final image. These signals must be processed by complex computer methods to allow the final image to be displayed.

During the 1970's, several innovations were introduced allowing broad application of the MRI technique. Paul Lauterbur demonstrated the generation of spatial maps by rotating the object to obtain a series of projections from which an image can be reconstructed. His method, called nmr zeugmatography, introduced a radically new approach to MRI. By superimposing a magnetic field gradient on the main magnetic field, it is possible to make the resonance frequency a function of the spatial origin of the signal. Later, Richard R. Ernst built on his earlier introduction of Fourier-transform NMR to develop methods of "two-dimensional nmr." Such techniques provide detailed information concerning the local structure of large molecules of biological importance. He was awarded the 1991 Nobel Prize in Chemistry because this same method laid the groundwork for the clinical use of MRI. Methods are now available for the creation of three- and four-dimensional MRI, which are important in protein studies and which will pave the way for future applications in nonchemical research.

USES AND COMPLICATIONS

MRI has been used in the evaluation of a wide variety of medical situations. The earliest uses involved the brain and the spinal cord, where it is absolutely necessary to avoid high-energy radiation or radioactivity. Since MRI is capable of providing excellent soft-tissue images and of penetrating bony and air-filled structures, it is also well suited to examination of the chest and abdomen. In these applications, it was first necessary to overcome problems associated with motion. A further important modification, the flow imaging technique, allows the use of MRI in studies of the vascular system and has led to magnetic resonance angiography. This latter approach has clear advantages over the invasive X-ray procedure. Additional modifications allow

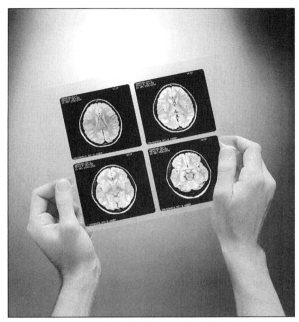

MRI scans of the head. (Digital Stock)

the direct study of tissues of various living organisms under physiological conditions.

Despite the broad applicability of MRI, there are limitations. Patients on life-support systems or with unstable physiological conditions must be evaluated with other imaging techniques. The presence of a magnetic metal apparatus in the body is another limitation. There have also been discussions concerning effects that might be related to the electrical currents induced by magnetic gradient fields.

—K. Thomas Finley, Ph.D.

See also Computed tomography (CT) scanning; Imaging and radiology; Neuroimaging; Noninvasive tests; Nuclear medicine; Positron emission tomography (PET) scanning; Radiopharmaceuticals; Ultrasonography.

FOR FURTHER INFORMATION:

Bongard, Frederick, and Darryl Y. Sue, eds. *Current Critical Care Diagnosis and Treatment.* 2d ed. New York: Lange Medical Books/McGraw-Hill, 2002. A medical text that combines medical and surgical perspectives with diagnostic and treatment knowledge. Covers forty topics in critical care basics, medical critical care, and essentials of surgical intensive care and includes information on imaging procedures.

Bushong, Stewart C. *Magnetic Resonance Imaging: Physical and Biological Principles.* 3d ed. St. Louis: Mosby, 2003. An introductory text that describes the fundamentals of electricity and magnetism, explains how the MRI system works, and reviews the latest imaging techniques.

Buxton, Richard B. *An Introduction to Functional Magnetic Resonance Imaging: Principles and Techniques.* New York: Cambridge University Press, 2002. Designed for the medical professional, this guide covers all aspects of magnetic resonance imaging.

Cahill, Donald R., Matthew J. Orland, and Gary M. Miller. *Atlas of Human Cross-Sectional Anatomy: With CT and MR Images.* 3d ed. New York: Wiley-Liss, 1999. Discusses such topics as X-ray computed tomography and magnetic resonance imaging. Includes bibliographical references and an index.

Griffith, H. Winter. *Complete Guide to Symptoms, Illness, and Surgery.* Revised and updated by Stephen Moore and Kenneth Yoder. Rev. 4th ed. New York: Perigee, 2000. Covers more than five hundred diseases and disorders and includes information about causes and risk factors, preventive techniques, and diagnostic tests such as the MRI.

Pagana, Kathleen Deska, and Timothy J. Pagana. *Mosby's Diagnostic and Laboratory Test Reference.* 7th ed. St. Louis: Elsevier Mosby, 2005. A clinical handbook that gives alphabetically organized laboratory and diagnostic tests for easy reference. Each listing includes such things as alternate or abbreviated test names, type of test, normal findings, possible critical values, test explanation and related physiology, and potential complications.

Smith, Michael B., K. Kirk Shung, and Timothy J. Mosher. "Magnetic Resonance Imaging." In *Principles of Medical Imaging,* edited by Shung, Smith, and Benjamin M. W. Tsui. San Diego, Calif.: Academic Press, 1992. A chapter in a text devoted to biophysics and diagnostic imaging. Includes bibliographical references and an index.

MALABSORPTION

DISEASE/DISORDER

ANATOMY OR SYSTEM AFFECTED: Gallbladder, gastrointestinal system, intestines, liver, pancreas, stomach

SPECIALTIES AND RELATED FIELDS: Biochemistry, biotechnology, family medicine, gastroenterology, genetics, neonatology, nutrition, pediatrics

DEFINITION: The impaired absorption of nutrients from food into the bloodstream.

CAUSES AND SYMPTOMS

The nutritive components of food—carbohydrates, protein, fats, vitamins, and minerals—must be digested in the gastrointestinal tract and absorbed into the circulatory system to be of use to the body. Malabsorption of these nutrients is caused by specific defects in any one of the many separate processes involved in the digestion and absorption of food. It is also the result of general impairment of the structure or function of the gastrointestinal tract.

Malabsorption leads to poor growth when it affects the uptake of any essential nutrient, which is one that must be obtained from the diet. It may cause diarrhea if one of the more abundant constituents of food is not absorbed; carbohydrate malabsorption will usually lead to a watery diarrhea, while protein and fat malabsorption will cause a foul-smelling diarrhea that is dark or whitish, respectively. Diarrhea itself may reduce the absorption of nutrients.

Cystic fibrosis is one of the most common causes of malabsorption in children. The mucus accompanying this disease is secreted into the gastrointestinal tract; it is largely indigestible and can obstruct the passage of nutrients.

TREATMENT AND THERAPY

Treatment for malabsorption depends entirely on its cause. In the case of bacterial infections that affect intestinal function, treatment with appropriate antibiotics will return this function to normal. In celiac sprue, an intolerance to the gluten found in wheat and other grains that alters the absorptive surface of the intestines, the removal of gluten from the diet restores normal activity. Some specific defects can be cured by the elimination or replacement of the dietary constituent that is not well digested or absorbed. In other cases, no curative treatment is known, as with cystic fibrosis.

PERSPECTIVE AND PROSPECTS

In 1825, William Beaumont, a U.S. Army surgeon, was the first to study human digestion in the stomach. Since then, the processes of digestion and absorption have become well understood, as have many of the causes of acquired and inherited malabsorption. Effective treatment has been developed in all but the most intractable cases. It is hoped that progress in understanding the genetic basis for inherited malabsorption will lead to earlier and definitive identification of affected individuals and eventually to suitable therapies.

—*James L. Robinson, Ph.D.*

INFORMATION ON MALABSORPTION

CAUSES: Cystic fibrosis, infection, physiological defects
SYMPTOMS: Diarrhea, poor growth
DURATION: Ranges from acute to chronic
TREATMENTS: Depends on form; may include antibiotics, dietary changes

---

See also Allergies; Bariatric surgery; Celiac sprue; Cystic fibrosis; Diarrhea and dysentery; Digestion; Gastroenterology; Gastroenterology, pediatric; Gastrointestinal system; Malnutrition; Nutrition.

FOR FURTHER INFORMATION:

Bonci, Leslie. *American Dietetic Association Guide to Better Digestion.* New York: Wiley, 2003.

Christian, Janet L., and Janet L. Greger. *Nutrition for Living.* 4th ed. Redwood City, Calif.: Benjamin/Cummings, 1994.

Jackson, Gordon, and Philip Whitfield. *Digestion: Fueling the System.* New York: Torstar Books, 1984.

Janowitz, Henry D. *Indigestion: Living Better with Upper Intestinal Problems.* New York: Oxford University Press, 1992.

Mayo Clinic. *Mayo Clinic on Digestive Health: Enjoy Better Digestion with Answers to More than Twelve Common Conditions.* 2d ed. Rochester, Minn.: Author, 2004.

Peikin, Steven R. *Gastrointestinal Health.* Rev. ed. New York: HarperCollins, 1999.

Sharon, Michael. *Complete Nutrition: How to Live in Total Health.* London: Prion, 2001.

MALARIA

DISEASE/DISORDER

ALSO KNOWN AS: Paludism

ANATOMY OR SYSTEM AFFECTED: Blood, immune system, liver, spleen

SPECIALTIES AND RELATED FIELDS: Biochemistry, immunology, internal medicine, pathology, public health

DEFINITION: One of the world's most serious and potentially fatal diseases, malaria is the result of a parasite transmitted into the bloodstream by mosquito bites. It is most common in subtropical zones, especially in Africa, Asia, and Latin America.

KEY TERMS:

Anopheles: the genus of mosquitoes that, by depositing infected saliva into the blood of humans, serves as a vector for transmission of the parasite that causes malaria

merozoites: products of a multistage reproductive process in the malarial parasite's life span; released into the bloodstream, where they destroy red blood cells

Plasmodium falciparum: one of several parasites that cause malarial symptoms; the species that is most dangerous, and lethal, for humans

---

INFORMATION ON MALARIA

CAUSES: Transmission of parasitic infection via mosquitoes

SYMPTOMS: Recurrent bouts of severe fever, chills, sweating, vomiting; damage to kidneys, blood, brain, and liver

DURATION: Acute to long-term

TREATMENTS: Drug therapy (chloroquine, mefloquine)

CAUSES AND SYMPTOMS

Malaria in humans is caused by transfer into the bloodstream, through the saliva of the *Anopheles* mosquito, of the protozoan (single-cell) *Plasmodium* parasite. There are several different strains of the malaria parasite, all belonging to the phylum Sporozoa, a classification connected with the importance of spores in the organism's reproductive cycle. Serious and potentially lethal malarial infections in humans are primarily associated with *P. falciparum*. Other *Plasmodium* parasites that can produce infection are *P. vivax* (formerly present in temperate climate zones but now found only in the subtropics), *P. malariae* (also only subtropical), and *P. ovale* (quite rare, and mainly limited to West Africa). Other *Plasmodium* parasites infect only non-human primates (*P. knowlesi* and *P. cynomolgi*, for example), only rodents (four different species), or only birds (*P. cathemerium* and *P. gallinaceum*). The latter two species have been used widely in experimental testing of antimalarial vaccines.

It is important to note that only one mosquito genus, *Anopheles*, and only the female *Anopheles* mosquito, serves the vector function in transmitting malaria. The explanation of the female's role is surprisingly simple: Only the female *Anopheles* nourishes itself (usually in the night hours) by piercing the skin of its victim and sucking small quantities of blood. The male of the species feeds mainly on fruit juices.

In the most common scenario, the mosquito ingests the *Plasmodium* parasite when it sucks the blood of an already infected human. This phase is followed by several others—all connected with the reproductive processes of the same organism (both sexual and asexual)—until subsequent generations of the parasite are passed on by the mosquito to another human host, who then becomes infected. The protozoan's first, sexual stage of reproduction occurs when male gametes emit flagella that seek out and join their female counterpart,

producing a fertilized zygote. Once lodged in the gut tissue of the mosquito in the form of an oocyst, a further, asexual stage of reproduction occurs through what is called sporogony: the release from the oocyst of myriad spores. They spread rapidly throughout the body of the mosquito. Many enter the insect host's salivary glands, from which they are transferred into the blood of the next human bitten by the mosquito. It is the further development of the spores in the human organism that produces the disease symptoms associate with malaria.

Once transmitted into the human host through the mosquito saliva, the parasite spores flow quickly through the blood, entering the liver. Their next transformation occurs once they lodge themselves in the cells of the liver, becoming what are called hepatic trophozoites. As they feed off of the liver cells, the trophozoites grow and burst open. This process of asexual multiplication in the liver is referred to as hepatic schozogony. At that stage, the parasite has multiplied many hundreds of times, producing the actual agent of malarial disease, merozoites. If the parasite is *P. vivax*, then this phase may not occur immediately, as a result of a state of dormancy in the parasitic trophozoites. In this case, months or even years can pass before the merozoites are released. Even then, the delayed release is still not final. This explains why some malaria-infected individuals experience a cyclical disappearance of symptoms, followed some time later by a resurgence of the latent disease.

When released from the trophozoites, the merozoites quickly invade the red blood cells of the host. The damage that they inflict leads to anemic reactions as the number of healthy blood cells in the organism decreases. It is not only the liver that is affected; the disease can also spread to the spleen.

Once the effects of malaria begin to take hold in the blood and various organs of the body, certain symptoms will appear. There is an onset of fever, probably caused by the release of a pyrogen (a fever-inducing agent) by the white blood cells reacting to the diseased situation of red blood cells that have been attacked by the malaria parasite. Since this release of pyrogens may follow an irregular pattern, fever can come and go, seemingly sporadically. Meanwhile, as the number of parasitized red blood cells increases, infected red blood cells begin to attach themselves to the inside tissue of capillaries of the internal organs. The effect is blockage of the necessary free flow of blood. If pressure builds because of this blockage, then blood vessels themselves may burst. Such internal hemorrhages allow the directionless dispersion of infected blood within the body, increasing the anemic symptoms that are characteristic of malaria. Perhaps the most dramatic sign of blocked blood vessels occurs if and when the parasitized cells affect the blood flow to the brain. In such cases, convulsions occur, eventually leading to coma.

TREATMENT AND THERAPY

Long before researchers were able to explain the causes of malaria, treatment of its symptoms, primarily manifested in spells of fever, involved giving the patient doses of quinine. As knowledge of the disease increased, different forms of treatment evolved. Such developments occurred not only as new discoveries emerged; they also became necessary as the malaria parasite itself evolved genetically, in effect developing its own immunity to quinine-based treatment.

Several compounds were developed in the later decades of the twentieth century to complement or, more recently, to replace completely dependence on quinine.

Depending on the *Plasmodium* species coming into contact with it, the alkaloid quinine could kill the parasitical organism at key stages in its reproductive activity. Sometimes, however, toxic side effects accompanied the use of quinine in malaria cases. These negative effects eventually sparked research aimed at producing

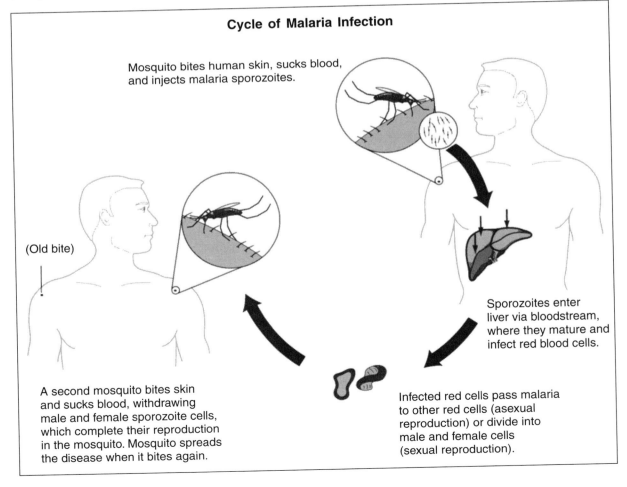

Cycle of Malaria Infection

Mosquito bites human skin, sucks blood, and injects malaria sporozoites.

(Old bite)

A second mosquito bites skin and sucks blood, withdrawing male and female sporozoite cells, which complete their reproduction in the mosquito. Mosquito spreads the disease when it bites again.

Sporozoites enter liver via bloodstream, where they mature and infect red blood cells.

Infected red cells pass malaria to other red cells (asexual reproduction) or divide into male and female cells (sexual reproduction).

synthetic drugs that could be as effective as quinine in preventing malaria, even though they might not be as effective in treating the disease once contracted. The earliest synthetic antimalarials, introduced between 1926 and the early 1950's, included pamaquine, the first synthetic; mepacrine; and chloroquine and primaquine, two well-known drugs from the mid-1940's through the 1950's. These synthetic agents intervened to stop reproduction of the malaria parasite at different points in its life span. Depending on which preventive drug was taken, treatment might have to begin well before expected exposure, during the period of exposure, or for a certain period after being present in a malaria-infected area. Several generations of antimalarial drugs are on the market, but such progress in pharmaceutical options has not effectively resolved the problem of endemic malaria in regions of the world where those most in need lack either public health information programs or the financial means to obtain necessary drugs.

Research involving vaccination to protect against malarial infection has tended to follow one of two main approaches: vaccines to combat the diffusion of spores directly, and vaccines to block one or several stages of in the parasite's life cycle. Some vaccines have been developed by extracting spores from the blood of infected patients and using methods such as radiation to reduce their potency. Injection of these weakened agents into the blood can induce formation of antibodies that are able to fight invasive spores coming from an outside source (mosquito saliva) into a potential host organism. Commercial production of such vaccines, however, would require finding an economically viable way of obtaining and treating large quantities of *Plasmodium* spores, not only from *P. falciparum* but also from other malaria parasites that are less deadly but an important threat to large numbers of people around the world. For this reason, researchers have tended to concentrate more on isolating antigens that the body produces naturally to fight invasive spores and merozoites, analyzing them, and attempting to use biotechnology to produce effective synthetic antigens.

Observation over a long period of time has provided statistical evidence that, in a number of subtropical areas where malaria is endemic, fatalities from the disease are more frequent among children than among adults. The reason for this is linked to the adult population's prior exposure to one or more nonlethal malarial infections. In essence, the adult body's production of natural antigens seems to neutralize the effects of blood cells that have become carriers. If they remain in the bloodstream, these antigens reduce the susceptibility to what, in children, takes the form of a sudden invasion of infected and (for the body's immune system) unrecognizable blood cells transmitted through *Anopheles* mosquito bites.

There is, therefore, an entire field of malaria research dealing with the body's own immune responses. Where malaria is concerned, researchers pay particular attention not only to the challenge of understanding how immunity can build in populations living in endemic zones but also to the possibility of increasing the efficiency of certain body organs that naturally affect the bloodstream in ways that can impede the spread of the parasite's damage. Attention has focused, for example, on the internal functions of the spleen. The spleen can prevent the progress of intravascular pathogens in general by reducing the flow of infected red blood cells to other organs and isolating them in a chemical state that renders them less directly dangerous to the body. This capacity is called splenic filtration. Although research has not yet identified an effective way to use externally applied medications to enhance this facet of the spleen's natural defense system, it is agreed that here there is a serious prospect for another area of treatment to complement, if not replace, preventive drugs and synthetic antigens.

Once it was clear that malaria was transmitted by mosquitoes, the most logical tactic to prevent spread of the disease involved campaigns to eradicate, or at least diminish the life chances of, *Anopheles*. Thus, drainage of swamp areas (a costly but effective measure where possible), public health measures to guard against insalubrious concentrations of stagnant water, and insecticide spraying have been practiced throughout the world to combat *Anopheles*. During World War II and until the late 1950's, DDT was the insecticide of choice. When the harmful side effects of DDT for humans and the environment became apparent, legislation in most but not all countries banned the chemical. Research has since aimed at, but not fully succeeded in, developing safer insecticides that can approach DDT's levels of efficiency.

PERSPECTIVE AND PROSPECTS

Research in the field of malarial disease and its biological origins advanced rather slowly, with most major advances occurring fairly late in the nineteenth century. It was in 1897 that a surgeon in the British Indian army, Sir Ronald Ross, following British tropical disease expert Sir Patrick Manson's suggestions, announced his discovery that malaria was transmitted to humans by mosquitoes. There had been earlier theories concerning the role of mosquitoes, some going back as far as the early eighteenth century in Italy (where the term "malaria," meaning "bad air," had originated). It took the work of a French military doctor in Algeria, Alphonse Laveran, to show, under a microscope, the ongoing activity of parasites in the blood of malaria patients. Laveran also did postmortem studies of malaria victims' blood and organs and found a dark pigment composed mainly of iron which came from the parasites' apparent digestion and waste disposal of vital hemoglobin in the red blood cells. He became the first to posit that malaria was a disease of red blood cells and that it was caused by an invasion of parasites.

From there, it was a question of finding how the parasites entered the human bloodstream. This was the result of Ross's observation in India of a particular variety of mosquito larvae (later identified as the small brown *Anopheles*, distinct from *Culex* varieties commonly observed in the daytime) collected from stagnant waters in the region. When Ross followed Manson's suggestion that mosquitoes hatched from these larvae should be induced to feed from a known malaria patient, he found that only a few insects survived the next few days. When these were dissected, he found oocysts embedded on the wall of the mosquitoes' gut. Microscopic analysis showed that they contained the same dark pigment that Laveran had found in the blood of malaria victims in Algeria.

Both Ross (in 1902) and Laveran (in 1907) received Nobel Prizes in recognition of their work, Ross in medicine and Laveran in physiology or medicine. Other contributors, notably the Italian Giovanni Batista Grassi, carried on significant work in the same first decade of the twentieth century that paralleled (or, according to Grassi, may have been accomplished before) Ross's studies. The most important suggestion by Grassi—which was correct but which took much more work to prove in the laboratory—was that there must be significant transformations, in fact multiple stages of reproduction, between the sporozoite phase of dissemination of the parasite via mosquito saliva and the merozoite phase, when the actual attacking parasite can destroy red blood cells in the human host. Later researchers finally provided, in 1934, convincing evidence that there was a sequence of sexual and asexual phases of reproduction (the later labeled schizogony) in the life cycle of the *Plasmodium* parasite.

Over the years, other researchers helped broaden the understanding of malaria, its causes, and treatment. Despite the obvious costs paid during the first half of the twentieth century involving debilitation and loss of human lives in areas where malaria was endemic, truly major breakthroughs occurred only during the extraordinary conditions created by World War II. The fact that large numbers of troops were sent to areas in East, South, and Southeast Asia as well as Africa meant that the danger of widespread malarial infection could hamper strategic operations. Distribution of all forms of preventive equipment, including both mosquito nets and insect repellents, was destined to become standard procedure in tropical zones. Doses of quinine were also part of each soldier's medical supply packet.

—*Byron D. Cannon, Ph.D.*

See also Bites and stings; Centers for Disease Control and Prevention (CDC); Epidemiology; Fever; Insect-borne diseases; Parasitic diseases; Protozoan diseases; Tropical medicine; Zoonoses.

FOR FURTHER INFORMATION:

Farmer, Paul. *Infections and Inequality*. Berkeley: University of California Press, 1999. This book surveys the past history of, and future prospects for, attempts to address the imbalance between malarial (and other disease) risk factors characteristic of developed and less developed tropical regions of the world.

Honigsbaum, Mark. *The Fever Trail: In Search of the Cure for Malaria*. New York: Farrar, Straus and Giroux, 2002. A popular science book that chronicles the history of malaria and its effect on the world.

Malaria Foundation International (MFI). http://www.malaria.org/. A group that funds global outreach projects designed to fight malaria and raises public awareness and provides education about the disease.

Rocco, Flammetta. *The Miraculous Fever-Tree: Malaria and the Quest for a Cure That Changed the World*. New York: HarperCollins, 2003. A historical view of scientific advances in the treatment of malaria since the centuries-old use of bark from the cinchona tree.

_____. "Corrections and Clarification: The Global Spread of Malaria in a Future, Warmer World." *Science* 289 (September, 2000): 2283-2284. This graphically illustrated article attempts to predict which areas of the globe now vulnerable to malarial infections may not be vulnerable by 2050, and, conversely, which areas now free of the disease may become malaria zones.

MALIGNANCY AND METASTASIS
DISEASE/DISORDER

ANATOMY OR SYSTEM AFFECTED: All

SPECIALTIES AND RELATED FIELDS: Internal medicine, oncology, pathology, plastic surgery

DEFINITION: "Malignancy" is the uncontrolled growth of tumor cells that invade and compress surrounding tissues and break through the skin or barriers within the body; "metastasis" describes the tendency of malignant cells to break loose from their tumor of origin to travel to other locations within the body.

KEY TERMS:

benign tumors: tumors that grow relatively slowly, do not interfere with normal body functions, and do not metastasize

carcinogen: a natural or artificial substance inducing the transformation of cells toward the malignant state

chemotherapy: the use of chemicals to kill or inhibit the growth of cancer cells

multistep progression: the typical pathway of induction of cancer, beginning with an initial alteration to a gene and progressing to the fully malignant state

oncogene: a gene directly or indirectly inducing the transformation of cells from the normal to the malignant state; most oncogenes have normal counterparts in body cells

retrovirus: a virus infecting mammalian and other cells that sometimes carries and introduces oncogenes into host cells

transfection: a technique used to introduce genes into cells by exposing the cells to fragmented deoxyribonucleic acid (DNA) under conditions that promote the uptake and incorporation of DNA

tumor suppressor gene: a gene that, in its normal form, inhibits cell division

CAUSES AND SYMPTOMS

Cancer cells are characterized by two primary features. One of these is uncontrolled cell division: Cells enter an unregulated, rapid growth phase by losing the controls that normally limit division rates to the amount required for normal growth and maintenance of body tissues. The second feature is metastasis, in which tumor cells lose the connections that normally hold them in place in body tissues, break loose, and spread from their original sites to lodge and grow in other body locations. Tumor cells with these characteristics are described as malignant.

The detrimental effects of solid malignant tumors result from the interference of rapidly growing masses of cancer cells with the activities of normal tissues and organs, or from the loss of vital functions because of the conversion of cells with essential functions to nonfunctional forms. Some malignant tumors of glandular tissue upset bodily functions by producing and secreting excessive quantities of hormones.

Solid malignant tumors, as they grow, compress surrounding normal tissues; they destroy normal structures by cutting off blood supplies and interrupting nerve function. They may also break through barriers that separate major body regions, such as internal membranes and epithelia or the gut wall. They may also break through the skin. Such breakthroughs cause internal or external bleeding and infection, and they destroy the organization and separation of body regions necessary for normal function. Both compression and breakthroughs can cause pain that, in advanced cases, may become extreme.

Malignant tumors of blood tissues involve cell lines that normally divide to supply the body's requirements for red and white blood cells. Cancer in these cell lines crowds the bloodstream with immature, nonfunctional cells that are unable to accomplish required activities, such as the delivery of oxygen to tissues or the activation of the immune response.

When the total mass of actively growing and dividing malignant cells becomes large, their demands for nutrients may deprive normal cells, tissues, and organs of their needed supplies, leading to generally impaired functions, fatigue, weakness, and weight loss.

Not all unregulated tissue growths are malignant. Some tumors, such as common skin warts, are benign—they do not usually interfere with normal body functions. They grow relatively slowly and do not metastasize. Often, benign tumors are surrounded by a closed capsule of connective tissue that prevents or retards expansion and breakup. Some initially benign tumors, however, including even common skin warts, may change to malignant forms.

Individual cells of a malignant tumor exhibit differences from normal cells in activity, biochemistry, physiology, and structure. First and foremost is the characteristic of uncontrolled division. Cancer cells typically move through the division cycle much more rapidly than normal cells. The rapid division is accompanied by biochemical changes characteristic of dividing cells such as high metabolic rates; increases in the rate of transport of substances across the plasma membrane; increases in protein phosphorylation; raised cytoplasmic concentrations of sodium, potassium, and calcium ions; and an elevated pH. Often chromosomal abnormalities are present, including extra or missing chromosomes, exchanges of segments between chromosomes, and breakage.

Cancer cells also typically fail to develop all the characteristics and structures of fully mature cells of their type. They may also lose mature characteristics if these were attained before conversion to the malignant state. Frequently, loss of mature characteristics involves disorganization or disappearance of the cytoskeleton. Alterations are also noted in the structure and density of surface carbohydrate groups. Cancer cells lose tight attachments to their neighbors or to supportive extracellular materials such as collagen; some cancer cells secrete enzymes that break cell connections and destroy elements of the extracellular material, aiding their movement into and through surrounding tissues. If removed from the body and placed in test-tube cultures, most cancer cells have the capacity to divide indefinitely. In contrast, most normal body cells placed in a culture medium eventually stop dividing.

The conversion of normal cells to malignant types usually involves multiple causes inducing a series of changes that occur in stages over a considerable length of time. This characteristic is known as the multistep progression of cancer. In most cases, the complete sequence of steps leading from an initiating alteration to full malignancy is unknown.

The initial event in a multistep progression usually involves the alteration of a gene from a normal to an aberrant form known as an oncogene. The gene involved is typically one that regulates cell growth and division or that takes part in biochemical sequences with this effect. The alteration may involve substitutions or the loss of DNA sequences, the movement of the gene to a new location in the chromosomes, or the movement of another gene or its controlling elements to the vicinity of the gene. In some cases, the alteration involves a gene that in normal form suppresses cell division in cells in which it is active. Loss or alteration of function of such genes, known as tumor suppressor genes, can directly or indirectly increase growth and division rates.

An initiating genetic alteration may be induced by a long list of factors, including exposure to radiation or certain chemicals, the insertion of viral DNA into the chromosomes, or the generation of random mutations during the duplication of genetic material. In a few can-

INFORMATION ON MALIGNANCY AND METASTASIS

CAUSES: Genetic factors, carcinogens, retroviruses

SYMPTOMS: Varies; can include loss or impairment of normal bodily functions, interrupted nerve function, internal or external bleeding and infection, pain, swelling, fatigue, weakness, weight loss

DURATION: Often chronic with recurrent episodes

TREATMENTS: Surgery, radiation, chemotherapy

cers, the initiating event involves the insertion of an oncogene into the DNA by an infecting virus that carries the oncogene as a part of its genetic makeup.

In some cases, about 5 percent in humans, an initiating oncogene or faulty tumor suppressor gene is inherited, producing a strong predisposition to the development of malignancy. Among these strongly predisposed cancers are familial retinoblastoma, familial adenomatous polyps of the colon, and multiple endocrine neoplasia, in which tumors develop in the thyroid, adrenal medulla, and parathyroid glands. In addition to the strongly predisposed cancers, some, including breast, ovarian, and colon cancers other than familial adenomatous polyps, show some degree of disposition in family lines—members of these families show a greater tendency to develop the cancer than individuals in other families.

Subsequent steps from the initiating change to the fully malignant state usually include the conversion of additional genes to oncogenic form or the loss of function of tumor suppressor genes. Also important during intermediate stages are further alterations to the initial and succeeding oncogenes that increase their activation. The initial conversion of a normal gene to oncogenic form by its movement to a new location in the chromosomes may be compounded at successive steps, for example, by sequence changes or the multiplication of the oncogene into extra copies. The subsequent steps in progression to the malignant state are driven by many of the sources of change responsible for the initiating step. Because genetic alterations often occur during the duplication and division of the genetic material, an increase in the cell division rate by the initiating change may increase the chance that further alterations leading to full malignancy will occur.

A change advancing the progression toward full malignancy may take place soon after a previous change or only after a long delay. Moreover, further changes may not occur, leaving the progression at an intermediate stage, without the development of full malignancy, for the lifetime of the individual. The avoidance of environmental factors inducing genetic alterations—such as overexposure to radiation sources such as sunlight, X rays, and radon gas and chemicals such as those in cigarette smoke—increases the chance that progressions toward malignancy will remain incomplete.

The last stage in progression to full malignancy is often metastasis. After the loss of normal adhesions to neighboring cells or to elements of the extracellular matrix, the separation and movement of cancer cells from a primary tumor to secondary locations may occur through the development of active motility or from breakage into elements of the circulatory system.

Relatively few of the cells breaking loose from a tumor survive the rigors of passage through the body. Most are destroyed by various factors, including deformation by passage through narrow capillaries and destruction by blood turbulence around the heart valves and vessel junctions. Furthermore, tumor cells often develop changes in their surface groups that permit detection and elimination by the immune system as they move through the body. Unfortunately, the rigors of travel through the body may act as a sort of natural selection for the cells that are most malignant—that is, those most able to resist destruction—and that can grow uncontrollably and spread by metastasis.

Many natural and artificial agents trigger the initial step in the progression to the malignant state or push cells through intermediate stages. Most of these agents, collectively called carcinogens, are chemicals or forms of radiation capable of inducing chemical changes in DNA. Some, however, may initiate or further this progression by modifying ribonucleic acids (RNAs) or proteins, or they may act by increasing the rate of DNA replication and cell division.

TREATMENT AND THERAPY

Cancer is treated most frequently by one or a combination of three primary techniques: surgical removal of tumors, radiation therapy, and chemotherapy. Surgical removal is most effective if the growth has remained localized so that the entire tumor can be detected and removed. Often, surgery is combined with radiation or chemotherapy in an attempt to eliminate malignant cells that have broken loose from a primary tumor and

lodged in other parts of the body. Surgical removal followed by chemotherapy is presently the most effective treatment for most forms of cancer, especially if the tumor is detected and removed before extensive metastasis has taken place. Most responsive to surgical treatments have been skin cancers, many of which are easily detected and remain localized and accessible.

Radiation therapy may be directed toward the destruction of a tumor in a specific body location. Alternatively, it may be used in whole-body exposure to kill cancer cells that have metastasized and lodged in many body regions. In either case, the method takes advantage of the destructive effects of radiation on DNA, particularly during periods when the DNA is under duplication. Because cancer cells undergo replication at higher rates than most other body cells, the technique is more selective for tumors than for normal tissues. The selection is only partial, however, so that body cells that divide rapidly, such as those of the blood, hair follicles, and intestinal lining, are also affected. As a consequence, radiation therapy often has side effects ranging from unpleasant to serious, including hair loss, nausea and vomiting, anemia, and suppression of the immune system. Because radiation is mutagenic, radiation therapy carries the additional disadvantage of being carcinogenic—the treatment, while effective in the destruction or inhibition of a malignant growth, may also initiate new cancers or push cells through intermediate stages in progression toward malignancy.

When possible, radiation is directed only toward the body regions containing a tumor in order to minimize the destruction of normal tissues. This may be accomplished by focusing a radiation source on the tumor or by shielding body regions outside the tumor with a radiation barrier such as a lead sheet.

Chemotherapy involves the use of chemicals that retard cell division or kill tumor cells more readily than normal body cells. Most of the chemicals used in chemotherapy have been discovered by routine screening of substances for their effects on cancer cells in cultures and test animals. Several hundred thousand chemicals were tested in the screening effort that produced the thirty or so chemotherapeutic agents available for cancer treatment.

Many of the chemicals most effective in cancer chemotherapy alter the chemical structure of DNA, produce breaks in DNA molecules, slow or stop DNA duplication, or interfere with the natural systems repairing chemical lesions in DNA. The effects inhibit cell division or interfere with cell functions sufficiently to kill the cancer cells. Because DNA is most susceptible to chemical alteration during duplication and cancer cells duplicate their DNA and divide more rapidly than most normal tissue cells, the effects of these chemicals are most pronounced in malignant types. Normal cells, however, are also affected to some extent, particularly those in tissues that divide more rapidly. As a result, chemotherapeutic chemicals can produce essentially the same detrimental side effects as radiation therapy. The side effects of chemotherapy are serious enough to be fatal in 2 to 5 percent of persons treated. Because they alter DNA, many chemotherapeutic agents are carcinogens and carry the additional risk, as with radiation, of inducing the formation of new cancers.

Not all chemicals used in chemotherapy alter DNA. Some act by interfering with cell division or other cell processes rather than directly modifying DNA. Two chemotherapeutic agents often used in cancer treatment, vinblastine and taxol, for example, slow or stop cell division through their ability to interfere with the spindle structure that divides chromosomes. The drugs can slow or stop tumor growth as well as the division of normal cells.

Tumors frequently develop resistance to some of the chemicals used in chemotherapy, so that the treatment gradually becomes less effective. Development of resistance is often associated with random duplication of DNA segments, commonly noted in tumor cells. In some, the random duplication happens to include genes that provide resistance to the chemicals employed in chemotherapy. The genes providing resistance usually encode enzymes that break down the applied chemical or its metabolic derivatives, or transport proteins of the plasma membrane capable of rapidly excreting the chemical from the cell. One gene in particular, the multidrug resistance gene (MDR), is frequently found to be duplicated or highly activated in resistant cells. This gene, which is normally active in cells of the liver, kidney, adrenal glands, and parts of the digestive system, encodes a transport pump that can expel a large number of substances from cells, including many of those used in chemotherapy. Overactivity of the MDR pump can effectively keep chemotherapy drugs below toxic levels in cancer cells. Cells developing resistance are more likely to survive chemotherapy and give rise to malignant cell lines with resistance. The chemotherapeutic agents involved may thus have the unfortunate effect of selecting cells with resistance, thereby ensuring that they will become the dominant types in the tumor.

Success rates with chemotherapy vary from negligible to about 80 percent, depending on the cancer type. For most, success rates do not range above 50 to 60 percent. Some cancer types, including lung, breast, ovarian, and colorectal tumors, respond poorly or not at all to chemotherapy. The overall cure rate for surgery, radiation, and chemotherapy combined, as judged by no recurrence of the cancer for a period of five years, is about 50 percent.

It is hoped that full success in the treatment of cancer will come from the continued study of the genes controlling cell division and the regulatory mechanisms that modify the activity of these genes in the cell cycle. An understanding of the molecular activities of these genes and their modifying controls may bring with it a molecular means to reach specifically into cancer cells and halt their growth and metastasis.

Perspective and Prospects

Indications that malignancy and metastasis might have a basis in altered gene activity began to appear in the nineteenth century. In 1820, a British physician, Sir William Norris, noted that melanoma, a cancer involving pigmented skin cells, was especially prevalent in one family under study. More than forty kinds of cancer, including common types such as cancer of the breast and colon, have since been noticed to occur more frequently in some families than in others. Another indication that cancer has a basis in altered gene activity was the fact that the chromosomes of many tumor cells show abnormalities, such as extra chromosomes, broken chromosomes, or rearrangements of one kind or another. These abnormalities suggested that cancer might be induced by altered genes with activities related to cell division.

These indications were put on a firm basis by research with tumors caused by viruses infecting animal cells, most notably those caused by a group of viruses infecting mammals and other animals, the retroviruses. Many retroviral infections cause little or no damage to their hosts. Some, however, are associated with induction of cancer. (Another type of pathogenic retrovirus is responsible for acquired immunodeficiency syndrome, or AIDS.) The cancer-inducing types among the retroviruses were found to carry genes capable of transforming normal cells to the malignant state. The transforming genes were at first thought to be purely viral in origin, but DNA sequencing and other molecular approaches revealed that the viral oncogenes had normal counterparts among the genes directly or indirectly regulating cell division in cells of the infected host. Among the most productive of the investigators using this approach were J. Michael Bishop and Harold E. Varmus, who received the 1989 Nobel Prize in Physiology or Medicine for their research establishing the relationship between retroviral oncogenes and their normal cellular counterparts.

The discovery of altered host genes in cancer-inducing retroviruses prompted a search for similar genes in nonviral cancers. Much of this work was accomplished by transfection experiments, in which the DNA of cancer cells is extracted and introduced into cultured mouse cells. Frequently, the mouse cells are transformed into types that grow much more rapidly than normal cells. The human oncogene responsible for the transformation is then identified in the altered cells. Many of the oncogenes identified by transfection turned out to be among those already carried by retroviruses, confirming by a different route that these genes are capable of contributing to the transformation of cells to a cancerous state. The transfection experiments also identified some additional oncogenes not previously found in retroviruses.

In spite of impressive advances in treatment, cancer remains among the most dreaded of human diseases. Recognized as a major threat to health since the earliest days of recorded history, cancer still counts as one of the most frequent causes of human fatality. In technically advanced countries, it accounts for about 15 to 20 percent of deaths each year. In a typical year, more persons die from cancer in the United States than the total number of Americans killed in World War II and the Vietnam War combined. Smoking, the most frequent single cause of cancer, is estimated to be responsible for about one-third of these deaths.

—*Stephen L. Wolfe, Ph.D.*

See also Biopsy; Cancer; Carcinogens; Carcinoma; Cytology; Cytopathology; Imaging and radiology; Laboratory tests; Lymphadenopathy and lymphoma; Mammography; Oncology; Pathology; Radiation therapy; Tumor removal; Tumors.

FOR FURTHER INFORMATION:

Alberts, Bruce, et al. *Molecular Biology of the Cell.* 4th ed. New York: Garland, 2002. Describes the development and characteristics of malignance and metastasis. The text is clearly written at the college level and is illustrated by numerous diagrams and photographs.

Dollinger, Malin, et al. *Everyone's Guide to Cancer Therapy.* 4th ed. Kansas City, Mo.: Andrews McMeel, 2002. An excellent source of medical information about cancer, written for the general public. Various cancer sites in the body are described. A helpful glossary of medical terminology is provided.

Eyre, Harmon J., Dianne Partie Lange, and Lois B. Morris. *Informed Decisions: The Complete Book of Cancer Diagnosis, Treatment, and Recovery.* 2d ed. Atlanta: American Cancer Society, 2002. This text from the American Cancer Society is intended for the layperson. It is exemplary in its discussion of cancer.

Lackie, J. M., and J. A. T. Dow, eds. *The Dictionary of Cell and Molecular Biology.* 3d ed. San Diego, Calif.: Academic Press, 1999. Encompasses cytology and molecular biology. Includes bibliographical references.

Lodish, Harvey, et al. *Molecular Cell Biology.* 5th ed. New York: W. H. Freeman, 2004. An excellent textbook written at the college level. Includes an unusually complete discussion of the characteristics and causes of malignancy and metastasis. Many highly illustrative diagrams and photographs are included.

Weinberg, Robert A. "Finding the Anti-Oncogene." *Scientific American* 259 (September, 1988): 44-51. A lucidly written description of tumor suppressor genes and their possible use as a means to inhibit tumor growth. Many innovative and informative illustrations are included with the article.

Wolfe, Stephen L. *Molecular and Cellular Biology.* Belmont, Calif.: Wadsworth, 1993. Chapter 22, "The Cell Cycle, Cell Cycle Regulation, and Cancer," describes the cellular factors and processes regulating the growth and division of both normal and malignant cells. Written at the college level, the book is readable and illustrated with many useful and informative diagrams and photographs.

MALNUTRITION

DISEASE/DISORDER

ANATOMY OR SYSTEM AFFECTED: Gastrointestinal system, intestines, nails, stomach, all bodily systems

SPECIALTIES AND RELATED FIELDS: Gastroenterology, nutrition, pediatrics, public health

DEFINITION: Impaired health caused by an imbalance, either through deficiency or excess, in nutrients.

KEY TERMS:

anemia: a condition in which there is a lower-than-normal concentration of the iron-containing protein in red blood cells, which carry oxygen *famine:* a lack of access to food in a population, the cause of which can be a natural disaster, such as a drought, or a situation created by humans, such as a civil war

kwashiorkor: the condition that results from consuming a diet that is sufficient in energy (kilocalories) but inadequate in protein content

marasmus: the condition that results from consuming a diet that is deficient in both energy and protein

osteoporosis: a bone disorder in which the bone's mineral content is decreased over time, resulting in a weakening of the skeleton and susceptibility to bone fractures

protein energy malnutrition (PEM): a deficient intake of energy (kilocalories) and/or protein, the most common type of undernutrition in developing countries; the two major types of PEM are kwashiorkor and marasmus

undernutrition: continued ill health caused by a long-standing dietary deficiency of the energy (kilocalories) and the nutrients that are required to maintain health and provide protection from disease

CAUSES AND SYMPTOMS

Malnutrition literally means "bad nutrition." It can be used broadly to mean an excess or deficiency of the nutrients that are necessary for good health. In industrialized societies, malnutrition typically represents the excess consumption characterized by a diet containing too much energy (kilocalories), fat, and sodium. Malnutrition is most commonly thought, however, to be undernutrition or deficient intake, the consumption of inadequate amounts of nutrients to promote health or to support growth in children. The most severe form of undernutrition is called protein energy malnutrition, or PEM. It commonly affects children, who require nutrients not only to help maintain the body but also to grow. Two types of PEM occur: kwashiorkor and marasmus.

Kwashiorkor is a condition in which a person consumes adequate energy but not enough protein. It usually is seen in children between one and four who are weaned so that the next baby can be breast-fed. The weaning diet consists of gruels made from starchy foods that do not contain an adequate supply of amino acids, the building blocks of protein. These diets do, however, provide enough energy.

Diets in many developing countries are high in bulk, making it nearly impossible for a child to consume a sufficient volume of foods such as rice and grain to obtain an adequate amount of protein for growth. The

outward signs of kwashiorkor are a potbelly, dry unpigmented skin, coarse reddish hair, and edema in the legs. Edema results from a lack of certain proteins in the blood that help to maintain a normal fluid balance in the body. The potbelly and swollen limbs often are misinterpreted as signs of being "fat" among the developing world cultures. Other signs requiring further medical testing include fat deposits in the liver and decreased production of digestive enzymes. The mental and physical growth of the child are impaired. Children with kwashiorkor are apathetic, listless, and withdrawn. Ironically, these children lose their appetites. They become very susceptible to upper respiratory infection and diarrhea. Children with kwashiorkor also are deficient in vitamins and minerals that are found in protein-rich foods. There are symptoms caused by these specific nutrient deficiencies as well.

Marasmus literally means "to waste away." It is caused by a deficiency of both Calories (kilocalories) and protein in the diet. This is the most severe form of childhood malnutrition. Body fat stores are used up to provide energy, and eventually muscle tissue is broken down for body fuel. Victims appear as skin and bones, gazing with large eyes from a bald head with an aged, gaunt appearance. Once severe muscle wasting occurs, death is imminent. Body temperature is below normal. The immune system does not operate normally, making these children extremely susceptible to respiratory and gastrointestinal infections.

A vicious cycle develops once the child succumbs to infection. Infection increases the body's need for protein, yet the PEM child is so protein deficient that recovery from even minor respiratory infections is prolonged. Pneumonia and measles become fatal diseases for PEM victims. Severe diarrhea compounds the problem. The child is often dehydrated, and any nourishment that might be consumed will not be adequately absorbed.

The long-term prognosis for these PEM children is poor. If the child survives infections and is fed, PEM returns once the child goes home to the same environment that caused it. Children with repeated episodes of kwashiorkor have high mortality rates.

Children with PEM are most likely victims of famine. Typically, these children either were not breast-fed or were breast-fed for only a few months. If a weaning formula is used, it has not been prepared properly; in many cases, it is mixed with unsanitary water or watered down because the parents cannot afford to buy enough to use it at full strength.

It is difficult to distinguish between the cause of kwashiorkor and that of marasmus. One child ingesting the same diet as another may develop kwashiorkor, while the other may develop marasmus. Some scientists think this may be a result of the different ways in which individuals adapt to nutritional deprivation. Others propose that kwashiorkor is caused by eating moldy grains, since it appears only in rainy, tropical areas.

Another type of malnutrition involves a deficiency of vitamins or minerals. Vitamin A is necessary for the maintenance of healthy skin, and even a mild deficiency causes susceptibility to diarrhea and upper respiratory infection. Diarrhea reinforces the vicious cycle of malnutrition, since it prevents nutrients from being absorbed. With a more severe vitamin A deficiency, changes in the eye and, eventually, blindness result. Night blindness is usually the first detectable symptom of vitamin A deficiency. The blood that bathes the eye cannot regenerate the visual pigments needed to see in the dark. Eventually, the tissues of the eye become infected and total blindness results. Vitamin A deficiency, the primary cause of childhood blindness, can result from the lack of either vitamin A or the protein that transports it in the blood. If the deficiency of vitamin A occurs during pregnancy or at birth, the skull does not develop normally and the brain is crowded. An older child deficient in vitamin A will suffer growth impairment.

Diseases resulting from B-vitamin deficiencies are rare. Strict vegetarians, called vegans, who consume no animal products are at risk for vitamin B_{12} deficiency resulting in an anemia in which the red blood cells are large and immature. Too little folate (folic acid) in the diet can cause this same anemia. Beriberi is the deficiency disease of thiamine (vitamin B_1) in which the heart and nervous systems are damaged and muscle wasting occurs. Ariboflavinosis (lack of riboflavin) describes a collection of symptoms such as cracks and redness of the eyes and lips; inflamed, sensitive eyelids; and a purple-red tongue. Pellagra is the deficiency disease of niacin (vitamin B_3). It is characterized by "the Four Ds of pellagra": dermatitis, diarrhea, dementia, and death. Isolated deficiency of a B vitamin is rare, since many B vitamins work in concert. Therefore, a lack of one hinders the function of the rest.

Scurvy is the deficiency disease of vitamin C. Early signs of scurvy are bleeding gums and pinpoint hemorrhages under the skin. As the deficiency becomes more severe, the skin becomes rough, brown, and scaly, eventually resulting in impaired wound healing, soft bones, painful joints, and loose teeth. Finally, hardening of the arteries or massive bleeding results in death.

Rickets is the childhood deficiency disease of vitamin D. Bone formation is impaired, which is reflected in a bowlegged or knock-kneed appearance. In adults, a brittle bone condition called osteomalacia results from vitamin D deficiency.

Malnutrition of minerals is more prevalent in the world, since deficiencies are observed in both industrialized and developing countries. Calcium malnutrition in young children results in stunted growth. Osteoporosis occurs when calcium reserves are drawn upon to supply the other body parts with calcium. This occurs in later adulthood, leaving bones weak and fragile. General loss of stature and fractures of the hip, pelvis, and wrist are common, and a humpback appears. Caucasian and Asian women of small stature are at greatest risk for osteoporosis.

Iron-deficiency anemia is the most common form of malnutrition in developing societies. Lack of consumption of iron-rich foods is common among the poor, especially in women who menstruate. This deficiency, which is characterized by small, pale red blood cells, causes weakness, fatigue, and sensitivity to cold temperatures. Anemia in children can cause reduced ability to learn and impaired ability to think and to concentrate.

Deficiencies of other minerals are less common. Although these deficiencies are usually seen among people in developing nations, they may occur among the

---

INFORMATION ON MALNUTRITION

CAUSES: Limited diet, possibly related to poverty, famine, or war; chronic diarrhea; vitamin and mineral deficiency; iron-deficiency anemia; certain diseases

SYMPTOMS: Varies; may include dry and unpigmented skin, coarse reddish hair, swollen limbs, impaired mental and physical development, apathy, listlessness, increased susceptibility to upper respiratory infection and diarrhea, gaunt appearance, muscle wasting

DURATION: Can be short-term or chronic

TREATMENTS: Refeeding with diet adequate in protein, calories, and other essential nutrients; fluid restoration; vitamin and mineral supplements poor, pregnant women, children, and the elderly in industrialized societies. Severe growth retardation and arrested sexual maturation are characteristics of zinc deficiency. With iodine deficiency, the cells in the thyroid gland enlarge to try to trap as much iodine as possible. This enlargement of the thyroid gland is called simple or endemic goiter. A more severe iodine deficiency results from a lack of iodine that leads to a deficiency of thyroid hormone during pregnancy. The child of a mother with such a deficiency is born with severe mental and/or physical retardation, a condition known as cretinism.

The causes of malnutrition, therefore, can be difficult to isolate, because nutrients work together in the body. In addition, the underlying causes of malnutrition (poverty, famine, and war) often are untreatable.

TREATMENT AND THERAPY

Treatment for PEM involves refeeding with a diet adequate in protein, Calories, and other essential nutrients. Response to treatment is influenced by many factors, such as the person's age, the stage of development in which the deprivation began, the severity of the deficiency, the duration of the deficiency, and the presence of other illnesses, particularly infections. Total recovery is possible only if the underlying cause that led to PEM can be eliminated.

PEM can result from illnesses such as cancer and acquired immunodeficiency syndrome (AIDS). Victims of these diseases cannot consume diets with enough energy and protein to meet their body needs, which are higher than normal because of the illness. Infections also increase the need for many nutrients. The first step in treatment must be to cure the underlying infection. People from cultures in which PEM is prevalent believe that food should not be given to an ill person.

Prevention of PEM is the preferred therapy. In areas with unsafe water supplies and high rates of poverty, women should be encouraged to breast-feed. Education about proper weaning foods provides further defense against PEM. Other preventive efforts involve combining plant proteins into a mixture of high-quality protein, adding nutrients to cereal products, and using genetic engineering to produce grains with a better protein mix. The prevention of underlying causes such as famine and drought may not be feasible.

Prekwashiorkor can be identified by regular plotting of the child's growth. If treatment begins at this stage, patient response is rapid and the prognosis is good. Treatment must begin by correcting the body's fluid

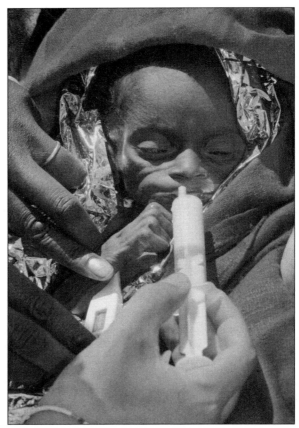

A seven-month-old child suffering from severe malnutrition is helped by a medic in Angola in 2002. (AP/Wide World Photos)

imbalance. Low potassium levels must be corrected. Restoration of fluid is followed by adequate provision of Calories, with gradual additions of protein that the patient can use to repair damaged immune and digestive systems. Treatment must happen rapidly yet allow the digestive system to recover—thus the term "hurry slowly." Once edema is corrected and blood potassium levels are restored, a diluted milk with added sugar can be given. Gradually, vegetable oil is added to increase the intake of Calories. Vitamin and mineral supplements are given. Final diet therapy includes a diet of skim milk and other animal protein sources, coupled with the addition of vegetables and fat.

The residual effects of PEM may be great if malnutrition has come at a critical period in development or has been of long duration. In prolonged cases, damage to growth and the digestive system may be irreversible. Mortality is very high in such cases. Normally, the digestive tract undergoes rapid cell replacement; therefore, this system is one of the first to suffer in PEM. Absorptive surfaces shrink, and digestive enzymes and protein carriers that transport nutrients are lacking.

Another critical factor in the treatment of PEM is the stage of development in which the deprivation occurs. Most PEM victims are children. If nutritional deprivation occurs during pregnancy, the consequence is increased risk of infant death. If the child is carried to term, it is of low birth weight, placing it at high risk for death. Malnutrition during lactation decreases the quantity, but not always the nutritional quality, of milk. Thus, fewer Calories are consumed by the baby. Growth of the child is slowed. These babies are short for their age and continue to be shorter later in life, even if their diet improves.

During the first two years of life, the brain continues to grow. Nutritional deprivation can impair mental development and cognitive function. For only minimal damage to occur, malnutrition must be treated in early stages. Adults experiencing malnutrition are more adaptive to it, since their protein energy needs are not as great. Weight loss, muscle wasting, and impaired immune function occur, and malnourished women stop menstruating.

Successful treatment of a specific nutrient deficiency depends on the duration of the deficiency and the stage in a person's development at which it occurs. Vitamin A is a fat-soluble vitamin that is stored in the body. Thus, oral supplements or injections of vitamin A can provide long-term protection from this deficiency. If vitamin A is given early enough, the deficiency can be rapidly reversed. By the time the child is blind, sight cannot be restored, and frequently the child dies because of other illnesses. Treatment also is dependent upon adequate protein to provide carriers in the blood to transport these vitamins. Treatment of the B-vitamin deficiencies involves oral and intramuscular injections. The crucial step in treatment is to initiate therapy before irreversible damage has occurred. Scurvy (vitamin C deficiency) can be eliminated in five days by administering the amount of vitamin C found in approximately three cups of orange juice. Treatment of vitamin D deficiency in children and adults involves an oral dose of two to twelve times the recommended daily allowance of the vitamin. Halibut and cod liver oils are frequently given as vitamin D supplements.

Successful treatment of a mineral deficiency depends on the timing and duration of the deficiency. Once the bones are fully grown, restoring calcium to optimal levels will not correct short stature. To prevent osteoporosis, bones must have been filled to the maximum with calcium during early adulthood. Estrogen replacement therapy and weight-bearing exercise retard calcium loss in later years and do more than calcium supplements can.

Iron supplementation is necessary to correct iron-deficiency anemia. Iron supplements are routinely prescribed for pregnant women to prevent anemia during pregnancy. Treatment also includes a diet with adequate meat, fish, and poultry to provide not only iron but also a factor that enhances absorption. Iron absorption is also enhanced by vitamin C. Anemias caused by lack of folate and vitamin B_{12} will not respond to iron therapy. These anemias must be treated by adding the appropriate vitamin to the diet.

Zinc supplementation can correct arrested sexual maturation and impaired growth if it is begun in time. In areas where the soil does not contain iodine, iodine is added to salt or injections of iodized oil are given to prevent goiter. Cretinism cannot be cured—only prevented.

In general, malnutrition is caused by a diet of limited variety and quantity. The underlying causes of malnutrition—poverty, famine, and war—are often untreatable. Overall treatment lies in prevention by providing all people with a diet that is adequate in all nutrients, including vitamins, minerals, and Calories. Sharing the world's wealth and ending political strife and greed are essential elements of the struggle to end malnutrition.

PERSPECTIVE AND PROSPECTS

Over the years, the study of malnutrition has shifted to include the excessive intake of nutrients. In developing countries, the primary causes of death are infectious diseases, and undernutrition is a risk factor. In industrialized societies, however, the primary causes of death are chronic diseases, and overnutrition is a risk factor. The excessive consumption of sugar is linked to tooth decay. Also, overnutrition in terms of too much fat and Calories in the diet leads to obesity, high blood pressure, stroke, heart disease, some cancers, liver disease, and one type of diabetes.

Historically, the focus of malnutrition studies was deficiencies in the diet. In the 1930's, classic kwashiorkor was described by Cicely Williams. Not until after World War II was it known that kwashiorkor was caused by a lack of protein in the diet. In 1959, Derrick B. Jelliffe introduced the term "protein-calorie malnutrition" to describe the nutritional disorders of marasmus, marasmic kwashiorkor, and kwashiorkor.

PEM remains the most important public health problem in developing countries. Few cases are seen in Western societies. Historically, the root causes have been urbanization, periods of famine, and the failure to breast-feed or early cessation of breast-feeding. Marasmus is prevalent in urban areas among infants under one year old, while kwashiorkor is prevalent in rural areas during the second year of life.

Deficiencies of specific nutrients have been documented throughout history. Vitamin A deficiency and its cure were documented by Egyptians and Chinese around 1500 B.C.E. In occupied Denmark during World War I, vitamin A deficiency, caused by dairy product deprivation, was common in Danish children. Beriberi, first documented in the Far East, was caused by diets of polished rice that were deficient in thiamine. Pellagra was seen in epidemic proportions in the southern United States, where corn was the staple grain, during World War I.

Zinc deficiency was first reported in the 1960's. The growth and maturation of boys in the Middle East were studied. Their diets were low in zinc and high in substances that prevented zinc absorption. Consequently, the World Health Organization recommended increased zinc intake for populations whose staple is unleavened whole grain bread. Goiter was documented during Julius Caesar's reign. Simply adding iodine to salt has virtually eliminated goiter in the United States.

If classic malnutrition is observed in industrialized societies, it usually is secondary to other diseases, such as AIDS and cancer. Hunger and poverty are problems that contribute to malnutrition; however, the malnutrition that results is less severe than that found in developing countries.

Specific nutrients may be lacking in the diets of the poor. Iron-deficiency anemia is prevalent among the poor, and this anemia may impair learning ability. Other deficiencies may be subclinical, which means that no detectable signs are observed, yet normal nutrient pools in the body are depleted. Homelessness, poverty, and drug or alcohol abuse are the major contributing factors to these conditions. In addition, malnutrition as a result of poverty is exacerbated by lack of nutritional knowledge and/or poor food choices.

—*Wendy L. Stuhldreher, Ph.D., R.D.*

See also Anemia; Anorexia nervosa; Appetite loss; Bariatric surgery; Beriberi; Breast-feeding; Bulimia; Celiac sprue; Cholesterol; Eating disorders; Failure to thrive; Food biochemistry; Fructosemia; Galactosemia; Goiter; Growth; Hirschsprung's disease; Hypercholesterolemia; Hyperlipidemia; Kwashiorkor; Lactose intolerance; Lead poisoning; Malabsorption; Metabolism; Nutrition; Osteoporosis; Scurvy; Supplements; Thyroid disorders; Vitamins and minerals; Weaning; Weight loss and gain; Weight loss medications.

FOR FURTHER INFORMATION:

Barasi, Mary E. *Human Nutrition: A Health Perspective.* 2d ed. New York: Oxford University Press, 2003. A text that emphasizes basic nutrition information and the application of this information to health maintenance and disease prevention.

Christian, Janet L., and Janet L. Greger. *Nutrition for Living.* 4th ed. Redwood City, Calif.: Benjamin/ Cummings, 1994. This introductory textbook of nutrition is easy to understand. It provides brief explanations of various vitamin and mineral deficiencies, as well as of PEM. Photographs showing symptoms are included.

Garrow, J. S., W. P. T. James, and A. Ralph, eds. *Human Nutrition and Dietetics.* 10th ed. New York: Churchill Livingstone, 2000. Several chapters in this book provide information on malnutrition, from PEM to specific nutrient deficiencies. History, causes, symptoms, and treatments of the disorders are covered. An excellent list of references is provided.

Kreutler, Patricia A., and Dorice M. Czajka-Narins. *Nutrition in Perspective.* 2d ed. Englewood Cliffs, N.J.: Prentice Hall, 1987. This textbook provides a chapter on the food supply, including issues for meeting the problem of undernutrition. It also describes the deficiency diseases for vitamins and minerals and PEM in various chapters.

Wardlaw, Gordon M., and Anne M. Smith. *Contemporary Nutrition.* 6th ed. New York: McGraw-Hill, 2006. One chapter of this text covers undernutrition and emphasizes the types of undernutrition and hunger found in the United States.

Whitney, Ellie, and Sharon Rady Rolfes. *Understanding Nutrition.* 10th ed. Belmont, Calif.: Thomson/ Wadsworth, 2005. This is an introductory nutrition textbook. Various chapters have information about the different nutrient deficiencies and malnutrition.

MALPRACTICE

ETHICS

DEFINITION: The failure to care for patients in accordance with professional standards, for which injured patients are allowed to sue for compensation.

KEY TERMS:

damages: compensation awarded to a plaintiff for an injury incurred because of a defendant's action or lack of action

defendant: a person or corporation alleged in a lawsuit to have committed a wrong

liability: responsibility for a wrongdoing

plaintiff: a person or corporation that brings legal action against another person or corporation

tort: an action or the result of an action that is defined by law to be a wrong or injury

CONTROVERSIES SURROUNDING MALPRACTICE LITIGATION

In the United States, few medical topics arouse more anger in physicians, more debate in state legislatures, or more confusion in the public than malpractice. In part, the media encourages this attention when it reports multimillion-dollar jury awards for damages, sensational stories that often make all the parties involved—lawyers, the defendant doctor, the plaintiff patient, and juries—look somehow reprehensible. In part, the rise in malpractice insurance, which has contributed to the increasing cost of medical care, has upset both doctors and the public. Yet inflation and the rare spectacular settlement obscure the value of a system that since the late eighteenth century has given patients legal redress for injury, has helped maintain professional standards of medical care, and has allowed state governments some control over the local health care industry.

As the word's elements imply, "malpractice" simply means the poor execution of duties. The definition bears close examination, however, on one key feature: what "poor" entails. The first recourse of a patient who feels inadequately cared for is to discuss the complaint with the doctor (or dentist, chiropractor, or other health care provider). This measure clears up many complaints, since most are based on simple misunderstandings. A patient receiving no satisfaction from the doctor may file a complaint with the state board of medical examiners, which is each state's official government body, staffed by doctors, that issues medical licenses and disciplines physicians and surgeons. In both cases, the doctor or a panel of peers will decide if the patient's complaint meets the professional standards of "poor." A patient who is not pleased with this decision may bring suit in civil court. No patient, however, can press a lawsuit for malpractice simply because he or she feels wronged. For legal action to have any chance of succeeding, the doctor must have injured the patient because of negligent care. Even then, lawyers for the patient must rely on expert testimony from other doctors to establish that the physician gave the patient poor care. All official avenues of redress therefore depend on the medical profession's own standards.

Four basic standards guide doctors in ethically performing their professional duties, and failure in any one of them may constitute malpractice. First, doctors must inform their patients about treatments for an ailment and receive their explicit consent. The patient must understand the doctor's plan of treatment and any procedure's potential risks and benefits; if a patient cannot understand because of age or mental condition, a guardian must consent, except in some emergency situations. The consent may be verbal unless an invasive technique, such as surgery, is involved, in which case the law requires a signed consent form. Without the patient's consent, a physician performing a medical procedure not only may be subject to a malpractice lawsuit but also can be charged with assault under criminal law. Second, a doctor must treat a patient with reasonable skill, as defined by accepted medical practice. This point is crucial. Doctors do not have to render the best aid possible, or even the best aid of which they are capable; they must only meet professional guidelines for any specific diagnostic, palliative, or corrective measure. Both the key terms in this standard—"reasonable" and "accepted medical practice"—have been notoriously hard to define in court because they vary from region to region and from school of medicine to school of medicine. Rural physicians, for example, cannot be expected to give the level of care available in cities, since cities have more specialists available and support technology; nor are general practitioners expected to have the skill of a specialist, such as a cardiologist. Third, physicians are responsible for what other health care workers under their charge do to patients. If other doctors (such as medical residents), nurses, physical therapists, or medical technicians act on a doctor's orders, that doctor is ultimately responsible for supervising their performance. Fourth, a doctor accepting responsibility for a patient enters a contractual obligation and may not abandon that obligation without either finding another physician to take his or her place or notifying the patient well in advance so the patient can engage another doctor. At the same time, however, the patient's obligation is to follow the doctor's medical advice.

Doctors are not the only health care workers who can be charged with malpractice. If other medical personnel act as a team with a doctor or surgeon, they may also be held liable. For example, during surgery a surgeon is assisted by an anesthesiologist and various nurses, any of whom may separately fail in his or her duties and be sued as a result. Thus, whenever a patient suffers at the hands of a medical team, the trend has been to sue each member. Furthermore, if the facilities or personnel employed by a hospital prove substandard, the hospital itself may be liable.

Tort liability and contractual responsibility govern the legal treatment of malpractice, both of which fall under civil law. (This classification assumes that doctors inadvertently cause harm; if they intentionally injure a patient, they are subject to charges under criminal law.) A patient may sue for breach of contract if his or her doctor has broken that contract—usually by abandoning the patient without proper notice. This sort of lawsuit is by far the least common. Tort liability means that the doctor is responsible for any injury (tort) caused to the patient through negligence. The patient may seek compensation for a tort by suing the doctor for damages. The presumption is that money, which is almost always the form of compensation sought, can make up for the harm done. Damages can be awarded for two types of injury. Concrete physical injury is the most typical, and damages may include money to cover medical bills, lost wages, convalescent care, and other expenses relating directly to the disability. A jury may also grant damages for pain and suffering, a difficult type of injury on which to place a price; such damages account for some of the largest monetary awards.

Because damages may amount to millions of dollars, most doctors who lose a malpractice suit cannot hope to pay them without help. Insurance provides that help, which usually takes one of three forms. First, for monthly payments (premiums), traditional insurance companies offer policies to doctors that will guarantee money up to a certain amount to pay damages. Also, if its client is sued, the insurance company assigns attorneys who handle the legal negotiations and the defense in court. Second, hospitals or other large organizations may pay for malpractice damages from a pool of money reserved for that purpose alone. Third, doctors and other health care providers may set up an insurance

company of their own for mutual coverage, often called "bedpan mutuals."

Malpractice litigation in the United States is a ponderous, expensive business. In the mid-1970's, malpractice insurance prices began to rise sharply; between 1983 and 1985 alone, the cost increased 100 percent. Malpractice premiums remained relatively flat during the 1990's. By the end of the decade, however, physicians began to be hit with unexpectedly large increases. In 2001, eight states saw two or more liability insurers raise rates by at least 30 percent, according to the American Medical Association, and doctors in more than a dozen states saw one or more insurers charge at least 25 percent more for medical malpractice insurance. The George W. Bush presidential administration released a report in 2002 that found the price of malpractice insurance for certain high-risk specialists increased about 10 percent in 2001 alone and was expected to rise another 20 percent between 2002 and 2003. From 1996 to 1999, jury awards for medical malpractice claims jumped 76 percent, according to Jury Verdict Research. Doctors pass on some or all of these costs to patients by charging higher fees. If a patient sues, however, the insurance cannot cover every type of loss. The amount of time that a doctor must spend with lawyers, the time in court, and the overall distraction from practicing mean reduced earnings. Yet the cost is not only to the doctor. The plaintiff pays attorneys by contingency fee, which means that the attorney receives a percentage (usually 20 to 30 percent) of money from any settlement. A patient losing a suit does not pay the attorney but still must pay court costs and expenses, which can quickly amount to thousands of dollars. Finally, when suits reach court, public funds contribute to the court's expenses, and those expenses climb if a decision is appealed or retried, as is sometimes the case.

Patients and doctors alike complain that soaring malpractice litigation in the United States since 1960 has been destructive, introducing suspicion into the doctor-patient relationship. In addition to its emotional impact, the suspicion concretely affects medical practice, most medical economists claim. Because physicians fear lawsuits, they perform more diagnostic tests than are called for by medical protocols. Often the chances are remote that these tests will reveal any useful information, yet doctors order them to show that they have done everything possible for the patient if they are sued. The extra tests cost money, which either the patient or the insurance company must pay. In either case, the expenditures inflate the cost of medicine. The practice of such "defensive medicine" has also led some doctors to refuse to perform high-risk procedures except in hospitals that have extensive facilities. Obstetricians provide a signal case in point. Fearing lawsuits for any complications that may arise, many obstetricians will not deliver babies at home or in small hospitals, forcing rural patients to rush long distances to the nearest big-city hospital for delivery.

One scholar of the malpractice system has remarked that it seems designed to protect the interests of everyone except the person who most needs help: the injured patient. While this is surely a rhetorical exaggeration, all studies have found that only a fraction of injuries are ever compensated. Moreover, the system, based on adversarial disputation, seems hostile and dauntingly complex to both patient and physician. Yet, although no one thinks it perfect, the system evolved in accordance with two widely held American attitudes toward regulation in general: It limits abuses, and it preserves professional autonomy.

TRIAL PROCEDURES IN MALPRACTICE CASES

Few malpractice claims actually end in jury awards for damages. Only about 10 percent of patients injured by doctors file lawsuits, of which about 20 percent end in payment to the plaintiff. Overwhelmingly the payments come from out-of-court settlements that win the plaintiff only a part of the money sought in the suit. Taking a suit all the way to a jury settlement is risky for plaintiffs; they win only about two in ten cases.

From the outset, then, the chances are against the injured patient, and for this reason malpractice litigation is not popular among lawyers. To have a reasonable chance to win a case in court, or at least to force the doctor's insurance company to offer a settlement out of court, the lawyer must first be sure that a causal connection can be made between the patient's injury and physician negligence. In other words, patients cannot sue simply on the hope of winning damages; courts try to reject such "frivolous" suits before they come to trial.

A lawyer believing that a reasonable causal link can be established will write up a summons and complaint on the client's behalf and send them to the doctor. The summons warns the doctor that the patient is filing a lawsuit. The complaint explains the patient's allegation of harm and the amount of damages that the patient demands in compensation. The doctor must answer in a specific time—about a month in most states—and the answer, issued through the doctor's lawyers or those of his or her insurance company, almost always denies responsibility for any injury. The legal battle is then joined.

During a pretrial period known as discovery, each side investigates the other, hoping to find facts that will support arguments in court. Lawyers rely on three investigative methods. The first is documentary disclosure. The plaintiff's lawyer will demand records, especially the patient's medical record, and the doctor must furnish them in a reasonable time. In the second method, written interrogatories, the plaintiff's lawyer sends the doctor a list of questions that must be answered in writing. Third is the deposition, a formal legal proceeding. Lawyers from both sides meet and together question, in separate sessions, the defendant, plaintiff, and key witnesses, all of whom answer the questions under oath, so that they are guilty of perjury if they lie. Many suits are dropped during discovery, with or without monetary settlement. If the suit continues but one side has little evidence on which to base arguments, the other side will probably file a motion for summary judgment, which essentially asks a judge to end the litigation by disqualifying the weak case. Discovery and pretrial motions may take years to complete.

Trials follow a pattern, with some variations, designed to allow each side to present claims and counterclaims systematically. A trial starts with opening statements in which the lawyers describe the general plan for their cases; no actual arguments are made. Next, to clarify matters for the jury, the judge may summarize the applicable legal principles for the case. Then witnesses are called and questioned, first by the plaintiff's lawyer. After he or she finishes with each witness, the defendant's lawyer may also ask questions, a procedure called cross-examination. When the plaintiff's side is done calling witnesses, then the defense lawyer calls and questions more, which the lawyer for the plaintiff may also cross-examine.

During the questioning, two types of evidence are admitted: testimony, the oral or written statements of what people have seen or heard, and "real" or "demonstrative" evidence, physical objects such as an X ray or a needle that have a bearing on the case. The testimony is crucial for the plaintiff, because at this point an expert witness must swear that the defendant was negligent to a "medical certainty" by failing to adhere to one or more medical standards of practice. Since only a doctor is qualified to make this judgment, expert witnesses are always physicians. Finally, the lawyers make closing statements, each insisting that the evidence supports the position of his or her client, and the jury retires to decide on a verdict. If the jurors decide in favor of the plaintiff, they can also lower or raise the amount of requested damages. If they decide for the defendant, the doctor, then the case ends without a monetary settlement. A victorious plaintiff cannot expect immediate payment. Appeals to higher courts may last years, and the appellate courts, after examining the trial records, can reverse a verdict, change the amount of damages, or order a new trial.

Even if a trial does get under way, however, it may not end in a verdict. At any point in the proceedings, one side or the other may give up. Insurance companies regularly send observers to malpractice trials who assess the progress of arguments objectively. An observer detecting a weakness in the defense or noticing that the jury favors the plaintiff for any reason will offer a settlement to the plaintiff's lawyer, because such a settlement will save court costs and probably involve less money than a jury award for damages. Likewise, the plaintiff's lawyer, recognizing that the chances of winning are slim, may try to make a deal with the insurance company. Such dickering may even continue after a verdict is announced, if it is appealed. Also, at any point in the trial the judge may end the case if he or she thinks that one side cannot possibly win; similarly, the judge may reverse a verdict or change the amount of damages if the jury's decision shocks his or her professional conscience.

PERSPECTIVE AND PROSPECTS

By the mid-1970's, the entire American health care system, in the view of most health care observers, was in a state of crisis. Costs had risen, and facilities, especially in urban areas, were strained, while rural areas were often underserved. Critics have blamed the problems on increasingly costly technology and drugs, government regulation, professional salaries, and inadequate preventive medicine. Few doubt that malpractice litigation has contributed significantly as well.

Estimates in 1993 claimed that defensive medicine alone had increased the annual cost of American health care from $10 billion to $36 billion. Combined with increasing fees for medical services and other costs, defensive medicine has helped drive up the cost of medical insurance. Because of these financing problems, legislatures around the country have tried to control the increasing numbers of malpractice suits with tort reform, arbitration or review panels, and legal fee limits.

In 2002, lawmakers in Ohio and other states began attempting to drive down premiums by passing laws that limit the jury awards injured patients can be given for pain and suffering. The Bush administration also supported a nationwide limit of $250,000 on these damages, although questions remain about how well the caps work.

Tort reforms include a number of measures that modify the procedures or awards of malpractice litigation. Two reforms are designed to shorten the process. One method is to reduce the statute of limitations for malpractice claims—the period after injury when a lawsuit can be started. The second involves limiting the rules governing the discovery phase of pretrial action. Two further reforms restrict the amount of damages. The most popular of these is to impose maximum amounts for types of injury, especially pain and suffering. In the second reform, jury damages must be reduced by the amount of money from other sources, such as health insurance, that a patient receives for the injury.

Several states have instituted review panels or required arbitration before a suit can proceed to court. Laypeople and judges, as well as doctors, make up the review panels, which try to identify and disallow frivolous suits. Arbitration panels actually decide on the amount of damages, if any, to be made, and their decisions cannot be appealed.

These reforms have only slowed the rate of lawsuits and the rise in the amount of money spent on paying damages and fees. Whatever its defects, the tort system has succeeded in making doctors wary of negligence. Critics insist, however, that the system for addressing malpractice has punished all physicians, not simply the incompetent, and has contributed to the increasingly litigious tenor of American society.

—Roger Smith, Ph.D.;
updated by Martha Oehmke Loustaunau, Ph.D.

See also American Medical Association (AMA); Autopsy; Critical care; Critical care, pediatric; Emergency medicine; Ethics; Euthanasia; Forensic pathology; Health maintenance organizations (HMOs); Hippocratic oath; Hospitals; Iatrogenic disorders; Law and medicine; Obstetrics; Pathology; Resuscitation.

FOR FURTHER INFORMATION:

Furrow, Barry R., et al. *Health Law: Cases, Materials and Problems.* 5th ed. St. Paul, Minn.: West, 2004. Covers a range of issues related to health and the law, including cost control, prospective payment, health care antitrust, and federal and state regulation of health care delivery; legal and ethical issues created by reproductive technology and by the dilemmas of death and dying; and the core topics of professional liability and the physician-patient relationship.

Groopman, Jerome E. *Second Opinions: Stories of Intuition and Choice in the Changing World of Medicine*. New York: Viking, 2000. Among other examples, Groopman describes the case of a woman with leukemia wrongly diagnosed as having asthma, a patient with melanoma who became the object of professional infighting about the availability and advisability of interferon treatment, and a young physicist told that he had fewer than six months to live and the ensuing tussle between specialists about the usefulness of bone marrow transplant.

Jonsen, Albert R., Mark Siegler, and William J. Winslade. *Clinical Ethics: A Practical Approach to Ethical Decisions in Clinical Medicine*. 6th ed. New York: McGraw-Hill, 2006. Discusses the whole range of medical ethics, including legal issues, confidentiality, care of the dying patient, and euthanasia and assisted suicide.

Merry, Alan, and Alexander McCall Smith. *Errors, Medicine, and the Law*. New York: Cambridge University Press, 2001. Argues that many medical accidents are linked to the complexity of modern health care and calls for a more informed alternative to the "blaming culture" in medicine.

Pence, Gregory. *Classic Cases in Medical Ethics: Accounts of Cases That Have Shaped Medical Ethics, with Philosophical, Legal, and Historical Backgrounds*. 4th ed. New York: McGraw-Hill, 2004. Surveys important cases that have defined and shaped the field of medical ethics. Each case is accompanied by careful discussion of pertinent philosophical theories and legal and ethical issues.

Sage, William M., and Rogan Kersh, eds. *Medical Malpractice and the U.S. Health Care System*. New York: Cambridge University Press, 2006. Examines medical liability with regard to U.S. health policy. Offers ideas for reform in the areas of patient safety, liability insurance, and tort litigation.

Sharpe, Virginia F., and Alan I. Faden. *Medical Harm: Historical, Conceptual, and Ethical Dimensions of Iatrogenic Illness*. New York: Cambridge University Press, 1998. Of the many seekers after a healthier life or of relief from suffering who rightfully expect benefit from the health care system, some are more harmed than helped. This book deals mostly with harmful medical events which happen in hospitals.

Zobel, Hiller B., and Stephen N. Rous. *Doctors and the Law: Defendants and Expert Witnesses*. New York: W. W. Norton, 1993. Zobel, a judge, and Rous, a physician, give advice to physicians on how best to endure a malpractice suit. The step-by-step account of the legal proceedings, evidential requirements, and possible psychological effects on the physician make insightful reading for nonphysicians as well.

MAMMOGRAPHY

PROCEDURE

ANATOMY OR SYSTEM AFFECTED: Breasts

SPECIALTIES AND RELATED FIELDS: Gynecology, oncology, preventive medicine, radiology

DEFINITION: The use of X rays of the female breast, primarily in the detection and diagnosis of malignant breast tumors

INDICATIONS AND PROCEDURES

X-ray mammography is a complicated procedure. The quality of the mammographic image is proportionately dependent upon the imaging equipment in use and the way in which it is utilized.

Critical factors include compression of the breast, positioning of the breast, the use of the right image receptor, and exposure of the X-ray tube. Improper use of equipment and procedures contributes to an image that is suboptimal. With proper care and thorough knowledge in the use of instruments designed for mammography, however, excellent image quality can be obtained.

In mammography, four physical constraints must be considered when evaluating the performance of the systems. First, contrast is of utmost importance because minute differences in soft tissue density are essential. Second, resolution is important because of the need to identify microcalcifications as small as 100 micrometers, which are often associated with abnormalities. Third, an adequate X-ray dose is vital to obtain an image with the proper signal-to-noise ratio. Too much radiation, however, means added risk for the patient. Fourth, a decrease in noise (background) is important to achieve an image with an adequate signal-to-noise ratio for proper diagnosis.

The examination can be conducted with the patient standing or sitting. To achieve the desired radiographic projection, the X-ray tube is set at an optimal angle. The mammography unit has a support plate onto which the breast is positioned. A plastic paddle assists in compressing the breast onto this plate. The pressure applied to achieve proper compression can be applied manually, but most mammography technicians prefer power-assisted compression, as this permits the radiographer to use both hands to position the breast properly. The shape, rigidity, and composition of the compression or support plate are crucial factors. The support plate is composed of a carbon-fiber composite capable of a high X-ray transmission. The support is in front of the tunnel, and the tunnel receives the image receptor. The standard image receptor uses a high-resolution mammographic screen-film combination. With receptor technology advancing rapidly, however, digital receptors are fast becoming available. The big advantage of digital receptors is that they offer either a limited field of view for stereotactical localization or a full field of view for standard mammographic imaging.

Since all mammography units are intended to show the soft tissue of the breast while displaying differences in contrast and since proper compression is vital, the natural mobility of the breast should be considered. The breast is easiest to compress from the inferior and lateral aspects. The preliminary automatic compression between the paddle and the support plate should never go beyond 45 pounds of pressure, and the patient should not be in pain. Nevertheless, the breast must be taut to the touch.

Improper compression can lead to erroneous results. The outcome of proper compression is a reduction of X-ray radiation to the breast by reducing tissue thickness; the bringing of lesions closer to the film, thus facilitating an accurate reading; a reduction in movement blurriness because the breast is held immobile; increased contrast as a result of flattened breasts, thereby decreasing thickness; elimination of confusion caused by superimposition shadows; and easier visualization of the borders of circumscribed lesions.

It is helpful if magnification of the image is possible, particularly if small areas are being examined. Magnification is of greater importance in areas of suspicious microcalcifications or at surgical sites. Unfortunately, the greater the magnification, the higher the patient's radiation dose because the breast is placed much closer to the source of radiation.

In addition to compression, image quality depends on a number of factors: positioning, radiation exposure, contrast, sharpness, noise, artifacts, and labeling. The craniocaudal position (compression of the breast from top to bottom) and the mediolateral oblique position (compression of the breast from side to side) are the two standard positions employed in mammography. Each position provides specific views, and proper positioning reveals as much of the tissue as possible for diagnosis. Any area that is omitted will result in false results that may endanger the patient's life. Adequate exposure to radiation is essential. If this is not acheived, then it is difficult to identify the skin and subcutaneous tissue. Usually, contrast is highest for thinner breasts and lowest for thicker breasts; this is primarily the result of more scattered radiation and greater tissue absorption of low radiation in thicker breasts. Without contrast, particularly in thicker breast tissue, different tissue densities will have very similar appearances.

Sharpness, or the visualization of fine details in the image, is one of the central factors in achieving a correct diagnosis. If the desired sharpness is not obtained, then the image is referred to as unsharp. Unsharpness may be the result of motion blur, poor screen-film contrast, or other technical factors. Noise and sharpness are closely linked. Noise is defined as increased background and a decreased ability to see tiny structures, such as calcifications. The major contributors of noise are scatter and quantum mottle, which is fluctuation in the number of X-ray photons needed to form the image. Examples of artifacts are scratches, fingerprints, dirt, lint, and dust. Standardized labeling in mammography to identify the left side from the right side, so that the films cannot be subject to misinterpretation, is vital, especially because mammograms can be legal documents.

A slightly different approach is used to screen women with breast implants. Two craniocaudal views are obtained, one with the implant in the field of view and one with the implant as much out of the field as possible. In a similar way, two mediolateral oblique views are imaged.

Digital mammography differs from regular mammography in that in the former electronic detectors capture and facilitate the display of the X-ray signals on a computer or laser-printed film. In all other aspects, it is still the same procedure—proper positioning and compression of the breast are still critical for obtaining quality digital images. The goal of digital mammography also remains the same, to detect and localize breast abnormalities.

As exposure to radiation is a major concern with traditional mammography, the primary force to developing digital X-ray mammography is the idea that it has the potential to enhance image quality, and therefore lesion detection (especially for dense breasts), with a lower dose of radiation. The greatest advantage in digital mammography is its ability to separate image acquisition from image display, thus providing the ability to manipulate contrast, brightness, and magnification with one exposure.

Dynamic or real-time imaging, especially with biopsies, is possible with digital mammography, providing a better understanding of breast tumors with regard to localization and boundaries. This procedure can also facilitate the direct use of computers for detection and diagnosis. In addition, with this technology it is possible to form three-dimensional images by combining images from all angles. The ease of digital image archiving, retrieval, and transmission is another advantage.

USES AND COMPLICATIONS

There are two basic types of mammographic examinations: screening mammography and diagnostic mammography. Screening mammography refers to examinations of women with no obvious symptoms to detect breast cancers. A standard screening examination includes two views of each breast, sometimes referred to as the standard views.

General agreement has been reached that screening mammography reduces mortality from breast cancer in women fifty years of age or older, but an ongoing debate exists over the effectiveness of screening mammography in women aged forty to forty-nine. Randomized clinical trials have confirmed the validity of screening mammography. Deaths attributable to breast cancer have been reduced. The American Cancer Society and most other well-known professional societies have continued to recommend mammography screening for women in the younger age group because of the results of several studies that advocate the benefits of screening in this age group. For example, a fourteen-year follow-up to the Edinburgh trial has shown a mortality reduction of 21 percent for women aged forty-five to forty-nine who were screened with mammography. A sixteen-year follow-up to the UK Trial of Early Detection of Breast Cancer revealed a 27 percent decrease in mortality in women who were screened with mammography, and no evidence was found that women aged forty-five to forty-six at the start of screening received less benefit than did older women. Breast self-examination alone does not bring down the rate of mortality.

A negative result produced by screening mammography would not include straight lines, unless there is a history of surgery or trauma, and would not show bulg-

A woman receives a mammogram. It is recommended that regular screenings take place beginning in middle age. (PhotoDisc)

ing contours from tissue into fatty areas. Characteristics in a screening view that suggest the need for follow-up diagnostic screening are masses, microcalcifications, architectural distortion, and parenchymal asymmetry. Palpable abnormalities described by the patient, focal tenderness, and spontaneous nipple discharge also warrant diagnostic screening.

As with all preventive measures, screening mammography cannot eliminate all deaths from breast cancer, for several reasons. It does not detect all types of cancers, including some that are actually detected by physical examination. Also some tumors may appear and develop too quickly to be detected and identified at an early, more curable stage. Mammograms are particularly difficult to interpret for women with dense breast tissue, which is especially common in young women. The dense tissue prevents the identification of abnormalities associated with tumors, thereby leading to a higher rate of false-positive and false-negative test results.

Diagnostic mammography, also referred to as consultative or problem-solving mammography, is the type of study preferred when there are clinical findings, such as a palpable lump or an abnormal screening mammogram requiring additional analysis. Additionally, each diagnostic mammography examination is performed to suit the individual patient who has symptoms or abnormal findings. Diagnostic mammography may warrant additional views of the breast, such as spot compression and magnification, a correlative clinical examination, and ultrasonography. In almost all instances, barring a few exceptions, a radiologist is present during the performance of a diagnostic mammography study.

Diagnostic mammography should be carried out when a biopsy is being considered for a palpable lump in a woman over thirty years of age. The reason for doing a mammogram preceding a biopsy is to define the nature of the clinical abnormality better and to find other unexpected lesions.

Mammographic characteristics of possible benign lesions are a cluster of small round or oval calcifications; nonpalpable, noncalcified, and solid round or oval, and predominantly well-circumscribed, masses; nonpalpable focal symmetry with concave margins and interspersed fat; asymptomatic single dilated duct (no nipple discharge); and multiple (three or more) similar findings, distributed randomly and often bilaterally. Mammographic characteristics of malignant lesions are a mass with no history of previous surgery, trauma, or mastitis that is ill-defined and microtubulated; malignant-type microcalcifications; skin thickening and retraction; nipple retraction; and architectural distortion with no history of previous surgery or trauma.

The ruling concern in mammography is the amount of radiation to which the patient is exposed. Therefore, an automatic radiation exposure control device is necessary to avoid overexposure. The radiation detector is placed behind the image receptor so that its image does not appear on the mammogram. Exposure is terminated when the signal recorded by the monitor reaches a predefined level. Unfortunately, the X-ray photons reaching the detector fluctuate considerably depending on the size and composition of the breast. As a result, the signal recorded by the detector is only an approximate indication of the energy absorbed. Therefore, it is unlikely that an accurate reading will be available.

In any therapeutic model that is considered a source of risk to the patient, it is essential to bear in mind the number of deaths caused by the technique as opposed to the number of deaths that it actually prevents. Fortunately, the benefits of mammography supersede the risk of radiation exposure. Furthermore, risk estimates have decreased following the adoption of a relative risk model and allowance for the variation of risk with age at exposure.

PERSPECTIVE AND PROSPECTS

Though much progress has been made in the field of cancer medicine, early detection is the best approach in the war against breast cancer. Ample clinical data have shown that women diagnosed with breast cancers in the early stages are more likely to survive than those diagnosed with more advanced stages of the same disease. A systematic physical breast examination by a clinician once a year and breast self-examination once a month can help in identifying tumors that are fairly small and that can go unnoticed in the absence of such examinations.

Nearly all medical experts agree that in women over fifty, routine X-ray mammography, with or without clinical examination, has been valuable in detecting tumors and at earlier stages. This has been very effectively shown in randomized clinical trials to reduce disease-specific mortality. In the United States, women undergo screening mammography as part of their routine health maintenance, and mammography is considered to be a necessary procedure in the annual physicals of women over fifty. Subsequently, routine, annual mammographic screening has been actively promoted in many countries and nongovernmental agencies.

Breast imaging technologies that are being developed are progressing with three distinct goals in mind: to identify the most minute tumor lesions; to localize abnormalities to aid further examination, analysis, or treatment; and to characterize the abnormalities and assist in the decision-making process following identification. Radiologists and patients alike dream of an ideal imaging modality that would achieve all three goals in a single use. In reality, most current technologies fail to do so; hence, many developers are intent on perfecting one goal at a time. In addition to these technical goals, developers hope to generate methods that are more practical, inexpensive, harmless, and appealing to the patient.

—Giri Sulur, Ph.D.

See also Breast biopsy; Breast cancer; Breast disorders; Breast surgery; Breasts, female; Cancer; Cyst removal; Cysts; Glands; Gynecology; Imaging and radiology; Mastectomy and lumpectomy; Mastitis; Noninvasive tests; Oncology; Pathology; Screening; Tumor removal; Tumors; Women's health.

FOR FURTHER INFORMATION:

Bassett, Lawrence W., et al. *Film-Screen Mammography: An Atlas of Instructional Cases*. New York: Raven Press, 1991. This teaching atlas is an anthology of high-quality mammograms with a wide variety of pathologically proved cases.

Gamagami, Parvis. *Atlas of Mammography: New Early Signs in Breast Cancer*. Cambridge, Mass.: Blackwell Science, 1996. Provides many examples of images that will help laypeople understand a mammogram.

Kopans, Daniel B. *Breast Imaging*. 3d ed. Baltimore: Lippincott Williams & Wilkins, 2007. Well written and comprehensive. An important reference in the field.

Love, Susan M., and Karen Lindsey. *Dr. Susan Love's Breast Book*. Rev. 4th ed. Cambridge, Mass.: Da Capo Press, 2005. One of the most influential books in women's health written for a general audience. Details breast development, changes with age, and breast cancer detection and treatment.

Mitchell, George W., Jr., and Lawrence W. Bassett, eds. *The Female Breast and Its Disorders*. Baltimore: Williams & Wilkins, 1990. A comprehensive text offers the expertise of representatives from obstetrics and gynecology, diagnostic radiology, pathology, surgery, medicine, therapeutic radiology, and psychiatry.

Sutton, Amy L., ed. *Cancer Sourcebook for Women: Basic Consumer Health Information About Leading Causes of Cancer in Women*. 3d ed. Detroit: Omnigraphics, 2006. An excellent overview of female cancers, including screening.

MANIC-DEPRESSIVE DISORDER. *See* BIPOLAR DISORDERS.

MAPLE SYRUP URINE DISEASE (MSUD)
DISEASE/DISORDER

ALSO KNOWN AS: Branched-chain ketoaciduria

ANATOMY OR SYSTEM AFFECTED: Nervous system

SPECIALTIES AND RELATED FIELDS: Family medicine, genetics, neonatology, pediatrics

DEFINITION: A recessive autosomal genetic disease resulting in the absence, partial activity, or inactivity of a multisubunit enzyme responsible for metaboliz-

---

INFORMATION ON MAPLE SYRUP URINE DISEASE (MSUD)

CAUSES: Genetic defect resulting in accumulation of amino acids leucine, isoleucine, and valine

SYMPTOMS: Within three to seven days after birth, poor weight gain, high-pitched cry, irritability, lethargy, characteristic maple syrup smell; if untreated, mental retardation, seizures, and death

DURATION: Lifelong

TREATMENTS: Diet with controlled amounts of isoleucine, leucine, and valine

---

ing the branched-chain amino acids leucine, isoleucine, and valine.

CAUSES AND SYMPTOMS

As a result of deficient branched-chain alpha-ketoacid dehydrogenase (BCKD), the essential branched chain amino acids leucine, isoleucine, and valine are not metabolized in patients with maple syrup urine disease (MSUD). The branched-chain amino acids and their ketoacid products accumulate in the blood and interfere with brain function. High levels of leucine are especially toxic. The classic form of the disease results in little (less than 2 percent) or no BCKD activity. Symptoms develop within three to seven days after birth and include poor weight gain, a high-pitched cry, irritability, lethargy, and a characteristic maple syrup smell to the urine. If the disease is untreated, then mental retardation, various neurological symptoms such as seizures, and even death can result.

Variant forms of the disease in which there is some (3 to 12 percent) BCKD activity result in milder symptoms. A rare variant form of the disease called thiamine-responsive MSUD responds to high doses of thiamine.

TREATMENT AND THERAPY

The treatment of severe MSUD, which should begin immediately after diagnosis, involves a special diet with controlled amounts of isoleucine, leucine, and valine to ensure metabolic control. Enfamil, a special dietary formula, provides leucine but may have to be supplemented with isoleucine and valine to provide adequate intake of all three amino acids and permit normal growth and development.

Treatment of the milder forms of MSUD also involves management through diet therapy. Diet therapy should be continued throughout life, and the levels of the branched-chain amino acids should be monitored often.

PERSPECTIVE AND PROSPECTS

MSUD was first described in 1954. The name derives from the sweet, maple syrup smell of the patient's urine. Because MSUD is caused by a recessive gene, there is a 1 in 4 chance that two heterozygous carriers will have an affected child. MSUD affects about 1 in 180,000 newborns in the United States, but in some populations, such as Mennonites, it may be as high as 1 in 176.

Some states test for the disease in their newborn screening programs. Testing should be done within the first twenty-four hours after birth, since early diagnosis is essential. Some of the milder variant forms are missed in the screening programs. The detection of alloisoleucine is diagnostic for MSUD but may not appear until the sixth day of life. Carrier testing is available for the Mennonite variant of the disease.

—*Charles L. Vigue, Ph.D.*

See also Enzyme therapy; Enzymes; Food biochemistry; Genetic counseling; Genetic diseases; Metabolic disorders; Metabolism; Neonatology; Nutrition; Screening.

FOR FURTHER INFORMATION:

Clarke, Joe T. R. *A Clinical Guide to Inherited Metabolic Diseases*. 3d ed. New York: Cambridge University Press, 2006.

Icon Health. *Maple Syrup Urine Disease: A Medical Dictionary, Bibliography, and Annotated Research Guide to Internet References*. San Diego, Calif.: Author, 2004.

Jorde, Lynn B., et al. *Medical Genetics*. Rev. 3d ed. St. Louis: Mosby, 2006.

Pritchard, Dorian J., and Bruce R. Korf. *Medical Genetics at a Glance*. Malden, Mass.: Blackwell Science, 2003.

MARBURG VIRUS

DISEASE/DISORDER

ALSO KNOWN AS: Green monkey fever

ANATOMY OR SYSTEM AFFECTED: Immune system

SPECIALTIES AND RELATED FIELDS: Epidemiology, virology

DEFINITION: Marburg hemorrhagic fever is a rare, highly lethal disease caused by Marburg filovirus.

CAUSES AND SYMPTOMS

Marburg hemorrhagic fever is caused by a filovirus. Filoviruses are separated into two distinct types, Marburg and Ebola. All filoviruses are classified as biohazard level 4 agents based on their high mortality rate, potential transmissibility, and absence of effective vaccines or treatments. The systemic nature of filovirus infections suggest they may have immunosuppressive effects.

Human-infecting viruses usually appear as small, round, or oval organisms. Filoviruses are unique among human viruses, appearing as long, cylindrical organisms with twists and loops. The natural reservoir for filoviruses is unknown but is presumed to be wild animals (zoonotic). Research suggests that filoviruses may possibly be linked to bats, from which the viruses are occasionally introduced into primate populations. The primary transmission of Marburg filovirus from its natural reservoir appears to occur only in sub-Saharan Africa within five degrees of the equator.

Human transmission of Marburg hemorrhagic fever is by direct contact with infected blood, semen, urine, mucus, and organs. Some evidence suggests that aerosol transmission may also occur. The virus enters the body through lesions and initially infects the lymph nodes, spleen, and liver. Marburg filovirus can survive several weeks in corpses and blood samples.

The incubation period of Marburg hemorrhagic fever is three to ten days after infection, and symptoms include high fever, severe headache, painful sore throat, rashes, muscle pain (myalgia), inflamed lymph nodes, dementia, and bloody vomiting and diarrhea from internal hemorrhaging. Symptoms usually include bleeding from the gums and nose, puncture openings in the skin, small hemorrhages in the whites of the eyes, and eventual red blood cell immobilization. Hair, skin, and nail loss, as well as searing body pain from inflamed nerves, occur in later stages of infection. The infection may last as long as three weeks and is often described as agonizing. In fatal cases, the patient's blood pressure undergoes a final severe drop resulting in surgical shock prior to death.

TREATMENT AND THERAPY

There is no vaccine or specific therapy available for filoviral infections. Specific symptoms are treated during the course of infection; the patient either re-

INFORMATION ON MARBURG VIRUS

CAUSES: Infection with a filovirus
SYMPTOMS: High fever, headache, sore throat, rashes, muscle pain, inflamed lymph nodes, dementia, bloody vomiting and diarrhea, bleeding from gums and nose, small hemorrhages in eyes
DURATION: Up to three weeks, often fatal
TREATMENTS: None; alleviation of symptoms

sponds or does not. Secondary prevention requires total isolation of infected patients. Primary infected patients show a higher mortality rate than do secondary infected patients. The mortality rate for humans infected with Marburg hemorrhagic fever ranges from 23 to 90 percent, with some outbreaks being more deadly than others.

PERSPECTIVE AND PROSPECTS

Marburg hemorrhagic fever was first described in 1967 during outbreaks at research laboratories in Marburg and Frankfurt, Germany, and Belgrade, Yugoslavia, and linked to African Green monkeys imported from Uganda. Since the initial outbreaks, sporadic cases of Marburg hemorrhagic fever have been identified in eastern and southern Africa, with the largest outbreak occurring in the Democratic Republic of the Congo in 1998. One of the most frightening aspects of Marburg hemorrhagic fever is its ongoing inclusion in some nations' biological weapons programs.

—*Randall L. Milstein, Ph.D.*

See also Bleeding; Centers for Disease Control and Prevention (CDC); Ebola virus; Epidemiology; Tropical medicine; Viral infections; Zoonoses.

FOR FURTHER INFORMATION:

Garrett, Laurie. *The Coming Plague: Newly Emerging Diseases in a World out of Balance*. New York: Penguin, 1995.

Klenk, Hans-Dieter, ed. *Marburg and Ebola Viruses*. New York: Springer, 1999.

Levy, Elinor, and Mark Fischetti. *The New Killer Diseases: How the Alarming Evolution of Mutant Germs Threatens Us All*. New York: Crown, 2003.

McCormick, Joseph B., Susan Fisher-Hoch, and Leslie Alan Horvitz. *Level 4: Virus Hunters of the CDC*. Rev. ed. New York: Barnes & Noble Books, 1999.

MARFAN SYNDROME

DISEASE/DISORDER

ANATOMY OR SYSTEM AFFECTED: Bones, eyes, heart, musculoskeletal system, spine
SPECIALTIES AND RELATED FIELDS: Cardiology, genetics, ophthalmology, orthopedics
DEFINITION: A condition in which the connective tissue does not form correctly and tends to be too flexible. The abnormal chemical composition, especially of the skeleton and heart, leads to major medical characteristics that are sometimes in evidence only at puberty.

CAUSES AND SYMPTOMS

Recent studies have located the gene that causes the inherited form of Marfan syndrome. About 25 percent of Marfan syndrome cases result from spontaneous mutation. While this knowledge promises better future recognition of the condition, the range and severity of the condition is so variable that diagnosis remains difficult.

Usually, Marfan syndrome is discovered through a detailed family history. The observation that a person is tall and slender and has unusually long fingers or arms is often an early clue. The presence of loose joints with great suppleness is characteristic of the disease. Manifestations of this condition may occur in any part of the body, but the heart, eyes, and spinal column are the most common.

TREATMENT AND THERAPY

Because a variety of organs may be involved in Marfan syndrome, it is essential that several specialists form a team to evaluate and monitor the patient during his or her lifetime. The most serious, and most common, problem area is the heart. Mitral valve problems may lead to leakage or regurgitation of blood. The aortic valve can develop a backflow into the heart.

INFORMATION ON MARFAN SYNDROME

CAUSES: Genetic mutation
SYMPTOMS: Tall and slender appearance, long fingers or arms, loose joints, heart problems, dislocation of eye lens, scoliosis, crowded teeth
DURATION: Lifelong
TREATMENTS: Dependent on severity and structures affected; may include surgery and medications

In the eyes, a characteristic sign is the dislocation of the lens. This symptom is difficult to detect and, like many others, can vary widely in intensity. Cataracts are also associated with this condition.

Other characteristics are found in the skeleton. Spinal curvature, or scoliosis, and a breastbone that either protrudes or indents are observed. Crowded teeth and an arched palate are not uncommon.

Any of these symptoms can lead to serious consequences and should be discovered as early as possible. Regular examinations by specialists in cardiology, ophthalmology, and orthopedics are essential. Most of the possible progressive aspects of the condition can be treated effectively.

—*K. Thomas Finley, Ph.D.*

See also Bones and the skeleton; Cardiology; Cardiology, pediatric; Eye infections and disorders; Eyes; Genetic diseases; Growth; Heart; Mitral valve prolapse; Optometry; Optometry, pediatric; Orthopedics; Orthopedics, pediatric; Scoliosis; Vision disorders.

FOR FURTHER INFORMATION:

Hetzer, R., P. Gehle, and J. Ennker, eds. *Cardiovascular Aspects of Marfan Syndrome*. New York: Springer, 1995.

National Marfan Foundation. http://www.marfan.org/.

Parker, James N., and Philip M. Parker, eds. *The Official Patient's Sourcebook on Marfan Syndrome*. San Diego, Calif.: Icon Health, 2002.

Pyeritz, Reed E., and Julia Conant. *Marfan Syndrome*. 4th ed. Port Washington, N.Y.: National Marfan Foundation, 1994.

Robinson, Peter N., and Maurice Godfrey, eds. *Marfan Syndrome: A Primer for Clinicians and Scientists*. New York: Kluwer Academic/Plenum, 2004.

MARIJUANA

DISEASE/DISORDER, TREATMENT

ALSO KNOWN AS: *Cannabis sativa*, hemp, various popular names (pot, ganja, weed)

ANATOMY OR SYSTEM AFFECTED: Brain, circulatory system, eyes, gastrointestinal system, heart, lungs, musculoskeletal system, nerves, nervous system, psychic-emotional system, respiratory system

SPECIALTIES AND RELATED FIELDS: Alternative medicine, ethics, neurology, pharmacology, psychiatry, psychology, public health

DEFINITION: A plant containing a psychoactive substance with the potential for both recreational abuse and medical use.

INTRODUCTION

The term "marijuana" refers to both the illegal drug and the plant itself. The hemp plant, *Cannabis sativa*, is a fast-growing (to fifteen feet), bushy annual with finely branched leaves further divided into lance-shaped, sawtooth-edged leaflets. The species was first classified in 1735 by the Swedish botanist Carolus Linnaeus. Both male and female plants produce tetrahydrocannabinol (THC), the psychoactive ingredient in the drug. THC collects in tiny droplets of sticky resin produced by glands located at the base of fine hairs covering most of the plant's surface, with the most highly concentrated THC found in the female flower heads. When pollinated, however, the female flower heads produce highly nutritious seeds containing no THC.

RECREATIONAL AND MEDICINAL USES

Marijuana ranks as the third most commonly used recreational drug in the Western world, behind alcohol and tobacco. It is usually smoked, but it can be eaten or brewed as tea. Responses vary according to dosage and experience using the drug, but most people experience a mild euphoria, or "high." Mood, short-term memory, motor coordination, thought, sensation, and time sense can all be affected. Hunger, known as "the munchies," frequently occurs soon after exposure. The heart rate increases, the blood pressure increases while supine but drops when standing, and the eyes can become bloodshot. The most rapid onset with most temporary effect occurs with smoked marijuana. Unlike alcohol or tobacco, no deaths have been directly attributed to marijuana use alone.

Marijuana has been cultivated and used as a medicine for thousands of years. The U.S. Food and Drug Administration (FDA) has approved a synthetic formulation of THC, Marinol (brand name of the generic drug dronabinol), that doctors can prescribe legally for the treatment of nausea and vomiting associated with cancer chemotherapy and the loss of appetite and weight loss characteristic of patients with acquired immunodeficiency syndrome (AIDS). In addition, both Marinol and marijuana are used to alleviate pain, muscle spasms, neurological disorders, and glaucoma. Many users of medicinal THC prefer to smoke marijuana despite its illegality rather than take the legal pill because orally delivered THC is not well absorbed by the body. Research is being conducted into a patch or some other method of delivering the legal drug more effectively. Previously classified among drugs such as cocaine and morphine with a high potential for abuse, Marinol was moved to a less restricted category that includes anabolic steroids in July, 1999.

PERSPECTIVE AND PROSPECTS

Despite the FDA's tacit acknowledgment of the medicinal value of marijuana by the approval of Marinol, marijuana itself is classified as a substance with high potential for abuse and no accepted medical use under federal drug laws, stifling research into other potential medical benefits. Scientific evidence, including the 1990 report of the National Academy of Sciences *Marijuana and Medicine: Assessing the Science Base*, strongly supports further research.

—*Sue Tarjan*

See also Addiction; Alcoholism; Alternative medicine; Club drugs; Eye infections and disorders; Glaucoma; Herbal medicine; Intoxication; Narcotics; Nausea and vomiting; Pain management; Pharmacology; Self-medication; Smoking; Tobacco.

FOR FURTHER INFORMATION:

Earleywine, Mitch. *Understanding Marijuana: A New Look at the Scientific Evidence*. New York: Oxford University Press, 2002.

ElSohly, Mahmoud A., ed. *Marijuana and the Cannabinoids*. Totowa, N.J.: Humana Press, 2007.

Iversen, Leslie L. *The Science of Marijuana*. New York: Oxford University Press, 2000.

Mack, Alison, and Janet Joy. *Marijuana as Medicine? The Science Beyond the Controversy*. Washington, D.C.: National Academy Press, 2001.

Onaivi, Emmanuel S., ed. *Marijuana and Cannabinoid Research: Methods and Protocols*. Totowa, N.J.: Humana Press, 2006.

Shohov, Tatiana, ed. *Medical Use of Marijuana: Policy, Regulatory, and Legal Issues*. New York: Nova Science, 2003.

MASSAGE
TREATMENT
ANATOMY OR SYSTEM AFFECTED: All

SPECIALTIES AND RELATED FIELDS: Alternative medicine, exercise physiology, geriatrics and gerontology, oncology, pediatrics, physical therapy, preventive medicine, sports medicine

DEFINITION: The intentional and systematic manipulation of the soft tissues of the body to promote health and healing.

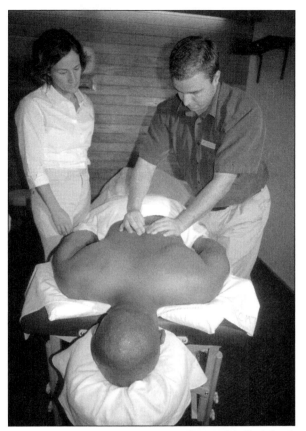

A patient receives massage therapy. (Custom Medical Stock Photo)

INDICATIONS AND PROCEDURES

Massage is used in both wellness and treatment models of health care. Wellness implies the achievement of an optimal state of well-being. The health enhancing effects of massage such as relaxation, stress reduction, and increased body conditioning or awareness contribute to general wellness. In the treatment model, massage is considered a modality indicated to alleviate the symptoms and/or pain of a specific condition. A particular massage technique can be more or less effective for each illness or injury. The treatment model includes the subspecialty of sports massage, a beneficial intervention for athletes and people engaged in strenuous physical activity.

Two men were instrumental in the development of classic Western massage: Per Henrik Ling (1776-1839) and Johann Mezger (1838-1909). Ling developed an approach for treating medical conditions called the Swedish movement cure in the nineteenth century. Mezger defined four categories of massage using

French terminology: *effleurage*, *petrissage*, *tapotement*, and *frictions*. The work of these men was further developed by their students and was incorporated into both regular and alternative medicine.

The physical effects of massage include healthy skin, relaxation, increased blood circulation and immune system functioning, metabolic balance in the muscles, connective tissue pliability, increased joint mobility and flexibility, and pain reduction. The mental and emotional benefits include increased mental clarity, reduced anxiety, and emotional release.

USES AND COMPLICATIONS

Massage has proven benefits for mind and body health. Research in the twentieth century showed a positive relationship between the reduction of pain and stress after massage. Other studies revealed that massage promoted weight gain in premature infants and reduced anxiety in adolescents hospitalized for psychiatric conditions. It can help slow the aging process among older adults and bring comfort to the terminally ill.

A basic tenet of massage practice is "Do no harm." Massage practitioners are trained to identify "endangerment sites." These are areas of the body which are less protected and more vulnerable to damage. "Contraindications" are conditions under which receiving massages are not advisable, such as when it could worsen a condition or spread infection. Health history information is essential for a safe massage session.

As of the year 2000, twenty-five states and the District of Columbia had licensing requirements for massage therapists. The American Massage Therapy Association (AMTA) had thirty thousand members who had to have a minimum of five hundred hours of training from a recognized school. Every practitioner must adhere to a code of ethics and standards of practice.

PERSPECTIVE AND PROSPECTS

Massage has been used for centuries in native and folk cultures all over the world. It has periodically lost and regained popularity in the Western world. After a decline in the 1950's, it experienced a revival of credibility and value during the human potential movement of the late 1960's. Since then, it has been increasingly incorporated into medical treatment and prevention programs. The Office of Alternative Medicine was established by the National Institutes of Health to explore alternative medical practices. Massage therapy was included in the comprehensive 1994 report.

—*Susan L. Sandel, Ph.D.*

See also Acupressure; Alternative medicine; Headaches; Muscle sprains, spasms, and disorders; Muscles; Pain; Pain management; Physical rehabilitation; Stress; Stress reduction.

FOR FURTHER INFORMATION:

American Massage Therapy Association. http://www.amtamassage.org/.

Beck, Mark F. *Theory and Practice of Therapeutic Massage*. Clifton Park, N.Y.: Thomson Delmar Learning, 2006.

Fritz, Sandy. *Mosby's Fundamentals of Therapeutic Massage*. 3d ed. St. Louis: Mosby Year Book, 2004.

Salvo, Susan G., and Maureen Pfeiffer, eds. *Massage Therapy: Principles and Practice*. 2d ed. Philadelphia: W. B. Saunders, 2003.

Trivieri, Larry, Jr., and John W. Anderson, eds. *Alternative Medicine: The Definitive Guide*. 2d ed. Berkeley, Calif.: Ten Speed Press, 2002.

Werner, Ruth. *A Massage Therapist's Guide to Pathology*. Philadelphia: Lippincott Williams & Wilkins, 2005.

MASTECTOMY AND LUMPECTOMY
PROCEDURES

ANATOMY OR SYSTEM AFFECTED: Breasts

SPECIALTIES AND RELATED FIELDS: General surgery, oncology, pathology, plastic surgery, radiology

DEFINITION: Mastectomy involves the surgical removal of one or both breasts, whereas lumpectomy involves the removal of one or more tumors and surrounding tissue from the breast.

KEY TERMS:

BRCA1: an abbreviation for breast cancer 1; the mutant chromosomal factor, when found in chromosome 17, which indicates that a woman is vulnerable to developing breast cancer

estrogen: any of several hormones produced by the ovaries that regulate some female reproductive processes and maintain secondary sex characteristics in the female

fibrocystic breasts: the lumpy breasts that some women routinely develop, particularly in the seven or eight days before menstruation

mammography: an X-ray examination of the breasts, the purpose of which is to reveal tumors and other abnormalities

metastasis: the spreading of cancer cells from the original site to other parts of the body *palpation:* a digital examination of affected parts of the body

quadrantectomy: a form of lumpectomy that removes more tissue than the usual lumpectomy, leaving little visible scarring but slightly diminishing the size of the affected breast

sonogram: an image of body organs produced through focusing sound waves on the part to be examined

ultrasound: a method of diagnostic imaging that focuses sound waves inaudible to humans on a given organ to produce detailed images of that organ

INDICATIONS AND PROCEDURES

The early indications of breast cancer are often quite subtle, although in this stage it may be revealed by routine mammograms. In some cases, no overt symptoms exist until the cancer is well advanced. Women between forty and fifty years of age without risk factors are advised to have a mammogram every two years. Women over fifty or in the high-risk category because of a family history of breast cancer should have a mammogram once every year. If palpation of the breast reveals a lump, then immediate mammography is indicated.

It is necessary to be constantly vigilant for any sign that an abnormality exists in the breast. Clear indications of possible breast cancer include lumps or thickening of the tissue in the breast or in the area under the arms. Symptoms such as discoloration of the breasts or dimpling, thickening, scaling, or puckering of one or both breasts may also arouse suspicion of breast cancer. A significant change in the shape of the breast or a swelling of it are also symptomatic. A bloody discharge from the nipple, scaly skin on the nipple or surrounding area, inversion of the nipple, or discoloration of the area surrounding the nipple may presage the presence of breast cancer.

Monthly palpation of the breasts, preferably seven or eight days after menstruation, may reveal lumps that could be harmless growths but that might be cancerous. This procedure is referred to as breast self-examination (BSE). Because the female breast contains many glands, it is not uncommon in some women for lumps to appear regularly—often profusely—particularly in the week prior to menstruation. Women with notably lumpy breasts are said to have fibrocystic breasts. Often, the lumps diminish in size in the week following menstruation. If they do not recede, however, then these lumps should be regarded with suspicion and the patient should be examined by a physician, preferably a surgeon, gynecologist, or oncologist.

Once a problem is detected, a number of procedures must be considered for dealing with it. The initial procedure in treating suspected breast cancer usually involves a mammogram to reveal irregularities in the breast. If the results of the mammogram are negative and the patient is still convinced that there is a lump in the breast, an ultrasound or sonographic examination may be indicated. In such tests, harmless sound waves are focused on the breast. These sound waves are reflected so that they create an image of formations within the breast. Although ultrasound cannot definitively indicate whether a lump is cancerous, it can at least verify whether a lump exists. It can also show whether the lump is hollow and filled with fluid, in which case it is usually a benign cyst rather than a cancerous growth.

If a growth is detected, the next, least-invasive means of determining whether it is cancerous is through a needle biopsy. In this procedure, the patient, under local anesthetic, has a hollow needle inserted into the growth. Fluids and cells are then harvested from it. If the growth is a cyst, a clear or light yellow fluid will be withdrawn, causing the cyst to collapse. This may be all the treatment required. In all cases, however, the substances withdrawn from the growth are examined by a pathologist for the presence of cancer cells.

Not all growths are so positioned that needle biopsies are possible. In such cases, a surgical biopsy is probably necessary. If the lump is small, then a lumpectomy, or the removal of the entire lump, may occur. Larger lumps often cannot be removed at this stage, so portions are excised for pathological examination. A pathologist carefully studies the tissue removed to determine whether it contains cancer cells.

In the past, biopsies often occurred while patients were anesthetized and, if the pathological report was positive for cancer, then a radical mastectomy was performed immediately while the patient was still under anesthetic. Since the late twentieth century, however, a two-step procedure has usually replaced this one-step method. If cancer is detected, then surgery is delayed, giving physicians the opportunity to consult with their patients about the treatments available to them.

The major decision in such cases usually is whether a total mastectomy or a partial mastectomy, commonly referred to as a lumpectomy, should be performed. Total mastectomy involves the total removal of the breast and the surrounding lymph nodes.

A radical mastectomy, done under general anesthetic, involves making a large, elliptical incision on the breast, including the nipple and often the entire breast. The incision normally extends into the armpit. All the breast tissue is excised, including the skin and the fat down to the chest muscles. The incision extends into the armpit to remove as much of the breast tissue as possible, including the lymph nodes, which may be cancerous. Once the bleeding has been controlled, a drainage tube is inserted and the incision is closed with sutures, clips, or adhesive substances.

This drastic form of treatment can be traumatic both physically and psychologically to patients. Many women fear the disfigurement that follows it. Some women, especially those with a family history of breast cancer, may decide that the total removal of the breast is their safest option. In some cases, to prevent future threats of breast cancer, they demand the removal of both breasts.

A lumpectomy, usually performed under local anesthetic, involves the removal only of cancerous tissue. The incision is made under the breast, and the lump, with surrounding tissue, is removed. The appearance of the breast remains much the same as it was before the surgery. In some cases, physicians recommend a quadrantectomy, which involves the removal of the cancerous tissue as well as significant amounts of the surrounding tissue. Quite often, the lymph nodes are removed as well. When this treatment is used, the breast will appear slightly smaller than it previously was, but it can be enhanced through plastic surgery.

Subcutaneous mastectomy is frequently indicated in situations where the tumor is small. In this procedure, the surgeon makes an incision under the breast. Most of the skin and the nipple remain intact, although the milk ducts that lead into the nipple are cut. Following the surgery, sometimes immediately, a breast implant can be inserted, restoring the breast to its normal appearance. Mastectomy and lumpectomy are routinely followed by a course of radiation and/or chemotherapy designed to kill any fugitive cancer cells that the surgery has missed.

Mastectomy is done with as little scarring as possible, but considerable scarring may occur, particularly with radical mastectomy, and the absence of one or both breasts usually requires significant psychological adjustments on the part of women who have undergone the procedure. The breast reconstruction performed by a plastic surgeon following a mastectomy is often accompanied by treatment from a psychologist or psychiatrist.

Some women with family histories of breast cancer, particularly if the disease has occurred in first-level relatives (mother or sisters), may opt for a mastectomy rather than a lumpectomy to relieve themselves of the fear of contracting the disease, although most oncologists make such women fully aware of other, less drastic procedures available to them.

Certainly a consideration in reaching a decision about whether to have a lumpectomy or the more drastic mastectomy must include many factors. High on the list of such factors is heredity. In many patients who suffer from this disease, BRCA1, a mutated gene found on chromosome 17, is an early indication that breast cancer may eventually occur. BRCA1 is a gene frequently present in the female members of families with histories of breast cancer and ovarian cancer. About 85 percent of women with the BRCA1 gene will develop breast cancer if they live a normal life span. Women who have the BRCA1 gene may decide to have a prophylactic mastectomy before symptoms occur, although many women in this situation prefer treatment with tamoxifen, which appears to hold breast cancer at bay.

Advances in treating cancers of all kinds progressed rapidly during the last half of the twentieth century, and even greater impetus characterizes current advances. The four major treatments—often used in combination with each other—are surgery, radiation therapy, chemotherapy, and hormonal therapy. In the treatment of breast cancer, radiation may be used initially to shrink existing tumors that, once reduced in size, will be removed surgically. Although, when surgeons remove cancerous tumors, they also remove large numbers of surrounding cells that might be affected, such a procedure is usually followed by additional radiation aimed at killing any lingering cancer cells the surgery has missed.

USES AND COMPLICATIONS

The salient use of surgery in cases of breast cancer is to remove its source, not only clearing away any tumors that may be found but also removing additional cancerous tissue as well as lymph nodes that might be affected.

Cancer cells can exist either in the breast's lobules, which contain the cells that produce milk, or in the ducts that carry the milk to the nipples. Cancer cells in either of these locations can be of two types, invasive or noninvasive (also called in situ). The major complication with invasive cancer is that it can and usually does metastasize, spreading often to the lymph nodes, into the lungs and to other parts of the body. In such cases, a radical mastectomy is indicated. It must be performed as quickly as possible and followed by a strenuous course that typically includes radiation or chemotherapy. Noninvasive cancer is less likely to metastasize, although it sometimes does. Lumpectomy or quadrantectomy is often used to treat such cancers, but these procedures must be followed by close monitoring over the rest of the patient's life and by radiation or chemotherapy following surgery.

Chemotherapy is used less often than radiation in the postsurgical treatment of breast cancer but is occasionally used along with it. Some physicians use anticancer drugs to reduce the possibility of recurrence. This treatment, as well as hormone treatment, is designed to kill any fugitive cancer cells that have strayed from the immediate site of the cancer that has been removed. Whereas surgery and radiation are local, affecting only the part of the body being focused upon, chemotherapy is systemic: The drugs used in chemotherapy travel through the bloodstream to all parts of the body. The disadvantage of chemotherapy is that it nearly always has significant side effects. In rare cases, complications are so extreme that they result in death. Usually, chemotherapy is indicated only for women who have not yet undergone the menopause and whose tumors are an inch or larger in size. It may also be employed in cases in which the patient's tumor shows signs of growing rapidly and aggressively invading and attacking other parts of the body.

Related to chemotherapy is hormonal therapy. Hormones are chemicals produced by the body for various purposes. For example, when one is under sudden, undue stress, the body produces adrenaline, which provides a rush of energy and causes the heartbeat to accelerate. In women, the body produces estrogen every month during the menstrual cycle. Estrogen causes the cells in the milk ducts and lobules to grow in preparation for pregnancy. This chemical stimulates the growth of normal cells but can also stimulate the growth of cancer cells. Hormonal therapy is systemic. It involves introducing into the bloodstream a synthetic chemical, usually tamoxifen, which makes it impossible for the body's natural estrogen to find its way to cancer cells that would be nourished by it. A complete biopsy report can determine whether hormonal therapy is appropriate in individual cases.

PERSPECTIVE AND PROSPECTS

Until the middle of the twentieth century, a diagnosis of cancer, particularly of breast cancer, was viewed as a death sentence. Diagnosis generally occurred after the cancer had metastasized. In the first half of the century, general practitioners were much more prevalent than the specialists who, working as a team, are now generally mustered to provide cancer treatment once a diagnosis is made.

With the proliferation of sophisticated medical equipment, including the highly sensitive X-ray machines used in mammography and the various forms of ultrasound and sonograph equipment that are part of nearly every hospital's arsenal of diagnostic equipment, an increasing number of cancers are discovered before they become symptomatic, so that they can be treated with considerable success.

Historically, mastectomies have been performed for centuries. President John Adams's daughter underwent this excruciating surgery early in the nineteenth century, enduring this procedure without the benefit of anesthesia. As was usually true in such cases, the surgery extended her life for only a little while because her cancer was discovered in an advanced stage and had metastasized.

By the late nineteenth and early twentieth centuries, accepted treatment for breast cancer was a radical mastectomy that involved the removal of the affected breast and of as many surrounding cancer cells and lymph nodes as possible. William Halsted, a pioneer in the field of breast cancer surgery and a professor of surgery at the highly respected Johns Hopkins University Medical School, championed the cause of the radical mastectomy, which he viewed as a procedure that could extend substantially the survival of his patients. Little was said about curing breast cancer patients of their cancers. The radical surgery that physicians across the country performed following Halsted's lead was viewed simply as a means of adding months or years to the life of the cancer patient. Until 1970, about 70 percent of women in the United States who had breast cancer were subjected to radical mastectomy.

Several factors brought about a major change in the treatment of breast cancer during the 1960's and 1970's, when social activism was very much in the forefront of American life. Feminists pointed out that most of the surgeons treating breast cancer were men. As an increasing number of women entered medical schools and eventually established medical practices, greater attention was paid to treating breast cancer in less disfiguring ways than had been common earlier.

Along with this change came advances in medical technology that made early diagnosis and more focused treatment a reality. As the chemical treatment of all cancers came to be better understood and more widely employed, the focus was more on preventing and curing cancer than on merely prolonging the lives of those who suffered from it.

Laboratory tests for detecting a woman's predisposition for breast cancer became increasingly sophisticated and accurate. Where the BRCA1 gene was present, the possibility of developing breast cancer was greatly increased, so that women shown to possess this gene were made more vigilant than ever before in monitoring their conditions and in seeking immediate medical intervention if even the slightest symptom appeared.

Shortly after the end of World War II, some oncologists rejected Halsted's emphasis on radical mastectomy. Surgeon Jerome Urban garnered numerous followers in his call for superradical surgeries in cancer cases. His procedures involved the removal of ribs, various internal organs, and even limbs in order to find and destroy every cancer cell. Surgeon Bernard Fisher stood in opposition to Urban, championing the effectiveness of smaller surgeries, such as the simple mastectomy, which involved the removal of one breast but not of all the lymph nodes and, in some cases, the lumpectomy, involving the removal only of the tumor and its surrounding cells.

The lumpectomy has gained acceptance through the intervening years. It is less disfiguring than either the radical or the simple mastectomy, leaving only a small scar on the underside of the breast. In cases where lumpectomy is viewed as a viable option, survival rates and cure rates are comparable to those of patients who have undergone more radical surgery.

Advances in medical science are accelerating substantially. Stem cell research offers great promise in the treatment and cure of diseases such as breast cancer. Researchers appear to be on the threshold of developing cells designed to destroy specific errant cells, such as those that cause cancer, while leaving healthy cells intact.

—*R. Baird Shuman, Ph.D.*

See also Breast biopsy; Breast cancer; Breast disorders; Breast surgery; Breasts, female; Cancer; Chemotherapy; Gynecology; Malignancy and metastasis; Mammography; Oncology; Plastic surgery; Radiation therapy; Sex change surgery; Tumor removal; Tumors; Women's health.

For Further Information:

Fowble, Barbara, et al. *Breast Cancer Treatment: A Comprehensive Guide to Management.* St. Louis: Mosby Yearbook, 1991. Although the presentations in this book are somewhat outdated, they do offer excellent general information, particularly in regard to specific means of performing breast surgery in minimally disfiguring ways.

Friedewald, Vincent, and Aman U. Buzdar, with Michael Bokulich. *Ask the Doctor: Breast Cancer.* Kansas City, Mo.: Andrews McMeel, 1997. Written at a level that laypersons can easily understand, this comprehensive presentation of causes, treatment, and overall outlook for people suffering from breast cancer is strongly recommended.

Hirshaut, Yashar, and Peter I. Pressman. *Breast Cancer: The Complete Guide.* 4th ed. New York: Bantam Books, 2004. This user-friendly book is thorough and accurate in its presentations of the diagnosis and pathology of breast cancer and in its extensive discussion of various means used to treat it. The chapter entitled "Prognosis" is especially cogent.

Judd, Sandra J., ed. *Breast Cancer Sourcebook: Basic Consumer Health Information About Breast Cancer.* 2d ed. Detroit: Omnigraphics, 2004. One of the most extensive treatments of the topic of breast cancer. Its glossary of terms relating to breast cancer is helpful.

Lange, Vladimir. *Be a Survivor: Your Guide to Breast Cancer Treatment.* Los Angeles: Lange Productions, 1999. Directed toward those who are dealing with breast cancer, this upbeat book focuses on managing the disease with an eye toward survival. It deals with the psychology of breast cancer victims and suggests coping mechanisms. A valuable and encouraging book for those who are in the early stages of dealing with their diagnoses. Its guide to cancer centers around the United States is helpful.

Lerner, Barron H. *The Breast Cancer Wars: Hope, Fear, and the Pursuit of a Cure in Twentieth-Century America.* New York: Oxford University Press, 2001. The author provides a medical and cultural history of how breast cancer was dealt with during the twentieth century. Lerner uses his extensive knowledge of the field to show the progress made over a hundred-year period.

Mayer, Musa. *Examining Myself.* London: Faber & Faber, 1994. This first-person account of a woman who has suffered from breast cancer is well written.

It presents valuable medical information at a level that the average reader will easily comprehend.

Morris, Peter J., and William C. Wood, eds. *Oxford Textbook of Surgery*. 2d ed. 3 vols. New York: Oxford University Press, 2000. Perhaps the most extensive and complete book available on surgery. It deals fully with every surgical aspect of breast cancer.

Phippen, Mark L., and Maryann Papanier Wells, eds. *Patient Care During Operative and Invasive Procedures*. Philadelphia: W. B. Saunders, 2000. Aimed primarily at nurses and other support staff, this book is thorough and offers excellent information about the instruments that must be available to surgeons for various procedures, including radical mastectomy and lumpectomy.

Sproul, Amy, ed. *A Breast Cancer Journey: Your Personal Guidebook*. Atlanta: American Cancer Society, 2001. This authoritative book is particularly valuable for its presentation of the options that breast cancer patients have available to them. The presentation is up to date and timely. Impeccably accurate.

MASTITIS

DISEASE/DISORDER

ANATOMY OR SYSTEM AFFECTED: Breasts, glands
SPECIALTIES AND RELATED FIELDS: Bacteriology, family medicine, gynecology, nutrition, obstetrics
DEFINITION: A bacterial infection of the mammary gland.

CAUSES AND SYMPTOMS

Mastitis is usually caused by a staphylococcal infection of the breast. The bacteria may enter the breast through a sore or crack in the nipple, although some patients do not have sore nipples. Generally, mastitis occurs in breast-feeding mothers, but women who are not breast-feeding may also experience the disease, as do small babies occasionally. Onset of the infection is often associated with stress, reduced immunity, or missed or increased intervals between breast-feedings of a baby.

Common symptoms of mastitis are swelling, redness, hotness, tenderness, an area of hardness, and pain in part or all of the infected breast. In some cases, there is a localized area of soreness in the breast, while in other cases, the entire breast may be inflamed. The victim typically has flulike symptoms, such as tiredness, aches, chills, fever, and fatigue. These feelings often occur prior to breast soreness. If the cause is simple engorgement with breast milk or a plugged duct, then the patient will start feeling better instead of worse.

> ### INFORMATION ON MASTITIS
>
> **CAUSES:** Bacterial infection (usually staphylococcal) typically through cracks in nipples during breast-feeding; also, engorgement with breast milk or plugged duct
> **SYMPTOMS:** Breast swelling, redness, hotness, tenderness, hard area, pain; typically begins with flulike symptoms (tiredness, aches, chills, fever, fatigue)
> **DURATION:** Two to five days for bacterial infection; one to two days for blocked duct
> **TREATMENTS:** Alternate hot and cold packs, gentle massage, acetaminophen or ibuprofen for fever; continued breast-feeding; antibiotics if necessary (cephalexin, cloxacillin, erythromycin, flucloxacillin)

Blocked ducts usually resolve themselves naturally within twenty-four to forty-eight hours, although a blocked duct may sometimes lead to mastitis.

TREATMENT AND THERAPY

Alternate hot and cold packs applied to the sore area of the infected breast help reduce the inflammation and pain and provide comfort. Gently massaging the tender area increases circulation and helps loosen any plugged ducts. Fever can be treated with acetaminophen or ibuprofen without any harm to a breast-feeding baby. Patients should also drink plenty of fluids. For nursing mothers, unless the pain is too intense, breast-feeding should be continued during the treatment of mastitis. If breast-feeding is discontinued, then the breast should be drained regularly with a breast pump.

Once a diagnosis of mastitis is made, proper antibiotics should be administered, if necessary. Cephalexin, cloxacillin, erythromycin, and flucloxacillin are effective drugs against the staphylococcus bacteria. Once they are administered, the soreness usually starts to disappear within two to five days. Redness may continue for up to a week or more. Bed rest helps relieve stress and builds up the immune system. If not treated properly and in a timely manner, mastitis can lead to a breast abscess that requires surgical draining.

PERSPECTIVE AND PROSPECTS

Mastitis is most common among nursing mothers during the first three months postpartum. The most important preventive measure against mastitis for these women is regular breast-feeding. Recurrent mastitis is associated with irregular breast-feeding patterns, fatigue, and stress. Frequent breast-feeding and lifestyle changes that promote good health and a strengthened immune system are key ingredients for reducing the occurrence of mastitis.

If antibiotics are prescribed for treatment, it is important that the full course be taken even though the patient improves quickly; otherwise, the risk of mastitis returning increases. Two newer drugs, clindamycin and ciprofloxacin, have proven effective in treating mastitis if the patient is allergic to penicillin-derived medication.

—*Alvin K. Benson, Ph.D.*

See also Abscess drainage; Abscesses; Antibiotics; Bacterial infections; Breast biopsy; Breast disorders; Breast-feeding; Breasts, female; Hormones; Mammography; Women's health.

FOR FURTHER INFORMATION:

Colson, Jenni Lynn, ed. *Breastfeeding Sourcebook.* Detroit: Omnigraphics, 2002.

Icon Health. *Mastitis: A Medical Dictionary, Bibliography, and Annotated Research Guide to Internet References.* San Diego, Calif.: Author, 2004.

Marz, Russell B. *Medical Nutrition from Marz.* 2d ed. Portland, Oreg.: Quiet Lion Press, 1999.

Reddy, Pavani. "Postpartum Mastitis and Community-Acquired Methicillin-Resistant *Staphylococcus aureus.*" *Emerging Infectious Diseases* 13, no. 2 (February 1, 2007): 298.

Swenson, Deborah E. *Telephone Triage for the Obstetric Patient: A Nursing Guide.* Philadelphia: W. B. Saunders, 2001.

MASTURBATION

DEVELOPMENT

ANATOMY OR SYSTEM AFFECTED: Genitals
SPECIALTIES AND RELATED FIELDS: Psychiatry
DEFINITION: A manual stimulation of one's own or another person's genital organs usually resulting in orgasm without engaging in sexual intercourse.

PHYSICAL AND PSYCHOLOGICAL FACTORS

Masturbation is the first sexual experience among a great majority of people. Some young people inadvertently stumble on sexual arousal and orgasm in the course of engaging in some other physical activity. Others purposefully stimulate themselves, aroused by curiosity after reading erotic literature, watching sexually explicit films, or listening to imaginary or real sexual adventures of their peers.

Most men and women practice masturbation to relieve sexual tension, achieve sexual pleasure, enjoy sexual stimulation in the absence of an available partner, and experience relaxation. When masturbating, men tend to focus on the stimulation of the penis. Stimulation of the clitoral shaft and clitoral area with a hand or an object is the method that women most commonly employ. Some women masturbate by using a vibrator. Mutual masturbation provides a satisfying and pleasurable form of sexual intimacy and release for many couples. It is also one of the most common techniques that gay and lesbian couples use during sexual intimacy.

DISORDERS AND EFFECTS

Under certain circumstances, masturbation may result in some undesirable consequences. If a child masturbates constantly, it may be an indication of excessive anxiety and tension. Compulsive and frenzied masturbation may reflect abuse or maltreatment in a child's home life. Frequent masturbation may be a child's way of relieving tension or unconsciously re-enacting past or present traumatic sexual episodes. Among adults, excessive masturbation may point toward a person's lack of self-esteem and the resultant fear and inability to develop healthy interpersonal relationships with persons of the opposite sex. Psychiatry, psychotherapy, and sex therapy have proven helpful in successfully alleviating these problems.

PERSPECTIVE AND PROSPECTS

Throughout history, attitudes toward the practice of masturbation have been riddled with misconceptions, guilt, and fear. Fear of masturbation and its supposed harmful effects, such as loss of memory and intelligence, was widespread in the nineteenth century. Semen was considered a vital fluid important for bodily functioning, and wasting it through masturbation was considered as contributing to weakening of the body and production of illness. Medical authorities today do not find any evidence of physical damage from masturbation. In fact, many modern sex therapists encourage self-stimulation as part of healthy sexuality. In modern sex therapy, masturbation has become part of the therapeutics used in treating certain sexual dysfunctions. Patients with difficulties or inability to have orgasm are encouraged by their therapists to engage in masturbation. It is widely believed that orgasm once achieved through masturbation will eventually generalize and transfer to satisfactory sexual intercourse.

—*Tulsi B. Saral, Ph.D.*

See also Aphrodisiacs; Domestic violence; Puberty and adolescence; Reproductive system; Sexual dysfunction; Sexuality.

FOR FURTHER INFORMATION:

Bockting, Walter, and Eli Coleman, eds. *Masturbation as a Means of Achieving Sexual Health.* New York: Haworth Press, 2003.

Dodson, Betty. *Sex for One: The Joy of Selfloving.* New York: Harmony Books, 1996.

Laqueur, Thomas Walter. *Solitary Sex: A Cultural History of Masturbation.* New York: Zone Books, 2003.

Marcus, Irwin M., and John J. Francis, eds. *Masturbation: From Infancy to Senescence.* New York: International Universities Press, 1975.

Rowan, Edward L. *The Joy of Self-Pleasuring: Why Feel Guilty About Feeling Good?* Amherst, Mass.: Prometheus Books, 2000.

Sarnoff, Suzanne, and Irving Sarnoff. *Masturbation and Adult Sexuality.* Bridgewater, N.J.: Replica Books, 2001.

MEASLES

DISEASE/DISORDER

ALSO KNOWN AS: Morbilli, rubeola

ANATOMY OR SYSTEM AFFECTED: Ears, lungs, mouth, nervous system, respiratory system, skin

SPECIALTIES AND RELATED FIELDS: Family medicine, internal medicine, pediatrics, public health, virology

DEFINITION: A highly contagious disease contracted through a virus transmitted in respiratory secretions and characterized by a spreading skin rash.

KEY TERMS:

desquamation: the sloughing off of the outer layers of skin

Koplik's spots: small red spots with white centers generally found in the mouth during early stages of measles

maculopapular rash: reddish skin eruptions characterized by small, flat discolorations that may progress into small pimples

otitis media: infection or inflammation of the middle ear, an occasional complication of measles infection

paramyxoviruses: a group of ribonucleic acid (RNA) viruses that includes the etiological agents for measles, mumps, and a variety of respiratory infections

pharyngitis: infection or inflammation of the pharynx, or throat

photophobia: abnormal sensitivity of the eyes to light, a condition common to a variety of illnesses, including measles

prodromal stage: the early stage of a disease during which symptoms first appear

viremia: a condition characterized by the presence of a virus in the bloodstream

CAUSES AND SYMPTOMS

Measles is a highly contagious viral disease characterized by a maculopapular (pimply) rash that develops on the skin and spreads rapidly over much of the cutaneous surface of the body. Measles virus is classified with the paramyxoviruses, a class of viruses in which ribonucleic acid (RNA) serves as the genetic material. Closely related viruses in the same group include rinderpest and distemper virus, agents associated with disease in ruminants such as cows and in dogs or cats, respectively. It is likely that measles originated when one of these other animal viruses became adapted to humans several thousand years ago.

In modern times but before the advent of measles vaccination, measles was a common disease of childhood, usually appearing between the ages of five and ten. The illness is among the most contagious of infections, and the virus was generally spread among children in schools. Widespread immunization of children, begun in the 1960's, tended to push the age of exposure into the teenage years. Most outbreaks since the 1980's have occurred among college students. Since recovery from the disease confers lifelong immunity, infection among older adults is infrequent. In developing or Third World nations, places where vaccination may be haphazard, measles is still a disease of early childhood; malnutrition and related problems of poverty have resulted in a significant level of mortality among infected children.

Exposure generally follows an oral-oral means of transmission, as the person inhales contaminated droplets from an infected individual. The incubation period for active measles ranges from seven to fourteen days. During this early stage, the infected individual becomes increasingly contagious. The lack of any obvious symptoms during these early stages lends itself to the spread of the disease.

Contact by the virus with the surface cells of the respiratory passages, or sometimes the conjunctiva (the outer surface of the eye), allows the infectious agent to enter the body. The virus spreads through the local lymph nodes into the blood, producing a primary viremia. During this period, the virus replicates both in the lymph nodes and in the respiratory sites through which the virus entered the body. The virus returns to the bloodstream, resulting in a secondary viremia and widespread passage of the virus throughout the body by the fifth to seventh day after the initial exposure. Viral levels in the blood reach their peak toward the end of the incubation period, some fourteen days after infection. Once symptoms begin, the virus is widely disseminated throughout the body, including sites in small blood vessels, lymph nodes, and even the central nervous system.

The initial incubation period is followed by a prodromal stage, in which active symptoms appear. This stage is characterized by a fever that may reach as high as 103 degrees Fahrenheit, coughing, sensitivity of the eyes to light (photophobia), and malaise. Koplik's spots appear on the buccal mucosa in the mouth one to two days prior to development of the characteristic measles rash.

The maculopapular rash first appears on the head and behind the ears and gradually spreads over the rest of the body during the course of twenty-four to forty-eight hours. Clear signs of respiratory infection appear, including a cough, pharyngitis, and occasional involvement of the bronchioles or even pneumonia. While malaise and anorexia (appetite loss) are common during the fever period, diarrhea and vomiting generally do not occur. Over time, the rash becomes increasingly dense, exhibiting a blotchy character. Desquamation is common in many affected areas of the skin. Gradually, over a period of three to five days, the rash begins to fade, usually following the sequence by which it first appeared. The rash fades first on the forehead, then on the extremities.

Complications, while they do occur, are unusual in otherwise healthy individuals. Most result from secondary bacterial infections. Occasionally, these complications may manifest themselves as infections of the ear. Pulmonary infections are common among cases of measles and account for most of the rare deaths that follow development of the disease. Photophobia is also common, accounting for the former belief that measles patients had to be kept in a dark room; as long as the patient is comfortable, this step is unnecessary.

The obvious manifestations of measles infection make the isolation of the virus unnecessary for diagnosis. Ironically, the near disappearance of measles in the United States has made most physicians unfamiliar with the disease; it is not unusual for an attending physician to mistake the rash for another illness. For this reason, laboratory diagnosis is often useful. Laboratory confirmation is generally based on a serological assay for measles antibodies in the blood of infected persons.

A rare sequela to measles infection is the development of subacute sclerosing panencephalitis, a disease characterized by progressive neurological deterioration. The specific mechanism by which measles infection may develop into this disease remains unclear, but it may be the result of a rare combination of events in the victim. Since spread of the virus into the central nervous system is common during measles infection whereas the development of subacute sclerosing panencephalitis is rare (approximately one case per 100,000 measles infections), it is likely that some form of immune impairment is at the root of this disease. Diagnosis of subacute sclerosing panencephalitis is difficult and is based on developing dementia accompanied by unusual levels of measles antibodies in cerebrospinal fluid.

TREATMENT AND THERAPY

No specific treatment for measles is available; therapy consists of symptomatic intervention. Bed rest is recommended, and the patient should not come into contact with persons not previously exposed to the virus through either natural infection or immunization.

Itching of the rash is common and may be treated with cool water or the standard regimen of cornstarch or baking soda applications. The most common complications result from secondary bacterial infections, which generally take the form of otitis media (middle-ear infection), pharyngitis, or pneumonia. Appropriate use of antibiotics is usually sufficient to prevent or treat such complications.

Immunization with the measles virus may be either passive or active. Children less than one year of age and patients who are immunocompromised or chronically ill may be protected if human immunoglobulin is administered within a week after exposure. While effective immunity is short term, it is capable of protecting these individuals during this period. Since no active disease or infection develops, however, immunity to future infection remains minimal in these cases.

During the early 1960's, an effective vaccine was developed to immunize children against measles. The vaccine consists of an attenuated form of the virus. Although early forms of the vaccine were inconsistent in producing a lifelong immunity, they were effective in decreasing the prevalence of the disease. Later generations of the attenuated vaccine proved more effective in developing long-term immunity among the recipients.

Since maternal antibodies are present in newborns, it is recommended that measles immunization begin between twelve and fifteen months of age. Often, this program is part of a combination MMR vaccine, for measles, mumps, and rubella (German measles). A second booster is given following elementary school. The American Academy of Pediatrics does not consider a third vaccination to be necessary if the approved routine has been followed. It is recommended that children who were first immunized prior to their first birthday should receive boosters at fifteen months of age and again at age twelve. Indications are that immunity from vaccination is long term, if not lifelong. Recovery from natural infection results in a lifelong immunity to measles.

Inconsistency of the first generation of vaccine resulted in ineffective immunity among some individuals vaccinated during the 1960's. A number of small outbreaks during the 1980's were the result. Most cases of measles, however, have occurred in individuals who failed to be immunized.

PERSPECTIVE AND PROSPECTS

The origin and early history of measles is uncertain, as the first authentic description of measles as a specific entity was that by the Arab physician al-Razi (Rhazes) in a 910 treatise on smallpox and measles. Rhazes quoted earlier work by the Hebrew physician El Yehudi, so it is likely that familiarity with these respective illnesses had existed for some time.

Measles is entirely a human disease, with no known animal reservoir. Consequently, the paucity of human populations of sufficient size to maintain transmission means that the spread of such an epidemic disease would have been unlikely before 2500 B.C.E. It is probable that the disease entered the human species through adaptation of the similar animal viruses of rinderpest or distemper. The absence of any description of a disease like measles in the writings of Hippocrates (c. fourth century B.C.E.) likewise renders it unlikely that the disease was widespread before that date.

Epidemic disease with a rash characteristic of measles is known to have spread through the Roman Empire during the early centuries of the common era. The difficulty in differentiating measles from smallpox by the physicians of the time contributes to the difficulty in understanding the history of the illness. It is certain that by the time of Rhazes, measles had become common in the population.

The terminology of measles lent further confusion during the Middle Ages. Measles was often referred to as *morbilli*, a Latin term meaning "little disease," to distinguish it from *il morbo*, or plague. The word "measles" first appeared in the fourteenth century treatise *Rosa Anglica*, by John of Gaddesden. The term may have been applied initially to the sores on the legs of lepers (*mesles*), and it was only later that illnesses char-

A child with measles. (CDC/Barbara Rice)

acterized by similar rashes (measles, smallpox, and rubella) were clearly differentiated by European physicians. The significance of a rash with a white center in the mouth was probably recognized by John Quier in Jamaica and Richard Haxeltine in New England during the latter portion of the eighteenth century, but it was in 1896 that the American pediatrician Henry Koplik firmly reported its role in early stages of the disease.

Measles followed the path of European explorers to the Americas during the sixteenth century. Repeated outbreaks of measles devastated the native populations, which had minimal immunity to the newly introduced disease. The most thorough epidemiological investigation of measles newly introduced into a population was that by Peter Panum in his study *Observations Made During the Epidemic of Measles on the Faroe Islands in the Year 1846* (1940). In the population of 7,864 persons, 6,100 became ill, with 102 deaths. Mortality rates as high as 25 percent were not unusual in previously unexposed populations. In Hawaii in 1848, 40,000 deaths occurred among the population of 150,000 persons following the introduction of measles. Even higher mortality rates probably occurred among the populations of Peru and Mexico in 1530-1531, following their exposure to infected Spanish explorers.

The earliest attempt at immunization was probably that of Francis Home of Edinburgh in 1758. Home soaked cotton in the blood of measles patients and placed it on the small cuts on the skin of children. The viral nature of measles was first demonstrated by John Anderson and Joseph Goldberger of the United States Public Health Service, who in 1911 induced the disease in monkeys using filtered extracts from human tissue. In 1954, the virus itself was isolated by John Enders, who grew the agent in human and monkey tissue in a laboratory.

The first effective vaccine was developed by Enders in 1958 using an attenuated (live) form of the virus. The vaccine was tested and then licensed in 1963. Several variations of the vaccine that proved superior in producing long-term immunity were developed in the decades that followed. In 1974, the World Health Organization introduced a widespread vaccination program within developing countries.

The absence of any natural reservoir for measles other than humans has made the eradication of the disease possible. Active immunization of children in the United States reduced the annual incidence of the disease from 482,000 reported cases in 1962 to fewer than

1,000 in the late 1990's. Widespread vaccination and worldwide surveillance has made global eradication of the disease a realistic possibility.

—Richard Adler, Ph.D.

See also Childhood infectious diseases; Fever; Immunization and vaccination; Mumps; Rashes; Rubella; Viral infections.

For Further Information:

American Medical Association. *American Medical Association Family Medical Guide*. 4th rev. ed. Hoboken, N.J.: John Wiley & Sons, 2004. An excellent general source for information about illnesses and questions about medical problems.

Bernstein, David, and Gilbert Schiff. "Viral Exanthems and Localized Skin Infections." In *Infectious Diseases*, edited by Sherwood L. Gorbach, John G. Bartlett, and Neil R. Blacklow. Philadelphia: W. B. Saunders, 2004. This book contains extensive discussions of bacterial and viral illnesses. The section addressing measles contains much information about the symptoms and progression of the disease.

Biddle, Wayne. *A Field Guide to Germs*. 2d ed. New York: Anchor Books, 2002. This comprehensive book is easily accessible to the nonspecialist and includes a discussion of nearly every virus, bacterium, and fungus known to cause human and nonhuman animal disease. The history of the microbe and the treatment of diseases are included.

Kiple, Kenneth F., ed. *The Cambridge World History of Human Disease*. New York: Cambridge University Press, 1993. In addition to being an encyclopedia describing human diseases, this book provides an epidemiological history of disease and discusses possible origins and treatments. The authors target a general population.

Madigan, Michael T., and John M. Martinko. *Brock Biology of Microorganisms*. 11th ed. Upper Saddle River, N.J.: Pearson Prentice Hall, 2006. A college textbook on the subject of microbiology. An extensive section on microbial diseases provides a concise description of measles and its prevention.

Wagner, Edward K., and Martinez J. Hewlett. *Basic Virology*. 2d ed. Malden, Mass.: Blackwell Science, 2004. A very readable undergraduate text covering issues of virology and viral disease, properties of viruses and virus-cell interaction, working with viruses, and replication patterns of specific viruses.

Woolf, Alan D., et al., eds. *The Children's Hospital Guide to Your Child's Health and Development*.

Cambridge, Mass.: Perseus, 2002. An authoritative and comprehensive guide to children's health, providing a guide to every common illness or condition that affects children and a carefully designed emergency section.

MEDICARE
PROGRAM
DEFINITION: A federal health insurance program for persons over sixty-five, persons with end-stage renal disease, and some disabled individuals. Medicare is part of the Social Security system, and participation is closely tied to Social Security eligibility.

KEY TERMS:

beneficiary: the person who receives the benefits of an insurance policy; for health insurance, the beneficiary is the patient receiving health care

coinsurance: an arrangement in which a percentage of the total bill for health services is paid by the insurer and the rest is paid by the beneficiary

deductible: the amount that the patient must pay before the insurance pays any amount

managed care organization: a health care organization that combines the functions of insurer and provider; it reduces redundancy of services and uses primary care providers as gatekeepers to reduce cost

medically necessary: services and supplies that are appropriate and needed for the diagnosis or treatment of the person's medical condition

Medicare Trust Fund: accumulated contributions from Social Security payroll taxes that are used to pay for the Medicare program

premiums: periodic payments for insurance coverage

primary care provider: a doctor or nurse practitioner who is trained to provide basic medical care

skilled nursing care: a level of care that requires the skills of a registered nurse

INTRODUCTION

Medicare is a federal health insurance program for individuals who are sixty-five or older, persons who have end-stage renal disease (irreversible kidney failure), and some individuals who have disabilities. In addition to age and special conditions, eligible individuals or their spouses must have been employed for at least ten years in a job where they paid Social Security payroll taxes and must be citizens or permanent residents of the United States. Medicare was passed into law as Title XVIII of the Social Security Act of 1965. The intent of the Medicare law was to provide financial protection to elderly individuals against the high cost of illness and hospitalization.

In 2002, more than forty million Americans were covered by Medicare services, making it the largest health insurance program in the United States. Medicare is administered through the Centers for Medicare and Medicaid Services (CMS), formerly the Health Care Financing Administration (HCFA). CMS is an agency of the Social Security Administration within the Department of Health and Human Services (DHHS).

Medicare is financed through a combination of Social Security payroll tax, premiums, and general revenue funds. Services for the Original Medicare Plan are available nationwide, and the insured person can go to any provider that accepts Medicare. The original program operates in the same way as other fee-for-service medical insurance plans, which means the insured person is charged a fee each time that person receives health care services. The person providing the service files a claim for payment. These fees, or claims, are paid fully or partially by Medicare. The Social Security Administration does not pay the claims directly; it has contractual arrangements with private insurance organizations that handle all payments. Fiscal intermediaries process claims from hospitals and other inpatient facilities, and carriers process claims from physicians and suppliers.

CMS has the responsibility to interpret and clarify the provisions of the laws and regulations governing Medicare. Its responsibility includes making determinations as to whether a particular service will be approved for payment by Medicare. However, the majority of decisions about whether a specific type of service will be covered are made at the local level by the fiscal intermediaries or carriers who process claims.

The structure of the Medicare program has remained basically unchanged since its inception. There are two parts to the Original Medicare Plan: Part A and Part B. Part A, called Hospital Insurance (HI), pays for inpatient services. Most people do not pay for Medicare Part A; it is financed through the Social Security payroll taxes that are earmarked for the Medicare Trust Fund. At age sixty-five, individuals receive Part A automatically if they are already receiving Social Security retirement benefits or retirement benefits through the Railroad Retirement Board, or if they are eligible to receive either of these benefits but have not yet filed for them. Individuals who had Medicare-covered government employment also receive Part A without paying premiums, as do their spouses. Individuals under sixty-five can receive Part A benefits without paying if they have had Social Security or Railroad Retirement Board disability benefits for twenty-four months. Other individuals entitled to Part A benefits without paying are those with end-stage renal disease (ESRD) who are receiving kidney dialysis or who have had a kidney transplant.

Part A benefits include a semiprivate room, in a hospital or skilled nursing facility, with related services and supplies including laboratory and diagnostic procedures, nursing care, surgical care, and rehabilitative services. Skilled nursing home services are paid for after the person has been hospitalized for three days for a related health condition. Medicare pays for medications given to the patient while in the hospital or skilled nursing facility. In situations of medical necessity, a private room is allowed. Part A pays for part-time skilled nursing care in the home, as well as for physical, occupational, and speech-language therapy. Hospice care for people with a terminal illness is paid for through Part A. Hospice care includes medical and support services such as drugs for the control of pain or other symptoms and skilled nursing care.

Part B, called Supplemental Medical Insurance (SMI), pays for outpatient services, including services from primary care providers, specialist physicians, clinical psychologists, and social workers. Part B also pays for outpatient mental health services, surgical services and supplies, diagnostic tests, procedures, outpatient therapies, and durable medical equipment such as canes, wheelchairs, walkers, and oxygen-delivery equipment. These services and supplies are covered when they are medically necessary. Medicare helps pay for ambulance services when other sources of transportation would endanger the person's health, artificial limbs and prosthetic devices, braces, chiropractic services, emergency care, immunosuppressive drugs for patients who have undergone organ transplantation, kidney dialysis, nutritional therapy services for diabetics or patients with ESRD, and telemedicine in rural areas. Medicare pays for approved medications that are administered as part of physicians' services.

Preventive services are also covered under Part B. These preventive services are bone density tests, colorectal cancer screening, diabetes services and supplies, glaucoma screening, mammography, clinical breast examinations, Pap smears and pelvic examinations, prostate cancer screening, and vaccinations. Rules apply as to who qualifies and the frequency of these services.

Under the Original Medicare Plan, neither Part A nor Part B will pay for any of the following: services that Medicare does not consider medically necessary, private-duty nursing, routine physical examinations, dental care or dentures, custodial care (basic maintenance care such as bathing and feeding), hearing aids and hearing examinations, outpatient medications (with some limited exceptions), cosmetic surgery, glasses (except following cataract surgery), orthopedic shoes, or alternative medicine such as acupuncture. Medicare does not pay for medical services outside the United States (with some very limited exceptions).

A provider or supplier must inform the beneficiary if a specific service will likely not be paid for by Medicare. If the person still chooses to receive the service, the person will be asked to sign an advance beneficiary notice (ABN). By signing the ABN, the person is agreeing to pay out-of-pocket if Medicare does not pay.

Part B is optional, and individuals have a choice of whether to enroll in Part B at the same time that they enroll in Part A. Most people do have to pay for coverage under Part B. In 2000, approximately 75 percent of eligible seniors had Part B. Approximately one-fourth of the total cost for these services is financed through premiums, and the remainder is financed through general federal revenue funds. The charge for the premium is adjusted yearly; in 2007, the monthly premium for Part B was $93.50, which is deducted from the person's Social Security, railroad retirement, or civil service retirement check. If individuals do not receive a retirement check, then Medicare bills them for the Part B premiums on a quarterly basis. Eligible persons can postpone enrolling in Part B if they or their spouses are working and have group health insurance through their employment. However, if they do not have group health insurance and delay enrolling in Part B, then their monthly payments will be increased by 10 percent for every year that they did not enroll but could have done so.

For services under both Part A and Part B, the insured person is responsible for paying the deductible, coinsurance, and copayment. The deductible for Part B is $131 per year. As an example, a patient has surgery on January 2 costing $531. Since he has not paid his deductible for the year, he must first pay that amount ($131); then Medicare pays its share, which is usually 80 percent, of the remaining amount ($320). The patient pays the remainder ($80). One exception to the usual 20 percent paid by beneficiaries is in the case of outpatient mental health services, in which beneficiaries pay 50 percent of the fees.

Private insurance can be purchased separately to help pay coinsurance amounts, deductibles, and other out-of-pocket expenses for individuals who have the Original Medicare Plan. They are called Medigap policies, since they are used to fill the gaps in the Original Medicare Plan. Medigap policies are regulated by federal and state laws. There are ten standard plans referred to as Plans A through J, each of which has a different set of benefits. Some Medigap policies pay a portion of prescription medication fees.

In 2007, Medicare Part A had a $992 deductible for a hospital stay for each benefit period. A benefit period begins the day the person becomes an inpatient in either a hospital or a skilled nursing facility and ends when the person has not received inpatient care for sixty consecutive days. If the person is hospitalized after one benefit period has ended, then a new benefit period begins. In 2007, for each benefit period the costs were an initial deductible of $992 for days one through sixty and $248 per day for days sixty-one through ninety. After ninety days, the person can use lifetime reserve days, which means that Medicare will pay all covered costs, except for a coinsurance payment of $496 a day, for up to sixty days. These reserve days can be used only once during the person's lifetime. For care in a skilled nursing facility, for each benefit period the beneficiary pays nothing for the first twenty days, up to $124 per day for days twenty-one through one hundred, and all costs after one hundred days.

Medicare beneficiaries sometimes have additional health care coverage that pays bills first, then Medicare pays the remainder; this is called Medicare Secondary Payer. Examples of primary payers are veterans' benefits, workers' compensation, union health coverage, or employer-sponsored insurance. In order to conserve Medicare funds, the Coordination of Benefits program monitors and manages the payment process when beneficiaries have more than one policy.

Physician services and supplies will cost more if the physician or supplier does not accept assignment. Assignment is an agreement from a physician, other health care provider, or supplier of medical equipment whereby they accept the Medicare-approved fee as full payment for rendered services. The approved fee is the cost that has been established by Medicare as reasonable for the particular service. Even if the physician or other providers do not accept assignment, a maximum is placed on what they can charge, called the limiting charge. The maximum, or limit, is 15 percent over Medicare's approved amount.

To reflect the changes occurring in health care delivery, Medicare law was amended in 1997 to allow beneficiaries to choose among several different health insurance plans based on their needs. The Original Medicare Plan remained as it was originally implemented. Another option, Medicare+Choice, enables beneficiaries to enroll in a managed care plan or private fee-for-service plan. In managed care plans, a specified group of providers render services to all members enrolled in the plan. All Medicare+Choice plans must include services covered by Parts A and B of the Original Medicare Plan. These plans can also provide additional services such as prescription medication, dental care, preventive care, and glasses. The cost for additional services depends on the specific plan. With Medicare private fee-for-service plans, no restriction is placed on which providers the beneficiary can use for services, as long as the provider is willing to accept the plan's payment. Under these plans, the beneficiary may be required to pay a premium, in addition to what is paid for Part B, and a copayment when services are rendered.

In order to enroll in a Medicare+Choice program, the individual must have Part A and B of the Original Medicare Plan, live in an area where a particular plan is available, and not have ESRD. Medicare pays a determined amount of money monthly to these private plans for beneficiaries' coverage. In 2002, 11 percent of Medicare beneficiaries were enrolled in a Medicare+Choice plan.

All Medicare beneficiaries, regardless of the type of plan, have the right to appeal a decision related to the amount of payment for a service, whether a particular service or item should be covered, or the length of time that a service should be provided. After filing an appeal, the beneficiary must receive a response within seventy-two hours if a delay would cause medical harm.

In addition to the right to appeal decisions, beneficiaries have a right to information, to know their treatment choices and be involved in treatment decisions, to file complaints, and to nondiscriminatory treatment that reflects sensitivity to cultural differences. Medicare is required by law to protect the privacy of medical information as set forth in the Health Insurance Portability and Accountability Act (HIPAA) of 1996.

If a person qualifies for Medicare but cannot afford to pay for Medicare deductibles and coinsurance, that person may be eligible for the Medicare Savings Programs available through the State Medical Assistance Office. If the person's income and resources are severely limited, then the individual may qualify for Medicaid in addition to Medicare.

In 2000, Medicare expenditures were $131.1 billion for Part A and $90.7 billion for Part B. Since 1965, benefits have expanded, and there has been an increase in both expenditures per person and the number of beneficiaries in the program. These factors have caused continuing concern in Congress regarding the cost and financing of Medicare. Cost-containment measures over the years have included instituting a prospective payment system for hospitals, nursing home care, and home care; providing more options through managed care organization; and shifting services previously covered by Part A to Part B.

PERSPECTIVE AND PROSPECTS

In June, 2003, both houses of Congress passed bills to amend Medicare to include coverage for prescription medications and give individuals more choice in the selection of health insurance plans. These bills reflected Congress's attempt to monitor and improve the quality of health care services for Medicare recipients while maintaining the integrity of the Medicare Trust Fund. The resulting Part D drug benefit received mixed reviews.

—*Roberta Tierney, M.S.N., J.D., A.P.N.*

See also Aging: Extended care; American Medical Association (AMA); Geriatrics and gerontology; Hospice; Hospitals; Terminally ill: Extended care.

FOR FURTHER INFORMATION:

Blevins, Sue A. *Medicare's Midlife Crisis.* Washington, D.C.: Cato Institute, 2001. The author provides a history of government-sponsored health insurance, the background leading to the passage of Medicare, the cost trends of Medicare, and the ongoing effort to maintain a sound and responsive program.

Medicare: The Official Government Site for People with Medicare. http://www.medicare.gov/. Provides information on the quality of care provided by health care facilities approved by Medicare.

Rettenmaier, Andrew J., and Thomas R. Saving. *The Economics of Medicare Reform.* Kalamazoo, Mich.: W. E. Upjohn Institute for Employment Research, 2000. An in-depth discussion of health insurance financing; examines present costs and alternative methods of financing as applied to the Medicare program.

U.S. Department of Health and Human Services. Centers for Medicare and Medicaid Services. *Medicare*

and You 2007. Washington, D.C.: Author, 2007. Updated yearly, this easy-to-understand booklet provides information about enrollment, coverage, options, and contact persons. Essential reading for anyone who is, or may be, eligible for Medicare benefits. Also available at http://www.medicare.gov/publications/pubs/pdf/10050.pdf.

MEDITATION

TREATMENT

ANATOMY OR SYSTEM AFFECTED: All

SPECIALTIES AND RELATED FIELDS: Alternative medicine, preventive medicine

DEFINITION: Techniques involving controlled breathing, visualization, and repeated words or phrases that are used to achieve relaxation and reduce muscle tension, which may have health benefits.

INDICATIONS AND PROCEDURES

One of the most popular techniques used in meditation is concentration, in which one focuses attention on a single object such as the function of breathing, a candle flame, or a visualized image. When attention wanders, the practitioner brings it gently back to the original focus. Sometimes a mantra, a chosen word or phrase given by a teacher or chosen by the practitioner, is repeated silently or aloud. Mantras are central to the practice of meditation. A typical mantra is the om mantra of Tibetan Buddhism.

Guided imagery utilizes listening to a voice, taped or live, that guides the practitioner to visualize a beautiful and peaceful place, where one feels calm and secure. Walking or dancing meditation focuses on movement and ritual, and the practice of yoga incorporates breathing and movement or physical postures to help relax body and mind. Soothing music may also be used with any of the techniques. Teachers recommend starting slowly with five-minute sessions, working up to twenty minutes once or twice a day.

USES AND COMPLICATIONS

Meditation techniques, which are thousands of years old, are being promoted as a benefit to health and well-being, primarily in stress-related conditions. Meditation traditionally has been and is used in a religious sense to deepen one's understanding and involvement with the spiritual, mystical, and sacred aspects of life. It is also used as an exercise in self-discovery and revelation, helping the practitioner turn inward, temporarily shutting out worldly cares and strife to find inner peace and calm. Being religious, however, is not essential to meditation; in fact, anyone can learn the techniques and reap the health benefits of this age-old practice.

Numerous studies confirm that prolonged or interpersonal stress can produce such conditions as constriction of blood vessels, pain and swelling in joints, suppression of the immune system, decreases in white blood cells and changes in their function, and high cholesterol levels. Chemicals such as adrenaline, produced when the body is under stress, can raise blood pressure, increase heart rate, and cause other harmful physiological responses when stress is persistent or sustained. Stress is also linked to many diseases and conditions, including heart attacks, diabetes, cancer, allergies, and skin disorders.

Meditation, in helping the patient to relax, reduces muscle tension and decreases the release of these harmful chemicals. A number of stress-related conditions have been shown to benefit from meditation, including chronic pain, arthritis, infertility, psoriasis, respiratory conditions such as asthma and emphysema, premenstrual syndrome (PMS), tension headaches, irritable bowel syndrome (IBS), ulcers, insomnia, and fibromyalgia.

—Martha Oehmke Loustaunau, Ph.D.

See also Alternative medicine; Anxiety; Biofeedback; Hypnosis; Stress; Stress reduction; Yoga.

FOR FURTHER INFORMATION:

Benson, Herbert, and Miriam Z. Klipper. *The Relaxation Response*. Updated and expanded ed. New York: Avon Books, 2000.

Harmon, Robert, and Mary Ann Myers. "Prayer and Meditation as Medical Therapies." *Physical Medicine and Rehabilitation Clinics of North America* 10, no. 3 (August, 1999): 651-662.

Kabat-Zinn, Jon. *Wherever You Go, There You Are: Mindfulness Meditation in Everyday Life*. 10th anniversary ed. New York: Hyperion, 2005.

Trivieri, Larry, Jr., and John W. Anderson, eds. *Alternative Medicine: The Definitive Guide*. 2d ed. Berkeley, Calif.: Ten Speed Press, 2002.

MELANOMA
DISEASE/DISORDER

ANATOMY OR SYSTEM AFFECTED: Skin

SPECIALTIES AND RELATED FIELDS: Dermatology, internal medicine, pathology

DEFINITION: A malignant disease which originates with the melanocytes in the skin. While there may be

---

INFORMATION ON MELANOMA

CAUSES: Exposure to ultraviolet light and resulting mutations

SYMPTOMS: Nevus (usually a mole) that changes in shape, size, or pigmentation; may spread to lymphatic system and other regions

DURATION: Chronic, sometimes fatal

TREATMENTS: Surgery, chemotherapy, radiation, biological therapy using protein extracts from the melanoma

---

a variety of causes, the primary risk factor is extent of exposure to sunlight.

KEY TERMS:

dysplasia: the aberrant growth or development of cells

melanocytes: cells in the upper layer of skin which produce the pigment melanin

metastasis: the spread of cells from a primary site of cancer to areas throughout the body

nevus: a pigmented site on the skin which is composed of melanocytes

CAUSES AND SYMPTOMS

Melanocytes are cells in the skin which produce the melanin, most commonly recognized as the basis of skin color. Following exposure to ultraviolet (UV) light, particularly that found in sunlight, melanocytes begin the synthesis of increased levels of pigment, some of which is transferred to the surrounding cells. The process is a response to the potential damage induced by UV light and helps disperse the damaging effects of the rays.

Ultraviolet light is relatively high in energy, and significant exposure, especially exposure sufficient to cause sunburn, is damaging to deoxyribonucleic acid (DNA), the genetic material in the cell. The genetic changes that result have the potential to produce mutations which develop into cancer. Much of current research into the biology of melanomas has involved an understanding of these molecular changes.

The first alteration in physical appearance of the site is the formation of a nevus, a benign lesion consisting of replicating melanocytes. Generally speaking, nevi do not often evolve beyond the benign stage, and they rarely progress to cancer. Depending upon the extent of mutation or the accumulation of genetic changes over time with continued exposure to sunlight, however, melanocytes within the lesion may grow increasingly

Melanoma. (National Cancer Institute)

dysplastic. Growth regulation is disrupted, and, on a microscopic level, they no longer appear normal. It is during this period that the first symptoms of an abnormal condition may appear.

Most melanomas start at the site of a mole. Often the initial indication a mole has progressed to a malignant form is a change in its shape, size, or pigmentation. The phrase "ABCD" is often recommended as a means to remember the symptoms: *a*symmetry, in which one side of the mole differs from the other; *b*order, in which the edge is no longer sharp and pigmentation begins to spread; *c*olor, in which the pigmentation may develop hues of different shades; and *d*iameter, in which the size of the mole increases.

Analysis of what have become malignant cells, and therefore the decision as to the course of treatment, is indicated by a staging designation ranging from stage 0 to stage IV. Stage 0 designates a melanoma that is limited to the outer layer of skin, the epidermis. Stage IV indicates that a cancer has undergone metastasis, spreading into the lymphatic system and other regions of the body.

TREATMENT AND THERAPY

Initial treatment remains the surgical removal of the melanoma itself. Since this is an aggressive form of cancer, early diagnosis, prior to the stage at which metastasis has begun, is critical. The National Cancer Institute has recommended four methods of treatment, the choice dependent upon the stage of the disease. If

surgery is insufficient, usually because of metastasis, then chemotherapy remains the second choice. Chemotherapeutic drugs are either taken orally or injected directly into the bloodstream. If the tumor is localized, then the drug may be perfused directly into the local tissue. The relatively nonspecific nature of the chemotherapy often produces severe side effects.

An alternative treatment may involve radiation. Radiation therapy may be directed into the cancer either externally or from an implanted radiation source within the cancerous region itself. This form of directed treatment may help avoid the side effects of chemotherapy, but it is most effective only if the cancer is in a limited area.

In recent years, some success has been achieved using new forms of biological treatment. A cancer "vaccine" is prepared using protein extracts from the melanoma itself, the idea being that by allowing the immune system to react against the vaccine, the cancer itself may also be targeted.

PERSPECTIVE AND PROSPECTS

Melanoma is a particularly deadly form of skin cancer. While only approximately 4 percent of skin cancers are actually melanomas, this form of cancer accounts for some 80 percent of skin cancer deaths.

While research into the molecular nature of melanoma has provided significant insight into the cause and progress of the disease, at least at the molecular level, prevention remains of primary importance. Most cases result from exposure to the UV light found in sunlight. Since sensitivity to sunlight is in part a function of the level of pigmentation of the skin, individuals, especially those with light skin, must be more cognizant of the danger of overexposure to the sun. If sun exposure cannot be avoided or is desired, then people must be careful to use proper sunscreens to at least limit the level of exposure to UV rays. Whether it is the myth of the "healthy tan" or simply the psychological desire to show a tanned body, however, people will continue to expose themselves to the sun. Until such behaviors change, it remains likely that the incidence of melanoma will remain at current levels.

Since the earlier the stage of development, the better the prognosis, recognition of the ABCD warning signs is critical for those who have had extensive exposure to the sun. Current treatments for advanced or recurrent melanoma are primarily palliative, an attempt to prolong and improve the quality of life. Improved prognosis depends upon the effectiveness of new and combined forms of therapy, most notably combinations of immune therapy and chemotherapy.

—*Richard Adler, Ph.D.*

See also Cancer; Carcinogens; Chemotherapy; Dermatology; Dermatopathology; Malignancy and metastasis; Oncology; Radiation therapy; Skin; Skin cancer; Skin disorders; Skin lesion removal.

FOR FURTHER INFORMATION:

Gilchrest, B., et al. "The Pathogenesis of Melanoma Induced by Ultraviolet Radiation." *New England Journal of Medicine* 340, no. 17 (April 29, 1999): 1341-1348.

Gore, Martin, and Julie Newton-Bishop. *Melanoma: Critical Debates*. Malden, Mass.: Blackwell, 2002.

Melanoma Patients' Information Page. http://www.mpip.org/.

Miller, Arlo, and Martin C. Mihm, Jr. "Melanoma." *New England Journal of Medicine* 355, no. 1 (July 6, 2006): 51-65.

Poole, Catherine. *Melanoma: Prevention, Detection, and Treatment*. 2d ed. New Haven, Conn.: Yale University Press, 2005.

MELATONIN

BIOLOGY

ANATOMY OR SYSTEM AFFECTED: Brain, endocrine system, glands

SPECIALTIES AND RELATED FIELDS: Alternative medicine, endocrinology, neurology, pharmacology, preventive medicine

DEFINITION: A substance produced by the pineal gland that has been used as a controversial therapeutic agent.

KEY TERMS:

endocrine system: the glands that produce hormones

hormone: a substance produced in one part of the body that has effects in other parts of the body

melatonin: the hormone produced by the pineal gland

pineal gland: a small organ inside the brain that produces melatonin

STRUCTURE AND FUNCTIONS

Melatonin, also known as N-acetyl-5-methoxytryptamine, is a hormone found in a wide variety of living organisms. In vertebrates (animals with backbones), including humans, it is produced by the pineal gland. The pineal gland is located deep within the center of the brain. Although it is inside the brain, it is considered part of the endocrine system rather than the nervous system. In humans, the pineal gland is a gray or white organ less than 1 centimeter long and shaped like a pinecone.

The pineal gland produces varying amounts of melatonin in response to changes in light. Light inhibits the production of melatonin, and darkness stimulates it. In some small animals, light reaches the pineal gland directly through the skull. In larger animals, including humans, information about light and darkness is transmitted by the nervous system from the eyes to the suprachiasmatic nucleus, a cluster of nerve cells in a region of the brain known as the hypothalamus. The suprachiasmatic nucleus regulates the secretion of melatonin by the pineal gland.

Melatonin is believed to be involved in regulating the sleep cycle in response to changes in light. Because the amount of melatonin produced by the pineal gland declines sharply at puberty, it is believed to be involved in the development of the reproductive system. Because melatonin production continues to decline with age, some researchers believe that it is associated with the process of aging.

DISORDERS AND DISEASES

Disorders of melatonin production other than its normal decline with age are rare. Tumors of the pineal gland may reduce melatonin production. Some evidence suggests that this may lead to premature aging. Children with tumors of the pineal gland may reach puberty at a very early age.

Some researchers suggest that the normal decline in melatonin production with age is associated with diseases of the elderly. Animal studies suggest that loss of melatonin is associated with increased cell damage. Melatonin is believed to act as an antioxidant, a substance that protects cells from free radicals, which are produced when cells use oxygen. Cell damage has been linked to a large number of diseases of the elderly, including various forms of cancer, heart disease, and Alzheimer's disease.

Based on this evidence, melatonin has been used to treat and prevent a wide variety of illnesses. In the 1990's, melatonin became widely used in the United States. Because it was classified as a dietary supplement rather than as a drug, it was available without a prescription and with little government regulation. While some researchers suggested caution until more was known about melatonin, others suggested taking small daily doses of the hormone to slow down the aging process. Popular books such as *The Melatonin Miracle* (1995), by Walter Pierpaoli, William Regelson, and Carol Colman, claim that melatonin can stimulate the immune system, prevent cancer and heart disease, improve sexual relations, reduce the effects of stress, act as a contraceptive, and add years to the human life span. Critics argue that these claims are greatly exaggerated.

The least controversial suggested use for melatonin is as a sleeping aid. Human studies have indicated that melatonin is safe and effective for this use. Unlike many other sleeping pills, melatonin seems to have no effect on normal sleep patterns and few side effects. Melatonin has also been shown to be effective in treating jet lag, the difficulty that travelers have adjusting to a new time zone.

Critics of routine melatonin use point out that little is known about its long-term effects. They also point to evidence that some people may experience short-term side effects such as nightmares, headaches, daytime sleepiness, and mild depression. A major concern is the lack of regulation of melatonin products, leading to the possibility that other, unknown substances may be present.

Even the most optimistic proponents of melatonin suggest certain precautions. Many products contain more melatonin than researchers believe is necessary, leading to the possibility of a greater risk of side effects with no increase in benefit. Melatonin should only be taken at bedtime to avoid unwanted sleepiness. It should not be used by children, who already produce high levels of melatonin. It should not be used by pregnant women because its effect on the fetus is unknown. Because it is believed to stimulate the immune system, melatonin should be avoided in people with severe allergies, autoimmune disorders, or cancer of the immune system.

PERSPECTIVE AND PROSPECTS

The pineal gland was known to exist in ancient times. It was first described scientifically by the Greek physician Galen in the second century. The French philosopher René Descartes (1596-1650) suggested that it was the location of the human soul. The true function of the pineal gland remained unknown until the middle of the twentieth century.

Melatonin was discovered in 1958 and first described as a hormone in 1963. Research into its effects began in the 1970's and 1980's. Interest in this hormone increased dramatically in 1995, with the publication of several books and articles publicizing its possible benefits. Research on melatonin is expected to continue for many years, particularly in regard to its long-term effects.

—Rose Secrest

See also Aging; Antioxidants; Brain; Chronobiology; Endocrine disorders; Endocrinology; Endocrinology, pediatric; Glands; Hormone replacement therapy (HRT); Hormones; Light therapy; Pharmacology; Sleep disorders.

FOR FURTHER INFORMATION:

Brook, Charles G. D., and Nicholas J. Marshall. *Essential Endocrinology*. Rev. 4th ed. Cambridge, Mass.: Blackwell Science, 2001. This text addresses the field of endocrinology, describing the physiology of the endocrine glands and the hormones that they produce. Includes an index.

Brzezinski, Amnon. "Melatonin in Humans." *New England Journal of Medicine* 336, no. 3 (January 16, 1997): 186-195. Discusses the evidence that melatonin has a role in the biologic regulation of circadian rhythms, sleep, and mood and perhaps reproduction, tumor growth, and aging.

Goodman, H. Maurice. *Basic Medical Endocrinology*. 3d ed. Boston: Academic Press, 2003. Focuses on research advances in the understanding of hormones involved in regulating most aspects of bodily functions. Includes coverage of the pineal gland and its regulatory principles.

"Melatonin: Questions, Facts, Mysteries." *University of California, Berkeley, Wellness Letter* 16, no. 8 (May, 2000): 1-2. Argues that too little is known about the dosage and health effects of melatonin.

Olcese, James, ed. *Melatonin After Four Decades: An Assessment of Its Potential*. New York: Kluwer Academic/Plenum, 1999. Nearly sixty contributions review the research advances made in the understanding of melatonin's role in health and disease and discuss the future uses of melatonin.

Pandi-Perumal, S. R., and Daniel P. Cardinali, eds. *Melatonin: Biological Basis of Its Function in Health and Disease*. Georgetown, Tex.: Landes Bioscience, 2006. Wide-ranging chapters explore the latest research on melatonin.

Memory loss

Disease/disorder

Anatomy or system affected: Brain, nervous system, psychic-emotional system

Specialties and related fields: Geriatrics and gerontology, neurology, psychiatry, psychology

Definition: Total or limited impairment of memory that may be sudden or gradual.

Causes and Symptoms

Memory impairment is a common problem, and often a concern among older individuals. Memory problems are not, however, restricted to older adults. They may occur at any age and may be attributable to numerous conditions and events. Memory loss occurs in various degrees and may be associated with other evidence of brain dysfunction and other physical and emotional problems. Memory loss may be partial, limited to events immediately before or after a traumatic event. Memory loss may also be complete. Amnesia is the term used to describe complete memory loss. Memory loss may also be permanent or temporary, or may vacillate, with a person slipping in and out of being able to remember appropriately.

Benign senescent forgetfulness. In this condition, the memory deficit affects mostly recent events, and although a source of frustration, it seldom interferes with the individual's professional activities or social life. An important feature of benign forgetfulness is that it is selective and affects only trivial, unimportant facts. For example, one may misplace the car keys or forget to return a phone call, respond to a letter, or pay a bill. Cashing a check or telephoning someone with whom one is particularly keen to talk, however, will not be forgotten. The person is aware of the memory deficit, and written notes often are used as reminders. Patients with benign forgetfulness have no other evidence of brain dysfunction and maintain their ability to make valid judgments.

Dementia. In dementia, the memory impairment is global, does not discriminate between important and trivial facts, and interferes with the person's ability to pursue professional or social activities. Patients with dementia find it difficult to adapt to changes in the workplace, such as the introduction of computers. They also find it difficult to continue with their hobbies and interests.

The hallmark of dementia is no awareness of the memory deficit, except in the very early stages of the disease. This is an important difference between de-

mentia and benign forgetfulness. Although patients with early dementia may write themselves notes, they usually forget to check these reminders or may misinterpret them. For example, a man with dementia who is invited for dinner at a friend's house may write a note to that effect and leave it in a prominent place. He may then go to his host's home several evenings in succession because he has forgotten that he already has fulfilled this social engagement. As the disease progresses, patients are no longer aware of their memory deficit.

In dementia, the memory deficit does not occur in isolation but is accompanied by other evidence of brain dysfunction, which in very early stages can be detected only by specialized neuropsychological tests. As the condition progresses, these deficits become readily apparent. The patient is often disoriented regarding time and may telephone relatives or friends very late at night or not realize the time of day. As the disease progresses, the disorientation affects the patient's environment: A woman with dementia may wander outside her house and be unable to find her way back, or she may repeatedly ask to be taken back home when she is already there. In later stages, patients may not be able to recognize people whom they should know: A man may think that his son is his father or that his wife is his mother. In fact, it is possible for the patient to not even recognize his or her own reflection in a mirror. This stage is particularly distressing to the caregivers. Patients with dementia may often exhibit impaired judgment. They may go outside the house inappropriately dressed or at inappropriate times, or they may purchase the same item repeatedly or make donations that are disproportional to their funds. Alzheimer's disease is one of the most common causes of dementia in older people.

Multiple infarct dementia. Multiple infarct dementia is caused by the destruction of brain cells by repeated strokes. Sometimes these strokes are so small that neither the patient nor the relatives are aware of their occurrence. When many strokes occur and significant brain tissue is destroyed, the patient may exhibit symptoms of dementia. Usually, however, most of these strokes are quite obvious because they are associated with weakness or paralysis in a part of the body. One of the characteristic features of multiple infarct dementia is that its onset is sudden and its progression is by steps. Every time a stroke occurs, the patient's condition deteriorates. This is followed by a period during which little or no deterioration develops until another stroke occurs, at which time the patient's condition deteriorates further. Very rarely, the stroke affects only the memory center, in which case the patient's sole problem is amnesia. Multiple infarct dementia and dementia resulting from Alzheimer's disease should be differentiated from other treatable conditions which also may cause memory impairment, disorientation, and poor judgment. It is important to recognize, however, that both conditions may exist in the same person.

Depression. Depression may cause memory impairment as a result of problems related to concentration and attention. This condition is quite common and at times is so difficult to differentiate from dementia that the term "pseudo-dementia" is used to describe it. One of the main differences between depression that presents the symptoms of dementia and dementia itself is insight into the memory deficit. Whereas patients with dementia are usually oblivious of their deficit and not distressed (except those in the early stages), those with depression are nearly always aware of their deficit and are quite distressed. Patients with depression tend to be withdrawn and apathetic and to show a marked disturbance of affect. In contrast, those with dementia demonstrate emotional blandness and some degree of emotional lability, or a lack of stableness in expressed emotion. One of the problems characteristic of depressed patients is their difficulty in concentrating. This is typified by poor cooperation and effort in carrying out tasks with a variable degree of achievement, coupled with considerable anxiety. Further, anxiety too may disrupt memory, compounding any other problems.

Head trauma. Amnesia is sometimes seen in patients who have sustained a head injury. The extent of the amnesia is usually proportional to the severity of the injury. In most cases, the complete recovery of the patient's memory occurs, except for the events just preceding and following the injury. With traumatic brain injury, however, amnesia may not be the only symptom. Other memory deficits can be observed and experienced. As such, following any head injury, evaluation is advisable, even if the injury is a closed head injury.

PERSPECTIVE AND PROSPECTS

Memory impairment is a serious condition that can interfere with one's ability to function independently, and sometimes at all. Any time that memory loss develops, identification of underlying causes should occur because a treatable cause may be found, preventing further memory loss or perhaps reducing the amount of memory loss. In some cases, proper treatment may even reverse memory loss, such as in some conditions related to alcohol-related memory loss. Research examining memory continues to differentiate among conditions involving memory loss. Efforts to better assess conditions and make distinctions earlier in the process of such conditions remain important. The earlier that problems such as dementia can be identified, for instance, the earlier treatment may be able to occur, potentially increasing quality of life.

Research has also identified ways to slow the progression of some diseases related to memory loss. As the root causes of memory impairment and brain changes are understood, future research may be able to arrest the progress of amnesia and memory loss and even to treat dementias now considered irreversible, such as Alzheimer's disease and multiple infarct dementia. Exciting research in the area of inflammation and immunological functioning may prove to be productive.

—Ronald C. Hamdy, M.D.,
and Louis A. Cancellaro, M.D.;
updated by Nancy A. Piotrowski, Ph.D.

See also Aging; Alzheimer's disease; Amnesia; Anxiety; Brain; Brain damage; Brain disorders; Concussion; Dementias; Depression; Geriatrics and gerontology; Head and neck disorders; Pick's disease; Psychiatry; Psychiatry, geriatric; Strokes.

FOR FURTHER INFORMATION:

Hamdy, Ronald C., et al., eds. *Alzheimer's Disease: A Handbook for Caregivers.* 3d ed. St. Louis: Mosby Year Book, 1998. This handbook offers nursing tips for people caring for Alzheimer's patients. Includes bibliographical references and an index.

Masoro, Edward J., and Steven N. Austad, eds. *Handbook of the Biology of Aging.* 6th ed. Boston: Else-

---

INFORMATION ON MEMORY LOSS

CAUSES: Aging, head trauma, certain diseases, repeated strokes, depression

SYMPTOMS: Varies; can include benign forgetfulness, disorientation and impaired judgment, weakness or paralysis in body part

DURATION: Acute to chronic

TREATMENTS: Varies; can include medication, surgery

vier Academic Press, 2005. This is part of a handbook on aging series. This edition significantly revises earlier versions of this work. Varied theories of aging are discussed, along with additions exploring whether diseases associated with aging are necessarily part of the aging process.

Mendez, Mario F., and Jeffrey L. Cummings. *Dementia: A Clinical Approach.* 3d ed. Philadelphia: Butterworth-Heinemann, 2003. This is a standard textbook, comprehensively presenting the clinical, diagnostic, therapeutic, and basic science aspects of the dementias. This edition has been revised and updated with nearly one thousand new references and revised descriptions of all major dementia syndromes.

O'Brien, John, David Ames, and Alistair Burns, eds. *Dementia.* 2d ed. New York: Oxford University Press, 2000. Text that covers advances in the research of degenerative disorders, current diagnostic criteria, rating scales, investigations, neurobiological mechanisms, therapeutic options and services, and all aspects of management, including psychosocial and psychological approaches, among other topics.

West, Robin L., and Jan D. Sinnott, eds. *Everyday Memory and Aging.* New York: Springer-Verlag, 1992. This work discusses the methodology of research into the human memory. Focuses on the changes in memory that occur naturally with age, as well as those that are brought about by various forms of dementia in the older individual.

MÉNIÈRE'S DISEASE
DISEASE/DISORDER

ALSO KNOWN AS: Endolymphatic hydrops

ANATOMY OR SYSTEM AFFECTED: Ears

SPECIALTIES AND RELATED FIELDS: Audiology, otorhinolaryngology

DEFINITION: A disease of the inner ear caused by excessive pressure in the cochlear fluid. Its symptoms are hearing loss, tinnitus (ringing in the ear), nausea, and episodes of vertigo.

CAUSES AND SYMPTOMS

Ménière's disease results from excess pressure caused by surplus fluids in the cochlea (inner ear) or the semicircular canals concerned with the sense of balance. Typically this condition results when the structure that reabsorbs excess fluid from the inner ear ceases to function properly. The cause may be an infection, aller-

---

INFORMATION ON MÉNIÈRE'S DISEASE

CAUSES: Excess fluid in inner ear as result of infection, allergies, blood vessel spasm, or small hemorrhage in cochlear duct

SYMPTOMS: Ringing and fullness in ears, dizziness, hearing impairment, rapidly progressing hearing loss, dizziness, vertigo, loss of equilibrium, nausea and vomiting, rhythmic jerking motion of eyes, sometimes deafness

DURATION: Often chronic with recurrent attacks lasting thirty minutes to several hours

TREATMENTS: Diuretics, blood vessel dilators, low-salt diet, motion sickness medications, antihistamines, bed rest; in severe cases, destruction of cochlea through surgery or ultrasound

---

gies, a spasm of one of the tiny blood vessels in the semicircular canal, or a small hemorrhage in the cochlear duct. Ménière's syndrome affects both the vestibular nerve (causing attacks of vertigo) and the auditory nerve (causing hearing impairment).

The classic symptoms of Ménière's disease are tinnitus, a sensation of fullness in the ears, dizziness, hearing impairment (including fluctuating distortions of sound), and a rapidly progressing loss of hearing. The attacks are typically abrupt and momentary, but recur frequently. Dizziness may range from a mild whirling sensation and unsteady balance to severe attacks of vertigo and complete loss of equilibrium accompanied by nausea and vomiting. The eyes often show a rhythmic jerking motion.

TREATMENT AND THERAPY

The treatment selected for Ménière's disease depends on the theoretical diagnosed cause, as no single remedy is universally successful. Infections and allergies can often be treated by diuretic drugs, sedative and blood vessel dilators, or low-salt diets, all intended to reduce cochlear fluid pressure. Motion sickness and antihistamine drugs may be used to treat the symptoms. Since attacks of violent dizziness can occur suddenly, the affected person must immediately lie down to avoid falling. During a severe attack, the patient should be confined to bed since any movement of the head produces the disturbing sensation that the room is rotating. A bout may last several weeks, during which time bed rest and medication are recommended. Attacks, which recur at irregular intervals of weeks, or months, may last a half hour to several hours. Mild attacks usually disappear within a year, but more severe cases require a medical regimen. In some cases surgery may be necessary to decompress the cochlea and/or semicircular canals. If all other medical measures fail, the disability is severe, and deafness is well advanced, destruction of the cochlea by surgery or ultrasound may be a last resort.

PERSPECTIVE AND PROSPECTS
Ménière's disease was first described and recorded in detail in 1861 by French physician Prosper Ménière. Formerly only the most severe and disabling cases were treated surgically because the operation required destruction of the hearing nerve. Since the advent of microsurgical instruments it has become possible to separate the hearing and balance filaments in the main nerve and clip only the balance filaments when the problem is in the semicircular canals. It is also now possible to utilize ultrasonic beams to selectively destroy balance filaments without damaging the sensitive auditory nerves.

—*George R. Plitnik, Ph.D.*

See also Audiology; Balance disorders; Dizziness and fainting; Ear infections and disorders; Ears; Hearing loss; Nausea and vomiting; Otorhinolaryngology.

FOR FURTHER INFORMATION:
Griffith, H. Winter. *Complete Guide to Symptoms, Illness, and Surgery*. Revised and updated by Stephen Moore and Kenneth Yoder. Rev. 4th ed. New York: Perigee, 2000.

Harris, Jeffrey P., ed. *Ménière's Disease*. The Hague, Netherlands: Kugler, 1999.

Paparella, Michael M., ed. *Pathogenesis of Ménière's Disease: Treatment Considerations*. Philadelphia: W. B. Saunders, 2002.

Weber, Peter C., ed. *Ménière's Disease*. Philadelphia: W. B. Saunders, 1997.

MENINGITIS
DISEASE/DISORDER

ANATOMY OR SYSTEM AFFECTED: Brain, head, nervous system, spine

SPECIALTIES AND RELATED FIELDS: Emergency medicine, neurology, public health

DEFINITION: An inflammation of the meninges of the brain and spinal cord.

INFORMATION ON MENINGITIS

CAUSES: Bacterial or viral infection
SYMPTOMS: Severe headaches, vomiting, pain and stiffness in the neck, upper-respiratory infection, lethargy, confusion, disorientation
DURATION: Acute
TREATMENTS: Antibiotics, surgery, supportive therapy (blood transfusions, subdural taps)

CAUSES AND SYMPTOMS
The meninges is the three-layered covering of the spinal cord and brain. The layers are the outer dura mater, inner pia mater, and middle arachnoid. Meningitis is the inflammation or infection of the arachnoid and pia mater. It is characterized by severe headaches, vomiting, and pain and stiffness in the neck. These symptoms may be preceded by an upper respiratory infection. The age of the patient may affect which signs and symptoms are displayed. Newborns may exhibit either fever or hypothermia, along with lethargy or irritability, disinterest in feeding, and abdominal distension. In infants, examination may find bulging of the fontanelles (the soft areas between the bones of the skull found in newborns). The elderly may show lethargy, confusion, or disorientation. As pressure in the skull increases, nausea and vomiting may occur. With meningococcal meningitis, a rash of pinpoint-sized or larger dots appears.

Most cases of meningitis are the result of bacterial infection. These cases are sometimes referred to as septic meningitis. The bacteria invade the subarachnoid space and may have traveled from another site of infection, having caused pneumonia, cellulitis, or an ear infection. It is unclear if the bacteria make their way from the original area of infection to the meninges by the bloodstream or the lymphatic system. Once they have entered the subarachnoid space, they divide without inhibition since there is no impediment posed by defensive cells. In other words, the cerebrospinal fluid (CSF) contains very few white blood cells to inactivate the bacteria. More rarely, some bacteria may be introduced into the area by neurological damage or surgical invasion.

The most common cause of bacterial meningitis in adults and older children is meningococcus (*Neisseria meningitidus*). It is a diplococcus that typically does its damage inside the cell. The incidence of meningococcal meningitis is 2 to 3 cases per 100,000 people per year, and it most often affects schoolchildren and military recruits. *Haemophilus influenzae* is the most common culprit infecting babies between two months and one year of age. Complications or residual effects often follow bacterial meningitis. These may include deafness, delayed-onset epilepsy, hydrocephalus, cerebritis, and brain abscess. In addition, for several weeks after resolution of the disease the patient may experience headaches, dizziness, and lethargy.

Aseptic meningitis is meningitis attributable to causes other than bacteria. These causes include neurotropic viruses, such as those that cause poliomyelitis or encephalitis; other viruses such as those that cause mumps, herpes, mononucleosis, hepatitis, chickenpox, and measles; spirochetes; bacterial products from brain abscesses or previous cases of bacterial meningitis; and foreign bodies, such as those found in the air or chemicals, in the CSF. Most cases of aseptic meningitis are viral in origin. The signs and symptoms are similar to those of bacterial meningitis. Onset is usually gradual, with symptoms starting mildly. The slight headache becomes worse over the course of several days, the neck becomes characteristically stiff, and photophobia (dislike of bright light) occurs.

Tuberculous meningitis is different from most other forms of meningitis because it lasts longer, has a higher mortality rate, and affects the CSF less. It mostly strikes children and is usually the result of a bacillus infection from the respiratory tract or the lymphatic system that has relocated to the meninges. When the bacilli are translocated to the central nervous system, they form tubercles that release an exudate. If tuberculous meningitis is left untreated, death may occur within three weeks. Even with treatment, it may result in neurologic abnormalities.

TREATMENT AND THERAPY

If meningitis is suspected, the first testing procedure is an examination of the CSF. To obtain CSF, a lumbar puncture, sometimes called a spinal tap, is made. Opening pressure, protein and glucose concentrations, total cell count, and cultures of microbes are determined. In cases of meningitis, the CSF is almost always cloudy and generally comes out under higher-than-normal pressure. An elevated white blood cell count in the CSF would be one indication that the patient has bacterial meningitis; another would be lowered serum glucose but slightly raised protein concentration, especially al-

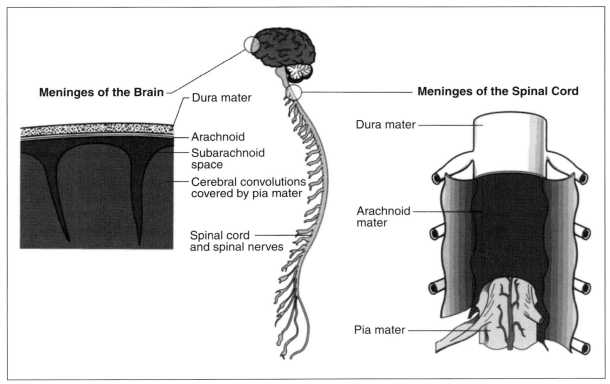

Meningitis attacks the meninges of the brain or the spinal cord or both.

bumin. About 90 percent of bacterial meningitis cases show gram-positive staining. The examination of this slightly atypical fluid, along with presenting symptoms and signs, gives the diagnostician some confidence in diagnosing meningitis accurately. Further cultures and a repeat puncture are necessary to pinpoint the kind of meningitis and to check the effect of the treatment.

Bacterial meningitis should be treated promptly with antibiotics specific for the causative bacteria. The success of treatment is contingent on the magnitude of the bacterial count and the quickness with which the bacteria can be controlled. Virtually all bacterial cases are treated with ampicillin or penicillin. Cases aggressively treated with very large doses of antibiotics are the most successful. If antibiotics do not destroy the areas of infection, surgery should be considered. Surgery is especially effective if meningitis is recurrent or persistent. Viral meningitis may be treated with adenine arabinoside if the cause is herpes simplex. No medication will kill other viruses causing the infection. The condition usually resolves itself in a few days, even without treatment. When necessary, supportive therapy should be employed, including blood transfusions. Young children with open fontanelles often undergo subdural taps to relieve pressure caused by CSF buildup.

Mortality rates in meningitis vary with age and the pathogen responsible. Those suffering from meningococcal meningitis (without overwhelming bacterial numbers) have a fatality rate of only 3 percent. Newborns suffering from gram-negative meningitis, however, have a 70 percent mortality rate. In addition, the younger the patient, the more likely the incidence of lasting neurological damage.

There are two basic ways to prevent meningitis: chemoprophylaxis for likely candidates of the disease and active immunization. Those exposed to a known case are usually treated with rifampin for four days; rifampin is especially useful in inactivating *H. influenzae*. Active immunization is suggested for toddlers eighteen to twenty-four months of age, especially for those in situations where there is a high risk of exposure (such as day care centers).

—*Iona C. Baldridge*

See also Abscesses; Bacterial infections; Brain; Brain damage; Brain disorders; Chickenpox; Encephalitis; Hepatitis; Herpes; Immunization and vaccination; Lumbar puncture; Measles; Mononucleosis; Mumps; Nervous system; Neuroimaging; Neurology; Neurol-

ogy, pediatric; Poliomyelitis; Spinal cord disorders; Spine, vertebrae, and disks; Viral infections; West Nile virus.

FOR FURTHER INFORMATION:

American Medical Association. *American Medical Association Family Medical Guide*. 4th rev. ed. Hoboken, N.J.: John Wiley & Sons, 2004.

Bloom, Floyd E., M. Flint Beal, and David J. Kupfer, eds. *The Dana Guide to Brain Health*. New York: Simon & Schuster, 2003.

Ferreiros, C. *Emerging Strategies in the Fight Against Meningitis*. New York: Garland Science, 2002.

Meningitis Research Foundation. http://www.meningitis.org/.

Shmaefsky, Brian. *Meningitis*. Rev. ed. Philadelphia: Chelsea House, 2005.

Tunkel, Allan R. *Bacterial Meningitis*. Philadelphia: Lippincott Williams & Wilkins, 2001.

Wilson, Michael, Brian Henderson, and Rod McNab. *Bacterial Virulence Mechanisms*. New York: Cambridge University Press, 2002.

MENOPAUSE

BIOLOGY

ANATOMY OR SYSTEM AFFECTED: Psychic-emotional system, reproductive system, uterus

SPECIALTIES AND RELATED FIELDS: Endocrinology, gynecology

DEFINITION: The time during a woman's life when her ability to conceive and bear children ends, marked by irregular, and eventually complete cessation of, menstruation, accompanied by hormonal changes such as the dramatic reduction in the body's production of estrogen.

KEY TERMS:

climacteric: that phase in the aging process of women marking the transition from the reproductive stage of life to the nonreproductive stage

estrogen: the female hormones estradiol and estrone, produced by the ovary and responsible for the development of secondary sex characteristics

exogenous: originating outside an organ or part

osteoporosis: a condition characterized by a loss of bone density and an increased susceptibility to fractures

progesterone: a hormone, released by the corpus luteum and placenta, responsible for changes in the uterine endometrium

PROCESS AND EFFECTS

The word "menopause" comes from two Greek words meaning "month" and "cessation." It is used medically to mean a cessation of, not a "pause" in, menstrual periods. Technically, the menopause begins the moment a woman has had her final menstrual period; until then, her menstrual periods may have shown a wide variety of irregularities, including missed periods.

Medical experts refer to the time when the body is noticeably preparing for the menopause as the perimenopause, which can begin anywhere from five to ten years before the menopause. While estrogen levels begin to decrease gradually, periods are normal but memory may be less sharp and mood swings may occur. During that time, a woman still experiences menstrual periods, but they are erratic. Some women stop menstruating suddenly, without irregularities; however, they are in the minority. For some women, signs of the menopause, such as hot flashes, may begin during the perimenopause. For even more women, such signs begin, or at least increase in intensity, at the menopause.

The term "climacteric" covers a longer span and includes all the years of diminishing estrogen production, both before and after a woman's last menstrual period. Some experts believe that women may undergo declines in their levels of estrogen even when they are in their late twenties; almost all experts believe that estrogen levels drop at least by a woman's mid-thirties, and the process accelerates in the late forties.

The average age at which the menopause occurs in women from the United States is 51.4 years, with the usual range between ages forty-five and fifty-five. For some it occurs much earlier, for others much later. Only 8 percent of women reach the menopause before age forty, and only 5 percent continue to menstruate after age fifty-three. A very few have menstrual periods until they are sixty.

Even after the menopause, the climacteric continues. Declining hormonal levels bring more changes, until the situation stabilizes. A decade or more of noticeable changes can take place before the climacteric is completed. Unlike the climacteric, the menopause itself is usually considered completed after one full year without a period. After two years, a woman can be reasonably certain that her periods have ceased permanently. The signs and symptoms of the menopause, however, can linger for years longer.

Starting in her mid-forties, a woman's ovaries gradually lose their ability to respond to the follicle-stimulating hormone (FSH), which is released by the pituitary into the blood, triggering the release of estrogen from the ovaries. A few eggs do remain even after menstrual flows have ceased, and the production of estrogen does not stop completely after the menopause; in much smaller amounts, it continues to be released by the adrenal glands, in fatty tissue, and in the brain. At the menopause, however, the blood levels of estrogen are drastically reduced—by about 75 percent.

About two to four years before the menopause, many women stop ovulating or ovulate irregularly or only occasionally. Although almost all the follicles enclosing the eggs are depleted by this time, the ovaries continue to produce estrogen. Estrogen continues to build up the endometrium (the lining of the uterus), but without ovulation no progesterone is produced to shed the extra lining. Therefore, instead of regular periods, a woman may bleed at unexpected times as the extra lining is shed sporadically.

During the perimenopause, menstrual periods may be late or early, longer than usual or shorter, and lighter than before or heavier. They may disappear for several months, then reappear for several more. It has been noted that in 15 to 20 percent of women the typical menopausal symptoms, sometimes accompanied by noticeable mood swings similar to premenstrual tension, begin during the perimenopausal period.

According to the National Institutes of Health (NIH), about 80 percent of women experience mild or no signs of the menopause. The rest have symptoms troublesome enough to seek medical attention. The two most important factors in determining how a woman will fare are probably the rate of decline of her female hormones and the final degree of hormone depletion. A woman's genes, general health, lifetime quality of diet, level of activity, and psychological acceptance of aging are also major influences. The most severe symptoms occur in women who lose their ovaries through surgery or radiation when they are perimenopausal.

When only the uterus is removed (hysterectomy) and the ovaries remain intact, menstrual periods stop but all other aspects of the menopause occur in the same way and at the same age. When only one ovary is removed, the menopause occurs normally. If both ovaries are removed, a complete menopause takes place abruptly, sometimes with intense effects. Women who have had a tubal ligation to prevent pregnancy will experience a normal menopause because tubal ligation does not affect ovaries, the uterus, or hormonal secretions.

Although experts disagree about the causes of a variety of symptoms that may appear at the menopause, there is no disagreement about the fact that the majority of women experience hot flashes, or flushes. For two out of three women, hot flashes can start well before the last menstruation. Generally, however, hot flashes increase dramatically at menopause and continue to occur, with intermittent breaks (sometimes lasting several months), for five years or so.

While hot flashes are not dangerous, they are uncomfortable. Many women have only three or four episodes a day—or even a week—and hardly notice them. Others have as many as fifty severe flashes a day. The intense waves of heat generally last several minutes, but some unusual flashes have been reported to last as long as an hour. Usually there is some perspiration; with a severe flash, there is heavy perspiration. Because the blood vessels dilate (expand) and then contract, the hot flash is often followed by chills, even intense shivering. Since the flashes are usually worse at night, they can cause insomnia.

Other vasomotor symptoms can also appear with the menopause. Experts believe that they are the result of disruptions of the same mechanisms—vasomotor instability—that are manifested as hot flashes. Palpitations, which are distinct and rapid heartbeats, may also occur. A woman may experience dizziness or may feel faint or nauseated at times. She may have peculiar sensations in her arms and hands, especially her fingers. Some feel these sensations as tingling, or pins and needles, while others say that their fingers occasionally feel numb. One of the oddest, most frightening sensations associated with the menopause is formication, a feeling of insects crawling over the skin.

Headaches, depression, mood swings, insomnia, and weight gain often affect women at the menopause and may be related to the body's hormonal readjustments. Insomnia is second only to hot flashes as the symptom that causes women to seek out their doctors' help at the menopause. The hypothalamus controls sleep as well as temperature and hormone production; insomnia is caused by changes in sleep patterns and brain waves from the same hypothalamic disturbances that result in the hot flashes and an overstimulated central nervous system.

COMPLICATIONS AND DISORDERS

During the menopause, the walls of the vagina become smooth and dry and produce less lubrication, producing a condition called atrophic vaginitis. It has been assumed that this condition is attributable to a lack of estrogen. Despite doubts concerning the relationship

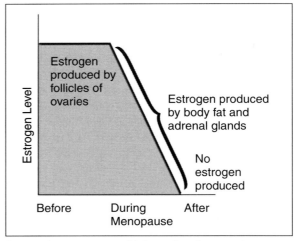

During the menopause, which may last for several years, estrogen production diminishes; after the menopause, estrogen is no longer produced by the body.

between circulating estrogen and objective measures of vaginal atrophy, estrogen (often topical) is frequently prescribed and effectively used in the alleviation or elimination of symptoms.

One of the problems that women encounter with the menopause is calcium deficiency. Many experts believe that before the menopause a woman requires a minimum of 1,000 milligrams of calcium a day in food or supplements. At the menopause, however, a woman who is not taking estrogen needs 1,500 milligrams of calcium a day. Since it is very difficult to obtain these daily allotments from food without consuming considerable amounts of milk or milk products, calcium supplements are often recommended for menopausal and postmenopausal women.

If the calcium deficiency is allowed to persist, osteoporosis, a loss of bone density that can lead to dangerous fractures, can result. Osteoporosis is known to have less of a damaging effect on women who are somewhat overweight because estrogen continues to be produced in fatty tissues after the menopause. Cigarettes, alcohol, and caffeine increase bone loss because they interfere with the body's ability to absorb calcium. A well-balanced diet, calcium supplements, and regular exercise—especially weight-bearing exercise—are effective ways of controlling osteoporosis. Hormone replacement therapy (HRT) is another means of coping with osteoporosis brought on by the menopause. Since nearly half of all women do not develop osteoporosis, however, many physicians do not believe that administering estrogen therapy to combat this disease is worth the risks except in women at high risk for osteo-porosis.

Although estrogen was isolated as a substance in the 1920's, the modern study of hormones—how they work, where they are produced, what their benefits are—began in the 1940's. Originally, estrogen was administered cautiously to women who had lost their ovaries through surgery and to those with severe distress after the menopause. It was not until the 1960's that estrogen replacement therapy became widespread, however, when books such as Robert A. Wilson's *Feminine Forever* (1966) promoted its use as the newfound fountain of youth for women. The replacement of estrogen was suddenly fashionable, with the hormone being viewed as a miracle drug that could keep women looking and feeling youthful well into their later years. Physicians began prescribing it for women well before the menopause, and it was recommended for use throughout life. Often, large doses were prescribed.

By the mid-1970's, twenty million American women were taking estrogen. A decade later, however, the number had fallen to four or five million. Beginning in 1975, research studies began documenting dramatic increases—sometimes as high as 500 percent—in cases of cancer of the lining of the endometrium among women taking estrogen, compared with those not taking it. Other studies at that time found higher rates of breast cancer as well as other problems, such as gallbladder conditions, among women taking estrogen.

Some studies found the overall risk of contracting uterine cancer increased 350 percent for women who took estrogen for a year or more. Some women who were on the therapy for long periods were judged to be as much as 100 percent more likely to contract uterine cancer. Furthermore, contrary to expectations, some studies claimed that the risk persisted even ten years after the estrogen use was discontinued. Other studies also found that the risk of cancer persisted, though for a shorter period.

These studies were based on replacement therapy using estrogen only. Estrogen stimulates the growth of cells in the endometrium, which is one of the aspects of the development of cancer. Consequently, a treatment was developed in which estrogen was combined with a form of progesterone in an effort to reduce the risk of uterine cancer and other diseases. Today, the most widely used regimen calls for estrogen in the lowest effective dose three weeks each month. During the last week to thirteen days of this therapy, a form of progesterone called progestin is added, and then both hor-mones are stopped. Uterine bleeding, similar to that of a menstrual period, may occur, allowing the progesterone to break down any excess buildup of cells in the endometrium.

Many women need only short-term HRT to alleviate menopausal symptoms. Other women, such as those at risk for developing osteoporosis, may choose long-term therapy. Some physicians prescribe estrogen therapy for women with severe symptoms after a surgical menopause. Other physicians have recommended HRT for the prevention of heart disease, as postmenopausal women are at increased risk.

In the early twenty-first century, however, the use of HRT—either long-term or short-term—was questioned. A study called the Women's Health Initiative, funded by the NIH, compared thousands of women who took combination HRT to women who were given placebos. Those on the combination treatment had an increased risk for heart disease, stroke, and blood clots in the lungs. As a result, organizations such as the American Heart Association (AHA), the American College of Obstetricians and Gynecologists (ACOG), and the North American Menopause Society (NAMS) recommended that combination therapy not be used for the prevention of cardiac disease. Moreover, other drugs can be used to prevent or treat osteoporosis, such as bisphosphonates and selective estrogen receptor modulators (SERMs), that do not carry the same risks as HRT.

Anecdotal evidence and some research studies suggest that stress reduction and exercise can relieve some of the symptoms of the menopause, including hot flashes and mood swings. In addition, a host of herbal remedies on the market claim to improve menopausal symptoms, although caution should be used in choosing these products. A double-blind pilot study of women using soy as a natural estrogen replacement therapy turned out positive; hot flashes decreased significantly in women taking soy powder for six weeks. The isoflavones in soy are chemically similar to estrogens. Vitamin E, which is structurally similar to estrogen at the molecular level, decreases hot flashes in some women, but the evidence so far is anecdotal and no large studies have been conducted. Black cohosh is the best documented of all the herbal remedies. Studies suggest that it can relieve menopause-related headaches, depression, anxiety, hot flashes, night sweats, heart palpitations, and vaginal dryness and thinning. Black cohosh suppresses the secretion of luteinizing hormone, a hormone that is believed to be at the root of many menopausal symptoms. One European study of eighty women found that black cohosh relieved menopausal symptoms more effectively than estrogen replacement therapy.

PERSPECTIVE AND PROSPECTS

The menopause, in various guises, was referred to in many early cultures and texts. Initially, an association was made between age and the loss of fertility. By the sixth century, written records on the cessation of menstruation were well documented. At that time, it was believed that menstruation did not cease before the age of thirty-five, nor did it usually continue after the age of fifty. It was thought that obese women ceased menstruation very early and that the periods remained normal or abnormal and increased in flow or became diminished depending on age, the season of the year, the habits and peculiar traits of women, the types of food eaten, and complicating diseases. Similar descriptions of menstrual cessation and its age of onset continued for another thousand years. It was not until the late eighteenth and early nineteenth centuries, however, that much advancement in the knowledge of the topic took place.

John Leake, influenced by William Harvey's historic description of the circulatory system, made one of the first reasonable attempts to explain the etiology of the menopause in his 1777 book *Medical Instructions Towards the Prevention and Cure of Chronic or Slow Diseases Peculiar to Women*. He believed that as long as the "prime of life" continued, along with the circulating force of the blood being more than equal to the resistance of the uterine vessels, the menses would continue to flow. When these vessels became firm from the effect of age, however, the diminished current of blood would be insufficient to force the uterine vessels open, and then periodic discharge would cease.

A later development in the history of menstruation studies was to link menstruation with all sorts of other problems, both emotional and organic. Leake commented that at the time of cessation of menses, women were often afflicted by various chronic diseases. He added that some women were prone to pain and lightheadedness, others were plagued by an intolerable itching at the neck of the bladder, and some were affected by low spirits and melancholy. Leake thought, because it seemed extraordinary that so many disorders should result from such a natural occurrence in a woman's life, that these symptoms could be explained away by indulgence in excesses, luxury, and an "irreg-

ularity" in the passions. Laying the blame for complications with the menopause on societal (in particular, female) excesses continued for some time.

Specific disease associations were also made; in 1814, John Burns announced that the cessation of menses seemed to cause cancer of the breast in some women. Edward John Tilt, a British physician, wrote one of the first full-length books on *The Change of Life in Health and Disease* (1857). Some of his views were that women should adhere to a strict code of hygiene during menstruation because they are often afflicted with cancer, gout, rheumatism, and nervous disorders.

These beliefs reflect a tendency from the mid-nineteenth century onward for medical literature to associate the menopause with many negative sociological features. For example, Colombat de l'Isère, in his book *Traité des maladies des femmes et de l'hygiène spéciale de leur sexe* (1838; *A Treatise on the Diseases and Special Hygiene of Females*, 1845), expressed his belief that during the menopause women ceased to live for the species and lived only for themselves. He thought that it was prudent for men to avoid having erotic thoughts about women in whom these feelings ought to have become extinct; he believed that after the menopause sexual enjoyment for women was ended forever.

Not all physicians, however, took such a negative attitude. Some believed that examining this phase in a woman's life presented a challenge. They believed that the boundaries between the physiological and the pathological in this field of study were ill-defined and that it was in the interest of the male gender that more research into this stage of a woman's life be done. The narrow boundary between normal physiology and pathology was not fully defined nearly a hundred years later, nor did the many negative and unsubstantiated theories cease. Well into the 1960's, the menopause was still considered "abnormal" and a "negative" state by some physicians.

Three major milestones exist in the history of menopause research in the twentieth century. The first event was the achievement of Adolf Butenandt, a Nobel Prize winner in chemistry. He succeeded in 1929 in isolating and obtaining, in pure form, a hormone from the urine of pregnant women which was eventually called estrone. The second development was the publication of *Feminine Forever* in 1966, which became an instant best seller. As a result of the book's publication, physicians were prompted to take sides in a heated and continuing debate. The third landmark was the publication of an editorial and two original articles in *The New England Journal of Medicine* of December 4, 1975, claiming an association between exogenous estrogens and endometrial cancer. This claim brought about legal action by initiating, at least in the United States, a series of health administration inquiries.

—*Genevieve Slomski, Ph.D.;*
updated by Karen E. Kalumuck, Ph.D.

See also Aging; Arteriosclerosis; Breast cancer; Cervical, ovarian, and uterine cancers; Endocrinology; Endometrial cancer; Gynecology; Heart disease; Herbal medicine; Hormone replacement therapy (HRT); Hormones; Hot flashes; Hysterectomy; Infertility, female; Menstruation; Midlife crisis; Obesity; Osteoporosis; Ovarian cysts; Sterilization; Women's health.

FOR FURTHER INFORMATION:

Corio, Laura E., and Linda G. Kahn. *The Change Before the Change: Everything You Need to Know to Stay Healthy in the Decade Before Menopause.* Rev. ed. London: Piatkus Books, 2005. An engaging and well-researched book that discusses what to expect during perimenopause, from the first sign of menstrual irregularity to the onslaught of physiological and emotional changes. Appendixes on herbs, phytoestrogens, and hormone therapy are particular strengths.

Doress-Worters, Paula B., and Diana Laskin Siegal. *The New Ourselves, Growing Older: Women Aging with Knowledge and Power.* New York: Simon & Schuster, 1994. In this updated version of a classic work developed in collaboration with the Boston Women's Health Book Collective, a host of issues related to maturing in women are addressed, including the menopause, osteoporosis, and estrogen replacement therapy. The positive aspects of changes are emphasized, and the book is filled with practical advice and resource lists.

Greenwood, Sadja. *Menopause, Naturally: Preparing for the Second Half of Life.* Updated ed. Volcano, Calif.: Volcano Press, 1996. This classic book gives a clear description of the natural changes in the menopause and up-to-date holistic approaches to its management.

Love, Susan, and Karen Lindsey. *Dr. Susan Love's Menopause and Hormone Book: Making Informed Choices.* Rev. ed. New York: Three Rivers Press, 2003. Renowned physician Love reviews recent research on HRT and offers advice about when such therapy is recommended. Also covers diet, exercise, stress management, alternative therapies, and medications other than hormones.

Maas, Paula, Susan E. Brown, and Nancy Bruning. *The Mend Clinic Guide to Natural Medicine for Menopause and Beyond.* New York: Dell, 1997. After giving a concise and lucid description of the physiological changes that occur during the menopause, this concisely written text addresses a host of symptoms and dispenses the current wisdom from a host of alternative medical traditions, including ancient Chinese medicine, acupressure, herbal therapy, and homeopathy.

North American Menopause Society (NAMS). http://www.menopause.org/. Web site run by a scientific research organization. Includes an excellent "consumers" section covering the range of menopause symptoms and treatments and providing referral lists and resource links, among other features.

Sheehy, Gail. *The Silent Passage: Menopause.* Rev. ed. New York: Pocket Books, 1998. Expanding on an article that she published in the October, 1991, issue of Vanity Fair, Sheehy draws from more than one hundred interviews conducted with women experiencing various stages of the menopause, as well as interviews with dozens of experts in many disciplines.

Stoppard, Miriam. *Menopause.* 2d ed. London: DK, 2002. A thorough exploration of the physiology, symptoms, medical complaints, and medical management of menopause, which also discusses maintaining sexuality, monitoring health, and preparing for the years beyond menopause.

MENORRHAGIA
DISEASE/DISORDER

ANATOMY OR SYSTEM AFFECTED: Blood, reproductive system, uterus
SPECIALTIES AND RELATED FIELDS: Gynecology
DEFINITION: Excessively heavy or prolonged menstrual flow.

CAUSES AND SYMPTOMS

Menorrhagia can be caused by many disorders: anatomic abnormalities of the uterus, hormonal imbalances, certain medical conditions, medications, and malignancy. Common anatomic causes are uterine fibroids and adenomyosis. Irregular menstrual cycles resulting from hormonal imbalances can be associated with menorrhagia. Medical conditions such as blood

INFORMATION ON MENORRHAGIA

CAUSES: Uterine abnormalities (fibroids, adenomyosis); hormonal imbalances; blood clotting disorders; liver or thyroid disease; blood thinners (coumadin, heparin); uterine and other reproductive tract cancers

SYMPTOMS: Excessive uterine bleeding, sometimes anemia

DURATION: Chronic

TREATMENTS: Depends on cause and severity; may include iron supplements, oral contraceptives or medroxyprogesterone, hormone injections to induce menopause, high-dose estrogens, dilation and curettage (D & C), thermal ablation, endometrial polyp or fibroid resection, placement of progesterone-impregnated IUD, myomectomy, hysterectomy

clotting disorders and liver or thyroid disease contribute to menorrhagia. Medications that prevent blood clotting, such as coumadin or heparin, can lead to increased menstrual flow. Uterine and other reproductive tract cancers can result in unusually heavy menstrual flow.

Symptoms of menorrhagia are uterine bleeding that is excessive (more than 80 milliliters) and/or bleeding that lasts for more than seven days. Unlike metrorrhagia, bleeding occurs at regular intervals. The patient can become anemic and exhibit symptoms of either acute or chronic blood loss. Symptoms and signs which suggest the cause of menorrhagia may be present, such as large palpable fibroids, or evidence of hypothyroidism or liver disease.

TREATMENT AND THERAPY

Menorrhagia can be treated via a medical or a surgical approach. The selection of treatment often depends on the cause and severity of the menorrhagia. If menorrhagia is the result of conditions amenable to medical treatment (such as a thyroid disorder), then control of these conditions may decrease the bleeding. If the patient has irregular cycles (for example, because of lack of ovulation), then hormones such as oral contraceptive pills or medroxyprogesterone may be used to regulate the cycles and decrease menstrual flow. A patient who is nearing the menopause can receive hormone injections that place her into an earlier artificial menopause, and hence eliminate menstrual bleeding altogether. If

the patient encounters acute and profuse bleeding, then high-dose estrogens may be given.

If menorrhagia is resistent to medical management, then surgical treatment may be necessary. Examples of procedural treatments for menorrhagia are dilation and curettage (D & C), for acute, profuse bleeding; thermal ablation of the endometrial lining; hysteroscopic resection of endometrial polyps or fibroids; and placement of a progesterone-impregnated intrauterine device (IUD). Hysterectomy is the definitive surgery for menorrhagia, no matter what the cause, since menstrual bleeding cannot occur without the uterus. Patients with large fibroids or adenomyosis often are not responsive to medical management. These patients would be candidates for hysterectomy. In patients with large fibroids and menorrhagia who wish to retain childbearing potential, a myomectomy may be performed instead of hysterectomy. If a patient is suspected or known to have a malignancy of the reproductive tract that is causing menorrhagia, then surgical management is the appropriate treatment.

Finally, patients can become severely anemic from menorrhagia, and blood transfusion may be necessary. Mild anemia can be treated with iron supplementation.

—*Anne Lynn S. Chang, M.D.*

See also Anemia; Bleeding; Dysmenorrhea; Endometriosis; Genital disorders, female; Hysterectomy; Menstruation; Myomectomy; Reproductive system; Women's health.

FOR FURTHER INFORMATION:

Golub, Sharon. *Periods: From Menarche to Menopause.* Newbury Park, Calif.: Sage Publications, 1992.

Icon Health. *Menorrhagia: A Medical Dictionary, Bibliography, and Annotated Research Guide to Internet References.* San Diego, Calif.: Author, 2004.

Kasper, Dennis L., et al., eds. *Harrison's Principles of Internal Medicine.* 16th ed. New York: McGraw-Hill, 2005.

O'Donovan, Peter, Paul McGurgan, and Walter Prendiville, eds. *Conservative Surgery for Menorrhagia.* San Francisco: Greenwich Medical Media, 2003.

Stenchever, Morton A., et al. *Comprehensive Gynecology.* 4th ed. St. Louis: Mosby, 2006.

Tierney, Lawrence M., Stephen J. McPhee, and Maxine A. Papadakis, eds. *Current Medical Diagnosis and Treatment 2007.* New York: McGraw-Hill Medical, 2006.

MEN'S HEALTH

OVERVIEW

ANATOMY OR SYSTEM AFFECTED: All

SPECIALTIES AND RELATED FIELDS: All

DEFINITION: Issues related to the health and well-being of men.

KEY TERMS:

colonoscopy: examination of the colon using an endoscope inserted into the rectum

digital rectal exam: examination in which a gloved finger is placed in the rectum to feel the prostate gland for lumps, enlargement, or irregularities

endoscope: a flexible tube with a camera device that is inserted into the body

epididymis: the coiled tube behind the testicles that stores and transports sperm

high-risk behaviors: behaviors that increase the chance of injury, disease, or harm

Klinefelter syndrome: a diseases in which an extra X chromosome in males causes abnormal development of the testicles

prostate diseases: diseases that affect the prostate gland

prostate-specific antigen (PSA): a glycoprotein produced by the prostate gland; its levels in the blood can indicate the presence of cancer

screening: tests to detect health problems and diseases

sexually transmitted diseases (STDs): contagious diseases that can be spread through sexual contact

sigmoidoscopy: examination of the lower portion of the colon (sigmoid) using an endoscope inserted in the rectum

MAJOR HEALTH CONCERNS

Men in the United States have a lower life expectancy than do women. Generally, men smoke, drink, and participate in more activities that may result in physical trauma. According to the Centers for Disease Control and Prevention (CDC), the ten leading causes of death among men are accidents, cancer, diabetes, heart disease, lung disease, liver disease, suicide, and homicide.

Accidents or unintentional injuries are the fifth leading cause of death in the United States. The risk of death as a result of a motor vehicle accident is twice as high among men and is highest within the age range of fifteen to twenty-four.

Cancer can occur in anyone at any age, but 76 percent of all cancers are diagnosed in those age fifteen and older. Nonmelanoma skin cancer is the most common cancer. Lung cancer is the leading cause of death among both men and women. Other cancers that affect men include prostate cancer, colon cancer, and testicular cancer.

Skin cancer may be identified as melanoma or nonmelanoma skin cancer. Skin cancers are more common in people with fair skin, hair, and eyes. The most important cause and risk factor for developing skin cancer is excessive sun exposure. Symptoms of skin cancer include skin areas that are crusty, scaly and rough, firm and red, shiny, or waxy, as well as nonhealing sores. The borders of cancerous areas are asymmetrical (uneven). The color is uneven, and the abnormal area is usually larger than six millimeters.

Lung cancer develops from abnormal cell growth in the lining of the lungs. Survival rates of lung cancer are poor. The earlier lung cancer is found, the better the chance for survival. Approximately one in ten survive five years after being diagnosed. Smoking is the number-one cause of lung cancer. Other risk factors include environmental pollution; exposure to radon, asbestos, and gases in closed areas, as in mining; and a family history of lung cancer. At first, one may have no symptoms, but as cancer grows, wheezing, shortness of breath, a persistent cough that worsens over time, coughing blood, chest pain, hoarseness, fatigue, decreased appetite, and neck and face swelling occur.

Colon cancer (colorectal cancer) develops from abnormal cell growth in the lining of the colon. It is the fourth most common cancer in men. About 90 percent of all colorectal cancers are diagnosed after age fifty. Risk factors and causes of colon cancer include a high-fat and low-fiber diet, alcohol abuse, smoking, lack of exercise, diabetes, colitis, irritable bowel, family history of colon cancer, and rectal polyps (growths on the lining of the colon). Polyps are common among those aged fifty and older. In the early stages, there may be no symptoms, but as the cancer grows, symptoms may include a change in bowel movements (diarrhea, constipation, bloody stools that are bright red or very dark, a feeling that the bowel does not empty completely, thin stools), abdominal discomfort (gas pains, cramping, bloating, sense of fullness), vomiting, weight loss, and fatigue.

Prostate cancer is caused by the growth of cancer cells in the prostate gland. Prostate cancer is the third most common cause of death from cancer in men, and it the most common cause of death from cancer in men over age seventy-five. A definitive cause of prostate cancer is still under investigation. It has been linked to a high-fat diet and elevated testosterone levels. African

American men older than age sixty, farmers, tire plant workers, painters, and those exposed to cadmium are at high risk for prostate cancer. Symptoms result from the blocking of urine flow because of prostate enlargement and include frequent urge to urinate (micturia), dribbling urine, painful or burning urination (dysuria), difficulty or inability to urinate, bloody urine or semen, painful ejaculation, and pain or stiffness in the thighs, hips, or lower back.

Testicular cancer is caused by the growth of cancer cells in one or both testicles. It is the most common cancer in men between ages fifteen and thirty-four and is most common in Caucasians. Approximately eight thousand men are diagnosed with testicular cancer annually in the United States. The causes of testicular cancer are still under investigation, but risks include cryptorchidism (undescended testicles) and a family history of testicular cancer. Symptoms of testicular cancer include a dull ache in the groin or low abdomen, pulling or heaviness in the scrotum, testicular or scrotal pain, and testicular enlargement.

Diabetes mellitus is a metabolic disorder in which the pancreas does not produce enough insulin to process and maintain proper blood sugar levels. Over time, poorly controlled diabetes can cause eye, heart, kidney, and nerve damage. About two-thirds of those with diabetes die of heart disease. There are two main types of diabetes. In Type I diabetes, the body produces no insulin. It affects 10 percent of those with diabetes and is most often seen in males under age thirty. Type I diabetes is more prevalent among North Europeans, African Americans, and Hispanics, respectively. The causes of Type I diabetes are not completely understood, but it is thought to be linked to an inherited, genetic predisposition that is activated by an environmental trigger from exposure to environmental chemicals or viruses that attack the immune system.

In Type II diabetes, the body either does not produce enough insulin or does not use insulin efficiently. Approximately 90 percent of those with diabetes have Type II diabetes. The risk of developing this type increases with age and most often affects those over age forty. One-third of men with Type II diabetes are unaware of it until problems such as erectile dysfunction (impotence), vision loss, or kidney disease develop. Causes and risk factors for developing Type II diabetes include a family history of diabetes, lack of exercise, a high-fat diet, elevated cholesterol levels, obesity, advancing age, high blood pressure, and being of African American, Hispanic, American Indian, Asian Ameri-

can, or Pacific Islander descent. Symptoms of both types of diabetes include blurred vision, headache, excessive thirst and hunger, unexplained weight loss, dry and itchy skin, slow-healing cuts and bruises, frequent urination, recurring infections, tingling in the hands and feet, mood swings, irritability, depression, and fatigue.

Cardiovascular disease refers to problems that affect the heart (heart disease) and circulation (vascular disease). Heart disease is the number-one killer of men. Being male increases the risk of developing heart disease. The mortality rate for African American men with heart disease is twice as high as for Caucasian men. Causes and risk factors include advancing age, family history, diabetes, elevated cholesterol, high blood pressure, a high-fat diet, lack of regular exercise, obesity, and smoking. Common cardiovascular diseases include coronary artery disease, cardiomyopathy, heart valve disease, heart failure, hyperlipidemia, high blood pressure, and stroke.

Coronary artery disease is the leading cause of heart attacks. In this condition, blood flow through the arteries of the heart is blocked. The most common cause is the buildup of fatty deposits (plaque) in the lining of an artery, called arteriosclerosis. Symptoms include shortness of breath, chest pain (angina), and/or a heart attack (myocardial infarction). Risk factors include smoking, elevated cholesterol, diabetes, high blood pressure, obesity, physical inactivity, and stress.

Cardiomyopathy involves conditions that enlarge the heart and weaken the heart muscle so that it does not pump efficiently. Causes and risk factors for developing cardiomyopathy are aging, alcoholism, high blood pressure, obesity, and smoking. Symptoms include chest pain, shortness of breath, irregular heartbeat, abdominal distention, swelling in the lower legs, fatigue, dizziness, and fainting.

Heart valve disease refers to conditions that damage the heart valves that may result in inadequate closure (prolapse), leaking (regurgitation), or narrowing (stenosis) of the valves so that blood does not circulate adequately. Causes and risk factors for the development of heart valve disease include rheumatic fever, heart attack (myocardial infarction), infections of connective tissue such as systemic lupus erthyematosus (SLE), poliomyelitis, rheumatoid arthritis, aging, congenital birth defects, medications, or radiation treatment. Symptoms of heart valve disease include shortness of breath, chest pain, irregular heart beat, high or low blood pressure, fatigue, and dizziness or faintness upon physical activity.

Heart failure is a condition in which the heart is unable to pump blood to organs and tissues efficiently. Heart failure may develop suddenly or gradually. Congestive heart failure is a condition in which the inability of the heart to pump blood to organs and tissues efficiently leads to a buildup of fluid in the body. Causes and risk factors for heart failure include coronary artery disease, heart valve disease, or cardiomyopathy. Symptoms of heart failure include shortness of breath, chest pain, heart palpitations, fluid retention that causes swelling in the lower legs and abdomen, weight gain (from fluid retention), weakness, dizziness, and fatigue.

Hyperlipidemia refers to elevated fats (lipids) in the blood that eventually form fatty deposits (plaque) on the walls of arteries that lead to coronary artery disease. The most common lipids include high-density lipoprotein (HDL) cholesterol, low-density lipoprotein (LDL) cholesterol, and triglycerides. Hypercholesterolemia refers to elevated blood cholesterol levels (higher than 200 milligrams) and is the leading risk factor for heart disease. High levels of HDL (higher than 60 milligrams) protect against heart disease. High levels of LDL (higher than 100 milligrams) can lead to heart disease. Hypertriglyceridemia refers to elevated triglyceride blood levels (higher than 150 milligrams). Hyperlipidemia increases the risk for heart attack, stroke, and diabetes. Causes and risk factors for hyperlipidemia include diabetes, high blood pressure, hypothyroidism, kidney or liver disease, aging, sex (men have a higher risk for elevated lipids), smoking, a high-fat diet, alcohol abuse, obesity, lack of exercise, heredity, stress, and medications such as corticosteroids, diuretics, and some blood pressure pills.

High blood pressure (hypertension) occurs when the pressure of the blood in the arteries is too high. High blood pressure is referred to as the silent killer because it often creates no symptoms. It is a major risk factor for heart disease. Untreated hypertension can lead to heart failure, heart attack, stroke, and kidney failure. A normal blood pressure is 120/80 or below. Blood pressure above 140/90 is considered high blood pressure. Prehypertension refers to blood pressures between 120/80 and 140/90. In those with diabetes and kidney disease, a blood pressure of 130/80 or higher is too high, and if it is not decreased, then high blood pressure is likely to develop. Causes and risk factors for high blood pressure include aging; race; sex (higher incidence in men); heredity; alcohol or drug abuse; obesity; stress; socioeconomic status; kidney, thyroid, or adrenal gland diseases, diabetes; sensitivity to salt; lack of

exercise, and some medications, such as cold, allergy, and migraine medications.

Stroke (also called a brain attack or cerebral vascular accident) can be either ischemic or hemorrhagic. Both prevent oxygen and nutrients from reaching the brain. Ischemic strokes are caused by blockage or narrowing of blood vessels leading to the brain, while hemorrhagic strokes are broken blood vessels that bleed into the brain. Causes and risk factors for a stroke include aging, arteriosclerosis, family history, race (higher incidence in African Americans), sex (higher incidence in men), diabetes, heart disease, high blood pressure, elevated blood lipids, a high-fat diet, lack of regular exercise, obesity, and smoking. Symptoms of a stroke include weakness or numbness of the face, arm, or leg on one side of the body; loss of vision; loss of speech; inability to understand what is being said; headache; dizziness; and walking problems or falling.

Pulmonary or lung diseases affect the health of the lungs. Common lung diseases are chronic obstructive pulmonary disease (COPD), bronchitis, emphysema, asthma, influenza, pneumonia, and lung cancer. Men are vulnerable to these diseases because they are more likely to smoke and to have jobs that involve exposure to hazardous materials.

COPD is the fourth leading cause of death in the United States. There is a strong link between COPD and lung cancer. Causes and risk factors for COPD include smoking; a history of childhood respiratory infections; asbestos, radon, and other air pollutants; and heredity. Symptoms of COPD include coughing, shortness of breath, chest tightness, and wheezing.

Chronic bronchitis occurs when the lining of the lungs become inflamed and swollen so that the airways become small and clogged with excess mucus and oxygen cannot be absorbed. Smoking and exposure to secondhand smoke are the main causes of bronchitis. Allergies, air pollution, infections, and pollutants from mining, farming, and working with textiles are also factors. Symptoms of chronic bronchitis include shortness of breath, coughing, and increased mucus that occurs most days for three months in a year over two consecutive years.

Emphysema occurs when the air sacs (alveoli) that exchange oxygen and carbon dioxide become damaged. Fifty-five percent of those with emphysema are men. Emphysema develops slowly over time, so symptoms do not become evident until it is well established. Smoking and exposure to secondhand smoke are the main causes of emphysema. Allergies, aging, heredity, air pollution, and pollutants from mining, farming, and working with textiles are also factors. Symptoms include a chronic cough with or without mucus production, fatigue, and loss of appetite.

Asthma results in inflammation and swelling in the airways that causes narrowing preventing air from passing through them. Causes and risk factors for developing asthma include smoking, gastric reflux disease, lung infections, exercise, heredity, allergies, pollution, cold air, and environmental triggers. Symptoms of asthma include wheezing, chest tightness, coughing, and shortness of breath.

Influenza is a contagious viral infection caused by the influenza virus that can be deadly. The elderly, young children, and those with weakened immune systems are at highest risk for serious complications. Symptoms include headache, fever, sore throat, dry cough, nausea, vomiting, diarrhea, fatigue, and muscle weakness and aching. Pneumonia is a deadly infection and/or inflammation of the lungs in which the airways become blocked by pus or fluid so that oxygen cannot be passed to and from the lungs. Individuals affected by heart disease, diabetes, age, or weakened immune systems are at a higher risk of dying from pneumonia. Risk factors and causes of pneumonia include chemicals, bacteria, viruses, and other microbes. Symptoms of pneumonia include fever, chills, sweating, shaking, cough, chest pain, and shortness of breath.

Chronic liver disease is the gradual failure of the liver to function effectively. Cirrhosis of the liver results from scar tissue that replaces healthy liver tissue and hinders the blood flow through the liver so that nutrients, hormones, and drugs are not processed normally. It is the eighth leading cause of death in the United States. Fibrosis of the liver is the overgrowth of scar tissue in the liver (usually from cirrhosis) that results from an infection, inflammation, or injury that prevents the liver from storing vitamins and minerals, regulating blood clotting, producing proteins and enzymes, maintaining hormone balance, and metabolizing or detoxifying substances. Risk factors for chronic liver disease include alcoholism, obesity, a low-fiber and high-fat diet, high blood pressure, elevated blood lipids, family history, and some medications. Symptoms include weakness, fatigue, confusion, loss of appetite, abdominal pain, excessive bruising, swelling in abdomen and legs, gastric bleeding, and yellow skin coloring (jaundice).

Suicide is the eighth leading cause of death among men in the United States. Men are four times more likely to commit suicide than are women. Suicide risk is related to depression, chronic illness, living alone, history of physical or sexual abuse, unemployment, age (highest among men in their twenties, sixties, and seventies), and marital status (higher among the never married, divorced, or recently widowed). Many men do not readily identify their depression and so do not seek treatment. It is estimated that each year more than six million men are affected with depression. Risk factors and causes of depression include loss of a loved one, stress, financial problems, relationship problems, positive or negative life changes, and heredity. Symptoms of depression include feelings of hopelessness, guilt, worthlessness, or helplessness; persistent sadness or anxiety; loss of interest in daily life activities and hobbies; difficulty concentrating; memory loss; indecisiveness; irritability; increased or decreased sleep; loss of energy; fatigue; weight loss or gain; physical ailments; and thoughts of death or suicide.

Men face unique diseases and disorders of the reproductive system. Testicular trauma is most often related to injuries acquired from contact sports or accidents. Symptoms of testicular trauma include pain, swelling, and bruising of one or both testes. Testicular rupture is rare, but it can cause blood to leak into the scrotum and requires surgical repair. Testicular torsion occurs when the spermatic cord twists and cuts the blood supply to the testicle. Adolescent males are often affected as a result of injuries sustained from strenuous activities. Symptoms of testicular torsion are sudden and severe testicular pain, tenderness, and testicular swelling.

Epididymitis is an inflammation of the epididymis. Males ages nineteen to forty are most often affected. Epididymitis is usually caused by an infection and can be the result of a sexually transmitted disease. Symptoms include scrotal pain and swelling, abscess (collection of pus), dysuria, frequent urination, urgency to urinate, abdominal pain, fever, and chills.

Hypogonadism occurs when the testicles do not produce enough testosterone. There are two types. Primary hypogonadism results from an abnormality in the testicles. Secondary hypogonadism results from a problem with the pituitary gland. Causes and risk factors of hypogonadism include undescended testicles, testicular trauma, hemochromatosis (excess iron in the blood), pituitary disorders from a head injury or pituitary tumor, mumps infection, Klinefelter syndrome, aging, chemotherapy or radiation therapy, and medications. Symptoms of hypogonadism include impaired growth of the penis and testicles, decreased muscle mass and body hair, enlarged breasts, infertility, erectile dysfunction, decreased sex drive, fatigue, difficulty concentrating, hot flashes, and depression.

Prostatitis is an inflammation in the prostate gland that is usually caused by a bacterial infection. Risk factors include urinary tract infections, medical procedure requiring insertion of objects into the penis, anal intercourse, or benign prostatic hyperplasia (BPH), or prostate enlargement. Symptoms of prostatitis include a tender and swollen prostate, fever; chills; low back, joint, and muscle pain; urinary frequency; dysuria; bloody urine (hematuria); difficulty starting the stream of urine (hesitancy); frequent urination at night (nocturia); and painful ejaculation.

BPH is an enlargement of the prostate gland. It naturally occurs with age and affects 50 percent of men after age sixty and 70 percent of men in their seventies and eighties. When an enlarged prostate presses against the urethra, it blocks the flow of urine. Symptoms of BPH include hesitant urination, frequent urination, urgency to pass urine, weak stream of urine, dribbling urine, dysuria, nocturia, straining to urinate, inability to pass urine (retention), and/or feeling that the bladder is not completely emptied.

Sexually transmitted diseases (STDs) are infections that are transferred through sexual acts such as intercourse, oral sex, sharing sexual objects such as vibrators, and intimate skin-to-skin contact. The United States has the highest number of STDs in the world, with more than 15 million cases reported each year. Almost two-thirds of all STDS occur in adults younger than age twenty-five. STDs include hepatitis B, genital herpes, human papilloma virus (HPV), chlamydia, gonorrhea, and syphilis. STDs can cause infertility and damage to the heart, kidneys, and brain, as well as an increased chance of contracting acquired immunodeficiency syndrome (AIDS). AIDS, the most serious STD, has no cure and can be fatal. STD symptoms may include discharge from the penis; painful sex; dysuria; sore throat from oral sex; pain in the anus from anal intercourse; chancres (painless red sores) on the genitals, tongue, throat, and anus; blisters or warts around the genitals; dark urine; light-colored bowel movements; and yellow skin (jaundice).

PREVENTION AND TREATMENT OPTIONS

The best way for men to manage these health concerns is prevention through education, healthy living, and screenings to identify diseases in their early stages, when they are most treatable.

Skin cancer can be prevented by minimizing sun exposure, wearing protective clothing that covers exposed skin, avoiding the sun during midday, and using sunscreen with SPF 15 or stronger year-round. Men should apply sunscreen at least one-half hour before going into the sun and then reapply it frequently. The American Academy of Dermatology recommends annual screening for skin cancer by a dermatologist. Treatment for skin cancer includes surgery to remove cancerous cells, radiation to shrink and kill cancerous cells, chemotherapy, and photodynamic therapy, in which a light-activated drug that targets cancerous cells is injected and then activated by lasers to destroy cancer cells.

Lung cancer is treated through the surgical removal of tumors, radiation therapy to shrink tumors, chemotherapy, photodynamic therapy, electrosurgery (which concentrates high-energy electromagnetic radiation to destroy tissue), and cryotherapy (which destroys cancerous tissue using extreme cold).

Colon cancer screening includes a rectal examination and stool test for blood every year, sigmoidoscopy every five years, barium enema every five years, and colonoscopy every ten years. Colon cancer screening should begin at age fifty, or sooner if there is a personal or family history of colon cancer or bowel disease. Treatment for colon cancer includes surgical removal of cancerous tissue, chemotherapy, and radiation therapy.

Prostate cancer screening recommendations are annual screenings after age fifty. For high-risk men, annual screenings should begin at age forty. Screenings include a digital rectal exam (DRE) and a prostate-specific antigen (PSA) test. The level of PSA is elevated when there are problems in the prostate. A biopsy may also show abnormal cells in the prostate. Treatment for prostate cancer includes prostatectomy (surgical removal of the prostate), radiation therapy, monthly hormone injections to shrink the prostate cancer cells, or "watchful waiting" until the tumor becomes larger.

Testicular self-examination (TSE) can help identify testicular cancer early. The American Cancer Society recommends that men over the age of fifteen perform monthly TSEs. These examinations are best done after a warm shower. Using both hands, the testicles should be rolled between thumbs and fingers to feel for any lumps. Abnormalities should be reported to a doctor. Treatment for testicular cancer includes orchiectomy (surgical removal of the testes), radiation therapy, and chemotherapy.

Diabetes is screened by a fasting blood glucose test, which measures blood glucose (sugar) after not eating for at least eight hours; a glucose tolerance test, which measures blood glucose two hours after drinking a concentrated sugar beverage; or a random blood glucose test, which checks the level of blood sugar without fasting. It is recommended that men over age forty-five be tested for diabetes every three years and those at high risk for diabetes be tested at age thirty. Treatment of diabetes may require taking hypoglycemic (low blood sugar) medications or insulin injections in addition to following a diabetic diet, monitoring blood glucose, and getting regular exercise.

Coronary artery disease is treated with lifestyle changes such as smoking cessation, exercise, medications, weight control, and a low-fat, high-fiber diet. Angioplasty (the opening of coronary arteries) or coronary artery bypass surgery may be needed. Cardiomyopathy and heart failure are treated with a low-salt, low-fat diet and medications to regulate and strengthen the heartbeat and decrease fluid retention. A cardiac pacemaker can improve the heart rhythm, while an implantable cardiac device (ICD) monitors heart rhythms and gives an electrical shock when a deadly heart rhythm occurs. Heart transplantation is a last resort when heart failure cannot be controlled. Heart valve disease can be treated with medication to regulate heart rhythm and strengthen the heartbeat, relax blood vessels (vasodilators), control blood pressure (antihypertensives), and reduce fluid retention (diuretics). A balloon valvuloplasty introduces an uninflated balloon into the heart valve that is then inflated to open the valve and then removed. If symptoms cannot be controlled, surgery may be necessary to repair or replace the affected valve.

Hyperlipidemia treatment includes lifestyle changes to reduce dietary fats and increase fiber in the diet, weight control, and regular exercise. Lipid-reducing medications may be used if lifestyle changes are not effective. If blood lipids are normal, then screening should be done at least every five years starting at age thirty-five. Screening should be done annually for elevated levels. Men who smoke, who have diabetes, or who have heart disease in their family should have their lipids checked starting at age twenty.

Blood pressure screenings should be done at each health care visit for men aged eighteen and older. Treatment for high blood pressure begins with lifestyle changes such as weight control, smoking cessation, limited alcohol consumption, regular exercise, and a low-fat, high-fiber diet. Antihypertensive medications are generally used if lifestyle changes are not effective.

Stroke can be treated with medications, surgical intervention and rehabilitation to restore optimum function. A carotid endarterectomy removes fatty deposits (plaque) in the artery that leads to the brain. Cerebral angioplasty opens the carotid artery by inflating a balloon into it to compress plaque, remove plaque with a rotating blade, or implant coils (stents) to keep the vessel open. Tissue plasminogen activator (TPA or tPA) is effective in treating strokes caused by blood clots by dissolving the clot and restoring circulation to the brain, but there is only a three-hour window of time in which it will be effective.

Bronchitis treatment is focused on reducing its symptoms, including avoiding smokers and air pollution, increasing fluids to keep mucus thin, humidifying the air to keep the airways open, deep breathing at least every hour to clear airways, and taking medications to open the airways, encourage coughing, and reduce inflammation, swelling, and mucus. If bronchitis worsens, then oxygen may be required to relieve shortness of breath and maintain adequate oxygen levels.

Emphysema treatment includes stopping smoking, avoiding smokers and air pollution, exercising to strengthen the lungs and diaphragm, maintaining a constant comfortable temperature in the home, increasing fluids to keep mucus thin, taking medications to open airways open the airways and thin mucus, and pursed lip breathing (lips partially closed while slowly breathing out to keep airways open). As emphysema worsens, supplemental oxygen may be required.

Asthma treatment begins with controlling the environment. Wearing a mask while cleaning; avoiding fur, feathers, and materials known to cause an attack; humidifying the air; and using an air conditioner in hot weather are some methods of avoiding an asthma attack. Medications for treating asthma include those that open the airways for quick relief; daily medications to control symptoms of inflammation, open airways, block release of chemicals that cause inflammation; and those that decrease the reaction to irritants. Desensitization is helpful in allergy-induced asthma, in which small amounts of substances that cause an allergic reaction are injected weekly over several months to develop immunity to them. Finally, anti-IgE monoclonal antibody medications help block antibodies that cause asthma attacks.

Men can lower the chances of developing influenza by getting a flu shot every year. Treatment for the flu is based on treating the symptoms and includes drinking adequate fluids, bed rest, and taking medications for fever, aches, cough, congestion, and nausea. Over-the-counter medications can minimize the discomfort of flu symptoms but do not treat the virus. Antiviral medications are helpful in preventing and treating the flu, but they must be given as soon as symptoms begin in order to be effective. Pneumonia can be prevented by having a pneumonia vaccination. It is 90 percent effective, and one dose prevents infection for five to ten years. Treatment for pneumonia includes drinking adequate fluids, bed rest, taking antibiotics for bacterial pneumonia, and taking medications to relieve fever, aches, cough, and congestion.

Liver disease treatment depends on the problem. Alcohol abuse is the primary cause of liver disease in men. Those at risk for exposure to hepatitis can be vaccinated against hepatitis B and hepatitis A. Treatment may include high blood pressure medication (antihypertensives), chemotherapy, radiation therapy, bile duct drainage, placing coils (stents) in the bile duct or blood vessels in the liver to keep them open, and liver transplantation.

Depression is most often treated by psychological counseling, cognitive behavioral therapy, interpersonal therapies, and antidepressant medications, with generally good results. Other treatments may include exercise, meditation, and light therapy. Treating depression in men can help to prevent suicide.

Testicular trauma can be evaluated by ultrasound or Doppler to identify the extent of injury. Treatment includes ice packs, scrotal support, anti-inflammatory medications, and bed rest for twenty-four hours. Surgical exploration may be warranted if the injury is severe. Testicular torsion is an emergency situation and should be evaluated by a urologist as soon after the injury as possible to prevent irreversible damage to the testicles. Treatment includes pain relief and manual rotation of the testicle to untwist the cord. This procedure is successful 70 percent of the time. If manual rotation does not work, then surgical intervention is necessary.

Treatment for epididymitis includes ice for swelling, a scrotal supporter, antibiotics, bed rest, and anti-inflammatory medicines (ibuprofen, naprosyn). Untreated epididymitis can cause scarring resulting in infertility. If the cause is related to a sexually transmitted disease, then any partners should be checked and provided treatment as well. Using condoms during sex can help to prevent infections.

Treatment for hypogonadism depends on its cause.

Testosterone replacement helps in sexual function, increases muscle strength, and prevents bone loss. Pituitary hormones may help increase testosterone levels and sperm production. Surgical removal of a pituitary tumor may help restore testosterone levels as well.

Benign prostatic hypertrophy is treated with medications to lower the tension in the valve under the bladder to allow urine to pass, or to decrease the amount of testosterone so that the prostate shrinks. Surgical removal of the prostate and radiation therapy to shrink the prostate are also optional treatments. There are no screening guidelines for BPH, and digital rectal examination is the only tool.

Prostatitis is not an easy diagnosis to make because symptoms are usually vague. Bacterial cultures of the urine and prostate secretions may or may not show an infection, but antibiotics are usually prescribed, along with medications to relax the prostate and relieve discomfort. Men are encouraged to increase their fluid intake for adequate hydration.

The only way to prevent STDs is through abstinence. Alternative means include education about STDs and their effects and using latex condoms during vaginal, anal, and oral sex. Polyurethane condoms are not as effective as latex, but they are the only alternative for those with latex allergies. Being with one partner (monogamy) who has tested negative for STDs is another way to prevent STDs. Regular screening for STDs are essential for those with multiple sexual partners. When diagnosed early, most STDs can be treated effectively.

PERSPECTIVE AND PROSPECTS

Men's health as a discrete subject within medicine began in the twenty-first century, modeled on the women's health movement. *The Journal of Men's Health and Gender* was founded in 2004. Its goals are to provide information and education about treatment and preventive care specifically for men. The Men's Health Act of 2005 established the Office of Men's Health in the Department of Health and Human Services.

Current men's health issues are in part attributable to the fact that men still tend to participate in risky activities, smoke, drink more alcohol, and be less likely to seek medical attention or participate in health screenings than are women. African American men are twice as likely to develop heart disease than the general population, one-third of men with Type II diabetes are not aware of it, suicide rates among men are four times higher than for women, and almost 69 percent of American men are overweight or obese.

In 2006, the National Center for Health Statistics reported that male life expectancy was seventy-five, about five years less than for women. Lifestyle changes play a large role in improving the life expectancy of men. Eating healthy, staying physically active, having regular medical checkups, and avoiding behaviors that are more prone to end in injury, illness, and death can increase men's life expectancy beyond the present average. Education and program development to engage more men in developing healthy lifestyles are essential for preventing disease and improving quality of life.

—*Sharon W. Stark, R.N., A.P.R.N., D.N.Sc.*

See also Accidents; Alcoholism; Asbestos exposure; Cancer; Cholesterol; Chronic obstructive pulmonary disease (COPD); Circumcision, male; Cirrhosis; Colon cancer; Color blindness; Concussion; Depression; Diabetes mellitus; Exercise physiology; Genital disorders, male; Gulf War syndrome; Gynecomastia; Hair loss and baldness; Hair transplantation; Heart attack; Heart disease; Heart valve replacement; Hemophilia; Hermaphroditism and pseudohermaphroditism; Hormones; Hydrocelectomy; Hypercholesterolemia; Hyperlipidemia; Hypertension; Hypertrophy; Hypospadias repair and urethroplasty; Incontinence; Infertility, male; Klinefelter syndrome; Lung cancer; Mumps; Occupational health; Orchitis; Penile implant surgery; Post-traumatic stress disorder; Proctology; Prostate cancer; Prostate enlargement; Prostate gland; Prostate gland removal; Puberty and adolescence; Pulmonary diseases; Screening; Sex change surgery; Sexuality; Sexually transmitted diseases (STDs); Skin cancer; Smoking; Sperm banks; Sports medicine; Steroid abuse; Suicide; Testicles, undescended; Testicular cancer; Testicular surgery; Testicular torsion; Vasectomy; Women's health.

FOR FURTHER INFORMATION:

Donatelle, Rebecca J. *Health: The Basics.* 7th ed. San Francisco: Benjamin Cummings, 2006. Provides information for lifestyle changes based in current health promotion and disease prevention trends for specific health issues.

Kasper, Dennis L., et al., eds. *Harrison's Principles of Internal Medicine.* 16th ed. New York: McGraw-Hill, 2005. Offers a comprehensive and detailed discussion of most diseases, symptoms, causes, diagnosis, treatment, and expected outcomes.

Litin, Scott C., ed. *Mayo Clinic Family Health Book.* 3d ed. New York: HarperResource, 2003. This handbook provides information regarding healthy living, diseases, and medical care from birth to old age.

Lunenfeld, Bruno, and Louis Gooren, eds. *Textbook of Men's Health.* Boca Raton, Fla.: Parthenon, 2002. Discusses the effects of hormone decline on aging and disease in men.

MedlinePlus. *Men's Health Issues.* http://www.nlm .nih.gov/medlineplus/menshealthissues.html#over views. This Web site provides links to news, overviews, and research into conditions affecting men.

National Institutes of Health. *Men's Health.* http:// health.nih.gov/search.asp/25. This Web site provides links to Internet sites with information and resources on a variety of issues related to men's health.

Simon, Harvey B. *The Harvard Medical School Guide to Men's Health.* New York: Free Press, 2004. Offers a comprehensive guide based on research for men to improve their health through healthy living and lifestyle changes.

U.S. Department of Health and Human Services. *Healthy People 2010: Understanding and Improving Health.* Rev. ed. Boston: Jones & Bartlett, 2001. A guide for reaching national goals to improve health in the United States. Specific areas of concern are identified, with discussions of physical, social, and psychological factors in disease and the means to address them.

MENSTRUATION

BIOLOGY

ANATOMY OR SYSTEM AFFECTED: Reproductive system, uterus

SPECIALTIES AND RELATED FIELDS: Endocrinology, gynecology, pediatrics

DEFINITION: The monthly discharge of blood and tissue (menses) by women of childbearing age, caused by changes in hormonal levels.

KEY TERMS:

endometrium: the layer of cells lining the inner cavity of the uterus; the source of menstrual discharge

feedback: a system in which two parts of the body communicate and control each other, often through hormones; can be either negative (inhibitory) or positive (stimulatory)

follicle: a spherical structure within the ovary that contains a developing ovum and that produces hormones; each ovary contains thousands of follicles

hormone: a chemical signal produced in some part of the body that is carried in the blood to another body part, where it has some observable effect *menstrual cycle:* the cycle of hormone production, ovulation, menstruation, and other changes that occurs on an approximately monthly schedule in women

ovary: the organ that produces ova and hormones; the two ovaries lie on either side of the uterus, within the abdominal cavity

ovulation: the process by which an ovum is released from its follicle in the ovary; occurs in the middle of each menstrual cycle

ovum (pl. ova): the egg or reproductive cell produced by the female, which when fertilized by a sperm from the male will develop into an embryo

prostaglandins: chemical signals that have local effects on the organ that produces them

uterus: the organ that nourishes and supports the developing embryo; also called the womb

PROCESS AND EFFECTS

Menstruation is the monthly discharge of bloody fluid from the uterus. It occurs in humans and in other primates (apes and monkeys), but not in all mammals; for example, horses, cats, and dogs do not menstruate. The menstrual fluid consists of blood, cells and debris from the endometrial lining of the uterus, and mucus and other fluids. The color of the discharge varies from dark brown to bright red during the period of flow. The menstrual discharge does not normally clot after leaving the uterus, but it may contain endometrial debris that resembles blood clots. The flow lasts from four to five days in most women, with spotting (the discharge of scant fluid) possibly continuing another day or two. The volume of fluid lost ranges from 10 to 80 milliliters, with a median of about 40 milliliters. The blood in the menstrual discharge amounts to only a small fraction of the body's total blood volume of about 5,000 milliliters, so normal physiological functioning is not usually impaired by the blood loss that occurs during menstruation.

The first menstruation (menarche) begins when a girl goes through puberty at the age of twelve or thirteen; the last episodes of menstruation occur some forty years later at the time of menopause. Menstruation does not occur during the months of pregnancy or for the first few months after a woman has given birth.

Menstruation is the most visible event of the woman's monthly menstrual cycle. The average length of the menstrual cycle in the population is about 29.1 days, but it may vary from 16 to 35 days, with variation occurring between different individuals and in one in-

dividual from month to month. Girls who have just gone through puberty and women who are approaching the menopause tend to have more variation in their cycles than do women in the middle of their reproductive years. There is also an age-related change in cycle length: Cycles tend to be relatively long in teenagers, then decrease in length until a woman is about forty years old, after which cycles tend to lengthen and become irregular.

Hormones cause menstruation to be coordinated with other events in the menstrual cycle. Uterine function is regulated by two hormones, estrogen and progesterone, that are produced in the ovaries. In turn, the production of estrogen and progesterone is controlled by follicle-stimulating hormone (FSH) and luteinizing hormone (LH), both of which are produced in the pituitary gland. The hormones from the ovaries and from the pituitary have mutual control over each other: They participate in a feedback relationship. The fact that females produce ova only once a month, in a cycle, rather than continuously, is the result of a change in the feedback relationships between the ovarian and pituitary hormones as the menstrual cycle proceeds.

In the first half of the cycle, the follicular phase, a predominant negative feedback effect keeps pituitary hormone levels low while allowing estrogen to increase. Day 1 of the menstrual cycle is defined as the day of the onset of the menstrual flow. During the days of menstrual bleeding, levels of estrogen and progesterone are low, but FSH levels are high enough to cause the growth of follicles in the ovary. As the follicles start to grow, they secrete estrogen, and increasing amounts are secreted as the follicles continue to enlarge over the next five to ten days. The estrogen exerts negative feedback control over the pituitary: FSH and LH production is inhibited by estrogen, so levels of these hormones remain low during the follicular phase. Besides producing estrogen, the growing follicles contain ova that are maturing and preparing for ovulation. Meanwhile, estrogen acts on the uterus to cause the growth of the endometrial lining. The lining becomes thicker and its blood supply increases; glands located in the lining also grow and mature. These uterine changes are known as endometrial proliferation.

As the woman nears the middle of her cycle, a dramatic change in hormonal feedback occurs. The increasing secretion of estrogen shifts the hormonal system into a positive feedback mode, whereby an increase in estrogen stimulates the release of LH and FSH from the pituitary instead of inhibiting it. Thus, at the middle

Menstrual Cycle

Days 1-6: Shedding of the endometrium; estrogen and progesterone low.

Days 7-12: Ripening of new egg; estrogen rising.

Days 13-18: Release of egg; estrogen and progesterone rising.

Days 19-23: Thickening of the endometrium.

Days 24-28: Unfertilized egg passes through uterus; estrogen and progesterone levels drop.

Exact timing varies from woman to woman; day 1 is defined as the day of onset of menstrual flow; ovulation occurs in mid-cycle (around day 14). Hormonal levels are rising and falling throughout the cycle.

of the cycle (around day 14), simultaneous peaks in levels of estrogen, LH, and FSH occur. The peak in LH triggers ovulation by causing changes in the wall of the follicle, allowing it to break open to release its ovum. Although a group of follicles had matured up to this point, usually only the largest one ovulates, and the remainder in the group die and cease hormone production.

Following ovulation, negative feedback is reestablished. The follicle that just ovulated remains as a functional part of the ovary; it becomes transformed into the corpus luteum, a structure which produces estrogen and progesterone throughout most of the second half of the cycle, the luteal phase. During this phase, the com-

bined presence of estrogen and progesterone reestablishes negative feedback over the pituitary, and LH and FSH levels decline. A second ovulation is prevented because an LH peak is not possible at this time. The combined action of estrogen and progesterone causes the uterus to enter its secretory phase during the second half of the cycle: The glands in the thickened endometrium secrete nutrients that will support an embryo if the woman becomes pregnant, and the ample blood supply to the endometrium can supply the embryo with other nutrients and oxygen. If the woman does in fact become pregnant, the embryo will secrete a hormone that will ensure the continued production of estrogen and progesterone, and because of these hormones, the uterus will remain in the secretory condition throughout pregnancy. Menstruation does not occur during pregnancy because of the high levels of estrogen and progesterone, which continually support the uterus.

If the woman does not become pregnant, the corpus luteum automatically degenerates, starting at about the twenty-fourth day of the menstrual cycle. As the corpus luteum dies, it fails to produce estrogen and progesterone, so levels of these hormones decrease. As the amounts of estrogen and progesterone drop, the uterus begins to produce prostaglandins, chemicals that act as local signals within the uterus. The prostaglandins cause a number of changes in uterine function: Blood flow to the endometrium is temporarily cut off, causing the endometrial tissue to die, and the uterine muscle begins to contract, causing further changes in blood flow. The decreased blood flow and the muscle contractions contribute to the cramping pain that many women feel just before and at the time of menstrual bleeding. Menstrual bleeding starts when the blood flow to the endometrium is reestablished and the dead tissue is sloughed off and washed out of the uterus. This event signals the start of a new menstrual cycle.

COMPLICATIONS AND DISORDERS

Many disorders involving menstruation exist. Toxic shock syndrome is a disease that, while not caused directly by menstruation, sometimes occurs during menstruation in women who use tampons to absorb the menstrual flow. The symptoms of toxic shock syndrome—fever, rash, a drop in blood pressure, diarrhea, vomiting, and fainting—are caused by toxins produced by the bacterium *Staphylococcus aureus*. This bacterium is normally present in limited numbers within the vagina, but the use of high-absorbency tampons is associated with a higher-than-normal bacterial growth and toxin production. Toxic shock syndrome requires immediate medical attention, since it may be fatal if left untreated. Women can reduce the risk of toxic shock syndrome by changing tampons often, using lower-absorbency types, and alternating the use of tampons and sanitary napkins.

Amenorrhea is defined as the absence of menstruation. It is usually, but not always, coincident with lack of ovulation. Amenorrhea may be primary (the woman has never menstruated) or secondary (menstrual cycles that were once normal have stopped). The condition is usually associated with abnormal patterns of hormone secretion, but the problem in hormone secretion may itself be merely the symptom of some other underlying disorder. One of the most common situations leading to both primary and secondary amenorrhea is low body weight, caused by malnutrition, eating disorders, or sustained exercise. Body fat has two roles in reproduction: It provides energy needed for tissue growth and cell functions, and it contributes to circulating estrogen levels. Loss of body fat may create a situation in which the reproductive system ceases to function because of low estrogen levels and because of lack of needed energy. The result is seen as amenorrhea. Emotional or physical stress may also cause amenorrhea, because stress results in the release of hormones that interfere with the reproductive hormones. Ideally, amenorrhea is treated by removing its cause; for example, a special diet or a change in an exercise program can bring about an increase in body fat stores, or stress level can be reduced through changes in lifestyle or with counseling. Ironically, sometimes birth control pills are prescribed for women with amenorrhea. The pills do not cure the amenorrhea, but they counteract some of the long-term problems associated with it, such as changes in the endometrial lining and loss of bone density.

Dysmenorrhea refers to abnormally intense uterine pain associated with menstruation. It is estimated that 5 to 10 percent of women experience pain intense enough to interfere with their school or work schedules. Dysmenorrhea may be primary (occurring in women with no known disease) or secondary (caused by a disease condition such as a tumor or infection). Studies have shown uterine prostaglandin levels to be correlated with the degree of pain perceived in primary dysmenorrhea, and drugs that interfere with prostaglandins offer an effective treatment for this condition. These drugs include aspirin, acetaminophen, ibuprofen, and naproxen; some formulas are available without a doctor's prescription, but the stronger drugs require one. Secondary dysmenorrhea is best managed by removing the underlying cause; if this is not possible, the antiprostaglandin drugs may be useful in controlling the pain.

Menorrhagia is excessive menstrual blood loss, usually defined as more than 80 milliliters of fluid lost per cycle. This condition can have serious health consequences because of the loss of red blood cells, which are essential for carrying oxygen to tissues. Women who have given birth to several children are more likely to suffer from menorrhagia, possibly because of enlargement of the uterine cavity and interference with the mechanisms that limit menstrual blood flow. Women who have diseases that interfere with blood clotting may also have menorrhagia. Although the menstrual discharge itself does not usually form clots after it leaves the uterus, clots do form within the uterine endometrium; these clots normally prevent excessive blood loss. Treatment for menorrhagia may begin with iron and vitamin supplements to induce increased red blood cell production, or transfusions may be used to replace the lost red blood cells. If this is unsuccessful, treatment with birth control pills, destruction of the endometrium by laser surgery, or a hysterectomy (surgical removal of the uterus) may be necessary.

Endometriosis is a condition in which endometrial cells from the uterus become misplaced within the abdominal cavity, adhering to and growing on the surface of internal organs. The outside of the uterus, the oviducts (Fallopian tubes), the surface of the ovaries, and the outer surface of the intestines can all support the growth of endometrial tissue. Endometriosis is thought to arise during menstruation, when endometrial tissue enters the oviducts instead of being carried outward through the cervix and vagina. Through the oviducts, the endometrial tissue has access to the abdominal cavity. Since the misplaced endometrial tissue responds to hormones in the same way that the normal endometrium does, it undergoes cyclic changes in thickness and attempts to shed at the time of menstruation. Endometriosis results in intense pain during menstruation and can cause infertility because of interference with ovulation, ovum or sperm transport, or uterine function. Endometriosis is treated with birth control pills or with drugs that suppress menstrual cycles, or the endometrial tissue may be removed surgically.

Premenstrual syndrome (PMS) is a set of symptoms that occurs in some women in the week before the start of menstruation, with the symptoms disappearing once menstruation begins. Researchers and physicians who study PMS have struggled to devise a standard definition for the disorder, but the list of possible symptoms is lengthy and varies from woman to woman and even within one woman from month to month. The possible symptoms include both psychological and physical changes: irritability, nervous tension, anxiety, moodiness, depression, lethargy, insomnia, confusion, crying, food cravings, fatigue, weight gain, swelling and bloating, breast tenderness, backache, headache, dizziness, muscle stiffness, and abdominal cramps. A diagnosis of PMS requires that the symptoms show a clear relation to the timing of menstruation and that they recur during most menstrual cycles. Researchers estimate that 3 to 5 percent of women have PMS symptoms that are so severe that they are incapacitating, but that

milder symptoms occur in about 50 percent of all women.

Because of the variability in symptoms between women, some researchers believe that there are several subtypes of PMS, each with its own cluster of symptoms. It is possible that each subtype has a unique cause. Suggested causes of PMS include an imbalance in the ratio of estrogen to progesterone following ovulation, changes in the hormones that control salt and water balance (the renin-angiotensin-aldosterone system), increased levels of prolactin (a hormone that acts on the breast), changes in amounts of brain chemicals, altered functioning of the biological clock that determines daily rhythms, poor diet or sensitivity to certain foods, and psychological factors such as attitude toward menstruation, stresses of family or professional life, and underlying personality disorders. Studies evaluating these theories have yielded contradictory results, so that no one cause of PMS has yet been found. Current treatments for PMS include dietary therapy, hormone administration, and psychological counseling, but no treatment has been found effective in all PMS patients.

An interesting phenomenon associated with menstruation is menstrual synchrony, also known as the "dormitory effect." Among women who live together, menstrual cycles gradually become synchronized, so that the women begin to menstruate within a few days of one another. Researchers have found that this phenomenon probably occurs because of pheromones, chemical signals that are produced by an individual and that have an effect on another individual. Pheromones act on the brain through the sense of smell, even though there may not be an odor that is consciously perceived.

PERSPECTIVE AND PROSPECTS

Early beliefs about menstruation were based on folk magic and superstition rather than on scientific evidence. Even today, some cultures persist in believing that menstruating women possess deleterious powers: that the presence of a menstruating woman can cause crops to fail, farm animals to die, or beer, bread, jam, and other foods to be spoiled. Some people believe that these incidents will occur even if the menstruating woman has no evil intention. Because of the possibility of these events, some cultures prohibit menstruating women from interacting with others. In the most rigorous example of such a taboo, some societies require that menstruating women live in special huts for the duration of the bleeding period.

Folk beliefs about menstruating women have been bolstered by religious views of menstruating women as "unclean" and in need of purification. In Orthodox Judaism, there are detailed proscriptions to be observed by a menstruating woman, including the avoidance of sexual intercourse. Seven days after her menstrual flow has stopped, the Orthodox Jewish woman undergoes a ritual purification, after which she may resume sexual relations with her husband. Early Christians absorbed the Jewish belief in the uncleanliness of a menstruating woman and prohibited her from entering church or receiving the sacraments. These injunctions were lifted by the seventh century, but the view of women as spiritually and bodily impure persists in some Christian groups to this day.

In the United States, most couples abstain from intercourse during the woman's menstrual period. There is no medical justification for this behavior; in fact, research has demonstrated that intercourse can alleviate menstrual cramping, at least temporarily. Still, surveys have shown that a majority of both men and women think that it is wrong for a woman to have intercourse while menstruating.

There are also persistent beliefs that women's physical and mental abilities suffer during menstruation. In fact, this was the predominant medical opinion up through the nineteenth and early twentieth centuries. Medical writings from this time are filled with injunctions for women to rest and refrain from exercise and intellectual strain while menstruating. It was a common belief that education could actually cause physical harm to women. Some men used this advice as justification for excluding women from equal opportunities in education and employment. Starting in the late 1800's, however, scientific studies clearly demonstrated that education has no harmful effects and that there is no diminution of intellectual or physical performance during menstruation. Nevertheless, the latter finding has been one that the general population finds difficult to accept.

The latest view of menstruation is that, far from being harmful, menstrual bleeding is directly beneficial to a woman's health. Margie Profet, an evolutionary biologist at the University of California, theorizes that menstruation evolved as a means of periodically removing disease-causing bacteria and viruses from the woman's uterus. These organisms might enter the uterus along with sperm after sexual activity. In Profet's view, the energetic cost of replacing the blood and tissue lost through menstruation is more than outweighed by the protective benefits of menstruation. Her theory implies that treatments which suppress menstruation, as birth control drugs sometimes do, are not always advantageous.

Nevertheless, pharmaceutical companies and some consumers have embraced the concept of suppressing menstruation. Users of the drug Seasonale, introduced in 2003, have menstrual bleeding every three months, and Wyeth sought approval for Lybrel, which would eliminate cycles altogether.

—Marcia Watson-Whitmyre, Ph.D.

See also Amenorrhea; Cervical, ovarian, and uterine cancers; Childbirth; Conception; Contraception; Dysmenorrhea; Endocrinology; Endometriosis; Genital disorders, female; Gynecology; Hormones; Hot flashes; Infertility, female; Menopause; Menorrhagia; Ovarian cysts; Pregnancy and gestation; Premenstrual syndrome (PMS); Puberty and adolescence; Reproductive system; Toxic shock syndrome; Women's health.

FOR FURTHER INFORMATION:

Ammer, Christine. *The New A to Z of Women's Health: A Concise Encyclopedia.* 5th ed. New York: Checkmark Books/Facts On File, 2005. A respected classic that covers the full spectrum of women's health issues, including the reproductive system, the aging process, methods of contraception, and childbearing. Helpful charts and illustrations.

Berek, Jonathan S., ed. *Berek and Novak's Gynecology.* 14th ed. Philadelphia: Lippincott Williams & Wilkins, 2007. A standard text covering all aspects of gynecology including biology and physiology, family planning, sexuality, and benign gynecologic conditions.

Covington, Timothy R., and J. Frank McClendon. *Sex Care: The Complete Guide to Safe and Healthy Sex.* New York: Pocket Books, 1987. Parts 1 and 2 deal with contraception and sexually transmitted diseases, but part 3 covers some topics directly related to menstruation: premenstrual syndrome, toxic shock syndrome, feminine hygiene, and various myths.

Golub, Sharon. *Periods: From Menarche to Menopause.* Newbury Park, Calif.: Sage Publications, 1992. An exceptionally complete book that presents information on all aspects of the menstrual cycle. The chapters dealing with scientific studies are accurate and easy to read. The author includes her thoughts on how society could make menstruation easier for women and on further research that needs to be done.

Loulan, JoAnne, and Bonnie Worthen. *Period: A Girl's Guide to Menstruation*. Rev. ed. Minnetonka, Minn.: Book Peddlers, 2001. A guide for young women that thoroughly covers questions about puberty and menstruation and includes diagrams to familiarize readers with the inner workings of their bodies.

Quilligan, Edward J., and Frederick P. Zuspan, eds. *Current Therapy in Obstetrics and Gynecology*. 5th ed. Philadelphia: Saunders, 2000. A standard medical reference on treatment for women's disorders, arranged in an encyclopedia format, with short articles on each topic. There is a particularly good description of premenstrual syndrome, written by Guy E. Abraham and Richard J. Taylor.

Rako, Susan. *No More Periods? The Risks of Menstrual Suppression and Other Cutting-Edge Issues in Women's Reproductive Health*. New York: Harmony Books, 2003. Argues that menstrual suppression and the manipulation of women's hormones for the purposes of birth control is "bad science" and can lead to bone loss, sexual dysfunction, sterility, and depression.

Weschler, Toni. *Taking Charge of Your Fertility*. Rev. ed. New York: HarperCollins, 2001. An excellent book that encourages women to become responsible for their own reproductive health. Includes discussions of menstrual cycles and the hormones involved.

MENTAL ILLNESS. *See* PSYCHIATRIC DISORDERS; *specific diseases.*

MENTAL RETARDATION
DISEASE/DISORDER

ANATOMY OR SYSTEM AFFECTED: Brain, nervous system, psychic-emotional system

SPECIALTIES AND RELATED FIELDS: Genetics, psychiatry, psychology

DEFINITION: Significant subaverage intellectual development and deficient adaptive behavior often accompanied by physical abnormalities.

KEY TERMS:

educable mentally retarded (EMR): individuals with mild-to-moderate retardation; they can be educated with some modifications of the regular education program and can achieve a minimal level of success

idiot: an expression which was formerly used to describe a person with profound mental retardation; such an individual requires custodial care

inborn metabolic disorder: an abnormality caused by a gene mutation that interferes with normal metabolism and often results in mental retardation

mental handicap: the condition of an individual classified as "educable mentally retarded"

mental impairment: the condition of an individual classified as "trainable mentally retarded" and typically distinguished from mentally ill

neural tube defects: birth defects resulting from the failure of the embryonic neural tube to close; usually results in some degree of mental retardation

trainable mentally retarded (TMR): individuals with moderate-to-severe retardation; only low levels of achievement may be reached by such persons

CAUSES AND SYMPTOMS

Mental retardation is a condition in which a person demonstrates significant subaverage development of intellectual function, along with poor adaptive behavior. Diagnosis can be made at birth if physical abnormalities also accompany mental retardation. An infant with mild mental retardation, however, may not be diagnosed until problems arise in school. Estimates of the prevalence of mental retardation vary from 1 to 3 percent of the world's total population.

Diagnosis of mental retardation takes into consideration three factors: subaverage intellectual function, deficiency in adaptive behavior, and early-age onset (before the age of eighteen). Intellectual function is a measure of one's intelligence quotient (IQ). Four levels of retardation based on IQ are described by the American Psychiatric Association. An individual with an IQ between 50 and 70 is considered mildly retarded, one with an IQ between 35 and 49 is moderately retarded, one with an IQ between 21 and 34 is severely retarded, and an individual with an IQ of less than 20 is termed profoundly retarded.

A person's level of adaptive behavior is not as easily determined as an IQ, but it is generally defined as the ability to meet social expectations in the individual's own environment. Assessment is based on development of certain skills: sensorimotor, speech and language, self-help, and socialization skills. Tests have been developed to aid in these measurements.

To identify possible mental retardation in infants, the use of language milestones is a helpful tool. For example, parents and pediatricians will observe whether children begin to smile, coo, babble, and use words during the appropriate age ranges. Once children reach school age, poor school achievement may identify those who are mentally impaired. Psychometric tests appropriate to the age of the children will help with diagnosis.

Classification of the degree of mental retardation is never absolutely clear, and dividing lines are often somewhat arbitrary. There has been debate about the value of classifying or labeling persons in categories of mental deficiency. On one hand, it is important for professionals to understand the amount of deficiency and to determine what kind of education and treatment would be appropriate and helpful to each individual. On the other hand, such classification can lead to low self-esteem, rejection by peers, and low expectations from teachers and parents.

There has been a marked change in the terminology used in classifying mental retardation from the early days of its study. In the early twentieth century, the terms used for moderate, severe, and profound retardation were "moron," "imbecile," and "idiot." In Great Britain, the term "feeble-minded" was used to indicate moderate retardation. These terms are no longer used by professionals working with the mentally retarded. "Idiot" was the classification given to the most profoundly retarded until the middle of the twentieth century. Historically, the word has changed in meaning, from William Shakespeare's day when the court jester was called an idiot, to an indication of psychosis, and later to define the lowest grade of mental deficiency. The term "idiocy" has been replaced with the expression "profound mental retardation."

Determining the cause of mental retardation is much more difficult than might be expected. More than a thousand different disorders that can cause mental retardation have been reported. Some cases seem to be entirely hereditary, others to be caused by environmental stress, and others the result of a combination of the two. In a large number of cases, however, the cause cannot be established. The mildly retarded make up the largest proportion of the mentally retarded population, and their condition seems to be a recessive genetic trait with no accompanying physical abnormalities. From a medical standpoint, mental retardation is considered to be a result of disease or biological defect and is classified according to its cause. Some of these causes are infections, poisons, environmental trauma, metabolic and nutritional abnormalities, and brain malformation.

Infections are especially harmful to brain development if they occur in the first trimester of pregnancy. Rubella is a viral infection that often results in mental

---

INFORMATION ON MENTAL RETARDATION

CAUSES: Often unknown; may include genetic factors, disease, infections, poisons, environmental trauma, metabolic and nutritional abnormalities, brain malformation

SYMPTOMS: Physical abnormalities, subaverage intellectual function, deficiency in adaptive behavior

DURATION: Lifelong

TREATMENTS: None; supportive therapy may include special education, physical therapy, family counseling

---

retardation. Syphilis is a sexually transmitted disease that affects adults and infants born to them, resulting in progressive mental degeneration.

Poisons such as mercury, lead, and alcohol have a very damaging effect on the developing brain. More recent concerns about mercury in the diets of those who frequently consume fish and other seafood have encouraged some individuals, such as pregnant women, to change their dietary behavior in an effort to avoid potential harm to fetal development. Lead-based paints linger in old houses and may cause poisoning in children or otherwise affect the mental functioning of all in the home. Children may eat paint and plaster chips or put them in their mouths, possibly causing mental retardation, cerebral palsy, and convulsive and behavioral disorders as a result of lead exposure.

Traumatic environmental effects that can cause mental retardation include prenatal exposure to X rays, lack of oxygen to the brain, or a mother's fall during pregnancy. During birth itself, the use of forceps can cause brain damage, and labor that is too brief or too long can cause mental impairment. After the birth process, head trauma or high temperature can affect brain function.

Poor nutrition and inborn metabolic disorders may cause defective mental development because vital body processes are hindered. One of these conditions, for which every newborn is tested, is phenylketonuria (PKU), in which the body cannot process the amino acid phenylalanine. If PKU is detected in infancy, subsequent mental retardation can be avoided by placing the child on a carefully controlled diet, thus preventing buildup of toxic compounds that would be harmful to the brain.

The failure of the neural tube to close in the early development of an embryo may result in anencephaly (an incomplete brain or none at all), hydrocephalus (an excessive amount of cerebrospinal fluid), or spina bifida (an incomplete vertebra, which leaves the spinal cord exposed). Anencephalic infants will live only a few hours. About half of those with other neural tube disorders will survive, usually with some degree of mental retardation. Research has shown that if a mother's diet has sufficient quantities of folic acid, neural tube closure disorders will be rare or nonexistent.

Microcephaly is another physical defect associated with mental retardation. In this condition, the head is abnormally small because of inadequate brain growth. Microcephaly may be inherited or caused by maternal infection, drugs, irradiation, or lack of oxygen at birth.

Abnormal chromosome numbers are not uncommon in developing embryos and will cause spontaneous abortions in most cases. Those babies that survive usually demonstrate varying degrees of mental retardation, and incidence increases with maternal age. A well-known example of a chromosome disorder is Down syndrome (formerly called mongolism), in which there is an extra copy of the twenty-first chromosome. Gene products caused by the extra chromosome cause mental retardation and other physical problems. Other well-studied chromosomal abnormalities involve the sex chromosomes. Both males and females may be born with too many or too few sex chromosomes, which often results in mental retardation.

Mild retardation with no other noticeable problems has been found to run in certain families. It occurs more often in the lower economic strata of society and probably reflects only the lower end of the normal distribution of intelligence in a population. The condition is probably a result of genetic factors interacting with environmental ones. It has been found that culturally deprived children have a lower level of intellectual function because of decreased stimuli as the infant brain develops.

TREATMENT AND THERAPY

Diagnosis of the level of mental retardation is important in meeting the needs of the intellectually handicapped. It can open the way for effective measures to be taken to help these persons achieve the highest quality of life possible for them.

Individuals with an IQ of 50 to 70 have mild-to-moderate retardation and are classified as "educable mentally retarded" (EMR). They can profit from the regular education program when it is somewhat modified. The general purposes of all education are to allow for the development of knowledge, to provide a basis for vocational competence, and to allow opportunity for self-realization. The EMR can achieve some success in academic subjects, make satisfactory social adjustment, and achieve minimal occupational adequacy if given proper training. In Great Britain, these individuals are referred to as "educationally subnormal" (ESN).

Persons with moderate-to-severe retardation generally have IQs between 21 and 49 and are classified as "trainable mentally retarded" (TMR). These individuals are not educable in the traditional sense, but many can be trained in self-help skills, socialization into the family, and some degree of economic independence with supervision. They need a developmental curriculum which promotes personal development, independence, and social skills.

The profoundly retarded are classified as "totally dependent" and have IQs of 20 or less. They cannot be trained to care for themselves, to socialize, or to be independent to any degree. They will need almost complete care and supervision throughout life. They may learn to understand a few simple commands, but they will be able to speak only a few words. Meaningful speech is not characteristic of this group.

EMR individuals need a modified curriculum, along with appropriately qualified and experienced teachers. Activities should include some within their special class and some in which they interact with students of other classes. The amount of time spent in regular classes and in special classes should be determined by individual needs in order to achieve the goals and objectives planned for each. Individual development must be the primary concern.

For TMR individuals, the differences will be in the areas of emphasis, level of attainment projected, and methods used. The programs should consist of small classes that may be held within the public schools or outside with the help of parents and other concerned groups. Persons trained in special education are needed to guide the physical, social, and emotional development experiences effectively.

A systematic approach in special education has proven to be the best teaching method to make clear to students what behaviors will result in the successful completion of goals. This approach has been designed so that children work with only one concept at a time. There are appropriate remedies planned for misconceptions along the way. Progress is charted for academic skills, home-living skills, and prevocational training. Decisions on the type of academic training appropriate for a TMR individual are not based on classification or labels, but on demonstrated ability.

One of the most important features of successful special education is the involvement of parents. Parents faced with rearing a retarded child may find the task overwhelming and have a great need of caring support and information about their child and the implications for their future. Parental involvement gives the parents the opportunity to learn by observing how the professionals facilitate effective learning experiences for their children at school.

Counselors help parents identify problems and implement plans of action. They can also help them determine whether goals are being reached. Counselors must know about the community resources that are available to families. They can help parents find emotional reconciliation with the problems presented by their special children. It is important for parents to be able to accept the child's limitations. They should not lavish special or different treatment on the retarded child, but rather treat this child like the other children.

Placing a child outside the home is indicated only when educational, behavioral, or medical controls are needed which cannot be provided in the home. Physicians and social workers should be able to do some counseling to supplement that of the trained counselors. Those who offer counseling should have basic counseling skills and relevant knowledge about the mentally retarded individual and the family.

EMR individuals will usually marry, may have children, and often become self-supporting. The TMR will live in an institution or at home or in foster homes for their entire lives. They will probably never become self-sufficient. The presence of a TMR child has a great impact on families and may weaken family closeness. It creates additional expenses and limits family activities. Counseling for these families is very important.

Sheltered employment provides highly controlled working conditions, helping the mentally retarded to become contributing members of society. This arrangement benefits the individual, the family, and society as the individual experiences the satisfaction and dignity of work. The mildly retarded may need only a short period of time in the sheltered workshop. The greater the degree of mental retardation, the more likely shelter will be required on a permanent basis. For the workshop to be successful, those in charge of it must consider both the personal development of the handicapped worker and the business production and profit of the workshop. Failure to consider the business success of these ventures has led to failures of the programs.

There has been a trend toward deinstitutionalizing the mentally retarded, to relocate as many residents as possible into appropriate community homes. Success will depend on a suitable match between the individual and the type of home provided. This approach is most effective for the mentally retarded if the staff of a facility is well trained and there is a fair amount of satisfactory interaction between staff and residents. It is important that residents not be ignored, and they must be monitored for proper evaluation at each step along the way. Top priority must be given to preparation of the staff to work closely with the mentally impaired and handicapped.

In the past, there was no way to know before a child's birth if there would be abnormalities. With advances in technology, however, a variety of prenatal tests can be done and many fetal abnormalities can be detected. Genetic counseling is important for persons who have these tests conducted. Some may have previously had a retarded child, or have retarded family members. Others may have something in their backgrounds that would indicate a higher-than-average risk for physical and/or mental abnormalities. Some come for testing before a child is conceived; others do not come until afterward. Tests can be done on the fetal blood and tissues that will reveal chromosomal abnormalities or inborn metabolic errors.

Many parents do not seek testing or genetic counseling because of the stress and anxiety that may result. Though most prenatal tests result in normal findings, if problems are indicated the parents are faced with what may be a difficult decision: whether to continue the pregnancy. It is often impossible to predict the extent of an abnormality, and weighing the sanctity of life in relation to the quality of life may present an ethical and religious dilemma. Others prefer to know what problems lie ahead and what their options are.

Finally, it is important to realize that problems such as mental retardation may not occur in isolation of other problems. Concurrent physical and mental illnesses may add complexity to managing treatment and services for individuals with more than one condition. Assessment to rule out other conditions remains an important step in ongoing and evolving care for individuals with mental retardation and similar conditions.

PERSPECTIVE AND PROSPECTS

Throughout history, the mentally retarded were first ignored, and then subjected to ridicule. The first attempts to educate the mentally retarded were initiated in France in the mid-nineteenth century. Shortly afterward, institutions for them began to spring up in Europe and the United States. These were often in remote rural areas, separated from the communities nearby, and were usually ill-equipped and understaffed. The institutions were quite regimented, and harsh discipline was kept. Meaningful interactions usually did not occur between the patients and the staff.

The medical approach of the institutions was to treat the outward condition of the mentally retarded and ignore them as people. No concern for their social and emotional needs was shown. There were no provisions for children to play, nor was there concern for the needs of the family of those with mental handicaps.

Not until the end of the nineteenth century were the first classes set up in some U.S. public schools for education of the mentally retarded. The first half of the twentieth century brought about the expansion of the public school programs for individuals with both mild and moderate mental retardation. After World War II, perhaps in response to the slaughter of mentally handicapped persons in Nazi Germany, strong efforts were made to provide educational, medical, and recreational services for the mentally retarded.

Groundbreaking research in the 1950's led to the normalization of society's attitude about the mentally retarded in the United States. Plans to help these individuals live as normal a life as possible were made. The National Association for Retarded Citizens was founded in 1950 and had a very strong influence on public opinion. In 1961, President John F. Kennedy appointed the Panel on Mental Retardation and instructed it to prepare a plan for the nation, to help meet the complex problems of the mentally retarded. The panel presented ninety recommendations in the areas of research, prevention, medical services, education, law, and local and national organization. Further presidential commissions on the topic were appointed and have had far-reaching effects for the well-being of the mentally retarded.

A "Declaration of the Rights of Mentally Retarded Persons" was adopted by the General Assembly of the United Nations in 1971, and the Education for All Handicapped Children Act was passed in the United States in 1975, providing for the development of educational programs appropriate for all handicapped children and youth. These pieces of legislation were milestones in the struggle to improve learning opportunities for the mentally retarded.

Changes continue to take place in attitudes toward greater integration of the retarded into schools and the community, leading to significant improvements. The role of the family has increased in emphasis, for it has often been the families themselves that have worked to change old, outdated policies. The cooperation of the family is very important in improving the social and intellectual development of the mentally retarded child. Because so many new and innovative techniques have been used, it is very important that programs be evaluated and compared to one another to determine which methods provide the best training and education for the mentally retarded.

—Katherine H. Houp, Ph.D.;
updated by Nancy A. Piotrowski, Ph.D.

See also Batten's disease; Birth defects; Brain; Brain damage; Cornelia de Lange syndrome; Cretinism; Down syndrome; Endocrine disorders; Fetal alcohol syndrome; Fragile X syndrome; Genetic diseases; Genetics and inheritance; Learning disabilities; Phenylketonuria (PKU); Prader-Willi syndrome; Pregnancy and gestation; Psychiatry; Psychiatry, child and adolescent; Rubinstein-Taybi syndrome.

FOR FURTHER INFORMATION:

American Association of Mental Retardation. http://www.aamr.org/index.shtml. A group for professionals in the mental health field that promotes progressive policies, research, effective practices, and universal human rights for people with intellectual disabilities.

Beirne-Smith, Mary, James R. Patton, and Shannon H. Kim, eds. *Mental Retardation.* 7th ed. Upper Saddle River, N.J.: Prentice Hall, 2006. Covers the causes and characteristics of individuals with mental retardation across the life span, explores the benefits of assistive technology, and surveys related legislation and policy issues.

Best Buddies International. http://www.bestbuddies .org/. Facilitates support among people with mental retardation and involving them in their communities.

Drew, Clifford J., ed. *Mental Retardation: A Lifespan Approach to People with Intellectual Disabilities.* 8th ed. Boston: Allyn & Bacon, 2003. An introductory and interdisciplinary text that examines all aspects of diagnosis and intervention, and discusses the treatment of multicultural issues related to as-

sessment bias, language differences, and mental retardation in all stages of life.

Dudley, James R. *Confronting the Stigma in Their
Lives: Helping People with a Mental Retardation
Label*. Springfield, Ill.: Charles C Thomas, 1997.
This book is written for anyone concerned about
combating the negative effects of being labeled as
having a mental disorder.

Glidden, Laraine Masters. *International Review of Research in Mental Retardation*. New York: Elsevier,
2006. An interdisciplinary text, updated regularly,
that surveys recent research into the causes, effects,
classification systems, and syndromes of mental retardation. Contributions from nutrition, genetics,
psychology, education, and other health and behavioral sciences are included.

Matson, Johnny L., and Rowland P. Barrett, eds. *Psychopathology in the Mentally Retarded*. 2d ed. Boston: Allyn & Bacon, 1993. This book addresses an
often-neglected topic: the psychological problems
that may be found in mentally retarded individuals.
Discusses special emotional problems of various
types of mentally retarded persons based on the causation of their deficiency.

MERCURY POISONING
DISEASE/DISORDER

ANATOMY OR SYSTEM AFFECTED: Nervous system

SPECIALTIES AND RELATED FIELDS: Environmental health, epidemiology, neurology, occupational
health, pediatrics

DEFINITION: Mercury is a naturally occurring element
that can cause neurological damage in humans exposed to it.

KEY TERMS:

neuropathy: any disease of the nervous system

methylmercury: a neurotoxin that is the form of mercury that accumulates most easily in biological tissues

CAUSES AND SYMPTOMS

Mercury is a metallic element once used in a wide variety of applications, ranging from industrial use in processing ore to serving as the indicator fluid in thermom-
eters. In its pure form, mercury is a soft silver-colored
metal with a melting point of a frigid −40 degrees
Celsius. Consequently, mercury is liquid at room temperature. Mercury and mercury compounds such as
methylmercury are known neurotoxins. Prolonged exposure to mercury, either through inhaling mercury va-

**INFORMATION ON MERCURY
POISONING**

CAUSES: Exposure to mercury through inhalation or ingestion

SYMPTOMS: Neurological damage; may include
tremors, slurred speech, cognitive problems

DURATION: Chronic

TREATMENTS: None; avoidance or limiting of
exposure

pors or through ingesting it as a contaminant in foodstuffs, will lead to permanent neurological damage.
Ingested mercury can also irritate the gastrointestinal
tract and has been known to damage kidneys.

Occupational neuropathy has long been anecdotally
associated with mercury exposure. The phrase "mad as a
hatter," for example, became common in the nineteenth
century when workers in the hat industry developed
tremors, slurred speech, and problems thinking clearly
following exposure to fumes produced by the felting
process. A mercury nitrate compound was used to remove animal hair from hides in hat factories. In some
cases of long-term exposure, neuropathy progressed to
the point where the sufferers experienced hallucinations.

Despite the widespread prevalence of occupational
illness among hatters, the nineteenth century medical
community did not recognize the dangers of mercury
exposure. Mercury was, in fact, used for a variety of
medical applications, ranging from treating syphilis to
being applied as a topical antiseptic in the form of
mercurochrome. Mercurochrome continued to be used
as late as the 1990's, although the Food and Drug Administration (FDA) ruled in 1998 that it would be
treated as a "new drug," meaning that any company
wishing to manufacture it for nationwide distribution
had to submit it for FDA review first.

The mining industry also used mercury extensively.
Mercury amalgamates readily with gold dust, making it
heavier and causing it to sink in to the bottom of rocker
boxes as ore is washed as part of placer mining. During
the California gold rush, at least 7,600 tons of mercury
were deposited into Sierra Nevada streams. Similar
amounts were used elsewhere globally, leading to large
quantities of mercury being deposited on stream beds
and ocean floors. That mercury is now making its way
back into the environment in the form of methylmercury, the organic form of mercury that causes most
concern among health care professionals today.

Methylmercury is formed when mercury forms a mercury-carbon compound through bacterial action. Manufactured methylmercury and dimethylmercury were common fungicides until the 1970's, when they were banned due to their toxicity.

TREATMENT AND THERAPY

With mercury poisoning, prevention is the best form of treatment. Occupational exposure to mercury rarely takes place, and the biggest risk of mercury poisoning today comes from its ingestion within the food chain. Methylmercury bioaccumulates readily and has been found in large concentrations in seafood such as tuna, swordfish, and shark. Numerous studies have shown that when pregnant women consume fish containing high levels of methylmercury the resulting mercury poisoning can cause permanent neurological damage to the developing fetus. Young children are also at risk of developing neuropathy if they eat fish with high mercury levels. This problem was first recognized in the 1970's, but did not become widely publicized until the early twenty-first century. Pregnant women, nursing mothers, and young children are all now advised to avoid some varieties of fish completely, while limiting their consumption of others.

PERSPECTIVE AND PROSPECTS

Although the use of mercury for many applications was discontinued as evidence mounted regarding the dangers of mercury exposure, thimerosal, a mercury compound, continued to be used as a preservative in vaccines used in human medicine into the twenty-first century. In the 1990's, many parents became convinced that thimerosal, which metabolizes readily to ethylmercury, was responsible for the rising rate of autism in American children. Autism is a cognitive disorder whose causes remain unknown, with researchers still uncertain about the roles that genetics, environmental exposures, and other factors may play in its development. Health activists argued that the increase in autism in the late twentieth century correlated with the increase in the number of vaccines that young children received in the first few years of life. Research into the question remains inconclusive, but the use of thimerosal as a preservative was discontinued by manufacturers for most vaccines, with the exception of influenza.

One use of mercury that does continue despite several decades of debate over its safety is the application of mercury amalgam tooth fillings in dentistry. The typical "silver" tooth filling is actually 50 percent mercury. Health activists argue that the practice should be stopped, as mercury leaching from the filling into the body could lead to mercury poisoning. In 2002, the FDA concluded that research to date had shown no evidence of ill effects other than rare cases of allergic reactions.

Given the widespread dispersion of mercury into the environment through pollution from numerous industries, mercury exposure will continue to be a health issue for many generations to come. Marine estuaries and ocean floors, as well as inland lakes and rivers, remain contaminated, and methylmercury will continue to work its way up the food chain.

—*Nancy Farm Mannikko, Ph.D.*

See also Autism; Cavities; Dentistry; Dentistry, pediatric; Environmental diseases; Environmental health; Food poisoning; Immunization and vaccination; Lead poisoning; Nervous system; Neurology; Neurology, pediatric; Occupational health; Poisoning; Toxicology.

FOR FURTHER INFORMATION:

Booth, Shawn. "Mercury, Food Webs, and Marine Animals: Implications of Diet and Climate Change for Human Health," *Environmental Health Perspectives* 113, no. 5 (May, 2005): 521-526. Discusses the effect of changes in diet on a specific population in the Faroe Islands, and shows how the amount of methylmercury exposure in utero affected cognitive development in children.

Davidson, Philip W., Gary J. Myers, and Bernard Weiss, eds. *Neurotoxicity and Developmental Disabilities.* London: Elsevier, 2006. An anthology that includes articles on mercury exposure as well as other environmental toxins.

Friberg, Lars. *Inorganic Mercury.* Geneva: World Health Organization, 1991. Looks at mercury and environmental pollution.

WHO Task Group on Environmental Health Criteria for Mercury. *Mercury: Environmental Aspects.* Geneva: World Health Organization, 1989. Discusses mercury toxicity and toxicology.

METABOLIC DISORDERS

DISEASE/DISORDER

ANATOMY OR SYSTEM AFFECTED: All

SPECIALTIES AND RELATED FIELDS: Biochemistry, endocrinology, genetics, nutrition, pediatrics, perinatology

DEFINITION: Disorders resulting from alterations in the pathways by which the body derives energy and synthesizes other molecules from carbohydrates, lipids, and proteins in food; usually caused by genetic defects that result in a missing or faulty enzyme.

KEY TERMS:

anabolic: the metabolic processes by which small molecules are combined together to produce larger molecules; used for energy storage or growth of the organism

catabolic: the metabolic processes by which food and stored products are broken down to release energy for use by the cell

enzyme: a protein whose job is to enable chemical reactions to occur in the cell in a timely manner; a biological catalyst

essential: referring to an amino acid, lipid, or vitamin that is necessary for proper cell functioning, but which the human body is ordinarily unable to produce on its own; must be supplied through the diet

metabolism: the process of extracting energy that can be used to power the cells of the body; includes both anabolic and catabolic processes

prenatal/neonatal screening: a tool whereby small volume fluid samples (prenatal) or blood samples (neonatal) are drawn and studied to determine the genetic traits carried by the child; neonatal screening is often mandated by law and used to find metabolic diseases as early in life as possible

CAUSES AND SYMPTOMS

Metabolic disorders of all types are usually inherited from one or both parents who carry a defective gene; the gene is one that codes for an enzyme responsible for a part of the metabolic pathway (either anabolic or catabolic). Much like an assembly line that takes raw material and produces a final product through multiple steps, the metabolism of proteins, lipids, and carbohydrates in the human body requires multiple steps, each with its own enzyme. In some cases, there are multiple pathways to metabolize a particular starting product. In this case, lack of one enzyme may not have a dramatic effect. Other pathways are exclusive, however, and any disruption of an enzyme will lead to disease. In addition to loss of a particular product, some enzyme defects lead to the accumulation of precursor molecules that may be toxic or may interfere with normal function of the cell.

When the deoxyribonucleic acid (DNA) coding for a particular gene is altered, one of three outcomes may be seen: no change (silent mutation), partial loss of ability

---

---

of the enzyme to do its job (mild disease), or complete loss of enzyme function (mild to severe disease). Diseases in the human are not known for all enzymes that could potentially be lost; this is most likely because disruption of an enzyme that is absolutely necessary in early development of the fetus will lead to early (and undetected) loss of the fetus.

Disorders of metabolism may be classified according to the pathways that are disrupted. Disorders associated with protein/amino acid metabolism may be seen when amino acids cannot be effectively broken down or when they cannot be transported into the cells of the body for use in building new proteins. Most of these disorders are seen early in life, since many proteins are essential for growth and development of the body. Examples of amino acid metabolism disorders are phenylketonuria (PKU) and maple syrup urine disease (MSUD). Other amino acid/protein disorders are homocystinuria, citrullinemia, alkaptonuria, and tyrosinemia.

Phenylalanine is an essential amino acid involved in the production of tyrosine, which in turn is converted to dopamine and serotonin. In PKU, the absence of this conversion means that phenylalanine accumulates in the body, causing toxic reactions within the brain and other organs. Mental retardation is the most obvious effect of this toxicity; other symptoms may include seizures, skin rashes, nausea and vomiting, and aggressive behavior. Phenylacetate (a by-product of excess phenylalanine) is secreted in sweat and urine, giving a distinctive odor to the child.

Leucine, isoleucine, and valine are amino acids that have a branched side chain. As a result of the presence of this special shape, an enzyme that can convert these enzymes is needed in order to metabolize food containing them. In MSUD, that enzyme is absent or deficient and these amino acids accumulate in the urine, giving a distinctive smell for which the disorder is named. If left untreated, this can lead to vomiting, staggering, confusion, coma, and eventual death from degeneration of the developing nerves early in life. A total of six different genes are responsible for production of the branched-chain alpha-ketoacid dehydrogenase enzyme complex, thus leading to some variation in the severity of the disease. While this disease is rare in the general population, the Mennonite community of Pennsylvania has a high rate of carriers for these mutations and thus is particularly affected.

Lipids (fats) are used in numerous ways in the human body, including for energy, temperature regulation, cell membrane structure, and nerve function. A variety of enzymes are responsible for breaking down and processing both stored and dietary lipids. In the absence of efficient processing of lipids, accumulations occur that can be extremely harmful to the organs of the body. Examples of lipid metabolism disorders are fatty acid oxidation disorders and Tay-Sachs disease. Other lipid metabolism disorders include Gaucher's disease, Refsum's disease, Niemann-Pick disease, Tangier disease, carnitine uptake defect, and trifunctional protein deficiency.

Several enzymes are involved in pathways that help stored lipids to be broken down and turned into energy. In the most common fatty acid oxidation disorder the enzyme deficient in this pathway is medium-chain acyl-coenzyme A dehydrogenase (MCAD). This is one of the most common errors of metabolism among people of northern European descent. A buildup of acyl-coenzyme A leads to delayed development, heart muscle weakness, and enlarged liver; death may occur. Symptoms develop shortly after birth and are most severe if the child goes without food for a prolonged period of time, or following exercise and the need for more energy to the cells (thus triggering the lipid breakdown pathways).

Perhaps the best known of the lipid metabolism disorders, Tay-Sachs disease results from errors in the enzyme β-hexosaminidase, which is responsible for breaking down the lipid GM2 ganglioside. The gene for this enzyme is known to reside on chromosome 15, and the absence of this enzyme allows large amounts of the ganglioside to accumulate in neurons. This accumulation leads to neurodegeneration that often results in floppy muscle tone, then paralysis, dementia, blindness, and death by age three or four. Less severe forms lead to long-term problems in the nervous system that progress throughout life. Tay-Sachs disease is most commonly seen in the Ashkenazi Jewish community but is also seen in the French Canadian population of Quebec and the Cajun population of Louisiana.

Carbohydrates (especially glucose) are the principal fuels for the body on a daily basis. Carbohydrate metabolism requires a variety of intracellular enzymes, as well as those responsible for transport and entry into the cell. Diseases or disorders of carbohydrate metabolism can be quite severe. Examples of carbohydrate metabolism disorders are Type I diabetes mellitus and glycogen storage diseases.

The ability to get glucose (the primary carbohydrate) into the cells of the body requires the hormone insulin. A lack in the production of insulin in the pancreas (Type I diabetes) leads to hyperglycemia (high blood levels of glucose) and a lack of glucose for energy within the cells. In addition to lack of cellular energy, this can lead to increased risk of blindness, heart disease, kidney failure, neurological diseases, and problems with circulation in the extremities. Type I diabetes may result from any one of several known mutations in DNA, the most common of which has been tracked to chromosome 6. In some forms of Type I diabetes, the body attacks either the insulin or the pancreatic cells that produce it, making this an autoimmune disease.

Glycogen is the branched-chain storage form of glucose in the liver and muscles of the body. Glycogen storage diseases are actually a group of eleven similar diseases that result in the inability of the body to produce sufficient glucose for the bloodstream to be used by cells of the body to produce energy. In addition to low blood sugar levels, children with this diseases often have with enlarged livers, swollen abdomens, and weak muscles. Elevated levels of lipids in the blood (taking the place of glucose as an energy source), may lead to acidosis and stress on the heart and kidneys.

In addition to the transport, storage, and breakdown of proteins, lipids, and carbohydrates, metabolism involves alterations in the use of elements such as iron and copper and the synthesis, storage, and use of the components of DNA and ribonucleic acid (RNA). Diseases and disorders in each of these areas are known as well. Examples include Wilson's disease, Menkes disease, hereditary hemochromatosis, and Lesch-Nyhan syndrome.

Copper is necessary in cells for energy metabolism, bone production, and nerve maturation. Wilson's disease and Menkes disease are disorders of copper transport and absorption that lead to a buildup of copper to toxic levels in the liver and the brain. Both liver disease and neurological damage can be present if they are not diagnosed early on; eventually, toxicity can be seen in many other organs as well. Menkes disease is usually fatal during infancy. Both diseases have been mapped to chromosome 13 and appear to be the result of proteins that are part of a transmembrane pump system. Menkes disease is transmitted as an X-linked recessive trait, while Wilson's disease is autosomal recessive.

Hereditary hemochromatosis is a disorder of iron metabolism seen predominantly in those of Northern European, Caucasian descent and traceable to a mutation on chromosome 6. Because iron is not adequately metabolized, the levels stored in the body grow over time, leading to symptoms that include cirrhosis of the liver, cardiomyopathy (heart muscle disease), alterations in skin pigmentation, joint damage, and decreased functioning of the gonads. Because men generally retain iron better than women do, symptoms often occur earlier in men. Symptoms also occur early in alcoholics, as alcohol consumption affects uptake of dietary iron.

Both DNA and RNA are constructed in part from nitrogen-containing bases; these bases are chemically grouped as purines and pyrimidines. The body can both make and recycle these bases. One of the genes involved in the recycling of purines (HPRT1) is located on the X chromosome. In Lesch-Nyhan syndrome, several known mutations result in low levels of the enzyme, and thus a lack of purine recycling. The resulting disease is seen almost exclusively in males and causes accumulation of uric acid (the starting point in purine synthesis). Uric acid leads to gout (painful deposits in the skin and joints) and kidney stones. For unknown reasons, this enzyme deficiency also leads to self-mutilation (biting of the fingers and tongue). Severe muscle weakness and mental retardation generally occur.

TREATMENT AND THERAPY

The most important diagnostic tool available for metabolic disorders is routine neonatal genetic screening. In 2005, a report by the American College of Medical Genetics recommended a core panel of twenty-eight metabolic disorders that should be screened for in all newborn children. This list includes disorders of protein metabolism, carbohydrate metabolism, and lipid metabolism, as well as a few multisystem disorders. Such screening does not prevent disorders but does allow early detection and therefore early intervention with diet, drugs, and other regimens that allow extended life spans for those afflicted.

Once detected, treatment of metabolic disorders is quite varied and is related to the underlying cause of the disorder. For protein/amino acid disorders, dietary restrictions are a key element in treatment. For instance, in PKU, phenylalanine intake must be restricted starting in the first few weeks of life. This means elimination of most forms of natural protein and substitution with phenylalanine-free foods. Patients with homocysteinuria often improve with vitamin B_6 (pyridoxine) or vitamin B_{12} (cobalamin). In maple syrup urine disease, restricting the dietary intake of the three branched-chain amino acids to the minimal amount required for growth and development allows for the best improvement. Vitamin B_1 (thiamine) is helpful in those with mild disease; dialysis is used in those with severe disease. Gene therapy is a possibility in the future.

In lipid disorders, control of diet is also essential. With fatty acid oxidation disorders it is important that patients eat often, never skip meals, and consume a diet high in carbohydrates and low in lipids. Treatment with intravenous glucose is helpful during attacks. The long-term outcome is very good in those who follow a strict dietary regimen. Likewise, in Refsum disease, a diet with little or no phytanic acid (carefully controlled plant products that contain no chlorophyll) is the key; plasmapheresis may be also be helpful. Other lipid disorders, including Gaucher's and Tay-Sachs, require drug intervention. Gaucher's type I patients (especially those without nervous system damage) can be treated with enzyme replacement therapy; the modified enzyme is given intravenously every two weeks. Enzyme therapy has been shown to stop, and even reverse, many of the symptoms of this disease. The late-onset (less severe) form of Tay-Sachs has seen some promise from treatment with a ganglioside synthesis inhibitor. Treatment of the infantile form has shown little promise, since much of the neurological damage occurs prior to birth and reversing neurological damage that has already occurred has proven to be extremely difficult.

Type I diabetes can usually be controlled well with daily insulin (artificial) and control of diet (to match the amount of energy needed for daily activities). Although islet cell transplantation or immunosuppression has been on the drawing board for several years, no real success has yet been obtained.

Other metabolic disorders run the gamut from easy to impossible to treat. Hereditary hemochromatosis, for instance, is easy to control, with therapeutic phlebotomy (blood-letting) to remove excess iron that has built up. Early diagnosis and treatment leads to a normal life span. By contrast, there is no cure for Niemann-Pick disease, and these children generally die of infection or degeneration of the central nervous system. For Menkes disease, administration of copper histidinate has shown promise, but it increases the patient's life span only by a few years (less than ten). In Lesch-Nyhan syndrome, medications are used to decrease the levels of uric acid; restraint against self-mutilation is commonly needed. Recent advances in gene therapy look promising for several of these conditions as well.

PERSPECTIVE AND PROSPECTS

Metabolic disorders have existed since the earliest humans roamed the earth, but it was not until the early twentieth century that the mechanism for these disorders was recognized. The term "inborn error of metabolism" was coined by Archibold Garrod, a British physician who published a classic text on the subject in 1923, following a study of children with alkaptonuria. This was the first such treatise to explain how symptoms often seen in sickly children could be explained on the basis of enzyme defects. Many of these diseases, such as diabetes, had been well established and named years before but not yet understood in terms of their biochemistry. The genetic basis for these disorders was not determined until much later—the 1970's and beyond.

Another early pioneer in this field was the German pediatrician Albert Niemann, who in 1914 described in detail a child with nervous system impairment. This condition later became known as Niemann-Pick disease, when Luddwick Pick took tissue samples from several such children after their deaths and provided chemical evidence of a distinct lipid storage problem.

The discovery of insulin in the 1920's provided the first opportunity to treat a metabolic disease in a standardized way, as insulin could be extracted and purified in a controlled laboratory setting. The availability of insulin has saved millions of lives since its discovery.

The hope for the future is gene therapy. The first gene therapy successes were recorded in children with enzyme deficiencies, and there are many trials throughout the world aimed at improving the chances of survival and healthy lives of those with similar metabolic disorders through correction of the genetic defect. In the future, such therapy might even be available in utero.

—*Kerry L. Cheesman, Ph.D.*

See also Arthritis; Diabetes mellitus; Digestion; Endocrinology; Endocrinology, pediatric; Enzyme therapy; Enzymes; Fatty acid oxidation disorders; Food biochemistry; Fructosemia; Gastroenterology; Gastroenterology, pediatric; Gastrointestinal system; Gaucher's disease; Genetic diseases; Glands; Glycogen storage diseases; Glycolysis; Gout; Hemochromatosis; Hormones; Insulin resistance syndrome; Kidney disorders; Lipids; Maple syrup urine disease (MSUD); Mental retardation; Metabolic syndrome; Metabolism; Mucopolysaccharidosis (MPS); Niemann-Pick disease; Nonalcoholic steatohepatitis (NASH); Obesity; Obesity, childhood; Phenylketonuria (PKU); Tay-Sachs disease; Wilson's disease.

FOR FURTHER INFORMATION:

Gilbert, Hiram F. *Basic Concepts in Biochemistry*. 2d ed. New York: McGraw-Hill, 2000. Although written as a review for medical students, its simple, nononsense approach to metabolism makes it a useful tool for anyone seeking an introduction to human metabolic systems.

Machalek, Alisa Zapp. *The Structures of Life*. Bethesda, Md.: U.S. Department of Health and Human Services, Public Health Service, National Institutes of Health, National Institute of General Medical Sciences, 2000. General introduction to proteins and how errors in manufacturing them can create problems in the body. Also discusses development of new drugs and other research. Also available at http://publications.nigms.nih.gov/structlife/.

Nussbaum, Robert L., Roderick R. McInnes, and Willard F. Huntington. *Thompson and Thompson Genetics in Medicine*. Rev. 6th ed. Philadelphia: W. B. Saunders, 2004. An excellent text meant primarily for medical students but readable by anyone with a background in basic biology, it describes many of the important metabolic diseases of the human and their basis in genetic defects.

Scriver, Charles R., et al., eds. *The Metabolic and Molecular Bases of Inherited Disease*. 8th ed. New York: McGraw-Hill, 2001. Probably the most important text in its field, this is an exhaustive look at metabolic diseases, their causes, and their treatment.

METABOLIC SYNDROME

DISEASE/DISORDER

ALSO KNOWN AS: Syndrome X, Deadly Quartet

ANATOMY OR SYSTEM AFFECTED: All

SPECIALTIES AND RELATED FIELDS: Cardiology, endocrinology, internal medicine, nutrition

DEFINITION: A constellation of metabolic changes that affect most major organ systems and may impinge on practically all systems of the body, beginning with excess weight or obesity.

KEY TERMS:

atherosclerosis: fat deposition and pathologic changes in the arterial surface and walls of major blood vessels of the body

diabetes mellitus Type II: peripheral resistance to insulin and increases in serum glucose and insulin concentrations, with damage to arteries in various organs

dyslipidemia: abnormal blood lipid levels, especially characterized by high serum triglycerides and very low-density lipoproteins (VLDL) and depressed serum high-density lipoprotein (HDL) cholesterol

hyperinsulinemia: abnormally high serum insulin concentration

overweight: having a body mass index (BMI), calculated as weight in kilograms divided by height in meters squared, that is between 25 and 29.9

obese: having a BMI that is greater than 30

steatohepatitis: an increased fat content in the liver independent of alcohol consumption

CAUSES AND SYMPTOMS

The metabolic syndrome, also known as Syndrome X, is a complex medical disorder characterized by the following clinical measures: dyslipidemia (high triglycerides and low HDL), insulin resistance, truncal (abdominal) obesity, and high blood pressure (hypertension). The metabolic syndrome may affect as many as forty-seven million adults in the United States, according to an estimate by the Centers for Disease Control and Prevention (CDC). The syndrome affects males more than females, and it is being recognized now even among children and adolescents. Key aspects of the metabolic syndrome are an energy imbalance and resultant altered metabolic pathways. The major diseases that result from the metabolic abnormalities are obesity, hypertension, diabetes mellitus Type II, and cardiovascular diseases (heart disease and stroke) because of abnormal lipid patterns. Several other diseases—colon cancer, nonalcoholic steatohepatitis (NASH), poly-cystic ovary disease, and chronic renal failure—may also be included as part of this syndrome.

The metabolic syndrome commonly features four major risk factors, sometimes referred to as the Deadly Quartet: dyslipidemia or blood lipid abnormalities (increased triglycerides and cholesterol), resistance to insulin or impaired glucose tolerance, overweight or truncal obesity, and elevated blood pressure. The underlying pathophysiology is speculated to be the poor utilization of glucose by muscle and fat tissues, coupled with an abnormality in the cellular metabolism of fat cells, muscle cells, and other peripheral or extrahepatic cells.

Increased rates of overweight and obesity in the United States had become widely recognized in the last decade of the twentieth century, and they serve as the beginning of the epidemic of this syndrome. This increase in the body mass index (BMI)—greater than 25 is defined as overweight and greater than 30 as obese—of American adults, coupled with the increasing prevalence of diabetes mellitus Type II among adults of all ethnicities, accentuated the extent of the problem by the early twenty-first century. Excessive intakes of macronutrients and insufficient physical activities in daily living in the affluent societies of the West are the bases of the metabolic syndrome, but adverse effects on micronutrient status may also result from the development of Type II diabetes. During its early onset period, urinary losses of several trace minerals may have an impact on other aspects of metabolism.

The pathophysiology of overweight/obesity relates to excess triglyceride (triacylglycerol, or TAG) accumulation in fat tissues scattered throughout the body, but especially apparent in the abdomen (android distribution) or buttocks and thighs (gynoid distribution). The defective steps that result from excessive fat stores in fat cells (adipocytes), however, are not clear. Peripheral resistance to insulin action occurs in both adipocytes and muscle cells; it involves gradually elevated blood levels of both glucose and insulin. The fat cells show resistance to insulin by reducing the distribution of glucose membrane transporters into cell membranes on the enveloping surfaces adjacent to extracellular fluids. This down-regulation results from a major shift in the metabolic steps leading to TAG synthesis. When fat cells shut down their synthesis of TAGs, the elevated blood glucose concentration permits glucose molecules to combine with diverse proteins in the body, including hemoglobin within red blood cells, by a process known as glycation or glycosylation. This

INFORMATION ON METABOLIC SYNDROME

CAUSES: Unknown; possibly poor utilization of glucose and abnormal cellular metabolism

SYMPTOMS: Lipid abnormalities, insulin resistance, abdominal obesity, high blood pressure; may result in diabetes, heart disease, stroke, colon cancer, nonalcoholic steatohepatitis (NASH), polycystic ovary disease, chronic renal failure

DURATION: Chronic

TREATMENTS: Weight loss, diet modification, drug therapy

glycosylation step becomes very significant and serves as a marker of poor control over blood glucose and, indirectly, of hyperinsulinemia.

Accompanying overweight/obesity and Type II diabetes are hypertension and abnormal lipid patterns. The atherosclerotic process is accelerated in the metabolic syndrome and in Type II diabetes because of the presence of multiple metabolic abnormalities. In insulin resistance, plaque formation may be enhanced because of the increased expression of adhesion molecules on endothelial cells and an increased rate of monocyte adhesion to endothelial cells. Circulating plasminogen is also more likely activated, which typically leads to increased clotting. In addition, hypertension may contribute to an increased risk of stroke in those with the metabolic syndrome.

TREATMENT AND THERAPY

Treatment strategies for the metabolic syndrome should focus on weight loss through a comprehensive program utilizing behavioral changes, including improved nutrition and an increase in physical activities. The long-term goal of therapy is a better balance between the intake of food energy sources and energy expenditure, so that a healthier body weight can be achieved.

The treatment of overweight and obesity is so difficult and inconsistent, however, that the other major components of the syndrome, dyslipidemia and hyperinsulinemia, often receive greater focus through both dietary modification and drug therapy. Dietary treatment typically requires the involvement of nutritionists and registered dieticians to provide educational information and institute changes in food selection. Physicians provide overall care, including the prescription of medications for one or more of the components of metabolic syndrome.

Since the emerging epidemic of the metabolic syndrome is expected to continue, both preventive and treatment strategies are needed. Prevention aimed toward reducing the development of this syndrome in children and adolescents should involve schools and community agencies.

PERSPECTIVE AND PROSPECTS

The metabolic syndrome has deadly consequences because of the nature of the chronic diseases that it spawns. This problem will worsen in the future in the United States because excessive eating and too little physical activity continue to dominate society. The epidemic nature of this syndrome requires that new public health measures be initiated and implemented as soon as possible. Preventive strategies need to be instituted to reduce the enormous impact of this syndrome anticipated in the United States in the early twenty-first century. The overall cost of treatment will be enormous.

Recognition of the metabolic syndrome essentially paralleled the increases in overweight and obesity in the United States in the early 1990's, but the epidemic of overweight actually began almost a decade earlier, although it was not detected by national survey data. Physicians were diagnosing many overweight and obese patients with the major components of the metabolic syndrome without linking them to a major health trend. Other countries of affluence were also reporting cases.

Now that the metabolic syndrome has been found to influence practically all bodily systems, it is likely that further research will identify may new variants of its effects in diverse organs beyond the ovaries and kidneys, which now are recognized to be targets of this disorder.

—*John J. B. Anderson, Ph.D.*

See also Arteriosclerosis; Diabetes mellitus; Endocrine disorders; Endocrinology; Endocrinology, pediatric; Hormones; Hyperlipidemia; Hypertension; Insulin resistance syndrome; Metabolic disorders; Obesity; Obesity, childhood; Weight loss and gain.

FOR FURTHER INFORMATION:

Byrne, Christopher D., and Sarah H. Wild, eds. *The Metabolic Syndrome*. Hoboken, N.J.: John Wiley & Sons, 2005.

Chrousos, George P., and Constantine Tsigos, eds. *Stress, Obesity, and Metabolic Syndrome*. Boston: Blackwell/New York Academy of Sciences, 2006.

Codario, Ronald A. *Type 2 Diabetes, Pre-diabetes, and the Metabolic Syndrome: The Primary Care Guide to Diagnosis and Management.* Totowa, N.J.: Humana Press, 2005.

Levine, T. Barry, and Arlene Bradley Levine. *Metabolic Syndrome and Cardiovascular Disease.* Philadelphia: Saunders/Elsevier, 2006.

Mokdad, A. H., et al. "The Continuing Epidemics of Obesity and Diabetes in the United States." *Journal of the American Medical Association* 286 (2001): 1195.

Reusch, J. E. "Current Concepts in Insulin Resistance, Type 2 Diabetes Mellitus, and the Metabolic Syndrome." *American Journal of Cardiology* 90, no. 5A (2002): 19G.

METABOLISM
BIOLOGY

ANATOMY OR SYSTEM AFFECTED: Gastrointestinal system, intestines, kidneys, liver, pancreas, spleen, stomach

SPECIALTIES AND RELATED FIELDS: Biochemistry, cytology, exercise physiology, gastroenterology, nutrition, pharmacology

DEFINITION: The processes by which the substance of plants and animals incidental to life is built up and broken down.

KEY TERMS:

adipose tissue: tissue that stores fat; occurs in humans beneath the skin, usually in the abdomen or in the buttocks

anabolism: the metabolic activity through which complex substances are synthesized from simpler substances

basal metabolic rate (BMR): the standardized measure of metabolism in warm-blooded organisms

calorie: a measurement of heat, particularly in measuring the value of foods for producing energy and heat in an organism

catabolism: the complete breaking down of molecules by an organism for the purpose of obtaining chemical building blocks

essential nutrients: molecules that an organism needs for survival but cannot manufacture itself

standard metabolic rate (SMR): the standardized measure of metabolism in cold-blooded organisms

storage compounds: areas in the body that store nutrients not immediately required by an organism

STRUCTURE AND FUNCTIONS

Metabolism is an ongoing process in living organisms. It is fundamentally concerned with the chemistry of life. An organism's metabolic rate is the rate at which it consumes the energy it derives from the nutrients that sustain it. Organisms consume energy by converting chemical energy to heat and external work; most of the latter is converted to heat also, as external work, such as walking or moving in any way, overcomes friction. A workable measure of metabolic rate, therefore, is the rate at which an organism produces heat. The food that organisms ingest is measured in Calories, each Calorie being the measure of what is required to raise one kilogram of water by one degree Celsius.

Metabolism consists of two essential underlying processes, anabolism and catabolism. In vertebrates, the food ingested is immediately mixed with digestive enzymes in the mouth. These enzymes are produced by the salivary glands. As a ball of food, a bolus, passes through the digestive system, additional enzymes found in the stomach, the pancreas, and the small intestine work upon it, accelerating the digestive process.

Some nonenzymes are also vital to the digestive process. Most notable are hydrochloric acid, which, in the stomach, is a necessary ingredient for the efficient use of the stomach's pepsin, and bile salts in the small intestine, nonenzymes essential to the digestive process. The action of the digestive apparatus results in catabolism, or the breaking down of the components of food, notably lipids, carbohydrates, and proteins, into small molecules used to build and repair cells. Such molecules, through absorption, traverse the wall of the small intestine to enter the blood or the lymph so that they can be distributed throughout the body to meet its immediate requirements.

Amino acids break down protein, permitting it to enter the bloodstream, whereas glucose and other enzymes act to break down the large carbohydrates into small molecules that are absorbed into the bloodstream. After they are catabolized into smaller molecules, the lipids or fats, unlike proteins and carbohydrates, enter the lymphatic system rather than the bloodstream, which they can enter only after they have passed through the lymphatic system.

Organisms typically cannot digest all the types of nutrients they ingest. Most vertebrates, for example, are incapable of digesting cellulose, the major carbohydrate component of most plants. This material, therefore, simply passes through the digestive system and is excreted. Fiber, which passes through the digestive tract essentially undigested, performs a valuable function in keeping the colon clear and, over the long term, in preventing colon cancer.

A remarkably complex biochemical process occurs when the circulatory system delivers its absorbed sugars, lipids, and amino acids to the parts of the body where they are needed to build new cells and repair existing cells. Sometimes, this process requires the conversion of sugar molecules to fat molecules or animo acids. For a cell to construct a protein, it must connect in a specific, complex order the many animo acid molecules that the process requires. While some of the requisite amino acids result directly from ingesting nutrients, others are not available in this way and must be obtained through the synthesis of sugar molecules.

Molecules that an organism needs for survival but that it cannot manufacture itself are obtained through ingestion. Such molecules are called essential nutrients. It takes twenty different kinds of amino acids, for example, to manufacture protein, but the body is capable of producing only half of these. Because green plants can synthesize all twenty forms of amino acids, they are a major and ready source of the essential nutrients required to sustain life.

Also, as part of a nutritional chain, one can note that although neither humans nor chickens can synthesize valine, a vital amino acid, chickens obtain valine by eating grain that is rich in it. Humans, in turn, eat chickens, through which they obtain valine. This amino acid is also available to humans through the green vegetables they eat.

The food that organisms ingest is used both to provide the necessary building blocks for the synthesis of membranes, enzymes, and other parts of cells and to provide energy. If the nutrients ingested are greater than the body's requirements for such synthesis and for the production of energy, then food molecules may be husbanded for future use in storage compounds within the organism. The excess stored in this way is usually in the form of lipids. In humans, such excesses are stored essentially around the abdomen and buttocks, where they can accumulate in considerable quantity.

If a human's food supply is severely reduced or completely cut off, the body draws on these reserves, using the stored fat cells until they have been completely depleted. Afterward, nutrients, mostly proteins, will be drawn from muscle mass, the sudden reduction of which can quickly eventuate in death.

The survival of organisms is usually dependent upon the work that they perform. Energy to carry out this work is derived through the splitting of the chemical bonds of adenosine triphosphate (ATP) and the splitting of the bonds of food molecules. Highly sophisticated and refined series of biochemical reactions called cellular respiration and aerobic catabolism permit most animals to transfer energy from the chemical bonds of nutrient molecules to the bonds of ATP.

Every cell in the body has the enzymes and cellular equipment to carry out aerobic catabolism and to manufacture its own ATP. Oxygen, carried through the blood, is the essential ingredient in aerobic catabolism, which results in the oxidization of nutrient molecules and their being broken up into small molecules composed largely of carbon dioxide and water. In this process, energy is released, some of it lost as heat and some of it conserved in the bonds of ATP.

As amino acids, lipids, and carbohydrates are catabolized in humans, the lipids and carbohydrates are used by the muscles, whereas the brain gains its energy almost exclusively through the glucose that catabolized carbohydrates produce. Excess amino acids are converted by the liver and, to a smaller extent, by the kidneys to carbohydrates or lipids.

In a process called anaerobic glycolysis, which involves the creation of ATP without the presence of oxygen, energy is produced by converting glucose or glycogen into lactic acid. The body cannot excrete lactic acid, thereby making impossible its accumulation in its original form in the body. Lactic acid is released into the bloodstream after exercise and, now subjected to oxygen, is metabolized by the liver and either converted to glucose or oxidized aerobically in order to release additional energy.

As vertebrates age, their metabolic rate often decreases. In humans, a decreased metabolic rate, reduced activity in old age, and a failure to reduce caloric intake can result in substantial weight gain. Therefore, as humans age, their physicians usually encourage them to engage in physical activity and to reduce the overall number of calories that they consume. Physical activity generally helps to sustain the basal metabolism at levels higher than those found among the sedentary.

DISORDERS AND DISEASES

All metabolic disorders stem either from genetic or environmental origins, or from a combination of the two. For example, a person with a predisposition for diabetes, an inherited genetic disorder, may exacerbate this predisposition by indulging in a diet high in fats and carbohydrates, by overindulging in alcoholic beverages, and by engaging in little physical activity.

Environmental factors such as diet and exercise can hasten the onset of a disease that lurks in one's genes. On the other hand, people with this predisposition who control diet and alcohol consumption and who make strenuous exercise regular parts of their daily activity

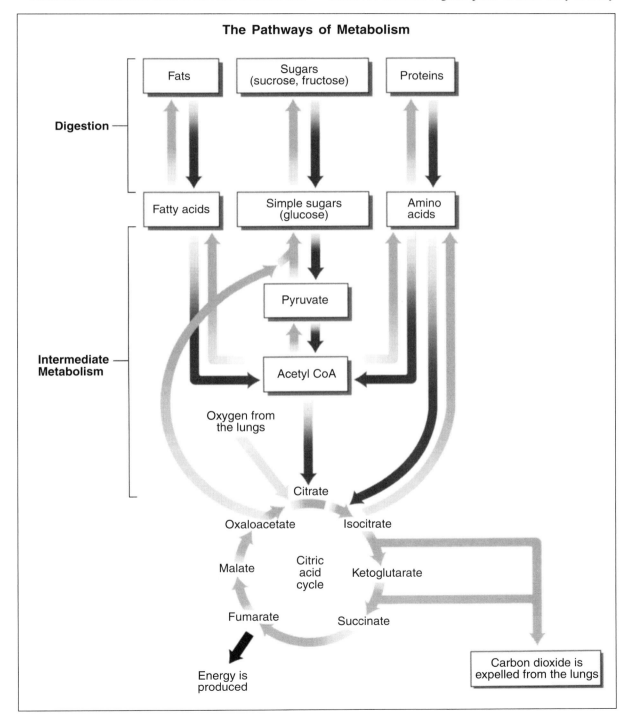

The Pathways of Metabolism

may forestall the onset of the disease, possibly keeping it at bay for their entire lifetimes.

Significant advances were first made in the 1960's in tracing the genetic origins of diseases. The discovery that deoxyribonucleic acid (DNA), the molecular basis of heredity, exists in the nucleus of every cell of living organisms was a major biochemical discovery. It has led to vastly increased insights into heredity and into metabolic disorders of genetic origin, certainly the overwhelming majority of all such disorders. Among the many metabolic disorders attributable to inheritance are diabetes, arthritis, gout, phenylketonuria (PKU), Tay-Sachs disease, Niemann-Pick disease, and hemochromatosis.

Microbiologists can detect a number of abnormalities in fetuses by analyzing the amniotic fluid that surrounds them in the womb. This process, known as amniocentesis, can identify more than twenty inherited metabolic disorders before an infant is born. Genetic manipulation in utero can alter some metabolic disorders, thereby bypassing or modifying faulty or abnormal genes. The genes of a person carrying a predisposition for a metabolic defect usually do not carry the information required for the synthesizing of a particular protein, usually an enzyme. This deficiency inhibits catalytic activity and blocks a metabolic pathway, resulting in a genetic abnormality.

In a minority of cases, the protein serves a role in transport or acts as a cell-surface receptor. Whatever role the protein in question serves, a delicate balance exists within the cells. When this balance is disturbed, metabolic problems ensue. For example, a gene may be responsible for producing an enzyme that converts one substance to another substance. If this gene is defective, the enzyme derived from it may be deficient and may fail to carry out the conversion or carry it out so slowly as to result in an inefficient conversion. While the first substance, a protein, accumulates in the cell, causing a surplus, it will be in short supply in the cell involved in the conversion, resulting in a deficiency. The surplus or the shortage may eventuate in a metabolic disorder, the genetic disbalance often revealing itself in overt symptoms.

Evidence of metabolic disorders can occur at any time in a person's life. They sometimes are detectable prenatally, but they may occur in early childhood, adolescence, adult life, or old age. In some cases, the onset of a serious metabolic disorder will be followed quickly by death. On the other hand, many people suffering from such disorders live long, active, full lives, many of them exceeding the average life span. Some metabolic disorders, such as diabetes, are manageable over long periods through diet and medication.

Some types of metabolic disorders can be treated successfully with massive doses of vitamins. At least twenty fairly common disorders respond favorably to such treatment. For example, Wilson's disease, which results in excessive amounts of copper being accumulated in the tissues, is generally treated successfully with D-penicillamine, a compound that removes copper from the tissues and deposits it into the urinary system for excretion as urine.

Certain nutrients trigger metabolic disorders in some organisms. The avoidance of these nutrients can prevent the triggering of the disorder on a permanent basis. Also, where the disorder results from a deficiency of an end product in a reaction, the disorder may be forestalled by replacing the end product.

Perspective and Prospects

The metabolism was scarcely understood until the 1770's, when Joseph Priestley discovered oxygen and set other researchers on the path to understanding its role in the biochemical aspects of all life. In the next decade, Antoine-Laurent Lavoisier and Adair Crawford were the first researchers to measure the heat produced by animals and to suggest convincingly that animal catabolism is a form of combustion.

These early, tentative steps toward understanding how organisms derive energy and how they expend it led to further research that, in 1828, resulted in Friedrich Wohler's synthesis of an organic compound, urea, from inorganic substances, demonstrating that the compounds that living organisms produce can be converted from inorganic to organic through metabolism.

It was not until 1842 that Justus von Liebig categorized foods as falling into three essential types, carbohydrates, lipids, and proteins. He measured the caloric values of nutrients and advanced considerably what was known about nutrition and its role in metabolism. At about the same time, Julius Robert von Mayer and James Joule discovered that motion, heat, and electricity are all forms of the same thing, energy. It was not until the 1890's, however, that Max Rubner and Wilbur Atwater demonstrated conclusively through empirical data that animals release energy according to thermodynamic and biochemical principles established through studies of inanimate systems.

Landmark discoveries about metabolism proceeded

into the twentieth century. In 1907, Walter Fletcher and Frederick Gowland Hopkins discovered that lactic acid results when glucose is subjected to the anaerobic contraction of muscles. Five years later, Hopkins discovered substances that are now recognized as vitamins, a term invented in 1912 by Casimir Funk. Ten years later, Frederick Banting and others pinpointed insulin as a substance that could be synthesized and used to reduce levels of blood sugar in humans, thereby making diabetes a manageable rather than a clearly fatal disorder.

A turning point in the understanding of metabolism and especially of metabolic disorders came in 1926 when James B. Sumner purified the first enzyme, showing it to be a protein, clearly leading to the realization that metabolic disorders result from a faulty protein in the genes. In 1941, Fritz Lipmann established the central role of ATP as a carrier of energy in living organisms, and the following year, Rudolf Schoenheimer demonstrated that the adult body's chemical constituents are in constant flux, suggesting that normal, healthy organisms are constantly renewing themselves.

As one surveys the future in terms of the rapidly increasing knowledge of metabolism and genetics, it is clear that genetic engineering offers daunting biological challenges. Birth defects can be detected well before birth, and many of them, through genetic manipulation, can be prevented. It is now within the capability of genetic engineering to predetermine the sex of a fetus and to control matters of gender. Amniocentesis can reveal abnormalities by the second trimester of pregnancy, revealing such conditions as metabolic disorders.

The capabilities that currently lie within reach pose substantial ethical problems and challenges. For example, if a fetus clearly shows evidence of being afflicted with a metabolic disorder, what use should be made of this information? Some parents would elect to terminate the pregnancy, given the challenges of raising such a child.

—R. Baird Shuman, Ph.D.

See also Acid-base chemistry; Arthritis; Caffeine; Cholesterol; Diabetes mellitus; Digestion; Endocrinology; Endocrinology, pediatric; Enzyme therapy; Enzymes; Exercise physiology; Fatty acid oxidation disorders; Food biochemistry; Fructosemia; Gastroenterology; Gastroenterology, pediatric; Gastrointestinal system; Gaucher's disease; Genetic diseases; Glands; Glycogen storage diseases; Glycolysis; Gout; Hemochromatosis; Hormones; Insulin resistance syndrome;

Kidney disorders; Lipids; Maple syrup urine disease (MSUD); Metabolic disorders; Metabolic syndrome; Mucopolysaccharidosis (MPS); Niemann-Pick disease; Nonalcoholic steatohepatitis (NASH); Obesity; Obesity, childhood; Phenylketonuria (PKU); Tay-Sachs disease; Wilson's disease.

FOR FURTHER INFORMATION:
Barasi, Mary E. *Human Nutrition: A Health Perspective.* 2d ed. New York: Oxford University Press, 2003. A text that emphasizes basic nutrition information, its role in metabolism, and the application of this information to health maintenance and disease prevention.
Becker, Kenneth L., et al., eds. *Principles and Practice of Endocrinology and Metabolism.* 3d ed. Philadelphia: Lippincott Williams and Wilkins, 2001. The treatment of metabolic disorders is extensive and accurate. The contributors are well informed and current in their information.
Devlin, Thomas M., ed. *Textbook of Biochemistry: With Clinical Correlations.* 6th ed. Hoboken, N.J.: Wiley-Liss, 2006. This college textbook presents considerable information on genetic engineering, hormones, and related topics. Includes chemical structures, diagrams, and references useful to the reader. All descriptions are simple but scholarly.
Edwards, Christopher R., and Dennis W. Lincoln, eds. *Recent Advances in Endocrinology and Metabolism.* 4th ed. New York: Churchill Livingstone, 1992. Particularly thorough in its treatment of such common metabolic disorders as diabetes, arthritis, and thyroid problems. The contributors also treat the less common metabolic disorders directly and clearly.
Feek, Colin, and Christopher Edwards. *Endocrine and Metabolic Disease.* New York: Springer-Verlag, 1988. This comprehensive volume presents information about every conceivable sort of metabolic disorder. The language is sometimes technical, but readers not specifically schooled in the field will be able to comprehend the salient points the authors make.
Hoffmann, Georg F., et al. *Inherited Metabolic Diseases.* Philadelphia: Lippincott Williams & Wilkins, 2002. A clinical text that details medical history, symptoms, the process of diagnosis and therapy, and organ-specific treatment of metabolic disorders.
Isaacs, Scott, and Neil Shulman. *The Hormonal Balance: Understanding Hormones, Weight, and Your Metabolism.* Boulder, Colo.: Bull, 2007. Details

how metabolic and hormonal imbalances can affect weight and perpetuate obesity. Examines diet and lifestyle changes to address menstrual irregularities and diseases such as diabetes.

King, Richard A., Jerome I. Rotter, and Arno G. Motulsky, eds. *The Genetic Basis of Common Diseases*. 2d ed. New York: Oxford University Press, 2002. Covers advances in the understanding of molecular processes involved in genetic susceptibility and disease mechanisms. Examines a range of diseases in detail and includes a chapter on genetic counseling.

Larsen, P. Reed, et al., eds. *Williams Textbook of Endocrinology*. 10th ed. Philadelphia: W. B. Saunders, 2003. Text that covers the spectrum of information related to the endocrine system, including thyroid disorders, diabetes, endocrinology and aging, female reproduction and fertility control, sexual function and dysfunction, kidney stones, and endocrine hypertension.

Whitehead, Roger G. *New Techniques in Nutritional Research*. San Diego, Calif.: Academic Press, 1990. This book provides the most thorough treatment of the nutritional aspects of metabolic disorders. It is especially strong in its presentation of disorders stemming from the accumulation of trace minerals, suggesting ways of treating such situations with vitamins or by other means.

METASTASIS. *See* CANCER; MALIGNANCY AND METASTASIS.

MICROBIOLOGY

SPECIALTY

ANATOMY OR SYSTEM AFFECTED: Cells, immune system

SPECIALTIES AND RELATED FIELDS: Bacteriology, environmental health, epidemiology, immunology, pathology, public health, virology

DEFINITION: The study of organisms too small to be seen by the unaided human eye, especially the identification, transmission, and control of microorganisms that cause disease.

KEY TERMS:

deoxyribonucleic acid (DNA): the genetic material of a cell that directs the synthesis of proteins; ribonucleic acid (RNA) is the intermediary needed to complete protein synthesis

flora: the microorganisms that are commonly found on or in the human body; also called microflora

infectious disease: an illness caused by a microorganism or its products, in contrast to diseases caused by factors such as heredity or poor nutrition

microorganism: an organism that is too small to be seen without a magnifying lens; also known as a microbe

pathogen: an organism that causes an infectious disease

SCIENCE AND PROFESSION

Microbiology is the field of science that focuses on microorganisms, living things that can be studied only by using microscopes and other special equipment. Microorganisms have an important place in the ecology of the planet. They form a basis for food chains and, as decomposers, recycle many materials in the environment. Because microbes are everywhere, humans come in contact with a wide variety every day; many live on or in the human body. Most of these organisms either are harmless or are prevented from multiplying by the immune system and other defenses. Others are able to penetrate these defenses and cause an illness. Medical microbiologists study microorganisms that cause these diseases. These pathogens come primarily from four groups: bacteria, fungi, protozoans, and viruses.

Bacteria, along with blue-green algae, belong to the Monera kingdom and are the simplest organisms that exist in cellular form. The bacterial chromosome consists of a loop of deoxyribonucleic acid (DNA) containing several hundred genes. Because it is unprotected by a nuclear membrane, bacterial DNA can be manipulated more easily than can DNA in plants and animals. Several traits are used to identify bacterial species. There are three basic shapes: coccus (round), bacillus (rod), and spirillum (spiral). Gram's stain procedure divides bacteria into two main groups based on their cell wall content. Other staining procedures can identify the presence of such structures as flagella, capsules, and endospores, which may have implications for control measures. For example, endospores are resistant to many common disinfectants, and boiling them for up to four hours may not destroy them. In addition to staining, chemical and metabolic tests are used to differentiate bacterial species.

Although the fungi kingdom includes larger organisms such as mushrooms, the ones of interest to medical microbiology are the yeasts, molds, and related microorganisms. Like plants, they have cell walls. They cannot manufacture their own food by photosynthesis, however, and must either be saprophytes, living on dead organic material, or parasites, obtaining nutrients from another living organism. Fungi reproduce by means of spores that are released and carried by the air to a suitable medium. They thrive in a warm, moist environment with a carbohydrate source of food.

Protozoa, members of the Protista kingdom, are often referred to as one-celled animals. They have no cell walls and must ingest or absorb their food. Their ability to move enables them to spread more quickly than can nonmotile microbes. Four main categories exist. The amoebas move by means of projections called pseudopodia. The flagellates move by means of long hairlike structures (flagella) that whip back and forth. Ciliates are covered with short hairlike structures (cilia) that beat in a synchronized way to cause movement. Sporozoans must move by means of the circulation of blood and tissue fluids within a host. Of all the microorganisms, protozoa are the ones that most resemble human cells. Treatment for a protozoal disease must be monitored closely; most chemicals that are effective against protozoa are also toxic to humans.

Viruses are on the borderline between living and nonliving things. They are not cellular in form, unlike all other forms of life. Each virus particle, called a virion, is made up of a protein coat and a nucleic acid core of either DNA or RNA. Viruses are classified by size, shape, type of nucleic acid in their core, and type of cell they invade or disease they cause.

In order to reproduce, a virion attaches itself to a living cell and injects its core into the cell. The nucleic acid then takes over the cell's protein-manufacturing apparatus to make new virus particles. The host cell ruptures as these viruses are released to infect other cells. Some viral DNA can incorporate itself into the host DNA and remain dormant until some factor triggers a new reproductive cycle. Viruses usually can attack only one type of cell or species; however, mutations can occur that allow them to infect other species. For example, human immunodeficiency virus (HIV), the cause of acquired immunodeficiency syndrome (AIDS), is believed to have mutated from simian immunodeficiency virus (SIV) in monkeys.

DIAGNOSTIC AND TREATMENT TECHNIQUES

When the type of microorganism causing an infectious disease is unknown, a medical microbiologist follows a series of procedures known as Koch's postulates. Named for Robert Koch, who proposed them, these procedures identify and confirm that a particular microorganism is the cause of the disease. First, the microorganism must be present in the tissues of all individuals who have the disease. This means that all the microorganisms in a sample of diseased tissue must be identified and classified so that a possible pathogen may be differentiated from the normal flora. Second, the suspected pathogen must be isolated and grown in a pure culture. Many microorganisms can be grown on a simple medium called nutrient agar. Some microorganisms may need specific nutrients added to the medium or may be obligate parasites—that is, they can grow only on or in living cells. Anaerobic organisms cannot grow at all if oxygen is present. Since these special needs are not known in advance, the detection of some pathogens may be difficult.

The third step the researcher takes is to inoculate an animal with the organism in an effort to duplicate the disease. In the case of human diseases, mammals—such as rabbits, guinea pigs, and mice—are used. Finding the right animal subject may also pose a problem, since not all animals are susceptible to human diseases. For example, armadillos must be used to study leprosy, because the more common laboratory animals are not susceptible to it. In the last of Koch's procedures, the organism must be reisolated from the diseased animal. This step verifies the identity of the pathogen and confirms that it is the same as the original form. If the organism has been identified correctly as the cause of the disease, researchers can then proceed to learn more about the microorganism and its role in the disease process.

The identification of a pathogen as the cause of a specific disease and knowledge of its biological characteristics aid medical researchers in finding prevention and treatment strategies. In order to cause illness, a microorganism must meet several criteria. First, it must survive transfer to the new host. Some pathogens can form protective structures, such as endospores, that will keep them alive outside a host for a long period of time. A pathogen that cannot survive outside a host must be passed directly in some way from an infected person to a healthy one. Second, a pathogen must overcome the host's defenses. Some may enter through a wound, bypassing the skin barrier that protects the human body from many infections. Some produce chemicals that damage cells and weaken the body. Still others may be able to cause illness only if the person's defenses are weakened by some factor such as age, malnutrition, or another existing illness. Finally, the organism must cause some damage to the host, resulting in the symptoms and signs associated with that illness. The disease process can best be understood by examining several examples of pathogens, the diseases they cause, and the strategies used against them.

The members of the genus *Clostridium* are all anaerobic, form endospores, and produce toxins. Among the bacteria in this group are the pathogens that cause gangrene, tetanus, and botulism. Gangrene usually occurs when a wound has cut off the blood supply to an area of the body. *Clostridium perfringens* enters the body and is able to survive because the lack of blood has created an anaerobic condition. It produces a toxin that destroys surrounding tissue, allowing it to spread. Antibiotics may be effective in preventing the bacteria from spreading to healthy tissue but, because drugs are transported in the blood, may not be able to reach the infected site. Placing the patient in a chamber containing oxygen under high pressure is one strategy used to destroy anaerobic bacteria. *Clostridium tetani* also enters the body through a wound—sometimes a very small one. Since this organism is common and a small wound may go unnoticed, regular immunizations with tetanus vaccine are recommended. Once *C. tetani* bacteria enter the body, they produce a neurotoxin. This nerve poison causes the muscles to stiffen, resulting in a condition called tetanus, or lockjaw. In addition to antibiotics, an antitoxin must be given to neutralize the poison. *Clostridium botulinum* causes botulism, a type of food poisoning. If proper canning techniques are not used, the endospores will germinate. The food then provides a medium on which they can grow, and the sealed can provides the perfect anaerobic conditions. *C. botulinum* produces a neurotoxin that, if it is not destroyed by adequate cooking, will produce neurological symptoms such as double vision and dizziness. This disease must be treated by an appropriate antitoxin or death from respiratory failure can occur in a matter of days.

The human intestine contains large numbers of microorganisms. Some of them provide benefits to their host by producing vitamins and inhibiting the growth of other, potentially harmful, microorganisms. Disease can result if the balance is changed. *Escherichia coli*, part of the normal intestinal flora, can cause infections when it is transferred to another part of the body, such as the urinary bladder. In developing countries, *E. coli* bacteria contaminate drinking water in such large numbers that they result in infantile diarrhea, a common cause of death in those countries. A 1993 epidemic in the United States involved a particularly virulent strain of *E. coli* that had been ingested in improperly cooked

ground beef. The characteristics of the strain, combined with the large number of bacteria in the meat, disrupted the intestinal balance of those who ingested it, caused hundreds of people to become ill, and resulted in the deaths of three young children.

The use of antibiotics can disrupt the natural balance by destroying beneficial bacteria as well as pathogens. *Candida albicans*, a yeastlike fungus, is part of the normal human flora. Its growth in the intestine is controlled by certain kinds of bacteria. When antibiotics are used, these beneficial bacteria are destroyed and the *Candida* begins to multiply. This may not only result in intestinal yeast infections but also contribute to yeast infections in the vagina and other areas where *Candida* can be found. Strategies used to restore the balance may involve eating yogurt or capsules containing *Acidophilus*, one of the beneficial bacteria. Sugars, an important source of food for yeast, should be eliminated from the diet. If these measures do not work, antifungal medication may have to be used.

Fungi that cause skin infections such as athlete's foot are called dermatophytes. When an infected person takes a shower, dermatophyte spores are left in the shower stall. The warm, moist environment then allows the spores to survive until a potential new host comes. Since feet are usually enclosed in shoes and socks, the dermatophytes are again provided with an ideal warm, moist environment. Prevention strategies involve using fungicidal disinfectants to kill the spores and wearing sandals in the shower to avoid coming in contact with the spores. Treatment includes antifungal medication and making the environment less suitable for fungi by keeping the feet dry.

Protozoa are also vulnerable to dry conditions. *Entamoeba histolytica*, the cause of amebic dysentery, is usually ingested in contaminated water. It can, however, form cysts, which allows it to resist drying and freezing. An individual can become ill after eating food rinsed in contaminated water or drinking a "safe" beverage that contained ice made from contaminated water.

Plasmodium species are responsible for malaria, which kills two million people in the world each year. Because this protozoan cannot live outside a host, it is dependent on the female *Anopheles* mosquito to transmit it from one person to another. When a mosquito "bites," it actually pierces the skin with a hypodermic-like mouth and injects a local anesthetic to prevent the host from feeling its presence. At the same time, if it is infected with *Plasmodium*, it will inject malarial parasites into the bloodstream. These parasites spend most of their life cycle inside red blood cells, where they are protected from normal immune defenses. When they have multiplied, they rupture the cells as they leave. Treatment involves maintaining sufficiently high levels of medicine, such as quinine, in the plasma that the parasites die. The most important public health strategy is to control the mosquito population and prevent transmission.

Other than bacteria, viruses are the most common pathogens. The mode of transmission of viruses from one host to another depends on the type of virus. Some can survive for a long period of time outside a host, others must be transferred quickly through the air or by contact, and others can survive only when passed directly into the host by body fluids or insect bites. The damage done to the host depends on the type of tissue that is infected by the virus. For example, the Epstein-Barr virus invades the lymphatic system. It causes the enlarged lymph nodes and abnormal lymphocytes that are characteristic of mononucleosis. It is also associated with Burkitt's lymphoma and Hodgkin's disease, both of which are cancers of the lymphatic system. The human immunodeficiency virus (HIV) invades the T lymphocytes, the white blood cells that are crucial to the functioning of the immune system. Damage to the immune system not only makes the individual vulnerable to disease organisms coming from outside the body but also disrupts the balance between the host and normal human flora. This allows other viruses, bacteria, protozoa, and fungi such as *Candida* to multiply and cause potentially fatal secondary infections.

PERSPECTIVE AND PROSPECTS

Infectious diseases have had devastating effects on human populations and societies. For example, during the eighty-year period starting in 1347, recurrent plague epidemics resulted in the deaths of 75 percent of the European population. For many centuries, some physicians and others hypothesized that invisible creatures were the cause of disease. In 1546, Girolamo Fracastoro suggested the presence of germs (seeds) of disease that could be passed from person to person. Because these creatures could not be seen, this "germ" theory was not widely accepted. Then, in 1673, Antoni van Leeuwenhoek began sending descriptions and pictures of what he called "animalcules" to the Royal Society of London. An amateur scientist, Leeuwenhoek made simple microscopes and systematically studied the objects and materials around him. His discoveries of what are now known to be protozoa and bacteria were verified, and they opened the field of microbiology as a science. Using their new knowledge of the microbial world, nineteenth century researchers began to reexamine the germ theory of disease. In 1857, Louis Pasteur, a chemist, discovered that certain bacteria caused wine to spoil. A few years later, he isolated a protozoan as a cause of a silkworm disease and predicted that microbes could cause human illness. In 1875, Robert Koch, a German physician, devised a procedure by which he demonstrated that anthrax was caused by a specific type of bacterium: *Bacillus anthracis*. His experiments led to widespread acceptance of the germ theory of disease, and his procedures provided a systematic method by which researchers could identify those germs. The twenty-five years that followed are referred to as the golden age of microbiology; one by one, nearly all the major bacterial pathogens were identified.

During this intense period of discovery, researchers soon found that, although fine porcelain filters were used to trap microorganisms, in some cases the liquid filtrate was capable of causing disease. The term "virus," meaning poison, was used because it was thought at first that the liquid contained a toxic substance. Pasteur hypothesized that there might be an organism too small to be seen using the light microscope. Later, this was verified, when researchers were able to remove the water from the filtrate, leaving crystals. After the invention of the electron microscope in 1933, individual virions could be seen.

The discovery of pathogens quickly led to research aimed at finding ways to prevent and treat infectious diseases. The contagious nature of disease was known in ancient times. This is illustrated by the practices of Greek physicians and Jewish hygiene laws. Prior to Koch's work, Ignaz Phillipp Semmelweis in the 1840's and Joseph Lister in the 1860's showed that antiseptic techniques could control transmission of diseases. In 1849, John Snow traced the source of a cholera epidemic to a water pump in London. The knowledge that a specific pathogen was involved made it possible for more specific means of prevention to be applied. Within ten years of Koch's report, Louis Pasteur developed vaccines for anthrax and rabies. Immunizations for many infectious diseases were developed, public sanitation measures were taken to reduce the contamination of food and water, and surgeons adopted techniques to control surgical and wound infection.

Although progress in disease prevention was being made, once a person became ill, treatment was still primarily a matter of keeping the patient alive until the disease ran its course. In the early 1900's, a German physician named Paul Ehrlich began to search for what he called a "magic bullet"—a chemical that would specifically treat a disease by killing the pathogens that caused it. After several years of work, compound 606, an arsenic derivative, was made available to treat syphilis. Sulfa drugs were developed in the 1920's. In 1929, Alexander Fleming discovered penicillin, a substance produced by the mold *Penicillium* that could destroy bacteria in cultures. In 1939, Ernst Chain and Howard Florey used penicillin successfully to treat bacterial infections. In 1944, Selman Waksman discovered streptomycin and used the term "antibiotic" to refer to a substance manufactured by a living organism that kills or inhibits the growth of a pathogen.

By the 1970's, it seemed that the end of infectious disease as a major medical problem was in sight. Several developments brought an end to this complacency. Strains of *Staphylococcus* appeared that were resistant to common antibiotics and caused an increase in postsurgical infections. Antibiotic-resistant strains of gonorrhea and syphilis also became widespread. Childhood diseases, once thought to be under control, reappeared as a result of neglected vaccination programs. Increased world travel also facilitated the spread of disease from country to country. Then, in 1981, AIDS was first described; within a few years, it became a worldwide health problem. As people with AIDS began to succumb to previously uncommon secondary diseases, these diseases had to be studied. A new antibiotic-resistant strain of tuberculosis also appeared as a direct result of the AIDS epidemic. These developments have reemphasized the study of microbiology and demonstrated its importance to human health.

—*Edith K. Wallace, Ph.D.*

See also Antibiotics; Bacterial infections; Bacteriology; Bionics and biotechnology; Cells; Cytology; Cytopathology; DNA and RNA; Drug resistance; Epidemiology; Fungal infections; Gastroenterology; Gastroenterology, pediatric; Gastrointestinal disorders; Gastrointestinal system; Genetic engineering; Gram staining; Immune system; Immunization and vaccination; Immunology; Laboratory tests; Microscopy; Mutation; Pathology; Pharmacology; Pharmacy; Prion diseases; Protozoan diseases; Serology; Toxicology; Tropical medicine; Urinalysis; Urinary system; Urology; Urology, pediatric; Viral infections.

FOR FURTHER INFORMATION:

Alcamo, I. Edward. *Microbes and Society: An Introduction to Microbiology.* Sudbury, Mass.: Jones and Bartlett, 2002. A nonscientific text for the liberal arts student that explores the importance of microbes to human life and their role in food production and agriculture, in biotechnology and industry, in ecology and the environment, and in disease and bioterrorism.

Biddle, Wayne. *A Field Guide to Germs.* 2d ed. New York: Anchor Books, 2002. This comprehensive book is easily accessible to the nonspecialist and includes a discussion of nearly every virus, bacterium, and fungus known to cause human and nonhuman animal disease. The history of the microbe and the treatment of diseases are included.

Crook, William G. *The Yeast Connection Handbook.* Jackson, Tenn.: Professional Books, 1999. Written for the general reader, this book explains the balance between the normal human flora and *Candida*, disrupting factors, and the correction of imbalances. Diagrams, recipes, questionnaires, and detailed references add to the value of this work.

Gallo, Robert. *Virus Hunting.* New York: Basic Books, 1991. Written for the general reader by one of the discoverers of the AIDS virus. It examines the field of virology and the methods used to study viruses, especially cancer-causing viruses. The search for the AIDS virus is detailed. Name and subject indexes are included.

Gladwin, Mark, and Bill Trattler. *Clinical Microbiology Made Ridiculously Simple.* 4th ed. Miami: Med Master, 2007. The authors explain the principles behind microbiology in easy-to-understand terms. Includes a bibliography and an index.

Jensen, Marcus M., and Donald N. Wright. *Introduction to Microbiology for the Health Sciences.* 4th ed. Englewood Cliffs, N.J.: Prentice Hall, 1997. An introductory college textbook that focuses on the field of medical microbiology. It reviews the general characteristics of microorganisms, but the emphasis is on pathogenic species, and the prevention and treatment of disease. Each chapter contains case histories illustrating the direct application of principles.

Madigan, Michael T., and John M. Martinko. *Brock Biology of Microorganisms.* 11th ed. Upper Saddle River, N.J.: Pearson Prentice Hall, 2006. An outstanding microbiology text. The authors provide a thorough description of bacteria and the means by which they are studied. Relevant to this topic are chapters on methods of isolation and characterization.

Murray, Patrick R., Ken S. Rosenthal, and Michael A. Pfaller. *Medical Microbiology*. 5th ed. Philadelphia: Elsevier/Mosby, 2005. Focuses on microbes that cause disease in humans. Each chapter consistently presents the etiology, epidemiology, host defenses, identification, diagnosis, prevention, and control of each disease.

MICROSCOPY
PROCEDURE

ANATOMY OR SYSTEM AFFECTED: Cells

SPECIALTIES AND RELATED FIELDS: Bacteriology, cytology, histology, microbiology, pathology, virology

DEFINITION: The use of a microscope to make extremely small objects appear larger in order to make them visible.

INDICATIONS AND PROCEDURES

Conventional microscopy uses a beam of light to illuminate a thin slice of material to be viewed. The material may be stained to provide contrast among its components. The visible light is aimed through the material and collected in a lens. Additional lenses magnify the image until it is visible to the eye of the viewer.

Electron microscopy is a procedure in which a beam of electrons, rather than visible light, is projected toward an object to be viewed. The object is prepared by coating it with a fine layer of metal, frequently gold, that is one or two atoms thick. The electrons reflect off the coated object and hit a screen. The image on the screen is magnified and becomes visible to the human eye. An alternative procedure involves a very thin section of material that is dried and put into a vacuum chamber. A beam of electrons is directed through the prepared specimen. A coated screen receives the electron beam and transforms the image into one visible to the human eye.

Fluorescence microscopy is a procedure that is based on the fact that fluorescent materials emit visible light when they are irradiated with ultraviolet light, which is outside the spectrum visible to the human eye. Some materials manifest this property naturally; others may have to be treated with fluorescent solutions in a process similar to staining. When the absorption of the specimen is in the relatively long ultraviolet range, two filters are also used. The first is placed over the light source to eliminate all but the desired long ultraviolet

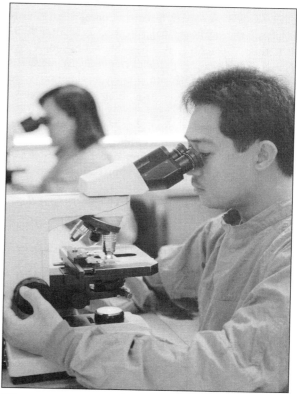

Microscopes are essential in the analysis of laboratory specimens. (PhotoDisc)

rays. The second is placed over the eyepiece. The result is a field that becomes dark and allows any red or yellow fluorescence to be visible.

USES AND COMPLICATIONS

Microscopy has extended the range of understanding for physical objects. Intracellular organelles are routinely made visible. Microscopy has made possible the science of microbiology. Fluorescence allows immunoglobulins to be routinely assayed. Viruses are too small to be seen with a light microscope, but electron microscopy has enabled virologists to view and classify viruses.

The drawbacks of current microscopy techniques are primarily that only small samples of material can be viewed at a time. Usually, the material must be destroyed while it is being prepared. Living tissue may be viewed, but only at levels of magnification below those possible at the limits of normal microscopy and far below those possible with electron microscopy.

Electron microscopy allows the greatest amount of magnification for objects. Because the wavelength of electrons is thousands of times shorter than that of visible light, the resulting magnification is several thousand times greater than that possible with visible light. The use of subatomic particles theoretically increases the potential of magnification, but a continuous source of subatomic particles is difficult and quite expensive to supply.

—L. Fleming Fallon, Jr., M.D., Ph.D., M.P.H.
See also Antibiotics; Bacteriology; Cells; Cytology; Cytopathology; Gram staining; Laboratory tests; Microbiology; Microscopy, slitlamp; Pathology.

FOR FURTHER INFORMATION:

Hawkes, Peter W., and John C. H. Spence, eds. *Science of Microscopy*. New York: Springer, 2007.

Madigan, Michael T., and John M. Martinko. *Brock Biology of Microorganisms*. 11th ed. Upper Saddle River, N.J.: Pearson Prentice Hall, 2006.

Murray, Patrick R., Ken S. Rosenthal, and Michael A. Pfaller. *Medical Microbiology*. 5th ed. Philadelphia: Elsevier/Mosby, 2005.

Singleton, Paul, and Diana Sainsbury. *Dictionary of Microbiology and Molecular Biology*. Rev. 3d ed. Hoboken, N.J.: John Wiley & Sons, 2006.

Spector, David L., and Robert D. Goldman, eds. *Basic Methods in Microscopy: Protocols and Concepts from Cells—A Laboratory Manual*. Cold Spring Harbor, N.Y.: Cold Spring Harbor Laboratory Press, 2005.

MICROSCOPY, SLITLAMP

PROCEDURE
ALSO KNOWN AS: Biomicroscope
ANATOMY OR SYSTEM AFFECTED: Eyes
SPECIALTIES AND RELATED FIELDS: Ophthalmology
DEFINITION: The use of a special instrument to examine the tissues of the eye.

INDICATIONS AND PROCEDURES

The slitlamp microscope, or biomicroscope, is used to examine and evaluate tissues of the eye with both stereopsis and multiple values of optical magnification. The anterior segment of the eye is observed with several types of illumination: diffuse, direct (both broad and narrow beam, the latter allowing an almost slide-like examination of the clear corneal layers), indirect (side illumination), retroillumination (in which abnormalities are back-illuminated with light reflected from more internal structures), specular (in which light is re-

The slitlamp microscope, or biomicroscope, is used by ophthalmologists to examine the health of the eye.

flected off various layers to show the detail of each surface), and sclerotic scatter (internal illumination). Various dyes (such as fluorescein or rose bengal) may be employed to help differentiate normal from abnormal tissues.

The instrument has two coaxial rotating arms controlled by a joystick level; one arm carries the adjustable slitlamp illumination system, with attendant filters and optical stops, and the other arm carries the observation optics (a binocular microscope). An adjustable chin and forehead rest positions the subject's head.

Auxiliary devices allow the measurement of intraocular pressure (tonometer) and corneal thickness (pacometer) and the evaluation of the angle between the cornea and iris (gonioscope lens). Cameras, both still and video, may be attached at various sites. High-powered auxiliary optical lenses have also been developed, which allow the clinician to use the slitlamp microscope to observe the posterior pole of the eye (through the pharmacologically dilated pupil), including the optic nerve and most of the retina. Ophthalmic lasers can also be attached to this system in order to treat the various structures of the eye as they are observed directly through the same optics, using the principle of the reversibility of the path of light.

Allvar Gullstrand received a Nobel Prize in 1911 for his contributions to optics, and the same year he introduced his refinement of the slitlamp microscope. Modern instruments and techniques are largely based on his work.

—Barry A. Weissman, O.D., Ph.D.
See also Eye infections and disorders; Eye surgery; Eyes; Laser use in surgery; Microscopy; Ophthalmology; Optometry; Vision disorders.

FOR FURTHER INFORMATION:

Kaufman, Paul L., and Albert Alm. *Adler's Physiology of the Eye: Clinical Application.* 10th ed. St. Louis: Mosby, 2003.

Ledford, Janice K., and Valerie N. Sanders. *The Slit Lamp Primer.* 2d ed. Thorofare, N.J.: SLACK, 2006.

Newell, Frank W. *Ophthalmology: Principles and Concepts.* 8th ed. St. Louis: C. V. Mosby, 1996.

Riordan-Eva, Paul, and John P. Whitcher. *Vaughan and Asbury's General Ophthalmology.* 16th ed. New York: Lange Medical Books/McGraw-Hill, 2004.

Sutton, Amy, ed. *Eye Care Sourcebook: Basic Consumer Health Information About Eye Care and Eye Disorders.* 2d ed. Detroit: Omnigraphics, 2003.

Wenzel, Martin. *Specular Microscopy of Intraocular Lenses: Atlas and Textbook for Slit-Lamp and the Specular Microscopic Examinations.* New York: Thieme Medical, 1993.

MIDLIFE CRISIS

DISEASE/DISORDER

ANATOMY OR SYSTEM AFFECTED: Psychic-emotional system

SPECIALTIES AND RELATED FIELDS: Psychiatry, psychology

DEFINITION: The emotional, psychological, physical, spiritual, and relationship crises that arise during the transition from early to later adulthood.

KEY TERMS:

development: a generally predictable process of physical, emotional, cognitive, and/or spiritual growth or differentiation

developmental stressors: the events or other characteristics associated with the developmental process, which may be experienced as causing subjective or objectively measurable discomfort

midlife crisis: a crisis resulting from stressors related to the transition from early adulthood to later adulthood

situational stressors: the events or characteristics that may be experienced unpredictably during life and that may cause subjective or objectively measurable discomfort

CAUSES AND SYMPTOMS

Before the nature of the midlife crisis can be explored, it is first helpful to identify what is meant by "midlife." As the average life expectancy has changed throughout history, so has the period termed midlife. For example, current human life expectancy in the United States had risen to 77.5 years of age; this breaks down to 74.8 years for men and 80.1 for women of all races. These figures are more than twice as long as the average life expectancy during the time of the Massachusetts Bay Colony, and more than three and a half times as long as someone in ancient Greece could have expected to live.

Life expectancy changes as it is influenced by any number of factors, including nutrition, health care and prevention, stress and lifestyle issues, historical period, culture, race, individual variability, gender, and social context. Consequently, there is no precise age at which midlife commences. It is also difficult to state unequivocally when the possibility for a midlife crisis ends. Nevertheless, some developmental theorists, such as D. J. Levinson, suggest the period from forty to forty-five is the time of the midlife transition or "crisis." Others have indicated that this time period may last until the age of fifty-three. Yet the results of these studies, collected primarily from Caucasian males in the United States, may not be applicable to the general population.

Other researchers, Carol Gilligan among them, have engaged in a critique of the assumptions underlying previous comments on midlife crises and theories of how human beings develop, pointing out how this research may be based on outdated and/or incomplete studies of human development and experience. Gilligan's line of research demonstrates, for example, how it may be that women have an experience of the aging process that is different from the one commonly experienced by men. As a result, the process of normal adult development and the nature of this crisis remain less than crystal clear.

Midlife crisis experiences seem to arise in response to a variety of precipitating factors, including both normal developmental changes and severe or numerous stressors. This variability raises another interesting challenge to the notion of a midlife crisis. Is experience of a midlife crisis a predictable event or an aberration? Some experts claim that the belief in a "midlife crisis" is one of the many myths about the aging process.

Some argue that that many adults do not experience an unusually severe crisis at midlife, or instead that midlife may be a tremendous period of growth. Others suggest that those who do experience a significant midlife crisis tend to have suffered similar crises throughout their adulthood. The stress involved in the transitions in midlife may be similar to, and not necessarily occurring more frequently than, those experienced by the same individual in any stage of life. If so, the adjective "midlife," as indicative of a qualitatively or quantitatively different kind of crisis, may be misleading.

On the other hand, some clinical studies reveal the male population in midlife to have a significant increase in mental health problems, including depression, alcoholism, and suicide. In fact, most studies of adulthood display something atypical among middle-aged men, whether dramatic or subtle. In addition, discussions around midlife changes for women are becoming more popular. With these discussions, however, the age range examined is advancing.

Caution is necessary when making general statements about a phenomenon such as midlife crisis, but for the sake of this discussion, a more general perspective is taken. It is assumed that midlife crises, however varied in form, intensity, or duration, do commonly occur. In addition, they are best understood from a holistic and contextual perspective on the individual's life.

A developmental framework which describes the cycle that an individual experiences in life further clarifies an understanding of midlife crises. The life changes of an individual may be seen as summative and consecutive. During this life cycle, one stage, with its tasks and crises, is lived and resolved before another is reached. Erik Erikson developed one framework for understanding the individual life cycle and its tasks, crises, and stages. Life crises are attributable in large part to the stress of transitioning from one part of life to another. The stage relevant to a discussion of midlife crises is termed generativity versus stagnation; in other words, midlife is the period of time during which individuals strive to come to terms with whether they are and may continue to be productive, or whether they will stagnate.

Development is also a physical experience. Therefore, an individual's psychological and emotional responses are influenced by changing physiology and health. One common midlife example in women is the menopause and its attendant hormonal changes. At few other times in a woman's life is there such a complex interaction between physical and psychological factors. Along with the physical stresses brought about by hormonal changes, the psychological and emotional reactions of each woman to this normal transition vary depending on her lifestyle, attitudes, self-image, and network of supportive relationships. This type of experience may contribute to crises in midlife.

In addition to the impact of changing physiology, the experience of midlife is emotional, cognitive, and spiritual. Midlife crises may be precipitated by an individual's reflection on or reevaluation of the meaning of life. Similarly, midlife may be a time during which people begin or intensify the process of spiritual evaluation and reckoning. It is a time during which people take stock of their lives and come to grips with their mortality.

A decline or change in physical functioning may trigger thoughts about mortality and death. A frequent phenomenon is evident in the change of one's perspective on time, from a focus on "time since birth" to one on "time left to live." Self-assessment may lead to greater emphasis on long-neglected aspects of the self or relationships with others.

All these issues are known as developmental issues or stressors, which are more or less predictable in life according to the person's stage of development. Situational stressors also contribute to the development of life crises. Situational stressors include such things as unexpected illness or injury, unemployment, and war—all things which are not necessarily related to the person's chronological age or development through time. Consequently, it is reasonable to conclude that these factors may be potent in midlife as well.

Typically, individuals live not in isolation from one another but within the context of relationships. The most common network of relationships is the family. A discussion of issues that have biological, emotional, psychological, and social components, therefore, must include an examination of what is happening with other family members and the family as a group. These factors, including what is termed the family life cycle, may influence the development or severity of the subjective experience of midlife crisis. In fact, the crises of midlife often arise from the interaction between individual and family factors.

Those experiencing midlife crisis are usually members of what has become known as the "sandwich generation"—a generation sandwiched be-

---

INFORMATION ON MIDLIFE CRISIS

CAUSES: Interrelated biological, emotional, psychological, and social components

SYMPTOMS: Anxious or depressed mood; loss of interest in normal activities; intensified reevaluation of life; sudden changes in relationships; difficulty with organic processes (sleeping, eating, concentration); spiritual reevaluation

DURATION: Ranges from short-term to long-term

TREATMENTS: Highly individualized; may include medication and/or psychotherapy tween, and with the responsibility for taking care of, those in two others. For example, a middle-aged woman may have responsibilities with aging parents on one hand and with an adolescent son on the other. The coincidence of adolescence, with her son's focus on the development of an identity and his constant evaluation of his own and his parents' values, beliefs, and behaviors, may only exacerbate her similar search for meaning. She also may be reevaluating her accomplishments and striving to do more of what she believes has been meaningful so far in life. In contrast, the elder generation may be struggling to find some sense of integrity about a life ending. Each individual in the family becomes a point of contact, contrast, or conflict with the other.

The various manifestations of a midlife crisis are much like the symptoms exhibited by people in response to stress. The symptoms include an anxious or depressed mood, loss of interest in normal activities, an intensified reevaluation of life (both past and future), sudden changes in relationships, difficulty with organic processes (such as sleeping, eating, and concentration), and a subjective feeling of the need for a change. Extreme reactions may be a function of the psychology and emotional makeup of a particular individual in the context of his or her life. In addition, people who have less social support or who are living a lifestyle which they have long been aware was unfulfilling are more likely to experience a more significant crisis.

Not only do people and family groups vary in their reactions to midlife stress, but different ethnic and cultural groups do as well. The meaning associated with life events is generated within the context of these various social groups. Each social group develops its own culture with its own rules and regulations regarding how to respond or behave. In other words, individuals understand and respond to stressors as they do because of their experience within larger social groups. For example, within the Caucasian culture in the United States, a certain mythology has developed around the midlife crisis. Midlife is sometimes seen as a time when a man will buy a sports car and leave his middle-aged wife for a younger woman, or when a woman will leave her husband for a younger man or to start a business. Someone else might give up her booming career and begin working with the underprivileged. As a result, within the context of this particular culture, dramatic lifestyle changes are predicted, explained, and possibly even supported. It must be understood, however, that not all the changes that occur are pathological; in fact, some may be signs of new and important growth.

In summary, midlife crises are those crises that may arise during the developmental stage associated with midlife. Like crises or other stress reactions, midlife crises vary in timing, intensity, duration, and character from one person, family, and social group to another. Crises in midlife seem to be no more frequent than crises at other stages of development.

TREATMENT AND THERAPY

Medical science has contributed to the understanding of the concept of midlife crisis through research, theory building, and the development and testing of treatment strategies, including the use of medication and psychotherapeutic techniques. Yet there are no specific treatments for a midlife or any other kind of crisis because the needs of the individual and the family group vary considerably. The range of possible treatments or clinical applications of medical science to this area are largely in the form of supporting the preexisting resources and coping skills of the individual and his or her family and other social support systems.

As with other life skills, an individual's ability to cope with and manage crises depends on the nature of one's character and personality, past experiences in managing crises, and degree of social support. The more well developed the person's character and coping mechanisms, the more numerous his or her experiences in successfully resolving past crises, and the greater amount of perceived support from family and friends, the more likely he or she will be able to resolve conflicts and crises in the present and future successfully.

Since midlife crises can differ from those in other stages, because of the particular tasks to be negotiated at this stage, resolution may involve the need to address certain tasks constructively. An individual may be called on to reevaluate or reassess his or her life, putting into perspective what is hoped for relative to what has transpired. An individual struggling with crises associated with midlife should be encouraged to explore the contributing situational and developmental issues openly. This process may involve cognitive reevaluation, working through feelings, or spiritual and existential reassessment.

Professionals often suggest that several tasks must be addressed in order to facilitate the successful resolution of a midlife crisis. The individual must reckon with his or her own mortality, go through a process of self-assessment, examine sex role obligations and expectations, and gain perspective on his or her generativity. Self-assessment involves taking stock and putting life into perspective. Life's polarities and contradictions must be examined and resolved in some manner.

One central polarity involves sex roles. The traditional differences between men and women often break down during the period of midlife. This process is facilitated by the life review accompanying a midlife crisis. For example, a woman may decide that she has devoted much of her life to the care and nurture of others while putting her own needs second. As a result, she may attempt to remedy the situation by developing the more stereotypical male characteristics of being assertive and goal-directed. Similarly, a male may turn away from his career as the primary source of self-esteem and gratification to developing richer interpersonal relationships.

Clinical and research evidence demonstrates a solid link between life crisis and disease onset. Consequently, medical health professionals may be called on to assist individuals struggling with the effects of a midlife crisis. These professionals, as well as other concerned individuals, may intervene in a variety of ways.

In a preventive fashion, helpers may offer what is termed anticipatory guidance to the individual approaching midlife transitions. In other words, conversations can include predictive or educative content orienting the person toward what to expect as he or she approaches or anticipates these changes. Individuals in the midst of midlife review and crisis may also need assistance, support, and/or direction in resolving generativity issues. The individual needs to resolve how he or she will make a significant contribution to others, rather than stagnate and become increasingly self-absorbed. Accomplishment of these tasks may involve repercussions in work, family, and social relationships.

Sometimes physicians are called to treat individuals exhibiting physical and/or psychological symptoms related to midlife crises. Antidepressant and antianxiety medications are very effective with some conditions, including those in which the symptoms are impairing the person's ability to function over an extended period.

Various forms of assistance also may be offered through informal conversation, in an office visit for brief counseling, or within the process of psychotherapy for a longer-term approach. Regardless of the context, however, being able to anticipate or come to grips with the issues involved helps individuals to feel less out of control and to believe that the problems are being handled constructively.

Family and social support are very helpful in times of crisis. The degree to which these relationship contexts are flexible and supportive can either exacerbate problems or ameliorate struggles. A balance between permission and validation, with encouragement for the individual to continue managing daily functioning and obligations, is important. In the absence of an individual's ability to negotiate and resolve successfully the conflicts associated with the crisis, and perhaps without the presence of a supportive network of family and friends, individual and/or family therapy or a support group may be of help. These modes of therapy and support provide helpful perspective, normalization of the experience, and training or advice regarding constructive problem-solving and conflict resolution techniques.

PERSPECTIVE AND PROSPECTS

In many areas of medical science pertaining to human behavior and emotional experience, important ideas from different theories are often integrated to yield a more comprehensive understanding. Congruently, several theoretical frameworks shape approaches to and perspectives on the understanding of midlife crises. Evolutionary theory, human growth and development, sociocultural theories, theories about the life cycle, behavior theory, family systems theory, learning theory, and theories of stress and coping all contribute to this understanding.

The theory of evolution proposed by Charles Darwin provides the understanding of human beings as living interdependently, as well as adapting to their changing environment. The development of effective coping strategies ensures survival and promotes human community. Midlife crises present the individual and his or her social context with an opportunity for testing the effectiveness of these strategies.

The work of psychologist Abraham Maslow emphasized the tendency of human beings to strive toward the maintenance of life and the promotion of growth. An individual negotiating transitions in life taps into this growth motivation in order to maximize and enrich personal experience. In the midst of crisis, basic necessities of life are the first priority. Once the fundamental needs for food, shelter, and physical survival are satisfied, an individual will strive toward fulfilling what Maslow termed higher-level goals, such as emotional security and spiritual enlightenment.

According to Rupolf H. Moos, crisis theory deals with the impact of disruptions on established patterns of personal and social identity. This framework suggests that, in addition to seeking to maximize human growth and potential, each individual first struggles to maintain a state of social and psychological equilibrium. In crisis, the midlife adult will seek homeostasis or balance prior to exploring opportunities for productive change. Thus, the similarity between crisis theory and theories of human growth and development may be apparent. The crises involved in midlife are more often related to the higher-level goals defined within each of these frameworks.

The stage or developmental theories described previously provide a framework within which to understand some of these transitions and the emotional, psychological, and physical changes that are involved. In addition, the perspective of the individual as developing, growing, evolving, and coping within the context of a family system enriches the view of midlife crisis. Further sociocultural theories help one to see how individuals within specific cultures may or may not view change at midlife as a crisis. Change is relative with regard to cultural mores. For instance, to the extent that individuals within a culture have a history of having one job or one spouse or one home throughout a lifetime, changes brought on by any number of factors that might change this could be viewed as a crisis. In other cultures, where such change is more the norm, such events may be seen not as crisis-related but more in accord with what is viewed as normal. In this way, the experience of midlife crises may be saying as much about a culture as it does about individuals within that culture.

The resulting context for an understanding of midlife crisis, then, is one of an integration of ideas and theories. This integration supports an understanding of midlife crisis as a product of the normative development and transitions in life. An individual's reaction to the required transitions depends on his or her personal characteristics, coping skills, family and social relationships, aspects of the transition or crisis itself, and other features of the physical and social environments.

—*Layne A. Prest, Ph.D.;*
updated by Nancy A. Piotrowski, Ph.D.

See also Aging; Antidepressants; Anxiety; Death and dying; Depression; Factitious disorders; Hypochondriasis; Menopause; Neurosis; Panic attacks; Psychiatric disorders; Psychiatry; Psychoanalysis; Psychosomatic disorders; Sexual dysfunction; Sexuality; Stress; Stress reduction.

FOR FURTHER INFORMATION:

Bee, Helen L., and Barbara L. Bjorklund. *The Journey of Adulthood*. 6th ed. Upper Saddle River, N.J.: Prentice Hall, 2008. A comprehensive text that explores the major theories of adult development and covers health and medicine, behavior genetics, cognitive development, social psychology, and social development in the context of adult development. Topics related to midlife crisis include dealing with stress, conceptualizing the transitions of adulthood, and adult anxiety and depression.

Berk, Laura E. *Development Through the Life Span*. 4th ed. Boston: Allyn & Bacon, 2002. This book examines basic theories, research findings, current applications of theory, and social policies as they relate to development across the life span.

Gaudette, Pat, and Gay Courter. *How to Survive Your Husband's Midlife Crisis*. New York: Berkley, 2003. Uses personal stories and an engaging sense of humor to explore the reasons for midlife crises and to offer resources for support.

Gilligan, Carol. "New Maps of Development: New Visions of Maturity." *American Journal of Orthopsychiatry* 52 (April, 1982): 199-212. In this article, Gilligan begins to map out her alternatives to previously accepted theories of adult development. These alternatives are based on comparative research that contrasts male and female experiences. The author suggests that a woman's development cannot be measured according to the same yardstick as a man's.

Holmes, Thomas H., and E. M. David, eds. *Life Change, Life Events, and Illness*. New York: Praeger, 1989. The editors of this book have compiled an important collection of research and clinical applications of stress and coping theories to practical and everyday experience. The authors of the various papers clarify the connection between life stressors and both psychological and physical illness.

Moos, Rudolf H., ed. *Coping with Life Crises*. Cambridge, Mass.: Springer, 1986. Moos is a pioneer in the field of stress, families, and development. The book and its authors provide a view of midlife crises within the larger context of life development and transitions, as well as of crises in general. The authors emphasize the perspective that many crises are normal or normative.

Schulz, Richard, and Robert B. Ewen. *Adult Development and Aging*. 3d ed. New York: Macmillan, 1999. This textbook can be easily understood by the general reader and includes a comprehensive view of the development and aging processes.

MIGRAINE HEADACHES

DISEASE/DISORDER

ANATOMY OR SYSTEM AFFECTED: Blood vessels, brain, eyes, head, nerves, nervous system

SPECIALTIES AND RELATED FIELDS: Family medicine, internal medicine, neurology, occupational health, pharmacology, vascular medicine

DEFINITION: Chronic, severe, and throbbing vascular headaches.

KEY TERMS:

armamentarium: the arsenal of drugs aimed at preventing or lessening the impact of a disease or disorder

aura: sensory symptoms that proceed and indicate the onset of a migraine

ergot: a fungal parasite on rye that contains ergoline alkaloid; ergot poisoning in the Middle Ages gave rise to dry gangrene, insanity, and St. Anthony's Fire, but derivatives of ergot may be medically prescribed to treat migraines

tyramine and tyrosine: amino acids that may trigger the onset of migraines in some patients

CAUSES AND SYMPTOMS

Migraine is the name given to a particularly severe, chronic, and painful headache that occurs often on one side but sometimes on both sides of the head, usually just behind or above one or both eyes. Until the early 2000's, migraines were medically described as vascular headaches resulting from the dilation of blood vessels that supply nervous tissue in the brain. Recent research indicates that the primary source of migraines may be neurological rather than vascular. It appears that neuron messages that control the size of blood vessels in the brain are interrupted as a result of chemical changes in the brain. The dilated vessels become swollen and press on adjacent nerves, neurons, and other brain tissue, which in turn become irritated and inflamed. The result is a throbbing headache that is often debilitating.

Between 18 and 28 percent of Americans suffer from migraines, although the number may be much higher as many cases remain undiagnosed or are mistaken for sinus headaches or bouts of colds or influenza. Migraines are three times more common in women than in men. More than half of the women experiencing migraines have more headaches near or during their menstrual cycle; these are referred to as menstrual migraines. The peak incidence of migraines occurs between the ages of thirty to forty and wanes after the age of fifty, but they also occur in some children and elderly people. The incidence of migraine headaches is increasing in all age groups, and it is estimated that at least one out of every four individuals suffers from migraines at some point in life. Some recent medical research has linked certain genes to migraines, indicating that the source might be genetic. This correlates with the fact that 70 to 80 percent of migraine sufferers have family members who also experience migraines.

At least fourteen distinct types of migraine headaches are recognized by the International Headache Society. They can be grouped broadly into three categories: classical migraines, which are preceded by a warning aura; common migraines, which are not preceded by an aura; and atypical migraines.

Migraine symptoms often vary greatly from patient to patient and sometimes from one migraine episode to another. Warning aura symptoms of classic migraines occur within an hour of migraine onset and may include sensitivity to bright lights and sound, especially flashing lights, strobe lights, and laser lights. Some people are disturbed by loud or unexpected noise. Other aura symptoms may include hallucinations, hot flashes, a tingling of limbs that may extend in the hands and feet, numbness or weakness on one side of the body, and cravings for certain kinds of foods. Women experience classic migraines less often than do men.

Aura symptoms are followed by the onset of migraine headache. In most types of migraines, the pain is concentrated on one side of the head and then may radiate into the face, eyes, and sinuses. As the migraine becomes increasingly severe, nausea, vomiting, and dizziness are manifested, along with increased urination and sometimes diarrhea. Some patients report vision problems including blind spots, sensitivity to bright and flickering lights, double vision, or tunnel vision.

Three types of migraines occur mostly in children: hemiplegic, basilar, and retinal migraines. Sufferers of hemiplegic migraines sometimes experience temporary paralysis on the same side of the head as the migraine pain. Basilar migraine may last several days, and the pain is centered in the eye and the nerves that control vision. The patient may experience double vision, hearing loss, vertigo, and a bulging, enlarged eye. In both basilar migraine and retinal migraine, temporary blindness or vision blurring may occur.

Two other atypical types of migraines are complicated migraines, in which both symptoms and aura persist for a week or more, and abdominal migraines, in which migraine pain is transferred to the abdominal area. Abdominal migraine is a recurrent disorder that occurs mainly in children. Moderate to severe abdominal pain and nausea may last for up to three days. The source of this type of migraine is unknown. Most children who experience abdominal migraines suffer migraine headaches later in life.

The causes of migraines are varied. Heredity, lifestyle, environmental factors, and changes in hormone levels have all been implicated, and probably all contribute to some degree to the onset and severity of migraines. Some specific migraine triggers include lights, weather changes, certain foods, food additives, certain beverages, odors, lack of sleep, loud noises, and stress. In many patients, a single factor may trigger a migraine, while in other patients several factors may work in tandem, each contributing to the onset of the migraine. It is recommended that migraine victims keep a headache log or diary. This will help to identify individual triggers and narrow down the causes. As much as possible, these triggers should be avoided or limited. A few patients report no obvious triggers that initiate their migraine headaches.

Bright or strong lights, especially when glaring or flickering, are incipient migraine triggers in some patients. In others, the flickering of a television or computer screen or strobe lighting may start a migraine. Changes in weather also initiate migraines, at least in some patients, especially the rapid temperature and humidity changes during the fall/winter and spring/summer transition periods.

Foods that trigger migraines in some patients include dairy products, eggs, red wines and other alcoholic drinks, and caffeinated and carbonated drinks. Preserved foods that contain high levels of nitrates, such as hot dogs or pepperoni, and pickled foods have also been implicated as migraine triggers. Some migraine sufferers also react to foods that contain a high content of specific amino acids such as tyramine and tyrosine.

Probably the most compelling correlation can be made between the amount of stress in a person's life and the onset and frequency of migraines. Emotional factors that have been implicated as migraine triggers include frustration, anger, and depression. In addition, emotional stress may exacerbate response to other migraine triggers as well.

Unlike tension headaches, migraines are so frequent and so painful that most patients seek medical attention. Migraines are clinically diagnosed by health care specialists who employ radiological and laboratory tests to ensure that other factors such as tumors or epilepsy are not the cause of headaches.

TREATMENT AND THERAPY

The treatment of migraines fall roughly into two categories: prescription drugs or changes in lifestyle to prevent migraines, and various strategies to alleviate the pain and duration of migraines. For many migraine sufferers, taking over-the-counter nonsteroidal anti-inflammatory drugs (NSAIDs) as needed (such as Advil, Motrin, Aleve, or Excedrin Migraine), drinking plenty of water, and eating regularly spaced meals helps to prevent or minimize the occurrence of migraines.

To prevent the onset of migraines, powerful antidepressants may be prescribed, particularly drugs that shut down terminal nerve receptors, thereby stopping further pain transmission sequences. Most effective are tricyclic antidepressants, such as amitriptyline, nortriptyline (Pamelor), and protriptyline (Vivactil). They appear to reduce the effect of migraines by changing the level of serotonin and other brain chemicals. These medications are considered to be first-line treatment agents. In some cases, these medical treatments have met with mixed success and have limited effectiveness.

Therapeutic strategies for sufferers of severe migraines employ some of the armamentarium of medically prescribed drugs now

---

INFORMATION ON MIGRAINE HEADACHES

CAUSES: Dilation of blood vessels related to heredity, lifestyle, environmental factors, hormones; may be triggered by lights, weather, certain foods or additives, certain beverages, odors, stress

SYMPTOMS: Severe throbbing pain on one side, sometimes nausea, vomiting, dizziness, and vision problems; may be preceded by aura (*e.g.*, sensitivity to bright light or sound, hallucinations, hot flashes, tingling in limbs, numbness or weakness on one side, food cravings)

DURATION: Chronic with acute episodes

TREATMENTS: Medications (beta-blockers, barbiturates, ergotamines, antidepressants, serotonin inhibitors, anticonvulsants); lifestyle changes (stress management, exercise, alternative therapies, fasting, psychotherapy); symptom relief (ice packs, pain medications)

available, including beta-blockers, barbiturates, ergotamines, triptans, botulinum toxin type A (Botox) injections, antidepressants, serotonin inhibitors, and anticonvulsants. Of these drugs, some of the most powerful are ergotamines, which are derivatives of ergot alkaloids. They are injected into the muscle or vein or placed under the tongue. Ergot-derived drugs are potentially dangerous, however, and should be taken with caution. They should never be taken if the patient is pregnant or has a blood disease. Any medication that constricts blood vessels can be very dangerous if the victim already suffers from narrowing of the blood vessels, such as high blood pressure or coronary artery disease.

The triptans, including sumatriptan (Imitrix), rizatriptan (Maxalt), zolmitriptan (Zomig), almotriptan (Axert), naratriptan (Amerge), frovatriptan (Frova), and eletriptan (Relpax), can help to lessen the effects of migraines quickly. The first of the triptans to be used, Imitrix, acts to balance chemicals in the brain by binding to serotonin receptors and causing blood vessels to constrict. The others act similarly. Imitrix can be administered orally, by nasal spray, or by injection. Since triptans are not addictive narcotics or barbiturates, migraine pain can be relieved while the victim is still alert and in control. Side effects of triptans can include nausea, dizziness, and muscle weakness. On rare occasion, they can lead to stroke or heart attack. The triptan drugs should not be used with ergotamines or with antidepressants, particularly monoamine oxidase inhibitors (MAOIs) or selective serotonin reuptake inhibitors (SSRIs) such as Prozac. When used with antidepressants, triptans can produce serotonin syndrome, an excessive release of serotonin, which can result in weakness, tremors, and lack of coordination. A physician should be consulted before mixing any migraine drugs.

Self-care remedies aimed at preventing migraines include stress management, aerobic exercise, yoga, meditation, acupuncture, anger management, fasting, psychotherapy aimed at developing a positive attitude, emotional repair and stabilization, biofeedback, and the use of herbal and flower extracts. Magnesium supplements help some migraine victims.

A few migraine sufferers resort to folk remedies such as vinegar compresses, warm salt packs, herbal or ice footbaths, or headache tonics. One popular headache tonic consists of fresh ginger root, coriander seeds, diced garlic, and honey. Folk remedies should never be substituted for medical attention.

During and immediately following a migraine, most patients attempt to lessen or alleviate pain by ice packs and aspirin, acetaminophen (Tylenol), or other nonprescription drugs.

Perspective and Prospects

Although the pain is sometimes debilitating for short periods following attacks, migraines are not life-threatening. Furthermore, there are typically no serious aftereffects of migraine headaches, although the individual is often wan, fatigued, and sometimes confused following a migraine episode. Some recent medical studies have shown that some migraine sufferers are at increased risk of stroke.

The incidence and intensity of migraine headaches wanes with age; most patients report that migraines either disappeared or become infrequent after the age of fifty. Many female patients also report that migraines stopped following the menopause.

—*Dwight G. Smith, Ph.D.;*
updated by Alvin K. Benson, Ph.D.

See also Auras; Brain; Brain disorders; Cluster headaches; Fatigue; Headaches; Multiple chemical sensitivity syndrome; Nausea and vomiting; Pain; Pain management; Stress; Stress reduction.

For Further Information:

American Council on Headache Education. *Migraine: The Complete Guide*. New York: Dell, 1994. A thorough account aimed for educating the general public.

Davidoff, Robert A. *Migraine: Manifestations, Pathogenesis, and Management*. 2d ed. New York: Oxford University Press, 2002. This comprehensive and scientific treatment is written by a clinician. Emphasizes the many different types and severity of migraines and their causes, pathophysiology, and treatment.

Evans, Randolph W., and Ninan T. Matthew. *Handbook of Headache*. 2d ed. Philadelphia: Lippincott Williams & Wilkins, 2005. Written by two medical doctors, this book contains a comprehensive discussion about migraines, including causes, symptoms, and treatments.

Henry, Katherine A, and Anthony P. Bossis. *One Hundred Questions and Answers About Migraine*. Sudbury, Mass.: Jones & Bartlett, 2005. A patient-oriented guide that covers causes, symptoms, diagnosis, treatments, and coping skills.

Milne, Robert D., and Blake More, with Burton Goldberg. *Definitive Guide to Headaches: An Alternative Medicine*. Tiburon, Calif.: Future Medicine, 1997. The authors emphasize the alternative therapy approach to eliminating migraines and other types of headaches.

Paulino, Joel, and Ceabert J. Griffith. *The Headache Sourcebook*. Chicago: McGraw-Hill/Contemporary Books, 2001. This paperback is billed as the complete guide to managing migraines and other sources of headache.

MISCARRIAGE

DISEASE/DISORDER

ALSO KNOWN AS: Spontaneous abortion

ANATOMY OR SYSTEM AFFECTED: Psychic-emotional system, reproductive system, uterus

SPECIALTIES AND RELATED FIELDS: Embryology, gynecology, obstetrics, perinatology, psychology

DEFINITION: A pregnancy that self-terminates within the first twenty weeks of gestation; the same condition occurring after twenty weeks is termed a stillbirth.

KEY TERMS:

abortion: the medical term for intended and unintended pregnancy loss

blighted ovum: a condition in which the gestational sac and placenta grow without a developing child inside

ectopic pregnancy: a pregnancy in which the implantation of the fertilized egg occurs anywhere outside the uterus, usually in the Fallopian tube

human chorionic gonadotropin (hCG): the hormone, produced only in pregnancy, that makes the uterine lining receptive for the developing embryo or fetus; pregnancy tests determine its presence

molar pregnancy: abnormal, cystlike placental tissue that grows either in place of the developing child (complete mole) or in addition to the developing child (partial mole)

recurrent miscarriage: a condition in which a woman experiences three consecutive miscarriages

threatened abortion: when the symptoms of a miscarriage first occur

CAUSES AND SYMPTOMS

Approximately 15 to 20 percent of all known pregnancies will end in miscarriage. Furthermore, it is estimated that 50 to 75 percent of all fertilized eggs fail to implant in the uterus—a situation generally unknown to the woman. The likelihood of a miscarriage drops during the pregnancy's duration: approximately 10 percent in the first four weeks after implantation, 5 percent for the next six weeks, and 3 percent for the following eight weeks. (The stillbirth rate is approximately 1 percent.)

The symptoms of a threatened abortion are usually fourfold: spotting of blood, which may turn into heavier bleeding; cramping, possibly accompanied by lower back pain; vaginal discharge of tissue, clots, or pinkish fluid; and nausea and loss of pregnancy signs, such as a decrease in breast sensitivity. A hormonal sign of a threatened abortion is the failure of human chorionic gonadotropin (hCG) levels to double every two days. A positive followed by a negative pregnancy test for hCG, and then gradually increasing lower abdominal pains, is symptomatic of an ectopic pregnancy, the leading cause of maternal death during the first trimester of pregnancy.

There are three conditions where a woman experiences a miscarriage and the developing child is missing in the sac. About 30 percent of miscarriages before the eighth gestational week are blighted ova, as an embryo has failed to develop. Complete molar pregnancies arise when a sperm (or two) fertilize an egg that has lost its genes. The resulting development of pregnancy tissues—absent the developing child—usually leads to the symptoms of a miscarriage in the first several gestational weeks, but expulsion of the placenta may not occur. Because of the higher likelihood of residual disease (including cancer) in the abnormal tissue, surgical removal of the molar tissue is often warranted. Finally, a woman may have a recognized pregnancy yet not realize that she was actually pregnant with twins and one died. This "vanishing twin syndrome" occurs in an estimated 3.5 percent of all twin pregnancies.

Analyses reveal the probability of the most common causes of miscarriages: 50 to 60 percent, genetic abnormalities; 10 to 15 percent, defects in the uterus (such as double or septal uterus) or the cervix (such as incomplete closure); and 10 to 15 percent, hormonal (such as low progesterone or thyroxin) and/or immune disorders (such as lupus or antiphosphid antibody syndrome). A woman's poor health, history of disease (such as endometriosis), history of miscarriages, and advanced age (a 75 percent miscarriage rate for women forty-five and older) also increase the probability of a miscarriage. Recent studies have indicated that the presence of bacterial vaginosis is associated with late-onset miscarriages and preterm deliveries. The presence of the bacteria known as beta strep in the mother's birth canal is tied to preterm labor when it goes untreated. Lifestyle choices that can compromise a successful pregnancy may involve the abuse of substances

INFORMATION ON MISCARRIAGE

CAUSES: Genetic abnormalities, uterine or cervical defects, hormonal or immune disorders; risks increase with poor health, history of reproductive tract disease or miscarriage, age over forty-five, certain substances (caffeine, cocaine, nicotine), radiation exposure, STDs

SYMPTOMS: Spotting that turns into heavier bleeding; cramping and lower back pain; vaginal discharge (tissue, clots, pinkish fluid); nausea; loss of pregnancy signs

DURATION: Acute

TREATMENTS: None in first two months of pregnancy; later, magnesium sulfate for preeclampsia or premature contractions, cervical stitch for incompetent cervix

such as caffeine, cocaine, or nicotine; the contraction of sexually transmitted diseases (STDs), such as chlamydia, human immunodeficiency virus (HIV), or human papillomavirus (HPV); or exposure to harmful agents, such as radiation.

TREATMENT AND THERAPY

Little can be done to stop a miscarriage in the first two months of pregnancy, though some effective interventions are possible in later gestational periods. Magnesium sulfate is effective in combating preeclampsia (high blood pressure during pregnancy) and premature labor contractions. A cervical stitch (cerclage) can rectify an incompetent cervix (premature dilation). Most medical efforts, however, are directed toward the prevention of future miscarriages—the treatment of disease, lifestyle changes, RhO shots for Rh problems—and recovery from the present miscarriage.

There are two aspects of recovery from a miscarriage. The physical part involves the natural or artificial removal of pregnancy tissue—either chemically, as with pitocin, or surgically, as with dilation and curettage (D & C)—and the establishment of a new menstrual cycle. A typical physical recovery ranges from a few days to a few weeks for the miscarriage itself and one to two months after the miscarriage for the next period. Women are usually advised to wait one to two normal periods before trying to conceive again. Approximately 60 percent of women trying to conceive will be successful within six months of the miscarriage.

The psychological recovery may take longer than the physical recovery. Social support, good mental health prior to the miscarriage, deeper religious faith, and successful grieving (mourning, not denying, the loss and then moving forward in life) are some of the factors correlated with a better psychological recovery. Support groups exist for individuals who have suffered miscarriage, stillbirth, or infant death. Similar groups exist to provide support to individuals who are pregnant after the loss of an earlier pregnancy. Such support is essential in decreasing anxiety.

PERSPECTIVE AND PROSPECTS

Until the latter half of the twentieth century, miscarrying women received little satisfaction from the medical community. In fact, many of the drugs introduced in the mid-twentieth century, such as diethylstilbestrol (DES) and its numerous estrogenic cousins, caused more harm than good. However, by the latter part of the twentieth century significant progress was made in diagnosing and preventing miscarriages.

In the early twenty-first century, three avenues of research appear to be promising. Studies are revealing certain genetic predispositions for miscarriages, such as the low production of nitric oxide, resulting in less blood to the uterus. Miscarriages are also being linked to autoimmune disorders and hormonal deficiencies. Use of hormone injections to women who are found to have a hormonal imbalance can help to prevent miscarriage. Finally, assisted reproductive technologies offer intriguing possibilities, such as the ethically controversial opportunity to screen preimplantation embryos for chromosomal abnormalities. In these and other areas of research, new hopes are being raised for old griefs.

—Paul J. Chara, Jr., Ph.D.,
and Kathleen A. Chara, M.S.;
updated by Robin Kamienny Montvilo, Ph.D.

See also Abortion; Addiction; Assisted reproductive technologies; Ectopic pregnancy; Fetal alcohol syndrome; Genetic diseases; Genetics and inheritance; Obstetrics; Placenta; Pregnancy and gestation; Premature birth; Stillbirth; Teratogens; Women's health.

FOR FURTHER INFORMATION:

Friedman, Lynn, and Irene Daria. *A Woman Doctor's Guide: Miscarriage—The Support and Facts You Need to Get Through Pregnancy Loss.* New York: Kensington, 2001.

Jutel, A. "What's in a Name? Death Before Birth." *Perspectives in Biology and Medicine* 49, no. 3 (2006): 425-434.

Lanham, Carol Cirruli. *Pregnancy After a Loss: A*

Guide to Pregnancy After a Miscarriage, Stillbirth, or Infant Death. New York: Berkley, 1999.

Murkoff, Heidi, Arlene Eisenberg, and Sandee E. Hathaway. *What to Expect When You're Expecting.* 3d ed. New York: Workman, 2002.

Ugwumadu, A. H., and P. Hay. "Bacterial Vaginosis: Sequelae and Management." *Current Opinions in Infectious Disease* 12, no. 1 (1999): 53-59.

MITES. *See* BITES AND STINGS; LICE, MITES, AND TICKS; PARASITIC DISEASES.

MITRAL VALVE PROLAPSE
DISEASE/DISORDER

ANATOMY OR SYSTEM AFFECTED: Circulatory system, heart

SPECIALTIES AND RELATED FIELDS: Cardiology, family medicine, internal medicine, vascular medicine

DEFINITION: The inability of the mitral valve in the heart to close properly.

Valves of the Heart

Pulmonary semilunar valve

Pulmonary artery

Aortic semilunar valve

Coronary artery

Opening of coronary artery

Aorta

Left ventricle

Right ventricle

Mitral valve

Tricuspid valve

CAUSES AND SYMPTOMS

The mitral valve connects the heart's left ventricle and left atrium. The oxygenated blood, having already passed through the right heart chambers and the lungs, arrives in the left atrium through the pulmonary veins and then passes through the mitral valve into the left ventricle. Compression of the left ventricle pumps the blood into the aorta and on to the rest of the body. A properly functioning mitral valve closes and prevents regurgitation or backflow into the left atrium. Mitral valve prolapse occurs when the two leaves of the mitral valve close imperfectly, allowing leakage. This condition, known also as mitral valve insufficiency prolapse, is the most common cardiac syndrome. Found in all

segments of society, it is most common in young adult women.

Mitral valve prolapse has several possible causes including rheumatic fever, inflammation of the heart lining (endocarditis), cardiac tumors, or most often, genetic error. Its symptoms are undue fatigue after exercise, shortness of breath, and chest pain. Other common complaints are anxiety, depression, and panic, all related to stress. The number of diagnosed cases in Western countries is rising markedly and may be the result of more sophisticated diagnostic techniques or the increasing stress in modern society.

PERSPECTIVE AND PROSPECTS

Until the 1960's, the detection of mitral valve prolapse was through a characteristic "click" heard by the physician when the mitral leaves attempted to close. Now the use of echocardiograms, allowing ultrasound images of the beating heart and blood flow, is standard practice.

People with mitral valve prolapse lead a normal life, and many are unaware that they have the condition. Repeated irregularity in breathing or an inexplicable shortness of breath is a sign to see one's physician. Regular exercise and good eating habits are recommended for this mild condition. Only in severe cases is mitral valve prolapse treated surgically or considered life-threatening.

—K. Thomas Finley, Ph.D.

INFORMATION ON MITRAL VALVE PROLAPSE

CAUSES: Rheumatic fever, inflammation of heart lining (endocarditis), cardiac tumors, genetic error

SYMPTOMS: Undue fatigue after exercise, shortness of breath, chest pain

DURATION: Chronic

TREATMENTS: Regular exercise; good eating habits; occasionally, surgery

See also Anxiety; Cardiology; Cardiology, pediatric; Circulation; Congenital heart disease; Echocardiography; Endocarditis; Fatigue; Heart; Heart disease; Rheumatic fever; Stress.

FOR FURTHER INFORMATION:

Alpert, Joseph S., James E. Dalen, and Shahbudin H. Rahimtoola, eds. *Valvular Heart Disease*. 3d ed. Philadelphia: Lippincott Williams & Wilkins, 2000. Discusses diseases of the heart valve and their treatments. Includes bibliographical references and an index.

Boudoulas, Harisios, and Charles F. Wooley, eds. *Mitral Valve: Floppy Mitral Valve, Mitral Valve Prolapse, Mitral Valvular Regurgitation*. 2d ed. Armonk, N.Y.: Futura, 2000. A thorough study of mitral valve insufficiency. Includes bibliographical references and an index.

Crawford, Michael, ed. *Current Diagnosis and Treatment in Cardiology*. 2d ed. New York: Lange Medical Books/McGraw-Hill, 2003. Discusses advances in cardiac diagnostics, treatments, and prognostic indicators and includes extensive information on prevention techniques.

Eagle, Kim A., and Ragavendra R. Baliga, eds. *Practical Cardiology: Evaluation and Treatment of Common Cardiovascular Disorders*. Philadelphia: Lippincott Williams & Wilkins, 2003. Details advances in cardiac medicine.

Frederickson, Lyn. *Confronting Mitral Valve Prolapse Syndrome*. New York: Warner Books, 1992. Designed for the lay reader, this guide offers concise coverage of mitral valve prolapse. Includes bibliographical references and an index.

Gersh, Bernard J., ed. *The Mayo Clinic Heart Book*. 2d ed. New York: William Morrow, 2000. One of the most respected texts for laypeople on heart disease. Covers all aspects of anatomy, physiology, diagnosis, treatment, and prevention.

MOLD AND MILDEW

BIOLOGY

ANATOMY OR SYSTEM AFFECTED: Immune system, lungs, nose, respiratory system, skin

SPECIALTIES AND RELATED FIELDS: Environmental health, microbiology, pediatrics, pulmonary medicine, toxicology

DEFINITION: Mold is a generalized term describing nonfruiting fungi, often microscopic and living in moist areas both outdoors and inside buildings,

---

INFORMATION ON MOLD AND MILDEW

CAUSES: Exposure to parasitic fungi

SYMPTOMS: Allergies, runny nose, sinus problems, coughing, rashes, asthma attacks, headaches, nausea, memory loss

DURATION: Acute to chronic

TREATMENTS: Frequent household cleaning, allowing air to circulate, keeping moisture levels in check

---

which consume nutrients and produce spores. Mold, which thrives in humid and closed spaces, has contributed to the development of effective pharmaceuticals but has also been blamed for various health problems and diseases.

KEY TERMS:

conidiophore: a spore-creating area on hyphae in fungi

conidium: spores

hyphae: thin tubes in fungi which secure food and grow, expanding mold size

mycelium: mold colonies consisting of numerous meshed hyphae

mycologists: scientists who study the biological field specializing in fungi and similar spore producers that do not undergo photosynthesis

mycotoxins: poisons released by fungi

STRUCTURE AND FUNCTIONS

Mold grows in wet environments where abundant food, primarily organic materials such as cellulose, provides nourishment. Although mycologists consider mildew to be an outdoor fungal plant disease, that term is popularly used to designate mold found indoors on cloth and wooden objects. Thousands of mold species and millions of strains exists. Scientists have found molds both on Earth and in space. Mold spores are always present in air, moving with currents and surrounding humans. They cannot totally be eliminated inside buildings.

Fungi release enzymes to digest food in hyphae to create cells and energy. Mold eats dust, paper, and leather products, living in basements and cooling and heating systems. It can be found in walls, in insulation, and on ceilings. Flooding intensifies mold growth. Mold perishes if food sources are completely devoured or if mites that eat mold spores are present.

Mold hyphae have conidiophores that make conidium. Shaped as spirals, ovals, or spheres, mold spores can be barbed or smooth. If spores have access to nutrients, moisture, air, and sufficiently warm temperatures, then germination starts within twelve to forty-eight hours of being discharged from the conidiosphore, and an initial hyphae emerges from the spore. As the hyphae consumes food, a mycelium forms in a period ranging from several days to almost two weeks later for *Stachybotrys chartarum*, also called black mold.

Although some molds such as penicillin are helpful, many molds are toxic. In their spores usually, but sometimes in hyphae, molds create mycotoxins, which protect them from bacteria and can cause sickness in other organisms. The access of molds to food and water affects their production of mycotoxins, which are not created by every mold. Molds do not discharge mycotoxins every place that they grow, nor do they always create toxic quantities of mycotoxins. Molds are mostly benign when outdoors because mycotoxins frequently scatter in the air. Inside, however, mycotoxins can accumulate in dangerous amounts.

DISORDERS AND DISEASES

Scientists have proven that outdoor molds can cause many human, plant, and animal illnesses. Some researchers have considered inside molds to be detrimental to human health, associating them with weakened immune systems and various ailments because people have suspected that exposure to indoor molds intensified their allergies and asthma. Some have blamed contact with molds in their homes and other buildings for triggering headaches, skin rashes, nosebleeds, and fevers.

Based on animal testing and cases of humans exposed to moldy agricultural products, medical researchers recognize known mold dangers. For example, black mold produces satratoxin, which can attack and destroy brain cells, particularly neurons, impeding the ability to smell and detect odors. *Trichothecenes* mycotoxins created by *Stachybotrys* and *Fusarium* molds can cause sore throats, blistered skin, and excessive bleeding. *Aspergillus flavus* produces aflatoxins, which can be carcinogenic. Aspergillosis, a disease affecting the lungs, is triggered by mycotoxins created by *Aspergillus* molds. *Claviceps purpurea*, referred to as ergot, produces mycotoxins that can be hallucinogenic. Some forms of that mycotoxin are useful, however, in soothing migraines or inducing childbirth.

Although individual mold mycotoxins might be harmless, mixtures of mycotoxins can be potentially damaging as their adverse effects combine. The degree

to which molds might cause health problems depends on the concentration of mycotoxins and how they invade body systems, specifically whether humans breathe or ingest spores and where the spores settle within their bodies. The size of spores influences their impact on people's health. Researchers hypothesize that some mycotoxins might reach vulnerable lung tissues because they are too tiny to be stopped by nasal defenses that block other harmful microorganisms.

PERSPECTIVE AND PROSPECTS

In 1837, scientists initially became aware that black mold existed when it was found in wallpaper in a Prague, Czechoslovakia, residence. By 1986, William Croft, B. B. Jarvis, and C. S. Yatawara presented the first scientific paper, published in *Atmospheric Environment*, discussing the toxicity of indoor mold. They suggested that black mold spores located in a Chicago house, which later proved lethal to laboratory animals, might be linked to health issues that the residents experienced.

During 1993 and 1994, physicians treated infants whose lungs bled at a Cleveland, Ohio, children's hospital. An investigation by hospital physicians and Centers for Disease Control and Prevention (CDC) personnel revealed that the infants lived in homes containing black mold spores. The media printed stories blaming black mold for the infants' sickness, while hospital officials emphasized the complexity of the situation and the need for a thorough investigation to verify if mold had caused the medical conditions.

The possible dangers of indoor molds again became news in 1999, when *USA Weekend* magazine warned of health hazards allegedly attributed to black mold. Lawsuits resulting in several million dollars in damages increased public awareness of the mold health issue as the media sensationalized the topic. Litigation and mold-related services escalated; con artists took advantage of people's fears of toxic mold. Some legislation relevant to mold and health concerns required house sellers to reveal whether mold had ever existed in structures for sale.

By the early twenty-first century, experts, including National Academy of Sciences representatives, emphasized that no scientific proof existed connecting inside mold and human diseases. Some researchers believed that the link was possible and continued studying how indoor mold might irrefutably be related to human respiratory problems and other illnesses.

—Elizabeth D. Schafer, Ph.D.

See also Allergies; Aspergillosis; Asthma; Blisters; Coughing; Environmental diseases; Environmental health; Fungal infections; Headaches; Immune system; Immunology; Lungs; Microbiology; Multiple chemical sensitivity syndrome; Nasopharyngeal disorders; Pulmonary diseases; Pulmonary medicine; Rashes; Respiration; Sinusitis; Skin; Skin disorders; Sore throat; Wheezing.

FOR FURTHER INFORMATION:

Lankarge, Vicki. *What Every Home Owner Needs to Know About Mold and What to Do About It*. New York: McGraw-Hill, 2003.

May, Jeffrey C., and Connie L. May. *Mold Survival Guide for Your Home and for Your Health*. Baltimore: Johns Hopkins University Press, 2004.

Money, Nicholas P. *Carpet Monsters and Killer Spores: A Natural History of Toxic Mold*. New York: Oxford University Press, 2004.

Shoemaker, Ritchie C. *Mold Warriors: Fighting America's Hidden Health Threat*. Baltimore: Gateway Press, 2005.

MOLES

DISEASE/DISORDER

ALSO KNOWN AS: Nevi pigmentosa

ANATOMY OR SYSTEM AFFECTED: Skin

SPECIALTIES AND RELATED FIELDS: Dermatology, family medicine, plastic surgery

DEFINITION: Nonmalignant marks, pigmented spots, or growths on the skin.

CAUSES AND SYMPTOMS

The common mole, also known as a nevus pigmentosus, is a mark, spot, or growth found on the skin that is generally benign and may be either congenital (present at birth) or developmental. Moles may be various colors, shapes, and sizes, and they can be flat or raised. Caucasian adults usually have about twenty pigmented

---

INFORMATION ON MOLES

CAUSES: Congenital and environmental factors, aging

SYMPTOMS: Flat or raised mark, spot, or growth on skin

DURATION: Short-term to chronic

TREATMENTS: Removal through cauterization, laser treatment

A mole on the chin. (Custom Medical Stock Photo)

nevi, the majority of which are less than 0.5 inch in diameter, with fewer pigmented ones evident at birth.

A mole is primarily the result of an accumulation of melanocytes, cells that form the skin pigment melanin. The greater the number of melanocytes, the darker the brown color of the mole. When the melanocytes are located deep below the skin surface, the mole appears dark bluish in color. Melanocytes also form the relatively larger vascular nevi (birthmarks) that derive from abnormal vascular construction in the skin. Types of birthmarks include the strawberry hemangioma and the port-wine stain, which arise from poorly developed blood vessels, and the nevus anemicus, which is attributed to a reduced blood flow.

TREATMENT AND THERAPY

In most cases, moles are benign, but occasionally they develop into malignant melanoma, especially after puberty. This transformation may be indicated by the development of a flat, pigmented zone around the base of a mole or the progressive enlargement of an existing mole. Other evidence of skin cancer involves increased darkening and loss of the hair surrounding a mole, as well as ulceration and bleeding.

A newly formed mole is usually flat. If it arises between the dermis and the epidermis, then the mole is called a junction nevus; this type may become malignant. A dermatologist's care in a timely manner is usually recommended. The main treatment involves removal of the mole by cauterization or laser treatment.

Moles occasionally disappear with age. Generally, however, more nevi form with aging, such as freckles, and they are usually permanent. The growth of new moles and darkening or other changes in existing ones should be monitored. New moles are usually dome-shaped and elevated slightly above the surrounding skin. Plucking the hair associated with moles is not recommended, as this may damage the skin and lead to ulceration and bleeding.

—*Soraya Ghayourmanesh, Ph.D.*

See also Birthmarks; Dermatology; Dermatology, pediatric; Melanoma; Skin; Skin cancer; Skin disorders; Warts.

FOR FURTHER INFORMATION:

Burns, Tony, et al., eds. *Rook's Textbook of Dermatology.* 7th ed. Malden, Mass.: Blackwell Science, 2004.

McClay, Edward F., and Jodie Smith. *One Hundred Questions and Answers About Melanoma and Other Skin Cancers.* Sudbury, Mass.: Jones & Bartlett, 2003.

Mackie, Rona M. *Clinical Dermatology.* 5th ed. New York: Oxford University Press, 2003.

Marks, James G., Jr., and Jeffrey J. Miller. *Lookingbill and Marks' Principles of Dermatology.* 4th ed. Philadelphia: Saunders Elsevier, 2006.

Schofield, Jill R., and William A. Robinson. *What You Really Need to Know about Moles and Melanoma.* Baltimore: Johns Hopkins University Press, 2000.

Turkington, Carol, and Jeffrey S. Dover. *The Encyclopedia of Skin and Skin Disorders.* New York: Facts On File, 2002.

Weedon, David. *Skin Pathology.* 2d ed. New York: Churchill Livingstone, 2002.

MONKEYPOX

DISEASE/DISORDER

ANATOMY OR SYSTEM AFFECTED: Immune system, respiratory system, skin

SPECIALTIES AND RELATED FIELDS: Dermatology, emergency medicine, internal medicine, public health, virology

---

INFORMATION ON MONKEYPOX

CAUSES: Viral infection transmitted by bite or direct contact with infected animal (primarily African rodents); also transmitted person-to-person through respiratory droplets, direct contact with body fluids or skin lesions

SYMPTOMS: Rash, fever, headache, lymph node enlargement, coughing; may spread to brain, causing encephalitis

DURATION: Two to four weeks

TREATMENTS: Protection with smallpox vaccine before or after exposure; antiviral drug cidofovir only in severe cases

---

DEFINITION: A rare disease, originating in the rain forests of Central and West Africa, that affects animals and humans and is caused by a virus.

CAUSES AND SYMPTOMS

Monkeypox is a poxvirus in the *Orthopoxvirus* genus, which contains three other species affecting humans: variola (smallpox), vaccinia (the current smallpox vaccine), and cowpox (the original smallpox vaccine). The virion is large and brick-shaped, containing double-stranded deoxyribonucleic acid (DNA) that has been decoded and comprises 196,858 base pairs. Since smallpox was declared eradicated in 1979, monkeypox is regarded as the most serious naturally occurring poxvirus infection.

Bites or direct contact with an infected animal may result in transmission. Person-to-person spread also occurs through respiratory droplets, requiring close contact with an infected host. Direct contact with body fluids or skin lesions may also transmit the virus. Less commonly, virus-contaminated objects from infected humans, pets, or laboratory animals may spread the disease indirectly.

The disease can affect persons of any age, but children are more common. The incubation period is about twelve days, and the illness commences with a fever which may be accompanied by headache and enlarged lymph nodes. One to three days later, a maculopapular rash develops. The rash primarily involves the periphery (head and extremities) and resembles smallpox more than chickenpox, which is more centrally (trunk) located. However, lymphadenopathy is not usually seen in smallpox. The rash of monkeypox may involve the palms and soles. The skin lesions progress through a vesiculopustular stage before finally crusting. Secondary infection and scarring may occur. Lesions may also be seen in the mouth and upper respiratory tract, producing a cough and occasionally respiratory distress. Spread of the infection to the brain, causing encephalitis, is a rare but serious complication. The illness typically lasts two to four weeks, and while mortality rates as high as 10 percent have been reported from Africa, fatal cases are rare with modern health care.

TREATMENT AND THERAPY

Smallpox vaccine is about 85 percent protective against monkeypox infection, and individuals at risk should receive the vaccine. Exposed individuals should receive vaccine within four days of exposure but may benefit up to two weeks after exposure. Vaccinia immunoglobulin may be considered for treatment or prophylaxis, although its effectiveness is unproven. The antiviral agent cidofovir is active against monkeypox in vitro and in animals. Unfortunately, the efficacy of cidofovir for human cases is unknown. Because cidofovir is a toxic drug, it should be considered for treatment only in severe cases and should not be used for prophylaxis.

PERSPECTIVE AND PROSPECTS

In 1958, monkeypox was first described in captive *Cynomolgous* monkeys in Copenhagen, Denmark. The first human case was identified in 1970 in the Democratic Republic of Congo. African squirrels are the main reservoir of monkeypox, but the virus has been found in a number of other African rodents.

A shipment of eight hundred African rodents from Ghana to an animal distributor in Texas during April, 2003, resulted in the infection of coinhabiting captive prairie dogs. Many of these animals were sold as pets, and the result was eighty-one human cases of monkeypox in six states. All patients survived, but 25 percent required hospitalization and two children had severe disease.

Low herd immunity, along with repeated introduction of monkeypox from the African wild reservoir, will likely produce more human illness, both in Africa and at distant sites. The use of smallpox vaccine in high-risk and exposed persons, along with antiviral agents such as cidofovir for severe cases, should limit disease and improve outcomes.

—*H. Bradford Hawley, M.D.*

See also Immunization and vaccination; Rashes; Smallpox; Viral infections; Zoonoses.

FOR FURTHER INFORMATION:

Bernard, Susan M. "Qualitative Assessment of Risk for Monkeypox Associated with Domestic Trade in Certain Animal Species, United States." *Emerging Infectious Diseases* 12, no. 12 (December 1, 2006): 1827.

Centers for Disease Control and Prevention. "Multistate Outbreak of Monkeypox—Illinois, Indiana, and Wisconsin, 2003." *Morbidity and Mortality Weekly Report* 52 (June 13, 2003): 537-540.

_____. "Update: Multistate Outbreak of Monkeypox—Illinois, Indiana, Kansas, Missouri, Ohio, and Wisconsin, 2003." *Morbidity and Mortality Weekly Report* 52 (July 2, 2003): 1-3.

Hutlin, Yvan J. F., et al. "Outbreak of Human Monkeypox, Democratic Republic of Congo, 1996-1997." *Emerging Infectious Diseases* 7 (May/June, 2001): 434-438.

Ježek, Zdeněk, and Frank Fenner, eds. *Human Monkeypox.* New York: S. Karger, 1988.

MONONUCLEOSIS
DISEASE/DISORDER

ALSO KNOWN AS: Infectious mononucleosis, the kissing disease

ANATOMY OR SYSTEM AFFECTED: Heart, lymphatic system, spleen, throat

SPECIALTIES AND RELATED FIELDS: Family medicine, pediatrics, virology

DEFINITION: An acute viral infectious disease that produces lymph node enlargement (hyperplasia).

KEY TERMS:

anorexia: loss of appetite

dysphagia: difficulty in swallowing

lymph nodes: glandlike masses or knots of lymphatic tissue that are distributed along the lymphatic vessels to filter bacteria or foreign bodies from the body

periorbital: referring to the region around the eyes

spleen: a large lymphatic organ in the abdominal cavity that forms lymphocytes and other blood cells and stores blood

splenomegaly: enlargement of the spleen

CAUSES AND SYMPTOMS

Mononucleosis is caused by the Epstein-Barr virus, which is transmitted through infected saliva or by blood transfusions. It has an incubation period of four to six weeks. The saliva may remain infective for as long as eighteen months, and after the primary infection, the virus may be present in the nasal secretions and shed periodically for the rest of the host's life.

INFORMATION ON MONONUCLEOSIS

CAUSES: Viral infection
SYMPTOMS: Fever, malaise, lymph node enlargement, sore throat, chills, rash, bleeding gums, red spots on tonsils
DURATION: Four to six weeks
TREATMENTS: Supportive therapy, including bed rest, limited activity, acetaminophen (Tylenol), increased fluid intake

Many cases occur in adolescents—hence the popular name "the kissing disease." The virus can be cultured from the throat of 10 to 20 percent of most healthy adults. The incidence of mononucleosis varies seasonally among high school and college students but does not vary among the general population. The disease is fairly common in the United States, Canada, and Europe and occurs in both sexes.

Mononucleosis is characterized by fever, fatigue, anorexia, a sore throat, chills, a skin rash, bleeding gums, red spots on the tonsils, malaise, and periorbital edema. Lymph nodes in the neck enlarge, and splenomegaly develops in about half of patients. In a small number of patients, liver involvement with mild jaundice occurs.

The diagnosis is made by several different tests, such as the differential white blood count. In mononucleosis, lymphocytes and monocytes make up greater than 50 percent of the blood cells, with a figure of more than 10 percent being atypical. The leukocyte count is normal early in the disease but rises during the second week. Serology studies show an increase in the heterophile antibody titer, although the monospot test is more rapid and can detect the infection earlier and is widely used. Children under four years of age often test negative for heterophil antibodies, but the test will identify 90 percent of cases in older children, adolescents, and adults.

TREATMENT AND THERAPY

The treatment of mononucleosis is mainly supportive, since the disease is self-limiting. The patient is usually placed on bed rest during the acute stage of the disease, and activity is limited to prevent rupture of the enlarged spleen, usually for at least two months. Acetaminophen (Tylenol) is given for the fever, and saline gargles or lozenges may be used for the sore throat. Patients need to increase their fluid intake. Many doctors use cortico-steriods such as prednisone during the course of the disease to lessen the severity of the symptoms. If rupture of the spleen occurs, emergency surgery is necessary to remove the organ.

Complications are uncommon but may include rupture of the spleen, secondary pneumonia, heart involvement, neurologic manifestations such as Guillain-Barré syndrome, meningitis, encephalitis, hemolytic anemia, and orchitis (inflammation of the testes).

PERSPECTIVE AND PROSPECTS

Viruses, such as the one responsible for mononucleosis, were first studied in the 1930's, and they remain a challenge to laboratory investigators. Most information about viruses has come from studying their effects, rather than the viruses themselves. The majority of methods for destroying or controlling viruses are ineffective. There is no prevention for many of the diseases caused by viruses, such as infectious mononucleosis. It may be reassuring to know that the disease seldom causes severe complications if the symptoms are treated and medical care is given to those infected with the Epstein-Barr virus.

—*Mitzie L. Bryant, B.S.N., M.Ed.*

See also Childhood infectious diseases; Chronic fatigue syndrome; Epstein-Barr virus; Fatigue; Fever; Hodgkin's disease; Immune system; Jaundice; Lymphadenopathy and lymphoma; Lymphatic system; Otorhinolaryngology; Sore throat; Viral infections.

FOR FURTHER INFORMATION:

Beers, Mark H., et al. *The Merck Manual of Diagnosis and Therapy.* 18th ed. Whitehouse Station, N.J.: Merck Research Laboratories, 2006. Contains a useful exposition of the characteristics, etiology, diagnosis, and treatment of mononucleosis. Designed for physicians, the material is also useful for less specialized readers.

Dreher, Nancy. "What You Need to Know About Mono." *Current Health 2* 23, no. 7 (March, 1997): 28-29. Infectious mononucleosis is an illness that is most common among young people ages fifteen to twenty-five. The infection is caused by the Epstein-Barr virus. Facts about mono are presented.

Harkness, Gail, ed. *Medical-Surgical Nursing: Total Patient Care.* 10th ed. St. Louis: C. V. Mosby, 1999. This textbook briefly covers the cause, symptoms, diagnosis, and treatment of infectious mononucleosis. The clinical pathology and possible complications of the disease are discussed as well.

Kimball, Chad. *Colds, Flu, and Other Common Ailments*. New York: Omnigraphics, 2002. A comprehensive guide for general readers covering treatment issues and controversies surrounding common ailments and injuries. Includes discussions on mononucleosis.

Litin, Scott C., ed. *Mayo Clinic Family Health Book*. 3d ed. New York: HarperResource, 2003. Perhaps the best general medical text for the layperson, this book covers the entire medical field. While the information is derived from a wide variety of highly technical sources, the articles are written to be easily understood by a general audience.

Shrader, Laurel, and John Zonderman. *Mononucleosis and Other Infectious Diseases*. Rev. ed. New York: Chelsea House, 1999. Part of the Twenty-first Century Health and Wellness series for young adults. Covers symptoms, diagnosis, treatment, historical perspective, and conditions that lead to the spread of mononucleosis and other infectious diseases.

Sompayrac, Lauren. *How Pathogenic Viruses Work*. 5th ed. Sudbury, Mass.: Jones & Bartlett, 2002. Engaging exploration of the basics of virology. The author uses twelve of the most common viral infections to demonstrate how viruses "devise" various solutions to stay alive.

Woolf, Alan D., et al., eds. *The Children's Hospital Guide to Your Child's Health and Development*. Cambridge, Mass.: Perseus, 2002. An authoritative and comprehensive guide to children's health, providing a guide to every common illness or condition that affects children and a carefully designed emergency section.

MOSQUITO BITES. *See* BITES AND STINGS; INSECT-BORNE DISEASES.

MOTION SICKNESS
DISEASE/DISORDER

ALSO KNOWN AS: Carsickness, airsickness, seasickness

ANATOMY OR SYSTEM AFFECTED: Ears, gastrointestinal system, head, nervous system, stomach

SPECIALTIES AND RELATED FIELDS: Family medicine, neurology, otorhinolaryngology

DEFINITION: A disorder characterized by nausea, vomiting, and vertigo and caused by a combination of repetitive back-and-forth and up-and-down movements.

KEY TERMS:

cranial: pertaining to the bones of the head

medulla oblongata: a continuation of the spinal cord that forms the lower portion of the brain stem; the site of many regulatory centers, as for cardiac rhythm, breathing, and the diameter of blood vessels

transdermal patch: a drug delivery system in which medication is slowly released from a patch and absorbed through the skin over a period of days

vertigo: a specific type of dizziness in which people feel as though either they themselves are spinning around or the room is spinning around them

CAUSES AND SYMPTOMS

Motion sickness appears to be caused by overstimulation of the balance centers of the inner ears by repeated back-and-forth and up-and-down movements. Messages are carried from this area of the inner ear, known as the vestibular apparatus, to the vomiting center in the medulla oblongata. The nerve pathways for this journey are not entirely known, but certainly the cranial nerve, which is responsible for hearing and balance, is involved. Responses in the medulla oblongata set into motion automatic motor reactions in the upper gastrointestinal tract, diaphragm, and abdominal muscles that lead to vomiting.

Individuals vary considerably in their susceptibility to motion sickness, and experts believe that there may be an inherited tendency toward the problem. Shifting visual input (such as watching waves on the horizon), a poorly ventilated environment, and fear and anxiety all seem to play a role in the development and severity of motion sickness.

The diagnosis of motion sickness is usually self-evident. Vertigo, nausea, and vomiting follow exposure to a repetitive and usually irregular rocking motion while in a moving vehicle or on an amusement park ride. The first indication of motion sickness may be yawning, excessive salivation, pale skin, and sweating. The person may begin to breathe deeply or complain of sleepiness. The patient may also develop a need for air, dizziness, or a headache. In most cases, nausea and vomiting occur sooner or later. On an extended trip, patients with motion sickness may eventually develop a tolerance to the motion and feel better, or they may continue to feel sick. If severe rocking motions develop once again, however, patients may also become sick again. Repeated vomiting may lead to dehydration and low blood pressure. Depression is another feature of prolonged motion sickness. As one patient with ex-

INFORMATION ON MOTION SICKNESS

CAUSES: Overstimulation of balance centers of inner ears, shifting visual input, poorly ventilated environment, fear and anxiety
SYMPTOMS: Yawning, excessive salivation, pale skin, sweating, nausea, vomiting, vertigo
DURATION: Acute
TREATMENTS: Over-the-counter or prescription medications; preventive measures

treme motion sickness has described it, "First you are afraid you are going to die, and then you are afraid you *won't* die."

TREATMENT AND THERAPY

This malady is far easier to prevent than to treat. People who suffer from motion sickness should avoid drinking liquids just before and during short trips. On longer trips, they should limit liquids and have only small, easy-to-digest foods at regular intervals. Plenty of fresh air may also help prevent sickness. Those prone to motion sickness should not read in a car or other moving vehicle. Focusing the eyes well above the horizon while riding in a car or on a boat may help. People who are susceptible to motion sickness should also avoid amusement park rides that involve swinging and rocking.

Sufferers may be treated with over-the-counter or prescription medications an hour before travel begins. Medications used for this purpose include diphenhydramine, promethazine, scopolamine, dimenhydrinate, cyclizine, buclizine, and meclizine. They are available in a variety of forms, including tablets, rectal suppositories, and transdermal patches. Many of these drugs cause sleepiness, which may be helpful during a trip but cause drowsiness or lack of alertness on arrival. Another common side effect of some of these drugs is dry mouth. In most cases, these medications are more effective when given before vomiting begins. An extract of ginger root has been recommended as a treatment using a natural substance, and so having fewer side effects. Some objective studies, however, have failed to demonstrate its efficacy.

If the person has already begun vomiting, medications must be given by injection, rectal suppository, or a transdermal patch. In cases of prolonged vomiting, where dehydration is a concern, the patient may require intravenous fluids. Of particular concern is the individual who is already ill with another disease and also suffers from motion sickness. Such patients may have serious complications related to the vomiting and resulting dehydration.

Nonpharmacologic treatments for motion sickness abound. The best known are acupressure wristbands. The autogenic-feedback training (AFT) exercise, designed by the National Aeronautics and Space Administration (NASA), is a self-regulation and biofeedback training scheme that has shown promise in studies of space motion sickness in astronauts. It requires a minimum of six hours of training and so is not the quick fix that drugs promise. NASA scientists have also explored devices for holding the astronaut's head steady, since head movement appears to exacerbate motion sickness. Such an apparatus might be applicable to the civilian population as well.

PERSPECTIVE AND PROSPECTS

Motion sickness is a common problem in children and some adults. New drugs to treat the problem are being explored. A number of chemicals showing promise are related to or interact with serotonin, a chemical that participates in a number of regulatory systems in the body. Drug companies are working on new drug delivery systems to make antinausea medications easier to take. Other advances include drug regimens that will provide antinausea effects without sleepiness.

—Rebecca Lovell Scott, Ph.D., PA-C;
updated by Carl W. Hoagstrom, Ph.D.

See also Acupressure; Acupuncture; Audiology; Balance disorders; Biofeedback; Dehydration; Dizziness and fainting; Ear infections and disorders; Ears; Gastrointestinal system; Nausea and vomiting; Nervous system; Neurology; Neurology, pediatric; Over-the-counter medications.

FOR FURTHER INFORMATION:

Canalis, Rinaldo, and Paul R. Lambert, eds. *The Ear: Comprehensive Otology.* Philadelphia: Lippincott Williams & Wilkins, 2000. A text covering all aspects of otology.

Crampton, George H., ed. *Motion and Space Sickness.* Boca Raton, Fla.: CRC Press, 1990. This state-of-the-art compendium, written by active researchers in the field, encompasses anatomical and physiological subjects, such as analyses of stimulus characteristics, prediction of sickness, and consideration of human factors.

Ferrari, Mario. *PDxMD Ear, Nose, and Throat Disor-*

ders. New York: Elsevier, 2002. A clinical yet accessible reference text that provides a comprehensive list of disorders, with a summary of the condition, background, diagnosis, treatment, outcomes, prevention, and resources.

Litin, Scott C., ed. *Mayo Clinic Family Health Book.* 3d ed. New York: HarperResource, 2003. Perhaps the best general medical text for the layperson, this book covers the entire medical field. While the information is derived from a wide variety of highly technical sources, the articles are written to be easily understood by a general audience.

Mendel, Lisa Lucks, Jeffrey L. Danhauer, and Sadanand Singh. *Singular's Illustrated Dictionary of Audiology.* San Diego, Calif.: Singular, 1999. A comprehensive reference guide to the field that provides numerous photographs, charts, and diagrams, including those of the inner ear. Appendixes cover acronyms, illustrations, topic categories, and physical quantities.

Spock, Benjamin, and Robert Needlman. *Dr. Spock's Baby and Child Care.* 8th ed. New York: Pocket Books, 2004. For more than a half a century, this book has been a virtual bible for parents seeking trustworthy information on child care. Informative, easy to use, and responsive to the changes in society.

Zajonc, Timothy P., and Peter S. Roland. "Vertigo and Motion Sickness, Part 1: Vestibular Anatomy and Physiology." *Ear, Nose, and Throat Journal* 84 (September, 2005): 581-584. Reviews the biological backdrop for motion sickness.

_____. "Vertigo and Motion Sickness, Part 2: Pharmacological Treatment." *Ear, Nose, and Throat Journal* 85 (January, 2006): 25-35. Reviews the drugs available for the treatment of motion sickness and some of the drugs under investigation for that purpose.

MOTOR NEURON DISEASES

DISEASE/DISORDER

ANATOMY OR SYSTEM AFFECTED: Muscles, musculoskeletal system, nerves, nervous system, spine

SPECIALTIES AND RELATED FIELDS: Neurology

DEFINITION: Progressive, debilitating, and eventually fatal diseases affecting nerve cells in muscles.

KEY TERMS:

Babinski's sign: an abnormal response to a neurological test involving a brisk stroke with a sharp object on the bottom of the foot; the normal response is for the toes to bunch together and curve downward, while the abnormal response is for the big toe to pull upward and not in unison with the other toes

corticospinal tracts: neurological pathways descending from the brain to the spinal cord that control and allow voluntary movement

fasciculations: spontaneous electrical impulses from neurons that result in irregular, involuntary muscular contractions; in motor neuron disease, these contractions indicate nerve death

lower motor neuron: a nerve cell whose cell body resides either in the brain stem (to form a cranial nerve) or in the spinal cord (to form a spinal motor neuron)

motor neuron: a nerve that functions either directly or indirectly to control a target organ

muscular atrophy: a wasting of muscle mass; a greatly reduced size of muscle cells caused by the lost innervation (neuron death) or disuse of muscles

spasticity: an abnormal condition in which the limbs demonstrate resistance to passive movement as a result of damage to the corticospinal tracts; the reflexes are hyperactive

tropic factors: chemicals released from nerve cells that have a vital influence on muscle health; in the absence of tropic factors, muscles atrophy

upper motor neuron: a nerve whose cell body resides within the brain but whose axon descends the brain stem and spinal cord to form a corticospinal tract

CAUSES AND SYMPTOMS

In motor neuron diseases, certain nerves die, specifically those that allow any and all body movement. The actual cause of spontaneous motor neuron death is unknown, but genetic defects, neurotoxins, viruses, autoimmune disruptions, and metabolic disorders are contributing factors.

The predominant features of motor neuron disorders are muscular weakness, muscular wasting, and the presence of fasciculations. As a nerve dies, it can no longer effectively innervate its target muscle, but neighboring nerves may sprout to keep the muscle active. A consequence of nerve sprouting is the onset of brief, spontaneous contractions, or twitches. These visible twitches are called fasciculations. Eventually, as increasing numbers of nerves die, fewer healthy nerves are left to sprout until, finally, all muscles are denervated. Dead nerves cannot prompt muscle movement, nor can they release tropic factors as they do in health. This loss of tropic input from the neuron causes muscular atrophy and renders the muscle useless.

Motor neuron diseases are usually first noticed in the

hands or upper limbs, where muscle weakness and decreased ability to use arms or hands cause problems. Unlike some disorders, motor neuron diseases fail to show stages of exacerbation or remission. Rather they progress—either rapidly or slowly, but relentlessly—until death, usually as a result of respiratory complications.

Although there are childhood forms, motor neuron diseases are more likely to strike between the ages of fifty and fifty-five, and they are seen in males more than females by a ratio of 1.5 to 1. Motor neuron diseases seem to occur rarely in the obese person and tend to afflict otherwise healthy, thin, and perhaps athletic persons. A famed person afflicted by the debilitating motor neuron disease amyotrophic lateral sclerosis (ALS) was baseball player Lou Gehrig, in whose memory it is often called Lou Gehrig's disease.

Motor neuron diseases are often subgrouped into three categories: ALS, progressive spinal muscular atrophy, and progressive bulbar (brain-stem) palsy. In the plural form, motor neuron diseases refer to all forms of the affliction, whereas the singular form, motor neuron disease, is synonymous with ALS.

Amyotrophic lateral sclerosis is the most familiar of the motor neuron diseases primarily because it accounts for a full 60 percent of all such disorders. The name has clinical meaning: "Amyotrophy" refers to the loss of muscle bulk as a result of missing tropic factors from dying or dead neurons, "lateral" refers to the locations within the spinal cord that are affected, and "sclerosis" refers to the hardened quality of the lateral regions of the diseased spinal cord, which otherwise would be soft tissue. The brain stem may also be sclerotic (hardened). ALS has an incidence of 1 or 2 persons per 100,000, although some Pacific islands, such as Guam, seem to have a higher incidence attributable to undetermined genetic factors. In addition, some populations show an autosomal dominant genetic component. ALS is fatal, and death generally occurs as a result of respiratory failure within three to five years after the onset of symptoms.

ALS is characterized by upper and lower motor neuron signs of neural death; thus the presence of both fasciculations and spasticity is required for a diagnosis. Spasticity is a medical term that describes a certain kind of muscular resistance (stiffness) to movement. In particular, spastic means a resistance that increases the more rapidly a muscle is extended; tendon reflexes are also hyperactive and Babinski's sign (abnormal re-

---

INFORMATION ON MOTOR NEURON DISEASES

CAUSES: Unknown; possibly genetic defects, neurotoxins, viruses, autoimmune disruptions, metabolic disorders

SYMPTOMS: Muscle weakness or wasting, twitching or spasticity, decreased ability to use arms or hands, increased clumsiness

DURATION: Chronic, sometimes progressive

TREATMENTS: None; management of symptoms and palliative care

---

flexes of the toes) must be present. Babinski's sign reveals the death of neurons in the corticospinal tracts, which signals the occurrence of upper motor neuron death. The presence of fasciculations reveals lower motor neuron death.

Progressive spinal muscular atrophy (SMA) will show only lower motor neuron signs—namely, muscular weakness, fasciculations, and atrophy. Babinski's sign or spasticity is not found. The early symptoms may include increased clumsiness in using the fingers for fine movements (including writing or using kitchen utensils), stiffness of the fingers and hands, and cramping of the upper and lower limbs. Once the brain-stem nerves become involved, difficulty in speaking and swallowing occur. Of all persons afflicted with one of the motor neuron diseases, 7 to 15 percent will have lower motor neuron signs only and are presumed to have the progressive spinal muscular atrophy form.

Progressive bulbar palsy literally means progressive brain-stem paralysis. This form of motor neuron disease accounts for 20 to 25 percent of all cases. The tongue is usually the first place to show muscular wasting and fasciculations. As the nerves controlling the tongue die, the tongue shrivels and shrinks so that speaking, chewing, and moving solids or liquids to the back of the mouth for swallowing become difficult or impossible.

Children can be afflicted with spinal muscular atrophy. This disease is believed by many experts to be completely unique from the adult form. The childhood form seems to be more associated with environmental and genetic factors. (This concept is greatly debated, however, since the actual cause of any of the motor neuron diseases is unknown.) Three forms of childhood SMA have been identified: type 1, or acute infantile SMA (also known as Werdnig-Hoffman disease); type 2, or intermediate SMA; and type 3, or juvenile SMA (also known as Kugelberg-Welander disease).

Of children afflicted with SMA, 25 percent have type 1. This form of the disease is an autosomal recessive genetic disorder that occurs in 1 of 15,000 to 25,000 births. In an experienced mother, there may be awareness of minimal fetal movement in the last trimester of pregnancy; the fetus tends to stay still as a result of muscular weakness. Upon birth, the newborn may be a "floppy" baby of great weakness and may immediately have trouble with nursing and breathing. In other cases, it may take three to six months before symptoms begin. Because of the eventual weakening of the muscles of respiration, the child becomes prone to respiratory infections that cannot be cleared because of a lost cough reflex. Death usually occurs at two to three years of age.

When a child fails to stand or walk between six to twelve months of age, the physician considers the possibility that the child has type 2 SMA. An abnormal curvature of the spine to the forward and sideways position (kyphoscoliosis) is often seen, but rarely is there any problem with feeding or breathing. It is generally the case that very fine tremors of the child's hands can be noticed, and sometimes contractures of the hips and knees can occur. There is no delay in terms of mental health or intellect for these children.

Type 3 SMA is most often seen in the adolescent, but this disease can be observed in some children as early as five years of age. The predominant feature is weakness of the hip muscles. Since these children have been walking for some time, a change in their walking gait to a waddle can be seen over the course of years. Most people with type 3 SMA must use wheelchairs in their mid-thirties, but some may lose their ability to walk earlier. Type 3 SMA has been shown to be an autosomal recessive disorder in many cases, but there are also reported cases of sporadic occurrences within families that have previously been unaffected. Clearly, there are unanswered questions about this disease.

It should be noted that controversy abounds on the assigned classifications of motor neuron diseases. This controversy arises from the fact that the origins of the diseases are not known. Since cause has not been established for any form of motor neuron disease, physicians must use clusters of symptoms to sort the differences in disease manifestation. This sorting is used to plan the best possible treatment programs for the circumstances; nevertheless, these distinctions may seem arbitrary once more is known about the causes of motor neuron death.

TREATMENT AND THERAPY

Perhaps one of the most frustrating attributes of motor neuron diseases is that neither prevention nor effective treatment and cures are available. For a person living with motor neuron disease, physicians and health care professionals must work as a team to manage the symptoms of the diseases and offer palliative care.

In general, patients are encouraged to use and exercise their muscles cautiously in order to avoid disuse atrophy, but activity to the point of fatigue is forbidden since it is believed to aggravate the progression of muscular wasting. In addition, exposure to cold may worsen muscular contractures. Physical therapy facilitates a delay in the total loss of willed body movement by allowing the use of braces, walkers, and wheelchairs as modes of locomotion. Adults are encouraged to continue nonexertive work for as long as possible; it aids both the body and the mind to maintain independence and a sense of wholeness, well-being, and dignity.

As muscular control of the voice wanes, sketch pads, word boards, and computers can aid the ill person in communicating with loved ones, doctors, nurses, and colleagues. In addition, respiratory therapy aids in maintaining healthy breathing in spite of ever-weakening respiratory muscles. Prophylactic immunizations for influenza and pneumococci are given, especially to those who are wheelchair-dependent or bedridden. Forced deep breathing and coughing are needed at least once every four hours to bring up any congestion that may otherwise lead to grave consequences. Almost all persons with motor neuron diseases die from respiratory insufficiency. For this reason, it is imperative that the patient and physician discuss respiratory care early after diagnosis to determine whether the patient wants to be placed on mechanical ventilators in the later stages of the disease. Other issues such as tube feedings should be discussed while the patient is still able to voice an opinion and express any concerns about the dying process associated with the disease.

PERSPECTIVE AND PROSPECTS

Life can be socially difficult for people with motor neuron diseases. Others tend to assume that persons who must use wheelchairs and are unable to control mouth movements (so that speech and swallowing are lost and drooling may occur) are not intelligent, thinking, or aware. This is a sad misperception.

Many persons suffering from a motor neuron disease rise above its physical challenges to conquer in spirit that which the body cannot. For example, former United States senator Jacob Javits labored hard to improve the awareness of and funding for ALS in spite of being on a ventilator and completely immobile because of his battle with the disease. Another example of how well the intellect is preserved in this physically tragic disease can be seen in the life and work of the world-renowned astrophysicist Stephen Hawking.

Until there is an established cause or causes for these diseases, effective treatments or cures are likely to remain hidden. The research continues in the hope of pinning down the ever-elusive motor neuron diseases.

—Mary C. Fields, M.D.

See also Amyotrophic lateral sclerosis; Aphasia and dysphasia; Huntington's disease; Muscle sprains, spasms, and disorders; Muscles; Nervous system; Neuralgia, neuritis, and neuropathy; Neurology; Neurology, pediatric; Palsy; Paralysis; Spinal cord disorders; Spine, vertebrae, and disks.

FOR FURTHER INFORMATION:

Bear, Mark F., Barry W. Connors, and Michael A. Paradiso. *Neuroscience: Exploring the Brain*. 3d ed. Philadelphia: Lippincott Williams & Wilkins, 2007. Undergraduate text that introduces the topics of neuroscience, neurobiology, neurodiseases, and physiological psychology.

Bloom, Floyd E., M. Flint Beal, and David J. Kupfer, eds. *The Dana Guide to Brain Health*. New York: Simon & Schuster, 2003. An easy-to-understand health guide to the brain from neuroscience, neurology, and psychiatry perspectives. More than seventy psychiatric and neurological disorders, their diagnoses, and their treatments are covered.

Calne, Donald B. *Neurodegenerative Diseases*. Philadelphia: W. B. Saunders, 1994. An excellent book with a section devoted to amyotrophic lateral sclerosis and related motor neuron diseases.

Heilman, Kenneth M. *Matter of Mind: A Neurologist's View of Brain-Behavior Relationships*. New York: Oxford University Press, 2002. A leading researcher in behavioral and cognitive neurology uses case studies to explore the knowledge about brain functions such as speaking, reading, writing, emotion, skilled movement, perception, attention, and motivation that has been gained from the study of patients with diseases of or damage to the brain. An excel-lent, accessible examination of neurological disorders.

Leigh, P. Nigel, and Michael Swash, eds. *Motor Neuron Disease: Biology and Management*. New York: Springer-Verlag, 1995. This text addresses motor neuron disease from the point of view of health care providers.

National Institute of Neurological Disorders and Stroke (NINDS). *Motor Neuron Diseases Information Page*. http://www.ninds.nih.gov/disorders/ motor_ neuron_diseases/. A section of the NINDS site that provides a good range of information about motor neuron diseases, scientific research, and organizations.

Parker, James N., and Philip M. Parker, eds. *Official Patient's Sourcebook on Amyotrophic Lateral Sclerosis*. San Diego, Calif.: Icon Health, 2003. Provides comprehensive information drawn from public, academic, government, and peer-reviewed research, and gives myriad sources for basic and advanced information on the disease.

Parsons, Malcolm, and Michael Johnson. *Diagnosis in Color: Neurology*. New York: Mosby, 2001. Impeccably assembled, this atlas shows the most distinguishing clinical features associated with motor neuron diseases, such as muscular wasting of the hands and tongue.

Thompson, Charlotte E. *Raising a Child with a Neuromuscular Disorder: A Guide for Parents, Grandparents, Friends, and Professionals*. New York: Oxford University Press, 1999. Although the field of neuromuscular disorders has grown, many of the guideposts have remained the same. In this rich resource, the author has kept sight of these guideposts, describing them and capturing the most current resources, references, and medical help available.

MOTOR SKILL DEVELOPMENT
DEVELOPMENT

ANATOMY OR SYSTEM AFFECTED: Bones, circulatory system, eyes, joints, muscles, musculoskeletal system, nerves, nervous system, psychic-emotional system

SPECIALTIES AND RELATED FIELDS: Exercise physiology, genetics, neonatology, neurology, orthopedics, pathology, pediatrics, perinatology, physical therapy, psychology, sports medicine

DEFINITION: The process of change in motor behavior with advancing age and the numerous physiological and psychological processes that underlie these changes, which describe the adjustments in posture, movement, and skillful manipulation of objects achieved through the coordination of several neurologic control structures.

KEY TERMS:

central nervous system: the brain and spinal cord, which process incoming information from the peripheral nervous system and form the main network of coordination and control in advanced organisms

motor control: the nature and cause of movement, which focuses on stability and movement of the body, and the manipulation of objects, which is achieved through the coordination of many structures organized both hierarchically and in a parallel manner

motor learning: the acquisition and modification of movement as a result of practice and experience, which leads to relatively permanent intrinsic changes in the ability to perform skilled activities; not directly measurable, but inferred from measures of motor performance

motor performance: the directly measurable extent to which the objective of a motor task is met, the scientific study of which originated as a branch of experimental psychology

motor skills: skills in which both movement and the outcome of actions are emphasized

peripheral nervous system: the system of nerves that link the central nervous system to the rest of the body; consists of twelve pairs of cranial nerves, thirty-one pairs of spinal nerves, and the autonomic nervous system

skeletal muscle: striated muscle that contracts voluntarily and involuntarily to carry out the functions of body support, posture, and locomotion

somatosensory system: the system by which muscle, joint, and cutaneous sensory receptors contribute to the perception and control of movement through ascending pathways

PHYSICAL AND PSYCHOLOGICAL FACTORS

Motor skill development, the process of change in motor behavior with increasing age, focuses on adjustments in posture, movement, and the skillful manipulation of objects. Early researchers attributed essentially all developmental changes to modifications occurring within the central nervous system, with increasing motor abilities reflecting increasing neural maturation. Contemporary researchers have determined that the central nervous system works in combination with other body systems (such as the musculoskeletal, cardiovascular, and respiratory systems) and the environment to influence motor development, with all systems interacting in an extremely complex fashion as the individual ages.

Prenatal development of motor behavior takes place between approximately seven weeks after conception and birth, as was first determined during the 1970's using technology to visualize the fetus in utero. Following approximately eight weeks of gestation, the fetus is able to exert reflex and reaction actions, as well as active spontaneous movement. It is currently believed that the ability to self-initiate movements within the womb is an integral part of development, as compared to the traditional view that the fetus is passive and reflexive.

Infancy, the period from birth until the child is able to stand and walk, lasts approximately twelve months. The neonate begins life essentially helpless against the force of gravity and gradually develops the ability to align body segments with respect both to other body segments and to the environment. The Bayley Scales of Infant Development measure the following milestones of motor skill development for the first year of life (with the average age of accomplishment listed in parentheses): erect and steady head holding (0.8 months), side to back turning (1.8 months), supported sitting (2.3 months), back to side turning (4.4 months), momentary independent sitting (5.3 months), rolling from back to stomach (6.4 months), steady independent sitting (6.6 months), early supported stepping movements (7.4 months), arm pull to standing position (8.1 months), assisted walking (9.6 months), independent standing (11.0 months), and independent walking (11.7 months). The transition from helplessness to physical independence during the first twelve months creates many changes for growing children and their caregivers. New areas of exploration open up for the baby as greater body control is gained, the force of gravity is conquered, and less dependence on holding and carrying by caregivers is required.

During the first three months after birth, the infant's motor skill development focuses on getting the head aligned from the predominating posture of flexion. Flexor tone, the tendency to maintain a flexed posture and to rebound back into flexion when the limbs are extended and released, probably results from a combination of the elasticity of soft tissues that were confined to a flexed position while in the womb and of central nervous system activity. As antigravity activity progresses, the infant develops the ability to lift the head. Movements during this period involve brief periods of stretching, kicking, and thrusting of the limbs, in addition to turning and twisting of the trunk and head. Infants tend to be the most active prior to feeding and more quiet and sleepy after feeding.

The third to sixth months after birth are marked by great strides in overcoming the force of gravity by both flexion and extension movements. The infant becomes more competent in head control with respect to symmetry and midline orientation with the rest of the body, is able to sit independently for brief periods, and can push up onto hands and knees. These major milestones enable considerably more independence and permit a much greater ability to interact with the rest of the world.

During the sixth to ninth months after birth, the infant is constantly moving and exploring the surrounding environment. As nine months is approached, most babies are able to pull themselves into a standing position using a support such as furniture. The child expends a great deal of energy to stand and often bounces up and down once standing is achieved. The up-and-down bouncing eventually leads to the shifting of body weight from side to side and the taking of first steps, with a caregiver assisting alongside the furniture; this is often called cruising.

The ninth to twelfth months involve forward creeping on hands and knees. This locomotor pattern requires more complicated alternating movements of the opposite arms and legs. Some infants have a preference for creeping even after they are able to walk independently, with many preferring plantigrade creeping (on extended arms and legs) to walking. The ease to which the child moves from sitting to creeping, kneeling, or standing is greatly improved and balance is developed to the point where the child can pivot around in circles while sitting, using the hands and feet for propulsion. The child begins to move efficiently from standing to floor sitting and can initiate rolling from the supine position using flexed legs. Unsupported sitting is accomplished with ease, and weight while sitting can be transferred easily from buttocks to hands.

The early childhood period lasts from infancy until about six years. It involves the child attaining new skills but not necessarily new patterns of movement, with the learning patterns that were acquired during the first year of life being put to use in more meaningful activities. The locomotor pattern of walking is refined, and new motor skills that require increased balance and control of force—such as running, hopping, jumping, and skipping—are mastered.

Running is usually begun between years two and four, as the child learns to master the flight phase and the anticipatory strategies necessary when there is temporarily no body contact with the ground. It is not until about age five or six that control during running with respect to starting, stopping, and changing directions is effectively mastered. Jumping develops at about age 2.5, as the ability and confidence to land after jumping from a height such as a stair is achieved. The ability to jump to reach an overhead object then emerges, with early jumpers revealing a shallow preparatory crouch that progresses to a deeper crouch. Hopping, an extension of the ability to balance while standing on one leg, begins at about age 2.5 but is not performed well until about age six, when a series of about ten hops can be performed consecutively and are incorporated into games such as hopscotch. Skipping, a step and a hop on one leg followed by a step and hop of the other leg, is generally not achieved until about six years, with the opportunity and encouragement for practice being a primary determining factor, as with other locomotor skills.

Throwing is typically acquired during the first year, but advanced throwing, striking (such as with a plastic baseball and bat), kicking (such as with a soccer ball), and catching are not developed until early childhood. Catching develops at approximately age three, with the child initially holding the arms in front of the body and later making anticipatory adjustments to account for the direction, speed, and size of the thrown object. Kicking, which requires balancing on one foot while transferring force to an object with the other foot, begins with little preparatory backswing and eventually develops to involve the knee, hip, and lean of the trunk at about age six.

Fine motor manipulation skills in the upper extremity that are important to normal activities of daily living such as feeding, dressing, grooming, and handwriting are greatly improved in early childhood. The key components include locating a target, which requires the coordination of eye-head movement; reaching, which requires the transportation of the hand and arm in space; and manipulation, which includes grip formation, grasp, and release.

During later childhood (the period from seven years to about eleven years), adolescence, and adult life throughout the remainder of the life span, changes in movement are influenced predominantly by age. Adolescence begins with the onset of the physical changes of puberty, at approximately eleven to twelve years of age in girls and twelve to thirteen years of age in boys, and ends when physical growth is curtailed. Most authorities believe that the growth spurt of adolescence leads to the emergence of new patterns of movement within the skills that have already been acquired. Most adolescents have strong drives to develop self-esteem and become socially acceptable with their peers in school and various recreational activities. Cooperation and competition become strong components of motor skill development, whereby many skills are stabilized prior to adolescence and preferences for various sports activities emerge. Boys typically demonstrate increased speed and strength as compared to girls, despite recent dramatic changes in available opportunities for girls in recreational and competitive sports activities. Even though age-related changes in motor behavior continue throughout adulthood, the physical skills that permit independence are primarily acquired during the first year of life.

Psychological factors that influence motor skill development include attention level, stimulus-response compatibility, arousal level, and motivation. The level of attention when attempting a motor task is critical, with humans displaying a relatively fixed capacity for concentration during different stages of development. Stimulus identification, response selection, and response programming stages—whereby an individual remembers or determines how to perform a task—affect skill development because the central nervous system takes longer to synthesize and respond to more complex skills. Also important are stimulus-response compatibility—the better the stimulus matches the response, the shorter the reaction time—and arousal, which is described as an "inverted U" by the Yerkes-Dodson model. The inverted U hypothesis implies that there exists an optimal level of psychological arousal to learn or perform a motor skill efficiently, with performance declining when the arousal level at a given moment in time is too great or too small. At a low level of arousal, the scope of perception is broad, and all stimuli (including irrelevant information) are being processed. As arousal level increases, perception narrows so that when the optimal level of arousal is reached and attention is sufficiently focused, concentration on only the stimuli relevant to successful skill learning and performance is enabled. If arousal level surpasses this optimal level, perception narrows to the point of tunnel vision, some relevant stimuli are missed, and learning

and skill performance are reduced. The influence of personal motivation during motor skill development encompasses the child's perceived relevance of the activity and also the child's individual ability to recognize the goal of the activity and desire to achieve it.

Three main factors that affect motor skill development in early and later childhood include feedback, amount of practice, and practice conditions. Feedback can be intrinsic, arising from the somatosensory system and senses such as vision and hearing, as information is gathered about a movement and its consequences rather then the actual achievement of the goal. In pathological conditions such as cerebral palsy, intrinsic feedback is often greatly impaired. Feedback can also be extrinsic and is often divided by researchers into knowledge of results, or information about the success of the movement in accomplishing the goal that is available after the skill is completed, and knowledge of performance, or information about skill performance technique or strategy. Knowledge of results provides information about errors as well as successes. True learning occurs by a process of trial and error, with the nervous system serving to detect and correct inappropriate or inefficient movements.

DISORDERS AND EFFECTS

Physical therapists, psychologists, teachers, and other professionals who work with pediatric patients often plan their treatment interventions and instructional lessons based on the normal age-related progression of motor skill development. Motor skill development is often significantly decreased as a consequence of a neurological impairment, however, with the child's resulting movement patterns revealing primary impairments such as inadequate activation of muscle, secondary impairments such as contractures, and compensatory strategies that are adopted to overcome the impairment and achieve mobility. The categories for impairments that have an impact on motor development can generally be divided into musculoskeletal, neuromuscular, sensory, perceptual, and cognitive.

Damage to various nervous system structures somewhat predictably reduces the motor control of movement via both positive symptoms (the presence of abnormal behavior) and negative symptoms (the loss of normal behavior). Positive symptoms include the presence of exaggerated reflexes and abnormalities of muscle tone. Negative symptoms include the loss of muscular strength and the inappropriate selection of muscles during task performance. The broad spectrum of muscle tone abnormalities ranges from flaccidity to rigidity, with muscle spasticity defined as the velocity-dependent increase in tonic stretch reflexes (also called muscle tone), with exaggerated tendon jerks resulting from changes in the threshold of the stretch reflex.

Secondary effects of central nervous system lesions are not directly caused by the lesions themselves but develop as a consequence of the lesions. For example, children with cerebral palsy often exhibit the primary problem of spasticity in muscles of the lower extremities, which causes the secondary problem of muscular and tendon tightness in the ankles, knees, and hips. The secondary problem of limited range of motion in these important areas for movement often impairs motor skills more than the primary problem of spasticity, with the resulting movement strategies reflecting the growing child's best attempt to compensate.

Another common compensatory strategy seen in children with a motor development dysfunction involves standing with the knee hyperextended because of an inability to generate enough muscular force to keep the knee from collapsing. Standing with the knee in hyperextension keeps the line of gravity in front of the knee joint. Contractures of joints are frequent consequences of disordered postural and movement patterns. For example, a habitual crouched sitting posture results in chronic shortening of the hamstring, calf, and hip flexor muscles, and a backward-tipped pelvis accommodates the shortened hamstrings. Chronic shortening of the calf muscles often results in toe walking (in which the heel does not strike the ground) and a reduced walking speed and stride length, because of decreased balance and leg muscle strength. Changes in the availability of sensory information and cognitive factors such as fear of falling and inattention may also contribute strongly to motor skill development in some pediatric patients.

PERSPECTIVE AND PROSPECTS

Interest in the scientific study of motor development was greatly enhanced by Myrtle B. McGraw's *The Neuromuscular Maturation of the Human Infant* (1945). It described four stages of neural maturation: a period in which movement is governed by reflexes as a result of the dominance of lower centers within the central nervous system; a period in which reflex expression declines as a result of maturation of the cerebral cortex and the inhibitory effect of the cortex over lower centers; a period in which an increase in the voluntary quality of activity as a result of increased cortical con-

trol produces deliberate or voluntary movement; and a period in which integrative activity of the neural centers takes place, as shown by smooth and coordinated movements.

Arnold Gesell then used cinematography to conduct extensive observations of infants during various stages of growth. He described the maturation of infants based on four behavior categories: motor behavior, adaptive behavior, language development, and personal-social development. Gesell identified six principles of development. The principle of motor priority and fore-reference states that the neuromotor system is laid down before it is voluntarily utilized. The principle of developmental direction states that development proceeds in head-to-foot and proximal-to-distal directions. The principle of reciprocal interweaving states that opposing movements such as extension and flexion show a temporary dominance over one another until they become integrated into mature motor patterns. The principle of functional asymmetry states that humans have a preferred hand, a dominant eye, and a lead foot, with this unilateral dominance being subject to change during development. The principle of self-regulation states that periods of stability and instability culminate into more stable responses as maturity proceeds. The principle of optimal realization states that the human action system has strong growth potential toward normal development if environmental and cultural conditions are favorable and if compensatory and regeneration mechanisms come into play when damage occurs to facilitate attainment of the maximum possible growth.

Esther Thelen suggested the dynamic systems theory. This theory argues that the maturing nervous system interacts with other biomechanical, psychological, and social environment factors to create a dimensional system whereby behavior represents a compression of the degrees of freedom.

A more refined systems theory of motor control developed by Anne Shumway-Cook and Marjorie Woollacott claims that the three main factors that interact in the development of efficient locomotion are progression (ability to generate rhythmic muscular patterns to move the body in the desired direction), stability (the control of balance), and adaptation (the ability to adapt to changing task and environmental requirements). These three factors generally appear sequentially, with muscular patterns appearing first, followed by equilibrium control, and finally adaptive capabilities. Although research on the emergence of human motor skills has primarily concentrated on the developmental milestones of infants and children, it appears that important changes in motor behavior continue throughout the human life span.

—Daniel G. Graetzer, Ph.D.

See also Cerebral palsy; Cognitive development; Developmental stages; Growth; Muscular dystrophy; Muscle sprains, spasms, and disorders; Muscles; Nervous system; Physical examination; Reflexes, primitive; Speech disorders; Well-baby examinations.

FOR FURTHER INFORMATION:

Berk, Laura E. *Child Development.* 7th ed. Boston: Pearson/Allyn and Bacon, 2006. A text that reviews theory and research in child development, cognitive and language development, personality and social development, motor skill development, and the foundations and contexts of development.

Feldman, Robert S. *Development Across the Life Span.* 4th ed. Upper Saddle River, N.J.: Pearson/Prentice Hall, 2006. Traces the physical, cognitive, and social and personality development of one's life span, focusing on basic theories, research findings, and current applications of theory.

Kalverboer, Alex F., Brian Hopkins, and Reint Geuze, eds. *Motor Development in Early and Later Childhood: Longitudinal Approaches.* New York: Cambridge University Press, 1993. An excellent text that reviews motor development in early and later childhood in a longitudinal fashion.

Nathanson, Laura Walther. *The Portable Pediatrician: A Practicing Pediatrician's Guide to Your Child's Growth, Development, Health, and Behavior from Birth to Age Five.* 2d ed. New York: HarperCollins, 2002. An engaging, easy-to-read guide for parents to assess their child's development, medical symptoms, and behavioral problems.

Newell, K. M. "Motor Skill Acquisition." *Annual Review of Psychology* 42 (1991): 213-237. This review focuses on the general laws of motor learning and the specifics of what is learned through repetitive practice.

Shumway-Cook, Anne, and Marjorie Woollacott. *Motor Control: Translating Research into Clinical Practice.* 3d ed. Philadelphia: Lippincott Williams & Wilkins, 2007. This excellent text provides a framework by which the various motor control theories can be incorporated into physical therapy clinical practice for a variety of patient populations.

Thelen, Esther, and Linda B. Smith. *A Dynamic Systems Approach to the Development of Cognition and Action.* Cambridge, Mass.: MIT Press, 1996. This text examines perceptual motor processes, motor abilities, and cognition in infants and children, in addition to describing various points of view of developmental psychobiology.

MOUTH AND THROAT CANCER
DISEASE/DISORDER

ANATOMY OR SYSTEM AFFECTED: Gums, mouth, neck, teeth, throat

SPECIALTIES AND RELATED FIELDS: Dentistry, general surgery, oncology, radiology

DEFINITION: A malignancy of the lips, tongue, gums, salivary glands, or pharynx.

KEY TERMS:

biopsy: the removal and examination of body tissue to determine whether it is cancerous

esophagus: a muscular tube connecting the pharynx and the stomach

pharynx: the area connecting the back of the throat to the esophagus

squamous cells: flat ephithelial cells that resemble scales

CAUSES AND SYMPTOMS

Often, dentists detect cancers of the mouth and throat during routine dental examinations. People who visit their dentists regularly, preferably twice a year, will likely have such cancers detected and diagnosed in their earliest stages when treatment is effective and the cure rate high.

Valid generalizations can be made about the causes of mouth and throat cancers. The most significant cause is the regular use of tobacco products. Cigarette smoking over long periods often results in these cancers or in lung cancer. Males, especially those over forty, have a higher rate of mouth and throat cancer than do females. Pipe and cigar smokers are at greater risk of cancer than are cigarette smokers, and a correlation also exists between the use of chewing tobacco and snuff and the development of mouth cancer. About 90 percent of people suffering from mouth and/or throat cancer have been consistent users of tobacco.

A second causal factor is the regular consumption of substantial quantities of alcoholic beverages, usually over four drinks a day. Some 80 percent of people suffering from mouth and/or throat cancer have used alcohol regularly and in substantial quantities. They are particularly subject to cancers on the floor of the mouth, the tonsils, the lower pharynx, and the tongue.

People who smoke two packs of cigarettes a day and consume over four drinks a day increase the likelihood that they will develop mouth and/or throat cancers by forty times. Other factors in such cancers are poor dental hygiene, ill-fitting dentures, or irregular teeth that cause irritations in the mouth. Those whose work brings them into direct contact with certain toxic chemicals are also at risk.

The most common symptom of lip cancer is the formation of a small, whitish patch (leukoplakia), usually painless, on the lip. It frequently consists of squamous cells. As it develops, it may become ulcerous, causing bleeding and compromising surrounding tissue. If the tongue becomes involved, then it may stiffen. As the malignancy advances, the tongue often becomes painful. Speech, chewing, and swallowing become progressively difficult.

Cancer of the oropharynx, the mid-section of the pharynx, is often accompanied by difficulty in swallowing and hoarseness. Such cancers may also cause patients to expectorate blood-stained sputum. A sore throat frequently accompanies this form of cancer, and earache may also occur, although both of these symptoms frequently result from other causes. People with severe and consistent stomach acid reflux are vulnerable to throat cancer.

TREATMENT AND THERAPY

The usual treatment of mouth and throat cancer is surgery to remove the affected tissue. Such surgery is almost always followed by a course of radiation, which may also precede such surgery to shrink any tumors that might be present. Sometimes, removal of the tongue is indicated, although this is a very drastic treatment because of the problems that it causes for the patient, whose ability to speak and to chew and swallow food will be drastically compromised. Cancer of the tongue is the most aggressive form of mouth cancer, which is justification for using drastic measures to deal with it. Facial disfiguration may also be involved in treating cancers of this sort, so extensive plastic surgery may be necessary following it.

Throat cancers usually require the surgical removal of cancerous tissue followed by radiation, but treatment with anticancer medications may also be involved in the management of such cancers. Often, a biopsy is performed in the operating room prior to surgery, usually in conjunction with invasive procedures that permit surgeons and oncologists to view the pharynx, the lungs, and the esophagus using laryngoscopes, bronchoscopes, or esophagoscopes.

PERSPECTIVE AND PROSPECTS

Cancer of the mouth and throat constitute about 8 percent of all the cancers diagnosed in the United States annually. When an early diagnosis is made and is followed by prompt treatment, a cure results in 75 percent of cases. More than half the people diagnosed with mouth cancer, even those for whom late diagnoses are made, survive for at least five years following treatment. As in all cancers, early detection is the key to effective management and desirable outcomes.

Perhaps the most important factor in reducing the incidence of mouth and throat cancer is to convince young people not to develop the habit of using tobacco products and not to abuse alcohol. People who are already smokers and drinkers are well advised to stop smoking and to limit their alcohol intake to two drinks a day or less.

No conclusive correlation has been made between mouth and throat cancer and secondhand smoke. As an increasing number of public venues and workplaces have become smoke-free, however, people who patronize or work in such places have been smoking less.

Most inveterate smokers want to overcome the habit, but nicotine addiction is so powerful that giving it up is difficult. Various methods have proved helpful in enabling people to control their habits, among them hypnosis, acupuncture, laser treatment, psychotherapy, and nicotine replacement through patches or nicotine chewing gum.

—*R. Baird Shuman, Ph.D.*

See also Addiction; Alcoholism; Biopsy; Cancer; Carcinogens; Carcinoma; Cells; Chemotherapy; Dental diseases; Dentistry; Dermatology; Dermatopathology; Glands; Laryngectomy; Malignancy and metastasis; Nasopharyngeal disorders; Oncology; Pharyngitis;

INFORMATION ON MOUTH AND THROAT CANCER

CAUSES: Tobacco, alcohol, dental problems, toxins, severe acid reflux disease

SYMPTOMS: May include whitish patches on lips, stiff tongue, bloody sputum, sore throat, earache

DURATION: Chronic

TREATMENTS: Surgery, radiation therapy, chemotherapy, plastic surgery

Plastic surgery; Radiation therapy; Skin cancer; Skin lesion removal; Smoking; Sore throat; Tumor removal; Tumors.

FOR FURTHER INFORMATION:

DeConno, Franco, et al. "Mouth Care." In *Oxford Textbook of Palliative Medicine*, edited by Derek Doyle et al. New York: Oxford University Press, 2004.

Hahn, Michael J., and Anne Jones. *Head and Neck Nursing*. Edinburgh, N.Y.: Churchill Livingstone, 2000.

Lydiatt, William M., and Perry J. Johnson. *Cancers of the Mouth and Throat: A Patient's Guide to Treatment*. Omaha, Nebr.: Addicus Books, 2001.

Mallet, Jane, and Lisa Dougherty, eds. *The Royal Marsden Hospital Manual of Clinical Nursing*. Malden, Mass.: Blackwell Science, 2004.

MRI. *See* MAGNETIC RESONANCE IMAGING (MRI).

MUCOPOLYSACCHARIDOSIS (MPS)

DISEASE/DISORDER

ALSO KNOWN AS: Diferrante syndrome, Hunter syndrome, Hurler's syndrome, Morquio syndrome

ANATOMY OR SYSTEM AFFECTED: All

SPECIALTIES AND RELATED FIELDS: Cardiology, embryology, genetics, pediatrics

DEFINITION: A genetic disorder characterized by accumulations of mucopolysaccharides in tissues.

CAUSES AND SYMPTOMS

Six distinct classes of mucopolysaccharidosis (MPS) have been described, with a number of subclasses. The basis for all mucopolysaccharidosis categories is found in recessive genetic defects of gene products associated with the metabolism of mucopolysaccharides, long chains of sugar molecule that are used to build connective tissue in the body. Specific symptoms are associated with each type, which is a function of which gene locus is at fault. All involve the degradation of specific mucopolysaccharides: dermatan sulfate, heparan sulfate, or keratan sulfate. At least ten enzymes are involved in these metabolic pathways.

The specific syndrome depends upon which enzyme, or which combination, is at fault. For example, MPS I, also called Hurler's syndrome, results from a deficiency of the enzyme alpha-L-iduronidase (IDUA) and is associated with early childhood defects in dis-

---

INFORMATION ON MUCOPOLYSACCHARIDOSIS (MPS)

CAUSES: Genetic enzyme defects

SYMPTOMS: Depends on type; may include defects in aorta or corneas, facial distortion, dwarfism, organ enlargement, mental deficiencies, shortened life span

DURATION: Progressive and fatal

TREATMENTS: None; alleviation of symptoms

---

parate sites such as the aorta or cornea. Other common symptoms include physical distortion of the face, dwarfism, organ enlargement, mental deficiencies, and shortened life span. MPS IV, also known as Morquio syndrome, is related to reduced activity of galactosamine-6-sulfatase and causes symptoms similar to those in other forms of the disorder.

Diagnosis has generally been based upon laboratory testing for the decreased presence of enzymes involved in the metabolic pathway, as well as the observed accumulation of intermediate polysaccharides such as heparan sulfate in cell lysosomes, reflecting the lack of breakdown. Recent procedures have taken advantage of more accurate laboratory tests, as in use of polymerase chain reaction (PCR) or deoxyribonucleic acid (DNA) blotting techniques for the analysis of specific genes. Fetal cells obtained by means of amniocentesis or chorionic villus sampling and grown in culture can also be tested for defects in the suspected pathways. Generally, symptoms begin to develop after the age of two.

The same tests can be useful for the detection of carriers who do not express the defective traits. The frequency of diagnosis in various populations has ranged from 1 in 25,000 to 1 in 125,000, with significant variation in the specific type.

TREATMENT AND THERAPY

All forms of MPS are progressive, resulting in physical or structural abnormalities of varying severity. Death usually occurs before the age of twenty, though in the most severe types, the child rarely reaches the teenage years. Treatment is primarily symptomatic. Bone marrow transplants have been attempted as a means to replace defective enzymes, with little success. Prospects are currently poor. Most recent advances have involved improved diagnosis as well as the detection of carriers for the various traits.

—Richard Adler, Ph.D.

See also Enzyme therapy; Enzymes; Gaucher's disease; Genetic counseling; Genetic diseases; Glycogen storage diseases; Lipids; Metabolic disorders; Metabolism; Neonatology; Niemann-Pick disease; Screening; Tay-Sachs disease.

FOR FURTHER INFORMATION:

Bach, G., et al. "The Defect in the Hunter Syndrome: Deficiency of Sulfoiduronate Sulfatase." *Proceedings of the National Academy of Sciences* 70 (1973): 2134-2138.

Beers, Mark H., et al., eds. *The Merck Manual of Medical Information, Second Home Edition.* Whitehouse Station, N.J.: Merck Research Laboratories, 2003.

Booth, C., and H. Nadler. "Demonstration of the Heterozygous State in Hunter's Syndrome." *Pediatrics* 53 (1974): 396-399.

Icon Health. *Hunter Syndrome: A Medical Dictionary, Bibliography, and Annotated Research Guide to Internet References.* San Diego, Calif.: Author, 2004.

_____. *Hurler Syndrome: A Medical Dictionary, Bibliography, and Annotated Research Guide to Internet References.* San Diego, Calif.: Author, 2004.

Scriver, Charles, et al., eds. *The Metabolic and Molecular Basis of Inherited Disease.* 8th ed. New York: McGraw-Hill, 2001.

MULTIPLE BIRTHS
BIOLOGY

ANATOMY OR SYSTEM AFFECTED: All

SPECIALTIES AND RELATED FIELDS: Embryology, genetics, neonatology, obstetrics, pediatrics

DEFINITION: The presence of two or more fetuses in the womb.

KEY TERMS:

chromosomes: the rod-shaped structures in the nucleus of a cell that carry genes

concordance: the condition among twins of having the same physical or psychological trait

dizygotes: fraternal twins; born from two ova separately fertilized by two sperm

embryo: the cells growing after conception until the eighth week of pregnancy

monozygotes: identical twins; born of a single ovum that divides after a single sperm fertilizes it

ovum: the egg cell released from the ovaries during ovulation

placenta: the membrane sac developed from the uterine wall that passes nutrients to the fetus through interconnected blood vessels

ultrasonography: an imaging technique that uses high-frequency sound waves to view fetuses in the womb, as well as other internal structures

zygote: a fertilized ovum before multicellular development begins

INTRODUCTION

Multiple births are rare events. The most common are twins; this occurs in approximately one out of every eighty complete pregnancies. Twins can come from a single egg or from two different eggs. Triplets occur once in approximately eight hundred completed pregnancies. Quadruplets occur once in every eight thousand completed pregnancies. Quintuplets occur naturally in approximately one out of every eighty thousand completed pregnancies.

As the number of fetuses increases, the chances that all will survive decreases. Multiple births are most commonly combinations of twins and single eggs. By reviewing the mechanics of twin formation, greater multiples can be understood.

THE DIFFERENT TYPES OF TWINS

Two types of twins are well known: fraternal twins and identical twins. Behind these general terms, however, lies considerable variation. This variation is based on the many changes that a human ovum can undergo after it is released by the ovary, is fertilized, travels along the Fallopian tube to the uterus, and implants there to develop into an embryo.

Fraternal twins are also known as dizygotic or binovular twins. In a normal menstrual cycle, only a single egg is released. When a sperm penetrates an ovum, the fertilized egg releases a chemical that prevents other sperm from penetrating the same egg. If a second egg has been released, however, it can also be fertilized. A newly fertilized egg is called a zygote. If both zygotes succeed in attaching to the uterine walls, a twin pregnancy begins. Usually, this dual insemination occurs during a single release of semen in a single copulation, so that the embryos have the same father. Occasionally, the two eggs may be fertilized in separate copulations during the same ovulation, a phenomenon called superfecundation. It is then possible for dizygotic twins to have different fathers. This possibility seems to have long been recognized. The Greek myth of Leda and the Swan derives from such a pregnancy.

Very rarely, an impregnated woman continues her monthly ovulation cycle. If a second ovulation occurs in the three months following conception, theoretically

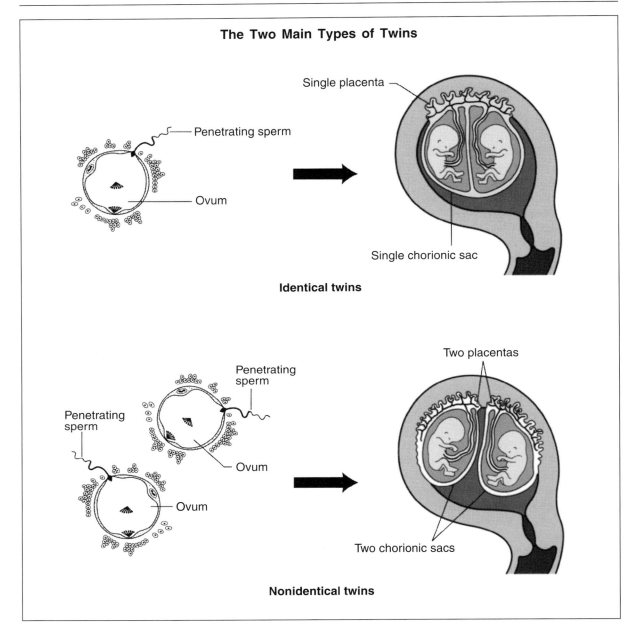

The Two Main Types of Twins

Single placenta

Penetrating sperm

Ovum

Single chorionic sac

Identical twins

Penetrating sperm

Penetrating sperm

Ovum

Ovum

Two placentas

Two chorionic sacs

Nonidentical twins

she could be impregnated again. This phenomenon is called superfetation and would result in twins who are one, two, or three months different in age. No unquestionable example of human superfetation has been documented because distinguishing the relative ages of twin fetuses is extremely difficult.

Fraternal twins have separate placentas and membranes in the womb. The placenta comprises maternal and fetal tissues interconnected by blood vessels. Nutrients pass from mother to the fetus through the pla-

centa. Waste products are removed from the fetus by a reverse process. Sometimes, the placentas press against each other in the womb and fuse. Having had separate placentas or one fused together, however, does not affect the nature of the twins after birth. Fraternal twins, even though they share the same birthday, are no more similar in appearance or manner than two siblings from separate births.

Identical twins are the result of different initial events. They are also called monozygotic or monovular twins. Identical or look-alike twins originate when a single egg spontaneously divides after penetration by a sperm cell. Each half develops separately. The reason for this division is not known. One theory holds that sometimes the fertilized ovum does not implant in the uterus right away as is normally the case. During the delay, the chromosomes double and the zygote halves, with each half then implanting and becoming a separate embryo.

Another theory suggests that early in the pregnancy, a genetic mutation occurs in one of the cells. Later, while the embryo is still no more than a few hundred cells, the unmutated cells recognize the genetic difference and reject the mutant cells, much as the immune system rejects substances foreign to it. The rejected group of cells develops separately. If this theory proves to be true, identical twins must not be completely identical after all. Cases in which one identical twin has a genetic disease and the other remains healthy appear to support this theory, although mutation in one twin may occur after splitting rather than causing the splitting.

Variation sometimes appears after birth in monozygotic siblings. Twins can vary in birth weight greatly (one may weigh twice as much), develop at different rates, and die from unrelated natural causes. As a rule, however, identical twins share an overwhelming majority of traits. When two (or more) siblings share a trait, they are considered to be concordant for that trait. Typically, body structures and coloration will be strikingly concordant. Features such as facial shape, hair texture and color, eye color, and height are typical examples of concordance. "Mirror" twins are an uncommon phenomenon. They show mirror image symmetry in some traits. For example, one may be left-handed while the other is right-handed. Whorls on the scalp may also occur as mirror images. In very rare cases, one mirror twin will have situs inversus: The placement of all internal organs is reversed. An individual with situs inversus will have the liver and appendix on the left side of the abdomen and the spleen on the right.

Genetic variation may account for the subtle variations in even the most concordant of twins. The internal environment of the womb also has an effect. Most identical twin fetuses share the same placenta but have different inner or chorionic sacs. They may have separate placentas (and separate chorions) depending on when the initial splitting of the zygote took place. Usually, those sharing a single placenta have separate chorions. In the rarest variation, the fetuses also share the same amnion. The degree of separation or number of barriers can influence the amount of oxygen or nutrients that each twin receives. Relatively minor differences can affect development.

A third type of twin is theoretically possible. During maturation and before becoming fertilized, the mature ovum could divide into a secondary oocyte (the cell to be fertilized) and a much smaller polar body. It is possible for the ovum to divide into roughly equal portions, both of which are viable and contain the same genetic material. If separate sperm then fertilize these ova, they would become two zygotes. Such twins would have exactly the same maternal genes, but a portion of the paternal genes would differ. They would be less identical than monozygotes but more so than dizygotes. Although this type of twinning has been described in rats and mice, no human case has been indisputably identified and reported.

A fourth variant of twinning is conjoined twins, popularly called Siamese twins. Conjoined twins share some tissue. This can range from simple joining of skin on the head or shoulder to having one heart or kidney or two torsos and a single pair of legs. Conjoined twins are identical (or monozygotic) twins created by incomplete cell division during early fetal life. The portion of cells that divide normally continue to develop in a normal fashion. The cells that did not divide completely also develop normally. The result is a portion of the body that is duplicated and a portion that is not. If the incomplete division occurred early in fetal development, the amount of shared tissue is likely to be greater than with an incomplete division that occurred later in fetal development.

About one-third of all twin births result in identical twins. The proportion of males and females is approximately equal. The incidence of identical twins remains constant throughout the world's diverse ethnic populations. Fraternal twins, however, show different proportions and distributions. About half the pairs have the same gender (with a nearly equal number of male-male and female-female pairs); about half are male-female pairs. Fraternal twin births occur most frequently among rural Nigerians (45 pairs per 1,000 births) and least frequently among Chinese and Japanese parents (4 pairs per 1,000 births). European and American rates, for both blacks and whites, are approximately halfway between these extremes.

Evidence suggests that women inherit a tendency to conceive fraternal twins from their mothers. There is little scientific evidence to support the belief that fathers possess a gene for monozygotic twins. Physiological factors can increase the likelihood of a woman having fraternal twins. Women who are tall and heavy and who have previously given birth to children have more twins than small women or those who have not been pregnant before. Women between thirty-five and forty years of age are the most likely to have twins, but the chances decrease thereafter.

Multiple pregnancies (triplets and more) are usually combinations of twins. Identical triplets do rarely occur, but triplets consisting of two identical and one fraternal sibling are the norm. Multiple births of four or more infants are almost always combinations of twins. Physicians can ascertain the status of multiple birth siblings by examining placentas and chorionic sacs.

POSSIBLE COMPLICATIONS

Multiple births create special problems for mothers. Specifically, they are more difficult to carry in the womb and to nurture through infancy than singletons. Multiples are smaller, so that vaginal deliveries are easier. Many physicians, however, recommend birth by Cesarean section to manage complications better. Most twins are born healthy, but they must be monitored carefully. As the number of fetuses increases, their size decreases. Because they are not fully mature, this increases the chances for medical problems.

Positively identifying multiple fetuses in the womb is not always an easy task, even though medical science has developed a variety of techniques. The traditional signs of considerable fetal movement, multiple heartbeats, and a large weight gain by the mother can be inaccurate and contradictory. Tests for the human chorionic gonadotropin hormone in the mother's blood or urine or alpha-fetoprotein in the blood may suggest the presence of multiple fetuses if the hormone or protein levels are unusually elevated. Nevertheless, imaging technologies provide the most reliable test. Ultrasonography has supplanted X rays, which declined in use because of the radiation hazard to fetuses. The images produced by ultrasonography can usually resolve multiple fetuses early in the pregnancy.

A multiple pregnancy itself strains the mother's body and is particularly subject to medical complications. Typically, a mother carrying multiple fetuses gains from 30 to 80 pounds, about twice the weight of a single pregnancy. The added weight can cause skeletal and muscular problems. The fetuses' demands on the mother's body may also worsen preexisting medical conditions, such as heart or kidney disease. As the multiple fetuses develop, their size stretches the uterus,

which can initiate early labor. For this reason, the premature birth rate is higher for multiple fetuses than for single fetuses. Twins occasionally reach full term; triplets and greater multiples do not.

Similarly, multiple pregnancies miscarry at more than three times the rate of singletons. Occasionally, one fetus will develop at the expense of the other by drawing a disproportionate amount of nutrients from the mother, a condition called twin transfusion syndrome. In cases of identical (monozygotic) twins who share a single placenta, a phenomenon known as a twin-twin transfusion can occur. When this occurs, one twin receives most of the blood, nutrients, and oxygen, in turn becoming much larger than the other twin. In some instances, the smaller twin (the donor) perishes due to lack of these vital substances. In other cases, the larger twin (the recipient) succumbs to heart failure as a result of having to pump the increased blood flow. A new surgical technique (ablation) is currently being used in the third trimester to sever the connection, stopping the twin-twin transfusion. If one fetus dies for any reason, then the mother's body may reabsorb it partially or completely, a phenomenon known as the vanishing twin. Some doctors believe that because of unobserved vanishing twins, miscarriages, and induced abortions, the number of twin conceptions has been underestimated.

Doctors carefully monitor the fetal development of multiple fetuses to ensure their health and, especially, to prepare for delivering them. Amniocentesis and genetic tests detect potential biochemical defects, genetic anomalies, and diseases. Ultrasonography allows doctors to identify defects in shape and the relative position of the fetuses in the womb. Their position is important during labor. Normally, babies are born headfirst. In multiples, one of the fetuses frequently lies crosswise or feetfirst. These positions greatly lengthen and complicate delivery, so that the second fetus runs a higher risk of dying during labor. Moreover, the mother's overdistended uterus, unable to contract properly after delivery, may begin to bleed. The fact that labor lasts too long may exhaust her dangerously. Because of such problems, many obstetricians recommend delivery by cesarean section—that is, by cutting a passage through the abdomen into the uterus—at the first sign of trouble to either mother or fetuses.

The prematurity and low birth weight common in multiple infants means that many are placed on life support. Studies have found that multiple infants suffer congenital defects as much as three times more often than singletons. Identical siblings are the most likely of all to have abnormalities. Heart malformations are most common. According to some studies, closed esophagus, clubfeet, excess fingers or toes, and forms of mental retardation such as Down syndrome occur at a slightly higher rate.

Conjoined twins are relatively rare, appearing approximately once in a hundred thousand pregnancies. Most are attached at the back or at the back of the head or neck. In an extreme rarity, one identical twin has a full set of chromosomes while the other has only the X chromosome from the mother and will be a female with a condition called Turner syndrome. Therefore, identical twins will be of opposite gender if the first twin has the XY chromosomes that defines a male and the other is a female with Turner syndrome.

That multiple birth siblings develop in the same environment and from a common origin allows researchers to trace the genetic and environmental influences on human development in general. Most of this research has been conducted on twins because of the relative rarity of triplets or larger groups of siblings. The reasoning is straightforward. In the case of identical twins, either their genetic heritage (nature) or the environment (nurture) dominates in determining how they grow mentally and physically. Researchers have tested the idea by tracking down identical twins who were separated while young, usually at birth, and reared separately. If genetics control development, then the separated twins should still look and behave similarly. If environment predominates, then separated twins should show variations in appearance and temperament.

The reported research results have been mixed. Some separated twins do not look and act any more alike than siblings separately born. Others show an uncanny degree of similarity throughout their lives—dressing the same way, marrying in the same year, having the same number of children, and dying nearly at the same time of the same disease. Their intelligence, which many scientists believe is heavily influenced by environment, nevertheless shows high concordance.

PERSPECTIVE AND PROSPECTS

Worldwide, superstitions and a strong moral overtone have traditionally accompanied multiple births. Some societies viewed one twin as automatically good and the other evil and treated them accordingly as they matured. Others thought twins shameful, a sign of corruption or promiscuity in the mother. These babies might be killed at birth or separated because of it. An African curse reflects the deep suspicion that some societies have held for twins: "May you be the mother of twins." On the other hand, some nations believed that twins have divine origin or power over the elements or special talents for prophecy and telepathy.

Multiple siblings enjoy a special advantage: They are rarely lonely. Some twins even share their own private language, a phenomenon known as idioglossa. Their common development means increased requirements of time and money for their families. It also provides continuous opportunities for sharing and relying on each other. The many national and international organizations created by and for twins and other multiple birth siblings reflect their pride in their status.

Triplets have historically had a reasonable chance for survival. Before the advent of support equipment for premature babies, lung immaturity was the factor that usually determined life or death. Surfactant is a chemical that is secreted in the seventh month of pregnancy. Without surfactant, lung tissues stick together and infants cannot breathe. Because of the combined size of all fetuses, many multiple infants are born before the seventh month of gestation. The Dionne quintuplets, who were born in the 1930's, were unusual in that for the first time in history, all five survived into adulthood. Modern support technology has helped several sets of sextuplets (six infants) to survive. In November, 1997, the same technology permitted all the McCaughey septuplets (seven infants) to survive. This was the first time such an event had occurred. (The chances of naturally conceiving septuplets are one in eight to ten million conceptions.)

Recent advances in the field of assisted reproduction have increased the odds of multiple pregnancies. Women who have difficulty conceiving are initially treated with drugs that cause more than one egg to be released during ovulation. This increases the chance of pregnancy but also increases the chance of carrying multiple fetuses. Couples who seek medical assistance to achieve pregnancy routinely use fertility drugs. A woman will have several eggs or zygotes implanted to improve the odds of successfully initiating a pregnancy. The result of this approach is an increased number of multiple births. In 1988, twelve fetuses, which were miscarried, resulted from a fertility drug. Artificially induced pregnancies have posed ethical dilemmas for many who believe that scientists should not manipulate human biological processes.

Multiple births raise other moral and ethical questions as well. Genetic tests can now identify potential fetal defects in the womb early enough that surgeons can remove a defective fetus without harming the healthy fetus, a procedure called selective birth, selective abortion, or selective fetocide. Those who hold abortions to be immoral have reservations about selective fetocide even when the defective fetus has little chance of surviving and may threaten the lives of the remaining healthy fetuses. That selective fetocide may be used simply because a mother does not want to rear more than one child has caused far greater concern. Since the procedure is tricky to perform and can result in the death of all fetuses, most doctors find selective fetocide for nonmedical reasons to be ethically indefensible.

Twin births bear witness to the successes of modern health care. In the United States, incidents of multiple births, both fraternal and identical, have increased slightly since the 1970's and more multiples are surviving to adulthood. Fertility drugs may account for part of the increase, as does the trend among American women to delay childbearing until their thirties. Nevertheless, prenatal care, better diet, improvements in neonatal intensive care, and education about pregnancy and birth are as important.

—Roger Smith, Ph.D.;
L. Fleming Fallon, Jr., M.D., Ph.D., M.P.H.;
updated by Robin Kamienny Montvilo, Ph.D.

See also Abortion; Amniocentesis; Assisted reproductive technologies; Birth defects; Cesarean section; Childbirth; Childbirth complications; Chorionic villus sampling; Conception; Embryology; Ethics; Gamete intrafallopian transfer (GIFT); Genetics and inheritance; In vitro fertilization; Miscarriage; Neonatology; Obstetrics; Pregnancy and gestation; Premature birth; Reproductive system; Sibling rivalry; Ultrasonography.

FOR FURTHER INFORMATION:

Bowers, Nancy A. *The Multiple Pregnancy Sourcebook.* New York: McGraw-Hill, 2001. The author, a perinatal nurse specializing in multiple birth education, provides an excellent guide to multiple pregnancy and birth, including topics such as infertility technology, prenatal testing, prenatal development, risk factors and complications, the birth of multiples, and adapting one's life to raise multiples.

Cunningham, F. Gary, et al., eds. *Williams Obstetrics.* 22d ed. New York: McGraw-Hill, 2005. This standard textbook in obstetrics would complement a similar text in gynecology. Provides wide coverage of events related to pregnancy and childbirth. A well-written text for the serious reader who wants in-depth information.

Malmstrom, Patricia Maxwell, and Janet Poland. *The Art of Parenting Twins.* New York: Random House International, 2000. Malmstrom and Poland cover the biology and causes of twinning; the emotional terrain of parenting multiples; the differences between twin and single pregnancies; twin development in babyhood, toddlerhood, the preschool and school-age years, and adolescence; and twins' relationships with each other from babyhood to adulthood.

Malone, J. A., S. P. Margevicius, and E. G. Damato. "Multiple Gestation: Side Effects of Antepartum Bed Rest." *Biological Research in Nursing* 8, no. 2 (2006): 115-128. An overview of problems encountered by pregnant women as a result of the bed rest that is often required to deal with multiples.

Moore, Keith L., and T. V. N. Persaud. *The Developing Human.* 7th ed. Philadelphia: W. B. Saunders, 2003. An outstanding textbook on human embryonic development, with information about the development of multiple embryos.

Noble, Elizabeth. *Having Twins and More: A Parent's Guide to Pregnancy, Birth and Early Childhood.* 3d ed. New York: Houghton-Mifflin, 2003. This book is well written and easy to understand. The author is a professional with many years of experience with multiple births.

Novotny, Pamela P. *The Joy of Twins and Other Multiple Births: Having, Raising, and Loving Babies Who Arrive in Groups.* Avenel, N.J.: Crown Books, 1994. The author provides interesting information for parents of multiple infants.

Rand, L., K. A. Eddleman, and J. Stone. "Long-Term Outcomes in Multiple Gestations." *Clinical Perinatology* 32, no. 2 (2005): 495-513. An in-depth look at problems for which multiples are at high risk and their likelihood of occurring.

Rothbart, Betty. *Multiple Blessings: From Pregnancy Through Childhood—A Guide for Parents of Twins, Triplets, or More.* San Francisco: Hearst Books, 1994. In a clear presentation of all the facts, the author helps parents through all stages of pregnancy, providing advice on feeding, home care, juggling hectic schedules, and other critical issues related to the raising of twins and triplets.

MULTIPLE CHEMICAL SENSITIVITY SYNDROME

DISEASE/DISORDER

ANATOMY OR SYSTEM AFFECTED: Eyes, immune system, lungs, muscles, nerves, nervous system, respiratory system, skin

SPECIALTIES AND RELATED FIELDS: Dermatology, environmental health, epidemiology, immunology, neurology, occupational health, public health, toxicology

DEFINITION: An increasing intolerance to commonly encountered chemicals at concentrations well tolerated by other people.

CAUSES AND SYMPTOMS

Multiple chemical sensitivity (MCS) syndrome, idiopathic environmental intolerance (IEI), reactive airway dysfunctions, and the "sick building" syndromes are overlapping disorders caused by intolerance of environmental chemicals. Exactly how many people are affected by MCS is unknown. The onset is often associated with initial acute chemical exposure; patients may report the onset of MCS after moving into a new home, after exposure to chemicals in the workplace, or following the use of pesticides in the home. Patients often describe an increasing intolerance to commonly encountered chemicals at concentrations well tolerated by other people. Diagnosis is made when the following six criteria are met: Repeated exposure reproduces symptoms, the condition is chronic, low chemical exposure levels cause symptoms, symptoms improve with the removal of offending chemicals, responses are triggered by multiple unrelated chemicals, and multiple systems are affected.

Symptoms usually wax and wane with exposure and are more likely to occur in patients with preexisting histories of migraine or classical allergies. Idiosyncratic medication reactions (especially to preservative chemicals) are common in MCS patients, as are dysautonomic symptoms (such as vascular instability), poor temperature regulation, and food intolerance. It is thought that patients with MCS have organ abnormalities involving the liver, the nervous system (including the brain and the limbic, peripheral, and autonomic systems), the immune system, and perhaps porphyrin metabolism, probably reflecting chemical injury to these systems. There is often a substantial overlap of MCS symptoms with fibromyalgia and chronic fatigue syndrome.

The common clinical symptoms may include head-aches (often migraine), chronic fatigue, musculoskeletal aching, chronic respiratory inflammation (rhinitis, sinusitis, laryngitis, asthma), attention-deficit disorder, and hyperactivity (affecting younger children). Less common complaints include tremor, seizure, and mitral valve prolapse. Agents associated with the onset of MCS include gasoline, kerosene, natural gas, pesticides (especially chlordane and chlorpyrifos), organic solvents, new carpet and other renovation materials, adhesives and glues, fiberglass, carbonless copy paper, fabric softener, formaldehyde and glutaraldehyde, carpet shampoo (lauryl sulfate) and other cleaning agents, isocyanates, combustion products (poorly vented gas heaters, overheated batteries), and medications (dinitrochlorobenzene for warts, intranasally packed neosynephrine, prolonged antibiotics, and general anesthesia with petrochemicals).

It is believed that the mechanisms that lead to MCS may be multifactorial and include neurogenic inflammation (respiratory, gastrointestinal, and genitourinary symptoms), kindling and time-dependent sensitization (neurologic symptoms), and immune activation or impaired porphyrin metabolism (multiple-organ symptoms). Pathological findings of MCS have rarely been examined. A preliminary study of nasal pathology in these patients indicates that they are characterized by defects in the junctions between cells, desquamation of the respiratory epithelium, glandular hyperplasia, lymphocytic infiltrates, and peripheral nerve fiber proliferation. A consistent physiologic abnormality in these patients has not been established.

Psychiatric, personality, cognitive/neurologic, immunologic, and olfactory studies have been conducted comparing MCS subjects with various control groups. Thus far, the most consistent finding is that patients

---

INFORMATION ON MULTIPLE CHEMICAL SENSITIVITY SYNDROME

CAUSES: Environmental exposure to chemicals

SYMPTOMS: Headaches (often migraine); chronic fatigue, musculoskeletal aching; chronic respiratory inflammation (rhinitis, sinusitis, laryngitis, asthma); attention-deficit disorder; hyperactivity (affecting younger children); food intolerance

DURATION: Acute to chronic

TREATMENTS: Alleviation of symptoms, supportive therapy

with MCS have a higher rate of psychiatric disorders across studies and relative to diverse comparison groups. Since these studies are cross-sectional, however, causality cannot be implied. Various working groups have proposed several research questions addressing the relationship between neurogenic inflammation and toxicant-induced loss of tolerance with the development of MCS.

TREATMENT AND THERAPY
The management of patients with MCS at present involves symptomatic and supportive therapy. There is a general consensus among researchers and clinicians that in order to treat patients with MCS effectively, a double-blind, placebo-controlled study performed in an environmentally controlled facility, with rigorous documentation of both objective and subjective responses, is needed to help elucidate the nature and origin of MCS.

—*Shih-Wen Huang, M.D.; updated by Sharon W. Stark, R.N., A.P.R.N., D.N.Sc.*

See also Allergies; Antihistamines; Asthma; Autoimmune disorders; Chronic fatigue syndrome; Dermatitis; Dermatology; Dizziness and fainting; Environmental diseases; Fatigue; Fibromyalgia; Hay fever; Headaches; Host-defense mechanisms; Immune system; Immunology; Laryngitis; Lungs; Migraine headaches; Mold and mildew; Nasopharyngeal disorders; Nausea and vomiting; Occupational health; Pulmonary medicine; Rashes; Seizures; Sinusitis; Skin; Skin disorders; Sore throat; Wheezing.

FOR FURTHER INFORMATION:
Baron-Faust, Rita, and Jill P. Buyon. *The Autoimmune Connection.* Chicago: Contemporary Books, 2003.

Barrett, Stephen J., and Ronald E. Gots. *Chemical Sensitivity: The Truth About Environmental Illness.* Amherst, N.Y.: Prometheus Books, 1999.

Delves, Peter J., et al. *Roitt's Essential Immunology.* 11th ed. Malden, Mass.: Blackwell, 2006.

Dwyer, John M. *The Body at War: The Miracle of the Immune System.* 2d ed. New York: J. M. Dent, 1993.

Kindt, Thomas J., Richard A. Goldsby, and Barbara A. Osborne. *Kuby Immunology.* 6th ed. New York: W. H. Freeman, 2007.

McCormick, Gail J. *Living with Multiple Chemical Sensitivity: Narratives of Coping.* Jefferson, N.C.: McFarland, 2000.

Morgan, Monroe T. *Environmental Health.* 3d ed. New York: Brooks Cole, 2002.

National Institute of Environmental Health Sciences (NIEHS). *Multiple Chemical Sensitivities Syndrome (MCSS).* http://www.niehs.nih.gov/external/faq/mcss.htm.

MULTIPLE SCLEROSIS
DISEASE/DISORDER

ANATOMY OR SYSTEM AFFECTED: Muscles, musculoskeletal system, nerves, nervous system, spine

SPECIALTIES AND RELATED FIELDS: Immunology, internal medicine, neurology, pediatrics

DEFINITION: A debilitating chronic inflammatory disease affecting the central nervous system.

KEY TERMS:

autoimmunity: a condition in which the immune system fails to recognize its own tissues as "self" and mounts an immune response against its own cells

demyelination: the destruction of myelin

disseminated sclerosis: another name for multiple sclerosis (MS)

myelin: a fatty substance wrapping nerves as a sheath that accelerates electric impulse propagation

primary progressive MS: the most aggressive form of MS, characterized by the absence of remissions and continual decline

relapsing-remitting MS: the most common form of MS, characterized by unpredictable attacks (relapses) followed by periods free of symptoms (remission)

remyelination: the repair of myelin

sclerosis: a process of hardening of tissues

secondary progressive MS: a form that occurs in patients who initially had relapsing-remitting MS and transition to a more aggressive MS

CAUSES AND SYMPTOMS
Multiple sclerosis (MS) is a chronic and disabling disease of the nervous system. Symptoms can be mild, such as limb numbness, or severe, such as paralysis and loss of vision. How the disease will progress and its severity in specific individuals are difficult to predict because it progresses differently in each of its victims.

Multiple sclerosis is caused by degeneration of the nervous system. A fatty substance called myelin surrounds and protects many nerve fibers of the brain and spinal cord. Myelin is important because it speeds up signals that move along the nerve fibers. In MS, the body attacks its own tissues, termed an autoimmune reaction, and a breakdown in the myelin layer along the nerves occurs. When any part of the myelin sheathing is

INFORMATION ON MULTIPLE SCLEROSIS

CAUSES: Genetic and environmental factors; possibly viral infection

SYMPTOMS: Tingling, numbness, slurring of speech, blurred or double vision, loss of coordination, muscle weakness and/or tightness, fatigue, bowel and bladder control difficulties, sexual dysfunction, paralysis, impaired cognitive functions

DURATION: Chronic with recurrent episodes

TREATMENTS: Steroids, human interferons, regular exercise

destroyed, nerve impulses to and from the brain are slowed, distorted, or interrupted. The disease is called "multiple" because it affects many areas of the brain. Scleroids are hardened, scarred patches that form over the damaged areas of myelin.

The initial symptoms of MS may include tingling, numbness, slurred speech, blurred or double vision, loss of coordination, and muscle weakness. Later manifestations include unusual fatigue, muscle tightness, bowel and bladder control difficulties, sexual dysfunction, and paralysis. The most common cognitive functions influenced are short-term memory, abstract reasoning, verbal fluency, and speed of information processing. All the mental and physical symptoms listed may come or go in any combination. The symptoms may also vary from mild to severe in intensity throughout the course of the disease.

The symptoms of MS not only vary from person to person but also may periodically vary within the same person. This makes the prognosis of the disease difficult to foresee. Although the general course of the disease may be anticipated, the symptoms and their severity seem to be quite unpredictable in most individuals. In the "classic" course of MS, as time progresses, chronic problems gradually accumulate over many years, slowly worsening the sufferer's quality of life. The total level of disability will vary from patient to patient.

The typical pattern of MS is marked by active periods of the disease during which the nerves are being ravaged by the immune system. These periods are called attacks, relapses, or exacerbations. The active periods of the disease are followed by calm periods called remissions. The cycle of attack and remission will differ from sufferer to sufferer. Some people have few attacks, and their MS disabilities slowly accumulate over time; in these sufferers, it takes decades to become truly debilitated. Most people with MS have what is known as the relapsing-remitting form of the disease. They suffer many attacks over time, and these attacks occur unpredictably; the attacks are then followed by complete remission which may last months or years. Again, the injuries may take many years to accumulate to complete disability.

The most aggressive form of the disease is primary progressive MS. In this type of MS, the disease follows a rapid course that steadily worsens from its first onset. Although there are still attacks and partial remission, the attacks are quite severe and occur more regularly in time. Full paralysis may develop in primary progressive MS in three to five years. Secondary progressive MS occurs in patients who initially have the relapsing-remitting type and later develop the more aggressive form.

Both genetic and environmental factors have been implicated in inducing the onset of MS. Viral infection has been suggested as a cause, but no single virus has ever been shown to be associated with MS. Although infections such as the common cold, flu, and gastroenteritis increase the risk of relapse, flu vaccination is safe in patients with MS. Risk may be conferred by exposure to a specific environment during adolescence, but that environment and the genetic risk factors have not yet been characterized. The support for the genetic component comes from examining identical twins. The likelihood of MS in the second identical twin, when the first twin has MS, is 30 percent.

Researchers Sharon Lynch and John Rose suggested that certain racial and geographic populations are less susceptible than others to the disease. MS is uncommon in Japanese people as well as among American Indians. The disease is more common among Northern European Caucasians as well as among North Americans of higher latitudes. There is an additional sexual dimorphism in the epidemiology of MS; the disease is found more frequently in women, by a ratio of 2:1.

The disease usually begins its first manifestations in late adolescence (around age eighteen) to early middle age (around age thirty-five). It is not clear how the interaction between the genetics of the sufferer and the environment may trigger onset. The progressive type of MS is more common over the age of forty, so those with late-onset MS often have the quickest deterioration of motor function. The reason that an older age predisposes someone to primary chronic progressive MS is still not clear.

Studies by Swiss researcher Avinoam Safran have shown that occasionally MS manifests after the age of fifty. This condition has been named late-onset multiple sclerosis. Late-onset MS is not rare. Nearly 10 percent of MS patients demonstrate their first symptom after the age of fifty. This type of MS is often not recognized by physicians, who do not expect it in the aged.

TREATMENT AND THERAPY

Scientists have been encouraged by recent advancements in MS diagnosis using the MRI brain scan. In 2002 they announced that these scans appear to detect damage around nerve fibers in patients with possible

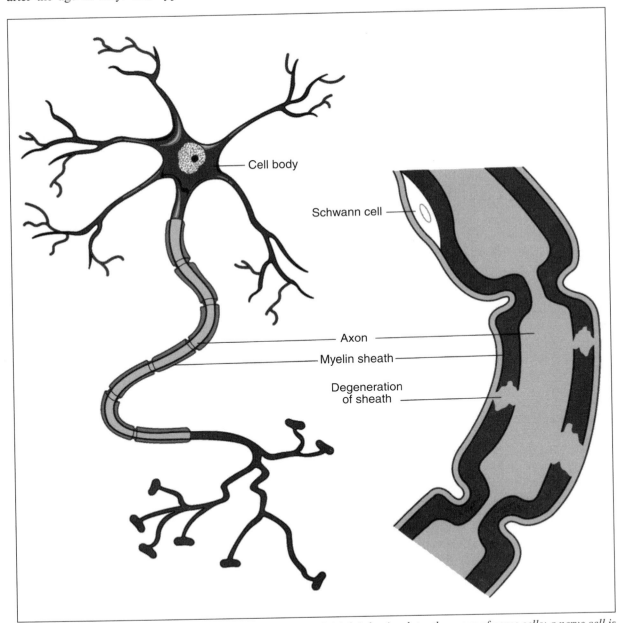

Multiple sclerosis is caused by degeneration of the myelin sheath (right) that insulates the axons of nerve cells; a nerve cell is shown on the left.

early signs of MS. This detection helps doctors predict those who will eventually develop MS and how severe one's experience with the disease might be. In turn, this allows a drug regimen to begin earlier. In the past, doctors did not officially diagnose MS or start treatment until patients had two episodes of nerve problems in different areas of the body—reoccurrences that could come years apart while damage nonetheless continued silently. New research has found that putting patients on MS drugs at the first sign of nerve inflammation drastically slows the chances of developing MS within a few years, although most will eventually still develop the disease.

While there is no cure for MS, there are many effective treatments. In most cases, steroidal drugs are used to treat relapses or attacks of the disease. Corticotropin was the first steroidal immunosuppressant to be used widely in MS treatment. The primary effect of the drug is to shorten the duration of an attack, although it does not appear to reduce the severity of the attack. Although it is still used with patients who respond well to it, corticotropin has been supplanted by other drugs. Methylprednisolone is an immunosuppressant and steroid that has replaced corticotropin. It has been shown to control the inflammation that accompanies demyelination. These steroids seem to work by sealing leaking blood vessels in the brain and reducing the responsiveness of the white blood cells of the immune system so that they cannot attack the myelin as easily.

Several federally approved drugs can slow the rate of attacks: Avonex, Rebif, and Betaseron are preparations of interferon (proteins regulating the immune system), and Copaxone is a mixture of small peptides that protects myelin. Although these drugs do not stop MS entirely, they actually limit the level of myelin destruction, as observed in magnetic resonance imaging (MRI) scans of the brain. Avonex slows down the rate of progression to disability, and all four slow down the natural course of

MS. University of Western Ontario researcher George Ebers was the first to perform experimental treatments on MS patients with interferons. The myelin sheath is actually produced by a special nerve cell called an oligodendrocyte; presumably the oligodendrocytes are stimulated to protect themselves by exposure to interferons. Patients treated with human interferons demonstrated a 34 percent reduction in frequency of attacks;

IN THE NEWS: NEW DRUG TREATMENTS FOR MULTIPLE SCLEROSIS

The neurodegeneration that characterizes multiple sclerosis (MS) results from the destruction of myelin that surrounds and protects nerves by the immune system. Myelin-specific T cells are required for this attack. Corticosteroids have been used as therapy because of their known immunosuppressive properties. They have proved to be effective against the symptoms of MS episodes, but they have serious side effects and can be taken only for short times. Because they suppress the immune system in a general, nonspecific way, they inhibit not only the destruction of myelin but also the body's ability to fight infection. This problem has led to the deaths of some MS patients. In addition, corticosteroids do not delay the long-term progression of MS. More recently, interferon-β has been used to treat MS. Although interferon-β therapy can be given for long periods and has been shown to reduce the frequency of relapses and to slow the progression of the disease, why it works is not known. One theory is that it reduces inflammation.

New drugs on the horizon aim to stop the progression of MS and eliminate all relapses. The theory behind them is that a drug should targeted to inhibit only the components of the immune system that destroy myelin. Such drugs, unlike the drugs currently available, would be attacking the underlying cause of MS, rather than its symptoms, and would be expected to cause few or no side effects.

Two of these new drugs, Tovaxin from Opexa Therapeutics and a not-yet named candidate, now called RTL1000, from Artielle ImmunoTherapeutics, act by specifically inactivating the patient's own myelin-specific T cells, while not interacting with other immune system cells. Myelin-specific T cells are required for the destruction of myelin, and when a large number of them are inactivated, myelin destruction slows down.

Another approach is being developed by Immune Response. Their drug NeuroVax acts by specifically stimulating patients' cells that down-regulate myelin-specific T cells. Clinical trials of NeuroVax are underway.

—Lorraine Lica, Ph.D.

that reduction was sustained over five years of treatment. More impressive was the 80 percent reduction of MS activity detected in their brains. Steroid treatment was rarely required in these patients.

In 2002, researchers announced that preliminary studies using mice and a class of statin drugs used to lower cholesterol in heart patients showed an improvement and some reversal of the debilitating symptoms of MS. The animal data were encouraging because of their demonstration that the statin drugs appear to reprogram the immune cells that attack myelin so they instead protect nerve coatings. Also in 2002, another parallel study using MS patients and the drug sold as Zocor—part of the statin class—showed early positive signs of similar anti-inflammatory effects in humans, but potential benefits in MS patients with normal cholesterol are currently under investigation. Another strategy using a monoclonal antibody, Natalizumab, was approved in 2006 for the treatment of the relapsing form of MS.

During the 1990's, in a study supported by the National Institutes of Health and conducted at the Mayo Clinic, plasma exchange, also called plasmapheresis, was proven to be an effective treatment for certain patients suffering from severe symptoms of multiple sclerosis who were not responsive to conventional methods of treatment. Plasma exchange involves the removal of the patient's blood; the elimination of the plasma-containing antibodies that target myelin, which is then replaced by a fluid with similar properties, usually containing albumin; and its subsequent return to the patient. This procedure has been used for treatment of other autoimmune diseases such as myasthenia gravis and Guillain-Barré syndrome in the past.

Investigators concluded that plasma exchange might contribute to recovery from an acute attack in people with MS who have not responded to standard steroid treatment. Therefore, they recommended that this treatment only be considered for individuals experiencing a severe, acute attack that is not responding to high-dose steroids. Since the vast majority (90 percent) of people experiencing acute attacks respond well to the standard steroid treatment, plasma exchange would be considered a treatment alternative only for the approximate 10 percent who do not. For those 10 percent, however, plasma exchange may offer an important and beneficial treatment option. Because the exact reasons for the effectiveness of plasmapheresis are not known, researchers feel that further studies are warranted based on the idea that some people may have antibodies in their plasma that are instrumental in certain disease activities which allow disabilities to occur.

As additional therapy, patients with MS should participate in a regular exercise program. Exercise is vital to the maintenance of functional ability in MS sufferers. It strengthens muscles, benefits gait, and generally improves coordination. The best type of exercise is aquatic in nature. Sufferers are often heat-intolerant, and participation in a regular aerobic program would be unpleasant. Also, aquatic exercise is a low-impact activity that puts less stress on chronically sore muscles. Exercise programs also encourage socialization of patients and engender peer support.

PERSPECTIVE AND PROSPECTS

The first written report of MS was published in 1400 when the famed Dutch skater Lydwina of Schieden was diagnosed. It was recognized initially as a wasting disease of unknown origin. The disease was described clinically by Jean-Martin Charcot in 1877. Charcot initially characterized the clinical signs and symptoms of MS. He recognized that the disease affected the nervous system and tried many remedies, without success. In 1890, the cause of MS was thought to be suppression of sweat; the treatment was electrical stimulation and bed rest. At the time, life expectancy for a sufferer was five years after diagnosis. By 1910, MS was thought to be caused by toxins in the blood, and purgatives were alleged the best treatment. In the 1930's, poor circulation was believed to cause MS, and blood-thinning agents became the treatment of choice. In the 1950's through the 1970's, MS was thought to be caused by severe allergies; treatments included antihistamines. Not until the 1980's was the basis of MS understood and effective treatment developed.

By the early twenty-first century, it was estimated that 400,000 Americans had this disorder of the brain and spinal cord, which causes disruption in the smooth flow of electrical messages from brain and nerves to the body. The progress of the disease is slow and may take decades to achieve complete nerve degeneration and paralysis. Although often considered a disease of youth, MS has the potential to become an increasing problem in aging populations. More cases of late-onset MS are coming to light in individuals over forty years of age, including such celebrities as comedian Richard Pryor, former Mouseketeer Annette Funicello, and talk-show host Montel Williams.

Several novel therapies are under investigation and include sphingosine receptor modulator (fingolimod), vitamin D, inosine (Axosine), and antimicrobial agents. Various combinations of drugs are also being examined and include mitoxantrone (an immunosuppressant) and Copaxone. Current clinical trials are likely to reveal treatment strategies that will further facilitate controlling symptoms and progression of MS.

—James J. Campanella, Ph.D.;
updated by W. Michael Zawada, Ph.D.

See also Amyotrophic lateral sclerosis; Muscle sprains, spasms, and disorders; Muscles; Nervous system; Neuralgia, neuritis, and neuropathy; Neuroimaging; Neurology; Paralysis; Spinal cord disorders; Spine, vertebrae, and disks.

FOR FURTHER INFORMATION:

Blackstone, Margaret. *The First Year—Multiple Sclerosis: An Essential Guide for the Newly Diagnosed.* 2d ed. New York: Avalon, 2007. Written by an MS patient, guides newly diagnosed patients step-by-step through their first year with MS and sets expectations by providing reliable and up-to-date information on the disease. The second edition includes new research on MS, updated medications, information on support groups, and more.

Halbreich, Uriel. *Multiple Sclerosis: A Neuropsychiatric Disorder.* Boston: American Psychiatric Press, 1993. Describes the psychological conditions that often accompany multiple sclerosis.

Iams, Betty. *From MS to Wellness.* Chicago: Iams House, 1998. An autobiography of an MS sufferer who outlines treatments that have helped her overcome the disease.

Kalb, Rosalind, ed. *Multiple Sclerosis: The Questions You Have, the Answers You Need.* 3d ed. New York: Demos Vermande, 2004. A guide for everyone concerned about multiple sclerosis.

Litin, Scott C., ed. "Multiple Sclerosis." In *Mayo Clinic Family Health Book.* 3d ed. New York: HarperResource, 2003. A chapter in a text that discusses both muscles and bones, underscoring the intimate relationship between disorders in the two systems. The text and illustrations are complete and easy to understand.

Matthews, Bryan. *Multiple Sclerosis: The Facts.* 4th ed. New York: Oxford University Press, 2001. Provides information on diagnosis, therapy, medications, and all stages of the disease.

National Multiple Sclerosis Society. http://www.nmss .org/. Provides services to persons with multiple sclerosis through local chapters and promotes research, educates, advocates on critical issues, and organizes a wide range of programs.

Polman, Chris H., et al. *Multiple Sclerosis: The Guide to Treatment and Management.* 6th ed. New York: Demos Vermande, 2006. An up-to-date guide to treatments available for MS and their effectiveness.

Russell, Margot. *When the Road Turns: Inspirational Stories About People with MS.* Deerfield Beach, Fla.: Health Communications, 2001. Gives the personal stories of seventeen MS patients and details their emotional and physical battles, their struggle to accept the illness, and their courage to create new lives.

Salter, Robert Bruce. *Textbook of Disorders and Injuries of the Musculoskeletal System.* 3d ed. Baltimore: Williams & Wilkins, 1999. Four sections of the book—"Basic Musculoskeletal Science and Its Applications," "Musculoskeletal Disorders: General and Specific," "Musculoskeletal Injuries," and "Research"—examine the diagnosis and treatment principles of disorders and trauma of the musculoskeletal system.

MUMPS

DISEASE/DISORDER

ALSO KNOWN AS: Epidemic parotitis

ANATOMY OR SYSTEM AFFECTED: Genitals, glands, nervous system, pancreas

SPECIALTIES AND RELATED FIELDS: Family medicine, pediatrics

DEFINITION: An acute, contagious childhood disease caused by a virus and characterized by swollen salivary glands.

KEY TERMS:

encephalitis: infection and inflammation of the brain

meningitis: infection and inflammation of the covering of the brain

orchitis: infection, inflammation, and swelling of a testicle or ovary; usually occurs only on one side and usually only in adults with mumps infection

parotitis: infection, inflammation, and swelling of the parotid gland, the major salivary gland located near the angle of the jaw; this swelling will often push out the earlobe

CAUSES AND SYMPTOMS

Mumps infection is acquired after contact with infected respiratory secretions. An infected person can spread the disease from twelve to twenty-two days after infection. One case in a family generally means that every family member has been infected. Mumps is most commonly transmitted in the winter and early spring. During the sixteen- to eighteen-day incubation period, the virus grows first in the nose and throat, moves to the regional lymph nodes and then into the bloodstream, and spreads to multiple organs and the central nervous system.

One-third of patients with mumps infection do not have symptoms or have very mild symptoms. Mumps is more severe after puberty. The first symptoms include fever, headache, stomach upset, loss of appetite, and a mildly congested nose. The most common finding is swelling of the salivary glands. This swelling usually starts on one side and then moves to both sides in three-quarters of cases. Salivary gland pain is most pronounced during the first few days and is associated with discomfort when eating or drinking acidic foods such as orange juice. Rarely, a thin red rash can occur. The fever usually resolves in three to five days, and the salivary gland swelling subsides within seven to ten days.

Between 1 and 10 percent of patients have clinical evidence of central nervous system infection, most commonly meningitis but very rarely encephalitis. Infection of the central nervous system is more common in males than in females. Central nervous system disease typically occurs one to three weeks after the onset of salivary gland swelling, but it can also precede or follow this swelling. Symptoms include headache, fever, lethargy, stiff neck, and vomiting. Seizures occur in 20 percent of hospitalized patients. Central nervous system infection is almost always limited, without any lasting effect or complications. Hearing loss occurs during mumps illness in 4 percent of patients but is not higher in those with central nervous system involvement. Higher-tone deficits are noted most frequently. Recovery from hearing loss usually occurs within a few

Mumps

Parotid gland

Mumps causes a characteristic swelling of the parotid (salivary) glands.

weeks following onset. Persistent hearing loss is usually only one-sided.

Orchitis, an infection of the testicles or ovaries, can also occur with mumps. The highest risk for this disease occurs after puberty, usually in males from fifteen to twenty-nine years of age. Between 14 and 35 percent of males with mumps infection develop orchitis. Fever, malaise, vomiting, and stomach pain are common symptoms. Testicular pain, swelling, and tenderness generally last for three to seven days. Involvement is one-sided in most cases. Symptoms usually began four to eight days following the onset of salivary gland swelling, but they can occur in the absence of gland swelling.

Mumps infection can cause other, less common complications. Infection of the kidney is almost always limited, but rare reports of kidney failure with mumps do exist. Multiple joint migratory arthritis with joint fluid has been described and is usually of short duration. Joint complaints are more common in males in their twenties. The usual signs of joint disease occur one to three weeks after the onset of salivary gland swelling. The large joints are more commonly affected.

Inflammation of the heart occurs in 4 to 15 percent of patients with mumps. It is most common in adults and generally resolves itself within two to four weeks. Infection and inflammation of the pancreas can occasionally occur. Pancreatitis can lead to fatty diarrhea and, very rarely, diabetes. Women who have mumps infection during pregnancy do not have an increased risk of delivering an infant with congenital malformation.

Very rarely, mumps will cause death. It is unclear why, prior to the advent of vaccination, mumps infec-

---

INFORMATION ON MUMPS

CAUSES: Viral infection

SYMPTOMS: Swollen salivary glands, fever, headache, stomach upset, loss of appetite, mildly congested nose, red rash; occasionally organ infection or joint inflammation

DURATION: Sixteen to eighteen days

TREATMENTS: Alleviation of symptoms with mild pain medications, adequate fluid and nutritional intake

In December, 2005, several students at an unnamed college in eastern Iowa displayed symptoms of illness that included glandular swelling in the salivary region. Antibody testing indicated that the students had active cases of mumps. Several weeks later, an additional case was diagnosed. In the following months, additional cases were reported in the surrounding states of Illinois, Kansas, Minnesota, and Nebraska; serotyping of isolated viruses indicated that all cases originated from a similar or identical strain. Since not all the cases were directly linked with each other—that is, involved known contact—the suspicion among health workers is that portions of the outbreak were maintained through inapparent infections.

The source of the illness remains unclear, but the initial case may have been contracted in Great Britain. During 2005, some 56,000 cases were diagnosed there, and the strain that first appeared in Iowa appears to be identical. It is likely that a student had either traveled to Great Britain during the period of the outbreak or had contact with someone who had.

By the time that the illness had run its course in the summer of 2006, more than 4,700 persons had been diagnosed with mumps, with cases reported as far away as California. Approximately 25 percent were college students. Mumps is generally a benign infection, and while there were no fatalities, pregnant women and persons with compromised immune systems, such as those who are HIV-positive, may be at risk for severe illness. An unusual feature of the outbreak was that more than two-thirds of the patients had already received the recommended two doses of the mumps vaccine in the form of the MMR (measles, mumps, rubella) vaccine, calling into question the long-term effectiveness of current immunization practices. In the light of the outbreak, health authorities recommended that all students be sure of prior immunization against mumps, or that they receive an additional two doses of the vaccine.

—Richard Adler, Ph.D.

acidic foods and should be light and generous in fluids. Occasionally, mild pain medications may be necessary for severe headaches or salivary gland discomfort. Stronger pain medications may be needed with testicular involvement. In unusual cases where vomiting is severe, intravenous fluids may be required. A spinal tap (lumbar puncture) is rarely indicated, but patients who have this procedure frequently find that it relieves their headaches.

Exposure to mumps infection may cause anxiety in adult family members or day care employees. A child with mumps should be isolated for nine days after the start of salivary gland swelling. Vaccine administration will probably not prevent infection after exposure, and a history of family exposure to mumps probably indicates past infection. The physician will reassure any adult exposed family members and indicate that it is unlikely that the vaccine will prevent this disease. Nevertheless, exposure may dictate the need to administer the vaccine, as determining immune status is generally not practicable.

Mumps is a self-limited illness and does not require the administration of antiviral medications, antibiotics, or antibody preparations. Mumps vaccine should be given to children to prevent this disease. The combined vaccine containing measles, mumps, and rubella (MMR) vaccines should be given routinely to children from twelve months to eighteen months of age. About 98 percent of children will respond to this vaccine and not acquire mumps infection.

tion killed forty persons in the United States each year. More than 50 percent of deaths are of adults.

Not all patients with salivary gland swelling have mumps. Swelling in this area of the face may be attributable to another disease of the salivary gland or another disease affecting other tissues in the face such as lymph nodes or bones. Persistent or recurrent swelling of the parotid gland should be evaluated by a physician.

TREATMENT AND THERAPY

Conservative therapy is indicated for mumps infection. No antiviral therapy is available. Adequate fluids and nutrition are important. A patient's diet should avoid

PERSPECTIVE AND PROSPECTS

The term "mumps" is derived from an English dialect meaning "grimace," attributed to the painful parotid gland swelling. The virus was first described in 1934, and a live vaccine was first licensed in 1967. Prior to 1980, the age group most affected by mumps was five-to nine-year-olds. In the 1980's, this group shifted to children and adolescents aged ten to nineteen. In the 1990's, most cases occurred in adults over twenty. This change was caused by the increased use of the mumps vaccine in children but not in adults.

Vaccination has been very successful, especially when combined with measles and rubella vaccine, given in the second year of life, and repeated prior to school. Side effects from mumps vaccine are extremely rare and can include anything that is seen in mumps infection. Recent research in the area has been directed toward determining whether the vaccine in its present form or in another form should be considered for administration both to decrease adverse reactions and to decrease its cost and improve its applicability to a broader population.

—*Peter D. Reuman, M.D., M.P.H.*

See also Childhood infectious diseases; Encephalitis; Fever; Glands; Immunization and vaccination; Infertility, male; Meningitis; Orchitis; Viral infections.

FOR FURTHER INFORMATION:

American Medical Association. *American Medical Association Family Medical Guide.* 4th rev. ed. Hoboken, N.J.: John Wiley & Sons, 2004. An excellent reference for the beginner. The scientific accuracy of the text is not compromised by its accessibility.

Beers, Mark H., et al. *The Merck Manual of Diagnosis and Therapy.* 18th ed. Whitehouse Station, N.J.: Merck Research Laboratories, 2006. Contains a useful exposition of the characteristics, etiology, diagnosis, and treatment of mumps.

Bellenir, Karen, and Peter D. Dresser, eds. *Contagious and Noncontagious Infectious Diseases Sourcebook.* Detroit: Omnigraphics, 1997. A handy reference source on infectious diseases. Includes bibliographical references and an index.

Gorbach, Sherwood L., John G. Bartlett, and Neil R. Blacklow, eds. *Infectious Diseases.* 3d ed. Philadelphia: W. B. Saunders, 2003. A thorough discussion of infectious diseases. Included is a brief history, an account of the mechanisms of disease and immunity, and a concise discussion of a broad range of infectious agents.

Litin, Scott C., ed. *Mayo Clinic Family Health Book.* 3d ed. New York: HarperResource, 2003. Perhaps the best general medical text for the layperson, this book covers the entire medical field. While the information is derived from a wide variety of highly technical sources, the articles are written to be easily understood by a general audience.

Sompayrac, Lauren. *How Pathogenic Viruses Work.* 5th ed. Sudbury, Mass.: Jones & Bartlett, 2002. Engaging exploration of the basics of virology. The author uses twelve of the most common viral infections to demonstrate how viruses "devise" various solutions to stay alive.

Woolf, Alan D., et al., eds. *The Children's Hospital Guide to Your Child's Health and Development.* Cambridge, Mass.: Perseus, 2002. An authoritative and comprehensive guide to children's health, providing a guide to every common illness or condition that affects children and a carefully designed emergency section.

MÜNCHAUSEN SYNDROME BY PROXY

DISEASE/DISORDER

ANATOMY OR SYSTEM AFFECTED: All

SPECIALTIES AND RELATED FIELDS: Ethics, family medicine, pediatrics, psychiatry, psychology

DEFINITION: A disorder in which a parent fabricates, simulates, or induces a medical condition in a child in order to receive attention and acknowledgment as the source of information about the child's health.

KEY TERMS:

covert video surveillance: the monitoring of a child using video equipment in which the parent is unaware of the taping

narcissistic personality disorder: a disorder characterized by maladaptive patterns of behavior that are used to deal with common life situations

CAUSES AND SYMPTOMS

Münchausen syndrome by proxy may occur in different forms. In its least invasive form, this syndrome involves lying about a child's medical problems. For example, a father may claim that his child stopped breathing or had a seizure. The harm to the child comes from the medical studies that are ordered by the physician in an attempt to evaluate and diagnose the condition. A second situation involves the simulation of symptoms in the child. For example, a mother may maintain that her child is experiencing hematuria, and examination of the urine reveals the presence of blood. The blood comes not from the child but from some external source, such as the mother's menstrual blood or animal blood from packaged meat. Again, the child is subjected to needless diagnostic tests, some of which can be invasive.

The most injurious form of Münchausen syndrome by proxy comes when a parent induces the symptoms in the child. This can be done in many ways: The parent can administer syrup of ipecac to induce vomiting, administer substances such as diphtheria-pertussis-tetanus (DPT) vaccine to cause a fever, or inject fecal materials into already existing intravenous lines to induce a bacterial bloodstream infection. Parental induction of an apparent life-threatening event (ALTE) has been documented through the use of covert video surveillance. Parents have been observed placing their hands or other objects over the infant's face. Many of these children demonstrated bleeding from the mouth or gums, a finding not reported in any of the control infants who were experiencing an ALTE.

In addition to being subjected to multiple and invasive diagnostic procedures, some children die as a direct result of their parents' actions. Some families have a history of sudden or unexplained deaths of siblings that may be attributable to Münchausen syndrome by proxy or other types of child abuse.

TREATMENT AND THERAPY

A physician should become concerned about the possibility of Münchausen syndrome by proxy in a child with multiple health care visits in whom an explanation for the problems is elusive. The most common complaints include bleeding, vomiting, apnea, seizures, and fever. In each case, the chronic nature of the problems and the constant switching of health care providers should be clues. Statements by experienced physicians such as "I've never seen anything like this" should also signal that the child may be the victim of Münchausen syndrome by proxy. Some physicians become trapped in the process of ordering multiple studies for fear of missing an exotic disease.

On the other hand, some parents represent the "worried well." These people bring their children in for many minor complaints: every runny nose, low-grade temperature, or nonapparent skin rash. Their motivation is not personal attention. Rather, they are fearful and view their children as vulnerable.

The psychologic profile of the parent helps to distinguish the overly concerned mother from the one with Münchausen syndrome by proxy. The usual perpetrator is the child's mother. The father is often detached, distant, and not involved in the child's care, although cases in which the father is the perpetrator have been documented. Most perpetrators are believed to have borderline personalities and narcissistic personality disorders. They enjoy the attention that they receive in a medical setting. Medical staff members often charac-

---

INFORMATION ON MÜNCHAUSEN SYNDROME BY PROXY

CAUSES: Psychological disorder
SYMPTOMS: Lying about or inducing a child's medical problems
DURATION: Chronic
TREATMENTS: Psychotherapy

---

terize these individuals as excellent parents because they are knowledgeable about their child's health, attentive to his or her needs, and cooperative with the staff. Many of the mothers have some type of medical or science background, which facilitates their understanding of medical conditions. Some have worked in physicians' offices, making them knowledgeable about medical terminology or procedures. Psychological assessment is needed to help define parental pathology. Members of the medical staff may be disbelieving of the diagnosis, since they often find the parent to be nice and helpful. Many parents deny the accusations and are resistant to psychiatric intervention.

The task of the medical team is to entertain the diagnosis, obtain evidence, and protect the child. In some institutions, covert video surveillance is used to catch the parent in the act of inflicting the symptoms. Although there is concern about issues of privacy, legal counsel at most institutions has supported the use of covert video surveillance because it assesses the situation of the child.

PERSPECTIVE AND PROSPECTS

Münchausen syndrome by proxy was initially described by Roy Meadow in 1977. In the twenty years after his initial report, more than three hundred cases were reported in the literature. The diversity of ways in which this syndrome is inflicted on children has expanded with each case report. In many cases, the prognosis for affected children is somewhat guarded because of the complexity of establishing the diagnosis on a legal level.

Once the child and the parent are separated, the symptoms resolve. Cases may be difficult to substantiate in court, without the presence of concrete evidence. Some children suffer from long-term sequelae, sometimes behaving like invalids because of the role in which they have been cast since childhood. There are reports of self-destructive behavior and Münchausen syndrome in some survivors. Psychological counseling is critical to ensure the well-being of these children. In most cases, the children cannot be returned to the parental perpetrator because of the intractable nature of the parent's problem.

—*Carol D. Berkowitz, M.D.*

See also Bacterial infections; Critical care; Critical care, pediatric; Domestic violence; Emergency medicine; Emergency medicine, pediatric; Fever; Hypochondriasis; Nausea and vomiting; Physical examination; Psychiatric disorders; Psychiatry; Psychiatry, child and adolescent; Psychosomatic illness.

FOR FURTHER INFORMATION:

Eminson, Mary, and R. J. Postlethwaite, eds. *Münchausen Syndrome by Proxy Abuse: A Practical Approach.* Boston: Butterworth-Heinemann, 2000. Aimed at the health professional, this book brings together a collection of essays discussing different aspects of this syndrome. Chapters deal with confirming factitious illness and the child protection process.

Feldman, Marc D. *Playing Sick? Untangling the Web of Munchausen Syndrome, Munchausen by Proxy, Malingering, and Factitious Disorder.* New York: Brunner-Routledge, 2004. Fascinating case histories of people whose conditions lead them to fake illnesses, in themselves and others, sometimes to the point of death.

Gregory, Julie. *Sickened: The Memoir of a Münchausen by Proxy Childhood.* New York: Bantam, 2003. A personal, engaging story in which the author details years of abuse due to her mother's disorder.

Rosenberg, D. A. "Münchausen Syndrome by Proxy." In *Child Abuse,* edited by Robert M. Reece. Philadelphia: Lea & Febiger, 1994. A discussion of the diagnosis and treatment of this abusive syndrome, in a text that includes bibliographical references and an index.

Southall, D. P., M. C. Plunkett, and M. W. Banks, et al. "Covert Video Recordings of Life-Threatening Child Abuse: Lessons for Child Protection." *Pediatrics* 100, no. 5 (November, 1997): 735-760. A descriptive, retrospective, partially controlled case study involving a total of thirty-nine children in whom hospital recordings were used to investigate suspicions of induced illness.

MUSCLE SPRAINS, SPASMS, AND DISORDERS

DISEASE/DISORDER

ALSO KNOWN AS: Myopathies

ANATOMY OR SYSTEM AFFECTED: Legs, ligaments, muscles, musculoskeletal system

SPECIALTIES AND RELATED FIELDS: Exercise physiology, family medicine, osteopathic medicine, physical therapy, sports medicine

DEFINITION: Injuries, defects, or disorders of the muscles of the body.

CAUSES AND SYMPTOMS

There are three kinds of muscle tissue in the human body: smooth muscle, cardiac muscle, and striated muscle. Smooth muscle tissue is found around the intestines, blood vessels, and bronchioles in the lung, among other areas. These muscles are controlled by the autonomic nervous system, which means that their movement is not subject to voluntary action. They have many functions: They maintain the airway in the lungs, regulate the tone of blood vessels, and move foods and other substances through the digestive tract. Cardiac muscle is found only in the heart. Striated muscles are those that move body parts. They are also called voluntary muscles because they must receive a conscious command from the brain in order to work. They supply the force for physical activity, and they also prevent movement and stabilize body parts.

Muscles are subject to many disorders: Muscle sprains, strains, and spasms are common events in everyone's life and, for the most part, they are harmless, if painful, results of overexercise, accidents, falls, bumps, or countless other events. Yet these symptoms can also signal serious myopathies, or disorders within muscle tissue.

Myopathies constitute a wide range of diseases. They are classified as inflammatory myopathies or metabolic myopathies. Inflammatory myopathies include infections by bacteria, viruses, or other microorganisms, as well as other diseases that are possibly autoimmune in origin (that is, resulting from and directed against the body's own tissues). In metabolic myopathies, there is some failure or disturbance in the body's ability to maintain a proper metabolic balance or electrolyte distribution. These conditions include glycogen storage diseases, in which there are errors in glucose processing; disorders of fatty acid metabolism, in which there are derangements in fatty acid oxidation; mitochondrial myopathies, in which there are biochemical and other abnormalities in the mitochondria of muscle cells; endocrine myopathies, in which an endocrine disorder underlies muscular symptoms; and the periodic paralyses, which can be the result of inherited or acquired illnesses. This is only a partial list of the myopathies, the symptoms of which include weakness and pain.

Muscular dystrophies are a group of inherited disorders in which muscle tissue fails to receive nourishment. The results are progressive muscular weakness and the degeneration and destruction of muscle fibers. The symptoms include weakness, loss of coordination, impaired gait, and impaired muscle extensibility. Over the years, muscle mass decreases and the arms, legs, and spine become deformed.

Neuromuscular disorders include a wide variety of conditions in which muscle function is impaired by faulty transmission of nerve impulses to muscle tissue. These conditions may be inherited; they may be attributable to toxins, such as in food poisoning (for example, botulism) or by pesticide poisoning; or they may be side effects of certain drugs. The most commonly seen neuromuscular disorder is myasthenia gravis.

The muscular disorders most often seen are those that result from overexertion, exercise, athletics, accidents, and trauma. Injuries sustained during sports and games have become so significant that sports medicine has become a recognized medical subspecialty. Besides the muscles, the parts of the body involved in these disorders include tendons (tough, stringy tissue that attaches muscles to bones), ligaments (tissue that attaches bone to bone), synovia (membranes enclosing a joint or other bony structure), and cartilage (soft, resilient tissue between bones). A sprain is an injury in which ligaments are stretched or torn. In a strain, muscles or tendons are stretched or torn. A contusion is a bruise that occurs when the body is subjected to trauma; the skin is not broken, but the capillaries underneath are, causing discoloration. A spasm is a short, abnormal contraction in a muscle or group of muscles. A cramp is a prolonged, painful contraction of one or more muscles.

Sprains can be caused by twisting the joint violently or by forcing it beyond its range of movement. The ligaments that connect the bones of the joint stretch or tear. Sprains occur most often in the knees, ankles, and arches of the feet. There is pain and swelling, and at least some immobilization of the joint.

A strain is also called a pulled muscle. When too great a demand is placed on a muscle, it and the surrounding tendons can stretch and/or tear. The main symptom is pain; swelling and muscle spasm may also occur.

Muscle spasms and cramps are common. Sometimes they occur spontaneously, such as the calf muscle cramps that occur at night. Sometimes they are attributable to muscle strain (the charley horse that tightens thigh muscles in runners and other athletes). Muscles that are used often will go into spasm, such as those in the thumb and fingers of writers (writer's cramp), as can muscles that have remained in one position for too long. Muscle spasms and cramps can also occur as direct consequences of dehydration; they are common in athletes who perspire excessively during hot weather.

Some injuries to muscles and joints occur so regularly that they are named for the activities associated with them. A good example is tennis elbow, a condition that results from repeated, vigorous movement of the arm, such as swinging a tennis racket, using a paintbrush, or pitching a baseball. Runners' knee can afflict joggers and other athletes. It is usually caused by sprains in the knee ligaments; there is pain and there may be partial or total immobilization of the knee. Achilles tendinitis, as the name suggests, is inflammation of the Achilles tendon in the heel. It is usually the result of excessive physical activity that causes small tears in the tendon. Pain and immobility are symptoms. Tendinitis can occur in other joints as well; elbows and shoulders are common sites. Tenosynovitis is inflammation of the synovial membrane that sheathes the tendons in the hand. It may be caused by bacterial infection or may be attributable to overexertion.

INFORMATION ON MUSCLE SPRAINS, SPASMS, AND DISORDERS

CAUSES: Injury, overexercise, disease, toxin or pesticide exposure, neurological or endocrine disorders, hereditary factors

SYMPTOMS: Varies; can include bruising, pain, inflammation, muscle spasms or cramps, progressive muscle weakness, loss of coordination, impaired gait

DURATION: Acute to chronic

TREATMENTS: Depends on condition; may include physical therapy, surgery, medications (analgesics, steroids and corticosteroids, anti-inflammatory drugs), rest-ice-compression-elevation (R-I-C-E) formula

Tumors and cancerous growths in muscle tissue are rare. If a lump appears in muscle, it is usually a lipoma, a fatty deposit that is benign. One tumor, called rhabdomyosarcoma, however, is malignant and can be fatal.

TREATMENT AND THERAPY

The myopathies are a wide group of diseases, and treatment varies considerably among them. The muscular dystrophies also vary in their treatment methods. Physical therapy is recommended to prevent contractures, the permanent, disfiguring muscular contractions that are a feature of the disease. Orthopedic appliances and surgery are also used. Because these diseases are genetic, it is sometimes recommended that people with a familial history of muscular dystrophy be tested for certain genetic markers that would suggest the possibility of disease in their children.

Myasthenia gravis is treated with drugs that increase the number of neurotransmitters available where nerves and muscles come together. The drugs help improve the transmission of information from the brain to the muscle tissue. In some cases, a procedure called plasmapheresis is used to eliminate blood-borne substances that may contribute to the disease. Surgical removal of the thymus gland is helpful in alleviating symptoms in some patients.

In treating the many muscle disorders that are caused by athletic activity and excessive wear and tear on the muscle, the R-I-C-E formula is recommended. The acronym stands for rest-ice-compression-elevation: The patient must rest and not use or exercise the limb or muscle involved; an ice pack is applied to the injury; compression is supplied by wrapping a moist bandage snugly over the ice, reducing the flow of fluids to the injured area; and the injured limb is elevated. If there is a fracture involved, the limb must be properly splinted or otherwise immobilized before elevation. The ice pack is held in place for twenty minutes and removed, but the bandage is held in place. Ice therapy can be resumed every twenty minutes.

Heat is also part of the therapy for strains and sprains, but it is not applied until after the initial swelling has gone down, usually after forty-eight to seventy-two hours. Heat raises the metabolic rate in the affected tissue. This brings more blood to the area, carrying nutrients that are needed for tissue repair. Moist heat is preferred, and it can be supplied by an electrical heating pad, a chemical gel in a plastic bag, or hot baths and whirlpools. In using pads and chemical gels, there should be a layer of toweling or other material between the heat source and the body. The temperature for a whirlpool or hot bath should be about 106 degrees Fahrenheit. Only the injured part should be immersed, if possible. As in the ice treatments, heat should be applied for twenty minutes and can be repeated after twenty minutes of rest.

Analgesics are given for pain. Over-the-counter preparations such as aspirin, acetaminophen, or ibuprofen are used most often. Sometimes, when pain is severe, more potent medications are required. Steroids are sometimes prescribed to reduce inflammation, and nonsteroidal anti-inflammatory drugs (NSAIDs) can alleviate both pain and inflammation. If a strained muscle or tendon is seriously torn or otherwise damaged, surgery may be required. Similarly, if a sprain involves torn or detached ligaments, they may have to be surgically repaired.

Muscle spasms and cramps may require both manipulation and the application of heat or cold. The affected limb is gently extended to stretch the contracted muscle. Massage and immersion in a hot bath are useful, as are cold packs.

Tennis elbow, runners' knee, and tendinitis respond to R-I-C-E therapy. Ice is applied to the injured site, and the limb is elevated and allowed to rest. When tenosynovitis is caused by bacterial infection, prompt antibiotic therapy may be necessary to avoid permanent damage. When it is attributable to overexertion, analgesics may help relieve pain and inflammation. Rarely, a corticosteroid is used when other drugs fail.

Often, the injured site requires physical therapy for the full range of motion to be restored. The physical therapist analyzes the patient's capability and develops a regimen to restore strength and mobility to the affected muscles and joints. Physical therapy may involve massage, hot baths, whirlpools, weight training, and/or isometric exercise. Orthotic devices may be required to help the injured area heal.

An important aspect of sports medicine and the treatment of sports-related muscle disorders is prevention. Many painful, debilitating, and immobilizing episodes can be avoided by proper training and conditioning, intelligent exercise practice, and restriction of exertion. Before undertaking any sport or strenuous physical activity, the individual is advised to warm up by gentle stretching, jogging, jumping, and other mild muscular activities. Arms can be rotated in front of the body, over the head, and in circles perpendicular to the ground. Knees can be lifted and pulled up to the chest. Shoulders should be gently rotated to relax upper-back muscles. Neck muscles are toned by gently and slowly moving the head from side to side and in circles. Back muscles are loosened by bending forward and continuing around in slow circles.

If a joint has been injured, it is important to protect it from further damage. Physicians and physical therapists often recommend that athletes tape, brace, or wrap susceptible joints, such as knees, ankles, elbows, or wrists. Sometimes a simple commercial elastic bandage, available in various configurations specific to parts of the body, is all that is required. Neck braces and back braces are used to support these structures.

Benign muscle tumors require no treatment, or may be surgically removed. Malignant tumors may require surgery, radiation, and chemotherapy.

PERSPECTIVE AND PROSPECTS

With the increased interest in physical exercise in the United States has come increasing awareness of the dangers of muscular damage that can arise from improper exercise, as well as of the cardiovascular risks that lie in wait for weekend athletes. Warm-up procedures are universally recommended. Individual exercisers, those in gym classes, professional athletes, and schoolchildren are routinely taken through procedures to stretch and loosen muscles before they start strenuous activity.

Greater attention is being paid to the special needs of young athletes, such as gymnasts. Over the years, new athletic toys and devices have constantly been developed for the young: Skateboards, skates, scooters, and bicycles expose children to a wide range of bumps, falls, bruises, strains, and sprains. Protective equipment and devices have been designed especially for them: Helmets, padding, and special uniforms give children more security in accidents. Similarly, adults should take the time and trouble to outfit themselves correctly for the sports and athletics in which they engage: Joggers should tape, wrap, and brace their joints; and cyclists should wear helmets.

Nevertheless, the incidence of sports- and athletics-related muscular damage is relatively high, pointing to the necessity for increased attention to prevention. The growth of sports medicine as a medical specialty helps considerably in this endeavor. Physicians and nurses in this area are trained to deal with the various problems that arise, and they are often expert commentators on the best means to prevent problems.

—C. Richard Falcon

See also Amyotrophic lateral sclerosis; Ataxia; Back pain; Bell's palsy; Beriberi; Botox; Cerebral palsy; Chronic fatigue syndrome; Exercise physiology; Fibromyalgia; Guillain-Barré syndrome; Hemiplegia; Hypertrophy; Kinesiology; Motor neuron diseases; Multiple sclerosis; Muscles; Muscular dystrophy; Myasthenia gravis; Neurology; Neurology, pediatric; Numbness and tingling; Osteopathic medicine; Overtraining syndrome; Palsy; Paralysis; Paraplegia; Parkinson's disease; Physical rehabilitation; Poliomyelitis; Ptosis; Quadriplegia; Rabies; Rheumatoid arthritis; Rotator cuff surgery; Seizures; Speech disorders; Sphincterectomy; Sports medicine; Tendon disorders; Tendon repair; Tetanus; Tics; Torticollis; Weight loss and gain; Whiplash.

FOR FURTHER INFORMATION:

Dragoo, Jason J. *Handbook of Sports Medicine.* Tempe, Ariz.: Renaissance, 1993. Dragoo covers the wide range of sports- and athletics-related disorders with clarity and precision. The text is intended for the general reader, and the illustrations are simple and clear.

Kirkaldy-Willis, William H., and Thomas N. Bernard, Jr., eds. *Managing Low Back Pain.* 4th ed. New York: Churchill Livingstone, 1999. This book covers the anatomy, biomechanics, pathophysiology, diagnosis, and management of low back pain from the perspective of a variety of disciplines. The aim of the book is to "help all those involved in the treatment of patients suffering from low back and leg pain."

Litin, Scott C., ed. *Mayo Clinic Family Health Book.* 3d ed. New York: HarperResource, 2003. Discusses both muscles and bones, underscoring the intimate relationship between disorders in the two systems. The text and illustrations are complete and easy to understand.

McArdle, William, Frank I. Katch, and Victor L. Katch. *Exercise Physiology: Energy, Nutrition, and Human Performance.* 6th ed. Philadelphia: Lippincott Williams & Wilkins, 2007. A wide-ranging text on exercise and the human body, covering topics such as nutrition, energy transfer, exercise training, systems of energy delivery and utilization, enhancement of energy capacity, the effect of environmental stress, and the effect of exercise on successful aging and disease prevention.

Marieb, Elaine N., and Katja Hoehn. *Human Anatomy and Physiology.* 7th ed. San Francisco: Pearson

Benjamin Cummings, 2007. This introductory anatomy and physiology textbook, easily accessible to those with little science background, is richly illustrated with diagrams and photographs, which help to illuminate body systems and processes.

Ryan, Allan J., and Fred L. Allman, eds. *Sports Medicine*. 2d ed. San Diego, Calif.: Academic Press, 1989. Directed to the professional, but the text can be understood by the layperson. Particularly useful in outlining the contemporary status of sports medicine and how it relates to the training and care of the athlete.

Salter, Robert Bruce. *Textbook of Disorders and Injuries of the Musculoskeletal System*. 3d ed. Baltimore: Williams & Wilkins, 1999. Four sections of the book—"Basic Musculoskeletal Science and Its Applications," "Musculoskeletal Disorders: General and Specific," "Musculoskeletal Injuries," and "Research"—examine the diagnosis and treatment principles of disorders and trauma of the musculoskeletal system.

MUSCLES

ANATOMY

ANATOMY OR SYSTEM AFFECTED: Arms, gastrointestinal system, legs, ligaments, musculoskeletal system

SPECIALTIES AND RELATED FIELDS: Cardiology, exercise physiology, orthopedics, osteopathic medicine, physical therapy, sports medicine

DEFINITION: Cardiac muscle, skeletal muscle, and smooth muscle—all of which have the ability to contract, making possible body movement, peristalsis (the movement of food through the gastrointestinal system), and the circulation of blood throughout the body.

KEY TERMS:

cardiac muscle: a type of muscle, found only in the heart, that makes up the major portion of the heart; involved in the movement of blood through the body

muscle contraction: the shortening of a muscle, which may result in the movement of a particular body part

muscle fibers: elongated muscle cells that make up skeletal, cardiac, and smooth muscles

musculature: the arrangement of skeletal muscles in the body

skeletal muscle: a type of muscle that attaches to bone and causes movement of body parts; the only type that is under conscious, voluntary control

smooth muscle: a type of muscle found in the walls of internal organs such as the stomach, intestines, and urinary bladder; involved in the movement of food through the digestive tract

STRUCTURE AND FUNCTIONS

More than half of the body weight of humans is made up of muscle. Three types of muscles are found in the body: skeletal muscle, cardiac muscle, and smooth muscle. These muscles are composed of different types of muscle cells and perform different functions within the body. The characteristics and functions of each of these three muscle types will be discussed separately, starting with skeletal muscle.

Skeletal muscles attach to and cover bones. This type of muscle is often referred to as voluntary muscle because it is the only muscle type that can be controlled or made to move by consciously thinking about it. Skeletal muscles perform four important functions: bringing about body movement, helping to maintain posture, helping to stabilize joints such as the knee, and generating body heat.

Nearly all body movement is dependent upon skeletal muscle. Skeletal muscle is needed not only to be able to run and jump but also to speak, to write, and to move and blink the eyes. These movements are brought about by the contraction or shortening of skeletal muscles. These muscles are attached to two bones or other structures by tough thin strips or cords of tissue known as tendons. When a muscle contracts or shortens, it pulls the tendons, which then pull on the bones or other structures to which they are connected. In this way, the desired movement is brought about.

Skeletal muscles also aid in the maintenance of posture. Posture is defined as the ability to maintain a position of the body or body parts: for example, the ability to stand or to sit erect. The constant force of gravity must be overcome in order to maintain a standing or seated posture. Small adjustments to the force of gravity are constantly being made through slight contractions of skeletal muscle.

Skeletal muscles—or, more appropriately, their tendons—help to maintain joint stability. Many of the tendons that connect muscles to bones cross movable joints such as the knee and the shoulder. These tendons are kept taut by the constant contraction of the muscles to which they are attached. As a result, they act as walls to prevent the joints from dislocating or shifting out of the normal positions.

More than 40 percent of the human body is composed of skeletal muscle. Skeletal muscles generate heat as they contract. As a result, skeletal muscles are of extreme importance in maintaining normal body temperature. When the body is exposed to cold temperatures, it begins to shiver. This shivering is the result of muscle contractions, which serve to generate body heat and maintain the body's normal temperature.

Skeletal muscles are made up of skeletal muscle cells. These cells are long and tube-shaped and therefore are referred to as skeletal muscle fibers. In some instances, these muscle fibers may be a foot long. When individual skeletal muscle fibers are viewed under a microscope, they display bands that are referred to as striations. For this reason, skeletal muscle is often called striated muscle.

Each skeletal muscle, depending upon its size, is made up of hundreds or thousands of skeletal muscle fibers. These muscle fibers are surrounded by a tough connective tissue that holds the muscle fibers together. These muscle fibers and their surrounding connective tissue form a skeletal muscle. In the human body, there are more than six hundred skeletal muscles. It is the arrangement of these muscles in the body that is referred to as the musculature, or muscle system.

Smooth muscles are often referred to as involuntary muscles because they cannot be made to contract by conscious effort. Smooth muscles are typically found in the walls of internal organs such as the esophagus, stomach, intestines, and urinary bladder. The primary function of smooth muscles in these organs is to enable the passage of material through a tube or tract. For example, the contraction of smooth muscles in the intestines helps to move digested materials through the digestive system.

Smooth muscle is composed of smooth muscle cells. These cells differ from skeletal muscle fibers in that they are short and spindle-shaped. They also differ from skeletal muscle cells in that they are not striated. Furthermore, smooth muscle cells usually are not surrounded by a tough connective tissue to form a muscle; instead, they are arranged in layers.

Cardiac muscle is found only in the heart. Like smooth muscle, cardiac muscle cannot be made to contract by means of conscious effort. Like skeletal muscle, however, cardiac muscle is striated. The contraction of cardiac muscle results in the contraction of the heart. This, in turn, results in the pumping of blood throughout the body.

Although many differences exist among skeletal, smooth, and cardiac muscle, all have one thing in common—their ability to contract. The methods by which this contraction is brought about in skeletal muscle, however, are different from those used by smooth muscle and cardiac muscle.

In order for skeletal muscles to contract, they must first be electrically stimulated. This electrical stimulation is brought about by nerves that are closely associated with the muscle fibers. Each muscle fiber has a branch of a nerve, known as an axon terminal, that lies very close to it. This axon terminal does not touch the muscle fiber, but is separated from it by a tiny space known as the synaptic cleft (or gap). An electrical impulse from the nerve causes the release of a chemical called a neurotransmitter into the synaptic cleft. The specific type of neurotransmitter for skeletal muscle is known as acetylcholine. The neurotransmitter will then pass through the synaptic cleft to the muscle fiber membrane, where it will bind to a special site known as a receptor. When the neurotransmitter binds to the receptor, it causes an electrical impulse to travel down the muscle fiber. This, in turn, causes the contraction of the muscle fiber. When most or all of the muscle fibers contract, the result is the contraction of the entire muscle.

The muscle fibers and muscle will remain in a contracted state as long as the neurotransmitter is bound to the receptor on the muscle fiber membrane. In order for the muscle fiber to relax, the neurotransmitter must be released from the receptor to which it is bound. This is accomplished by the destruction of the neurotransmitter. Another chemical, known as an enzyme, is released into the synaptic cleft. This enzyme destroys the neurotransmitter; thus, the neurotransmitter is no longer bound to the receptor. In skeletal muscle, this enzyme is called acetylcholinesterase, because it destroys the neurotransmitter acetylcholine.

The contraction of cardiac muscle differs from that of skeletal muscle in that each cardiac muscle fiber does not have an axon terminal associated with it. Cardiac muscle is capable of making its own electrical impulse; it does not need a nerve to initiate the electrical impulse for every cardiac muscle fiber. An impulse is started in a particular place in the heart, called the atrioventricular (A-V) node. This impulse spreads from muscle fiber to muscle fiber. Thus, each cardiac muscle fiber stimulates those fibers next to it. The electrical impulse spreads so fast that nearly all the cardiac muscle fibers contract at the same time. As a result, the single impulse that began in the A-V node causes the entire heart to contract.

DISORDERS AND DISEASES

Any type of muscle disorder has the ability to disrupt the normal functions performed by muscles. Skeletal muscle disorders can disrupt body movement and the ability to maintain posture. If these disorders affect the diaphragm, the principal breathing muscle, they can also be fatal.

Perhaps the most common and least detrimental muscle disorder is disuse atrophy. When muscles are not used, the muscle fibers will become smaller, a process called atrophy. As a result of the decrease in the diameter of the muscle fibers, the entire muscle also becomes smaller and therefore weaker.

Disuse atrophy occurs in such circumstances as when an individual is sick or injured and must remain in bed for prolonged periods of time. As a result, the muscles are not used and begin to atrophy. Disuse atrophy is also fairly common in astronauts. This occurs as a result of the lack of gravity against which the muscles must work. If a muscle does not work against a load or force, such as gravity, it will tend to decrease in size.

In general, disuse muscle atrophy is easily treated. The primary treatment is to exercise the unused muscle. Physical activity, particularly those activities in which the muscle must work to lift or pull a weight, will result in an enlargement in the diameter of the skeletal muscle fibers, and thus of the entire muscle. The increase in the diameter of the muscle fibers and muscle is referred to as hypertrophy.

Another common muscle disorder is a muscle cramp. A muscle cramp is a spasm in which the muscle undergoes strong involuntary contractions. These involuntary contractions, which may last for as short a time as a few seconds or as long as a few hours, are extremely painful. Muscle cramps appear to occur more frequently at night or after exercise, but their cause is unknown. Treatment for cramps involves rubbing and massaging the affected muscle.

Muscles are often overused or overstretched. When this is the case, it is possible for the muscle fibers to tear. When the muscle fibers are torn, the result is a muscle strain, more often referred to as a pulled muscle. Although pulled muscles may be painful, they are usually not serious. Treatment for pulled muscles most often involves the resting of the affected muscle. If the muscle fibers are torn completely apart, surgery may be required to reattach the muscle fibers.

Among the more serious skeletal muscle disorders is muscular dystrophy. The term "muscular dystrophy" is used to define those muscle disorders that are genetic or inherited. These diseases most often begin in childhood, but a few cases have been reported to begin during adult life. Muscular dystrophy results in progressive muscle weakness and muscle atrophy. The most common form of muscular dystrophy is known as Duchenne muscular dystrophy. This form of muscular dystrophy primarily affects males. In those affected with Duchenne muscular dystrophy, muscular weakness and atrophy begin to appear at three to five years of age. There is a progressive loss of muscle strength and muscle mass such that, by the age of twelve, those individuals afflicted with the disorder are confined to a wheelchair. Usually between the ages of fourteen and eighteen, the patients develop serious and sometimes fatal respiratory diseases as a result of the impairment of the diaphragm, the primary breathing muscle. The progressive deterioration of the muscles cannot be stopped, but it may be slowed with exercise of the affected muscles.

Myasthenia gravis is also a severe muscle disorder. This disease results in excessive weakness of skeletal muscles, a condition known as muscle fatigue. Those with myasthenia gravis complain of fatigue even after performing normal everyday body movements. Although severe, myasthenia gravis is usually not fatal unless the diaphragm is affected.

Myasthenia results from a decrease in the availability of the receptors for acetylcholine. If fewer acetylcholine receptors are available on the muscle fibers, less acetylcholine binds to the muscle fiber receptors; this binding is needed for contraction to occur. As a result, fewer muscle fibers within the muscle contract. The fewer muscle fibers within the entire muscle that contract, the weaker the muscle.

Myasthenia gravis affects about one in every ten thousand individuals. Unlike Duchenne muscular dystrophy, myasthenia gravis may affect any group, and, overall, women are affected more frequently than men. Myasthenia gravis is usually first detected in the facial muscles, particularly those of the eyes and eyelids. Those afflicted have droopy eyelids and experience difficulty in keeping the eyes open. Other symptoms are weakness in those muscles involved in chewing and difficulty swallowing as a result of weakening of the tongue muscles. In most patients, there is also some weakening of the muscles of the legs and arms.

The prognosis for the treatment of myasthenia gravis is very good. The most important treatment for the disorder is the use of anticholinesterase drugs. These drugs inhibit the breakdown of acetylcholine. As a result, there is a large amount of acetylcholine in the neuromuscular junction to bind with the limited number of acetylcholine receptors. This, in turn, increases the ability and number of the muscle fibers that are able to contract, resulting in an increase in muscle strength and the ability to use the muscles without fatigue.

Also of interest is the effect of pesticides and the way in which they affect muscle function. Some pesticides are classified as organic pesticides that inhibit the enzyme acetylcholinesterase. If acetylcholinesterase is inhibited, it will no longer break down the acetylcholine that is bound to the receptor on the skeletal muscle membrane. If the acetylcholine is not removed from the receptor, the muscle cannot relax and is therefore in a constant state of contraction. As a result, the respiratory muscles are unable to contract and relax, a process required for breathing. Thus, organic pesticides function to prevent the respiratory muscles from working, and an affected animal will die as a result of not being able to breathe.

Muscle fibers also require a blood supply in order to keep them alive. If the blood supply to the muscle fibers is inhibited, death of the muscle fibers can result. If enough muscle fibers are affected, death of the muscle can result. This most commonly occurs in cardiac muscle. If the blood supply to the cardiac muscle making up the heart is reduced or cut off, the result is a decrease in the ability of the cardiac muscle to contract. This, in turn, leads to heart failure.

PERSPECTIVE AND PROSPECTS

The study of muscles and musculature is as old as the study of anatomy itself. The first well-documented study of muscles was done by Galen of Pergamum in the first century. Galen made drawings of muscles and described their functions. In all, Galen described more than three hundred muscles in the human body, almost half of all the muscles now known.

The first refined drawings and descriptions of the skeletal muscles of the body were made in the late fifteenth century. Among those who stood out as muscle anatomists during this period was Leonardo da Vinci. Leonardo's drawings of the skeletal muscles of the body were magnificent. His chief interest in the muscles of the body, like Galen's, was their function. He accurately described, among many other muscles, the muscles involved in the movement of the lips and cheeks.

A major step to the understanding of muscle physiology did not occur until the late eighteenth century.

Luigi Galvani in 1791 discovered the relationship between muscle contraction and electricity when he found that an electrical current could cause the contraction of a frog leg. The use of electrical stimulation to study muscle contraction and function was fully utilized in the mid-1800's by Duchenne de Boulogne. The actual measurement of the electrical activity in a muscle came about in 1929, with the invention by Edgar Douglas Adrian and Detlev Wulf Bronk of the needle electrode, which could be placed into the muscle to record the muscle's electrical activity. This recording of the electrical activity of the muscle is known as an electromyogram, or EMG. Electromyograms are important in the evaluation of the electrical activity of resting and contracting muscles. Since the discovery of EMGs, they have been used by anatomists, muscle physiologists, exercise physiologists, and orthopedic surgeons to study and diagnose muscle diseases. Furthermore, the knowledge gained from EMGs has led to the making of artificial limbs that can be controlled by the electrical impulses of the existing muscles.

Knowledge of muscle names, muscle anatomy, and movement, as well as muscle physiology, is needed for many medical fields. These fields include kinesiology, the study of movement; physical and occupational therapy; the treatment and rehabilitation of those who are disabled by injury; exercise physiology and sports medicine, in which the effects of exercise on muscle and the damage of muscle as a result of sports injuries are studied; and, finally, orthopedic surgery, which is the surgical repair of damaged bones, joints, and muscles.

—*David K. Saunders, Ph.D.*

See also Acupressure; Amyotrophic lateral sclerosis; Anesthesia; Anesthesiology; Ataxia; Bed-wetting; Bell's palsy; Botox; Breasts, female; Cells; Cerebral palsy; Chronic fatigue syndrome; Exercise physiology; Fibromyalgia; Glycolysis; Guillain-Barré syndrome; Head and neck disorders; Hemiplegia; Kinesiology; Lower extremities; Mastectomy and lumpectomy; Motor neuron diseases; Multiple sclerosis; Muscle sprains, spasms, and disorders; Muscular dystrophy; Myasthenia gravis; Myomectomy; Orthopedic surgery; Orthopedics; Orthopedics, pediatric; Osteopathic medicine; Overtraining syndrome; Palsy; Paralysis; Paraplegia; Parkinson's disease; Physical rehabilitation; Poisoning; Poliomyelitis; Ptosis; Quadriplegia; Rabies; Respiration; Rotator cuff surgery; Seizures; Speech disorders; Sphincterectomy; Sports medicine; Steroid abuse; Tendon disorders; Tendon repair; Tetanus;

Tics; Torticollis; Trembling and shaking; Upper extremities; Weight loss and gain; Whiplash.

FOR FURTHER INFORMATION:

Blakey, Paul. *The Muscle Book*. Honesdale, Pa.: Himalayan Institute, 2000. A very accessible guide to the body's muscles. Identifies all major muscles of the human body, reviews how they work, and discusses first aid by massage and common injuries.

Burke, Edmund. *Optimal Muscle Performance and Recovery*. Rev. ed. New York: Putnam, 2003. A leading exercise physiologist provides a training guide for athletes that details exercise regimens and stresses healthy muscle development and recovery after injury.

Cash, Mel. *Pocket Atlas of the Moving Body*. New York: Crown, 2000. An excellent reference guide that covers information about movement and posture of the human body. Full-page anatomical illustrations; tables of muscles, joints, posture, and movement patterns; definitions of technical terms; and a listing of common types of injury are included.

Guyton, Arthur C., and John E. Hall. *Textbook of Medical Physiology*. 11th ed. Philadelphia: Elsevier Saunders, 2006. This textbook gives many examples of diseases and pathological conditions of skeletal and cardiac muscle. The text does an excellent job of describing how diseases and pathologies affect the normal functioning of the muscle. Although somewhat technical at times, the text is well written and understandable.

Marieb, Elaine N. *Essentials of Human Anatomy and Physiology*. 8th ed. San Francisco: Pearson/Benjamin Cummings, 2006. An excellent place to begin the study of muscles and musculature. This text uses little technical jargon and explains the jargon it does use. Provides good descriptions and drawings of the most important muscles.

Shier, David N., Jackie L. Butler, and Ricki Lewis. *Hole's Essentials of Human Anatomy and Physiology*. 9th ed. New York: McGraw-Hill, 2004. An introductory college anatomy and physiology book that is easy to read and understand. Provides a good general overview of skeletal, cardiac, and smooth muscle anatomy and function.

Tortora, Gerard J., and Bryan Derrickson. *Principles of Anatomy and Physiology*. 11th ed. Hoboken, N.J.: John Wiley & Sons, 2006. This text clearly explains the functions of many individual muscles. Furthermore, it provides many examples of clinical applications involving muscles, including diseases and the use of medical tests for the diagnosis of muscle disease.

MUSCULAR DYSTROPHY

DISEASE/DISORDER

ANATOMY OR SYSTEM AFFECTED: Legs, muscles, musculoskeletal system

SPECIALTIES AND RELATED FIELDS: Genetics, pediatrics, physical therapy

DEFINITION: A group of related diseases that attack different muscle groups, are progressive and genetically determined, and have no known cure.

KEY TERMS:

disease: an interruption, cessation, or disorder of a body function or system, usually identifiable by a group of signs and symptoms and characterized by consistent anatomical alterations

distal: situated away from the center of the body; the farthest part from the midline of the body

DNA (deoxyribonucleic acid): a type of protein found in the nucleus of a cell comprising chromosomes that contain the genetic instructions of an organism

dystrophin: both the gene and the protein that are defective in Duchenne muscular dystrophy

dystrophy: an improper form of a tissue or group of cells (literally, "bad nourishment")

enzyme: a protein secreted by a cell that acts as a catalyst to induce chemical changes in other substances, remaining apparently unchanged itself in the process

fiber: a slender thread or filament; the elongated, threadlike cells that collectively constitute a muscle

genetic: imparted at conception and incorporated into every cell of an organism

muscle: a bundle of contractile cells that is responsible for the movement of organs and body parts

muscle group: a collection of muscles that work together to accomplish a particular movement

CAUSES AND SYMPTOMS

Muscles, attached to bones through tendons, are responsible for movement in the human body. In muscular dystrophy, muscles become progressively weaker. As individual muscle fibers become so weak that they die, they are replaced by connective tissue, which is fibrous and fatty rather than muscular. These replacement fibers are commonly found in skin and scar tissue and are not capable of movement, and the muscles become progressively weaker. There are several different recognized types of muscular dystrophy. These have in common degeneration of muscle fibers and their replacement with connective tissue. They are distinguished from one another on the basis of the muscle group or groups involved and the age at which individuals are affected.

The most common type is Duchenne muscular dystrophy. In this disease, the muscles involved are in the upper thigh and pelvis. The disease strikes in early childhood, usually between the ages of four and seven. It is known to be genetic and occurs only in boys. Two-thirds of affected individuals are born to mothers who are known to carry a defective gene; one-third are simply new cases whose mothers are genetically normal. Individuals afflicted with Duchenne muscular dystrophy suffer from weakness in their hips and upper thighs. Initially, they may experience difficulty in sitting up or standing. The disease progresses to involve muscle groups in the shoulder and trunk. Patients lose the ability to walk during their early teens. As the disease progresses, portions of the brain become affected, and intelligence is reduced. Muscle fibers in the heart are also affected, and most individuals die by the age of twenty.

The dystrophin gene normally produces a very large protein called dystrophin that is an integral part of the muscle cell membrane. In Duchenne muscular dystrophy, a defect in the dystrophin gene causes no dystrophin or defective dystrophin to be produced, and the protein will be absent from the cell membrane. As a result, the muscle fiber membrane breaks down and leaks, allowing fluid from outside the cell to enter the muscle cell. In turn, the contents of affected cells are broken down by other chemicals called proteases that are normally stored in the muscle cell. The dead pieces of muscle fiber are removed by scavenging cells called macrophages. The result of this process is a virtually empty and greatly weakened muscle cell.

A second type is Becker's muscular dystrophy, which is similar to the Duchenne form of the disease. Approximately 3 in 200,000 people are affected, and it too is found only among males. The major clinical difference is the age of onset. Becker's muscular dystrophy typically first appears in the early teenage years. The muscles involved are similar to those of Duchenne muscular dystrophy, but the course of the disease is slower. Most individuals require the use of a wheelchair in their early thirties and eventually die in their forties.

Myotonic dystrophy is a form of muscular dystrophy that strikes approximately 5 out of 100,000 people in a population. Myotonia is the inability of a muscle group to relax after contracting. Individuals with myotonic dystrophy experience this difficulty in their hands and feet. On average, the disease first appears at the age of nineteen. The condition is benign, in that it does not shorten an affected person's life span. Rather, it causes inconveniences to the victim. Affected persons also experience a variety of other problems, including baldness at the front of the head and malfunction of the ovaries and testes. The muscles of the stomach and intestines can become involved, leading to a slowing down of intestinal functions and diarrhea.

Another type is limb girdle muscular dystrophy. The muscles of both upper and lower limbs—the shoulders and the pelvis—are involved. The onset of this dystrophy form is variable, from childhood to middle age. While the disorder is not usually fatal, it does progress, and victims experience severe disability about twenty years after the disease first appears. While this variant is also genetically transmitted, men and women are about equally affected.

One type of muscular dystrophy found almost exclusively among individuals of Scandinavian descent is called distal dystrophy. It first appears relatively early in adult life, between the thirties and fifties. The muscles of the forearm and hand become progressively weaker and decrease in size. Eventually, the muscles of the lower leg and foot also become involved. This form of muscular dystrophy is not usually fatal.

Oculopharyngeal muscular dystrophy is a particularly serious form that involves the muscles of the eyes and throat. In this disease, victims are affected in their forties and fifties. There is progressive loss of control

---

INFORMATION ON MUSCULAR DYSTROPHY

CAUSES: Genetic defect

SYMPTOMS: Ranges widely; may include progressive muscle weakness, loss of coordination, impaired gait, reduced intelligence, malfunction of ovaries or testes, slowed intestinal functions, impaired swallowing, impaired eye movement

DURATION: Chronic

TREATMENTS: None; supportive care (physical therapy, braces, orthopedic surgery, drug therapy)

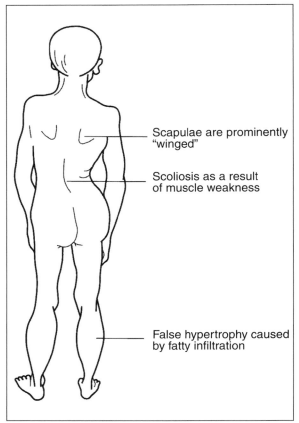

Scapulae are prominently "winged"

Scoliosis as a result of muscle weakness

False hypertrophy caused by fatty infiltration

Duchenne muscular dystrophy, the most common type, is characterized by prominently "winged" scapulae, scoliosis, false hypertrophy of the calves, and other less visible effects; children are the victims, usually not surviving beyond age twenty.

of the muscles that move the eyes and loss of the ability to swallow. Death usually results from starvation or from pneumonia acquired when the affected individual accidentally inhales food or drink.

A type of muscular dystrophy for which the location of the genetic abnormality is known is facioscapulohumeral muscular dystrophy; the defect is confined to the tip of the fourth chromosome. This disease initially involves the muscles of the face and later spreads to the muscles of the posterior or back of the shoulder. Eventually, muscles in the upper thigh are involved. The affected person loses the ability to make facial expressions and assumes a permanent pout as a result of loss of muscle function. As the condition advances, the shoulder blades protrude when the arms are raised. Weakness and difficulty walking are eventually experienced. As with other forms of muscular dystrophy,

there is some variability in the degree to which individuals are affected. Occasionally, a variety of deafness occurs involving the nerves that connect the inner ear and the brain. Less commonly, victims become blind.

There are other variants of muscular dystrophy that have been recognized and described. These forms of the disease, however, are rare. The main problem facing physicians is differentiating accurately the variety of muscular dystrophy seen in a particular patient so as to arrive at a correct diagnosis.

Treatment and Therapy

The diagnosis of muscular dystrophy is initially made through observation. Typically, parents notice changes in their affected children and bring these concerns to the attention of a physician. The physician takes a careful family history and then examines a suspected victim to make a tentative or working diagnosis. Frequently, knowledge of other family members with the condition and observations are sufficient to establish a firm diagnosis. Occasionally, a physician may elect to order physiological or genetic tests to confirm the tentative diagnosis. As Duchenne muscular dystrophy is the most common form of muscular dystrophy, it provides a convenient example of this process.

A diagnosis of Duchenne or any other form of muscular dystrophy is rarely made before the age of three. This form of the disease almost always occurs in boys. (Variants, rather than true Duchenne muscular dystrophy, are seen in girls, but this situation is extremely rare.) The reason for this finding is that the genetic defect occurs on the X chromosome, of which males only possess one. Approximately two-thirds of all victims inherit the defective chromosome from their mothers, who are asymptomatic carriers; thus, the condition is recessive and said to be X-linked. The disease occurs in the remaining one-third of victims as a result of a fresh mutation, in which there is no family history of the disease and the parents are not carriers.

Victims usually begin to sit, walk, and run at an older age than normally would be expected. Parents describe walking as waddling rather than the usual upright posture. Victims have difficulty climbing stairs. They also have apparently enlarged calf muscles, a finding called muscular hypertrophy. While the muscles are initially strong, they lose their strength when connective and fatty tissues replace muscle fibers. The weakness of muscles in the pelvis is responsible for difficulties in sitting and the unusual way of walking. Normal children are able to go directly from a sitting position to standing erect. Victims of Duchenne muscular dystrophy first roll onto their stomachs, then kneel and raise themselves up by pushing their hands against their shins, knees, and thighs; they literally climb up themselves in order to stand. These children also have a pronounced curvature of their lower backs, an attempt by the body to compensate for the weakness in the muscles of the hips and pelvis.

There is frequently some weakness in the muscles of the shoulder. This finding can be demonstrated by a physician, but it is not usually seen by parents and is not an early problem for the victim. A physician tests for this weakness by lifting the child under the armpits. Normal children will be able to support themselves using the muscles of the shoulder. Individuals with Duchenne muscular dystrophy are unable to hold themselves up and will slip through the physician's hands. Eventually, these children will be unable to lift their arms over their heads. Most victims of Duchenne muscular dystrophy are unable to walk by their teen years. The majority die before the age of twenty, although about one-quarter live for a few more years. Most victims also have an abnormality in the muscles of the heart that leads to decreased efficiency of the heart and decreased ability to be physically active; in some cases, it also causes sudden death. Most victims of Duchenne muscular dystrophy suffer mental impairment. As their muscles deteriorate, their measured intelligence quotient (IQ) drops approximately twenty points below the level that it was at the onset of the disease. Serious mental handicaps are experienced by about one-quarter of victims.

Other forms of muscular dystrophy are similar to Duchenne muscular dystrophy. Their clinical courses are also similar, as are the methods of diagnosis. The critical differences are the muscles involved and the age of onset.

Laboratory procedures used to confirm the diagnosis

IN THE NEWS:
THE PATH TOWARD GENE THERAPY FOR MUSCULAR DYSTROPHY

Gene therapy in the treatment of Duchenne muscular dystrophy (DMD), the gravest and most common form of muscular dystrophy, has been a subject of intensive research. The goal of such therapy is to introduce the normal gene for dystrophin, which is defective in DMD, into diseased muscle cells so that their ability to withstand the wear and tear of contractile activity is restored. Significant progress in this effort was reported in the October, 2002, issue of the *Proceedings of the National Academy of Science of the United States of America* by collaborating groups at the University of Washington in Seattle and the University of Michigan in Ann Arbor.

The researchers used as their model system the transgenic *mdx* mouse, which carries a truncated dystrophin gene and therefore produces virtually no dystrophin protein. The leg muscles of such mice are susceptible to contraction-induced injury and subsequent deterioration, much as in human DMD.

To deliver functionally effective levels of normal full-length dystrophin, the gene was engineered into an adenovirus, which was then injected directly into the *mdx* leg muscles. This viral vector, which is related to the family of viruses that cause the common cold, is an excellent choice as a genetic vehicle because of its efficiency at infecting muscle cells. However, the researchers needed to make significant changes to the adenoviral deoxyribonucleic acid (DNA) in order to overcome two major problems. First, the dystrophin gene is extremely large and therefore is not amenable to being inserted into a viral DNA sequence. Second, the immune systems of the mice tend to reject the adenoviral DNA. To solve both of these problems, the viral vector was stripped of all unnecessary DNA ("gutted") so that it would accommodate the entire cDNA sequence of dystrophin while not being rejected.

The gutted adenoviral vector made it possible for the first time to introduce full-length dystrophin into adult *mdx* leg muscles without eliciting an immune response. One month later, the muscle tissue near the injection sites was making 25 to 30 percent of normal dystrophin levels; furthermore, there was a 40 percent improvement in contraction-induced injury. These findings constitute an important step toward the use of adenoviral vector-based gene therapy to treat DMD. For the therapy to be truly effective, it will be necessary to develop systemic techniques for delivering the normal gene to all muscles.

—Mary A. Nastuk, Ph.D.

of muscular dystrophy include microscopic analysis of muscle tissue, measurement of enzymes found in the blood, and measurement of the speed and efficiency of nerve conduction, a process called electromyography. Some cases have been diagnosed at birth by measuring a particular enzyme called creatinine kinase. It is possible to diagnose some types of muscular dystrophy before birth with chorionic villus sampling or amniocentesis.

There is no specific treatment for any of the muscular dystrophies. Physical therapy is frequently ordered and used to prevent the remaining unaffected muscles from losing their tone and mass. In some stages of the disease, braces, appliances, and orthopedic surgery may be used. These measures do not reverse the underlying pathology, but they may improve the quality of life for a victim. The cardiac difficulties associated with myotonic dystrophy may require treatment with a pacemaker. For victims of myotonic dystrophy, some relief is obtained by using drugs; the most commonly used pharmaceuticals are phenytoin and quinine. The inability to relax muscles once they are contracted does not usually present a major problem for sufferers of myotonic dystrophy.

More useful and successful is prevention, which involves screening individuals in families or kinship groups who are potential carriers. Carriers are persons who have some genetic material for a disease or condition but lack sufficient genes to cause an apparent case of a disease or condition; in short, they appear normal. When an individual who is a carrier conceives a child, however, there is an increased risk of the offspring having the disease. Genetic counseling should be provided after screening, so that individuals who have the gene for a disease can make more informed decisions about having children.

Chemical tests are available for use in diagnosing some forms of muscular dystrophy. Carriers of the gene for Duchenne muscular dystrophy can be detected by staining a muscle sample for dystrophin; a cell that is positive for Duchenne muscular dystrophy will have no stained dystrophin molecules. The dystrophin stain test is also used to diagnose Becker's muscular dystrophy, but the results are not quite as consistent or reliable. Approximately two-thirds of carriers and fetuses at risk for both forms of muscular dystrophy can be identified by analyzing DNA. Among individuals at risk for myotonic dystrophy, nine out of ten who carry the gene can be identified with DNA analysis before they experience actual symptoms of the disease.

Perspective and Prospects

Muscular dystrophy has been recognized as a medical entity for several centuries. Initially, it was considered to be a degenerative disease only of adults, and it was not until the nineteenth century that the disease was addressed in children with Guillaume-Benjamin-Amand Duchenne's description of progressive weakness of the hips and upper thighs. An accurate classification of the various forms of muscular dystrophy depended on accurate observation and on the collection of sets of cases. Correct diagnosis had to wait for the development of accurate laboratory methods for staining muscle fibers. The interpretation of laboratory findings depended on the development of biochemical knowledge. Thus, much of the integration of knowledge concerning muscular dystrophy is relatively recent.

Genes play an important role in the understanding of muscular dystrophy. All forms of muscular dystrophy are hereditary, although different chromosomes are involved in different forms of the disease. The development of techniques for routine testing and diagnosis has also occurred relatively recently. Specific chromosomes for all forms of muscular dystrophy have not yet been discovered. Considering initial successes of the Human Genome Project, an effort to identify all human genes, it seems likely that more precise genetic information related to muscular dystrophy will emerge.

There still are no cures for muscular dystrophies, and many forms are relentlessly fatal. Cures for many communicable diseases caused by bacteria or viruses have been discovered, and advances have been made in the treatment of cancer and other degenerative diseases by identifying chemicals that cause the conditions or by persuading people to change their lifestyles. Muscular dystrophy, however, is a group of purely genetic conditions. Many of the particular chromosomes involved are known, but no techniques are yet available to cure the disease once it is identified.

The availability of both a mouse model and a dog model of Duchenne muscular dystrophy, however, has facilitated the testing of gene therapy for this disease. Dystrophic mouse early embryos have been cured by injection of a functional copy of the dystrophin gene; however, this technique must be performed in embryos and is not useful for human therapy. Two avenues of research under way in these animal models are the introduction of normal muscle-precursor cells into dystrophic muscle cells and the direct delivery of a functional dystrophin gene into dystrophic muscle cells. It is hoped that these studies will lead to a cure for the disease.

In the meantime, muscular dystrophy continues to cause human suffering and to cost victims, their families, and society large sums of money. The disease is publicized on an annual basis via efforts to raise money for research and treatment, but there is little publicity on an ongoing basis. For these reasons, muscular dystrophy remains an important medical problem in contemporary society.

—L. Fleming Fallon, Jr., M.D., Ph.D., M.P.H.;
updated by Karen E. Kalumuck, Ph.D.

See also Genetic counseling; Genetic diseases; Genetics and inheritance; Hypertrophy; Muscle sprains, spasms, and disorders; Muscles; Pediatrics; Physical rehabilitation; Screening.

FOR FURTHER INFORMATION:

Beers, Mark H., et al. *The Merck Manual of Diagnosis and Therapy.* 18th ed. Whitehouse Station, N.J.: Merck Research Laboratories, 2006. The more common forms of muscular dystrophy are discussed in clear, relatively nontechnical language. The entries are brief and succinct. This work is useful for an overview of muscular dystrophy; the more unusual and rarer forms of muscular dystrophy are not included.

Behrman, Richard E., Robert M. Kliegman, and Hal B. Jenson, eds. *Nelson Textbook of Pediatrics.* 17th ed. Philadelphia: Saunders, 2004. The forms of muscular dystrophy found in children are discussed in a logical and complete format. Pictures clearly depict the difficulties in movement experienced by victims of Duchenne muscular dystrophy.

Brown, Susan S., and Jack A. Lucy, eds. *Dystrophin: Gene, Protein, and Cell Biology.* New York: Cambridge University Press, 1997. This compilation of the latest research into the causes of muscular dystrophy at the molecular level is suitable for the nonspecialist with an introductory background in biology, as well as the specialist and clinician dealing with patients and their families affected by the disorder.

Emery, Alan E. H. *Muscular Dystrophy: The Facts.* 2d ed. New York: Oxford University Press, 2000. Covers all aspects of the disease in a question-answer format.

Goldman, Lee, and Dennis Ausiello, eds. *Cecil Textbook of Medicine.* 22d ed. Philadelphia: W. B. Saunders, 2004. The descriptions of muscular dystrophy are clear and detailed. The language used in the book is precise. Using multiple authors, each sec-tion is written by an internationally recognized expert.

Kumar, Vinay, Abul K. Abbas, and Nelson Fausto, eds. *Robbins and Cotran Pathologic Basis of Disease.* 7th ed. Philadelphia: Elsevier Saunders, 2005. A complete discussion about the pathology of several forms of muscular dystrophy. Technical language is employed, but the book is well written. Photographs of microscopic sections of muscle are included, as well as descriptions of the clinical course of muscular dystrophy.

Tierney, Lawrence M., Stephen J. McPhee, and Maxine A. Papadakis, eds. *Current Medical Diagnosis and Treatment 2007.* New York: McGraw-Hill Medical, 2006. In a brief and concise format, the diagnosis and management of muscular dystrophy are discussed. The section authors are recognized experts in their fields. Treatment protocols are included.

Wolfson, Penny. *Moonrise: One Family, Genetic Identity, and Muscular Dystrophy.* New York: St. Martin's Press, 2003. A personal memoir of a mother and her son, who suffers from Duchenne muscular dystrophy, which details the early days of her son's life, the diagnosis, and the impact on her family. Questions about scientific advances and their implications, special education, giftedness, prenatal testing, and familial genetic links are covered in the narrative.

MUTATION

BIOLOGY

ANATOMY OR SYSTEM INVOLVED: Cells, immune system

SPECIALTIES AND RELATED FIELDS: Cytology, genetics, pathology

DEFINITION: An error in the process that copies genetic information for each new generation, resulting in an alteration in the organism that can be beneficial, harmful, or neutral.

KEY TERMS:

alleles: alternate forms of a gene; each person has two alleles of each gene, and these alleles may be the same or different; a person inherits one allele from each parent

chromosomes: the parts of a cell that contain genetic information, made of DNA covered with protein; each human cell has twenty-three pairs of chromosomes

deoxyribonucleic acid (DNA): a long, spiral-shaped molecule that makes up the bulk of chromosomes;

the sequence of subunits contains the genetic information of the cell and organism

gene: the basic unit of inheritance; at the molecular level, a gene consists of a segment of DNA that codes for a particular protein

genotype: the genetic makeup of an individual; it is usually expressed as a list of alleles

heterozygous: having two different alleles for a particular gene

homozygous: having two identical alleles of a particular gene

meiosis: a special kind of cell division whereby four cells are produced; each cell has only half of the original number of chromosomes; meiosis produces the sex cells (eggs and sperm)

nucleotides: the subunits from which DNA is made

THE FUNCTION OF GENES

An individual is not a random assortment of characteristics. The way individuals look, their physiological makeup, their susceptibility to disease, and even how long they may live are determined by information received from their parents. The smallest unit of information for inherited characteristics is the gene. For each characteristic, an individual has two copies of the gene controlling that characteristic. The gene can have two forms, called alleles. For example, the alleles for eye color can be designated using the letters B and b, with the B allele carrying the information for brown eyes and the b allele specifying blue eyes. Thus the genotype, or genetic makeup, of an individual can be one of three types: BB, bb, or Bb. A BB individual will have brown eyes. A bb person will have blue eyes. A Bb individual will have brown eyes since the brown allele is dominant over the blue one. The dominant allele will always be expressed, whether present as two copies or only one. For a recessive allele to be expressed, an individual must have two recessive alleles (bb).

When a person reproduces, he or she passes on one allele for each gene to the child. Therefore, the child also has two alleles for each gene, one from each parent. A person with two identical alleles for a given gene is said to be homozygous for that trait and can pass on only one kind of allele. Someone with two different alleles for a particular gene is said to be heterozygous. A heterozygous person will pass on the dominant allele to 50 percent of his or her children, on average; the other 50 percent will receive the recessive allele. Alleles are passed on in the sex cells— the eggs and sperm. Eggs and sperm are produced by a special type of cell divi-

sion, meiosis, that reduces by half the amount of genetic information carried by the cell. When an egg is fertilized by a sperm cell, the amount of genetic information is once again doubled. In "normal" cell division, called mitosis, the amount of genetic material in each cell is kept constant. After fertilization, the egg cell divides repeatedly by mitosis to produce the millions of cells that make up the embryo and later the adult organism.

If the genetic makeup of a couple for a given trait is known, the probable characteristics of their children for this trait can be predicted. For example, one can predict the eye color for children of a brown-eyed husband and blue-eyed wife. Assuming that the husband comes from a family of only brown-eyed people, one can be fairly certain that he is homozygous for this trait (BB). Since his wife has blue eyes, and blue is recessive, she must be homozygous for the other allele (bb). Their children will each have a brown allele from their father and a blue allele from their mother; they will all be heterozygous (Bb). Since brown is dominant, they will all have brown eyes.

One can take this example a step further and predict the outcome for the next generation. If one of this couple's brown-eyed sons marries a blue-eyed woman, then one can predict the eye colors of their children using a simple diagram called a Punnett square. (Reginald Crundall Punnett contributed much to the early study of genetics.)

Using this simple tool, with the possible alleles in the sperm cells along the top and those from the eggs down the side, one can show all the possible combinations of inherited alleles (see figure 1). These boxes represent the genotypes of the fertilized eggs. In this case, one would expect about half of their children to have brown eyes (the Bb boxes) and half to have blue eyes (the bb

FIGURE 1. A PUNNETT SQUARE SHOWING ALLELES FOR EYE COLOR

		Father's Sperm Cells	
		B	b
Mother's	b	Bb	bb
Egg Cells	b	Bb	bb

boxes). Since chance determines exactly which sperm actually fertilizes the egg in every conception event, however, such a prediction is not always accurate. Nevertheless, the more children they have, the closer the actual percentage of brown-eyed or blue-eyed children will come to half.

Actually, the inheritance of eye color is somewhat more complicated than it is described above. Several genes contribute to eye color. Depending on the mix of dominant and recessive alleles for each gene involved, eye color can range from pale blue to dark brown. Other combinations produce green eyes.

In addition, many genes do not show complete dominance. For example, evidence shows that height is controlled by several genes that exhibit incomplete dominance. One homozygous individual (TT) will be tall, the other (tt) will be short, and the heterozygous individual (Tt) will be of medium height. The laws that determine how the alleles may be passed on from generation to generation, however, are exactly the same. One can use a simplified example of two people who are heterozygous for a hypothetical height gene (see figure 2).

Since both parents are heterozygous, each will be able to produce two kinds of sex cells, those with "tall" alleles and those with "short" alleles. From all the possible outcomes shown in the boxes of the Punnett square, one would predict 25 percent tall (TT), 25 percent short (tt), and 50 percent medium-height (Tt) children.

If several genes are involved, a wide range of heights is possible. A person who is homozygous for the "tall" alleles in most of the height genes will be very tall. Someone homozygous for most of the "short" alleles will be short. Someone who is heterozygous in most of these genes will be of medium height. Since even relatively short people will have some "tall" alleles, and since chance determines which sex cells are actually used, it is possible for two short people to have a tall child: By chance, the egg and sperm that united had more than the usual share of "tall" alleles.

The preceding examples have used genes that have only two alleles: brown or blue, tall or short. There are genes, however, for which more than two alleles are possible—although any one individual may have only two alleles in his or her genetic makeup. A good example of such a gene is the one that controls human

FIGURE 2. A PUNNETT SQUARE SHOWING ALLELES FOR HEIGHT

		Father's Sperm Cells	
		T	t
Mother's Egg Cells	T	TT	Tt
	t	Tt	tt

blood type. There are three blood type alleles: A, B, and O. The A and B alleles are dominant, while the O allele is recessive. This allows for the various types of blood (see table).

This table allows one to see the mechanism of dominance. A person with an A allele produces a particular chemical in the blood. Similarly, the B allele causes the production of a different chemical. The O allele produces no chemical at all. If a chemical not already present in the blood is introduced, such as in a blood transfusion, the body will react against it, destroying the new blood. Since people with type O blood produce neither chemical, they are sometimes referred to as "universal donors." Their blood can be given safely to anyone. Similarly, people with AB blood can receive any other blood type because their bodies already contain both types of chemical.

THE RELATIONSHIP BETWEEN GENOTYPE AND BLOOD TYPE

Genotype	Blood Type	Comments
AA	A	These two genotypes produce identical blood types.
AO	A	
BB	B	These two genotypes produce identical blood types.
BO	B	
AB	AB	Both dominant alleles are expressed.
OO	O	With no dominant alleles, the recessive allele is expressed.

FIGURE 3. A PUNNETT SQUARE SHOWING ALLELES FOR BLOOD TYPE

Father's Sperm Cells

		B	O
Mother's Egg Cells	A	AB (AB blood)	AO (A blood)
	O	BO (B blood)	OO (O blood)

One can also use a blood type example to show how parents can produce children who are genetically un-like both parents. The mother has type A blood and is heterozygous (AO), while the father has type B blood and is also heterozygous (BO). Their child could have any of the four blood types (see figure 3).

Although blood type is not an obvious visible fea-ture, many genes that express themselves in an individ-ual's appearance behave in a similar manner. There-fore, one should not be surprised to see two parents with a child who resembles neither of them.

The genes that control heredity actually consist of strands of deoxyribonucleic acid (DNA) that make up the chromosomes. Humans have twenty-three pairs of chromosomes in each cell. This explains how an indi-vidual can have two alleles for each gene, one on each chromosome of a pair. The exception is the sex chro-mosomes, which are different in males and females. Sex chromosomes come in two kinds, a relatively large X and a small Y. The X chromosomes can carry many more genes than the Y. Females have two X chromo-somes and thus have two alleles for every gene found on the X chromosome. Males have only one X chromo-some; therefore, they only have one allele for those genes carried on the X. The Y chromosome of the male has been shown to carry very little, although important, genetic information. Genes carried on the X chromo-some are called sex-linked, since they typically are ex-pressed in only one sex—the male. Females may be merely carriers of a sex-linked trait.

One sex-linked trait is the disorder called hemo-philia. A hemophiliac fails to produce a chemical which allows the blood to clot. This disorder is usually fatal if the hemophiliac is not constantly supplied with the clotting factor. Such an individual would simply bleed to death following even the slightest injury. Suppose that a woman who carries the trait for hemophilia mar-ries a man who does not have the disorder. Hemophilia is a recessive condition; therefore, the woman has one normal X chromosome and one bearing the recessive allele (denoted by Xh). Since the normal allele directs the production of the clotting factor, her blood can clot and she is perfectly normal. Since her husband is not a hemophiliac, his one X chromosome must bear the nor-mal allele. One can use a Punnett square to predict the likelihood of their children inheriting the disease (see figure 4). From this figure, one can see that their daugh-ters should all be normal. About half of them will be carriers for the trait, but there is no way of knowing which ones they are. Of the sons, one half will be nor-mal and the other half will suffer from hemophilia.

FIGURE 4. A PUNNETT SQUARE SHOWING ALLELES FOR HEMOPHILIA

Father's Sperm Cells

		X	Y
Mother's Egg Cells	X	XX Normal Girl	XY Normal Boy
	X_h	XX_h Normal Girl (carrier)	X_hY Hemophiliac Boy

HOW MUTATIONS OCCUR

There is a variety of genetic information in the human population, leading to a diversity of internal and exter-nal features. The process of sexual reproduction ran-domly selects among that variety for each new individ-ual who is born. Mutation is the process that created the variety originally, and it can continue to add to it today.

A human being begins as a single fertilized cell. That cell contains two copies of the genetic information in its twenty-three pairs of chromosomes. The cell divides constantly during growth and development to produce the millions of cells that make up an adult. Each one of those cells, with very few exceptions, also has twenty-three pairs of chromosomes. In order for each cell to have its own double copy of information, the DNA that makes up the chromosomes must replicate, once for each cell division. This process of replication must ensure that the information contained in the DNA is copied exactly, and for the most part, it is.

To understand how a mistake can occur, one must look at the structure of DNA, the genetic blueprint. The DNA molecule resembles a spiral staircase. The outside rails are strings of sugar molecules hooked together by phosphate groups. The steps are made of bases that project from each sugar-phosphate backbone toward the middle. The information is contained in the sequence of base pairs that make up the steps of the staircase. The bases that can form such a pair are determined by their shape and bonding properties. Of the four bases, only two pairs are possible. Adenine (A) always pairs with thymine (T), leaving cytosine (C) and guanine (G) to form the other pair. This structure explains the accuracy with which DNA replicates. During replication, the original molecule unwinds from its spiral structure. The two strands separate, and a new complementary strand forms on each of the original strands. The order of bases on the new strand is determined by the original strand and the base-pairing rules. Where there is an A in the old strand, there must be a T in the new one. The other bases will not fit because they do not have the correct shape or bonding properties. Similarly, where the old strand has a C, the new one must have a G. Each base is attached to a deoxyribose sugar and a phosphate group, all three forming a nucleotide. Once all proper nucleotides are linked together, the new strand is complete, the original DNA is rewound, and there are two molecules where there once was one.

The accuracy with which the DNA template is copied is impressive. It has been estimated that an error occurs only once for every 100,000 nucleotides copied. The replication of DNA is a chemical process which relies on random movements of molecules to put the correct ones together. There are enzymatic systems to make sure that only the correct nucleotides end up as part of the new DNA strand. There are also error detection and correction mechanisms that can remove an incorrect nucleotide and replace it with the correct one. This correction process reduces the error rate to one in 10 billion. Nevertheless, with the amount of DNA that has to be copied, mistakes do occur. If a mistake is made in a cell that produces an X or Y chromosome, the mistake will be passed on to future generations as a mutation.

The mistake will not be detected until the section of DNA that contains it is actually used by the cell to make a specific protein molecule. At the molecular level, a gene is a section of DNA that has the information necessary to make a particular protein molecule. Proteins are the working molecules of the body: They make up flesh and bone and the enzymes that speed up chemical reactions. The sequence of bases on a DNA molecule codes for the sequence of amino acids that makes up a protein molecule. Since there are twenty commonly used amino acids, and a protein can contain thousands of amino acids, there is an almost infinite number of different protein molecules. A mutation on a DNA molecule will usually mean that one amino acid in the protein for which it codes is changed.

Changing one unit in a thousand may not seem very significant, and usually it is not. Such a small change in a protein molecule generally has very little effect on the functioning of that molecule. Perhaps this mutation will make the molecule able to withstand a slightly higher temperature before breaking down. If the protein is an enzyme, the change may speed or slow its reaction time by a little bit. During human evolution, an individual may have been able to live slightly longer if the mutated protein was slightly improved in function. The longer that he or she lived, the greater was the chance that the individual could produce offspring—who would also have the mutated gene. In this way, positive, useful mutations became more common in the population. A change that made the protein less functional was less likely to be reproduced since the individual possessing the mutation may not have lived long enough to have children.

A slight change in a protein can make a very big difference. The hemoglobin (the oxygen-carrying protein in red blood cells) of a person with sickle cell disease differs from normal hemoglobin by one amino acid. The amino acid, however, is in a critical position. With the changed amino acid, the hemoglobin clumps uselessly in the cell and does not carry oxygen. This is a lethal mutation, as a person afflicted with sickle cell disease cannot live very long. One would assume that this mutation would not survive in the human population. Yet, in some parts of Africa, the mutant allele is carried by as much as 20 percent of the black population. To understand how this can be, one must consider the heterozygous individual. With one normal allele and one mutant one, such an individual makes both kinds of hemoglobin, including enough normal hemoglobin to be able to live comfortably under normal conditions.

Moreover, the presence of the altered hemoglobin confers significant resistance to malaria. Because the heterozygous individual has a selective advantage over the other two genotypes, this mutant allele not only has been maintained but even has increased in the black population in Africa.

PERSPECTIVE AND PROSPECTS

The modern study of genetics is conducted mostly at the molecular level. One project has identified every human gene and its location on a specific chromosome. Dubbed the Human Genome Project, it was a cooperative venture among scientists worldwide. This map tells researchers where each gene is located, and it is hoped that the defective copies in people with genetic diseases can be repaired using this knowledge. Genetic engineering techniques have already isolated many genes. For example, the gene for the production of insulin has been identified and extracted from human cells in culture. The gene has been inserted into the chromosomes of bacteria, and the bacteria are then grown in large quantities in commercial cultures. The insulin that they produce is harvested, purified, and made available to diabetics. This genuine human insulin is more potent than the insulin extracted from animals. In addition, such a process is essential for diabetics who suffer adverse reactions to the inevitable impurities that are found in insulin extracted from animals.

Ultimately, it should be possible to insert a functioning gene, like the one for insulin, directly into an afflicted person's chromosomes—thus curing the genetic disease. The cured individual, however, would still be able to pass the defective allele on to his or her children. The possibility of splicing genes into the chromosomes of sex cells does not seem likely in the near future.

More traditional genetics is also of value to prospective parents. A woman with a history of hemophilia in her family would want to know the chances that her children could inherit the disease. A genetic counselor would analyze the family tree of the woman and calculate a statistical probability. Some other genetic diseases can be detected in a fetus still in the womb. For example, a condition called phenylketonuria (PKU) can cause severe mental retardation and other medical problems. A genetic analysis of prospective parents with a family history of the condition could indicate the likelihood of PKU occurring in their children. If the chances are high, cells of the couple's child can be ex-

tracted and tested early in pregnancy. In the case of PKU, early detection can be used to prevent the effects of the disease. If the diet of the mother and then the newborn are carefully regulated, the toxic chemical that causes the disease will not accumulate in the fetus or newborn.

Genetic mutations have not stopped occurring in modern society. In fact, they are more likely. Many environmental factors have been shown to increase the mutation rate in animals. Several types of radiation and many chemicals can increase the mutation rate. This is why an X-ray technician will place a lead apron over the abdomen of a patient being X-rayed. Lead prevents the X rays from penetrating to the genital organs, where actively dividing DNA is particularly sensitive to the radiation. Such care should always be taken to protect the genetic makeup of future generations.

—*James Waddell, Ph.D.*

See also Bacteriology; Biostatistics; Cancer; Carcinogens; DNA and RNA; Embryology; Environmental diseases; Environmental health; Genetic counseling; Genetic diseases; Genetic engineering; Genetics and inheritance; Genomics; Microbiology; Oncology; Pathology; Radiation sickness; Screening.

FOR FURTHER INFORMATION:

Campbell, Neil A., et al. *Biology: Concepts and Connections*. 5th ed. San Francisco: Pearson/Benjamin Cummings, 2006. Chapters cover classical and molecular genetics, respectively. The text is accessible, and the many diagrams are useful.

Lewin, Benjamin. *Genes IX*. 9th rev. ed. Sudbury, Mass.: Jones & Bartlett, 2007. A college textbook that discusses the entire field of molecular biology and genetics, with many references to the structure and activity of the cell nucleus. Although written at the college level, it is readable and accessible to a general audience. Many highly informative illustrations and diagrams are included.

Lewis, Ricki. *Human Genetics: Concepts and Applications*. 7th ed. New York: McGraw-Hill, 2007. A very accessible undergraduate text that covers the fundamentals, transmission genetics, DNA and chromosomes, and the latest genetic technology, among other topics.

Radman, Mirislav, and Robert Wagner. "The High Fidelity of DNA Duplication." *Scientific American* 259 (August, 1988): 40-46. Provides a readable account of the "proofreading" and error-correcting mechanisms that make mutations so rare. The author

is careful to point out what is fact and what is speculation. The bibliography refers the reader to more
technical articles on the subject.

Rusting, Ricki L. "Why Do We Age?" *Scientific American* 267 (December, 1992): 130-135. A review of
contemporary research into the genetics of aging.
Evidence is presented for the presence of genes that
determine how long animals and humans may expect
to live.

Stahl, Franklin W. "Genetic Recombination." *Scientific American* 256 (February, 1987): 90-101. This
article describes how genes are constantly shuffled
to make new genetic combinations for each generation. This process occurs when chromosomes exchange pieces during the cell divisions that produce
the sex cells.

MYASTHENIA GRAVIS
DISEASE/DISORDER

ANATOMY OR SYSTEM AFFECTED: Immune system,
musculoskeletal system, nervous system

SPECIALTIES AND RELATED FIELDS: Immunology,
neurology

DEFINITION: A disorder characterized by selective
muscle fatigue following repeated use; it is caused
by an abnormal immune reaction to specific receptors on the muscle surface.

KEY TERMS:

acetylcholine: a chemical released by motor neuron
terminals; it causes muscle contraction

acetylcholine receptor: a protein on the surface of muscle cells; binding of acetylcholine to this receptor
causes muscle cells to contract

acetylcholinesterase: an enzyme that degrades acetylcholine

antibody: a protein produced by the immune system to
inactivate substances detected as foreign

autoimmune disease: a disorder in which the immune
system targets proteins that are normal components
of body tissues

thymus: a gland located at the base of the neck; part of
the immune system

CAUSES AND SYMPTOMS

Myasthenia gravis is a neuromuscular disorder characterized by weakness of skeletal muscles following repeated use. The prevalence of the disease in the United
States is approximately 14 in 100,000. It occurs in both
genders of all ethnic groups, and the average age of onset is under forty for women and over sixty for men.

Normally, body movements result from the contraction of skeletal muscles, which are voluntary muscles
attached to bone. These muscles are stimulated to contract by motor neurons in the brain and spinal cord.
Nerve impulses travel down the motor neurons to their
terminals, where a small amount of a substance known
as a neurotransmitter is released onto the muscle's surface. In this case, the neurotransmitter is the chemical
acetylcholine. When acetylcholine binds to specific receptors on the muscle surface, contraction results.

In myasthenia gravis, an autoimmune disease, the
patient's immune system fails to recognize the acetylcholine receptors on skeletal muscle as part of "self";
thus, antibodies are erroneously produced against these
receptors. Antibody binding to acetylcholine receptors
causes the total number of functional receptors to be reduced because they are internalized and degraded by
the muscle cells. With fewer remaining receptors, the
muscle's contractile response is weakened.

The root cause of this aberrant immune response remains unknown. The thymus, a gland involved in immune function, is abnormal in about 75 percent of patients with the disease. Two distinct thymic anomalies
may occur in myasthenia gravis: thymic hyperplasia
(an increase in the number of certain immune cells in
the thymus) or thymoma (a thymic tumor). In some
late-onset cases of myasthenia gravis, however, the
thymus appears normal or even shrunken—yet these
cases are also accompanied by elevated levels of antibodies recognizing acetylcholine receptors. Such in-
consistencies are part of the reason that the relationship
between the thymus and myasthenia gravis is not fully
understood.

Skeletal muscle weakness is a symptom common to
all forms of myasthenia gravis. Because this weakness
is exacerbated with muscle use, it is not surprising that
the first muscles to be affected are those used most often. Thus, the earliest signs of the disease often involve
the muscles of the eye, including drooping of the eyelids and double vision. As other muscle groups become
affected, advancing symptoms may include difficulty
in chewing and swallowing, slurred speech, limb weakness, and breathing difficulties. Although symptoms
are highly variable from patient to patient, they often
fluctuate in severity with a similar daily pattern: Weakness is usually more pronounced in the evening than in
the morning. Factors other than exertion that can provoke symptoms include viral illness, excitement, elevated temperature, menses, and pregnancy.

Although the long-term course of the disease can

INFORMATION ON MYASTHENIA GRAVIS

CAUSES: Autoimmune disorder in which immune system fails to recognize muscle receptors as "self"

SYMPTOMS: Weakness of muscles following repeated use, resulting in visual disorders, difficulty chewing and swallowing, slurred speech, limb weakness, breathing difficulties; in most cases, abnormal thymus gland

DURATION: Chronic, usually progressive

TREATMENTS: Alleviation of symptoms; may include medications (neostigmine, prednisone, azathioprine), surgery (removal of thymus), plasma exchange

vary, it is usually progressive. In a minority of patients, weakness affects only the eye muscles. In other cases, progression is often most rapid within the first three years and may be punctuated with spontaneous temporary remissions. Treatment can help keep the symptoms under control.

Early symptoms are not always recognized as being linked to myasthenia gravis. A definitive diagnosis includes testing for the presence of antibodies that bind acetylcholine receptors. In addition, impaired nerve-muscle communication should be demonstrated in the form of specific muscle weakness elicited by repetitive nerve stimulation. Finally, it should be shown that muscle weakness is briefly relieved following the administration of edrophonium. This drug blocks the breakdown of acetylcholine, temporarily increasing the amount of the neurotransmitter available to act on muscle receptors.

TREATMENT AND THERAPY

Several treatment options have been developed with the goal of symptomatic control of myasthenia gravis. Treatment must be individually tailored depending on disease history and severity. Therapies include medications, surgery, and plasma exchange.

To improve neuromuscular transmission, drugs can be given to inhibit the action of acetylcholinesterase, the naturally occurring enzyme that degrades acetylcholine, thus prolonging the availability of acetylcholine so that its contractile effect is enhanced. Such drugs include neostigmine. Another pharmacological approach is to suppress the immune system with drugs such as prednisone and azathioprine; as a result, the production of abnormal antibodies is reduced.

Thymectomy, the surgical removal of the thymus, is commonly recommended as a treatment for myasthenia gravis. In general, this procedure is considered the most effective approach for obtaining sustained relief or remission. Maximum postsurgical improvement may take several years to occur, and results are usually best in younger patients early in their disease.

Plasma exchange is used as an immediate intervention to combat the sudden onset of severe symptoms such as respiratory failure, or in cases where the patient has not responded to other treatments. In this procedure, abnormal antibodies are removed from the blood plasma.

PERSPECTIVE AND PROSPECTS

Myasthenia gravis was first described by the British physician Thomas Willis in 1685. Although relatively rare, it was the first neurological disease to be identified as having an autoimmune basis. The understanding of the disease was aided by converging research among neurophysiologists, neurologists, and immunologists; as such, these combined approaches have helped to elucidate other autoimmune diseases.

Although patients undergoing treatment for myasthenia gravis can expect a normal life span marked by significant improvement of their symptoms, as of 2003 there was no cure for the disease. Research is aimed at gaining a better understanding of the factors triggering the autoimmune response in myasthenia gravis, elucidating the relationship between the thymus and the disease, and fully understanding the molecular basis of normal and aberrant nerve-muscle transmission. This research should guide developments in treatment strategy, with a key goal being to cure the immune abnormality that underlies the disease.

—*Mary A. Nastuk, Ph.D.*

See also Autoimuune disorders; Glands; Immune system; Immunology; Immunopathology; Muscle sprains, spasms, and disorders; Muscles; Muscular dystrophy.

FOR FURTHER INFORMATION:

Icon Health. *Myasthenia Gravis: A Medical Dictionary, Bibliography, and Annotated Research Guide to Internet References.* San Diego, Calif.: Author, 2004.

Kaminski, Henry J., ed. *Myasthenia Gravis and Related Disorders.* Totowa, N.J.: Humana Press, 2003.

Kasper, Dennis L., et al., eds. *Harrison's Principles of Internal Medicine*. 16th ed. New York: McGraw-Hill, 2005.

Vincent, Angela. "Unravelling the Pathogenesis of Myasthenia Gravis." *Nature Reviews Immunology* 2 (October, 2002): 797-804.

MYOCARDIAL INFARCTION. *See* HEART ATTACK.

MYOMECTOMY
PROCEDURE

ANATOMY OR SYSTEM AFFECTED: Reproductive system, uterus

SPECIALTIES AND RELATED FIELDS: Gynecology

DEFINITION: The removal of a uterine myoma, also known as a fibroid or leiomyoma.

INDICATIONS AND PROCEDURES

The most common indication for a myomectomy is a fibroid which causes symptoms. In many cases, these fibroids are large (greater than 8 centimeters). A myomectomy is chosen over a hysterectomy (removal of the uterus) if the patient desires future childbearing and if there is no evidence of malignancy of the uterus. A myomectomy can be performed using abdominal, laparoscopic, vaginal, or hysteroscopic approaches. The choice of approach depends on the location and size of the fibroids, as well as on the experience of the surgeon.

The most common type is abdominal myomectomy. This procedure is performed in the operating room with the patient under general anesthesia. The abdomen is incised and entry into the pelvic cavity is obtained. The uterus is then identified and inspected for fibroids. Some surgeons apply a tourniquet to the uterine arteries for hemostasis. A vasocontrictive agent is injected into the myometrium surrounding the fibroid to minimize blood loss. The myometrium over the fibroid is then incised, and the fibroid is dissected out. Finally, the myometrial defect is closed with a suture to stop blood flow. In patients desiring fertility, care is taken to minimize entry into the endometrial cavity, as the procedure may increase the risk of uterine rupture with pregnancy.

In laparoscopic and vaginal myomectomies, access to the fibroids is obtained using endoscopic instruments and through an incision in the vagina, respectively. In hysteroscopic myomectomies, access to fibroids in the endometrial cavity is obtained using a hysteroscope inserted through the cervical canal. The hysteroscope holds an instrument that shaves away fibroids in the endometrial cavity.

USES AND COMPLICATIONS

The primary use of myomectomy is the relief of symptoms caused by fibroids. These symptoms can be any of the following: pressure sensation, pelvic pain, dyspareunia (painful intercourse), menorrhagia (excessive menstruation), dysmenorrhea (painful menstruation), urinary urgency or frequency, urinary incontinence, and constipation.

The short-term risks of abdominal myomectomies are the same as those for most pelvic surgeries. These risks are small but include infection, damage to internal organs such as the bowel or bladder, blood loss requiring transfusion, and complications from anesthesia. Long-term consequences include an increased risk of uterine rupture with future pregnancy, the recurrence of fibroid growth, and pelvic adhesion (scar tissue) formation. Laparoscopic myomectomies are less invasive than abdominal myomectomies, but the same short-term and long-term risks are present. Hysteroscopic myomectomies carry less risks than abdominal procedures, since no incision is made on the abdomen and there is no entry into the pelvic cavity, but the risks unique to hysteroscopy exist, such as uterine perforation and fluid overload.

—*Anne Lynn S. Chang, M.D.*

See also Dysmenorrhea; Genital disorders, female; Gynecology; Hysterectomy; Menorrhagia; Menstruation; Muscles; Reproductive system; Tumor removal; Tumors; Women's health.

FOR FURTHER INFORMATION:

Bieber, Eric J., and Victoria M. Maclin, eds. *Myomectomy*. Malden, Mass.: Blackwell Science, 1998.

Falcone, T., and M. A. Bedaiwy. "Minimally Invasive Management of Uterine Fibroids." *Current Opinion in Obstetrics and Gynecology* 14, no. 4. (August, 2002): 401-407.

Rock, John A., and Howard W. Jones III, eds. *Te Linde's Operative Gynecology*. 9th ed. Philadelphia: Lippincott Williams & Wilkins, 2003.

Stenchever, Morton A., et al. *Comprehensive Gynecology*. 4th ed. St. Louis: Mosby, 2006.

Tulandi, Togas, ed. *Uterine Fibroids: Embolization and Other Treatments*. New York: Cambridge University Press, 2003.

MYOPIA

DISEASE/DISORDER

ALSO KNOWN AS: Nearsightedness

ANATOMY OR SYSTEM AFFECTED: Eyes

SPECIALTIES AND RELATED FIELDS: Ophthalmology, optometry

DEFINITION: A visual defect that impairs the perception of distant objects.

CAUSES AND SYMPTOMS

Nearsightedness (myopia) occurs when light from distant objects reaches a focal point in front of the retina, the photoreceptive tissue of the eye. Consequently, vision of distant objects is blurred on the retina. The primary cause of myopia is an eyeball that is too long from front to back. Higher testosterone levels in the womb and a genetic predisposition have been advanced as possible causes of this condition. Research has also found that prolonged eyestrain, especially that which often accompanies long periods of reading, can distort

> ### INFORMATION ON MYOPIA
>
> **CAUSES:** Unknown; possibly higher testosterone levels in womb, genetic predisposition, prolonged eyestrain
> **SYMPTOMS:** Impaired perception of distant objects
> **DURATION:** Varies
> **TREATMENTS:** Wearing concave lenses, correction through laser surgery

the shape of the eye. This is one reason why well-educated people manifest higher rates of nearsightedness than less-educated individuals.

All children are born nearsighted; by the age of six months, however, vision begins to improve. Myopia is an uncommon problem in younger school-age children but begins to increase in prevalence as children move into their teenage years. From the twenties until the late sixties, the rate of visual deterioration tends to slow down. By the time people reach their seventies, however, the rate of visual decline accelerates again. People past the age of seventy are fourteen times as likely to experience myopia resulting in legal blindness as those in their twenties.

TREATMENT AND THERAPY

For several centuries, nearsightedness has been corrected by the use of a concave lens, which moves the focal point of light in myopic eyes closer to the retina. The first evidence for the use of concave lenses is found in a 1517 painting of Pope Leo X by Italian artist Raphael. As the twentieth century drew to a close, innovative surgical approaches were developed. Most of these procedures, such as laser surgery, move the focal point of light closer to the retina by changing the shape of the cornea.

—*Paul J. Chara, Jr., Ph.D.*

See also Aging; Blurred vision; Cataracts; Glaucoma; Eye infections and disorders; Eye surgery; Eyes; Laser use in surgery; Ophthalmology; Optometry; Optometry, pediatric; Sense organs; Vision disorders.

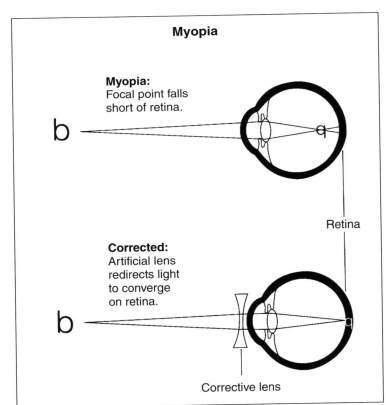

Myopia

Myopia:
Focal point falls short of retina.

Retina

Corrected:
Artificial lens redirects light to converge on retina.

Corrective lens

Myopia is commonly termed "nearsightedness" because most light rays entering the eye will not resolve, or focus, on the retina unless they are coming from a very near distance; corrective lenses or surgery can solve this problem.

FOR FURTHER INFORMATION:

Buettner, Helmut, ed. *Mayo Clinic on Vision and Eye Health: Practical Answers on Glaucoma, Cataracts, Macular Degeneration, and Other Conditions.* Rochester, Minn.: Mayo Foundation for Medical Education and Research, 2002.

Icon Health. *Myopia: A Medical Dictionary, Bibliography, and Annotated Research Guide to Internet References.* San Diego, Calif.: Author, 2004.

National Foundation for Eye Research (NFER). http://www.nfer.org/.

Riordan-Eva, Paul, and John P. Whitcher. *Vaughan and Asbury's General Ophthalmology.* 16th ed. New York: Lange Medical Books/McGraw-Hill, 2004.

Sutton, Amy, ed. *Eye Care Sourcebook: Basic Consumer Health Information About Eye Care and Eye Disorders.* 2d ed. Detroit: Omnigraphics, 2003.

MYRINGOTOMY

PROCEDURE

ANATOMY OR SYSTEM AFFECTED: Ears

SPECIALTIES AND RELATED FIELDS: Family medicine, otorhinolaryngology

DEFINITION: The creation of an opening in the eardrum (tympanic membrane) to allow drainage of accumulated fluid in the middle ear.

INDICATIONS AND PROCEDURES

Fluid can collect in the middle ear as a result of infection or allergy; this fluid consists of blood, pus, water, and debris. An ear, nose, and throat specialist may surgically insert small tubes into the middle ear to facilitate drainage. Usually, local anesthesia is administered, particularly if the patient is a young child.

This procedure, called myringotomy, is used to relieve pain caused by pressure and to prevent temporary or permanent hearing loss. Physiologically, the problem involves blockage of the Eustachian tube, a narrow canal that connects the middle ear to the back of the nasal cavity. This tube regulates air pressure in the middle-ear cavity, allowing the hearing mechanism to function properly and helping to maintain a sense of balance.

Prior to performing a myringotomy, medical treatment may involve the prescription of antihistamines, decongestants, and perhaps steroids, which usually reduce the swelling of the Eustachian tube and sometimes preclude a myringotomy. After the procedure, improvement in hearing is usually immediate, and the middle-ear infection should heal. Antibiotic eardrops may be prescribed; three or four drops should be placed in each ear twice a day for five days. In approximately six to twelve months, the myringotomy tube will be expelled into the outer ear canal automatically and can be removed by a physician. Treatment may include follow-up visits every two months.

USES AND COMPLICATIONS

Postoperatively, it is not unusual for the patient to experience a certain amount of pulsation, popping, clicking, and other sounds in the ear. It is important during the postoperative period to make certain that the patient does not get water in his or her ear, especially when the tube is in place. When washing the hair or face, cotton covered with petroleum jelly may be placed in the outer part of the ear. For long-term protection, earplugs may be used during showering, bathing, and swimming. Diving, deep swimming, and any other activities that may place pressure on the eardrum are not recommended.

—*John Alan Ross, Ph.D.*

See also Deafness; Ear infections and disorders; Ears; Hearing loss; Surgery, pediatric.

FOR FURTHER INFORMATION:

American Medical Association. *American Medical Association Family Medical Guide.* 4th rev. ed. Hoboken, N.J.: John Wiley & Sons, 2004.

Canalis, Rinaldo, and Paul R. Lambert, eds. *The Ear: Comprehensive Otology.* Philadelphia: Lippincott Williams & Wilkins, 2000.

Ferrari, Mario. *PDxMD Ear, Nose, and Throat Disorders.* New York: Elsevier, 2002.

Pender, Daniel J. *Practical Otology.* Philadelphia: J. B. Lippincott, 1992.

Sataloff, Robert T., and Joseph Sataloff. *Hearing Loss.* 4th ed. New York: Taylor & Francis, 2005.

Turkington, Carol, and Allen E. Sussman. *The Encyclopedia of Deafness and Hearing Disorders.* Rev. 2d ed. New York: Facts On File, 2004.

Woolf, Alan D., et al., eds. *The Children's Hospital Guide to Your Child's Health and Development.* Cambridge, Mass.: Perseus, 2002.

NAIL REMOVAL

PROCEDURE

ANATOMY OR SYSTEM AFFECTED: Feet, hands, nails

SPECIALTIES AND RELATED FIELDS: Emergency medicine, family medicine, internal medicine, pediatrics, podiatry, sports medicine

DEFINITION: The partial or total removal of either fingernails or toenails.

INDICATIONS AND PROCEDURES

Nail removal is one of the most common office procedures seen in primary care. Nail disorders leading to removal occur most often in toenails, but they can also occur in fingernails. Common reasons for removal are infection, ingrown nail, or trauma. Patients usually experience pain and inability to function in their normal activities. Rarely are there any systemic signs or symptoms such as fever, chills, or nausea, unless the cause is serious infection.

The patient's foot or hand is first cleansed and draped. Sterile techniques are used throughout the procedure. Patients undergoing partial or total nail removal require adequate anesthesia, which is usually done through a digital block. A digital block is performed at the base of the digit with lidocaine or similar anesthetic to numb the entire finger or toe. The provider should wait five minutes for the anesthesia to become effective. A tourniquet may be applied to minimize bleeding and enhance anesthesia. An instrument is then used to separate the nail from the nailbed with the least trauma possible. In a complete removal, the nail is then gently pulled away from the nailbed. In a partial removal, scissors are used to cut the desired amount of nail away from the intact nail. Some providers will also chemically destroy the nail matrix in the area of the partial removal to prevent recurrent ingrown nails, if clinically indicated. Compression for a few minutes may be needed to slow any bleeding from the nail removal. Topical antibiotic ointment may be applied with gauze and a compression dressing. When a toenail is removed, patients may walk immediately after the procedure and resume any activity as tolerated. Local wound care instructions are given, and, if the procedure is performed secondary to an infected digit, oral antibiotics may be ordered. The procedure usually takes approximately fifteen minutes to complete.

USES AND COMPLICATIONS

Partial nail removal or trimming may also be performed in diabetic patients or those unable to perform routine nail care. Fungal infections cannot be cured with nail removal.

Nail removal has few complications if performed properly. Pain is one of the most common complications of the procedure, especially if the digit was already infected. Bacterial infection may also occur after the procedure without proper wound care management. Bleeding may occur, as epinephrine is not used in digital blocks. Adequate compression or cautery usually stops any continued bleeding after the procedure. Patients must also be warned that the nail may not grow back with the exact same shape prior to removal. Nails should be cut straight across without curvature to prevent any ingrown nail recurrence.

—*Jeffrey R. Bytomski, D.O.*

See also Bacterial infections; Feet; Lower extremities; Nails; Podiatry; Upper extremities; Wounds.

FOR FURTHER INFORMATION:

Clark, Robert E., and Whitney D. Tope. "Nail Surgery." In *Cutaneous Surgery*, edited by Roland G. Wheeland. Philadelphia: W. B. Saunders, 1994.

Zuber, Thomas J. "Ingrown Toenail Removal." *American Family Physician* 65, no. 12 (June 15, 2002): 2547.

NAILS

ANATOMY

ANATOMY OR SYSTEM AFFECTED: Hands, feet, skin

SPECIALTIES AND RELATED FIELDS: Dermatology, histology

DEFINITION: The thin, horny plates covering the dorsal ends of the fingers or toes.

KEY TERMS:

cuticle: cutaneous or skin tissue that surrounds the nail plate on its proximal sides and provides a protective barrier to the nail bed; it is attached to the proximal nail fold and to the nail plate

hyponychium: cutaneous tissue underlying the free nail at its point of separation from the nail bed; structurally similar to the cuticle

keratinocytes: matrix basal epithelial cells that differentiate, fill with keratin, and form the dead horny substance making up the nail plate

lunula: a whitish, crescent-shaped area at the end of the proximal nail fold that marks the end of the nail matrix and is the site of mitosis and nail growth

onychomycosis: common nail disorder in which fungal organisms invade the nail bed causing progressive changes in the color, texture, and structure of the nail

STRUCTURE AND FUNCTIONS

Nails function to protect fingers and toes against bumps and trauma. Fine touch is amplified and skillful manipulation of small objects with the fingers is enabled by the presence of nails. Nails also provide the ability to scratch, both as a temporary relief of an itch or in personal defense. Nails are important social communicators of beauty and sexuality and hence are the focus of a major cosmetic industry.

Biologically, nails are characterized as plates of tightly packed, hard epidermis cells filled with a protein called keratin. Nails are normally seen on the dorsal side (the side opposite the palm or sole) of all fingers and toes. The anatomy of the normal nail consists of a nail plate, proximal nail fold, nail bed, matrix, and hyponychium. These components are epithelial derived structures, like skin and hair, which emerge from the live germinative zone of the epidermis. These cells differentiate and form the horny layer, which is considered to be dead.

The nail plate is a relatively hard and flat, transparent, horny structure that is rectangular in shape. It rests on the underlying nail bed but typically extends beyond the bed as an unattached, free-growing edge reaching beyond the tip of the finger or toe. In the fingers, the thickness of the plate in adults increases from the proximal edge to the distal edge from about 0.7 millimeter to 1.6 millimeters. The terminal tip thickness varies considerably between persons.

Normally, a pinkish nail bed is seen through the transparent nail plate. Frequently in the thumb nail and sometimes in the other fingers, a whitish, semimoon-shaped structure called the lunula is seen that extends under the proximal nail fold. The borders of the nail plate are covered by skin structures: two lateral folds and a single proximal fold.

The proximal nail fold or the cuticle is the cutaneous or skin structure that is in continuity with the visible proximal border of the nail but overlies part of the nail root. The ventral side (underside) of the proximal nail fold provides physical protection to the germinative zone of the nail and aids in the physical attachment of the nail plate. About a fourth of the total surface area of the nail plate is located under the proximal fold. The cuticle is a layer of epidermis extending from the proximal nail fold and attached to the dorsal side of the nail. The cuticle functions to provide a physical seal against microbes and chemical irritants, which may otherwise enter the matrix and affect nail production.

The nail bed is the portion of the digit upon which the nail rests. The nail bed is highly vascular, with numerous capillaries, consists of epithelial tissue, and extends from the lunula to the point where the bed separates from the nail. A series of fine longitudinal folds in the nail bed corresponds to the undersurface structure of the nail. This arrangement enhances the adherence of the nail plate to the nail bed.

The nail matrix generally is considered the most proximal part of the nail bed and is bordered by the proximal nail fold. On the distal end it is bordered by the distal margin of the lunula. The nail matrix epithelium cells consist predominantly of keratinocytes in both a basal and spinous layer. Melanocytes and Langerhans' cells are intermingled with keratinocytes. It is within the matrix that the germinating center of nail growth is found. Basal epithelial cells increase in number through mitosis or division and then differentiate into keratinocytes, which are epithelial cells filled with keratin protein. These keratinocytes condense their cytoplasm, lose their nucleus, and form flat, horny-looking cells which are dead. As further cell division occurs in the nail matrix, the more distal keratinocytes are pushed out to form the nail plate.

The hyponychium consists of epidermis tissue that underlies the edge of the nail plate and extends from the nail bed to the distal groove. It functions to provide a defense against entry of bacteria under the free edge of the nail plate. Excessively vigorous cleaning may dam-

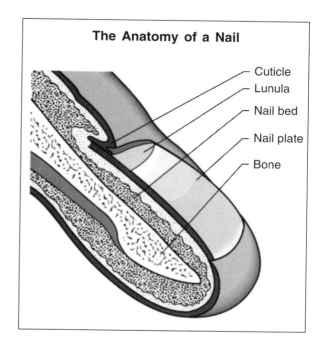

The Anatomy of a Nail

Cuticle
Lunula
Nail bed
Nail plate
Bone

age the hyponychium and allow for bacteria to enter more readily under the nail plate.

The turnover rate of matrix cells determines the growth rate of the nail. This rate varies with age, environmental conditions, nutritional status, and the specific digit. The growth rate proportionately increases with the length of the digit; thus the middle finger nail grows the fastest while the growth rate in the little finger is the slowest. Fingernails grow three times as rapidly as toenails. The growth rate is more rapid in the winter than in the summer. Furthermore, nails grow faster in young children than in older adults. It takes about six months for a fingernail to completely grow in. Male nails grow faster than female nails. Nails on the dominant hand grow faster than those on the other hand.

If nails are protected and untrimmed, they can grow to considerable lengths. Such long nails were prized by the wealthy classes in imperial Chinese culture as an indication of status. The practice of painting toenails red may have originated in the Ottoman seraglio, where it was a signal of menstrual status.

Nails continue to grow throughout life without a resting phase. Contrary to folk belief, nails cease growing when an individual dies. The matrix cells stop producing deoxyribonucleic acid (DNA) and dividing soon after death and thus the nail bed cannot grow longer. The appearance of nail growth after death is due to a retraction or shrinkage of nail matrix tissue, resulting in the apparent lengthening of the nail plate.

Professional grooming of the nails for both men and women is termed a manicure. Manicure procedures include cutting the nails according to fashion standards to improve their cosmetic appearance. A pedicure is the term applied to grooming the toenails. Typically, the nails are first soaked in a soapy solution to soften the nail plate and to remove dirt and debris. Currently it is fashionable to trim the nails to a delicate arc at the middle of the fingertip. The corners of the nail are typically filed. While this shape is attractive in creating the illusion of longer, slender fingers, it heightens the probability of nail plate fractures, hangnails, or ingrown nails. The cuticle, considered to be unattractive by manicurists, is typically minimized, partially removed, or traumatized. This may increase the incidence of fungal invasion and disease. Most of the problems associated with a manicure arise from excessive manipulation of the cuticle.

Nail polish typically consists of pigments suspended in a volatile solvent that also contains a film-forming agent. When the polish is applied to the finger, a covering film develops over the nail. The film is permeable to oxygen, which allows gas exchange to occur between the atmosphere and the nail plate. Resins and plasticizers are added to the polish to increase the flexibility of the film and to minimize chipping. The variety in nail polish color is due to the addition of coloring agents. Deep red nail polishes can cause a temporary yellowish staining of the nail plate.

Nail adornments are sometimes used. Frequently, small nail jewels or ribbons are applied to the fingernails immediately before the nail polish dries, allowing the decoration to adhere to the nail plate. Since some people frequently develop contact dermatitis to nickel, gold or nickel-free jewels should be selected. Artificial nail tips made of plastic also are glued to the nail tip to create the illusion of an elongated natural nail tip. The gluing may cause nail problems, since a portion of the natural nail is occluded by the glue. This occlusion inhibits oxygen transfer and stresses the nail plate. Frequently, the nail may thin and be unable to support its own weight after the plastic tip is removed. Removal of the plastic tip may result in nail pitting.

DISORDERS AND DISEASES

Nails are useful indicators of skin disease as well as of internal disorders. An abnormally pigmented band in the nail may indicate a malignant melanoma. A yellow nail may indicate psoriasis or a fungal infection. Pulmonary disease or smoking may also cause yellow or brownish nails. Antimalarial drugs may cause the nail to darken in appearance. Frequently, psoriasis causes pitting of nails and an acceleration in their growth rate. Chronic chest disease or a cyanotic congenital heart disorder is frequently associated with club-shaped deformity of the nail plate. Beau's lines, which are transverse depressions in the nail plates, are associated with illnesses such as coronary thrombosis, pneumonia, and severe injuries. Drug treatment may cause nail breakdown or destruction or complete shedding of the nail plate.

An unexplained aspect of nail physiology is its relationship to lung physiology. Hippocrates first described a connection between lung parenchymal disorders and an edema in the connective tissue beneath the lunula that results in clubbing. The relationship has long been recognized, but the causal link is still unexplained.

An ingrown nail results when a deformed nail grows improperly into the skin, or when the skin around the nails engulfs part of the nail. Wearing narrow, tight shoes can cause or worsen this pathology. Initially, symptoms may be slight or mild, but with time may come increasing pain. The affected area becomes reddish and, if not treated, may become infected. If infected, the area becomes swollen, inflamed, and painful. Blisters may develop. Treatment involves trimming away the nail from the infected area, allowing the inflammation to decline and the area to heal.

Clubbing is a disorder characterized by a bulblike enlargement of the nail with increased horizontal and longitudinal curvatures. Clubbing involves both fingers and toes and commonly begins at puberty. The disorder may be genetically inherited or acquired. Clubbed nails often have a spongy feel when pressure is placed on the proximal nail fold. This is due to the expanded soft tissue that underlies the nail. Acquired clubbing is often associated with another clinical pathology, most commonly pulmonary or cardiovascular disease. However, at times it is also associated with gastrointestinal inflammatory disease or cystic fibrosis.

A fungal infection is the cause of onychomycosis, which is the most common nail disorder. About half of all nail problems can be linked to this disease, which affects as many as 15 to 20 percent of people in North America. It is uncommon in children but more frequently seen in aged adults.

Several fungi may be the causal agents, although most belong to the group called dermatophytes. The fungi are present in soil, and indirect transmission to humans frequently occurs through public swimming pools and shower floors. Some yeasts and molds are also thought to cause this clinical condition. Alternatively, this infection is associated with athlete's foot infection. Typically this condition is found in toenails more frequently than fingernails. The presence of the fungus is furthered evidenced by scaling on the plantar surface of the foot, where it is often harbored.

In onychomycosis, the fungal organism invades the nail bed, causing a progressive change in the color, texture, and structure of the nail. The nail may turn white, thicken, and even detach from the nail bed. Debris from the infected nail often collects under its free edge. If untreated, the pathology may involve the entire nail plate, and rarely will the nail unit spontaneously heal itself.

Since several organisms may induce the pathology, effective treatment depends on matching the curative with the causal agent. Topically applied antifungals seldom are effective because most cannot penetrate the nail plate barrier to reach the causal organism. Sys-

temically (orally) administered antifungal therapy frequently uses one of several drugs such as griseofulvin, thiabendazole, or ketoconazole. These drugs are generally effective in halting further invasion of the fungus. While treatment continues the new growing nail is usually normal. Thus treatment typically continues until the old nail is replaced by new nail, and then the treatment is discontinued.

More than seventy tumors associated with parts of the nail have been found. Their origins may be from the epidermis, dermis, subcutaneous tissues, or the bone. The tumors may be found in the nail bed, nail matrix, hyponychium, or nail fold. The tumors may take various forms such as warts, erosion or ulceration of the nail bed, malignant neoplasms from underlying melanocytes, benign fibromas of the connective tissue, or squamous cell carcinomas. Diagnosis usually is made by taking a biopsy of the affected area. Treatment typically involves surgical removal of the tumor.

PERSPECTIVE AND PROSPECTS

The earliest cellular growth leading to nail formation can be seen histologically at eight weeks of human development, the end of the embryonic period. Microscopically, the cells forming the proximal edge of the nail field and the future matrix can be distinguished at this time. The earliest gross anatomical appearance of nails is seen on the finger digit surface at about nine weeks of development, the very early fetal stage. By eleven weeks of age, the nail field is seen clearly on the hand digits of the fetus. By twenty weeks of age, the fetus shows a nail plate and bed and a proximal cuticle. By thirty-two weeks, the third trimester of pregnancy, adult type nail structures are visible in the fetus, including a nail plate, matrix, and bed and a forming hyponychium.

Aging results in changes and disorders in nails. When people get older the color, contour, growth rate, surface texture, and thickness of the nail plate change. Some disorders are more prevalent with aging, such as brittle nails, splitting or fissuring of the nail plate, and increased infections. Aged nails appear dull and opaque, with a color varying from yellow to gray. Frequently in older persons, the lunula is decreased in size or is absent. The growth rate of nails decreases with aging. The most rapid period of growth is during the first thirty years; thereafter the rate steadily declines. With older persons, the nail plate thickness frequently increases, paralleled with discoloration and a loss of translucency of the nail plate.

For many years, blood and urine specimens have been used to detect and measure body concentrations of therapeutic drugs or drugs of abuse. During the past decade, alternative biological specimens, nails and hair, have been frequently used as the basis for drug detection. The basis for drug detection in nail clippings is that the dividing epidermal cells that form the nail plate also incorporate drugs from the systemic circulation. The subsequent cornification of these cells traps the drug within the forming nail plate. Drug detection methods involve taking a sample of nail clippings, and extracting and identifying drug molecules by using immunochemical or chromatographic techniques that are extremely sensitive and capable of detecting minute quantities of drug in the samples. As little as ten milligrams of nail clippings is required to detect the presence of drugs. Twenty-first century drug screening methods have detected amphetamines and cocaine in nail clippings. Using nail clippings for drug analysis and screening provides a long-term measure of drug exposure that potentially may represent months of drug use. Furthermore, nail clippings are relatively easy to collect and involve a noninvasive procedure; samples are easily stored, and once incorporated in the nail tissue most of the drugs are presumably stable.

Modern medicine in the early twenty-first century still lacks adequate descriptive science as well as understanding of the molecular mechanisms that control nail development and growth. To date, the specific genes or gene products that initiate nail growth have not been identified. The molecular basis for brittle nails, clubbing, and other nail pathologies is not known. Is onychomycosis affected by a systemic immune deficit? What causes yellow nail syndrome? Answers to these questions as well as additional information about the molecular control of nail physiology will greatly increase understanding and lead to better treatments for nail disorders.

—*Roman J. Miller, Ph.D.*

See also Fungal infections; Lower extremities; Nail removal; Pulmonary diseases; Skin; Skin disorders; Upper extremities.

FOR FURTHER INFORMATION:

Baran, R., et al., eds. *Baran and Dawber's Diseases of the Nails and Their Management.* 3d ed. Malden, Mass.: Blackwell Science, 2001. Describes the normal physiology and pathology of nails. Superb color photographs vividly illustrate various nail diseases.

Beers, Mark H., et al., eds. *The Merck Manual of Medical Information, Second Home Edition.* Whitehouse Station, N.J.: Merck Research Laboratories, 2003. This manual, written for home use, describes several common nail disorders. Symptoms, characteristics, and possible treatments are given.

Du Vivier, Anthony. *Atlas of Clinical Dermatology.* 3d ed. Edinburgh: Churchill Livingstone, 2002. Along with a comprehensive survey of skin pathologies, this atlas also covers nail disorders.

Hordinsky, Maria K., Marty E. Sawaya, and Richard K. Scher, eds. *Atlas of Hair and Nails.* Philadelphia: Churchill Livingstone, 2000. This vividly illustrated atlas emphasizes nail disorders and special issues affecting nail physiology. Numerous colored photographs.

Mix, Godfrey F. *Salon Professional's Guide to Foot Care.* Clifton Park, N.Y.: Delmar Learning, 1999. Written by a podiatrist for those in the beauty profession, making this an accessible guide to foot care and foot anatomy, including toenails.

Standring, Susan, et al., eds. *Gray's Anatomy.* 39th ed. New York: Elsevier Churchill Livingstone, 2005. This classic anatomy text uses simple line drawings to illustrate the parts of a nail. The accompanying text accurately describes the parts of a nail and is well recognized as authoritative by health care professionals.

Zaias, Nardo. *The Nail in Health and Disease.* 2d ed. Norwalk, Conn.: Appleton & Lange, 1992. Describes in detail the anatomy and physiology of nails, specific disorders, and cosmetic care. Written for the health care professional, this well-illustrated text is also understandable for the average reader.

NARCOLEPSY

DISEASE/DISORDER

ANATOMY OR SYSTEM AFFECTED: Brain, nervous system, psychic-emotional system

SPECIALTIES AND RELATED FIELDS: Neurology

DEFINITION: An apparently inherited disorder of the nervous system characterized by brief, numerous, and overwhelming attacks of sleepiness throughout the day.

KEY TERMS:

cataplexy: brief periods of partial or total loss of skeletal muscle tone, usually triggered by emotional stimuli, which can cause the person to collapse

electroencephalogram (EEG): a recording of brain wave activity using electrodes attached to the scalp *excessive daytime sleepiness:* a strong tendency to fall asleep, accompanied by reduced energy and lack of alertness during the entire day

hypnogogic hallucination: a bizarre, sometimes frightening, dreamlike occurrence just as one is falling asleep or just after waking

maintenance of wakefulness test: a polysomnographic technique to measure a person's ability to remain awake during repeated trials throughout the day

multiple sleep latency test: a polysomnographic technique to measure how quickly one falls asleep during repeated trials throughout the day

polysomnography: the continuous recording of brain waves, eye movements, skeletal muscle movements, and other body functions to determine bodily changes during the stages of sleep

REM sleep: a period of intense brain activity, often associated with dreams; named for the rapid eye movements that typically occur during this time

sleep paralysis: an inability to move voluntarily, occurring just at the beginning of sleep or upon awakening

CAUSES AND SYMPTOMS

Narcolepsy (*narco* meaning "numbness" and *lepsy* meaning "seizure") consists primarily of attacks of irresistible sleepiness in the daytime. The sleepiness is extreme; it has been described as the feeling that most people would experience if they tried to add columns of numbers in the middle of the night after forty-eight hours without sleep.

The narcoleptic's day is broken up by a series of brief and repetitive sleep attacks, perhaps even two hundred attacks in a single day. These transient, overpowering attacks of sleepiness may last from a few seconds to thirty minutes, with an average spell lasting two minutes. It is excruciatingly difficult, and frequently impossible, to ignore the urge to sleep, no matter how inconvenient or inappropriate. Narcoleptics typically fall asleep suddenly, on the job, in conversation, standing up, and even while eating, driving, or making love.

These sleep attacks result from an abrupt failure in resisting sleep, as opposed to a sudden surge in sleepiness, because narcoleptics are actually sleepy all day. The misconception that their daytime sleepiness is caused by insufficient nighttime sleep prompts undiagnosed patients to spend inordinately long hours in bed. Narcoleptics will be sleepy during the day regardless of how much sleep they get at night.

One of the most prominent and troubling features of

> ### INFORMATION ON NARCOLEPSY
>
> **CAUSES:** Genetic factors
> **SYMPTOMS:** Attacks of irresistible sleepiness in daytime, episodes of cataplexy, hypnogogic hallucinations, sleep paralysis, memory difficulties, eye fatigue, sleep apnea
> **DURATION:** Chronic with acute episodes
> **TREATMENTS:** Stimulant medications (dextroamphetamine, pemoline, Ritalin), tricyclic antidepressants, supportive counseling

narcolepsy is cataplexy, a sudden loss of muscle tone which causes the person to collapse. Cataplexy occurs during the daytime while the person is awake. It may involve all the muscles at once or only a select few, so the severity may range from total collapse to the ground to partial collapse of a limb or the jaw. The cataplectic sometimes remains conscious, able to think, hear, and see, although vision may be blurred. At other times, there is a brief loss of consciousness, associated with an experience of dreaming. Although most attacks of cataplexy last less than a minute, occasionally they go on for as long as twenty minutes. Cataplexy is often triggered by enjoyable feelings, laughter, or excitement during which the person suddenly crumples into a heap. For other patients, a strong negative emotion, such as fear or anger, precipitates an attack.

Many narcoleptics notice the symptom of excessive daytime sleepiness for as much as a year before the onset of cataplexy. After many years of experiencing cataplexy, some patients find that less emotional stimulus is required to induce the muscle collapse and that increasingly more muscles are involved. Others find that this symptom diminishes, possibly because they have become adept at anticipating and avoiding the situations that trigger attacks. It has been noted that other hypersomnias—that is, other diseases of excessive sleepiness—do not include cataplexy; only narcoleptics suffer from this embarrassing and troubling symptom of muscle collapse.

Many narcoleptics also experience hypnogogic hallucinations, dreams that intrude into the waking state. In normal sleep, dreaming generally occurs approximately ninety minutes after falling asleep; narcoleptics begin their sleeping episodes with vivid dreams. These hallucinations are extremely realistic and often violent. The patient sees someone else in the room or hears someone calling his or her name, for the hallucinations are nearly always visual and are usually auditory. The vivid sights, sounds, and feelings characteristic of hypnogogic hallucinations are thought to occur while the person is awake, both during the day and just at the edges of nighttime sleep. Since narcoleptics typically fall asleep dozens if not hundreds of times a day, they can experience these disturbing hallucinations with great frequency. Somewhat more than 50 percent of daytime sleep attacks include hallucinations, while only about 7 percent are usually marked by cataplexy.

Approximately 40 to 60 percent of narcoleptics suffer another frightening symptom: sleep paralysis. This condition occurs at the beginning or end of sleep and renders immobile virtually every voluntary muscle, except those around the eyes. During sleep paralysis, the mind is awake and one is aware of the external surroundings, but the muscles refuse to move. The paralysis usually lasts only a few seconds, but it may continue for as long as twenty minutes. Sleep researchers find that almost everyone has an episode of sleep paralysis that lasts a few seconds sometime during his or her lifetime. When the paralysis continues for more than a few seconds, however, it is usually a sign of narcolepsy. Although either sleep paralysis or hypnogogic hallucinations alone are distressing enough, they often happen simultaneously.

Because of their frequent, irresistible sleep attacks, narcoleptics often wobble back and forth between sleep and wakefulness in a state that has been likened to sleepwalking and is termed automatic behavior. When in this state, the person seems to behave normally but later does not remember extended periods of time. For example, narcoleptics might find themselves in a different building or several exits farther down a highway than they last remembered. Obviously, automatic behavior is very anxiety-producing; it is very troubling to narcoleptics to be unable to remember what they have done in the minutes or hours that have just passed.

In addition to these memory difficulties, some narcoleptics experience constant eye fatigue, difficulty focusing, and double vision. They also have a higher incidence of the heart abnormality called mitral valve prolapse, which affects blood flow to the left ventricle. The reason for this association is not clear.

Although narcolepsy is an illness of excessive daytime sleepiness, the nighttime sleep of those afflicted is far from normal as well. It is often troubled by restlessness and frequent awakenings, which are brief or may last for hours. Patients also experience many nightmares about murder and persecution. Many narcoleptics talk, cry out, or thrash about periodically during the night.

One narcoleptic in ten has the added complication of suffering from sleep apnea. This sleep disorder consists of recurrent interruptions in breathing during sleep. This further disturbance of nighttime sleep aggravates the narcoleptic's tendency to excessive daytime sleepiness.

Narcolepsy was once thought to be extremely rare. By the late twentieth century, however, the United States Department of Health estimated that 250,000 Americans suffer from this disease, which is more than the number afflicted by multiple sclerosis. The American Medical Association considers 250,000 to be a very conservative estimate and believes the number to be between 400,000 and 600,000.

Males and females are equally affected by narcolepsy. Although the disorder has been diagnosed in a five-year-old, its symptoms most frequently appear for the first time during adolescence. In about 75 percent of cases, the attacks begin between the ages of fifteen and twenty-five; only 5 percent of cases begin before the age of ten. Onset is rare after the age of forty; if narcolepsy seems to appear in an older person, it has probably existed undiagnosed for years. Sleep researchers believe that the extra need for sleep characteristic of adolescence may make this stage of development particularly vulnerable for the onset of narcolepsy. Thus, this disorder may typically begin in adolescence because it is somehow triggered by the brain changes associated with sexual maturation.

Between two and five persons in one thousand in the general population of the United States have scattered episodes of excessive daytime sleepiness but are not considered narcoleptics. It is not until a person has one to several attacks each day that narcolepsy is suspected.

TREATMENT AND THERAPY

Narcolepsy is now known to be a disease of the nervous system. Although incurable, it can be successfully treated with various medications once it has been diagnosed. The diagnosis of narcolepsy, however, is often slow to occur. The average interval between the first appearance of symptoms and diagnosis is often as long as thirteen years. Because early symptoms are usually mild, narcoleptics typically spend years wondering whether they are sick or whether they merely lack initiative. They are often called lazy because they repeatedly nap during the day and are lethargic even when awake. Diagnosis is made more difficult by the wide range of severity of symptoms. For example, excessive daytime sleepiness may trouble a person for ten or twenty years before cataplexy appears. Patients may even occasionally experience a temporary or partial remission in their condition. Narcoleptics often fight off their sleep attacks by ingesting large amounts of caffeine and never realize that they have an actual disease until years later.

If narcolepsy is suspected, a polysomnographic study is done at a sleep disorders center to confirm the diagnosis. The most reliable confirmation of narcolepsy can be obtained by what is called the multiple sleep latency test (MSLT). The MSLT is easy, convenient, inexpensive, and very informative. The person is given four or five opportunities to lie down and fall asleep during the daytime. Normal individuals take fifteen to thirty minutes to fall asleep. In the MSLT, falling asleep in less than five minutes is considered abnormal. Those afflicted with narcolepsy always fall asleep in less than five minutes and often within a minute. The maintenance of wakefulness test (MOWT) is also used in the confirmation of narcolepsy. In the MOWT, the person is kept all day in a comfortable reclining position. Polysomnography is used to measure the patient's ability to stay awake and how many times he or she falls asleep.

Along with the MSLT and the MOWT, a thorough physical examination is needed to discover if the person has some other disorder that can mimic narcolepsy; an underactive thyroid gland, diabetes, chronic low blood sugar, anemia, and a malfunctioning liver can each cause excessive daytime sleepiness. Similarly, drug use, poor nutrition, emotional frustration, dissatisfaction, or poor motivation can also result in the type of sleepiness that a narcoleptic experiences.

When the diagnosis of narcolepsy is confirmed, treatment usually consists of stimulant medications such as dextroamphetamine, pemoline, or methylphenidate (Ritalin) during the daytime. These stimulant drugs can increase alertness and cut down the number of sleep attacks from perhaps several per day to several per month. Unfortunately, patients can quickly develop tolerance to these medications.

Even on low doses, some patients become irritable, aggressive, or nervous, or they may develop obesity and sexual problems. It is very important, therefore, to monitor a narcoleptic carefully, determining the lowest effective dose and the best times of day to take it. It may be months before the positive effects of drug therapy are fully experienced. The MSLT will often be given on a day that one takes the medication and on another

when it is not taken, in order to evaluate the success of a given treatment.

Because specific drug and dosage schedules may have to be altered frequently, patients may repeatedly have to face drug withdrawal symptoms such as intensified sleepiness and disturbing dreams. To prevent adverse reactions, narcoleptics must often avoid certain foods and common medications. Their use of stimulant drugs may even be viewed as morally wrong, in these days of widespread drug abuse, by neighbors or coworkers who do not comprehend that narcolepsy is a disabling disease.

If cataplexy is present, medications other than amphetamines or Ritalin are required and useful. The class of drugs called tricyclic antidepressants, including protriptyline and imipramine, or the class of drugs called monoamine oxidase inhibitors may alleviate cataplexy. These medicines can often reduce attacks—for example, from three a day to three a month. In addition, effective treatment for cataplexy usually also relieves sleep paralysis and hypnogogic hallucinations.

Since the development of tolerance is common and these drugs can aggravate the symptom of sleepiness, determining the best timing and dose is critical. Another side effect of cataplexy drugs is impaired sexual function in males. Some men even discontinue these medications periodically for a day or two in order to sustain sexual relations. In addition, none of the drugs used for any symptoms of narcolepsy are safe to take during pregnancy.

In some cases, narcoleptics can be treated without medication if they carefully space naps during the day to relieve excessive sleepiness. Patients keep nap diaries to rate their alertness at regular intervals during the day. They then schedule short, strategically timed naps during those daytime periods when their sleep attacks are most likely to occur.

Naps are particularly valuable in treating children with narcolepsy because the consequences of a lifetime of medication on their development or on the course of their illness is unknown. Some children who show hyperactive behavior actually have narcolepsy; they are working frantically to overcome their persistent sleepiness and to keep themselves awake. Children with narcolepsy may also justifiably fear falling asleep, day or night, because of hallucinations and sleep paralysis.

It is evident that supportive counseling must be a strong component of treatment, whatever the patient's age. Sensitive medical monitoring can offer narcoleptics a measure of satisfactory daily living, but the use of stimulants to improve alertness may also make them more aware of their limitations and, therefore, more frustrated. Depression is not the cause of narcolepsy but may result primarily from the disruption in their lives and the feeling that they are denied the right to a "normal" life. Their constant sleepiness engenders feelings of inferiority and inadequacy. Narcoleptics usually refrain from mentioning their hallucinations and try to hide their automatic behavior for fear of being labeled insane. Loss of work, broken marriages, and social isolation are often witnesses to the crippling effects of narcolepsy.

Of all the people with narcolepsy seen at major sleep disorders centers, more than one-half have been completely disabled with respect to regular employment by the age of forty. With part-time, homebound, or self-employment, however, most narcoleptics can gain self-respect and help support themselves through work that is safe and tailored to their needs. They must be given tasks that can be divided into parts performed in relatively short time periods.

Drug and nap therapy can do little for narcoleptics without education of their families, friends, acquaintances, employers, and coworkers about the reality of this neurological disease. Most people find it hard to accept the notion that sleepiness cannot be controlled and insist that narcoleptics could be more alert if they tried harder. Narcoleptics are often stigmatized as slackers or incompetents, or assumed to be drug abusers or closet drinkers. It is most important that patients and all the people in their lives comprehend that excessive daytime sleepiness is not the patients' "fault."

Further help for narcoleptics seems to lie in animal studies, which may fill in many important pieces of the narcolepsy puzzle. The effects of the disease on behavior, the way in which it is inherited, and the benefits and risks of specific drugs continue to be evaluated in narcoleptic dogs.

PERSPECTIVE AND PROSPECTS

Once viewed as "all in the mind," narcolepsy is now recognized as a neurological disorder. Its origin is unknown, but research has already discovered evidence of possible causes. An understanding of narcolepsy both depended on and advanced the understanding of normal sleep and of other sleep disorders. Scientists define sleep as a reduction in awareness of and interaction with the environment, lowered movement and muscle activity, and partial or complete suspension of voluntary behavior and consciousness.

Although narcolepsy was named and described in 1880, it could not be genuinely studied until the 1930's, when the electroencephalograph (EEG) was developed to record brain activity during the various stages of sleep. By the 1940's, this advancement led to a description of the narcoleptic tetrad, the four usual symptoms of narcolepsy: excessive daytime sleepiness, cataplexy, sleep paralysis, and hypnogogic hallucinations.

In the 1950's, narcolepsy still only rated a paragraph in one neurology textbook, which mistakenly called it a rare variety of epilepsy. A major discovery occurred in 1960: Narcoleptics bypass the normal stages of light and deep sleep and fall directly into rapid eye movement (REM) sleep. Thus, sudden-onset REM period (or SOREMP) became the major distinguishing feature of this brain disorder.

It was soon noted that relatives of narcoleptics are sixty times more likely to have the disease than members of the general population. Clearly, there is a hereditary factor involved, and geneticists have joined the hunt for narcolepsy's cause. The hereditary aspects of the disease are particularly important to counselors because parents with narcolepsy may feel guilty if their child develops it. (Indeed, some patients abandon plans to have children.) Geneticists have found a gene which may be responsible for narcolepsy. Since the gene produces an antigen called DR2 on patients' white blood cells, which is not found in nonnarcoleptics, immunologists have also begun to search for the origins of narcolepsy.

Rapid advances have been made in the last few years in determining the cause of narcolepsy. The disease is thought to arise from a biochemical imbalance in the brain which disturbs the mechanism that activates the on/off cycle of sleep. Biochemists are studying the possible relationship of various brain chemicals called neurotransmitters to narcolepsy. A defect in the way in which the body produces or uses dopamine, acetylcholine, or some other neurotransmitter is suspected to precipitate narcolepsy, which never spontaneously disappears once it is developed. The newest discovery has been the finding of abnormalities in the structure and function of a particular group of nerve cells, called hypocretin neurons, in the brains of patients with narcolepsy. The molecules implicated in narcolepsy are neuropeptides known as orexins (originally described as hypocretins). Researchers discovered that changes in the hypocretin receptor 2 and preprohypocretin genes are able to produce narcolepsy in animals. In one study involving nine human subjects, hypocretin could not be detected in seven of the subjects. Other studies have produced hypocretin knockout mice, which have symptoms that are quite similar to those found in human narcoleptics. Hypocretins have been found to occur normally in the regions of the central nervous system that appear to be involved in the regulation of sleep. An autosomal recessive mutation has been discovered in narcoleptic dogs that alters the hypocretin receptor 2 gene. In humans, a similar disruption or deficiency in hypocretin is associated with most cases of narcolepsy, although it is still unclear as to what underlies the exact genetic predisposition to the disease. Scientists speculate that they one day may cure narcolepsy or reduce its effects with drugs mimicking secretions of the missing nerve cells or even with brain-cell transplants.

Two interesting discoveries may help in the diagnosis of narcolepsy even before the classical clinical symptoms develop. There is some evidence that REM sleep is entered with abnormal rapidity years before the disorder develops. The drug physostigmine salicylate has no effect on normal dogs but elicits cataplexy in puppies with narcolepsy. Both these discoveries may be useful in screening the children of narcoleptics.

Because narcolepsy involves the fundamental processes of sleep, the combined efforts of neuroscientists, geneticists, biochemists, immunologists, and other scientists to unravel its mysteries will continue to yield important information about the basic mechanism of sleep—that state in which humans spend almost one-third of their lives.

—Grace D. Matzen

See also Apnea; Brain; Electroencephalography (EEG); Hallucinations; Memory loss; Nervous system; Neurology; Neurology, pediatric; Paralysis; Sleep; Sleep disorders; Sleeping sickness; Unconsciousness.

FOR FURTHER INFORMATION:

Bassetti, Claudio L., Michel Billiard, and Emmanuel Mignot, eds. *Narcolepsy and Hypersomnia.* New York: Informa Healthcare, 2007. Discusses narcolepsy as an autoimmune disease. Covers diagnostic procedures, criteria, genetics, and epidemiological surveys.

Caldwell, J. Paul. *Sleep: The Complete Guide to Sleep Disorders and a Better Night's Sleep.* Rev. ed. Toronto: Firefly Books, 2003. A thorough examination of sleep disorders constitutes a good portion of this book, including such topics as what causes sleep apnea, sleep disorders in children and seniors, what drugs interfere and help with sleep, and treatment guidelines.

Dement, William C. *The Sleepwatchers.* Stanford, Calif.: Stanford Alumni Association, 1992. A lively and often amusing book by the chair of the National Commission on Sleep Disorders Research. Traces the story of such research since the 1950's, when Dement first studied narcolepsy. Solid science that reads like a novel.

Hartmann, Ernest. *The Sleep Book: Understanding and Preventing Sleep Problems in People over Fifty.* Glenview, Ill.: Scott, Foresman, 1987. An easily understood discussion by a well-known pioneer in normal sleep and sleep disorders research. Contains a forty-page appendix of sleep disorders classification, centers, and specialists.

Kryger, Meir H., Thomas Roth, and William C. Dement, eds. *Principles and Practices of Sleep Medicine.* 4th ed. Philadelphia: Elsevier/Saunders, 2005. Covers normal sleep and abnormal sleep, including narcolepsy and the diagnostic and therapeutic aspects of sleep problems.

Narcolepsy Network. http://www.narcolepsynetwork .org/. Provides referral service, support group meetings, and communication among members.

Poceta, J. Steven, and Merrill Mitler, eds. *Sleep Disorders: Diagnosis and Treatment.* Totowa, N.J.: Humana Press, 1998. This volume fills an important need by making this field accessible to primary care physicians and giving them the tools and confidence to diagnose and treat those cases that do not need specialized help. It also makes clear which patients should be referred to a sleep disorder service and when.

Reite, Martin, John Ruddy, and Kim E. Nagel. *Concise Guide to Evaluation and Management of Sleep Disorders.* 3d ed. Washington, D.C.: American Psychiatric Press, 2002. Goals of this book are to provide a portable and practical approach to the diagnosis and treatment of sleep problems and a current summary of the classification of sleep disorders.

Walsleben, Joyce A., and Rita Baron-Faust. *A Woman's Guide to Sleep: Guaranteed Solutions for a Good Night's Rest.* New York: Crown, 2001. Writing in an informal, easily comprehensible style, Walsleben, director of the Sleep Disorders Center at New York University School of Medicine, and freelancer Baron-Faust cover nearly every sleep disorder suffered by women.

Narcotics

Treatment

Anatomy or system affected: Brain, nervous system, psychic-emotional system

Specialties and related fields: Pharmacology

Definition: The use of drugs from the opiate family, which mimic the action of the body's own painkilling substances, to treat pain, anxiety, coughing, diarrhea, and insomnia.

Key terms:

agonist: a drug which acts in a fashion similar to that of a hormone or neurotransmitter normally found in the body

analgesia: the absence of pain; analgesics are compounds that stop the neurotransmission of pain messages

antagonist: a drug which acts to block the effects of a hormone or neurotransmitter normally found in the body

brain stem: the region between the brain and spinal cord that controls such functions as respiration and heart rate

central nervous system: the brain and spinal cord

dependence: a craving for a drug

endogenous: something naturally found in the body, such as neurotransmitters

exogenous: something originating outside the body and administered orally or by injection

neuron: a nerve cell that can conduct electrical impulses from one region of the body to another; it is capable of releasing neurotransmitters

neurotransmitter: a chemical substance released by one nerve cell to stimulate or inhibit the function of an adjacent nerve cell; a chemical message released from a neuron

opioids: drugs derived from opium; also known as narcotics or opiates

tolerance: the ability to endure ever-increasing amounts of a drug

The Effects of Narcotics

Narcotics are drugs commonly used to treat pain (analgesics), suppress coughing, control diarrhea, and aid in anesthesia. These drugs are some of the oldest and most used agents. Most drugs are able to alter the effects of body functions by mimicking naturally occurring chemicals (as with agonists) or by blocking the physiological effects of these chemicals (as with antagonists).

Researchers have examined the many effects of the substances derived from the opium poppy, including morphine, codeine, and heroin. They have identified endogenous opioid-like chemicals called endorphins, dynorphins, and enkephalins that act as neurotransmitters; that is, some opioid compounds are normally found in the human nervous system as substances that allow nerve cells to communicate with one another. The synthetic opioid morphine mimics the actions of endorphins, dynorphins, and enkephalins by taking the place of these neurotransmitters. Scientists and physicians now know that morphine and related compounds produce their major effects by acting on the central nervous system, which includes the brain and spinal cord. In order to understand how opioids affect the body's response to pain, one must first understand the physiology of pain.

Any time tissues are damaged, they release chemical substances into the space outside the damaged cell, known as the extracellular space. Sensory neurons that have the ability to detect these chemicals are known as pain neurons. Once the chemicals bind to receptors on a pain neuron, the neuron is stimulated to send an electrical message to the spinal cord. Two actions occur once this message arrives. The first is an immediate initiation of a reflex which attempts to remove the tissue from the source of injury. For example, when one accidentally places an arm on a hot stove, a neural reflex causes the muscles of the limb to retract the arm from the burner. This is accomplished when the pain neuron releases a chemical message (neurotransmitter) in the spinal cord to stimulate neurons that control the muscles of the affected limb. This neurotransmitter is known as substance P. The second action of the sensory pain neuron is to inform the brain of the tissue damage, so that appropriate behavioral modification can take place. For example, one may become more cautious around the kitchen after burning one's arm on the stove. Notification of the brain is also accomplished by activating a second neuron using the neurotransmitter substance P, which will carry this electrical message toward the brain. Morphine and related opioids are very effective analgesics that seem to alter this pathway, thus dampening the transmission of pain messages.

Morphinelike drugs act at several sites in the nervous system. One of the most clinically important places is within the spinal cord at the region where the pain neurons release substance P. Opioids are known to reduce the amount of substance P that is released and thereby to decrease the stimulatory message in the neural pathway to the brain. If the pain impulses traveling to the brain are reduced, so is one's perception of pain. The second area of the nervous system known to be involved in regulating the perception of pain is a diffuse area of neurons located between the brain and spinal cord referred to as the brain stem. When researchers stimulate a region of the brain stem, the pain impulses traveling to the brain are reduced. Opioid peptides have been identified in this area which, as in the spinal cord, are probably responsible for reducing the pain message.

Because exogenous opioids must act to mimic endogenous opioids, one may wonder why there is a need for narcotic drugs if the body already produces the opioid-like endorphins and enkephalins. The reason is that every individual has a different degree of pain tolerance. How much pain one can endure also changes with certain circumstances. For example, one hardly notices the pain of a cut when participating in an exciting outdoor game. If the same wound occurs while one's attention is focused on it, however, the cut becomes noticeably painful. Perhaps the best explanation for the differing interpretation of pain during these activities and among different people is the endogenous opioid system. It is likely that the acupuncture pins used to block pain messages cause neurons to release increasing amounts of endorphins, enkephalins, and dynorphins. In the same way, with the administration of narcotics, one artificially increases the amount of opioids in the body in order to block pain impulses.

Opioids act on the brain stem to affect several systems other than the one associated with pain. They suppress coughing in a way that is similar to their effect on neural signals to decrease pain messages to the brain. Narcotics seem to inhibit release of the neurotransmitters responsible for the cough reflex. Unfortunately, opioids can activate another area in the brain stem to produce nausea and vomiting. This unwanted effect is related to the dose and type of drug used. Therefore, physicians can usually diminish the vomiting response with appropriate treatment selections. Perhaps the most dangerous problem with opioid usage is the effect that opioids have on the brain stem's regulation of respiration. When the brain stem senses that the level of carbon dioxide is too high, breathing is increased to rid the body of this excess waste gas. Narcotics decrease the responsiveness of the brain stem to carbon dioxide. Therefore, breathing rates tend to be inappropriately low, causing a buildup of carbon dioxide.

Constriction of the pupils of the eyes is a very common effect of opioids on the visual system. In fact, this constriction serves as an important diagnostic clue in examining a patient who has taken an overdose of a narcotic.

Opioids have a constipating effect, indirectly through the central nervous system and directly through their influence on the intestines. Opioids cause a decrease in peristalsis, the series of muscular contractions of the intestinal wall that would normally move food toward the anus.

Most opioid analgesics have no direct effect on the heart and blood vessels. Thus, they do not alter heart rate or rhythm or blood pressure to any significant degree. The only noticeable effect of narcotics on the cardiovascular system is a flushing and warming of the skin because of a slight increase in blood flow to the skin. Occasionally, this is accompanied by sweating. Kidney function tends to be depressed by opioids, which may be attributable to a decrease in the amount of blood that is filtered through the kidneys. There is also a decrease in the ability to urinate, as these drugs increase contraction of the muscle that prevents urine from leaving the bladder.

USES AND COMPLICATIONS

Medical personnel use this knowledge of how narcotics alter the body to the patient's advantage. Narcotics are used in the relief of pain and anxiety, as sedatives and anesthetics, to reduce coughing, and as a way to control diarrhea.

Opioid analgesics are among the most effective and valuable medications for the treatment of serious pain. Morphinelike drugs dampen the pain response but do not affect to a great extent other senses such as vision and hearing. They are often used to treat pain in the postoperative period, in which they effectively reduce or eliminate the short-term pain from tissue trauma that is caused by surgery. When pain is reduced, patients tend to eat, sleep, and recover much more rapidly. Physicians often prescribe narcotics such as meperidine (Demerol) or codeine on an as-needed basis. In this way, the patient, who knows firsthand the effectiveness of the drug, can control the frequency of analgesic administration. In fact, patients are usually advised to administer a small dose before the pain becomes too intense, thus decreasing the pain message before it reaches a high level and requires a relatively high dose to make the patient comfortable again.

A painful sensation consists of the neural response to the tissue damage and the patient's reaction to the stimulus. The analgesic properties of narcotics are related to their ability to diminish both pain perception and the reaction of the patient to pain. These drugs effectively raise the threshold for pain, perhaps because of the euphoria experienced by patients given opioids. For example, a patient in pain who is given morphine experiences a pleasant floating sensation with a great reduction in distress and anxiety. It is interesting to note, however, that subjects who are not in pain do not experience euphoria when given morphine. In fact, they tend to have an unpleasant response known as dysphoria, which often includes restlessness and a feeling of general discomfort.

Physicians and other health care workers must achieve a delicate balance between alleviating pain from known causes and masking pain as a warning signal from unexpected sources. For example, a patient having abdominal surgery would likely require relatively high doses of narcotic analgesics to reduce the postoperative pain. Yet the administration of an analgesic could mask the pain from an unexpected abdominal infection. Therefore, if used excessively, narcotics may prevent the early recognition of complications.

In addition to their analgesic effects, opioids tend to have a sedative effect and are often used as a preanesthetic drug or as an anesthetic. Potent opioids are used in relatively large doses to achieve general anesthesia, particularly in patients undergoing heart surgery. These narcotics are also commonly used during other surgeries in which it is important that heart function be affected only minimally. Examples of narcotic agents used in anesthesia include fentanyl (Sublimaze), sufentanil, and alfentanil.

Suppression of the cough reflex is a clinically useful effect of narcotics. The therapeutic doses of opioids needed to reduce coughing are much lower than the doses to achieve analgesia. The opioid derivatives most commonly used to suppress the cough reflex are codeine, dextromethorphan, and noscapine. How these agents work to reduce coughing is not known, but they are thought to act on the brain stem.

Diarrhea from almost any cause can be controlled with opioids. Diphenoxylate (Lomotil) and loperamide (Imodium), narcotics commonly used to treat diarrhea, do not possess analgesic properties. These drugs appear to act on the nerves within the intestinal tract to decrease muscular activity.

Like all drugs, narcotics have both beneficial and undesired effects. The toxic effects of an opioid depend on the dosage, the agent used, the clinical condition in which it is used, and an individual patient's response to the drug. Some of the more common unwanted effects include restlessness and hyperactivity instead of sedation, respiratory depression, nausea and vomiting, increased pressure within the brain, low blood pressure, constipation, urinary retention, and itching around the nose. Most of these conditions are of short duration and resolve themselves after the drug has been discontinued.

Patients, or more often narcotic drug abusers, may become tolerant and dependent upon these agents. These individuals, such as heroin abusers, have a strong craving for the drugs. These agents are abused for their euphoric effect at relatively high doses. The human body is very efficient in tolerating the effects of opioids. Their effects lessen somewhat with each succeeding dose, so that a higher dose must be taken to achieve the same effect. Physiological adaptation to the long-term use of opioids (two to three weeks) causes the development of tolerance for these drugs.

Exogenous opioids take the place of endogenous ones. Therefore, the nervous system and other physiological systems attempt to bring the levels of these neurotransmitters back to normal. First, the liver speeds up its metabolism of the drugs to eliminate them from the system more rapidly. Second, the regions of the nervous system that respond to opioids become desensitized by reducing the number of neural receptors that are available. Finally, after a few weeks of high levels of opioids, changes in other areas of the brain attempt to compensate for the rising opioid levels. Individuals who abruptly stop taking the drugs enter a period of withdrawal in which the symptoms are similar to a bad case of influenza. Morphine and heroine withdrawal symptoms usually start within twelve hours of the last dose. Peak symptoms of narcotic withdrawal occur after one to two days. Most symptoms gradually subside and are usually gone after one week. It should be emphasized that, under a physician's direction, the abuse potential of narcotics is very low.

There are certain clinical conditions in which opioid drugs should not be used or should be used with extreme caution. Because of the potential for respiratory depression with opioid treatment, these drugs should not be administered to patients with head injuries or impaired lung function. Most opioid drugs can cross the placenta and therefore should be avoided during pregnancy; with long-term use, the infant can be born addicted to narcotics.

Fortunately, some drugs can reverse the effects of narcotics. Three opioid antagonists are nalmefene, naloxone (Narcan), and naltrexone (Trexan). When these agents are given in the absence of an opioid agonist, they have no noticeable effect. When administered to a morphine-treated patient, however, they completely reverse the opioid effects almost immediately. These narcotic antagonists are particularly useful in treating patients who have taken an overdose of opioids. Such patients often arrive in the hospital emergency room not breathing and in a coma. These antagonists will normalize respiration, restore consciousness, and counteract other opioid effects. Interestingly, individuals who have become tolerant to and dependent upon opioids will immediately experience withdrawal symptoms when given naloxone or naltrexone.

PERSPECTIVE AND PROSPECTS

Narcotic drugs were originally found in the opium poppy five thousand years ago. Opium is obtained from the milky fluid of the unripe seed capsules of the poppy plant. The juice is dried in the air and forms a brown, sticky substance. With continued drying, the mass can be pulverized into powder. It is this powder that contains opioids. Morphine, codeine, and papaverine are the natural opioids that are used clinically. Most other narcotics are chemically derived.

The opium poppy, *Papaver somniferum*, was named after the Roman god of sleep, Somnis. Ancient Egyptian medical texts listed opium as a cure for illness and as a poison. Although opium was used extensively, the abuse potential was low because the poppy has a very bitter taste. Smoking opium became popular in eighteenth century China as a treatment for severe diarrhea and was also used as a socially acceptable drug mainly for its euphoric effects.

The opium poppy contains more than twenty distinct agents with a variety of potencies and unwanted effects. In 1806, a pharmacist refined opium into one active substance, morphine, which was found to be ten times as potent. Morphine was named after Morpheus, the Greek god of dreams, because the drug has powerful sedative effects. The discovery of other medically active agents quickly followed. Codeine and papaverine were identified next and found to be slightly less potent than morphine. At this time, clinicians used these purified products rather than the crude opium juice.

Shortly after purified narcotics became available, so did the widespread use of hypodermic needles. This allowed physicians to administer narcotics directly into the bloodstream. The injected opioids would travel via the blood to the brain in as short a time as twenty seconds. In the United States, morphine found widespread use as an analgesic for wounded soldiers during the Civil War. It was one of the most powerful painkillers available to physicians, but its unrestricted availability created great potential for addiction with long-term use.

Opioids became so popular that hundreds of medications became available to the public. These tonics promised to cure everything from "tired blood" to common aches and pains. Their widespread, unregulated use produced a large number of addicts. At the beginning of the twentieth century, the U.S. government attempted to reduce the number of addicts by making it illegal to buy any opioid-containing compound without a prescription. Medical scientists tried to synthesize compounds with morphinelike characteristics but without the addictive effects.

Physicians now have available to them a wide range of narcotics with different pharmacological properties. For example, there are drugs without addictive, euphoric, or sedative properties that can treat coughing or diarrhea. Some of these are available without a prescription for the treatment of occasional coughing and diarrhea. Narcotic analgesics, however, are given only under the direction of a physician. For example, morphine is still used as a potent pain reliever; when it is used appropriately, there is little chance of addiction. It is likely that other clinical uses will be found for narcotic drugs as researchers learn more about the human body's own endogenous narcotics, the endorphins.

—*Matthew Berria, Ph.D.*

See also Addiction; Anesthesia; Anesthesiology; Coughing; Diarrhea and dysentery; Marijuana; Over-the-counter medications; Pain; Pain management; Pharmacology; Self-medication.

FOR FURTHER INFORMATION:

Acker, Caroline Jean. *Creating the American Junkie: Addiction Research in the Classic Era of Narcotic Control.* Baltimore: Johns Hopkins University Press, 2002. A fascinating examination of how the construction of addiction in the early twentieth century was influenced by a nexus of actors and events: psychiatrists, pharmacologists, and the American Medical Association's campaign to reduce prescriptions of opiates.

Davenport-Hines, J. P. *The Pursuit of Oblivion: A Global History of Narcotics.* New York: W. W. Norton, 2002. Blends social, political, and cultural history to trace the evolution of drugs, their role in society, and addiction.

Griffith, H. Winter. *Complete Guide to Prescription and Nonprescription Drugs.* Revised and updated by Stephen Moore. New York: Penguin Group, 2006. A complete guide to both prescription and nonprescription drugs, including major uses, unwanted effects, precautions, and interactions with other drugs. A highly organized, useful tool for the nonscientist.

Inaba, Darryl S., William E. Cohen, and Michael E. Holstein. *Uppers, Downers, All Arounders: Physical and Mental Effects of Psychoactive Drugs.* 5th ed. Ashland, Oreg.: CNS, 2003. Mainly covers drug abuse, but also contains brief descriptions of the history and medical uses for drugs with abuse potential. A reader-friendly book that offers numerous statements from drug addicts regarding their addiction and, in some cases, their recovery.

Ling, W., and D. R. Wesson. "Drugs of Abuse: Opiates." *Western Journal of Medicine* 152 (May, 1990): 565-572. This article reviews the ways that addiction can be treated. Also addresses the use of narcotic antagonists in the treatment of drug overdose.

Liska, Ken. *Drugs and the Human Body, with Implications for Society.* 7th ed. Upper Saddle River, N.J.: Prentice Hall, 2004. Examines the use of drugs in the North American culture by discussing such topics as what constitutes a drug and where drugs come from, federal laws, drug metabolism, and the different classifications of drugs.

Voth, Eric A., Robert L. Dupont, and Harold M. Voth. "Responsible Prescribing of Controlled Substances." *American Family Physician* 44 (November, 1991): 1673-1680. This article details some of the important problems in prescribing narcotics. Gives a description of characteristics that both health care workers and nonprofessionals can watch for in their attempts to identify drug abusers.

NASAL POLYP REMOVAL

PROCEDURE

ANATOMY OR SYSTEM AFFECTED: Head, nose

SPECIALTIES AND RELATED FIELDS: Family medicine, general surgery, otorhinolaryngology

DEFINITION: The excision of benign growths that project from the mucous membrane lining the nasal cavity.

INDICATIONS AND PROCEDURES

Nasal polyps are swollen masses that project from the nasal wall. These benign structures are commonly found in patients with allergies. They may cause chronic nasal obstruction, which results in diminished air flow through the nasal cavity.

Once a polyp is detected, the physician may prescribe a nasal spray to reduce its size, such as the corticosteroids beclomethasone or flunisolide. This treatment is usually effective for small nasal polyps that cause only minor symptoms. When pharmacological management is not successful, however, the polyps should be removed surgically.

Surgical removal of nasal polyps (nasal polypectomy) is typically done as an outpatient procedure. It requires either general anesthesia or local anesthesia with sedation. After the patient is asleep or sedated, the lining of the nasal cavity is injected with a combination of local anesthesia and epinephrine to control pain and bleeding. The surgeon (usually an otorhinolaryngologist) visualizes the polyps with a headlight, and the polyps are removed with specialized, long surgical instruments inserted into the nasal cavity. After the polyps are removed, the nasal passages are packed with ointment-coated gauze to help control bleeding and aid in the healing of the nasal mucosa. The gauze is removed in

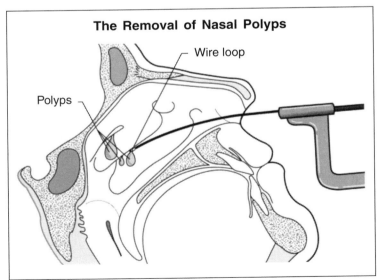

The Removal of Nasal Polyps

Wire loop

Polyps

Allergies or chronic sinus infections can lead to the development of nasal polyps, distended areas of the nasal lining. If they interfere with breathing or the sense of smell or if they cause frequent nosebleeds, the polyps may be removed with a wire loop.

the physician's office a few days after the surgery. Once the packing is removed, the patient enjoys improved breathing through the nasal passages.

USES AND COMPLICATIONS

There are relatively few complications associated with nasal polyp removal. Some of the more common complications include bleeding from the surgical site, nasal and ear discomfort or anxiety as a result of the packing, and nausea from the anesthesia. The recurrence of nasal polyps after polypectomy is not unusual. Patients with cystic fibrosis have a high rate of occurrence of nasal polyps and often have recurrent problems.

—Matthew Berria, Ph.D., and Douglas Reinhart, M.D.

See also Allergies; Nasopharyngeal disorders; Otorhinolaryngology; Sense organs; Sinusitis; Smell.

FOR FURTHER INFORMATION:

Adelman, Daniel C., et al., eds. *Manual of Allergy and Immunology.* 4th ed. Philadelphia: Lippincott Williams & Wilkins, 2002.

Benjamin, Bruce, et al. *A Color Atlas of Otorhinolaryngology.* Edited by Michael Hawke. Philadelphia: J. B. Lippincott, 1995.

Bull, P. D. *Lecture Notes on Diseases of the Ear, Nose, and Throat.* 9th ed. Malden, Mass.: Blackwell Science, 2002.

Ferrari, Mario. *PDxMD Ear, Nose, and Throat Disorders.* New York: Elsevier, 2002.

Icon Health. *Nasal Polyps: A Medical Dictionary, Bibliography, and Annotated Research Guide to Internet References.* San Diego, Calif.: Author, 2004.

Kimball, Chad T. *Colds, Flu, and Other Common Ailments.* Detroit: Omnigraphics, 2002.

Morelock, Michael, and J. B. Vap. *Your Guide to Problems of the Ear, Nose, and Throat.* Philadelphia: Lippincott Williams & Wilkins, 1985.

Settipane, Guy A., et al., eds. *Nasal Polyps: Epidemiology, Pathogenesis, and Treatment.* Providence, R.I.: OceanSide, 1997.

NASOPHARYNGEAL DISORDERS
DISEASE/DISORDER

ANATOMY OR SYSTEM AFFECTED: Nose, respiratory system, throat

SPECIALTIES AND RELATED FIELDS: Family medicine, occupational health, otorhinolaryngology

DEFINITION: Disorders of the nose, nasal passages (sinuses), and pharynx (mouth, throat, and esophagus).

KEY TERMS:

acute disease: a short and sharp disease process

chronic disease: a lingering illness

esophagus: the tube that leads from the pharynx to the stomach

larynx: the organ that produces the voice, which lies between the pharynx and the trachea; commonly called the voice box

nasopharyngeal: referring to the nose and pharynx (the upper part of the throat that leads from the mouth to the esophagus)

trachea: a tube that leads from the throat to the lungs; commonly called the windpipe

CAUSES AND SYMPTOMS

Nasopharyngeal disorders include all the diseases that can be present in the nasal cavity and the pharynx. These include the common cold, pharyngitis (sore throat), laryngitis (inflammation of the larynx), epiglottitis (inflammation of the lid over the larynx), tonsillitis (inflammation of the lymph nodes at the rear of the mouth), sinusitis (inflammation of the sinus cavities that surround the nose), otitis media (earache that is often associated with nasopharyngeal infection), nosebleed, nasal obstruction, halitosis (bad breath), and various other disorders.

The common cold is one of the most prevalent diseases that afflict humankind. Pharyngitis, or sore throat, often accompanies the common cold, or it may appear by itself. Acute infections can be caused by viruses or bacteria, often by certain streptococcus strains—hence the common term for the disorder, strep throat. Acute pharyngitis can also be caused by chemicals or radiation. As a chronic disorder, pharyngitis can be caused by lingering infection in other organs such as the lungs and sinuses, or it can be attributable to constant irritation from smoking, drinking alcohol, or breathing polluted air. The usual symptoms of pharyngitis include sore throat, difficulty in swallowing, and fever. The infected area appears red and swollen. Ordinarily, pharyngitis is not serious. If certain strains of streptococcus are the cause, however, then the infection may progress to rheumatic fever. This disease appears to be the result of an immune system reaction to some streptococcus bacteria. It can have painful effects in many parts of the body, such as in joints, and can do permanent damage to parts of the heart. In rare cases, rheumatic fever can be fatal.

Acute laryngitis is usually caused by a viral infection, but bacteria, outside irritants, or misuse of the voice are other causes. Ordinarily, the vocal cords produce sounds by vibrating in response to the air passing over them. When inflamed or irritated, they swell, causing distortion in the sounds produced. The voice becomes hoarse and raspy and may even diminish to a soft whisper. This distortion of sound is the main symptom of laryngitis, but there may also be a sore throat and congestion that causes constant coughing. The condition generally resolves itself and requires no treatment. Chronic laryngitis has the same symptoms but does not go away spontaneously. It may be caused by an infectious agent but more likely is attributable to some irritant activity, such as constantly misusing the voice, smoking, drinking alcohol, or breathing contaminated air.

The epiglottis is a waferlike tissue covered by a mucous membrane that sits on top of the larynx. It can become infected by such microorganisms as the bacteria *Haemophilus influenzae* type b in a condition called epiglottitis. Although the symptoms of epiglottitis can resemble those of pharyngitis, the infection can quickly progress to a very serious, life-threatening disorder. Epiglottitis usually afflicts children from two to four years of age, but adults can also be affected. The infection can begin rapidly, causing the epiglottis to swell and obstruct the airway to the lungs, creating a major medical emergency. Within twelve hours of the onset of symptoms, 50 percent of patients require hospitalization and intubation (insertion of a breathing tube into the trachea). The symptoms are high fever, severe sore throat, difficulty in breathing, difficulty in swallowing, and general malaise. As the airway becomes more and more occluded, the patient begins to gasp for air. The lack of oxygen may cause cyanosis (blue color in the lips, fingers, and skin), exhaustion, and shock.

Another disease associated with the larynx is croup, or laryngotracheobronchitis. As the medical name indicates, croup involves the larynx, the trachea, and the bronchi (the large branches of the lung). It is usually caused by a virus, but some cases are attributable to bacterial infection. Children from three to five years of age are the usual victims. This disease causes the airways to narrow because of inflammation of the inner mucosal surfaces. Inflammation causes coughing, but the narrowed airway causes the cough to be sharp and brassy, like the barking of a seal. Croup is usually relatively benign, but sometimes it progresses to a severe disease requiring hospitalization.

Various other disorders can afflict the larynx, such as damage to the vocal cords because of infection by bacteria, fungi, or other microorganisms. The vocal cords can also be damaged by misusing the voice, smoking, or breathing contaminated air. Polyps (masses of tissue growing on the surface), nodes (little knots of tissue), or "singers' nodules" may develop. Sores called contact ulcers may form on the vocal cords.

Tonsillitis is an inflammation of two large lymph nodes located at the back of the throat, the tonsils. It may also involve the adenoids, lymph nodes located at the top of the throat. The function of these lymph nodes is to remove harmful pathogens (disease-causing organisms) from the nasopharyngeal cavity. At times, the load of microorganisms that they absorb becomes more than they can handle, and they become infected. The tonsils and adenoids may then become enlarged. A sore throat develops, along with a headache, fever, and chills. Glands of the neck and throat feel sore and may become enlarged. Young adults can also suffer from quinsy, or peritonsillar abscess. In this condition, one of the tonsils becomes infected and pus forms between the tonsil and the soft tissue surrounding it. Quinsy is characterized by pain in the throat and/or the soft palate, pain on swallowing, fever, and a tendency to lean the head toward the affected side.

The nasal sinuses are four pairs of cavities in the bone around the nose. There are two maxillary sinuses, so called because they are found in the maxilla, or upper jaw. Slightly above and behind them are the ethmoid sinuses, and behind them are the sphenoid sinuses. Sitting over the nose in the lower part of the forehead are the two frontal sinuses. All these sinuses are lined with a mucous membrane and have small openings that lead into the nasal passages. Air moves in and

---

INFORMATION ON NASOPHARYNGEAL DISORDERS

CAUSES: May include bacterial or viral infection, nasal obstruction (polyps), environmental allergens or toxins

SYMPTOMS: Sore throat; inflamed lymph nodes, larynx, and sinus cavities; earache or ear infection; nosebleeds; nasal obstruction; fever; difficulty breathing or swallowing; general malaise; bad breath

DURATION: Acute to chronic

TREATMENTS: Antibiotics, over-the-counter medications, surgery; if severe, emergency intubation out of the sinuses and allows mucus to drain into the nose. In acute sinusitis, infection builds up in the mucous membrane of any or all of the sinuses. The membrane lining the sinus swells and shuts the opening into the nasal passages. At the same time, membranes of the nose swell and become congested. Mucus and pus build up inside the sinuses, causing pain and pressure. Most often, sinusitis accompanies the common cold: The mucous membrane that lines the nose extends into the sinuses, so the infection of a cold can readily spread into the sinuses. The various viruses responsible for the common cold may be involved, as well as a wide group of bacteria. Chronic sinusitis can be caused by repeated infections that have allowed scar tissue to build up, closing the sinus openings and impeding mucus drainage, or may be the result of allergies.

According to the Centers for Disease Control and Prevention, chronic sinusitis is the most common long-term illness in the United States, surpassing the rates for asthma, arthritis, and congestive heart disease and causing nearly 14 million doctor office visits per year. For reasons that are not yet understood, sinusitis sufferers are often beset with inflammation of the ducts, trapping mucus, bacteria, and viruses inside. Nasal polyps can then develop. Thus, researchers have been very interested in finding causes and effective treatments for sinusitis. In the late twentieth century, most chronic cases of sinusitis were treated with fiber optic surgery that allowed access to the cramped sinus passageways. However, patients often returned within weeks or months with ongoing problems. This fact recently has prompted a reconsideration of the problem and its underlying causes as well as a struggle to redefine sinusitis. Some medical experts suspect that inflammation or the responses of the immune system are the culprit but note that additional research must be completed before any definitive answers are found.

Tissues in the nasopharyngeal cavity may be affected by conditions occurring in other parts of the body. For example, vocal cord paralysis may be caused by vascular accidents, certain cancers, tissue trauma, and other events.

Some infections in the nasopharyngeal cavity can spread to the ear through the Eustachian tubes that connect the two areas. Chief among the diseases of the ear that can be associated with nasopharyngeal disorders are the various forms of acute otitis media, an earache occurring in the central part of the ear. There are four basic types of otitis media. With the first type, serous otitis media, there is usually no infection, but fluid ac-

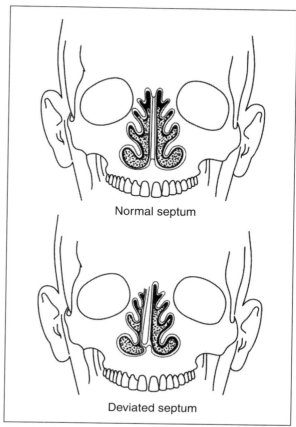

A deviated septum is a malformation in the cartilage between the nostrils, either present at birth or caused by a blow to the nose.

cumulates inside the middle ear because of the blockage of the Eustachian tube or the overproduction of fluid; the condition is usually mild, with some pain and temporary loss of hearing. The second type is otitis media with effusion; with this condition comes both infection and accumulation of fluid. The third form is acute purulent otitis media, the most serious type. Pus builds up inside the middle ear, and its pressure may rupture the eardrum, allowing discharge of blood and pus. The fourth type is secretory otitis media, which usually occurs after several bouts of otitis media. Cells within the middle ear start producing a fluid that is thicker than normal and produced in greater amounts.

Chronic otitis media is bacterial in origin. It is characterized by a perforation of the eardrum and chronic pus discharge. The eardrum is a flat, pliable disk of tissue that vibrates to conduct sounds from the outside to the inner-ear structures. The perforation that occurs in chronic otitis media can be one of two types: a relatively benign perforation occurring in the central part of the eardrum or a potentially dangerous perforation occurring near the edges of the eardrum. The latter perforation can be associated with loss of hearing, increased discharge of pus and other fluids, facial paralysis, and the spread of infection to other tissues. When the perforation of chronic otitis media is near the edges of the eardrum, something called a cholesteatoma develops. This accumulation of matter grows in the inner ear and can be destructive to bone and other tissue.

The same organisms that cause otitis media can be responsible for a condition called mastoiditis. The mastoid process is a bone structure lined with a mucous membrane. Infection from otitis media can spread to this area and in severe cases can destroy the bone. Mastoiditis used to be a leading cause of death in children.

Nosebleeds are common and most often result from a blow to the nose, but they can also be caused by colds, sinusitis, and breathing dry air. The septum (the cartilaginous tissue that separates the nostrils) and the surrounding intranasal mucous membrane contain many tiny blood vessels that are easily ruptured. If an individual receives a blow to the nose, these vessels can break and bleed. They can also rupture because of irritation from a cold or other condition. Breathing very dry air sometimes causes the nasal mucous membrane to crust over, and bleeding can follow. Nosebleeds are not usually serious, but sometimes they are indicative of an underlying condition, such as hypertension (high blood pressure), a tumor, or another disease.

Nasal obstruction is common during colds and allergy attacks, but it can also be caused by a deviated septum, a malformation in the cartilage between the nostrils that can be congenital or caused by a blow to the nose. Also, nasal obstruction can be attributable to nasal polyps, nasal tumors, or swollen adenoids. A common source of nasal obstruction is overuse of nasal decongestants. These agents relieve nasal congestion by reducing intranasal inflammation and swelling. If used too often or too long, however, they can cause the very problem that they were intended to cure: Intranasal blood vessels dilate, the area swells, secretions increase, and the nose becomes blocked. This is known as rebound congestion, or in medical terminology, rhinitis medicamentosa (nasal inflammation that is caused by a medication).

Halitosis, or bad breath, can be considered a nasopharyngeal disorder in the sense that it can originate in the mouth. It can be caused by diseases of the teeth and/ or gums, but the most common causes are smoking or eating aromatic foods such as onions and garlic. Bad breath may also be a sign of disease conditions in other parts of the body, such as certain lung disorders or cancer of the esophagus. Hepatic failure, a liver dysfunction, may be accompanied by a fishy odor on the breath. Azotemia, the retention of nitrogen in the blood, may give rise to an ammonia-like odor. A sweet, fruity odor on the breath of diabetic patients may accompany ketoacidosis, a condition that occurs when there are high levels of glucose in the blood. Sometimes, young children stick foreign objects or other materials into their noses; it has been reported that these materials can fester, causing severe halitosis. Bad breath is rarely apparent to the individual who has it, however offensive it may be to others. A good way to check one's breath is to lick the back of one's hand and smell the spot; malodor, if it exists, will usually be apparent.

TREATMENT AND THERAPY

Nasopharyngeal disorders are most often mild illnesses that can be treated at home. For example, acute pharyngitis or sore throat is easily managed most of the time. The patient is advised to rest, gargle with warm salt water several times a day, and soothe the pain with lozenges or anesthetic gargles. If the infection is caused by a virus, it usually will clear without further treatment. If the physician suspects, however, that the infection is bacterial in origin, throat smears may be taken so that the organism can be identified. If bacteria are discovered, antibiotic therapy will be undertaken to eradicate the pathogens. This is particularly important if the infection is caused by certain strains of streptococcus bacteria. In this case, it is vital to destroy the organism in order to avoid the development of rheumatic fever.

In acute laryngitis caused by viral infection, the patient is advised to rest the voice, inhale steam, and drink warm liquids. If bacteria are the cause of the laryngitis, antibiotic therapy is undertaken. In treating chronic laryngitis, the physician must discover the cause and remove it. If allergy is the cause, antihistamine therapy could help. If the cause is bacterial, antibiotic therapy is used. If smoking or drinking alcohol is the problem, the patient should be counseled to stop. The simple palliative measures used for acute laryngitis—resting the voice, drinking warm liquids, and breathing steam— are also useful for chronic laryngitis.

Symptoms of epiglottitis are often similar to those of sore throat. If there is any evidence of difficulty in breathing, however, the patient should be seen by a physician quickly because an emergency situation may be developing. If epiglottitis is obstructing the airway, the patient should be treated in an intensive care setting. It is important to make an airway for the patient, and it may be necessary to insert a tube into the trachea to allow the patient to breathe.

Before the age of antibiotics, tonsillitis was often treated surgically, with both tonsils and adenoids removed. This procedure is now rare because the infection usually responds to antibiotic therapy. Similarly, in peritonsillar abscess or quinsy, antibiotics usually clear the condition satisfactorily. In some cases, accumulations of pus may be removed surgically. If the abscesses return, it may be advisable to remove the tonsils.

As a rule, the child with croup is treated at home. Because the disease is usually caused by viruses, antibiotics are not used unless bacteria are known to be involved. Steam is often used to help liquefy mucus deposits on the interior walls of the trachea, the larynx, and the bronchi. The patient is given warm liquids to drink and is closely watched so that any signs that the condition is getting worse will be detected. The following symptoms should alert the caregiver to the possibility that an emergency situation is developing and that medical help is needed quickly: drooling, difficulty in swallowing, difficulty in breathing, inability to bend the neck forward, blue or dark color in the lips, high-pitched sounds when inhaling, rapid heartbeat, and loss of consciousness.

The main goals of therapy for sinusitis are to control infection, relieve the blockage of the sinus openings to permit drainage, and relieve pain. When sinusitis is known to be of bacterial origin, an appropriate antibiotic will be used to eradicate the organism. Often, however, sinusitis is attributable to viral infection, and other procedures are used to treat it. Inhaling steam is useful for reducing swelling and promoting drainage, as are decongestant sprays and oral decongestants. Analgesics can be given for pain. In certain circumstances, the sinuses are drained surgically.

Acute otitis media is most often diagnosed with the aid of an otoscope, an instrument that the doctor uses to look at the eardrum and surrounding tissues. The eardrum will be a dull red color, bulging, and perhaps perforated. While a viral infection may precede otitis media, the causative microorganisms for this and related ear infections, such as mastoiditis, are usually bacteria. Antibiotics are used both to treat the infections and to prevent the spread of disease to other areas. The drugs are usually taken orally, although antibiotic ear drops

are often given as well. Penicillin and its derivatives are used, as are erythromycin and sulfisoxazole. Antibiotic therapy for acute otitis media is usually continued for ten days to two weeks. Sometimes, pus and other fluids and solid matter build up in the inner ear. It may be necessary to pierce the eardrum in order to remove these deposits. To help relieve blockage of the Eustachian tubes, a topical vasoconstrictor may be used in the nose to reduce the swelling of blood vessels. Antihistamines could be helpful to patients with allergies, but otherwise they are not indicated.

For chronic otitis media, it is necessary to clean both the outer ear canal and the middle ear thoroughly. A mild acetic acid solution with a corticosteroid is used for a week to ten days. Meanwhile, aggressive oral antibiotic therapy is undertaken to eradicate the pathogen. The perforated eardrum associated with chronic otitis media can usually be repaired surgically with little or no loss of function, and the cholesteatoma must be surgically removed.

Simple nosebleed can be treated by pinching the nose with the fingers and breathing through the mouth for five or ten minutes, to allow the blood to clot. Also, a plug of absorbent paper or cloth can be inserted into the bleeding nostril. A nosebleed that does not stop easily should be seen by a physician.

Nasal obstruction resulting from colds or allergies is treated by appropriate medications, decongestants for colds, and antihistamines for allergies. A deviated septum may require surgery. The only therapy for rhinitis medicamentosa, or rebound congestion caused by overuse of nasal decongestants, is to stop the medication and endure the congestion for as long as it takes the condition to clear. Sometimes, it is necessary to consult a physician.

For simple halitosis caused by smoking or food, breath fresheners (with or without "odor-fighting" chemicals) are often used, even though they usually simply replace a "bad" odor with a "good" one. Some people firmly believe that chewing parsley or other leaves rich in chlorophyll will counteract the smell of garlic. When halitosis is attributable to tooth or gum disease, it will persist until the condition is cured. Halitosis may be of diagnostic value in certain situations where a characteristic odor could alert the physician to the possibility of a disease condition.

PERSPECTIVE AND PROSPECTS

Diseases and infections of the nasal cavity and throat have always been common among human populations, as have therapies to deal with them. Until the advent of antibiotics, some of these disorders were quite serious, especially in young children, but modern medications and surgeries, where appropriate, have greatly lessened the danger. Many over-the-counter drugs are now used to combat sore throats, sinus congestion, and other nasopharyngeal symptoms of the common cold, although colds themselves remain incurable because of the hundreds or thousands of different microorganisms that may be responsible. Despite the numerous medications that can be taken, however, more serious infections or diseases, such as chronic tonsillitis or laryngitis, require a doctor's care, with more potent, prescription drugs and surgery if needed. The treatments available to physicians and patients for the symptoms of nasopharyngeal disorders are many, but the search continues for better drugs and perhaps preventive measures such as vaccinations to address the causes of these conditions.

—*C. Richard Falcon*

See also Allergies; Antihistamines; Choking; Common cold; Decongestants; Ear infections and disorders; Ears; Halitosis; Hearing loss; Laryngectomy; Laryngitis; Mouth and throat cancer; Multiple chemical sensitivity syndrome; Nasal polyp removal; Otorhinolaryngology; Pharyngitis; Plastic surgery; Respiration; Rhinoplasty and submucous resection; Sinusitis; Smell; Sore throat; Strep throat; Taste; Tonsillectomy and adenoid removal; Tonsillitis; Voice and vocal cord disorders.

FOR FURTHER INFORMATION:

Ferrari, Mario. *PDxMD Ear, Nose, and Throat Disorders.* New York: Elsevier, 2002. A clinical yet accessible reference text that provides a comprehensive list of disorders, with a summary of the condition, background, diagnosis, treatment, outcomes, prevention, and resources.

Friedman, Ellen M., and James M. Barassi. *My Ear Hurts! A Complete Guide to Understanding and Treating Your Child's Ear Infections.* New York: Simon & Schuster, 2001. Reviews current research on ear infections and reviews a range of treatment approaches from both conventional and alternative medicine.

Greene, Alan R. *The Parent's Complete Guide to Ear Infections.* Reprint. Allentown, Pa.: People's Medical Society, 1999. Every parent who has ever had a child with recurrent otitis will appreciate this book. It explains the anatomy of normal ears, causes of in-

fections, prevention, symptoms, evaluation, initial and ongoing treatment, antibiotics, the pros and cons of surgical intervention, hearing loss, tubes, and complications.

Kimball, Chad T. *Colds, Flu, and Other Common Ailments.* Detroit: Omnigraphics, 2002. A comprehensive guide for general readers covering treatment issues and controversies surrounding common ailments and injuries. Includes discussions on ailments of the nose, throat, lungs, ears, eyes, and head.

Litin, Scott C., ed. *Mayo Clinic Family Health Book.* 3d ed. New York: HarperResource, 2003. A thorough and up-to-date medical text for the layperson. The section on nasopharyngeal diseases is quite complete and offers excellent anatomic illustrations.

Wagman, Richard J. *The New Complete Medical and Health Encyclopedia.* 4 vols. Chicago: J. G. Ferguson, 2002. The chapters on upper respiratory diseases in this work are thorough and clear, with good illustrations.

NATIONAL CANCER INSTITUTE (NCI)

ORGANIZATION

DEFINITION: A federal agency devoted to the study of cancer, as well as communication and education about this condition.

KEY TERMS:

carcinogenesis: the biological process of the initiation, promotion, and progression of cancer

epidemiology: the study of the relationships between a host, an agent, and an environment that lead to a condition or disease

OVERVIEW

The U.S. Department of Health and Human Services (DHHS) is the federal agency responsible for public health. The DHHS includes twelve divisions, one of which is the National Institutes of Health (NIH). The National Cancer Institute (NCI) is one of seventeen institutes within NIH. The NCI was established under the National Cancer Act of 1937 and is the principal federal agency for cancer research and training. Following special legislation in 1971, the scope of the NCI has continued to broaden through new initiatives and legislation.

The purpose of the NCI is to eliminate cancer as far as possible and to discover treatment for those cancers which cannot be eradicated. The NCI approaches these goals by supporting research, coordinating efforts in prevention and treatment, facilitating the movement of research findings into medicine, and providing education and resources for patients and their families, health educators, and scientists. The NCI conducts research in its own laboratories and clinics in Bethesda, Maryland, but also supports and coordinates research projects conducted by universities, hospitals, research foundations, and businesses throughout the United States and many other countries.

THE ORGANIZATION AND FOCUS OF THE NCI

The NCI is organized into the Office of the Director of NCI and eight divisions. Each division specializes in a different aspect of cancer research, although there is overlap among them. The divisions include the Division of Basic Sciences, the Division of Cancer Biology, the Division of Cancer Control and Population Sciences, the Division of Cancer Epidemiology and Genetics, the Division of Cancer Prevention, the Division of Cancer Treatment and Diagnosis, the Division of Clinical Sciences, and the Division of Extramural Activities.

The Division of Basic Sciences focuses on research relating to cellular, molecular, genetic, biochemical, and immunological mechanisms critical to the understanding, diagnosis, and treatment of cancer. Research in cancer cell biology, such as carcinogenesis and cancer immunology, falls within the realm of the Division of Cancer Biology. This division also examines the biological and health effects of exposures to ionizing and nonionizing radiation. The Division of Cancer Epidemiology and Genetics focuses on the special interests of genetic predisposition, lifestyle factors, environmental contaminants, occupational exposures, medications, radiation, and infectious agents, as well as epidemiological methods development. The efforts of the Division of Cancer Prevention center on early detection methods and the efficacy of nutritional or lifestyle changes on cancer prevention. The results of research in this area led to the 5 a Day for Better Health program. Initiated in 1991, this program is a collaborative effort between the food industry and the NCI, which encourages Americans to eat five or more servings of vegetables and fruits each day as part of a low-fat, high-fiber diet. The Division of Cancer Treatment and Diagnosis includes programs in biomedical imaging, cancer diagnosis, cancer therapy evaluation, developmental therapeutics, and radiation research.

The mission of the Division of Clinical Sciences is to take the scientific discoveries to the medical clinic. It has five major research areas: cancer genetics, cancer

vaccines and immunotherapy, molecular therapeutics, experimental transplantation, and advanced technology. The clinical cancer genetics program integrates all aspects of clinical and laboratory medicine, particularly in studies of breast, colon, renal, and prostate cancer. Processes include molecular diagnostics, novel imaging techniques, and the molecular assessment of normal tissues in at-risk populations. The cancer vaccines and immunotherapy program investigates the clinical feasibility of using vaccines against known conditions associated with cancer, such as the human papillomavirus and human immunodeficiency virus (HIV), as well as with cancer-specific products, such as in melanoma and in lymphomas. The molecular therapeutics program is concerned with most clinical trial experiments. Important recent discoveries include the development of Taxol as an effective anticancer agent, the development of AZT as an important anti-HIV drug, and the use of adoptive immunotherapy in the treatment of malignant melanoma. The scientific thrust of the molecular therapeutics program is the belief that the analysis of the molecular profile of individual cancers will help determine the most effective chemotherapeutic approaches. The experimental transplantation program examines bone marrow biology in order to advance transplantation techniques and the effectiveness of this approach.

Integrating many programs and divisions is the advanced technology program. New technology is an essential key to identifying genetic elements involved in cancer initiation and progression, as well as in drug efficacy and drug resistance. Although many drugs have been discovered that inhibit the growth of cancer cells successfully, they also affect healthy cells. This causes side effects that have a negative impact on patients' health and quality of life. New therapeutics and technology are being investigated to minimize or eliminate these side effects and enhance the effectiveness of therapy.

The eighth division of the NCI is the Division of Extramural Activities, which is responsible for handling all applications for funding and for monitoring research that has received funding from the NCI. Extramural activities also include the oversight of scientific communications. To enhance communication, the NCI has a number of advisory boards and groups that provide the institute with input from the public, medical, and research communities.

In 1998, the Office of Cancer Complementary and Alternative Medicine was established to coordinate research and communication activities in the arena of complementary and alternative medicine, both within the NCI and with other agencies.

The NCI is strengthening the information base for cancer care decision making. Researchers, medical providers, and patients seek to understand better what constitutes quality cancer care. The NCI is concerned with both geographic and racial or ethnic disparities in who receives quality care. The Cancer Information Service, established in 1976, is the section of the NCI that is the link to the public, attempting to explain research findings in a clear, timely, and understandable manner. To this end, the Cancer Information Service helps develop education efforts targeting minority audiences and people with limited access to health care information or services.

PERSPECTIVE AND PROSPECTS

To be successful in managing this range of responsibilities and breadth of mission, the NCI has a budget in the billions of dollars. Through the years, the work of the NCI has led to a decline in deaths due to cancer, even though advances in the treatment of infectious diseases have made cancer the second leading cause of death in the United States. Creative and dedicated scientists at the NCI have goals to lower its numbers even further in the near future. The NCI will enhance collaborations among institutions and researchers so that priorities are targeted and goals are achieved. An important path to achieving these goals is a program to increase access to clinical trials. Achievement of research goals may also be expedited through a program of extraordinary opportunities for scientific areas of recent importance and promise.

—*Karen Chapman-Novakofski, R.D., L.D., Ph.D.*
See also Cancer; Chemotherapy; Clinical trials; Environmental diseases; Environmental health; Epidemiology; Genetics and inheritance; Nutrition; Oncology; Preventive medicine; Radiation therapy.

FOR FURTHER INFORMATION:

Hewitt, Maria Elizabeth, et al., eds. *Ensuring Quality Cancer Care.* Washington, D.C.: National Academy Press, 1999.

Lerner, Barron H. *The Breast Cancer Wars: Fear, Hope, and the Pursuit of a Cure in Twentieth-Century America.* New York: Oxford University Press, 2003.

National Cancer Institute. *The Cancer Information Service: A Fifteen-Year History of Service and Research.* Bethesda, Md.: Author, 1993.

_____. *National Cancer Institute's Research Programs: Pursuing the Central Questions of Cancer Research.* Bethesda, Md.: Author, 1999.

_____. *NCI Fact Book.* Bethesda, Md.: Author, 1979- .

Reuben, Suzanne H. *Assessing Progress, Advancing Change: 2005-2006 Annual Report.* Bethesda, Md.: U.S. Department of Health and Human Services, National Institutes of Health, National Cancer Institute, 2006.

NATIONAL INSTITUTES OF HEALTH (NIH)

ORGANIZATION

DEFINITION: The National Institutes of Health (NIH), composed of more than twenty-five separate institutes, centers, and offices, is one of eight agencies constituting the United States Department of Health and Human Services.

KEY TERMS:

AIDSLINE: a database that is part of the National Library of Medicine (NLM) and is devoted to the topic of research on acquired immunodeficiency syndrome (AIDS)

CATLINE: the on-line catalog of books and manuscripts in the NLM

grant proposals: research plans that outline scientific methods to pursue new knowledge, the required budget, and the resulting products and significance of that work

institute: a specific subagency of the NIH that has the charge of advancing scientific discovery and clinical practice in a specific area of medical science

MEDLINE: a database that is available via the Internet featuring current and historical medical literature, research articles, monographs, presentations, and abstracts

HISTORY AND MISSION

The National Institutes of Health (NIH) is a U.S. federal agency that occupies a multibuilding campus in Bethesda, Maryland. It consists of a variety of offices, institutes focused on specific medical problems, research laboratories and centers, a center for scientific review, and a national medical library. Its main goal is to discover knowledge that will improve the state of public health for all persons, especially those in the United States. This goal extends to all medical conditions afflicting men, women, and children of all ethnic backgrounds. It also extends to seeking knowledge in areas of basic biological research, clinical research, and research on policy and practice in health care.

The National Institute of Health (precursor to the NIH) was formally established by the Ransdell Act of 1930, which bestowed the name on what was formerly called the Hygienic Laboratory (HL) of the Marine Hospital Service (MHS) in New York. The Ransdell Act also allowed for the establishment of fellowships for basic medical and biological research. The very beginnings of the NIH extend back to 1887, however, when basic laboratory work into medical problems was pursued by the MHS, the founding body of the United States Public Health Service (PHS). The MHS was formed in 1798 to provide hospital care for seamen, but by the 1880's it had shifted its focus to screening ship passengers for infectious diseases capable of starting epidemics.

New European research in the 1880's suggesting that microorganisms caused such diseases spurred American interest in medical research and helped form the original HL. Work by the HL continued, with the laboratory eventually moving from the MHS to its own Washington, D.C., campus. The study of microorganisms continued, extending from study of individual persons to studying the effects of bacteria on water and air pollution. Progress for such work was rewarded in 1901 with governmental money for the construction of a building (completed in 1904) to house the HL and further foster work focused on advancing the public health. Because the value of such work was not well established, however, no permanent funding was provided, leaving the organization subject to ongoing evaluation and supplemental funding.

In 1902 the MHS was reorganized and renamed the Public Health and Marine Hospital Service (PHMHS); in 1912 it adopted the shortened name of the Public Health Service (PHS). During the intervening time, the HL continued its work and expanded to work in chemistry, pharmacology, zoology, immunology, and the regulation and production of vaccines and antitoxins. Additionally, new scientific staff were added to the staff of medical doctors already on board. Changes in the mission of the organization in 1912 also opened the door for the pursuit of research on noncontagious diseases and water pollution. This work continued during World War I in the form of examining sanitation, anthrax outbreaks, smallpox, tetanus, influenza, and other combat-related conditions. The success of the PHS's work in these areas caught the attention of legislators and resulted in the Ransdell Act of 1930, which

established both the National Institute of Health and the practice of setting aside public monies for funding medical research. In 1937, the National Cancer Institute (NCI) was created. In 1944, the PHS formally designated the NCI as a component of the NIH, setting the pattern of a problem-focused structure within the NIH that continues to the present.

World War II led the NIH to focus almost exclusively on war-related problems. This involved examinations of fitness for military service and issues such as dental problems and syphilis. The effects of hazardous substances and conditions on workers in war industries; risks armed service professionals faced from lack of oxygen, cold temperatures, and blood clots while flying; burns, shock, bacterial infections, and fever; and the development of vaccines and therapies for tropical diseases such as malaria also composed much of its work during this time.

Successes established during the wars by such medical research led the PHS to take the 1944 Public Health Service Act to Congress. This act led to grant-funding mechanisms being extended from the NCI alone to the entire National Institute of Health. Additionally, an increasing public interest in health organizations caused Congress to create additional institutes for research on mental health, dental diseases, and heart disease between 1946 and 1949. In 1948, the National Heart Act allowed for the formal pluralization of the National Institutes of Health, rather than a singular institute with the NCI as a subinstitute. The Public Health Service Act of 1944 also provided funding for the Warren Grant Magnuson Clinical Center, which opened in 1953 to focus exclusively on clinical research on health.

From this point forward, each of the individual institutes now composing the NIH came into being. By 1960 there were ten institutes, by 1970 there were fifteen, and by 1998 there were twenty-four institutes and centers. As different health interests develop and advances in medical knowledge are needed, the NIH has responded by allocating its resources to pursue goals in those areas. This has been done both by developing institutes and also by creating specialized offices to pursue contemporary medical problems.

Illness and medicine know no boundaries, however, so the NIH has also maintained an interest in global public health issues. Such interest was formally shown in 1947, when grants were first awarded to investigators abroad. Similarly, in 1968, the John E. Fogarty International Center (FIC) was created to coordinate international research efforts, involving liaisons with the

World Health Organization and a variety of international research organizations. The FIC also supports language translation, documentation, and reviews of new health findings. It facilitates biomedical communications through its maintenance of the National Library of Medicine (NLM), MEDLINE, CATLINE, AIDSLINE, and numerous other databases for researchers, physicians, and the public at large. Similarly, focused consensus development conferences, where investigators and clinicians from around the world can meet to evaluate new and existing therapies, are another way that international interests are pursued. Since these conferences were initiated in 1977, more than one hundred such conferences have been held.

In keeping with its practical focus, the NIH has strived to seek out knowledge that yields new drugs, devices, and procedures that are useful not just for the government but for the public at large as well. In 1986, the Technology Transfer Act allowed for a partnership between NIH-funded research and the private sector. Encouraging researchers to examine possible commercial and practical applications of basic medical research to wide-reaching clinical or research use benefits overall scientific and health progress. Partnering with business allows private industries to take over the process of marketing and developing products in a manner more affordable to them than to the government, allowing the government to focus on development while benefiting through the use of the eventual marketed products.

ORGANIZATIONAL STRUCTURE AND METHOD

The NIH is organized to accomplish its goals by using its offices, institutes, and research centers. Research is conducted on the NIH campus in its own funded laboratories, as well as in the labs of scientists supported by NIH funding, who are stationed in institutes of higher education, teaching hospitals, and free-standing research institutions in the United States and other countries. In addition to supporting ongoing research, the NIH also supports research infrastructure by maintaining a library and a variety of printed and electronic resources to facilitate communication among its researchers, the larger scientific community, policymakers, and the public. Scientific research also is supported by developing one of the most valuable resources known to medicine: new researchers. The NIH sponsors a variety of training programs focusing on medical training and research in order to keep a large body of high-quality scholars and investigators in develop-

ment. Such programs extend from career development for postdoctoral researchers and predoctoral training, to high school level learning in the sponsoring of internships and other learning experiences for teenagers interested in medical science careers.

Funding for research and training programs outside of the NIH campus and research centers is facilitated through grant proposal programs that distribute federal tax monies devoted to such endeavors. Applicants to such programs are able to submit independent proposals for work related to the goals of the NIH that they believe is demanded by the state of science and knowledge. They are also able to submit proposals in response to program announcements and calls for proposals on specific topics as outlined by the institutes and offices of the NIH. Many different grant mechanisms exist for such proposals, including grants supporting the work of individual trainees, training programs for cohorts of researchers at different stages of career development, the ongoing work of career scientists, small grants for new or experimental work, focused projects, and even centers of research excellence where many researchers focus on the same topic of study. In addition, grant support is offered to sponsor conferences and academic meetings on special topics in health research and training.

In order to receive this funding, those wishing to be considered for receiving such grant monies need to submit proposals for confidential peer review through the Center for Scientific Review (CSR), which is part of the NIH structure. Proposals are reviewed by panels of experts who evaluate the research plans, goals, staff, environment, and overall innovation and merit of the work proposed. In addition, ethical considerations about the proposed research are reviewed and considered for both animal welfare and the welfare of human research participants. Emphasis on ethical issues has been a long-standing issue for medical research. It was, however, highlighted in the 1960's, when grantees receiving NIH grant monies were required to state the ethical principles guiding their research on humans, and in 1979, when written guidelines for research on human subjects were established. Once through peer review, proposals are reviewed again by a national advisory council to determine the priority of the work in addressing the goals of the NIH and its institutes and offices. After the proposals are approved by this council for advancement, the individual institutes (sometimes cooperating with specific NIH offices) work to fund them with the monies allotted. Unfortunately, not all proposals can be funded. It should be noted that even after funding, the work of the NIH Office for Protection from Research Risks continues so as to ensure that proper research ethics are followed through the life of the research.

Each year the CSR reviews more than thirty-eight thousand applications, while the NIH supports nearly thirty-five thousand grants nationally and internationally. Such work is facilitated by the various institutions and research offices that fall under the organizational umbrella of the NIH, each focusing on a discrete area of health interest. Some of the institutions involved include the NCI; the National Eye Institute; the National Heart, Lung, and Blood Institute; and the National Human Genome Research Institute. Also included are the National Institutes on Aging, Alcohol Abuse and Alcoholism, Allergy and Infectious Diseases, Arthritis and Musculoskeletal and Skin Diseases, Child Health and Human Development, Deafness and Other Communication Disorders, Dental and Craniofacial Research, Diabetes and Digestive and Kidney Diseases, Drug Abuse, Environmental Health Sciences, Mental Health, and Neurological Disorders and Stroke.

In addition to these institutes, the NIH has numerous offices focusing on specific issues or populations that need to be addressed in health research. These offices focus on contemporary issues of importance for research and include the Offices of Technology Transfer, AIDS Research, Research on Minority Health, Research on Women's Health, Behavioral and Social Sciences Research, Dietary Supplements, Medical Applications of Research, Rare Diseases, Science Policy, Biotechnology Activities, Science Education, and Information Technology. There are also offices that focus on the management of research, specific organizational issues at the NIH, or the communication of information from the NIH to members of the public. These include the Offices of Intramural Research, Extramural Research, Evaluation, Equal Opportunity, Human Resource Management, Financial Management, Procurement Management, Logistics Management, Contracts Management, Management Assessment, Communications and Public Liaison, and General Counsel, as well as the NIH Legal Advisor, and the Freedom of Information Act Office.

Perspective and Prospects

The NIH has been responsible for supporting some very influential research for more than one hundred years, garnering more than eighty Nobel Prizes for NIH-supported work. More vaccines against infectious diseases are available than ever before. The successful mapping of the human genome has set the stage for enhanced genetic testing and the development of gene therapies. Substantial decreases in mortality rates have been achieved for heart disease and strokes. Survival rates for individuals afflicted by cancer have increased, as have survival rates for infants with respiratory distress syndrome. Recovery from spinal cord injuries has been enhanced so as to lessen the probability of long-term disability. Advances in the pharmacological and behavioral treatment of mental health problems such as depression, anxiety, bipolar disorders, and schizophrenia have been achieved. Preventive approaches in dentistry have been highly successful in stopping and slowing dental problems.

Given such successes, billions of dollars of federal tax monies continue to be devoted to the NIH budget to foster continued scientific advances. New work focused on improving prevention, screening, assessment, diagnosis, and treatment for conditions such as AIDS, alcoholism and drug dependence, Alzheimer's disease, arthritis, blindness, communication disorders, diabetes, heart disease, kidney disease, lung cancer, lupus, mental illnesses, Parkinson's disease, stroke, and other persisting conditions continues on a daily basis. While great successes have been achieved to date with the majority of the population, new research is needed that will focus on specialized approaches that may enhance health for women, minorities, youth, and the elderly. The combination of these needs, past successes, and governmental commitment to improving the state of the public health ensures that the NIH will continue onward with its mission for the foreseeable future.

—*Nancy A. Piotrowski, Ph.D.*

See also Childhood infectious diseases; Disease; Environmental diseases; Environmental health; Epidemiology; Immunization and vaccination; National Cancer Institute (NCI); Occupational health; World Health Organization.

For Further Information:

Desalle, Rob. *Epidemic! The World of Infectious Disease*. New York: New Press, 1999. A book designed to accompany the American Museum of Natural History's exhibit of the same title, an accessible book that details the world of infectious disease from the perspective of science and medicine. Examines what is understood about bacteria, viruses, parasites, and their remedies.

Eberhart-Philips, Jason. *Outbreak Alert: Responding to the Increasing Threat of Infectious Diseases*. Oakland, Calif.: New Harbinger, 2000. Emphasizes the importance of public health to national health; defines and identifies infectious diseases posing a public health threat and how the current way that society functions relates to this threat.

Garrett, Laurie. *Betrayal of Trust: The Collapse of Global Public Health*. New York: Hyperion, 2000. Discusses global public health, putting the status of health in the United States in perspective on some very basic matters related to public health.

Institute of Medicine. *Scientific Opportunities and Public Needs: Improving Priority Setting and Public Input at the National Institutes of Health*. Washington, D.C.: National Academy Press, 1998. Provides an overview of scientific and popular perceptions of the needed long-term health interests of the United States, as well as other global health concerns.

Lee, Philip R., and Carroll L. Estes, eds. *The Nation's Health*. 7th ed. Sudbury, Mass.: Jones & Bartlett, 2003. A compendium of articles compiled by two preeminent American health policy analysts. Chapters discuss the complex web of issues, policies, controversies, and proposed solutions that surround health policy, public health, community health, and health care in the United States.

Shnayerson, Michael. *The Killers Within: The Deadly Rise of Drug Resistant Bacteria*. New York: Little, Brown, 2002. Traces the evolution of drug-resistant bacteria and how physicians are trying to combat it.

Tulchinsky, Theodore H., and Elena A. Varavikova. *The New Public Health: An Introduction for the Twenty-first Century*. San Diego, Calif.: Academic Press, 2000. Discusses global perspectives on how organizational structures of health care and other public activities affect the state of public health and health care service delivery.

NATIVE AMERICAN HEALTH. *See* AMERICAN INDIAN HEALTH.

NAUSEA AND VOMITING

DISEASE/DISORDER

ANATOMY OR SYSTEM AFFECTED: Brain, gastrointestinal system, nervous system, stomach

SPECIALTIES AND RELATED FIELDS: Gastroenterology, otorhinolaryngology

DEFINITION: Nausea is an unpleasant subjective sensation, accompanied by epigastric and duodenal discomfort, which often culminates in vomiting, the regurgitation of the contents of the stomach.

KEY TERMS:

affect: the emotional reactions associated with experience

antiemetics: drugs that prevent or relieve the symptoms of nausea and/or vomiting

chemoreceptor trigger zone: a sensory nerve ending in the brain which is stimulated by and reacts to certain chemical stimulation localized outside the central nervous system

emesis: the act of vomiting

psychogenic: of mental origin

psychotropics: drugs that affect psychic function, behavior, or experience

CAUSES AND SYMPTOMS

Nausea is defined as a subjectively unpleasant sensation associated with awareness of the urge to vomit. It is usually felt in the back of the throat and epigastrium and is accompanied by the loss of gastric tone, duodenal contractions, and reflux of the intestinal contents into the stomach. Retching is defined as labored, spasmodic, rhythmic contractions of the respiratory muscles (including the diaphragm, chest wall, and abdominal wall muscles) without the expulsion of gastric contents. Vomiting, or emesis, is the forceful expulsion of gastric contents from the mouth and is brought about by the powerful sustained contraction of the abdominal muscles, the descent of the diaphragm, and the opening of the gastric cardia (the cardiac orifice of the stomach).

Nausea and vomiting are important defense mechanisms against the ingestion of toxins. The act of emesis involves a sequence of events that can be divided into three phases: preejection, ejection, and postejection. The preejection phase includes the symptoms of nausea, along with salivation, swallowing, pallor, and tachycardia (an abnormally fast heartbeat). The ejection phase comprises retching and vomiting. Retching is characterized by rhythmic, synchronous, inspiratory movements of the diaphragm, abdominal, and external intercostal muscles, while the mouth and the glottis are kept closed. As the antral (cavity) portion of the stomach contracts, the proximal (nearest the center) portion relaxes and the gastric contents oscillate between the stomach and the esophagus. During retching, the hiatal portion of the diaphragm does not relax, and intraabdominal pressure increases are associated with a decrease in intrathoracic pressure.

In contrast, relaxation of the hiatal portion of the diaphragm (near the esophagus) permits a transfer of intraabdominal pressure to the thorax during the act of vomiting. Contraction of the muscles of the anterior abdominal wall, relaxation of the esophageal sphincter, an increase in intrathoracic and intragastric pressure, reverse peristalsis (movement of the contents of the alimentary canal), and an open glottis and mouth result in the expulsion of gastric contents. The postejection phase consists of autonomic and visceral responses that return the body to a quiescent phase, with or without residual nausea.

The complex act of vomiting, involving coordination of the respiratory, gastrointestinal, and abdominal musculature, is controlled by what researchers label the emetic center. This center in the brain stem has access to the motor pathways responsible for the visceral and somatic output involved in vomiting, and stimuli from several areas within the central nervous system can affect this center. These include afferent (inward-directed) nerves from the pharynx and gastrointestinal tract, as well as afferents from the higher cortical centers (including the visual center) and the chemoreceptor trigger zone (CTZ) in the area postrema (a highly vascularized area of the brain stem). The CTZ can be activated by chemical stimuli received through the blood or the cerebrospinal fluid. Direct electrical stimulation of the CTZ, however, does not result in emesis.

Clinical assessment of nausea and vomiting usually focuses on the occurrence of vomiting, that is, the frequency and number of episodes. Nausea, however, is a subjective phenomenon unobservable by another. Few data collection instruments that measure separately the patient's experience of nausea and vomiting and his or her symptom distress have been reported in the literature. In fact, the Rhodes Index of Nausea and Vomiting (INV) Form 2 is the only available tool that measures the individual components of nausea, vomiting, and retching. This index measures the patient's perception of the duration, frequency, and distress from nausea; the frequency, amount, and distress from vomiting; and the frequency, amount, and distress from retching (dry heaves). The INV score provides a measurement of the total symptom experience of the patient.

While the causes of nausea and vomiting are numerous—they include gastrointestinal diseases, infections, intracranial disease, toxins, radiation sickness, psychological trauma, migraines, and circulatory syncope—

INFORMATION ON NAUSEA AND VOMITING

CAUSES: May include gastrointestinal diseases, infections, intracranial disease, toxins, radiation sickness, migraines, motion sickness, pregnancy, anesthesia, psychological trauma

SYMPTOMS: Increased salivation and swallowing, pallor, rapid heartbeat, sweating

DURATION: Typically acute; can be recurrent with acute episodes

TREATMENTS: Depends on cause; may include drug therapy, diet regulation, lifestyle change, emotional support

---

three of the most common causes are motion sickness (air, sea, land, or space), pregnancy, and anesthesia administered during operative procedures.

The sequence of symptoms and signs that constitute motion sickness is fairly characteristic. Premonitory symptoms often include yawning or sighing, lethargy, somnolence, and a loss of enthusiasm and concern for the task at hand. Increasing malaise is directed toward the epigastrium, a sensation best described as "stomach awareness," which progresses to nausea. Diversion of the blood flow from the skin toward the muscles results in pallor. A feeling of warmth and a desire for cool air is often accompanied by sweating. Frontal headache and a sensation of disorientation, dizziness, or lightheadedness may also occur. As symptoms progress, vomiting occurs early in the sequence of symptoms for some; in others, malaise is severe and prolonged and vomiting is delayed. After vomiting, there is often a temporary improvement in well-being; however, with continued provocative motion, symptoms build again and vomiting recurs. The symptoms may last for minutes, hours, or even days.

The most coherent explanation for the development of motion sickness is provided by sensory conflict theory. Motion sickness is generally thought to occur as the result of a "sensory conflict" between information arising from the semicircular canals and organs of the vestibular system, visual and other sensory input, and the input that is expected on the basis of past experience or exposure history. It is argued that conflicts between current sensory inputs are by themselves insufficient to produce motion sickness since adaptation occurs even though the conflicting inputs continue to be present. Visual input alone, however, can produce symptoms of motion sickness, such as watching motion pictures shot from a moving vehicle or looking out of the side window (as opposed to the front window) of a moving vehicle.

Nausea and/or vomiting in the early morning during pregnancy, so-called morning sickness, is so common that it is accepted as a symptom of normal pregnancy. Occurring soon after waking, it is often retching rather than actual vomiting and usually does not disturb the woman's health or her pregnancy. The symptoms nearly always cease before the fourteenth week of pregnancy. In a much smaller proportion of cases, approximately 1 in 1,000 births, the vomiting becomes more serious and persistent, occurring throughout the day and even during the night. The term "hyperemesis gravidarum" is given to this serious form of vomiting. Theories on the etiology of morning sickness have tended to be grouped under four main areas: endocrine (caused by estrogen and progesterone levels), psychosomatic (a conscious or unconscious wish not to be pregnant), allergic (a histamine reaction), and metabolic (a lack of potassium).

Nausea and vomiting occur frequently as unpleasant side effects of the administration of anesthesia in many clinical procedures. Most postoperative vomiting is mild, and only in a few cases will the problem persist so as to cause electrolyte disturbances and dehydration. The factors affecting postoperative nausea and vomiting may be divided into two categories: by the type of patient and surgery, and by the anesthetic and preoperative and postoperative medication uses. Patients with a history of motion sickness have a predisposition to postoperative vomiting. Nearly 43 percent of patients who vomited following previous surgery vomited again, whereas slightly more than 14 percent of those who did not vomit previously had an emetic episode at their next operation. Patients undergoing their first anesthetic procedure had an incidence of vomiting of approximately 30 percent.

No direct association between vomiting and age has been found. That vomiting may be hormonally related, however, is suggested by the higher incidence of nausea and vomiting in the latter half of the menstrual cycle. Other factors that may affect nausea and vomiting associated with anesthesia include patient weight (female obese patients being particularly more vulnerable), amount of hydration, metabolic status, and psychological state.

With regard to the type of surgery performed, the highest incidence of nausea and vomiting appears to be associated with abdominal surgery, as well as ear, nose, and throat surgery, with middle-ear surgery being the major category. The length of surgery, and therefore the duration of anesthesia, also has a direct effect on nausea and vomiting. Short (thirty-minute to sixty-minute) operations using cyclopropane had an emetic incidence of 17.5 percent, while operations lasting one and a half to three and a half hours had an incidence of 46.4 percent.

Most of the causes of vomiting associated with general anesthesia are expected to be eliminated with regional or spinal anesthesia. The type of anesthesia used also has an effect on nausea and vomiting. Research indicates that cyclopropane, ether, and nitrous oxide are potent emetics.

TREATMENT AND THERAPY

Since the generation of sensory conflict underlies all motion environments that give rise to motion sickness, practical measures that reduce conflict are likely to reduce motion sickness incidence. Motion sickness can be minimized if the subject has the widest possible view of a visual reference in which the earth is stable. Passengers aboard ships are less likely to be seasick if they remain on deck at midship, where vertical motion is minimized, and view the horizon. In a car or bus, individuals should be in a position to see the road directly ahead, since the movement of this visual scene will correlate with the changes in the direction of the vehicle. While head movements in a rotating environment are known to precipitate motion sickness, there is no clear experimental evidence that they elicit nausea in mild linear oscillation. Thus, some nonpharmacologic remedies for motion sickness are restricting head movements, lying in a supine position, or closing the eyes. In addition, the use of acupressure wrist bands has proven effective in combating motion sickness.

Pharmacologically, the drug hyoscine hydrobromide (also called hyoscine or scopolamine) emerged as a valuable prophylactic drug following extensive research during World War II into the problems of motion sickness in troops transported in aircraft, ships, and landing craft. It remains one of the most effective drugs for short-duration exposures to provocative motion. Doses in excess of 0.6 milligram, however, are very likely to lead to drowsiness, and there is much experimental evidence that hyoscine impairs short-term memory. Hyoscine can be absorbed transdermally, and in order to extend the duration of action, a controlled-release patch was developed to deliver 1.2 milligrams on application and 0.01 milligram hourly thereafter. There is substantial evidence of its sustained effectiveness, but, perhaps as a result of variable absorption rates, there is an increased risk of blurred vision after more than twenty-four hours of use.

Amphetamines, ephedrine, and a number of antihistamines (such as dimenhydrinate) have been found to be clinically useful in motion sickness. Following oral administration, these drugs are generally slower than hyoscine in reaching their peak efficacy, but they have a longer duration of action.

For most susceptible subjects whose exposure to motion sickness-inducing stimuli is infrequent, prophylactic drugs offer the only useful treatment. When exposure to provocative stimuli is more frequent, as for example in professional aircraft pilots, spontaneous adaption occurs during training and an initially high incidence of motion sickness decreases with time.

In medical conditions in which the cause is relatively unknown, it is usual to find a wide variety of suggested therapies; nausea and vomiting during pregnancy and hyperemesis gravidarum (the serious, persistent form of vomiting in pregnancy) are no exception. Prior to 1968, treatments numbered approximately thirty. In subsequent years, however, suggested therapy has been mainly drugs of the antiemetic variety. Yet since the thalidomide tragedy (in which severe deformities occurred in the children of women who took this drug), there has been a reluctance to use drugs of any kind during early pregnancy. Probably the only value of drug therapy is at the stage of morning sickness, when antiemetics or mild sedatives may counter the feeling of nausea and prevent women from experiencing excessive vomiting and entering the vicious cycle of dehydration, starvation, and electrolyte imbalance. Once the patient has reached the stage of hyperemesis gravidarum, much more basic therapy is required, and the regimen calls for correction of dehydration, carbohydrate deficiency, and ionic deficiencies. This program is best managed by intravenous therapy, with or without the addition of vitamin supplements and sedative agents.

Nonpharmacologic self-care actions for morning sickness fall into the three broad categories of manipulating diet, adjusting behavior, and seeking emotional support. Some of the most effective self-care actions are getting rest, eating several small meals rather than three large ones, avoiding bad smells, avoiding greasy or fried foods, avoiding cooking, and receiving extra attention and support.

In terms of postoperative nausea and vomiting caused by anesthesia, it has been found that routine antiemetic prophylaxis of patients undergoing elective surgical procedures is not indicated, since fewer than 30 percent of patients experience postoperative nausea and vomiting. Of those who develop these symptoms, many have transient nausea or only one or two bouts of emesis and do not require antiemetic therapy. In addition, commonly used antiemetic drugs can produce significant side effects, such as sedation. Nevertheless, antiemetic prophylaxis may be justified in those patients who are at greater risk for developing postoperative nausea and/or vomiting. Such therapy is often given to patients with a history of motion sickness or to those undergoing gynecologic procedures, inner-ear procedures, oral surgery (in which the jaws are occluded by wires, causing a high risk of breathing in vomitus), and operations on the ear or eye and plastic surgery operations (in order to avoid disruption of delicate surgical work).

Many different antiemetic drugs are available for the treatment of postoperative nausea and vomiting. Researchers have found it difficult to interpret the results of antiemetic drug studies because the severity of postoperative vomiting and the response to therapeutic agents can be influenced by many variables in addition to the antiemetic drug being studied. Even with the use of the same drugs in a homogeneous population undergoing the same procedure, the severity of emesis varies from individual to individual.

Because antiemetic drugs have differing sites of action, better results can be obtained by using a multidrug approach. If a combination of drugs with a similar site of action is used, however, the incidence of side effects may be increased. There are few data regarding combination antiemetic prophylaxis or therapy for postoperative nausea and emesis. Drug combinations have been avoided in postsurgical patients because of concerns about additive central nervous system toxicity. An exception is the combination of low-dose droperidol and metoclopramide, which appears to be more effective than droperidol alone for outpatient gynecologic procedures.

Although a full stomach is best avoided before any operative procedure, with situations such as emergencies, in which danger from vomiting is acute, a rapid sequence of administering anesthesia (induction) and clearing the air passage (intubation) remains the method of choice to avoid nausea and vomiting in patients with a full stomach. After the procedure, it is recommended that the patient minimize movement in order to avoid nausea and vomiting. Also, it has been found that avoiding eating solid food for at least eight hours after a surgical procedure is helpful in preventing postoperative nausea and vomiting.

Perspective and Prospects

Though it has existed for as long as there have been human beings, the symptom of nausea has never received much attention in health care practice or research. In fact, until the early 1970's the sensation of nausea was frequently dismissed as merely a passing phenomenon. The rationale for this dismissal was most likely the understanding that nausea is self-limiting (it always passes with time), is never life-threatening in itself, is probably psychogenic in nature (at least to some degree), and, being subjective, is very difficult to measure. In addition, in the past the most predictable nausea was related to pregnancy, which may also explain the lack of attention given to it.

Until the late 1980's, there was still little research being conducted on the nausea associated with pregnancy, although it is a common symptom. The historical lack of interest in nausea and vomiting during pregnancy may be traced to the fact that, since the symptoms generally persist only through the first trimester, health care professionals have viewed the problem as relatively insignificant. As more pregnant women work outside the home in demanding positions, however, these women have exhibited less tolerance for illness. Demands upon the health care industry and upon personal physicians for more research and effective treatment have become more widespread.

While it is surprising that nausea has received scant attention in the history of clinical research, it is even more astonishing that vomiting, an observable behavior, has received so little attention as well. Although vomiting is a primitive neurologic process that has remained almost unchanged in the evolution of animals, the mechanisms that regulate the behavior remain virtually unknown.

One reason for the paucity of information on the subject of nausea in particular stems from the lack of a reliable animal model. This fact has hampered research aimed at establishing the etiological basis for nausea and its relationship to vomiting. While some species of lower animals, for example rats, cannot vomit, it is not known whether rats experience the phenomenon of nausea. Thus no effective means of measuring nausea in lower animals has been devised.

Since the early 1970's, there has been a noticeable increase in research on nausea as a drug side effect because it was so frequently seen in cancer chemotherapy clinical trials sponsored by the National Cancer Institute and the American Cancer Society. As more powerful chemotherapy agents and aggressive combinations were clinically investigated, patients began to experience severe, potentially life-threatening nausea and vomiting. Yet it was still the symptom of vomiting that began to receive attention; nausea was either coupled with the investigation of vomiting, with the two treated as a unit, or it was ignored. Nevertheless, efforts continued to improve antiemetic drugs until nausea began to be seen as a separate but related symptom.

Aside from the pharmacological investigations of new drugs and drug combinations in the treatment of nausea and vomiting, an interesting branch of scientific investigation has begun the process of exploring alternative ways of managing these symptoms. Behavioral interventions, such as progressive muscle relaxation, biofeedback, imagery, or music therapy, have been used to alleviate postchemotherapy anxiety. These methods may also be used to treat other patients suffering from the symptoms of nausea and vomiting, such as pregnant women.

Another noninvasive, nonpharmacologic measure that has been considered in the relief of nausea and vomiting is transcutaneous electrical nerve stimulation (TENS). Several research studies indicate that TENS may be useful in alleviating chemotherapy-related nausea and vomiting, including delayed nausea and vomiting. Side effects from using TENS units are negligible, and with further study they may prove to be an acceptable, helpful relief measure.

—*Genevieve Slomski, Ph.D.*

See also Acid reflux disease; Anesthesia; Appetite loss; Botulism; Bulimia; Colitis; Crohn's disease; Digestion; Eating disorders; Food biochemistry; Food poisoning; Gastroenterology; Gastroenterology, pediatric; Gastrointestinal disorders; Gastrointestinal system; Heartburn; Indigestion; Influenza; Lactose intolerance; Motion sickness; Multiple chemical sensitivity syndrome; Noroviruses; Poisoning; Poisonous plants; Pregnancy and gestation; Radiation sickness; Rotavirus; Salmonella infection; Stomach, intestinal, and pancreatic cancers; Ulcer surgery; Ulcers; Vagotomy.

For Further Information:

Blum, Richard H., and W. LeRoy Heinrichs. *Nausea and Vomiting: Overview, Challenges, Practical Treat-*

ments and New Perspectives. Philadelphia: Whurr, 2000. Discusses such topics as drugs to prevent and control nausea and vomiting, pregnancy nausea and vomiting, allergy and immunology, anesthesiology, and gastroenterology.

Edmundowicz, Steven A., ed. *Twenty Common Problems in Gastroenterology.* New York: McGraw-Hill, 2002. Surveys common problems with the gastrointestinal tract, examining nausea and vomiting as both symptom and disorder.

Funk, Sandra G., et al., eds. *Key Aspects of Comfort: Management of Pain, Fatigue, and Nausea.* New York: Springer, 1989. This work, which discusses the management of pain, fatigue, and nausea, functions both as an introduction to these topics and as a sourcebook for treatment.

Hesketh, Paul J., ed. *Management of Nausea and Vomiting in Cancer and Cancer Treatment.* Sudbury, Mass.: Jones and Bartlett, 2005. Reviews the therapies available to prevent nausea and vomiting in cancer patients.

Kucharczyk, John, David J. Stewart, and Alan D. Miller, eds. *Nausea and Vomiting: Recent Research and Clinical Advances.* Boca Raton, Fla.: CRC Press, 1991. After an introductory chapter on pioneers in emesis research, discusses the mechanisms of emesis, including respiratory muscle control, digestive tract activity, and neural mechanisms; the clinical characteristics and consequences of vomiting; and antiemetic therapies.

Litin, Scott C., ed. *Mayo Clinic Family Health Book.* 3d ed. New York: HarperResource, 2003. Perhaps the best general medical text for the layperson, this book covers the entire medical field. While the information is derived from a wide variety of highly technical sources, the articles are written to be easily understood by a general audience.

Sleisenger, Marvin H., ed. *The Handbook of Nausea and Vomiting.* New York: Caduceus Medical/Parthenon, 1993. A short manual for dealing with the symptoms and causes of nausea and vomiting. Includes a bibliography and an index.

NECK INJURIES AND DISORDERS. *See* **HEAD AND NECK DISORDERS.**

NECROSES. *See* **FROSTBITE; GANGRENE.**

NECROTIZING FASCIITIS
DISEASE/DISORDER

ANATOMY OR SYSTEM AFFECTED: Blood vessels, muscles, skin

SPECIALTIES AND RELATED FIELDS: Bacteriology, critical care, dermatology, emergency medicine, epidemiology, histology, plastic surgery, vascular medicine

DEFINITION: An invasive bacterial infection that occurs in the connective tissue between the skin and muscle known as the fascia, cutting off blood flow; it must be urgently treated surgically and, even in the best circumstances, has a high mortality rate.

CAUSES AND SYMPTOMS

Although it had been identified in the past, in 1994 there were numerous headline newspaper reports describing a new "flesh-eating bacteria." These articles detailed the devastating effect of seemingly minor wounds infected with streptococcal bacteria. Patients quickly become very sick, with a rapidly progressive downward course, even from trauma resulting in a deep muscle bruise or muscle strain or in "minor" cuts and scrapes.

In the former nonpenetrating injuries, it is likely that the bacteria were already present in the blood and then seeded the site of damage. Most of these patients, however, did not recall any prior recent infection that may have made them susceptible. Penetrating injuries, where the normally protective barrier of the skin has been broken, were often minor and not originally treated as contaminated or infected. Other cases of necrotizing fasciitis are caused by surgical infections and bowel contamination. These cases are more rare and often found to have a mixture of bacteria, such as staphylococci or *Escherichia coli* (*E. coli*).

Patients with necrotizing fasciitis have fever, inflammation, severe pain, and blistering at the site of in-

---

INFORMATION ON NECROTIZING FASCIITIS

CAUSES: Bacterial infection

SYMPTOMS: Fever, inflammation, severe pain, blistering at site of infection, tissue death

DURATION: Acute

TREATMENTS: Emergency care, extensive surgical debridement, antibiotics fection. If this cellulitis is not recognized and urgently treated, the infection will quickly spread in the layers of connective tissue just under the skin known as the fascia. As the bacteria multiply, they cause blood vessels supplying the skin to form clots and thus cut off blood flow to the skin. Without nutrients, oxygen, and the ability to remove waste products, the skin dies. Once this occurs, the nerves are destroyed and the patient no longer has the excruciating pain. The skin at this point appears to be "eaten away." The possibility exists that the underlying muscle adjacent to the fascia will become infected. Thus, the potential for muscle death as well as skin death is of great concern, particularly if the infection begins in the arms, legs, abdomen, or back, as these areas have large muscle groups directly underlying the skin. In necrotizing fasciitis, the extremities and the area around the genitals and anus (perineum) are most commonly and extensively involved. Multiplication and movement of these streptococcal bacteria and their toxins into the bloodstream produces a shocklike state.

TREATMENT AND THERAPY

The patient with necrotizing fasciitis must be stabilized quickly in an intensive care unit, where fluids can be administered and heart and lung condition can be closely monitored. The only lifesaving treatment available is extensive surgical debridement to remove the necrotic (dead) tissue and slow the spread of the bacteria. Antibiotics including penicillins, clindamycin, and gentamicin are given to help eradicate the pathogen. Because the infection spreads so rapidly, death often results even with heroic surgical and drug therapy unless the condition is diagnosed and treated early. Fortunately, these infections remain relatively rare.

—*Matthew Berria, Ph.D.*

See also Antibiotics; Bacterial infections; Bacteriology; Dermatology; Epidemiology; Shock; Skin; Skin disorders; Streptococcal infections; Toxic shock syndrome; Wounds.

FOR FURTHER INFORMATION:

Biddle, Wayne. *A Field Guide to Germs.* 2d ed. New York: Anchor Books, 2002.

Forbes, Betty A. Daniel F. Sahm, and Alice S. Weissfeld. *Bailey and Scott's Diagnostic Microbiology.* 11th ed. St. Louis: Mosby, 2002.

Roemmele, Jacqueline A., and Donna Batdorff. *Surviving the Flesh-Eating Bacteria: Understanding, Preventing, Treating, and Living with the Effects of Necrotizing Fasciitis.* Garden City Park, N.Y.: Avery, 2000.

Salyers, Abigail, and Dixie D. Whitt. *Bacterial Pathogenesis: A Molecular Approach.* 2d ed. Washington, D.C.: ASM Press, 2000.

Snyder, Larry, and Wendy Champness. *Molecular Genetics of Bacteria.* 2d ed. Washington, D.C.: ASM Press, 2002.

Wilson, Michael, Brian Henderson, and Rod McNab. *Bacterial Virulence Mechanisms.* New York: Cambridge University Press, 2002.

NEONATOLOGY

SPECIALTY

ANATOMY OR SYSTEM AFFECTED: All

SPECIALTIES AND RELATED FIELDS: Cardiology, critical care, embryology, genetics, obstetrics, pediatrics, perinatology

DEFINITION: A subspecialty of pediatrics that involves the care of newborn infants from birth through the first month of life, especially those infants with life-threatening conditions such as prematurity, genetic defects, and serious illnesses.

KEY TERMS:

congenital disorders: abnormalities present at birth that occurred during fetal development as a result of genetic errors, exposure to toxins and microorganisms, or maternal illness

incubator: in the nursery, a plexiglass unit that encloses the premature or sick infant to allow strict temperature regulation

intrauterine growth retardation: the condition of infants who are born significantly smaller than the standard for the number of weeks that they have spent in the uterus

neonatal intensive care unit: a hospital nursery with advanced equipment and specially trained staff to maintain the vital functions of sick newborns and to monitor their progress closely

neonatal period: the first month of life; derived from the Greek *neo* (meaning "new") and the Latin *natum* (meaning "birth")

prematurity: strictly defined, birth before a full-term pregnancy (thirty-eight weeks); more commonly associated with birth before thirty-five weeks

respirator: a machine that inflates and deflates the lungs, imitating normal breathing; connected to the patient through a tube placed into the windpipe (endotracheal tube)

NUMBER OF INFANT DEATHS IN THE UNITED STATES, 2004

Cause of Death

Congenital malformations, deformations, and chromosomal abnormalities	5,622
Disorders related to short gestation and low birth weight	4,642
Sudden infant death syndrome (SIDS)	2,246
Newborn affected by maternal complications of pregnancy	1,715
Accidents (unintentional injuries)	1,052
Newborn affected by complications of placenta, cord, and membranes	1,042
Respiratory distress	875
Bacterial sepsis	827
Neonatal hemorrhage	616
Diseases of the circulatory system	593
All other causes	8,706
Total	**27,936**

Source: National Center for Health Statistics.

respiratory distress syndrome: a life-threatening illness primarily of premature infants; immature lungs lack surfactant, a vital substance that keeps the tiny air sacs (alveoli) from collapsing upon exhalation

SCIENCE AND PROFESSION

Neonatology has grown dramatically since its beginnings in the late 1960's, and neonatologists have become an integral part of the obstetric-pediatric team at major medical centers throughout the world. In large part because of an ever-expanding technological base and marked advances in scientific research, these health care professionals have greatly changed the outlook for premature and sick newborns. The last decades of the twentieth century saw a dramatic reduction in infant mortality in industrialized nations, where better prenatal care and advanced neonatal care significantly improved the chances of survival for millions of infants.

As a subspecialty of pediatrics, neonatology is concerned with the most critical time of transition and adjustment—the first four weeks of life, or the neonatal period—whether the infant is healthy (a normal birth) or sick (as a result of genetic problems, obstetric complications, or medical illness). By the early 1970's, it became increasingly clear to health administrators that hospitals throughout the United States had varying abilities to care for medical and pediatric cases requir-

ing the most sophisticated staff and equipment. Consequently, they developed a system that designated hospitals as either level I (small, community hospitals), level II (larger hospitals), or level III (major regional medical centers, also called tertiary care centers). It was in the last group that the most advanced neonatal care could be delivered. In these major centers, there are two types of nurseries, separating the normal healthy infant from the sick or high-risk infant: the routine nursery and the neonatal intensive care unit (NICU).

Routine nurseries are the temporary home of the vast majority of newborns. The services of the neonatologist are rarely needed here, and the general pediatrician or family practitioner observes and examines the infant for twenty-four to forty-eight hours to be sure that it has made a smooth transition from intrauterine to extrauterine life. These babies soon leave the hospital for their homes. Those neonates with minor problems arising from multiple births, difficult deliveries, mild prematurity, and minor illness are easily managed by their primary care physician in consultation with a neonatologist, perhaps at another hospital. It is in the neonatal intensive care unit, however, that the most difficult situations present themselves. Here several teams of pediatric subspecialists—surgeons, cardiologists, anesthesiologists, and highly trained nurses, along with many other health professionals—are led by a neonatologist, who coordinates the team's efforts. These newborns have life-threatening conditions, often as a result of extreme prematurity (more than six weeks earlier than the expected date of delivery), major birth defects (genetic or developmental), severe illness (such as overwhelming infections), or being born to drug- or alcohol-addicted mothers. They require the most advanced technological and medical interventions, often to sustain life artificially until the underlying problem is corrected. It is in this setting that the most dramatic successes of neonatology are found.

After hours of being inside a forcefully contracting uterus and sustaining the stress of passing through a narrow birth canal, the newborn emerges into a dry, cold, and hostile environment. The umbilical cord, which has provided oxygen and nutrients, is clamped and cut; the fluid-filled lungs must now exchange air instead, and the respiratory center of the infant's brain begins a lifetime of spontaneous breathing, usually heralded by crying. The vast majority of neonates make this extraordinary adjustment to extrauterine life without difficulty. At one minute and again at five minutes, the newborn is evaluated and scored on five physical signs: heart rate, breathing, muscle tone, reflexes, and skin tone. The healthy infant is vigorously moving, crying, and pink regardless of race. These Apgar scores, named for founder Virginia Apgar, evaluate the need for immediate resuscitation. A brief physical examination follows, which can identify other life-threatening abnormalities.

It is essential to remember that the medical history of a neonate is in fact the medical and obstetric history of its mother, and seemingly normal infants may develop problems shortly after birth. Risk factors include very young or middle-aged mothers; difficult deliveries; babies with Rh-negative blood types; mothers with diabetes mellitus, kidney disease, or heart disease; and concurrent infections in either the mother or the baby. Anticipating these problems of the healthy newborn by using the Apgar scores and the results of the physical examination allows the proper assignment of the infant to the nursery or NICU.

The NICU is a daunting place containing high-tech equipment, a tangle of wires and tubes, the sounds of beeps and alarms, and tiny, fragile infants. All this technology serves two simple purposes: to monitor vital functions and to sustain malfunctioning or nonfunctioning organ systems. Looked at individually, however, the machines and attachments become much more understandable. The incubator, perhaps the most common device, maintains a warm, moist environment of constant temperature at 37 degrees Celsius. Small portholes with rubber gloves allow people to stroke the child safely. Generally, the infants will have small electrodes taped on their chests, connected to video monitors that record the heart and breathing rates and that will sound alarms if significant deviations occur. These monitors will also record blood pressure through an arm or thigh cuff. In order to ensure immediate access to the blood, for delivering medications and taking blood for testing, catheters (plastic tubes) are placed into larger arteries or veins near the umbilicus, neck, or thigh (in adults, intravenous access is found in the arms).

The remaining equipment is used for the very serious business of life support, in particular the support of the respiratory system. Maintaining adequate oxygenation is critical and can be accomplished in several ways, depending on the baby's needs. The least stressful are tubes placed in the nostrils or a face mask, but these methods require that breathing be spontaneous although inadequate. More often, unfortunately, neonates with the types of problems that bring them to an intensive care unit cannot breathe on their own. In these cases, a tube must be connected from the artificial respirator into the windpipe (the endotracheal tube). Warm, moistened, oxygen-rich air is delivered under pressure and removed from the lungs rhythmically to simulate breathing. Tranquilizers and paralytic agents are used to calm and immobilize the infant. Sick or premature infants are also generally unable to feed or nurse naturally, by mouth. Again, several methods of feeding can be employed, depending on the problems and the length of time that such feedings will be needed. For the first few days, simple solutions of water, sugar, and protein can be given through the intravenous catheters. These lines, because of the very small, fragile blood vessels of the newborn, are seldom able to carry more complex solutions. A second method, known as gavage feeding, employs tubing that is inserted through the nose directly into the stomach. Through that tube, infant formula (water, sugar, protein, fat, vitamins, and minerals) and, if available, breast milk can be given.

As the underlying problems are resolved, the infant is slowly weaned, first feeding orally and then breathing naturally. Next, the infant will be placed in an open crib, and gradually the tangled web of tubes and wires will clear. With approval from the neonatologist, the baby is transferred to the routine nursery, a transitional home until discharge from the hospital is advisable.

Diagnostic and Treatment Techniques

Neonatology has amassed an enormous body of knowledge about normal neonatal anatomy and physiology, disease processes, and, most important, how to manage the wide variety of complications that can occur. Specific treatment protocols have been developed that are practiced uniformly in all neonatal intensive care units. Approximately 12 percent of all neonates in the United States require admission to the NICU. Short-term stays (twenty-four to forty-eight hours) are meant to observe and monitor the infant with respiratory distress at birth that required immediate intervention. Long-term stays, lasting from several weeks to months, are the case for the sickest newborns, most commonly those with severe prematurity and low birth weight (less than 1,500 grams), respiratory distress syndrome (also known as hyaline membrane disease), congenital defects, and drug or alcohol addictions.

Infants born prematurely make up the major proportion of all infants at high risk for disability and death, and each passing decade has seen younger and younger babies being kept alive. While many maternal factors can lead to preterm delivery, often no explanation can be found. The main problem of prematurity lies in the functional and structural immaturity of vital organs. Weak sucking, swallowing, and coughing reflexes lead to an inability to feed and the danger of choking. Lungs that lack surfactant, a substance that coats the millions of tiny air sacs (alveoli) in each lung to keep them from collapsing and sticking together after air is exhaled, cause severe breathing difficulty as the infant struggles to reinflate them. An immature immune system cannot protect the newborn from the many viruses, bacteria, and other microorganisms that exist. Inadequate metabolism causes low body temperature and inadequate use of food or medications. Neurological immaturity can lead to mental retardation, blindness, and deafness.

Aggressive management of the preterm baby begins in the delivery room, with close cooperation between the obstetrician and the neonatologist. Severely preterm infants, some born after only twenty weeks of pregnancy, require immediate respiratory and cardiac support. Placement of the endotracheal tube, assisted ventilation with a handheld bag, and delicate chest compressions similar to the cardiopulmonary resuscitation (CPR) done on adults to stimulate the heartbeat are each accomplished quickly. Once the respiratory

and circulatory systems have been stabilized, excess fluid will be suctioned, while a brief physical examination is performed to note any abnormalities that require immediate attention. As soon as transport is considered safe, the newborn is sent to the NICU. If the infant has been delivered at a small, community hospital, this may involve ambulance or even helicopter transport to the nearest tertiary care center.

Once in the unit, the neonate will be placed in an incubator and attached to video monitors that record heart rate, breathing, and blood pressure. The endotracheal tube can now be attached to the respirator machine, and intravenous or intra-arterial catheters will be placed to allow the fluid and medication infusions and the blood drawing for the battery of tests that the neonatologist requires. Feeding methods can be set up as soon as the infant has stabilized. Within a short time after delivery, the premature newborn has had a flurry of activity about it and is surrounded by the most sophisticated equipment and staff available. Supporting the immature organs becomes the first priority, although the ethical issues of saving very sick infants must soon be addressed as complications begin to occur. Nearly 15 percent of surviving preterm infants whose birth weights were less than 2,000 grams have serious physical and mental disabilities after discharge. The majority, however, grow to lead normal, healthy lives.

Congenital defects are common, with nearly 7 percent of the American population having some physical or cosmetic deformity, although most are not serious. Unfortunately, nearly 2 percent of all newborns have life-threatening abnormalities that require immediate attention and admission to the NICU. It is estimated that the majority of miscarriages are a direct result of congenital defects that are incompatible with life. Many infants that do survive development and delivery die shortly after birth despite the most sophisticated and heroic attempts to intervene. The causes of such defects are arbitrarily assigned to two broad categories, although a combination of these factors is the most likely explanation: genetic errors (such as breaks, doubling, and mutations) and environmental insults (such as chemicals, drugs, viruses, radiation, and malnutrition). In the United States, among the most common birth defects that require immediate intervention are heart problems, spina bifida (an open spine), and tracheoesophageal fistulas and esophageal atresias (wrongly connected or incomplete wind and food pipes).

The birth of a malformed infant is rarely expected, and the neonatologist's team plays a key role in its survival. Congenital heart disease is the most prevalent life-threatening defect. During development in utero, the umbilical cord supplies the necessary oxygen; it is not until birth, when that lifeline is cut, that the neonate's circulatory and respiratory systems acquire full responsibility. At delivery, all may appear normal, and the one-minute Apgar score may be high. Several minutes later, however, the pink skin color may begin to darken to a purplish blue (cyanosis), indicating that insufficient oxygen is being extracted from the air. Immediately, the infant receives rescue breathing from the bag mask. Upon admission to the neonatal unit, the source of the cyanosis must be determined. A chest X ray may provide significant information about the anatomy of the heart and lungs, but special tests are usually needed to pinpoint the problem. Catheters that are threaded from neck or leg vessels into the heart can reveal the pressure and oxygen content of each chamber in the heart and across its four valves. Echocardiograms, video pictures similar to sonograms generated by sound waves passing through the chest, enhance the data provided by the X rays and catheterizations, and a diagnosis is made. Based on the physical signs and symptoms of the newborn, a treatment plan is devised.

Because of the nature of congenital defects and structural abnormalities, their correction generally requires surgery. Openings between the heart's chambers (septal defects), valves that are too narrow or do not close properly, and blood vessels that leave or enter the heart incorrectly are all common defects treated by the pediatric heart surgeon. Because of the delicacy of the operation and the vulnerability of the newborn, surgery may be postponed until the baby is larger and stronger while it is provided with supplemental oxygen and nutrients. The risk of such operations is high, and depending on the degree of abnormality, several operations may be required.

Another group of infants who have benefited from advances in neonatology are those born to drug-addicted women. The lives of these infants are often complicated by congenital defects and life-threatening withdrawal symptoms. For example, heroin-addicted

Newborns at risk may require a special environment such as an incubator. (Digital Stock)

babies are quite small, are extremely irritable and hyperactive, and develop tremors, vomiting, diarrhea, and seizures. The newborn must be carefully monitored in the unit, and sedatives and antiseizure medications are given, sometimes for as long as six weeks. Cocaine and its derivatives frequently cause premature labor, fetal death, and maternal hemorrhaging during delivery. Infants that do survive often have serious congenital defects and suffer withdrawal symptoms. The risk of acquired immunodeficiency syndrome (AIDS) adds another dimension to an already complicated picture.

PERSPECTIVE AND PROSPECTS

Throughout human history, maternal and neonatal deaths have been staggering in number. Ignorance and unsanitary conditions frequently resulted in uterine hemorrhaging and overwhelming infection, killing both mother and baby. Highly inaccurate records at the beginning of the twentieth century in New York City show maternal death averaging 2 percent; in fact, the rate was probably greater, since most births occurred at home. Neonatal deaths from respiratory failure, congenital defects, prematurity, and infection loom large in these medical records. The expansion of medical, obstetric, and pediatric knowledge and technology that began after World War II has dramatically lowered maternal and infant mortality. It should not be forgotten, however, that nonindustrialized nations, the majority in the world, remain devastated by the neonatal problems that have plagued civilization for thousands of years.

Ironically, the problems associated with neonatology in Western nations are now at the other end of the spectrum: saving and prolonging life beyond what is natural or "reasonable." As neonatology advanced scientifically and technically, saving life took precedence over ethical issues. The famous and poignant story of "Baby Doe" in the early 1980's illustrates the dilemmas that occur daily in neonatal intensive care units. Baby Doe was a six-pound, full-term male born with Down syndrome and three severe congenital defects of the heart, trachea, and esophagus. These malformations were deemed surgically correctable, although the underlying problem of Down syndrome, a disease characterized by mental retardation and particular facial and body features, would remain. The parents would not agree to any operations and requested that all treatment be withheld. He was given only medication for sedation and died within a few days. The case was related by the attending physician in a letter to *The New England Journal of Medicine*. Enormous controversy was sparked. On July 5, 1983, a law was passed in effect stating that all handicapped newborns, no matter how seriously afflicted, should receive all possible life-sustaining treatment, unless it is unequivocally clear that imminent death is inevitable or that the risks of treatment cannot be justified by its benefit. The legislators believed that Baby Doe had been allowed to die because of his underlying condition (Down syndrome).

Since then, attorneys, ethicists, juries, and the courts have used the example of Baby Doe, and the law that grew from it, to interpret many cases that have come to light. Life-and-death decisions are made on a daily basis in the neonatal care unit. They are always difficult, but they usually remain a private matter between the parents and the neonatologist. These cases become public matters, however, when the family disagrees with the medical staff. Then the question of what is in the best interest of the child is compounded by who will pay for the treatments and who will care for the baby after it is discharged.

Such ethical dilemmas will continue as expertise and technology grow. A multitude of questions, previously relegated to philosophy and religion, will arise, and the benefits of saving a life will have to be weighed against its quality and the resources necessary to maintain it.

—Connie Rizzo, M.D., Ph.D.;
updated by Alexander Sandra, M.D.

See also Apgar score; Birth defects; Blue baby syndrome; Bonding; Cardiology, pediatric; Cesarean section; Childbirth; Childbirth complications; Chlamydia; Circumcision, male; Cleft lip and palate; Cleft lip and palate repair; Cognitive development; Colic; Congenital heart disease; Craniosynostosis; Critical care, pediatric; Cystic fibrosis; Developmental stages; Down syndrome; Embryology; Endocrinology, pediatric; Failure to thrive; Fetal alcohol syndrome; Fetal surgery; Gastroenterology, pediatric; Genetic diseases; Genetics and inheritance; Hematology, pediatric; Hemolytic disease of the newborn; Hydrocephalus; Intraventricular hemorrhage; Jaundice, neonatal; Metabolic disorders; Motor skill development; Multiple births; Nephrology, pediatric; Neurology, pediatric; Obstetrics; Orthopedics, pediatric; Pediatrics; Perinatology; Phenylketonuria (PKU); Premature birth; Pulmonary medicine, pediatric; Rh factor; Shunts; Sudden infant death syndrome (SIDS); Surgery, pediatric; Tay-Sachs disease; Teratogens; Toxoplasmosis; Urology, pediatric; Well-baby examinations.

FOR FURTHER INFORMATION:

Behrman, Richard E., Robert M. Kliegman, and Hal B. Jenson, eds. *Nelson Textbook of Pediatrics*. 17th ed. Philadelphia: Saunders, 2004. This bible of pediatrics is notable not only for its breadth and scope but also for its clarity and accessibility. The several chapters devoted to neonatology, intensive care, prematurity, and congenital defects provide a good overview in the context of pediatrics as a whole.

Bradford, Nikki. *Your Premature Baby: The First Five Years*. Toronto: Firefly Books, 2003. Guides the logistics of care for premature infants from birth into the preschool years and sets expectations for hospital care by describing hospital terms, procedures, treatments, and equipment.

Cunningham, Nicholas, ed. *Columbia University College of Physicians and Surgeons: Complete Guide to Early Child Care*. New York: Crown, 1990. A very well written and organized book meant for health professionals as well as parents; the finest of this type. Its material is thorough but not too technical, so it is accessible to a wider audience. A good place to start for an overview before turning to more difficult texts.

Levin, Daniel L., and Frances C. Morriss, eds. *Essentials of Pediatric Intensive Care*. 2d ed. New York: Churchill Livingstone, 1997. This superb paperback focuses on the daily routine of the neonatal intensive care unit. Good photographs and diagrams explain the technology and the procedures used. Often used as a supplement to hardcover neonatology texts, but it can be used alone.

MacDonald, Mhairi G., Mary M. K. Seshia, and Martha D. Mullett, eds. *Avery's Neonatology: Pathophysiology and Management of the Newborn*. 6th ed. Philadelphia: Lippincott Williams & Wilkins, 2005. This excellent text, used as a main reference for neonatologists, provides a thorough scientific background, including the anatomy, physiology, and biochemistry of all known abnormal conditions. As one of the most respected sources in the field, it can be technical and involved at times, but it is well worth the effort.

Martin, Richard J., Avroy A. Fanaroff, and Michele C. Walsh, eds. *Fanaroff and Martin's Neonatal-Perinatal Medicine: Diseases of the Fetus and Infant*. 2 vols. 8th ed. Philadelphia: Mosby Elsevier, 2006. This classic reference work is one of the most comprehensive to date and features discussions on the diverse practice of neonatal-perinatal medicine, pregnancy disorders and their impact on the fetus, delivery room care, provisions for neonatal care, and the development and disorder of organ systems.

Moore, Keith L., and T. V. N. Persaud. *The Developing Human*. 7th ed. Philadelphia: W. B. Saunders, 2003. An outstanding textbook on human embryonic development, with specific information about the causes of congenital malformations and common defects occurring in each of the body's systems.

Ruhlman, Michael. *Walk on Water: Inside an Elite Pediatric Surgery Unit*. New York: Viking-Penguin, 2003. A fascinating foray into life in a pediatric heart center—Cleveland Clinic—specializing in neonatal open-heart surgery, focusing on the daily experiences of world-renowned surgeon Dr. Roger Mee.

Sadler, T. W. *Langman's Medical Embryology*. 10th ed. Philadelphia: Lippincott Williams & Wilkins, 2006. Text that covers the fundamentals of embryology, with a chapter devoted to birth defects.

Woolf, Alan D., et al., eds. *The Children's Hospital Guide to Your Child's Health and Development*. Cambridge, Mass.: Perseus, 2002. An authoritative and comprehensive guide to children's health, providing a guide to every common illness or condition that affects children and a carefully designed emergency section.

NEPHRECTOMY

PROCEDURE

ANATOMY OR SYSTEM AFFECTED: Abdomen, kidneys, urinary system

SPECIALTIES AND RELATED FIELDS: General surgery, nephrology, oncology, urology

DEFINITION: The removal of the kidney, which may be performed to treat disorders and disease or for the purpose of transplantation.

KEY TERMS:

adrenal gland: a small hormone-producing gland which is adjacent to the upper pole of the kidney

donor nephrectomy: a procedure in which a kidney is removed for transplantation into another patient; the kidney can be removed from a person who is brain-dead but whose heart is still beating (cadaveric donor nephrectomy) or from a relative of the recipient (a living related donor)

nephroureterectomy: a procedure similar to a radical nephrectomy, with the additional removal of the ureter and a cuff of the bladder; performed to treat transitional cell carcinomas of the ureters and the pelvis of the kidneys *radical nephrectomy:* a procedure in which a kidney is removed along with the covering layers of tissue and the adjacent adrenal gland; performed with cancerous conditions

renal cell carcinoma (RCC): cancer of the small tubules of the kidney; generally known as kidney cancer

simple nephrectomy: a procedure in which a kidney is removed but the covering layers of tissue and the adjacent adrenal gland are left intact; usually performed to treat benign (noncancerous) conditions

transitional cell carcinoma (TCC): cancer arising from the lining of the urine-collecting system of the kidneys, ureters, and bladder

ureters: the tubes that drain urine from the kidneys to the bladder

INDICATIONS AND PROCEDURES

A kidney may be removed for several reasons, including congenital defects, trauma, cancer, inflammation, and transplantation. Congenital problems, or birth defects, associated with the kidneys include abnormal development, nonfunctional cysts, blockage, tumors, and cysts that are functional but which cause difficulty in breathing because of their large size. A kidney may be removed if the organ or its main blood vessels have been damaged beyond repair by trauma, such as a gunshot wound. Cancer is one of the most common reasons for nephrectomy; kidney cancers include renal cell carcinomas, transitional cell carcinomas, and tumors in the capsules of the kidneys or in surrounding layers of tissue. Infections or abscesses in the kidney that are beyond medical treatment and that become life-threatening also necessitate a nephrectomy. Finally, a kidney may be removed from a donor for transplantation.

Depending on the underlying disease and the surgeon's preference and experience, the kidney can be approached from the front, side, or back. In certain situations, the chest is also opened. The incisions used to reach the kidney are similar for simple, radical, and donor nephrectomies, but the steps that follow differ once the abdomen has been entered. For nephroureterectomy, in which the kidney, the connecting ureter, and a part of the bladder are removed, the surgeon makes either one long, S-shaped incision starting in the flank and ending near the bladder, or two separate incisions.

In the frontal approach to nephrectomy, the patient lies on his or her back and the abdomen and peritoneal cavity are opened. The intestines near the kidney are pushed to the side, and the kidney is approached from the front. The advantage of this approach includes better evaluation of the liver and the structures surrounding the kidney, better control of the blood vessels, and easy removal of clots from veins if necessary. The disadvantages of this approach are the possibility of adhesions developing in the intestines and lung complications after the surgery.

In the side approach, the patient is placed on his or her side and the incision is made through the eleventh or twelfth ribs. The kidney is approached from behind. This type of incision involves cutting into muscle and results in significant postoperative pain. The main advantage is that the peritoneal cavity is not entered.

In the back approach, known as dorsal lumbotomy, the patient is placed facedown and a muscle-splitting incision is used. The kidney is approached from be-

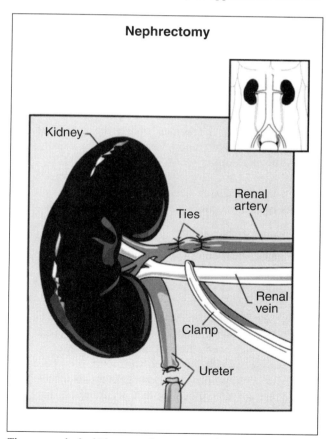

Nephrectomy

Kidney

Ties

Renal artery

Renal vein

Clamp

Ureter

The removal of a kidney may be necessary because of disease or because the kidney is intended for transplantation into another patient; the inset shows the location of the kidneys.

hind. This method is usually used for simple nephrectomy. Its primary advantages are less postoperative pain and avoidance of the peritoneal cavity. Its main disadvantage is a limited view of the surgery site.

In simple nephrectomy, after the kidney has been exposed, Gerota's fascia (the covering envelope of the kidney) is opened, and the fat around the kidney is dissected. The adjacent blood vessels and the connecting ureter are tied and cut, and the kidney is removed. In radical nephrectomy, the adjacent adrenal gland and surrounding lymph glands are also removed in the one block. For nephroureterectomy, the ureter is not cut close to the kidney but is dissected all the way down to the bladder. A 2-centimeter cuff of bladder is cut off, the entire specimen is removed, and the hole in the bladder is closed.

The techniques used with kidney transplantation differ for cadaveric donor nephrectomy and living related donor (LRD) nephrectomy. For cadaveric donor nephrectomy, the abdominal aorta (the main artery bringing blood to the kidney) and the inferior vena cava (the main vein taking blood away from the kidney) are isolated above and below the kidneys and cannulated with pipes to irrigate both kidneys with cold preservation fluid. Both kidneys and ureters, along with their related blood vessels, are removed. For LRD nephrectomy, the kidney is dissected along with its blood vessels and ureter. Great care is taken to obtain the maximum length of ureter and blood vessels without causing damage to the donor.

USES AND COMPLICATIONS

The major complications of nephrectomy during surgery are bleeding, damage to surrounding structures, and problems related to anesthesia. Therefore, there is significant evaluation of the patient before surgery. A battery of tests may be performed, including blood testing, urinalysis, electrocardiography, and X rays. A thorough medical examination is done to determine whether the patient can be placed under anesthesia safely. The patient's blood is also typed and cross-matched in the event that a transfusion is required. Good surgical skills, the availability of blood for transfusion, and proper anesthesia techniques usually ensure that any complications that occur are not life-threatening. Nevertheless, the patient may also experience complications during the procedure that are not directly related to the surgery, such as a heart attack.

After a nephrectomy, the patient is at some risk for other problems. These complications may include bleeding, infection, intestinal obstruction, blood clots in the legs or lungs, or a heart attack.

PERSPECTIVE AND PROSPECTS

Significant advances have been made in nephrectomy since the first such procedure was performed by Gustav Simmons in 1869. Thorough preoperative evaluation; improved anesthesia techniques; a greater understanding of anatomy, physiology, and pathology (including the nature of infections and microorganisms); and the discovery of antibiotics have all led to better surgical techniques. As a result, the death rate for nephrectomy operations is only 1 percent.

—*Saeed Akhter, M.D.*

See also Adrenalectomy; Dialysis; Hemolytic uremic syndrome; Kidney cancer; Kidney disorders; Kidney transplantation; Kidneys; Nephritis; Nephrology; Nephrology, pediatric; Transplantation.

FOR FURTHER INFORMATION:

Brenner, Barry M., and Samuel A. Levine, eds. *Brenner and Rector's The Kidney*. 7th ed. Philadelphia: W. B. Saunders, 2004. This treatise, at more than two thousand pages, is a comprehensive and authoritative source on the normal and diseased human kidney.

Danovitch, Gabriel, ed. *Handbook of Kidney Transplantation*. 4th ed. Philadelphia: Lippincott Williams & Wilkins, 2005. A clinical handbook that gives a practical overview of renal transplantation and includes up-to-date coverage of topics such as immunosuppressive drugs, short- and long-term post-transplant management, complications, and ethical/legal issues.

Hinman, Frank, Jr.. *Atlas of Urologic Surgery*. 2d ed. Philadelphia: W. B. Saunders, 1998. This is an excellent book with very useful diagrammatic and graphic details of operations and good descriptions of both old and new procedures.

Marshall, Fray F., ed. *Textbook of Operative Urology*. Philadelphia: W. B. Saunders, 1996. This book presents the most current information on indications for operation, preoperative management, operative technique, postoperative management, and complications specific to each procedure.

Novick, Andrew C., and Stevan B. Streem. "Surgery of the Kidney." In *Campbell's Urology*, edited by Patrick Walsh et al. 7th ed. Philadelphia: W. B. Saunders, 1998. A chapter in a classic urology text, which maintains its encyclopedic approach while following a new organ systems orientation. Halftone illustrations and contributions by multiple authors.

Schrier, Robert W., ed. *Diseases of the Kidney and Urinary Tract*. 8th ed. Philadelphia: Wolters Kluwer Health/Lippincott Williams & Wilkins, 2007. Covers full range of the biochemical, structural, and functional correlations in the kidney, as well as hereditary diseases, urological diseases and neoplasms of the genitourinary tract, acute renal failure, and nutrition, drugs and the kidney, among many additional topics.

Nephritis
Disease/disorder

Anatomy or system affected: Blood vessels, immune system, kidneys

Specialties and related fields: Immunology, internal medicine, nephrology

Definition: An inflammatory response of the kidneys, particularly of the glomeruli, to infectious agents or immunological challenges.

Key terms:

albuminuria: excretion in the urine of the protein albumin, usually as a result of changes occurring in the glomeruli

amyloidosis: the deposition of immunoglobulin fibrils in various tissues, including the kidneys

dialysis: the use of artificial membranes to remove metabolites from the blood when the kidneys fail; the peritoneum can also be used (peritoneal dialysis)

filtration rate: the amount of fluid passing per minute from blood across the glomerular capillaries to form glomerular fluid

glomeruli: structures consisting mainly of capillary blood vessels contained in a capsule, across whose walls water and solutes pass (filter) to form glomerular fluid

glomerulonephritis: inflammation of glomeruli

hematuria: the presence of red blood cells or red blood cell casts in the urine

immunoglobulins: proteins associated with immune responses

nephrotic syndrome: a condition involving edema, the retention of water and of sodium and chloride ions, urinary protein losses greater than 3 grams per day, and hypoalbuminemia

proteinuria: the presence of proteins, including globulins, in the urine; usually considered a sign of changes in the glomerular structures

renal blood flow: the amount of whole blood entering the renal arteries per minute; a fraction of water and solutes is removed to form urine

renal failure: severe kidney insufficiency requiring the use of dialysis or transplantation to return and maintain composition of body fluids at or near normal values

renal insufficiency: the inability of the kidneys to maintain a normal internal environment of the body and its fluids

streptococci: bacteria responsible for the development of some cases of acute glomerulonephritis, but without infection of the kidneys

tubules: hollow structures conducting glomerular fluid to the collecting ducts and the renal pelvis; they produce composition and volume changes of glomerular fluid passing through them and may reabsorb some of the protein that crosses the glomerular capillaries

Causes and Symptoms

Nephritis means any inflammatory responses of the kidney, whether the cause is infectious or immunological. Generally, it involves mainly the glomeruli, where the initial formation of urine takes place. The term is therefore equivalent in meaning to glomerulonephritis. Pathological changes may also occur in the interstitium (the extravascular, extracellular domain in which the tubules are embedded) and affect tubular functions. This condition, referred to as tubulointerstitial nephritis, is associated with localized cellular infiltrates and the accumulation of fluid.

The classic cause of acute glomerulonephritis is an infection in the throat or of the skin by a nephritogenic strain of Group A streptococci. The clinical presentation can be dramatic and can be associated not only with a sore throat but also with headaches, shortness of breath, and swelling of the ankles. Physical examination may find hypertension, rales in the lungs, peripheral pitting edema, and changes in the retinal vessels. In the chronic form, the onset is usually insidious; an infection may have been forgotten or ignored, without specific complaints except for some ankle edema, tiredness, and perhaps pallor. The physical findings for chronic glomerulonephritis are similar to but less striking than in the acute form.

The diagnosis in each type of nephritis is presumed on the basis of urinalysis, with a finding of blood (hematuria) in the acute form; proteinuria (actually mainly albuminuria, although globulins may also be

Information on Nephritis

Causes: Inflammation of kidney from bacterial infection (often streptococcal) or immune disorder

Symptoms: In acute form, sore throat, headache, shortness of breath, ankle swelling, hypertension, edema; in chronic form, ankle swelling, fatigue, pallor; either may lead to nephrotic syndrome (loss of albumin in urine, decreased serum albumin, water retention, sodium and chloride ion retention, massive edema and ascites)

Duration: Acute or chronic

Treatments: Usually none needed for acute form; for nonresolving or chronic form, dietary control (decreased protein and potassium), steroids, hemodialysis or peritoneal dialysis, kidney transplantation

present); and a decreased glomerular filtration rate. Diagnosis is established on the basis of renal biopsy with examination by both light and electron microscopy. Throat cultures and streptococcal group determination are appropriate if an infection is suspected.

Both conditions may be followed by the development of nephrotic syndrome, which is characterized by major losses of albumin in the urine, decreased serum albumin concentrations (hypoalbuminemia), the retention of water and of sodium and chloride ions, and massive edema and ascites (fluid leakage from blood vessels into the abdomen). Nephrotic syndrome may also appear without any history or evidence of a preceding episode of acute glomerulonephritis. On renal biopsy, essentially no changes or only minimal changes may be noted on inspection by light microscopy (minimal change disease), although characteristic changes are found with electron microscopy affecting particularly the foot processes (podocytes) of the glomeruli.

Acute glomerulonephritis resolves spontaneously and rapidly in about 95 percent of cases, without detectable residual damage to kidney functions. Apart from control of hypertension, no specific treatment is available. The edema is rarely sufficient to warrant the use of diuretics. Antibiotics are not indicated unless there is evidence of an infection. Patients can be considered to be cured but should nonetheless be followed in the event of a reappearance of symptoms or manifestations.

In nonresolving acute glomerulonephritis and in chronic glomerulonephritis, there can be progression of damage to the glomeruli so that the number of functioning glomeruli (normally, about one million in each kidney) diminishes. This process may be gradual or may occur as a part of acute exacerbations that subside but leave the patient with diminished renal functions. As a result, glomerular filtration is decreased and the accumulation of metabolic end-products, particularly urea, occurs in the blood and tissue fluids. Abnormalities of acid-base regulation appear with decreased blood pH (acidemia), decreased serum bicarbonate concentration, and increased potassium concentration. Generally, a significant anemia exists, and renal blood flow is decreased so that the metabolic activities of the renal tubule cells are affected. Renal insufficiency is established, and dietary control is instituted, with decreased intakes of protein and potassium. Paradoxically, with decreased glomerular function, proteinuria decreases, serum albumin increases, and edema decreases or disappears.

Unfortunately, the progression of glomerular dysfunction continues, and dietary measures provide insufficient control of metabolic abnormalities. Resort is then made to hemodialysis or peritoneal dialysis to control the metabolic abnormalities and lift dietary restrictions to some degree while the patient awaits kidney transplantation. During this waiting period, stimulants of the bone marrow, such as erythropoietin, are administered in the expectation of maintaining the red cell count and the hematocrit at a satisfactory level. Transplants will require the use of immunosuppressive agents to prevent rejection unless an identical twin is the donor.

Other diseases in which glomerular damage can occur include diabetes mellitus, amyloidosis, systemic lupus erythematosus (SLE), Wegener's granulomatosis, Goodpasture's syndrome, syphilis, and human immunodeficiency virus (HIV) infection. Common problems associated with glomerular damage of any etiology are hypertension, strokes, heart failure, pulmonary edema, arteriolar vasoconstriction and sclerosis, impaired vision from exudates, pericarditis, and pericardial effusions.

Treatment and Therapy

Acute glomerulonephritis is characterized by the disappearance of signs and symptoms, or at least their marked reduction, in most patients. In 90 to 95 percent of cases, there is no progression and no recurrence. In some patients, the problems may reappear after apparent complete remission, while in others the disease progresses, often to nephrotic syndrome. This phase, too, disappears as the disease worsens, reaching the stage where hemodialysis or peritoneal dialysis becomes necessary. A renal biopsy can aid in determining the appropriate treatment. For example, if the biopsy confirms that poststreptococcal nephritis is present, then no specific treatment is available. If progressive glomerulonephritis is the diagnosis, then steroids may be indicated.

Hemodialysis depends on an arteriovenous shunt being created, usually in the forearm, so that the patient's blood can pass through a dialysis machine, which functions in a manner similar to glomeruli. Usually, several sessions, two or three times per week for several hours at a time, are required. Peritoneal dialysis involves the introduction of large amounts of fluid into the peritoneal cavity and its withdrawal after adequate exchanges with body fluids across the peritoneal surfaces have occurred. Hemodialysis requires going to a hospital or specialized facility, while pertoneal dialysis can be performed at home. Both procedures require careful and frequent monitoring of the patient's acid-base, electrolyte, and metabolic statuses.

While arrangements can usually be made for local dialysis, patients on dialysis lose a significant degree of mobility and independence. This independence can be regained to a considerable degree through kidney transplantation. Kidneys may be obtained from cadavers, unrelated living donors, and related living donors, such as identical twins. Except with the latter group, rejection phenomena may occur. Infections can occur with the use of immunosuppressive agents. Rarely, malignancies can be introduced with transplanted kidneys.

A low protein intake is recommended in the later stages of glomerulonephritis because too high a protein intake may accelerate the progression of the disease. Lack of control of water intake may lead to edema. Anemia is common in the later stages and may require the administration of erythropoietin.

In the nephrotic phase and in minimal change disease, control of edema is sought through one or more of the following measures: salt restriction, diuretics, intravenous (IV) administration of concentrated human serum albumin, corticosteroids (such as prednisone, which is more likely to be effective in minimal change disease), and other immunosuppressive agents. Nephrotic syndrome may occur in the presence of other underlying diseases, such as lupus, diabetes mellitus, HIV infection, syphilis, amyloidosis, and microvascular angiopathies. Specific treatments should be used when applicable.

Perspective and Prospects

The monograph *Reports of Medical Cases* by Richard Bright, published in 1827, marks the first clear description of nephritis through clinical findings (edema), laboratory assessment (proteinuria), and gross structural changes in the kidneys at postmortem. For many years, nephritis was referred to as Bright's disease. Apart from the measurement of blood constituents such as urea and creatinine, functional assessment was limited until the development, by Donald D. Van Slyke, of the clearance concept, defined as the amount of a given substance excreted in the urine per unit time relative to its concentration in plasma or blood. Van Slyke focused on the clearance of urea, while P. B. Rehberg in Denmark proposed that the clearance of creatinine could be used as a measure of the glomerular filtration rate. Glomerular fluid had been shown by Newton Richards to have the same composition as an ultrafiltrate of plasma. Accordingly, if creatinine was neither secreted nor reabsorbed by the tubules, then its clearance would be equivalent to the glomerular filtration rate.

The assumptions with respect to creatinine were shown to be incorrect, and inulin, a polyfructoside studied by Homer Smith, was found to be a reliable and correct indicator for measuring the glomerular filtration rate. Smith and his collaborators systematized and advanced knowledge of the kidney as a whole organ in a quantitative manner. Detailed understanding of the components of the whole organ progressed rapidly with the discovery of the significance of countercirculation in establishing the solute concentration gradient from cortex to medulla reported by H. Wirz and B. Hargitay. Functions of limited segments of the tubules (and later of individual cells) have provided additional important information on transport and metabolic processes in the kidneys.

On the clinical side, the introduction of renal biopsies and of hemodialysis (and later peritoneal dialysis) by way of an arteriovenous shunt made for more accurate diagnoses and longer life expectancies for patients with chronic renal disease. Further encouragement was provided by the development of techniques for successful renal transplants, first from identical twins, then from living donors and cadavers. Problems of rejection remain. Another major challenge is to find the means of delaying or arresting the progression of chronic renal disease before dialysis and transplants become necessary.

—*Francis P. Chinard, M.D.*

See also Hemolytic uremic syndrome; Kidney cancer; Kidney disorders; Kidneys; Nephrectomy; Nephrology; Nephrology, pediatric; Pyelonephritis; Renal failure; Stone removal; Stones; Systemic lupus erythematosus (SLE); Transplantation.

For Further Information:

Brenner, Barry M. "Retarding the Progression of Renal Disease." *Kidney International* 64 (2003): 370-378. Addresses the control of various manifestations of renal disease (proteinuria, hyperlipidemia) through dietary and pharmacologic approaches. The goal is to prevent progression to end-stage renal disease (ESRD) when dialysis or a transplant is required.

Brenner, Barry M., and Samuel A. Levine, eds. *Brenner and Rector's The Kidney.* 7th ed. Philadelphia: W. B. Saunders, 2004. A multiauthored text reviewing the anatomy, physiology, and responses to injury of the kidneys.

Cameron, J. Stewart, and Richard J. Glassock, eds. *The Nephrotic Syndrome.* New York: Marcel Dekker, 1988. Reviews clinical aspects as well as pathophysiology. Contains an excellent historical account.

D'Amico, G., and C. Bazzi. "Pathophysiology of Proteinuria." *Kidney International* 63 (2003): 809-825. A critical review of the roles of the glomerular capillary walls and of the tubule cells in determining the identities and quantities of the proteins excreted in the final urine.

Eddy, A. A., and J. M. Symons. "Nephrotic Syndrome in Children." *Lancet* 362 (2003): 629-639. Nephrotic syndrome is trying for children, their families, and their physicians. Steroids are successful in reversing the problem in many but not all patients. The underlying pathogenesis, clinical presentations, treatment, and possible outcomes are well and critically addressed.

Hricik, D. E., M. Chung-Park, and J. R. Sedor. "Glomerulonephritis." *New England Journal of Medicine* 339 (1998): 888-899. Focuses on immunological and cellular responses, risk factors for progression, genetic factors, and absence of specific therapies.

Nephrology

Specialty

Anatomy or system affected: Abdomen, blood, kidneys, urinary system

Specialties and related fields: Biochemistry, biotechnology, endocrinology, genetics, hematology, internal medicine, urology

Definition: The field of medicine that deals with the anatomy and physiology of the kidneys.

Key terms:

analyte: any chemical substance undergoing measurement; includes charged electrolytes found in the blood, such as sodium or potassium

creatinine: a nitrogen-containing by-product of metabolism; levels of creatinine may be indicative of kidney function

endocrine: referring to a process in which cells from an organ or gland secrete substances into the blood; these substances in turn act on cells elsewhere in the body

glomerulonephritis: inflammation of the glomeruli, the clusters of blood vessels and nerves found throughout the kidney

nephritis: any disease or pathology of the kidney that results in inflammation

nephron: the structural and functional unit of the kidney; composed of the renal corpuscle, the loop of Henle, and renal tubules

nephrotic syndrome: an abnormal condition of the kidneys characterized by a variety of conditions, including edema and proteinuria; often accompanies glomerular dysfunction and diabetes

renal: pertaining to the kidney

urea: a waste product of protein metabolism which represents the form in which nitrogen is eliminated from the body

Science and Profession

Nephrology is the branch of medicine that deals with the function of the kidneys. As a consequence, a nephrologist frequently deals with problems related to homeostasis, that is, the maintenance of the internal environment of the body. The most obvious function of the kidneys is their ability to regulate the excretion of water and minerals from the body, at the same time serving to eliminate nitrogenous wastes in the form of urea. While such waste material, produced as by-products of cell metabolism, is removed from the circulation, essential nutrients from body fluids are retained within the renal apparatus. These nutrients include proteins, carbohydrates, and electrolytes, some of which help maintain the proper acid-base balance within the blood. In addition, cells in the kidneys regulate red blood cell production through the release of the hormone erythropoietin.

The human excretory system includes two kidneys, which lie in the rear of the abdominal cavity on opposite sides of the spinal column. Urine is produced by the kidneys through a filtration network composed of 2 million nephrons, the actual functional units within each kidney. Two ureters, one for each kidney, serve to remove the collected urine and transport this liquid to the urinary bladder. The urethra drains urine from the bladder, voiding the liquid from the body.

Each adult human kidney is approximately 11 centimeters in length, with a shape resembling a bean. When the kidney is sectioned, three anatomical regions are visible: a light-colored outer cortex; a darker inner region, called the medulla; and the renal pelvis, the lowest portion of the kidney. The cortex consists primarily of a network of nephrons and associated blood capillaries. Tubules extending from each nephron pass into the medulla. The medulla, in turn, is visibly divided into about a dozen conical masses, or pyramids, with the base of the pyramid at the junction between the cortex and medulla and the apex of the pyramid extending into the renal pelvis. The loops (such as the loop of Henle) and tubules within the medulla carry out the reabsorption of nutrients and fluids that have passed through the capsular network of the nephron. The tubules extend through the medulla and return to the cortical region.

There are approximately 1 million nephrons in each kidney. Within each nephron, the actual filtration of blood is carried out within a bulb-shaped region, Bowman's capsule, which surrounds a capillary network, the glomerulus. In most individuals, a single renal artery brings the blood supply to the kidney. Since the renal artery originates from a branch of the aorta, the body's largest artery, the blood pressure within this region of the kidney is high. Consequently, hypotension, a significant lowering of blood pressure, may also result in kidney failure.

The renal artery enters the kidney through the renal pelvis, branching into progressively smaller arterioles and capillaries. The capillary network serves both to supply nutrition to the cells that make up the kidney and to collect nutrients or fluids reabsorbed from the loops and tubules of the nephrons. Renal capillaries also enter the Bowman's capsules in the form of balls or coils,

the glomeruli. Since blood pressure remains high, the force filtration in a nephron pushes about 20 percent of the fluid volume of the glomerulus into the cavity portion of the capsule. Most small materials dissolved in the blood, including proteins, sugars, electrolytes, and the nitrogenous waste product urea, pass along within the fluid into the capsule. As the filtrate passes through the series of convoluted tubules extending from the Bowman's capsule, most nutrients and salts are reabsorbed and reenter the capillary network. Approximately 99 percent of the water that has passed through the capsule is also reabsorbed. The material which remains, much of it waste such as urea, is excreted from the body.

Nephrology is the branch of medicine that deals with these functions of the kidney. Loss of kidney function can quickly result in a buildup of waste material in the blood; hence kidney failure, if untreated, can result in serious illness or death. Within the purview of nephrology, however, is more than the function of the kidneys as filters for the excretion of wastes. The kidneys are also endocrine organs, structures that secrete hormones into the bloodstream to act on other, distal organs. The major endocrine functions of the kidneys involve the secretion of the hormones renin and erythropoietin.

Renin functions within the renin-angiotensin system in the regulation of blood pressure. It is produced within the juxtaglomerular complex, the region around Bowman's capsule in which the arteriole enters the structure. Cells within the tubules of the nephron closely monitor the blood pressure within the incoming arterioles. When blood pressure drops, these cells stimulate the release of renin directly into the blood circulation.

Renin does not act directly on the nephrons. Rather, it serves as a proteolytic enzyme that activates another protein, angiotensin, the precursor of which is found in the blood. The activated angiotensin, called angiotensin II, has several effects on kidney function that involve the regulation of blood pressure. First, by decreasing the glomerular filtration rate, it allows more water to be retained. Second, angiotensin II stimulates the release of the steroid hormone aldosterone from the adrenal glands, located in close association with the kidneys. Aldosterone acts to increase sodium retention and transport by cells within the tubules of the nephron, resulting in increased water reabsorption. The result of this complex series of hormone interactions within the kidney is a close monitoring of both salt retention and blood pressure and volume. In this manner, nephrology also relates to the pathophysiology of hypertension—high blood pressure.

The kidneys also regulate the production of erythrocytes, red blood cells, through the production of the hormone erythropoietin. Erythropoietin is secreted by the peritubular cells associated with regions outside the nephrons in response to lowered oxygen levels in the blood, also monitored by cells within the kidney. The hormone serves to stimulate red cell production within the bone marrow. Approximately 85 percent of the erythropoietin in blood fluids is synthesized within the kidneys, the remainder by the liver.

Since proper kidney function is related to a wide variety of body processes, from the regulation of nitrogenous waste disposal to the monitoring and control of blood pressure, nephrology may deal with a number of disparate syndromes. The kidney may represent the primary site of a disease or pathology, an example being the autoimmune phenomenon of glomerulonephritis. Renal failure may also result from the indirect action of a more general systemic syndrome, as is the case with diabetes mellitus. In many cases, the decrease in kidney function may result from any number of disorders, which poses many problems for the nephrologist.

Proper function of the kidney is central to numerous homeostatic processes within the body. Thus nephrology by necessity deals with a variety of pathophysiological disorders. Renal dysfunction may involve disorders of the organ itself or pathology associated with individual structures within the kidneys, the glomeruli or tubules. Likewise, the disorder within the body may be of a more general type, with the kidney being a secondary site of damage. This is particularly true of immune disorders such as lupus (systemic lupus erythematosus) or diabetes. Conditions that affect proper kidney function may result from infection or inflammation, the obstruction of tubules or the vascular system, or neoplastic disorders (cancers).

Immune disorders are among the more common processes that result in kidney disease. They may be of two types: glomerulonephritis or the more general nephrotic syndrome. Glomerulonephritis can result either from a direct attack on basement membrane tissue by host antibodies, such as with Goodpasture's syndrome, or indirectly through deposits of immune (antigen-antibody) complexes, such as with lupus. Nephritis may also be secondary to high blood pressure. In any of these situations, inflammation resulting from the infiltration of immune complexes and/or from the activation of the complement system may result in a de-

creased ability of the glomeruli to function. Treatment of such disorders often involves the use of corticosteroids or other immunosuppressive drugs to dampen the immune response. Continued recurrence of the disease may result in renal failure, requiring dialysis treatment or even kidney transplantation.

Activation of the complement system as a result of immune complex deposition along the glomeruli is a frequent source of inflammation. Complement consists of a series of some dozen serum proteins, many of which are pharmacologically active. Intermediates in the complement pathway include enzymes that activate subsequent components in a cascade fashion. The terminal proteins in the pathway form a "membrane attack complex," capable of significantly damaging a target (such as the basement membrane of a Bowman's capsule). Activation of the initial steps in the pathway begins with either the deposition of immune complexes along basement membranes or the direct binding of antibodies on glomerular surfaces. The end result can be extensive nephrotic destruction.

Nephrotic syndrome, which can also result in extensive damage to the glomeruli, is often secondary to other disease. Diabetes is a frequent primary disorder in its development; approximately one-third of insulin-dependent diabetics are at risk for significant renal failure. Other causes of nephrotic syndrome may include cancer or infectious agents and toxins.

DIAGNOSTIC AND TREATMENT TECHNIQUES

Nephrologists can measure glomerular function using a variety of tests. These tests are based on the ability of the basement membranes associated with the glomeruli to act as filters. Blood cells and large materials such as proteins dissolved in the blood are unable to pass through these filters. Plasma, the liquid portion of the blood containing dissolved factors involved in blood-clotting mechanisms, is able to pass through the basement membrane, the driving force for filtration being the hydrostatic pressure of the blood (blood pressure).

The glomerular filtration rate (GFR) is defined as the rate by which the glomeruli filter the plasma during a fixed period of time. Generally, the rate is determined by measuring either the time of clearance of the carbohydrate inulin from the blood or the rate of clearance of creatinine, a nitrogenous by-product of metabolism. Though the rate may vary with age, it generally is about 125 to 130 milliliters of plasma filtered per minute.

Any significant decrease in the GFR is indicative of renal failure and can result in significant disruptions of acid-base or electrolyte balance in the blood. A decrease in the GFR can sometimes be observed through measurements of urine output. Healthy individuals usually excrete from 1 to 2 liters of urine per day. If the urine output drops to less than 500 milliliters (0.5 liter) per day, a condition known as oliguria, the body suffers a diminished capacity to remove metabolic waste products (urea, creatinine, or acids). Taken to an extreme, in which the filtering capacity is completely shut down and urine formation drops below 100 milliliters per day (anuria), the resulting uremia may cause death in a matter of days.

Anuria may have a variety of causes: kidney failure; hypotension, in which blood pressure is insufficient to maintain glomerular filtration; or a blockage in the urinary tract. As waste products, fluids, and electrolytes (especially sodium and potassium) build up, the person may appear puffy, be feverish, and exhibit muscle weakness. Heart arrhythmia or failure may also occur. Mediation of the problem, in addition to attempts to alleviate the reasons for kidney dysfunction, include regulation of fluid, protein, and electrolyte uptake. Medications are also used to increase the excretion of potassium and tissue fluids, assuming that the cause is not a urinary blockage.

The nephrologist or other physician may also monitor kidney function through measurements of serum analytes or through observation of certain chemicals within the urine. The levels of blood, urea, and nitrogen (BUN), nitrogenous substances in the blood, present a rough measure of kidney function. Generally, BUN levels change significantly only after glomerular filtration has been significantly disrupted. The levels are also dependent on the amount of protein intake in the diet. When changes occur as a result of renal dysfunction, BUN levels can be a useful marker for the progression of the disease. A more specific indicator of renal function can be the creatinine concentration within the blood. Serum creatinine, unlike BUN levels, is not related to the diet. In the event of renal failure, however, changes in BUN levels usually can be detected earlier than those of creatinine.

As the glomeruli lose their ability to distinguish large from small molecules during filtration, protein can begin to appear in the urine, the condition known as proteinuria. Usually, the level of protein in the urine is negligible (less than 250 milligrams per day). A transient proteinuria can result from heavy exercise or minor illness, but persistent levels of more than 1 gram per day may be indicative of renal dysfunction or even

complications of hypertension. Generally, if the problem resides in the loss of tubular reabsorption, levels of protein generally are below 1 to 2 grams per day, with that amount usually consisting of small proteins. If the problem is a result of increased glomerular permeability caused by inflammation, levels may reach greater than 2 grams per day. In cases of nephrotic syndrome, excretion of protein in the urine may exceed 5 grams per day.

Measurement of urine protein is a relatively easy process. A urine sample is placed on a plastic stick with an indicator pad capable of turning colors, depending on the protein concentration. Analogous strips may be used for detection of other materials in urine, including acid, blood, or sugars. The presence of either red or white blood cells in urine can be indicative of infection or glomerulonephritis.

In addition to the filtration of blood fluids through the nephrons, the reabsorption of materials within the tubules results in increased urine concentration. A normal GFR within a healthy kidney produces a urine concentration three or four times as great as that found within serum. As kidney failure progresses, the concentration of urine begins to decrease, with the urine becoming more dilute. The kidneys compensate for the decreased concentration by increasing the amount of urine output: The frequency of urination may increase, as well as the volume excreted (polyuria). In time, if renal failure continues, the GFR will decrease, resulting in the retention of both analytes and water.

Determination of urine concentration is carried out following a brief period of dehydration: deprivation of fluids for about fifteen hours prior to the test. This dehydration will result in increased production by the hypothalamus of antidiuretic hormone (ADH), or vasopressin, a chemical which decreases the production of urine through increased renal tubule reabsorption of water. The result is a more concentrated urine. Following the dehydration period, the patient's urine is collected over a period of three hours and assessed for concentration. Significantly low values may be indicative of kidney disease.

A battery of tests in addition to those already described may be utilized in the diagnosis of kidney disease. These may include intravenous pyelography (in which a contrast medium is injected into the blood and followed as it passes through the kidneys), kidney biopsy, and ultrasound examinations. Diagnosis and course of treatment depend on an evaluation of these tests.

PERSPECTIVE AND PROSPECTS

The roots of modern nephrology date from the seventeenth century. In the early decades of that century, the English physician William Harvey demonstrated the principles of blood circulation and the role of the heart in that process. Harvey's theories opened the door for more extensive analysis of organ systems, both in humans and in other animals. As a result, in 1666, Italian anatomist Marcello Malpighi, while exploring organ structure with the newly developed microscope, discovered the presence of glomeruli (what he called Malpighian corpuscles) within the kidneys. Malpighi thought that these structures were in some way connected with collecting ducts in the kidneys that had recently been found by Lorenzo Bellini. Malpighi also suspected that these structures played a role in urine formation.

Sir William Bowman, in 1832, was the first to describe the true relationship of the corpuscles discovered by Malpighi to urine secretion through the tubules. Bowman's capsule, as it is now called, is a filter which allows only the liquid of the blood, as well as dissolved salts and urea within the blood, into the tubules, from which the urine is secreted. It remained for Carl Ludwig, in 1842, to complete the story. Ludwig suggested that the corpuscles function in a passive manner, in that the filtrate is filtered by means of hydrostatic pressure through the capsule into the tubules and from there concentrated as water and solutes are reabsorbed.

The first definitive work on urine formation, *The Secretion of the Urine*, was published by Arthur Robertson Cushny in 1917. In the monograph, Cushny offered a thorough analysis of the data published on kidney function. Though Cushny was incorrect in some of his conclusions, the work catalyzed intensive research activity on the functions of the kidney. A colleague of Cushny, E. Brice Mayrs, made the first attempt to determine the glomerular filtration rate, measuring the clearance of sulfate in rabbits. In 1926, the Danish physiologist Poul Brandt Rehberg demonstrated the superiority of creatinine as a marker for glomerular filtration; the "guinea pig" for the experiment was Rehberg himself.

A pioneer in renal physiology, Homer William Smith, began his research while serving in the United States Army during World War I. Until he retired in 1961, Smith was involved in much of the research related to renal excretion. It was Smith who developed inulin clearance as a measure of the GFR; his later years dealt with studies on mechanisms of solute excretion.

With the newer technology of the late twentieth century, more accurate methods for analysis became available. These have included ultrasound scanning, intravenous pyelography, and angiography. In addition, better understanding of immediate causes of many kidney problems has served to control or prevent some forms of renal failure.

—*Richard Adler, Ph.D.*

See also Abdomen; Abdominal disorders; Adrenalectomy; Blood and blood disorders; Cysts; Diabetes mellitus; Dialysis; Edema; Hemolytic uremic syndrome; Internal medicine; Kidney cancer; Kidney disorders; Kidney transplantation; Kidneys; Lithotripsy; Nephrectomy; Nephritis; Nephrology, pediatric; Polycystic kidney disease; Pyelonephritis; Renal failure; Stone removal; Stones; Systemic lupus erythematosus (SLE); Terminally ill: Extended care; Transplantation; Urinalysis; Urinary system; Urology; Urology, pediatric.

FOR FURTHER INFORMATION:

Brenner, Barry M., and Samuel A. Levine, eds. *Brenner and Rector's The Kidney*. 7th ed. Philadelphia: W. B. Saunders, 2004. This treatise, at more than two thousand pages, is a comprehensive and authoritative source on the normal and diseased human kidney.

Cameron, Stewart. *Kidney Disease: The Facts*. 2d ed. New York: Oxford University Press, 1990. A brief but thorough discussion of types of kidney disease. Written in a style that falls between detailed analysis and cursory treatment. Some knowledge of biology is helpful.

Hricik, Donald E., R. Tyler Miller, and John R. Sedor, eds. *Nephrology Secrets*. 2d ed. Philadelphia: Hanley & Belfus, 2003. Written by leading nephrology clinicians, covers "the seventy most important topics in nephrology" in a question-answer format.

Legrain, Marcel, et al. *Nephrology*. Translated by M. Cavaillé-Coll. New York: Masson, 1987. A basic text on the function of the kidney. The book provides an overview of kidney structure, diseases of the kidney, and their treatment. Also included is a chapter dealing with appropriate diets for the prevention or alleviation of kidney disease.

Marieb, Elaine N. *Essentials of Human Anatomy and Physiology*. 8th ed. San Francisco: Pearson/Benjamin Cummings, 2006. This introductory anatomy and physiology textbook, easily accessible to those with little science background, is richly illustrated with diagrams and photographs, which help to illuminate body systems and processes.

O'Callaghan, Chris A., and Barry M. Brenner. *The Kidney at a Glance*. Boston: Blackwell Scientific, 2000. Covers a range of topics related to the kidneys, presenting text on one page and accompanying illustrations on the facing page. Covers basic anatomy and physiology and the pathologies and presentations of renal and urinary tract disease.

Tanagho, Emil A., and Jack W. McAninich, eds. *Smith's General Urology*. 16th ed. New York: Lange Medical Books/McGraw-Hill, 2004. A text within the Appleton and Lange series of medical publications. An outstanding overview of kidney structure and function. Written at a level appropriate for readers with a basic knowledge of biology, but contains enough detail that it can also serve as a reference work.

Wallace, Robert A., Gerald P. Sanders, and Robert J. Ferl. *Biology: The Science of Life*. 4th ed. New York: HarperCollins, 1996. Included in the chapter on excretion is a fine description of the human excretory system. Written on a basic level, the section includes useful diagrams and a concise discussion of kidney function written for those with only rudimentary knowledge of the field.

Whitworth, Judith A., and J. R. Lawrence, eds. *Textbook of Renal Disease*. 2d ed. New York: Churchill Livingstone, 1994. A detailed analysis of kidney anatomy and function, with an emphasis on types of disease. The book provides a fine description of the effects of systemic problems on renal dysfunction. Also included are sections on imaging and diagnosis.

NEPHROLOGY, PEDIATRIC

SPECIALTY

ANATOMY OR SYSTEM AFFECTED: Abdomen, blood, kidneys, urinary system

SPECIALTIES AND RELATED FIELDS: Biochemistry, biotechnology, endocrinology, genetics, hematology, internal medicine, neonatology, pediatrics, urology

DEFINITION: The specialty involving the diagnosis and treatment of kidney disorders and diseases in children and adolescents.

KEY TERMS:

dialysis: the process of separating crystalloid molecules in solution by diffusion through a semiperme-

able membrane (essentially, a machine performing the function of the nephrons in the kidney)

glomerulus: one of the very small units in the kidney, where blood is filtered through a membrane

immunology: the science concerned with various phenomena of immunity, increased sensitivity, and allergy

nephrology: the medical science of the kidneys and their function

nephron: the basic functioning unit of the kidney, consisting of the glomerulus plus a series of collecting and transport tubules; there are approximately one million nephrons in each kidney

renal: referring to the kidneys

urea: a nitrogenous molecule found in the blood and urine; the largest component of urine besides water

SCIENCE AND PROFESSION

Pediatric nephrology is a major subspecialty limited to children and adolescents that involves the study of normal and abnormal kidney (renal) function. This discipline not only relates to kidney diseases and renal dysfunction but also places heavy emphasis on the kidneys' adaptive role in many diseases and disorders of nonrenal origin. Pediatric nephrologists are doctors of medicine or osteopathy who have completed three years of pediatric residency training, followed by two or three years in a pediatric nephrology fellowship.

The kidneys are among the most interesting and complex organs in the human body. Kidney diseases often involve the fields of immunology, oncology, genetics, chemistry, physiology, biotechnology, and both gross anatomy and microanatomy (histology). While the cognitive aspects of nephrology dominate the day-to-day work of its specialists, hands-on procedures such as renal biopsies and renal dialysis add variety and interest. Pediatric nephrologists spend approximately 60 percent of their time dealing with primary renal disease, while 40 percent of their time is spent with diseases and conditions of nonrenal origin, especially in critically ill children.

While the kidneys have many functions, their main role is filtering metabolic wastes from the blood and eliminating them via the urinary tract. The process of filtering blood, concentrating its wastes, and reabsorbing water and useful metabolic components (such as protein, sodium, and potassium salts) is accomplished with an elaborate system of passive and active mechanisms in the nephrons in each kidney. The kidneys respond to many factors, including blood volume, blood pressure, the salt and acid content of the blood, nitrogenous wastes (urea), and even hormonal and neural (nerve) stimuli. The kidneys deliver feedback to other vital organs with chemical messengers via the bloodstream and also through the nervous system.

Several key areas in pediatric nephrology make it unique from adult nephrology: immature renal function in infancy, growth retardation in chronic renal disease, and the role of genetics.

Diagnostic and Treatment Techniques

The patient's history, a physical examination, and routine urinalysis are the cornerstones of diagnosis in nephrology. Urinalysis is one of the most available, fastest, and least expensive tests in clinical medicine. Frequently, diagnosis is made or suspected from a routine urinalysis done in screening or as part of a routine physical. The test can reveal evidence of infection; microscopic traces of blood, protein, or sugar; and many other abnormalities. Often, early diagnosis of silent renal disease will aid in early intervention, treatment, and the prevention of advanced disease and morbidity. In addition to blood chemistry tests—such as for sodium, potassium, glucose (sugar), and blood, urea, and nitrogen (BUN)—many quantitative tests are available to measure other aspects of renal function.

Dramatic advances in imaging techniques have been made. X rays, ultrasound, computed tomography (CT) scans, magnetic resonance imaging (MRI), and nuclear scans are making detailed anatomical diagnosis possible in noninvasive ways. Very small tumors and structural abnormalities can be identified. Some scans can provide useful information on renal function.

Renal biopsy with a percutaneous (through-the-skin) technique, using a large-bore needle, was developed in the 1960's. The samples allow detailed examination at microscopic and submicroscopic (electron microscopy) levels. Since many renal diseases reveal a characteristic thickening from immunoglobulin deposits and inflammation of membranes in the glomerulus, exact diagnoses are often made by biopsy alone or in conjunction with immunological tests.

In the early part of the twentieth century, the treatment of renal diseases was limited to symptomatic and supportive measures. By the 1940's and 1950's, the advent of antibiotics allowed definitive treatment of kidney and urinary tract infections. Since that era, chemotherapy and immunotherapy have developed rapidly, and many primary renal diseases are now being treated successfully by such methods. Immuno-

therapy also plays a major role in renal transplantation.

In chronic renal disease, in which the total renal function becomes inadequate to sustain life, children can be treated successfully with renal dialysis. Evolving from pioneer efforts in the 1960's and early 1970's, dialysis is now done routinely for such children, including infants. The effectiveness, safety, and efficiency of the procedure have improved dramatically. Now infants and toddlers usually have peritoneal (abdominal cavity) dialysis conducted at home. Older children usually have hemodialysis about three times a week at a dialysis center. The dialysis machine is connected to a cannula (tubing) that is placed in the patient's arm.

Severe growth retardation is a major problem associated with chronic renal disease in children, often compounded by psychological problems such as severe depression. A combination of improved aggressive nutritional and metabolic support plus treatment with growth hormone has improved the health and mental well-being of these children.

By the early 1970's, kidney transplantation was being done on children. This operation is performed by urologists and pediatric surgeons. Originally, rejection rates and other complications were very high. Results have improved dramatically, and in the United States a national collaborative database reported in 1993 that five years after live donor grafts, 75 percent of the kidneys had not been rejected. This procedure allows thousands of children to lead healthy, normal lives.

The study of renal function in newborns, especially premature ones, has led to sophisticated intensive care for critically ill infants. Pediatric nephrologists may also act as consultants for older children with critical illnesses, injuries, poisonings, and even trauma. Such cases often involve sophisticated intravenous (IV) fluid therapy. Because of temporary renal failure, some of these cases require dialysis.

Perspective and Prospects

The progress in renal dialysis and transplantation has been remarkable. Continued advances in effectiveness, success rates, safety, and convenience are certain. The gene that causes familial polycystic kidney disease has been identified. Such discoveries, coupled with advances in genetics, may revolutionize therapy and even prevent some renal diseases through genetic engineering.

—*C. Mervyn Rasmussen, M.D.*

See also Abdomen; Abdominal disorders; Adrenalectomy; Blood and blood disorders; Diabetes mellitus; Dialysis; Edema; Hemolytic uremic syndrome; Internal medicine; Kidney disorders; Kidney transplantation; Kidneys; Nephrectomy; Nephritis; Nephrology; Pediatrics; Polycystic kidney disease; Pyelonephritis; Renal failure; Systems and organs; Transplantation; Urinalysis; Urinary system; Urology; Urology, pediatric.

FOR FURTHER INFORMATION:

Bock, Glenn H., Edward J. Ruley, and Michael P. Moore. *A Parent's Guide to Kidney Disorders.* Minneapolis: University of Minnesota Press, 1993. A good overview. Nicely organized, with a glossary.

Faris, Mickie Hall. *When Your Kidneys Fail: A Handbook for Patients and Their Families.* 3d ed. Los Angeles: National Kidney Foundation of Southern California, 1994. A handbook for patients and their families. Easy to read and contains an excellent glossary.

Frank, J. David, John P. Gearhart, and Howard M. Snyder, eds. *Operative Pediatric Urology.* 2d ed. New York: Churchill Livingstone, 2002. A technical clinical text that documents open reconstructive urologic procedures for congenital anomalies of the genitourinary tract.

O'Callaghan, Chris A., and Barry M. Brenner. *The Kidney at a Glance.* Boston: Blackwell Scientific, 2000. Covers a range of topics related to the kidneys, presenting text on one page and accompanying illustrations on the facing page. Covers basic anatomy and physiology and the pathologies and presentations of renal and urinary tract disease.

Orsini, Jenoveva. "Comprehensive Care for Children with Renal Disease." *The Exceptional Parent* 29, no. 9 (September, 1999): 36, 38. With commitment, patience, and the support of an outstanding pediatric nephrology team, parents of children with kidney disease and renal failure can provide the care and attention that will enhance the health of their children. Topics such as nutrition, medication, dialysis, and transplantation are addressed.

Webb, Nicholas J. A., and Robert J. Postlethwaite, eds. *Clinical Paediatric Nephrology.* 3d ed. New York: Oxford University Press, 2003. Discusses kidney diseases in infants and children. Includes a bibliography and an index.

NERVOUS SYSTEM

ANATOMY

ANATOMY OR SYSTEM AFFECTED: Ears, nerves, spine

SPECIALTIES AND RELATED FIELDS: Neurology

DEFINITION: The major control system of the body, which synchronizes physiologic activity by interpreting incoming stimuli and which is responsible for memory and reasoning; it is composed of the central nervous system (the brain and spinal cord) and the peripheral nervous system (nerve processes, sensory receptors, and ganglia).

KEY TERMS:

cerebrospinal fluid (CSF): the extracellular fluid of the central nervous system; it flows through the ventricles of the brain and the central canal of the spinal cord, circulating nutrients and providing a cushion for the brain

effector: a general term referring to skeletal, smooth, and cardiac muscles or glands that respond to impulses produced by the nervous system

glial cells: nonexcitable cells of the nervous system; they include astrocytes, microglial cells, oligodendrocytes, and Schwann cells

receptors: membrane-bound proteins with specific binding sites for neurotransmitters

synapse: a juncture between neurons or between neurons and muscle

STRUCTURE AND FUNCTIONS

The nervous system serves as the major control system of the human body. It is responsible for the synchronization of body parts, the integration of physiologic activity, the interpretation of incoming stimuli, and all intellectual activity, including memory and abstract reasoning. The nervous system regulates these activities by communication between various nerve cells; by controlling the actions of skeletal, smooth, and cardiac muscle; and by stimulating the secretion of products from various glands of the body.

Anatomically, the nervous system is divided into the central nervous system, which is composed of the brain and the spinal cord, and the peripheral nervous system, which includes all nervous structures outside the central nervous system—primarily, nerve processes, sensory receptors, and a limited number of cells of the nervous system that are located in special structures known as ganglia. Ganglia are found at various locations throughout the body. They are the only locations of neurons outside the central nervous system. Information from incoming cells can be transmitted to the ganglion cells, which in turn can transmit that information to other locations.

Although the brain and the spinal cord contain several different types of cells that are morphologically unique, there is only one functional cell present, which by convention is always referred to as the neuron. The neuron is one of the few cells in the body that cannot reproduce; a fixed number of these cells develop in infancy, and the number never increases. The number of neurons can, however, decrease in the event of injury or disease.

The neuron consists of a cell body that is similar to that of the typical animal cell familiar to most people. In addition, the neuron has extensions called processes. In the typical neuron, there are two types of processes: dendrites and axons.

Usually a neuron has many dendrites. Dendrites are very short, receive information from nearby cells, and relay that information to the cell body. Each cell has only a single axon, which may be very long, extending up and down the spinal cord or from the spinal cord to the ends of the fingers or toes. The axons conduct information from the cell bodies to the effectors—that is, the muscles and glands—or to other neurons.

Functionally, the nervous system is divided into two areas: the somatic nervous system and the autonomic nervous system. The somatic system controls posture and locomotion by stimulating the skeletal muscles. It is responsible for knowing where the body is in space and for ensuring that there is sufficient muscle contraction (tone) to maintain posture. Responses of the somatic system occur through the motor neurons.

The autonomic nervous system regulates the internal activities through the innervation, or nerve stimulation, of the smooth muscles or the glands. It is anatomically different from the somatic nervous system in that the stimulation of body parts always involves two neurons. The cell body of the second neuron in the sequence is located in a ganglion outside the central nervous system.

The autonomic nervous system is broken down further into two divisions: the sympathetic and the parasympathetic. The sympathetic system is also known as the "fight or flight" reaction, since it evolved from the mechanism in lower animals by which an animal would prepare to fight a predator or run from it. More commonly, it is referred to in humans as the adrenaline response, which is active during stressful situations, strenuous physical activity, public performance, or competition.

The parasympathetic system, which is responsible for the digestive functions of the body, controls stimulation of salivary gland secretions, increased blood flow to digestive organs, and movement of materials through the digestive system. The sympathetic and parasympathetic systems usually function in balance; the parasympathetic system predominates

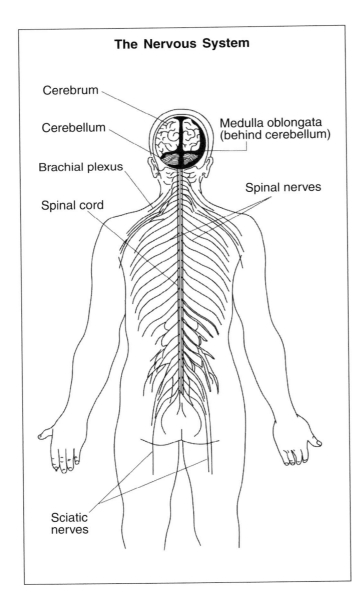

The Nervous System

Cerebrum

Cerebellum

Brachial plexus

Spinal cord

Medulla oblongata
(behind cerebellum)

Spinal nerves

Sciatic
nerves

after meals, and the sympathetic system predominates during periods of stress or physical activity.

Neurons communicate with other neurons or effectors through the release of chemical messengers known as neurotransmitters. At the termination of the axon, there is a widened area known as the synaptic knob. It produces and/or stores neurotransmitters. The effects of neurotransmitters are always localized and of short duration. There are many types of neurotransmitters, some of which are well known, such as acetylcholine and norepinephrine.

Neurotransmitters are released in response to an electrical impulse that is conducted along the axon. Once released, a neurotransmitter binds to cells that have appropriate receptors on their dendrites. Neurotransmitters may either stimulate or inhibit the activity of the second cell. If there is significant stimulation of the second cell, it will conduct the information along its axon and release a neurotransmitter from the axon terminal, which will in turn stimulate or inhibit the next neuron or effector. There must be a mechanism for the immediate removal of neurotransmitters from the synaptic cleft if the stimulation of the second neuron is to cease and if other impulses are to be conducted.

Neurotransmitters can influence only those cells that have the appropriate receptors on their surfaces. It is through the neurotransmitter-receptor complex that neurotransmitters are able to influence cells, and any alteration of the number of receptors or type of receptors on a cell membrane will lead to an alteration of cellular functioning.

The axons of some neurons are covered with multiple layers of a cell membrane known as myelin. The myelin is produced by specialized cells in the brain known as oligodendrocytes and by cells in the peripheral axons known as Schwann cells. Myelin serves as an insulator for axons and is effective in speeding up the conduction of nerve impulses. It is essential for the normal functioning of the nervous system.

The brain and spinal cord are enclosed by three membranes of dense connective tissue called the meninges. The meninges separate the nervous system from other tissue and from the skull and spinal cord. The meninges are, from the outside inward, the dura mater, the arachnoid mater, and the pia mater. Many of the blood vessels of the brain travel through the meninges; therefore, the surface of the brain is very vascular and is subject to bleeding or clotting after trauma.

DISORDERS AND DISEASES

Diseases of the nervous system can be arranged into several general categories: infections, congenital diseases, seizure disorders, circulatory diseases, traumatic injury, demyelinating diseases, degenerative diseases, mental diseases, and neoplasms.

Infections of the nervous system are described according to the tissues infected. If the meninges are infected, the disease is known as meningitis; if the brain tissue is infected, the disease is referred to as encephalitis. The development of abscesses in the nervous tissue can also occur. The conditions described can be caused by viruses, bacteria, protozoa, or other parasites.

In most cases, the organism that causes meningitis is spread via the bloodstream. It is also possible, however, for infections to be spread from an infected middle ear or paranasal sinus, a skull fracture, brain surgery, or a lumbar puncture. The infectious agent can usually be determined by analyzing the spinal fluid. Bacterial infections are treated with antibiotics, while viral infections receive only supportive treatment.

An abscess of nervous tissue is usually a complication resulting from an infection at some other anatomical site, particularly from middle-ear infections or sinus infections. Abscesses may also occur following penetrating injuries. The abscess can create pressure inside the skull, and, if left untreated, it may rupture and lead to death.

Viral encephalitis is an acute disease that is often spread to humans by arthropods from animal hosts. After a carrier insect bites a human, the virus is spread to the brain of the human via the bloodstream. The specific causative agent often goes undiagnosed. Some well-known forms of encephalitis are herpes simplex encephalitis, poliomyelitis, rabies, and cytomegalovirus encephalitis. In addition, some forms of encephalitis fall into the category of slow virus infections, which have latent periods as long as several years between the time of infection and the development of encephalitis.

Other serious infections include neurosyphilis, which occurs in the late stages of untreated syphilis infections; toxoplasmosis, a protozoan infection that is extremely dangerous to fetuses but rarely causes serious problems in adults; cerebral malaria; and African trypanosomiasis, which is also known as sleeping sickness.

Congenital diseases of the brain vary in the degree of malfunction they produce. Spina bifida is a general term for a group of disorders in which the vertebrae do not develop as they should. As a result, the spinal cord may protrude from the lower back. In some cases, the effects may be so minimal as to produce no symptoms; in other cases, however, these malformations may lead to major neurologic impairment.

Hydrocephalus is another congenital malformation. It may lead to an increase in the size of the ventricles of the brain. It may be caused by blockage of the flow of spinal fluid, which in the fetus may lead to expanded brain size. In some cases, the spinal fluid produced by the nervous system fills the ventricles and limits the space available for the growing brain and nervous tissue. The result under these conditions is the presence of larger-than-normal ventricles and a smaller-than-normal amount of nervous tissue.

A seizure disorder is any sudden burst of excess electrical activity in the neurons of the brain. Epilepsy is a general term for seizure disorders. The condition may be mild and have only minimal effects, or it may be severe, leading to convulsions. The cause is often unknown, but epilepsy may result from infection, trauma, or neoplasms.

Cerebrovascular accident (CVA) is the term used to describe a variety of malfunctions of the blood circulation in the nervous system that are not a result of trauma. More commonly, the term "stroke" is used to describe the condition. Strokes have many causes that generally fall into two categories: ischemic and hemorrhagic.

Ischemic strokes are those in which the nervous tissue is deprived of oxygen as a result of an impairment of blood flow to the area. An ischemic stroke is often the result of a blood clot that blocks the blood vessels leading to the brain or the blood vessels in the brain itself. Although there are other causes, these are the most common. Since the cells can live for only a few minutes without oxygen, the consequence of an ischemic stroke can be neurological impairment or even death.

In hemorrhagic strokes, there is bleeding in the brain itself. It may be caused by hypertension or by the rupture of a weakened blood vessel, which is known as an aneurysm. Both ischemic and hemorrhagic strokes lead to the death of neurons in the affected area. The degree of damage to the brain is determined by the number of cells destroyed by the oxygen deprivation.

Traumatic injury to the brain can generally be classified as penetrating or nonpenetrating. Penetrating injuries produce a risk of infection as well as bleeding at the site of the wound. Since many large blood vessels are located in the meninges, even injuries that penetrate only into the meninges may be sufficient to cause serious injury. Nonpenetrating injuries may also cause bleeding of the meninges, which can limit blood flow to the nervous tissue or put excessive pressure on the tissue.

Injury to the spinal cord may result in severing the spinal cord from the brain. If this should occur, communications between the brain and any structures below the area of the injury are lost, as is all sensory and motor function in those areas. Since neurons are unable to regenerate and axon repair is limited, there is little hope for reversal of this condition, although extensive research is being conducted in this area.

Demyelinating diseases are those that result in changes in the myelin sheaths of neurons. The most common example is multiple sclerosis, which affects myelin in the central nervous system but not in the peripheral nervous system. Although there are varying degrees of severity, the condition causes limb weakness, impaired perception, and optic neuritis, among other things. Some cases present only mild symptoms, while others are degenerative and can lead to death—in some patients, within months. Many patients, however, survive for more than twenty years. The cause of the disease is not yet clear, although viral infections have been associated with some demyelinating diseases.

Degenerative diseases are those in which there is a gradual decline in nervous function. The disease may be hereditary, as in the case of Huntington's disease, or may occur without any apparent genetic basis, as in the case of Parkinson's disease. Parkinson's disease involves the death of certain neurons in the brain and a decreased concentration of neurotransmitters. As the disease progresses, there is a gradual loss of motor ability and, ultimately, a complete loss of motor function. Not much is known about neurotransmitter replacement or mechanisms to stop degenerative diseases.

Little is known about mental diseases such as schizophrenia and manic depression. They appear to involve abnormal levels of neurotransmitters or errors in the membrane receptors associated with those neurotransmitters. Success in localizing the causes of these diseases has been slow in coming; there has been much more success in the development of medications to treat them.

Cancer of the brain can be primary or metastatic. Metastatic tumors, the more common variety, can arise from any source. Of the primary neoplasms, the most common are those derived from glial cells, which are responsible for more than 65 percent of all primary neoplasms. The second most common are neoplasms resulting from transformation of cells of the meninges. Since neurons cannot divide, neuron tumors are almost nonexistent except in children.

PERSPECTIVE AND PROSPECTS

When the control system of the body experiences a malfunction, the effects are wide ranging. Since the nervous system has the responsibility of regulating so many diverse activities, nervous system injury or disease must be treated immediately if the patient is to survive. This problem is further complicated by the fact that the brain is a difficult organ to study, because of its location within the skull and because its cells are vital and can be studied only after they have died.

Disease or injury of the cells of the nervous system—especially the brain—creates problems that are unique to that organ for several reasons, including the facts that those cells cannot repair themselves and cannot divide. In addition, the cells of the brain are restricted to a limited area. The cells of the nervous system are unique in that they are so highly specialized that they are not capable of cell division. As a result, humans have the greatest number of neurons during early childhood. Any neural injury or disease that kills cells results in a decreased number of neurons. In addition, neurons are not very good at repairing themselves. Furthermore, the space in the skull is tightly packed with cells and cerebrospinal fluid. There is no room for the blood that might appear as the result of an injury or the fluid accumulation that might be caused by tissue infection or tumors. Any of these conditions will increase the pressure within the skull and will also increase the extent of the injury to the nervous tissue.

Although there is no mechanism for replacing cells that have died, the prognosis is not totally bleak. There are cells in the brain that can, in the event of disease or injury, assume the responsibilities of the dead cells. For example, a person who has lost the capacity to speak following a stroke may be retaught to speak using cells that previously did not perform that function.

Among the problems with which the nervous system must cope, there are many things that can go wrong at the synapse of a neuron. The cell may produce too little or too much neurotransmitter. It is possible that the neurotransmitter may not be released on cue or that, if it is released, the postsynaptic cells will not have the appropriate receptors. There also may be no mechanism for removal of the neurotransmitter from the synaptic cleft. These are only a few of the problems that can interfere with communication between neurons and between neurons and other effectors. As science learns more about the communication system of neurons, efforts to correct these problems will intensify. Already there are many drugs available that can alter activity at the synapse. Correcting these errors can lead to methods for the treatment of mental diseases.

Someday it may be possible to transplant healthy neurons from one person to another. This procedure may permit physicians to prevent total paralysis in a person who has suffered a broken neck or total loss of motor function in an individual who suffers from Parkinson's disease. In 1990, normal neurons were grown in tissue culture for the first time. Such scientific breakthroughs will lead to more and better treatments for individuals who suffer from diseases of the nervous system.

—*Annette O'Connor, Ph.D.*

See also Acupressure; Acupuncture; Alzheimer's disease; Amnesia; Amputation; Anesthesia; Anesthesiology; Aneurysmectomy; Aneurysms; Anxiety; Aphasia and dysphasia; Apnea; Aromatherapy; Ataxia; Autism; Balance disorders; Behçet's disease; Bell's palsy; Biofeedback; Botox; Brain; Brain damage; Brain disorders; Brain tumors; Caffeine; Carpal tunnel syndrome; Cells; Cerebral palsy; Cluster headaches; Coma; Computed tomography (CT) scanning; Concussion; Craniotomy; Cysts; Deafness; Dementias; Disk removal; Dizziness and fainting; Dyslexia; Ear infections and disorders; Ear surgery; Ears; Electrical shock; Electroencephalography (EEG); Encephalitis; Epilepsy; Fetal alcohol syndrome; Fetal tissue transplantation; Ganglion removal; Guillain-Barré syndrome; Hallucinations; Head and neck disorders; Headaches; Hearing loss; Hemiplegia; Huntington's disease; Hydrocephalus; Intraventricular hemorrhage; Laminectomy and spinal fusion; Lead poisoning; Learning disabilities; Leprosy; Leukodystrophy; Lower extremities; Lumbar puncture; Memory loss; Meningitis; Mental retardation; Migraine headaches; Motor neuron diseases; Motor skill development; Multiple sclerosis; Narcolepsy; Neuralgia, neuritis, and neuropathy; Neurofibromatosis; Neuroimaging; Neurology; Neurology, pediatric; Neurosurgery; Numbness and tingling; Paget's disease; Palsy; Paralysis; Paraplegia; Parkinson's disease; Physical rehabilitation; Poisoning; Poliomyelitis; Porphyria; Premenstrual syndrome (PMS); Quadriplegia; Rabies; Reflexes, primitive; Sciatica; Seizures; Sense organs; Shingles; Shock therapy; Skin; Sleep disorders; Snakebites; Spina bifida; Spinal cord disorders;

Spine, vertebrae, and disks; Strokes; Sympathectomy; Systems and organs; Tetanus; Tics; Touch; Toxicology; Transient ischemic attacks (TIAs); Trembling and shaking; Unconsciousness; Upper extremities; Vagotomy.

FOR FURTHER INFORMATION:

Afifi, Adel K., and Ronald A. Bergman. *Functional Neuroanatomy: Text and Atlas.* 2d ed. New York: Lange Medical Books/McGraw-Hill, 2005. Written by a physician and an anatomist, this book is designed to be an integrated neuroscience textbook and atlas covering the regions of the central nervous system. The peripheral nervous system, however, is not covered.

Barondes, Samuel H. *Molecules and Mental Illness.* New York: Scientific American, 1999. A well-written book that describes the chemistry and physiology of mental illness. Provides a good background for understanding the pathology of mental illness.

Bear, Mark F., Barry W. Connors, and Michael A. Paradiso. *Neuroscience: Exploring the Brain.* 3d ed. Philadelphia: Lippincott Williams & Wilkins, 2007. Undergraduate text that introduces the topics of neuroscience, neurobiology, neurodiseases, and physiological psychology.

Bloom, Floyd E., M. Flint Beal, and David J. Kupfer, eds. *The Dana Guide to Brain Health.* New York: Simon & Schuster, 2003. An easy-to-understand health guide to the brain from neuroscience, neurology, and psychiatry perspectives. More than seventy psychiatric and neurological disorders, their diagnoses, and their treatments are covered.

McCance, Kathryn L., and Sue M. Huether. *Pathophysiology: The Biologic Basis for Disease in Adults and Children.* 5th ed. St. Louis: Elsevier Mosby, 2006. This book, which was written for nurses, describes the physiologic basis of diseases. There is an extensive section on diseases of the nervous system.

McLendon, Roger E., Marc K. Rosenblum, and Darell D. Bigner, eds. *Russell and Rubinstein's Pathology of Tumors of the Nervous System.* 7th ed. 2 vols. London: Hodder Arnold, 2006. This classic work of neuroscience has been completely redesigned from its previous edition. Collected together are the writings of thirty different authors, who approach neuro-oncology from a number of different perspectives.

Nicholls, John G., A. Robert Martin, and Bruce G. Wallace. *From Neuron to Brain: A Cellular and Molecular Approach to the Function of the Nervous System.* 4th ed. Sunderland, Mass.: Sinauer Associates, 2000. An excellent and detailed undergraduate neurobiology text that describes how nerve cells transmit signals, how signals are put together, and how higher functions emerge from this integration.

Underwood, J. C. E., ed. *General and Systematic Pathology.* 4th ed. New York: Churchill Livingstone, 2004. A well-developed pathology book written for students that contains illustrations and tables. Although some terms will be unfamiliar to the layperson, most of the material is presented in a straightforward manner.

Woolsey, Thomas A., Joseph Hanaway, and Mokhtar Gado. *Brain Atlas: A Visual Guide to the Human Central Nervous System.* 2d ed. New York: Wiley, 2002. This book provides an overview of modern neuroimaging. Particularly helpful is the display of magnetic resonance images and photographs of sections of fixed brain on facing pages.

MAGILL'S
MEDICAL GUIDE

ENTRIES BY ANATOMY OR SYSTEM AFFECTED

Varicose veins
Vascular medicine
Vascular system
Venous insufficiency
Von Willebrand's disease

BONES
Amputation
Arthritis
Bone cancer
Bone disorders
Bone grafting
Bone marrow transplantation
Bones and the skeleton
Bowlegs
Bunions
Cells
Cerebral palsy
Chiropractic
Cleft lip and palate
Cleft lip and palate repair
Craniosynostosis
Craniotomy
Disk removal
Dwarfism
Ear surgery
Ears
Ewing's sarcoma
Failure to thrive
Feet
Foot disorders
Fracture and dislocation
Fracture repair
Gaucher's disease
Gigantism
Hammertoe correction
Hammertoes
Head and neck disorders
Heel spur removal
Hematology
Hematology, pediatric
Hip fracture repair
Hip replacement
Histiocytosis
Hormone replacement therapy
 (HRT)
Jaw wiring
Kneecap removal
Knock-knees
Kyphosis
Laminectomy and spinal fusion
Lower extremities
Marfan syndrome
Motor skill development

Neurofibromatosis
Niemann-Pick disease
Nuclear medicine
Nuclear radiology
Orthopedic surgery
Orthopedics
Orthopedics, pediatric
Osgood-Schlatter disease
Osteochondritis juvenilis
Osteogenesis imperfecta
Osteomyelitis
Osteonecrosis
Osteopathic medicine
Osteoporosis
Paget's disease
Periodontitis
Physical rehabilitation
Pigeon toes
Podiatry
Prader-Willi syndrome
Rheumatology
Rickets
Rubinstein-Taybi syndrome
Sarcoma
Scoliosis
Slipped disk
Spinal cord disorders
Spine, vertebrae, and disks
Sports medicine
Teeth
Temporomandibular joint (TMJ)
 syndrome
Tendon disorders
Tendon repair
Upper extremities

BRAIN
Abscess drainage
Abscesses
Addiction
Alcoholism
Altitude sickness
Alzheimer's disease
Amnesia
Anesthesia
Anesthesiology
Aneurysmectomy
Aneurysms
Angiography
Antidepressants
Aphasia and dysphasia
Aromatherapy
Attention-deficit disorder (ADD)
Auras

Batten's disease
Biofeedback
Brain
Brain damage
Brain disorders
Brain tumors
Caffeine
Chronic wasting disease (CWD)
Cluster headaches
Cognitive development
Coma
Computed tomography (CT)
 scanning
Concussion
Cornelia de Lange syndrome
Corticosteroids
Craniotomy
Creutzfeldt-Jakob disease (CJD)
Cytomegalovirus (CMV)
Dehydration
Dementias
Developmental stages
Dizziness and fainting
Down syndrome
Drowning
Dyslexia
Electroencephalography (EEG)
Embolism
Emotions: Biomedical causes and
 effects
Encephalitis
Endocrinology
Endocrinology, pediatric
Epilepsy
Failure to thrive
Fetal alcohol syndrome
Fetal surgery
Fetal tissue transplantation
Fibromyalgia
Fragile X syndrome
Galactosemia
Gigantism
Gulf War syndrome
Hallucinations
Head and neck disorders
Headaches
Huntington's disease
Hydrocephalus
Hypertension
Hypnosis
Hypotension
Intraventricular hemorrhage
Jaundice
Kinesiology

Pacemaker implantation
Pityriasis rosea
Pleurisy
Pneumonia
Pulmonary diseases
Pulmonary medicine
Pulmonary medicine, pediatric
Respiration
Respiratory distress syndrome
Resuscitation
Sneezing
Thoracic surgery
Tuberculosis
Wheezing
Whooping cough

CIRCULATORY SYSTEM
Aneurysmectomy
Aneurysms
Angina
Angiography
Angioplasty
Antihistamines
Apgar score
Arrhythmias
Arteriosclerosis
Biofeedback
Bleeding
Blood and blood disorders
Blood testing
Blue baby syndrome
Bypass surgery
Cardiac arrest
Cardiac rehabilitation
Cardiology
Cardiology, pediatric
Cardiopulmonary resuscitation
 (CPR)
Catheterization
Chest
Cholesterol
Circulation
Claudication
Congenital heart disease
Decongestants
Dehydration
Diabetes mellitus
Dialysis
Disseminated intravascular
 coagulation (DIC)
Dizziness and fainting
Ebola virus
Echocardiography
Edema

Electrocardiography (ECG or EKG)
Electrocauterization
Embolism
Endarterectomy
Endocarditis
Ergogenic aids
Exercise physiology
Facial transplantation
Heart
Heart attack
Heart disease
Heart failure
Heart transplantation
Heart valve replacement
Heat exhaustion and heat stroke
Hematology
Hematology, pediatric
Hemorrhoid banding and removal
Hemorrhoids
Hormones
Hyperbaric oxygen therapy
Hypercholesterolemia
Hypertension
Hypotension
Ischemia
Juvenile rheumatoid arthritis
Kidneys
Kinesiology
Klippel-Trenaunay syndrome
Liver
Lymphatic system
Marburg virus
Marijuana
Mitral valve prolapse
Motor skill development
Nosebleeds
Obesity
Obesity, childhood
Osteochondritis juvenilis
Pacemaker implantation
Palpitations
Phlebitis
Phlebotomy
Placenta
Preeclampsia and eclampsia
Resuscitation
Reye's syndrome
Rheumatic fever
Scleroderma
Septicemia
Shock
Shunts
Smoking
Sports medicine

Stents
Steroid abuse
Strokes
Sturge-Weber syndrome
Systems and organs
Testicular torsion
Thrombocytopenia
Thrombolytic therapy and TPA
Thrombosis and thrombus
Transfusion
Transient ischemic attacks (TIAs)
Transplantation
Typhus
Varicose vein removal
Varicose veins
Vascular medicine
Vascular system
Venous insufficiency

EARS
Altitude sickness
Antihistamines
Audiology
Auras
Biophysics
Cornelia de Lange syndrome
Cytomegalovirus (CMV)
Deafness
Decongestants
Dyslexia
Ear infections and disorders
Ear surgery
Ears
Fragile X syndrome
Hearing aids
Hearing loss
Hearing tests
Histiocytosis
Leukodystrophy
Ménière's disease
Motion sickness
Myringotomy
Nervous system
Neurology
Neurology, pediatric
Osteogenesis imperfecta
Otoplasty
Otorhinolaryngology
Plastic surgery
Quinsy
Rubinstein-Taybi syndrome
Sense organs
Speech disorders
Wiskott-Aldrich syndrome

ENDOCRINE SYSTEM

EYES

FEET

GALLBLADDER

Fistula repair
Gallbladder cancer
Gallbladder diseases
Gastroenterology
Gastroenterology, pediatric
Gastrointestinal disorders
Gastrointestinal system
Internal medicine
Laparoscopy
Liver transplantation
Malabsorption
Nuclear medicine
Stone removal
Stones
Typhoid fever
Ultrasonography

GASTROINTESTINAL SYSTEM
Abdomen
Abdominal disorders
Acid reflux disease
Allergies
Anthrax
Appendectomy
Appendicitis
Appetite loss
Bacterial infections
Bariatric surgery
Botulism
Bulimia
Burping
Bypass surgery
Candidiasis
Celiac sprue
Childhood infectious diseases
Cholera
Cholesterol
Colic
Colitis
Colon and rectal polyp removal
Colon and rectal surgery
Colon cancer
Colon therapy
Colonoscopy and sigmoidoscopy
Constipation
Crohn's disease
Cytomegalovirus (CMV)
Diabetes mellitus
Diarrhea and dysentery
Digestion
Diverticulitis and diverticulosis
E. coli infection
Eating disorders
Ebola virus

Emotions: Biomedical causes and
  effects
Endoscopy
Enemas
Enterocolitis
Fistula repair
Food biochemistry
Food poisoning
Gallbladder cancer
Gallbladder diseases
Gastrectomy
Gastroenterology
Gastroenterology, pediatric
Gastrointestinal disorders
Gastrointestinal system
Gastrostomy
Giardiasis
Glands
Gulf War syndrome
Halitosis
Heartburn
Hemorrhoid banding and removal
Hemorrhoids
Hernia
Hernia repair
Hirschsprung's disease
Histiocytosis
Host-defense mechanisms
Ileostomy and colostomy
Incontinence
Indigestion
Internal medicine
Intestinal disorders
Intestines
Irritable bowel syndrome (IBS)
Klippel-Trenaunay syndrome
Kwashiorkor
Lactose intolerance
Laparoscopy
Lipids
Liver
Malabsorption
Malnutrition
Marburg virus
Marijuana
Metabolism
Motion sickness
Muscles
Nausea and vomiting
Nonalcoholic steatohepatitis
  (NASH)
Noroviruses
Nutrition
Obesity

Obesity, childhood
Obstruction
Pancreas
Pancreatitis
Peristalsis
Pinworm
Poisoning
Poisonous plants
Polycystic kidney disease
Premenstrual syndrome (PMS)
Proctology
Protozoan diseases
Pyloric stenosis
Radiation sickness
Reiter's syndrome
Rotavirus
Roundworm
Salmonella infection
Scleroderma
Sense organs
Shigellosis
Shunts
Soiling
Stomach, intestinal, and pancreatic
  cancers
Systems and organs
Tapeworm
Taste
Teeth
Toilet training
Trichinosis
Tumor removal
Tumors
Typhoid fever
Ulcer surgery
Ulcers
Vagotomy
Vitamins and minerals
Weaning
Weight loss and gain
Worms

GENITALS
Aphrodisiacs
Assisted reproductive technologies
Behçet's disease
Candidiasis
Catheterization
Cervical, ovarian, and uterine
  cancers
Cervical procedures
Chlamydia
Circumcision, female, and genital
  mutilation

HANDS

Amputation
Arthritis
Bones and the skeleton
Bursitis
Carpal tunnel syndrome
Cerebral palsy
Cornelia de Lange syndrome
Corns and calluses
Cysts
Fracture and dislocation
Fracture repair
Fragile X syndrome
Frostbite
Ganglion removal
Nail removal
Nails
Neurology
Neurology, pediatric
Orthopedic surgery
Orthopedics
Orthopedics, pediatric
Osteoarthritis
Rheumatoid arthritis
Rheumatology
Rubinstein-Taybi syndrome
Scleroderma
Skin lesion removal
Sports medicine
Tendinitis
Tendon disorders
Tendon repair
Thalidomide
Upper extremities
Warts

HEAD

Altitude sickness
Aneurysmectomy
Aneurysms
Angiography
Antihistamines
Botox
Brain
Brain disorders
Brain tumors
Cluster headaches
Coma
Computed tomography (CT)
    scanning
Concussion
Cornelia de Lange syndrome
Craniosynostosis
Craniotomy

Dizziness and fainting
Electroencephalography (EEG)
Embolism
Epilepsy
Facial transplantation
Fetal tissue transplantation
Fibromyalgia
Hair loss and baldness
Hair transplantation
Head and neck disorders
Headaches
Hydrocephalus
Lice, mites, and ticks
Meningitis
Migraine headaches
Nasal polyp removal
Nasopharyngeal disorders
Neuroimaging
Neurology
Neurology, pediatric
Neurosurgery
Rhinoplasty and submucous
    resection
Rubinstein-Taybi syndrome
Seizures
Shunts
Sports medicine
Strokes
Sturge-Weber syndrome
Temporomandibular joint (TMJ)
    syndrome
Thrombosis and thrombus
Unconsciousness
Whiplash

HEART

Aneurysmectomy
Aneurysms
Angina
Angiography
Angioplasty
Anxiety
Apgar score
Arrhythmias
Arteriosclerosis
Biofeedback
Bites and stings
Blue baby syndrome
Bypass surgery
Caffeine
Cardiac arrest
Cardiac rehabilitation
Cardiology
Cardiology, pediatric

Cardiopulmonary resuscitation (CPR)
Catheterization
Circulation
Congenital heart disease
Cornelia de Lange syndrome
DiGeorge syndrome
Echocardiography
Electrical shock
Electrocardiography (ECG or EKG)
Embolism
Endocarditis
Exercise physiology
Fatty acid oxidation disorders
Glycogen storage diseases
Heart
Heart attack
Heart disease
Heart failure
Heart transplantation
Heart valve replacement
Hemochromatosis
Hypertension
Hypotension
Internal medicine
Juvenile rheumatoid arthritis
Kinesiology
Lyme disease
Marfan syndrome
Marijuana
Mitral valve prolapse
Nicotine
Obesity
Obesity, childhood
Pacemaker implantation
Palpitations
Prader-Willi syndrome
Respiratory distress syndrome
Resuscitation
Reye's syndrome
Rheumatic fever
Rubinstein-Taybi syndrome
Scleroderma
Shock
Sports medicine
Stents
Steroid abuse
Strokes
Thoracic surgery
Thrombolytic therapy and TPA
Thrombosis and thrombus
Toxoplasmosis
Transplantation
Ultrasonography
Yellow fever

Enterocolitis
Fistula repair
Food poisoning
Gastroenterology
Gastroenterology, pediatric
Gastrointestinal disorders
Gastrointestinal system
Hemorrhoid banding and removal
Hemorrhoids
Hernia
Hernia repair
Hirschsprung's disease
Ileostomy and colostomy
Indigestion
Internal medicine
Intestinal disorders
Intestines
Irritable bowel syndrome (IBS)
Kaposi's sarcoma
Kwashiorkor
Lactose intolerance
Laparoscopy
Malabsorption
Malnutrition
Metabolism
Nutrition
Obesity
Obesity, childhood
Obstruction
Peristalsis
Pinworm
Proctology
Rotavirus
Roundworm
Salmonella infection
Soiling
Sphincterectomy
Stomach, intestinal, and pancreatic
   cancers
Tapeworm
Toilet training
Trichinosis
Tumor removal
Tumors
Typhoid fever
Ulcer surgery
Ulcers
Worms

JOINTS
Amputation
Arthritis
Arthroplasty
Arthroscopy

Braces, orthopedic
Bursitis
Carpal tunnel syndrome
Chlamydia
Corticosteroids
Cyst removal
Cysts
Endoscopy
Exercise physiology
Fracture and dislocation
Fragile X syndrome
Gout
Gulf War syndrome
Hammertoe correction
Hammertoes
Hip fracture repair
Juvenile rheumatoid arthritis
Klippel-Trenaunay syndrome
Kneecap removal
Lyme disease
Motor skill development
Orthopedic surgery
Orthopedics
Orthopedics, pediatric
Osteoarthritis
Osteochondritis juvenilis
Osteomyelitis
Osteonecrosis
Physical rehabilitation
Reiter's syndrome
Rheumatoid arthritis
Rheumatology
Rotator cuff surgery
Scleroderma
Spondylitis
Sports medicine
Systemic lupus erythematosus (SLE)
Temporomandibular joint (TMJ)
   syndrome
Tendinitis
Tendon disorders
Tendon repair
Von Willebrand's disease

KIDNEYS
Abdomen
Abscess drainage
Abscesses
Adrenalectomy
Corticosteroids
Cysts
Dialysis
Galactosemia
Hantavirus

Hemolytic uremic syndrome
Hypertension
Hypotension
Internal medicine
Kidney cancer
Kidney disorders
Kidney transplantation
Kidneys
Laparoscopy
Lithotripsy
Metabolism
Nephrectomy
Nephritis
Nephrology
Nephrology, pediatric
Nuclear medicine
Nuclear radiology
Polycystic kidney disease
Preeclampsia and eclampsia
Pyelonephritis
Renal failure
Reye's syndrome
Scleroderma
Stone removal
Stones
Toilet training
Transplantation
Ultrasonography
Urinalysis
Urinary disorders
Urinary system
Urology
Urology, pediatric

KNEES
Amputation
Arthritis
Arthroplasty
Arthroscopy
Bone disorders
Bones and the skeleton
Bowlegs
Braces, orthopedic
Bursitis
Endoscopy
Exercise physiology
Fracture and dislocation
Kneecap removal
Knock-knees
Liposuction
Lower extremities
Orthopedic surgery
Orthopedics
Orthopedics, pediatric

MUSCULOSKELETAL SYSTEM

Kyphosis
Lower extremities
Marfan syndrome
Marijuana
Mastectomy and lumpectomy
Motor neuron diseases
Motor skill development
Multiple sclerosis
Muscle sprains, spasms, and
    disorders
Muscles
Muscular dystrophy
Myasthenia gravis
Neurology
Neurology, pediatric
Nuclear medicine
Nuclear radiology
Numbness and tingling
Orthopedic surgery
Orthopedics
Orthopedics, pediatric
Osteochondritis juvenilis
Osteogenesis imperfecta
Osteomyelitis
Osteonecrosis
Osteopathic medicine
Osteoporosis
Paget's disease
Palsy
Paralysis
Paraplegia
Parkinson's disease
Periodontitis
Physical rehabilitation
Pigeon toes
Poisoning
Poliomyelitis
Prader-Willi syndrome
Precocious puberty
Quadriplegia
Rabies
Respiration
Rheumatoid arthritis
Rheumatology
Rickets
Sarcoma
Scoliosis
Seizures
Sleepwalking
Slipped disk
Speech disorders
Sphincterectomy
Spinal cord disorders
Spine, vertebrae, and disks

Sports medicine
Systemic lupus erythematosus (SLE)
Systems and organs
Teeth
Tendinitis
Tendon disorders
Tendon repair
Tetanus
Tics
Tourette's syndrome
Trembling and shaking
Trichinosis
Upper extremities
Weight loss and gain
Yellow fever

NAILS
Anemia
Dermatology
Fungal infections
Malnutrition
Nail removal
Nails
Nutrition
Podiatry

NECK
Asphyxiation
Back pain
Botox
Braces, orthopedic
Choking
Cretinism
Endarterectomy
Goiter
Hashimoto's thyroiditis
Head and neck disorders
Heimlich maneuver
Hyperparathyroidism and
    hypoparathyroidism
Laryngectomy
Laryngitis
Mouth and throat cancer
Otorhinolaryngology
Paralysis
Parathyroidectomy
Quadriplegia
Spine, vertebrae, and disks
Sympathectomy
Thyroid disorders
Thyroid gland
Thyroidectomy
Tonsillectomy and adenoid
    removal

Tonsillitis
Torticollis
Tracheostomy
Whiplash

NERVES
Anesthesia
Anesthesiology
Back pain
Bell's palsy
Biofeedback
Brain
Carpal tunnel syndrome
Cells
Creutzfeldt-Jakob disease (CJD)
Cysts
Emotions: Biomedical causes and
    effects
Epilepsy
Facial transplantation
Fibromyalgia
Guillain-Barré syndrome
Hemiplegia
Huntington's disease
Leprosy
Leukodystrophy
Lower extremities
Marijuana
Motor neuron diseases
Motor skill development
Multiple chemical sensitivity
    syndrome
Multiple sclerosis
Nervous system
Neuralgia, neuritis, and neuropathy
Neuroimaging
Neurology
Neurology, pediatric
Neurosurgery
Numbness and tingling
Palsy
Paralysis
Paraplegia
Parkinson's disease
Physical rehabilitation
Poliomyelitis
Ptosis
Quadriplegia
Sciatica
Seizures
Sense organs
Shock therapy
Skin
Spina bifida

Endocrinology, pediatric
Facial transplantation
Factitious disorders
Failure to thrive
Fibromyalgia
Grief and guilt
Gulf War syndrome
Hallucinations
Headaches
Hormone replacement therapy
  (HRT)
Hormones
Hydrocephalus
Hypnosis
Hypochondriasis
Kinesiology
Klinefelter syndrome
Learning disabilities
Light therapy
Marijuana
Memory loss
Menopause
Mental retardation
Midlife crisis
Migraine headaches
Miscarriage
Motor skill development
Narcolepsy
Narcotics
Neurology
Neurology, pediatric
Neurosis
Neurosurgery
Nicotine
Nightmares
Obesity
Obesity, childhood
Obsessive-compulsive disorder
Overtraining syndrome
Palpitations
Panic attacks
Paranoia
Pharmacology
Pharmacy
Phobias
Pick's disease
Postpartum depression
Post-traumatic stress disorder
Prader-Willi syndrome
Precocious puberty
Psychiatric disorders
Psychiatry
Psychiatry, child and adolescent
Psychiatry, geriatric

Psychoanalysis
Psychosis
Psychosomatic disorders
Puberty and adolescence
Rabies
Schizophrenia
Seasonal affective disorder
Separation anxiety
Sexual dysfunction
Sexuality
Shock therapy
Sibling rivalry
Sleep
Sleep disorders
Sleepwalking
Soiling
Speech disorders
Sperm banks
Stammering
Steroid abuse
Stillbirth
Stress
Strokes
Stuttering
Suicide
Tics
Toilet training
Tourette's syndrome
Weight loss and gain
Wilson's disease

REPRODUCTIVE SYSTEM
Abdomen
Abdominal disorders
Abortion
Acquired immunodeficiency
  syndrome (AIDS)
Amenorrhea
Amniocentesis
Anatomy
Anorexia nervosa
Assisted reproductive technologies
Breast-feeding
Breasts, female
Candidiasis
Catheterization
Cervical, ovarian, and uterine
  cancers
Cervical procedures
Cesarean section
Childbirth
Childbirth complications
Chlamydia
Chorionic villus sampling

Circumcision, female, and genital
  mutilation
Circumcision, male
Conception
Contraception
Culdocentesis
Cyst removal
Cysts
Dysmenorrhea
Eating disorders
Ectopic pregnancy
Electrocauterization
Endocrinology
Endometrial biopsy
Endometriosis
Episiotomy
Fetal alcohol syndrome
Fistula repair
Gamete intrafallopian transfer
  (GIFT)
Genetic counseling
Genital disorders, female
Genital disorders, male
Glands
Gonorrhea
Gynecology
Hermaphroditism and
  pseudohermaphroditism
Hernia
Herpes
Hormone replacement therapy
  (HRT)
Hormones
Hot flashes
Human immunodeficiency virus
  (HIV)
Human papillomavirus (HPV)
Hydrocelectomy
Hypospadias repair and
  urethroplasty
Hysterectomy
In vitro fertilization
Infertility, female
Infertility, male
Internal medicine
Klinefelter syndrome
Laparoscopy
Menopause
Menorrhagia
Menstruation
Miscarriage
Multiple births
Mumps
Myomectomy

Nicotine
Obstetrics
Orchitis
Ovarian cysts
Pap smear
Pelvic inflammatory disease (PID)
Penile implant surgery
Placenta
Precocious puberty
Preeclampsia and eclampsia
Pregnancy and gestation
Premature birth
Premenstrual syndrome (PMS)
Prostate cancer
Prostate enlargement
Prostate gland
Puberty and adolescence
Reproductive system
Sex change surgery
Sexual differentiation
Sexual dysfunction
Sexuality
Sexually transmitted diseases
    (STDs)
Sperm banks
Sterilization
Steroid abuse
Stillbirth
Syphilis
Systems and organs
Testicles, undescended
Testicular cancer
Testicular surgery
Testicular torsion
Trichomoniasis
Tubal ligation
Turner syndrome
Ultrasonography
Urology
Urology, pediatric
Vasectomy
Von Willebrand's disease
Warts

RESPIRATORY SYSTEM
Abscess drainage
Abscesses
Altitude sickness
Amyotrophic lateral sclerosis
Antihistamines
Apgar score
Apnea
Asbestos exposure
Aspergillosis

Asphyxiation
Asthma
Bacterial infections
Bronchiolitis
Bronchitis
Cardiopulmonary resuscitation
    (CPR)
Chest
Chickenpox
Childhood infectious diseases
Choking
Chronic obstructive pulmonary
    disease (COPD)
Common cold
Corticosteroids
Coughing
Croup
Cystic fibrosis
Decongestants
Diphtheria
Drowning
Edema
Embolism
Emphysema
Epiglottitis
Exercise physiology
Fetal surgery
Fluids and electrolytes
Fungal infections
Halitosis
Hantavirus
Head and neck disorders
Heart transplantation
Heimlich maneuver
Hiccups
Hyperbaric oxygen therapy
Hyperventilation
Influenza
Internal medicine
Interstitial pulmonary fibrosis (IPF)
Kinesiology
Laryngectomy
Laryngitis
Legionnaires' disease
Lung cancer
Lung surgery
Lungs
Marijuana
Measles
Monkeypox
Mononucleosis
Multiple chemical sensitivity
    syndrome
Nasopharyngeal disorders

Nicotine
Niemann-Pick disease
Obesity
Obesity, childhood
Otorhinolaryngology
Oxygen therapy
Pharyngitis
Plague
Pleurisy
Pneumonia
Poisoning
Pulmonary diseases
Pulmonary hypertension
Pulmonary medicine
Pulmonary medicine, pediatric
Respiration
Resuscitation
Rheumatic fever
Rhinitis
Roundworm
Severe acute respiratory syndrome
    (SARS)
Sinusitis
Sleep apnea
Smallpox
Sneezing
Sore throat
Strep throat
Systems and organs
Thoracic surgery
Thrombolytic therapy and TPA
Thrombosis and thrombus
Tonsillectomy and adenoid removal
Tonsillitis
Toxoplasmosis
Tracheostomy
Transplantation
Tuberculosis
Tularemia
Tumor removal
Tumors
Voice and vocal cord disorders
Wheezing
Whooping cough
Worms

SKIN
Abscess drainage
Abscesses
Acne
Acupressure
Acupuncture
Age spots
Albinos

Entries by Specialties and Related Fields

Shigellosis
Staphylococcal infections
Strep throat
Streptococcal infections
Syphilis
Tetanus
Tonsillitis
Tropical medicine
Tuberculosis
Tularemia
Typhoid fever
Typhus
Whooping cough

BIOCHEMISTRY

Acid-base chemistry
Antidepressants
Autopsy
Bacteriology
Caffeine
Cholesterol
Corticosteroids
Digestion
Endocrinology
Endocrinology, pediatric
Enzyme therapy
Enzymes
Ergogenic aids
Fatty acid oxidation disorders
Fluids and electrolytes
Fluoride treatments
Food biochemistry
Fructosemia
Gaucher's disease
Genetic engineering
Genomics
Glands
Glycogen storage diseases
Glycolysis
Gram staining
Histology
Hormones
Leptin
Leukodystrophy
Lipids
Malabsorption
Metabolism
Nephrology
Nephrology, pediatric
Niemann-Pick disease
Nutrition
Pathology
Pharmacology
Pharmacy

Respiration
Stem cells
Steroids
Toxicology
Urinalysis
Wilson's disease

BIOTECHNOLOGY

Assisted reproductive technologies
Bionics and biotechnology
Biophysics
Cloning
Computed tomography (CT)
  scanning
Dialysis
Echocardiography
Electrocardiography (ECG or EKG)
Electroencephalography (EEG)
Fatty acid oxidation disorders
Gene therapy
Genetic engineering
Genomics
Glycogen storage diseases
Huntington's disease
Hyperbaric oxygen therapy
In vitro fertilization
Magnetic resonance imaging
  (MRI)
Pacemaker implantation
Positron emission tomography
  (PET) scanning
Prostheses
Severe combined immunodeficiency
  syndrome (SCID)
Sperm banks
Stem cells
Xenotransplantation

CARDIOLOGY

Aging
Aging: Extended care
Aneurysmectomy
Aneurysms
Angina
Angiography
Angioplasty
Anxiety
Arrhythmias
Arteriosclerosis
Biofeedback
Blue baby syndrome
Bypass surgery
Cardiac arrest
Cardiac rehabilitation

Cardiology
Cardiology, pediatric
Cardiopulmonary resuscitation
  (CPR)
Catheterization
Chest
Cholesterol
Circulation
Congenital heart disease
Critical care
Critical care, pediatric
DiGeorge syndrome
Dizziness and fainting
Echocardiography
Electrocardiography (ECG or EKG)
Emergency medicine
Endocarditis
Exercise physiology
Fetal surgery
Geriatrics and gerontology
Heart
Heart attack
Heart disease
Heart failure
Heart transplantation
Heart valve replacement
Hematology
Hemochromatosis
Hypercholesterolemia
Hypertension
Hypotension
Internal medicine
Ischemia
Kinesiology
Leptin
Marfan syndrome
Metabolic syndrome
Mitral valve prolapse
Mucopolysaccharidosis (MPS)
Muscles
Neonatology
Nicotine
Noninvasive tests
Nuclear medicine
Pacemaker implantation
Palpitations
Paramedics
Physical examination
Polycystic kidney disease
Prader-Willi syndrome
Progeria
Prostheses
Pulmonary hypertension
Rheumatic fever

Phlebotomy
Rh factor
Septicemia
Serology
Sickle cell disease
Stem cells
Thalassemia
Thrombocytopenia
Thrombolytic therapy and TPA
Thrombosis and thrombus
Transfusion
Vascular medicine
Vascular system
Von Willebrand's disease

HISTOLOGY
Autopsy
Biopsy
Cancer
Carcinoma
Cells
Cytology
Cytopathology
Dermatology
Dermatopathology
Fluids and electrolytes
Forensic pathology
Healing
Histology
Laboratory tests
Microscopy
Nails
Necrotizing fasciitis
Pathology
Tumor removal
Tumors

IMMUNOLOGY
Acquired immunodeficiency
    syndrome (AIDS)
Allergies
Antibiotics
Antihistamines
Arthritis
Aspergillosis
Asthma
Autoimmune disorders
Bacterial infections
Biological and chemical weapons
Bionics and biotechnology
Bites and stings
Blood and blood disorders
Boils
Bone cancer

Bone grafting
Bone marrow transplantation
Breast cancer
Cancer
Candidiasis
Carcinoma
Cervical, ovarian, and uterine
    cancers
Childhood infectious diseases
Chronic fatigue syndrome
Colon cancer
Corticosteroids
Cytology
Cytomegalovirus (CMV)
Dermatology
Dermatopathology
DiGeorge syndrome
Endocrinology
Endocrinology, pediatric
Epstein-Barr virus
Facial transplantation
Fungal infections
Grafts and grafting
Healing
Hematology
Hematology, pediatric
Histiocytosis
Hives
Homeopathy
Host-defense mechanisms
Human immunodeficiency virus
    (HIV)
Hypnosis
Immune system
Immunization and vaccination
Immunodeficiency disorders
Immunology
Immunopathology
Impetigo
Juvenile rheumatoid arthritis
Kawasaki disease
Laboratory tests
Leprosy
Liver cancer
Lung cancer
Lymphatic system
Microbiology
Multiple chemical sensitivity
    syndrome
Myasthenia gravis
Nicotine
Noroviruses
Oncology
Oxygen therapy

Pancreas
Prostate cancer
Pulmonary diseases
Pulmonary medicine
Pulmonary medicine, pediatric
Rheumatology
Sarcoma
Scleroderma
Serology
Severe combined immunodeficiency
    syndrome (SCID)
Skin cancer
Stem cells
Stomach, intestinal, and pancreatic
    cancers
Stress
Stress reduction
Systemic lupus erythematosus (SLE)
Thalidomide
Transfusion
Transplantation
Tropical medicine
Wiskott-Aldrich syndrome
Xenotransplantation

INTERNAL MEDICINE
Abdomen
Abdominal disorders
Anatomy
Anemia
Angina
Anti-inflammatory drugs
Antioxidants
Anxiety
Appetite loss
Arrhythmias
Arteriosclerosis
Aspergillosis
Autoimmune disorders
Bacterial infections
Bariatric surgery
Behçet's disease
Beriberi
Biofeedback
Bleeding
Bronchiolitis
Bronchitis
Burkitt's lymphoma
Burping
Bursitis
Candidiasis
Chickenpox
Childhood infectious diseases
Cholecystitis

Tetanus
Thrombosis and thrombus
Toxic shock syndrome
Tumor removal
Tumors
Ulcer surgery
Ulcers
Ultrasonography
Viral infections
Vitamins and minerals
Weight loss medications
Whooping cough
Wilson's disease
Worms
Wounds

MICROBIOLOGY
Abscesses
Anthrax
Antibiotics
Aspergillosis
Autopsy
Bacterial infections
Bacteriology
Bionics and biotechnology
Drug resistance
E. coli infection
Epidemiology
Fluoride treatments
Fungal infections
Gangrene
Gastroenterology
Gastroenterology, pediatric
Gastrointestinal disorders
Gastrointestinal system
Genetic engineering
Genomics
Gram staining
Immune system
Immunization and vaccination
Immunology
Impetigo
Laboratory tests
Microbiology
Microscopy
Pathology
Pharmacology
Pharmacy
Protozoan diseases
Serology
Severe acute respiratory syndrome
  (SARS)
Smallpox
Toxic shock syndrome

Toxicology
Tropical medicine
Tuberculosis
Urinalysis
Urology
Urology, pediatric
Viral infections

NEONATOLOGY
Apgar score
Birth defects
Blue baby syndrome
Bonding
Cardiology, pediatric
Cesarean section
Childbirth
Childbirth complications
Chlamydia
Cleft lip and palate
Cleft lip and palate repair
Congenital heart disease
Critical care, pediatric
Cystic fibrosis
Disseminated intravascular
  coagulation (DIC)
Down syndrome
E. coli infection
Endocrinology, pediatric
Failure to thrive
Fetal alcohol syndrome
Fetal surgery
Gastroenterology, pediatric
Genetic diseases
Genetics and inheritance
Hematology, pediatric
Hemolytic disease of the newborn
Hydrocephalus
Intraventricular hemorrhage
Jaundice
Jaundice, neonatal
Karyotyping
Malabsorption
Maple syrup urine disease
  (MSUD)
Motor skill development
Multiple births
Neonatology
Nephrology, pediatric
Neurology, pediatric
Nicotine
Nursing
Obstetrics
Orthopedics, pediatric
Pediatrics

Perinatology
Phenylketonuria (PKU)
Physician assistants
Premature birth
Pulmonary medicine, pediatric
Respiratory distress syndrome
Rh factor
Shunts
Sudden infant death syndrome
  (SIDS)
Surgery, pediatric
Tay-Sachs disease
Toxoplasmosis
Transfusion
Trichomoniasis
Tropical medicine
Umbilical cord
Urology, pediatric
Well-baby examinations

NEPHROLOGY
Abdomen
Cysts
Diabetes mellitus
Dialysis
E. coli infection
Edema
Hemolytic uremic syndrome
Internal medicine
Kidney cancer
Kidney disorders
Kidney transplantation
Kidneys
Lithotripsy
Nephrectomy
Nephritis
Nephrology
Nephrology, pediatric
Polycystic kidney disease
Preeclampsia and eclampsia
Pyelonephritis
Renal failure
Stone removal
Stones
Transplantation
Urinalysis
Urinary disorders
Urinary system
Urology
Urology, pediatric

NEUROLOGY
Altitude sickness
Alzheimer's disease

NURSING

Aging: Extended care
Allied health
Anesthesiology
Cardiac rehabilitation
Critical care
Critical care, pediatric
Emergency medicine
Emergency medicine, pediatric
Geriatrics and gerontology
Holistic medicine
Hospitals
Immunization and vaccination
Neonatology
Noninvasive tests
Nursing
Nutrition
Pediatrics
Physical examination
Physician assistants
Surgery, general
Surgery, pediatric
Surgical procedures
Surgical technologists
Well-baby examinations

NUTRITION

Aging: Extended care
Anorexia nervosa
Antioxidants
Appetite loss
Bariatric surgery
Beriberi
Breast-feeding
Bulimia
Cardiac rehabilitation
Cholesterol
Digestion
Eating disorders
Exercise physiology
Fatty acid oxidation disorders
Food biochemistry
Fructosemia
Galactosemia
Gastroenterology
Gastroenterology, pediatric
Gastrointestinal disorders
Gastrointestinal system
Geriatrics and gerontology
Gestational diabetes
Glycogen storage diseases
Hyperadiposis
Hypercholesterolemia
Irritable bowel syndrome (IBS)

Jaw wiring
Kwashiorkor
Lactose intolerance
Leptin
Leukodystrophy
Lipids
Malabsorption
Malnutrition
Metabolic disorders
Metabolic syndrome
Metabolism
Nursing
Nutrition
Obesity
Obesity, childhood
Osteoporosis
Phytochemicals
Scurvy
Sports medicine
Supplements
Taste
Tropical medicine
Ulcers
Vagotomy
Vitamins and minerals
Weaning
Weight loss and gain
Weight loss medications

OBSTETRICS

Amniocentesis
Apgar score
Assisted reproductive technologies
Birth defects
Breast-feeding
Breasts, female
Cervical, ovarian, and uterine
  cancers
Cesarean section
Childbirth
Childbirth complications
Chorionic villus sampling
Conception
Cytomegalovirus (CMV)
Disseminated intravascular
  coagulation (DIC)
Down syndrome
Ectopic pregnancy
Embryology
Emergency medicine
Episiotomy
Family medicine
Fetal alcohol syndrome
Fetal surgery

Gamete intrafallopian transfer
  (GIFT)
Genetic counseling
Genetic diseases
Genetics and inheritance
Genital disorders, female
Gestational diabetes
Gonorrhea
Growth
Gynecology
Hemolytic disease of the newborn
In vitro fertilization
Incontinence
Invasive tests
Karyotyping
Miscarriage
Multiple births
Neonatology
Nicotine
Noninvasive tests
Obstetrics
Perinatology
Placenta
Postpartum depression
Preeclampsia and eclampsia
Pregnancy and gestation
Premature birth
Pyelonephritis
Reproductive system
Rh factor
Rubella
Sexuality
Sperm banks
Spina bifida
Stillbirth
Teratogens
Toxemia
Toxoplasmosis
Trichomoniasis
Ultrasonography
Urology

OCCUPATIONAL HEALTH

Altitude sickness
Asbestos exposure
Asphyxiation
Back pain
Biofeedback
Blurred vision
Carcinogens
Cardiac rehabilitation
Carpal tunnel syndrome
Environmental diseases
Environmental health

Keratitis
Laser use in surgery
Macular degeneration
Marfan syndrome
Microscopy, slitlamp
Myopia
Ophthalmology
Optometry
Optometry, pediatric
Prostheses
Ptosis
Refractive eye surgery
Reiter's syndrome
Rubinstein-Taybi syndrome
Sense organs
Strabismus
Sturge-Weber syndrome
Styes
Trachoma
Vision disorders

OPTOMETRY
Aging: Extended care
Astigmatism
Biophysics
Blurred vision
Cataracts
Eye infections and disorders
Eyes
Geriatrics and gerontology
Glaucoma
Keratitis
Myopia
Ophthalmology
Optometry
Optometry, pediatric
Ptosis
Refractive eye surgery
Sense organs
Styes
Vision disorders

**ORGANIZATIONS AND
   PROGRAMS**
Allied health
American Medical Association
   (AMA)
Blood banks
Centers for Disease Control and
   Prevention (CDC)
Clinical trials
Education, medical
Food and Drug Administration
   (FDA)

Gates Foundation
Health maintenance organizations
   (HMOs)
Hospice
Hospitals
Medicare
National Cancer Institute (NCI)
National Institutes of Health
   (NIH)
Sperm banks
Stem cells
World Health Organization

ORTHODONTICS
Bones and the skeleton
Dental diseases
Dentistry
Dentistry, pediatric
Jaw wiring
Nicotine
Orthodontics
Periodontal surgery
Teeth
Teething
Tooth extraction
Wisdom teeth

ORTHOPEDICS
Amputation
Arthritis
Arthroplasty
Arthroscopy
Back pain
Bariatric surgery
Bone cancer
Bone disorders
Bone grafting
Bones and the skeleton
Bowlegs
Braces, orthopedic
Bunions
Bursitis
Cancer
Chiropractic
Craniosynostosis
Disk removal
Dwarfism
Ewing's sarcoma
Feet
Flat feet
Foot disorders
Fracture and dislocation
Fracture repair
Geriatrics and gerontology

Growth
Hammertoe correction
Hammertoes
Heel spur removal
Hip fracture repair
Hip replacement
Jaw wiring
Juvenile rheumatoid arthritis
Kinesiology
Kneecap removal
Knock-knees
Kyphosis
Laminectomy and spinal fusion
Lower extremities
Marfan syndrome
Motor skill development
Muscle sprains, spasms, and
   disorders
Muscles
Neurofibromatosis
Orthopedic surgery
Orthopedics
Orthopedics, pediatric
Osgood-Schlatter disease
Osteoarthritis
Osteochondritis juvenilis
Osteogenesis imperfecta
Osteomyelitis
Osteonecrosis
Osteopathic medicine
Osteoporosis
Paget's disease
Physical examination
Physical rehabilitation
Pigeon toes
Podiatry
Prostheses
Reiter's syndrome
Rheumatoid arthritis
Rheumatology
Rotator cuff surgery
Rubinstein-Taybi syndrome
Scoliosis
Slipped disk
Spina bifida
Spinal cord disorders
Spine, vertebrae, and disks
Sports medicine
Tendinitis
Tendon disorders
Tendon repair
Upper extremities
Whiplash

Gigantism
Glycogen storage diseases
Growth
Gynecomastia
Hand-foot-and-mouth disease
Hematology, pediatric
Hemolytic uremic syndrome
Hirschsprung's disease
Hives
Hormones
Hydrocephalus
Hypospadias repair and
    urethroplasty
Juvenile rheumatoid arthritis
Kawasaki disease
Klippel-Trenaunay syndrome
Kwashiorkor
Learning disabilities
Leukodystrophy
Malabsorption
Malnutrition
Maple syrup urine disease (MSUD)
Massage
Measles
Menstruation
Metabolic disorders
Motor skill development
Mucopolysaccharidosis (MPS)
Multiple births
Multiple sclerosis
Mumps
Münchausen syndrome by proxy
Muscular dystrophy
Neonatology
Nephrology, pediatric
Neurology, pediatric
Niemann-Pick disease
Nightmares
Nosebleeds
Nursing
Nutrition
Obesity, childhood
Optometry, pediatric
Orthopedics, pediatric
Osgood-Schlatter disease
Osteogenesis imperfecta
Otoplasty
Otorhinolaryngology
Pediatrics
Perinatology
Phenylketonuria (PKU)
Pigeon toes
Pinworm
Poliomyelitis

Porphyria
Prader-Willi syndrome
Precocious puberty
Premature birth
Progeria
Psychiatry, child and adolescent
Puberty and adolescence
Pulmonary medicine, pediatric
Pyloric stenosis
Rashes
Reflexes, primitive
Respiratory distress syndrome
Reye's syndrome
Rheumatic fever
Rickets
Roseola
Rotavirus
Roundworm
Rubella
Rubinstein-Taybi syndrome
Safety issues for children
Scarlet fever
Seizures
Severe combined immunodeficiency
    syndrome (SCID)
Sexuality
Sibling rivalry
Soiling
Sore throat
Steroids
Strep throat
Streptococcal infections
Sturge-Weber syndrome
Styes
Sudden infant death syndrome
    (SIDS)
Surgery, pediatric
Tapeworm
Tay-Sachs disease
Teething
Testicles, undescended
Testicular torsion
Thumb sucking
Toilet training
Tonsillectomy and adenoid removal
Tonsillitis
Trachoma
Tropical medicine
Urology, pediatric
Weaning
Well-baby examinations
Whooping cough
Wiskott-Aldrich syndrome
Worms

PERINATOLOGY
Amniocentesis
Assisted reproductive technologies
Birth defects
Breast-feeding
Cesarean section
Childbirth
Childbirth complications
Chorionic villus sampling
Cretinism
Critical care, pediatric
Embryology
Fatty acid oxidation disorders
Fetal alcohol syndrome
Glycogen storage diseases
Hematology, pediatric
Hydrocephalus
Karyotyping
Metabolic disorders
Motor skill development
Neonatology
Neurology, pediatric
Nursing
Obstetrics
Pediatrics
Perinatology
Pregnancy and gestation
Premature birth
Reflexes, primitive
Shunts
Stillbirth
Sudden infant death syndrome
    (SIDS)
Trichomoniasis
Umbilical cord
Well-baby examinations

PHARMACOLOGY
Acid-base chemistry
Aging: Extended care
Anesthesia
Anesthesiology
Antibiotics
Antidepressants
Antihistamines
Anti-inflammatory drugs
Bacteriology
Blurred vision
Chemotherapy
Club drugs
Corticosteroids
Critical care
Critical care, pediatric
Decongestants

Bunions
Corns and calluses
Feet
Flat feet
Foot disorders
Fungal infections
Hammertoe correction
Hammertoes
Heel spur removal
Lower extremities
Nail removal
Orthopedic surgery
Orthopedics
Physical examination
Pigeon toes
Podiatry
Tendon disorders
Tendon repair
Warts

PREVENTIVE MEDICINE
Acupressure
Acupuncture
Aging: Extended care
Alternative medicine
Aromatherapy
Biofeedback
Braces, orthopedic
Caffeine
Cardiology
Chiropractic
Cholesterol
Chronobiology
Disease
Echocardiography
Electrocardiography (ECG or EKG)
Environmental health
Exercise physiology
Family medicine
Genetic counseling
Geriatrics and gerontology
Holistic medicine
Host-defense mechanisms
Hypercholesterolemia
Immune system
Immunization and vaccination
Immunology
Mammography
Massage
Meditation
Melatonin
Noninvasive tests
Nursing
Nutrition

Occupational health
Osteopathic medicine
Over-the-counter medications
Pharmacology
Pharmacy
Physical examination
Phytochemicals
Preventive medicine
Psychiatry
Psychiatry, child and adolescent
Psychiatry, geriatric
Screening
Serology
Spine, vertebrae, and disks
Sports medicine
Stress
Stress reduction
Tendinitis
Tropical medicine
Yoga

PROCTOLOGY
Bladder removal
Colon and rectal polyp removal
Colon and rectal surgery
Colon cancer
Colonoscopy and sigmoidoscopy
Crohn's disease
Diverticulitis and diverticulosis
Endoscopy
Fistula repair
Gastroenterology
Gastrointestinal disorders
Gastrointestinal system
Genital disorders, male
Geriatrics and gerontology
Hemorrhoid banding and removal
Hemorrhoids
Hirschsprung's disease
Internal medicine
Intestinal disorders
Intestines
Irritable bowel syndrome (IBS)
Physical examination
Proctology
Prostate cancer
Prostate gland
Prostate gland removal
Reproductive system
Urology

PSYCHIATRY
Addiction
Aging

Aging: Extended care
Alcoholism
Alzheimer's disease
Amnesia
Amyotrophic lateral sclerosis
Anorexia nervosa
Antidepressants
Anxiety
Appetite loss
Asperger's syndrome
Attention-deficit disorder (ADD)
Auras
Autism
Bariatric surgery
Bipolar disorders
Bonding
Brain
Brain damage
Brain disorders
Breast surgery
Bulimia
Chronic fatigue syndrome
Circumcision, female, and genital
  mutilation
Club drugs
Corticosteroids
Delusions
Dementias
Depression
Developmental stages
Domestic violence
Eating disorders
Electroencephalography (EEG)
Emergency medicine
Emotions: Biomedical causes and
  effects
Factitious disorders
Failure to thrive
Family medicine
Fatigue
Grief and guilt
Gynecology
Hallucinations
Huntington's disease
Hypnosis
Hypochondriasis
Incontinence
Intoxication
Light therapy
Marijuana
Masturbation
Memory loss
Mental retardation
Midlife crisis

Münchausen syndrome by proxy
Neurosis
Neurosurgery
Nicotine
Nightmares
Obesity
Obesity, childhood
Obsessive-compulsive disorder
Pain
Pain management
Panic attacks
Paranoia
Penile implant surgery
Phobias
Pick's disease
Postpartum depression
Post-traumatic stress disorder
Prader-Willi syndrome
Psychiatric disorders
Psychiatry
Psychiatry, child and adolescent
Psychiatry, geriatric
Psychoanalysis
Psychosis
Psychosomatic disorders
Schizophrenia
Seasonal affective disorder
Separation anxiety
Sex change surgery
Sexual dysfunction
Sexuality
Shock therapy
Sleep
Sleep disorders
Speech disorders
Steroid abuse
Stress
Stress reduction
Sudden infant death syndrome
  (SIDS)
Suicide
Toilet training
Tourette's syndrome

PSYCHOLOGY
Addiction
Aging
Aging: Extended care
Alcoholism
Amnesia
Amyotrophic lateral sclerosis
Anorexia nervosa
Anxiety
Appetite loss

Aromatherapy
Asperger's syndrome
Attention-deficit disorder (ADD)
Auras
Bariatric surgery
Bed-wetting
Biofeedback
Bipolar disorders
Bonding
Brain
Brain damage
Brain disorders
Bulimia
Cardiac rehabilitation
Cirrhosis
Club drugs
Cognitive development
Death and dying
Delusions
Depression
Developmental stages
Domestic violence
Dyslexia
Eating disorders
Electroencephalography (EEG)
Emotions: Biomedical causes and
  effects
Environmental health
Factitious disorders
Failure to thrive
Family medicine
Forensic pathology
Genetic counseling
Grief and guilt
Gulf War syndrome
Gynecology
Hallucinations
Holistic medicine
Hormone replacement therapy
  (HRT)
Huntington's disease
Hypnosis
Hypochondriasis
Juvenile rheumatoid arthritis
Kinesiology
Klinefelter syndrome
Learning disabilities
Light therapy
Marijuana
Meditation
Memory loss
Mental retardation
Midlife crisis
Motor skill development

Münchausen syndrome by proxy
Neurosis
Nightmares
Nutrition
Obesity
Obesity, childhood
Obsessive-compulsive disorder
Occupational health
Overtraining syndrome
Pain management
Panic attacks
Paranoia
Phobias
Pick's disease
Plastic surgery
Postpartum depression
Post-traumatic stress disorder
Psychosomatic disorders
Puberty and adolescence
Separation anxiety
Sex change surgery
Sexual dysfunction
Sexuality
Sibling rivalry
Sleep
Sleep disorders
Sleepwalking
Speech disorders
Sports medicine
Steroid abuse
Stillbirth
Stress
Stress reduction
Sturge-Weber syndrome
Stuttering
Sudden infant death syndrome
  (SIDS)
Suicide
Temporomandibular joint (TMJ)
  syndrome
Tics
Toilet training
Tourette's syndrome
Weight loss and gain
Yoga

PUBLIC HEALTH
Acquired immunodeficiency
  syndrome (AIDS)
Aging: Extended care
Allied health
Alternative medicine
Anthrax
Asbestos exposure

Prader-Willi syndrome
Pulmonary diseases
Pulmonary hypertension
Pulmonary medicine
Pulmonary medicine, pediatric
Respiration
Respiratory distress syndrome
Severe acute respiratory syndrome
 (SARS)
Sleep apnea
Smoking
Thoracic surgery
Thrombolytic therapy and TPA
Tuberculosis
Tumor removal
Tumors
Wheezing

RADIOLOGY
Angiography
Biophysics
Biopsy
Bladder cancer
Bone cancer
Bone disorders
Bones and the skeleton
Brain tumors
Cancer
Catheterization
Computed tomography (CT)
 scanning
Critical care
Critical care, pediatric
Emergency medicine
Ewing's sarcoma
Gallbladder cancer
Imaging and radiology
Kidney cancer
Liver cancer
Lung cancer
Magnetic resonance imaging (MRI)
Mammography
Mouth and throat cancer
Noninvasive tests
Nuclear medicine
Nuclear radiology
Oncology
Positron emission tomography
 (PET) scanning
Prostate cancer
Radiation sickness
Radiation therapy
Radiopharmaceuticals
Sarcoma

Stents
Surgery, general
Testicular cancer
Ultrasonography

RHEUMATOLOGY
Aging
Aging: Extended care
Anti-inflammatory drugs
Arthritis
Arthroplasty
Arthroscopy
Autoimmune disorders
Behçet's disease
Bone disorders
Bones and the skeleton
Bursitis
Corticosteroids
Fibromyalgia
Geriatrics and gerontology
Gout
Hip replacement
Hydrotherapy
Inflammation
Lyme disease
Orthopedic surgery
Orthopedics
Orthopedics, pediatric
Osteoarthritis
Osteonecrosis
Physical examination
Rheumatic fever
Rheumatoid arthritis
Rheumatology
Rotator cuff surgery
Scleroderma
Sjögren's syndrome
Spondylitis
Sports medicine

SEROLOGY
Anemia
Blood and blood disorders
Blood testing
Cholesterol
Cytology
Cytopathology
Dialysis
Fluids and electrolytes
Forensic pathology
Hematology
Hematology, pediatric
Hemophilia
Hodgkin's disease

Host-defense mechanisms
Hyperbaric oxygen therapy
Hypercholesterolemia
Hyperlipidemia
Hypoglycemia
Immune system
Immunology
Immunopathology
Jaundice
Laboratory tests
Leukemia
Malaria
Pathology
Rh factor
Septicemia
Serology
Sickle cell disease
Thalassemia
Transfusion

SPEECH PATHOLOGY
Alzheimer's disease
Amyotrophic lateral sclerosis
Aphasia and dysphasia
Audiology
Autism
Cerebral palsy
Cleft lip and palate
Cleft lip and palate repair
Deafness
Dyslexia
Ear infections and disorders
Ear surgery
Ears
Electroencephalography (EEG)
Hearing loss
Hearing tests
Jaw wiring
Laryngitis
Learning disabilities
Lisping
Paralysis
Rubinstein-Taybi syndrome
Speech disorders
Strokes
Stuttering
Thumb sucking
Voice and vocal cord disorders

SPORTS MEDICINE
Acupressure
Anorexia nervosa
Arthroplasty
Arthroscopy

Athlete's foot
Biofeedback
Blurred vision
Bones and the skeleton
Braces, orthopedic
Cardiology
Critical care
Dehydration
Eating disorders
Emergency medicine
Ergogenic aids
Exercise physiology
Fracture and dislocation
Fracture repair
Glycolysis
Head and neck disorders
Heat exhaustion and heat stroke
Hydrotherapy
Kinesiology
Massage
Motor skill development
Muscle sprains, spasms, and
    disorders
Muscles
Nutrition
Orthopedic surgery
Orthopedics
Overtraining syndrome
Oxygen therapy
Physical examination
Physical rehabilitation
Physiology
Psychiatry
Rotator cuff surgery
Safety issues for children
Spine, vertebrae, and disks
Sports medicine
Steroid abuse
Steroids
Tendinitis
Tendon disorders
Tendon repair

TOXICOLOGY
Biological and chemical weapons
Bites and stings
Blood testing
Botulism
Club drugs
Critical care
Critical care, pediatric
Cyanosis
Dermatitis
Eczema

Emergency medicine
Environmental diseases
Environmental health
Food poisoning
Forensic pathology
Gaucher's disease
Hepatitis
Herbal medicine
Homeopathy
Intoxication
Itching
Laboratory tests
Lead poisoning
Liver
Mold and mildew
Multiple chemical sensitivity
    syndrome
Nicotine
Occupational health
Pathology
Pharmacology
Pharmacy
Poisoning
Poisonous plants
Rashes
Snakebites
Toxicology
Toxoplasmosis
Urinalysis

UROLOGY
Abdomen
Abdominal disorders
Bed-wetting
Bladder cancer
Bladder removal
Catheterization
Chlamydia
Circumcision, male
Cystitis
Cystoscopy
Dialysis
E. coli infection
Endoscopy
Fetal surgery
Fluids and electrolytes
Genital disorders, female
Genital disorders, male
Geriatrics and gerontology
Gonorrhea
Hemolytic uremic syndrome
Hermaphroditism and
    pseudohermaphroditism
Hydrocelectomy

Hypospadias repair and
    urethroplasty
Incontinence
Infertility, male
Kidney cancer
Kidney disorders
Kidney transplantation
Kidneys
Lithotripsy
Nephrectomy
Nephritis
Nephrology
Nephrology, pediatric
Pediatrics
Pelvic inflammatory disease (PID)
Penile implant surgery
Polycystic kidney disease
Prostate cancer
Prostate enlargement
Prostate gland
Prostate gland removal
Pyelonephritis
Reiter's syndrome
Reproductive system
Schistosomiasis
Sex change surgery
Sexual differentiation
Sexual dysfunction
Sexually transmitted diseases
    (STDs)
Sterilization
Stone removal
Stones
Syphilis
Testicles, undescended
Testicular cancer
Testicular surgery
Testicular torsion
Toilet training
Transplantation
Trichomoniasis
Ultrasonography
Urethritis
Urinalysis
Urinary disorders
Urinary system
Urology
Urology, pediatric
Vasectomy

VASCULAR MEDICINE
Amputation
Aneurysmectomy
Aneurysms

Angiography
Angioplasty
Anti-inflammatory drugs
Arteriosclerosis
Biofeedback
Bleeding
Blood and blood disorders
Bruises
Bypass surgery
Catheterization
Cholesterol
Circulation
Claudication
Dehydration
Diabetes mellitus
Dialysis
Embolism
Endarterectomy
Exercise physiology
Glands
Healing
Hematology
Hematology, pediatric
Hemorrhoid banding and removal
Hemorrhoids
Histology
Hypercholesterolemia
Hyperlipidemia
Ischemia
Klippel-Trenaunay syndrome
Lipids
Lymphatic system
Mitral valve prolapse
Necrotizing fasciitis
Nicotine
Osteochondritis juvenilis
Phlebitis
Podiatry
Preeclampsia and eclampsia

Progeria
Shunts
Smoking
Stents
Strokes
Sturge-Weber syndrome
Thrombolytic therapy and TPA
Thrombosis and thrombus
Toxemia
Transfusion
Transient ischemic attacks (TIAs)
Varicose vein removal
Varicose veins
Vascular medicine
Vascular system
Venous insufficiency
Von Willebrand's disease

VIROLOGY
Acquired immunodeficiency
    syndrome (AIDS)
Biological and chemical weapons
Chickenpox
Childhood infectious diseases
Chlamydia
Chronic fatigue syndrome
Common cold
Creutzfeldt-Jakob disease (CJD)
Croup
Cytomegalovirus (CMV)
Drug resistance
Ebola virus
Encephalitis
Epstein-Barr virus
Fever
Hantavirus
Hepatitis
Herpes

Human immunodeficiency virus
    (HIV)
Human papillomavirus (HPV)
Infection
Influenza
Laboratory tests
Marburg virus
Measles
Microbiology
Microscopy
Monkeypox
Mononucleosis
Mumps
Noroviruses
Parasitic diseases
Pelvic inflammatory disease
    (PID)
Poliomyelitis
Pulmonary diseases
Rabies
Rheumatic fever
Rhinitis
Roseola
Rotavirus
Rubella
Serology
Severe acute respiratory syndrome
    (SARS)
Sexually transmitted diseases
    (STDs)
Shingles
Smallpox
Tonsillitis
Tropical medicine
Viral infections
Warts
Yellow fever
Zoonoses